Essentials of Modern Hearing Aids

Selection, Fitting, and Verification

Editor-in-Chief for Audiology
Brad A. Stach, PhD

Essentials of Modern Hearing Aids

Selection, Fitting, and Verification

Todd A. Ricketts, PhD
Ruth Bentler, PhD
H. Gustav Mueller, PhD

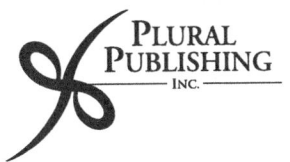

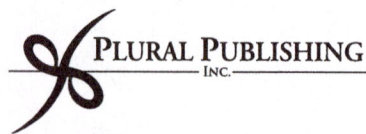

5521 Ruffin Road
San Diego, CA 92123

e-mail: information@pluralpublishing.com
website: https://www.pluralpublishing.com

Copyright © 2019 by Plural Publishing, Inc.

Typeset in 10½/13 Minion Pro by Flanagan's Publishing Services, Inc.
Printed in the United States of America by McNaughton & Gunn
24 23 22 21   3 4 5 6

All rights, including that of translation, reserved. No part of this publication may be reproduced, stored in a retrieval system, or transmitted in any form or by any means, electronic, mechanical, recording, or otherwise, including photocopying, recording, taping, Web distribution, or information storage and retrieval systems without the prior written consent of the publisher.

For permission to use material from this text, contact us by
Telephone: (866) 758-7251
Fax: (888) 758-7255
e-mail: permissions@pluralpublishing.com

Every attempt has been made to contact the copyright holders for material originally printed in another source. If any have been inadvertently overlooked, the publishers will gladly make the necessary arrangements at the first opportunity.

Library of Congress Cataloging-in-Publication Data:

Names: Ricketts, Todd, author. | Bentler, Ruth A., author. | Mueller, H. Gustav, author.
Title: Essentials of modern hearing aids : selection, fitting, and verification / Todd A. Ricketts, Ruth Bentler, H. Gustav Mueller.
Description: San Diego, CA : Plural Publishing, [2019] | Includes bibliographical references and index.
Identifiers: LCCN 2017041447| ISBN 9781597568531 (alk. paper) | ISBN 1597568538 (alk. paper)
Subjects: | MESH: Hearing Aids | Hearing Tests | Evidence-Based Practice | Quality Control
    Classification: LCC RF300 | NLM WV 274 | DDC 617.8/9--dc23
LC record available at https://lccn.loc.gov/2017041447

Contents

Preface — vii
Acknowledgments — ix

1 Evidence-Based Practice — 1

2 The Audiologist and Hearing Aid Provision — 27

3 Understanding the Hearing Aid Candidate — 53

4 Speech Acoustics — 75

5 Pre-Fitting Tests Using Frequency-Specific Measures — 101

6 Pre-Fitting Testing Using Speech Material — 135

7 Self-Assessment Scales for Pre-Fitting Testing — 197

8 Hearing Aid Styles and Fitting Applications — 225

9 Ear Impressions, Earmolds, and Associated Plumbing — 273

10 Hearing Aid Hardware and Software: The Basics — 307

11 Signal Classification and Sound Cleaning Technologies — 383

12 More Hearing Aid Features and Algorithms — 427

13 Electroacoustic and Other Quality Control Techniques — 473

14 Prescriptive Formulas and Programming — 517

15 Behavioral Assessment During Clinical Fittings — 559

16 Probe Microphone Measures: Rationale and Procedures — 603

17 Probe-Microphone Measures: Clinical Uses — 647

18 Hearing Aid Orientation and Troubleshooting — 709

19 Validation: Self-Report Outcomes — 735

20 Supplemental Information: Corrections, Conversions, and Calculations — 781

References — 819
Index — 857

Preface

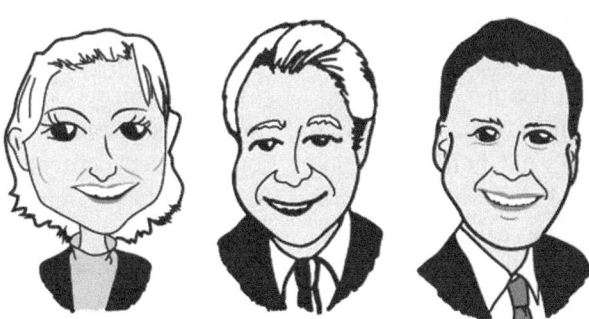

Expertise is sometimes an elusive concept when applied to clinical skills. In the 1950s famed psychologist Paul Meehl demonstrated that expert clinical opinion can often be less accurate than a simple unbiased algorithm. This led to his introduction (along with Lee Crohnbach) of construct validity, which in part provided the foundation for evidence-based practice. Later work by Daniel Kahneman and others demonstrated that clinical opinion can be important too, but it must be given limited weight and considered along with more heavily weighted unbiased data. Importantly, the more a clinical opinion is a guess that is not supported by evidence (limited validity), the more likely it is to lead to an erroneous conclusion. For example, Kahneman describes the error that wine experts make when tasting immature wine when trying to predict the quality when it will be mature. It turns out the two are unrelated, and that ignoring the actual taste—and focusing instead on valid and objectively measurable factors like temperature, moisture patterns, and soil conditions—provides a more accurate prediction.

So how much expertise is needed for selecting and fitting hearing aids? At the most basic level, provision of amplification is rather simple. Provide enough gain but not too much, so that patients have improved audibility without loudness discomfort. Programming a hearing aid using the automated manufacturer-recommended first fit, based on the patient's audiogram, will likely improve audibility for at least some sounds, and generally will keep loud sounds from being too loud. Application of a little science and expertise, however—and the addition of the probe microphone verification of modern, validated prescriptive gain methods—will lead to significantly better outcomes.

We have an incredible myriad of advanced hearing aid features, many of which provide benefits only in specific situations, and a few of which have some pro and con tradeoffs. Making things even more challenging is that many features interact with listening differently, depending on the manufacturer and the specific setting chosen. In addition, emerging data demonstrates that some features can have differential effects on speech recognition, localization, sound quality, listening effort, and other facets of the listening experience. Consequently, we believe evaluating individual listening needs, and then selecting, fitting, adjusting and counseling based on those listening needs are necessary to optimize patient benefits from hearing aids. In other words, assuming good patient rapport and people skills, the greater the expertise, the better chance at optimal outcomes. Of course, we must accomplish all this as efficiently as possible.

There have been around 2000 research articles published in the last decade related to the selection and fitting of hearing aids, and countless additional white papers and other manufacturer documents produced. In the last few years, we have authored three other textbooks that have focused on individual sections of the provision of hearing aids including hearing needs assessment, hearing aid selection, verification, counseling and outcomes. In this text, we put it all together in an updated form and add discussions of hardware, signal processing, and hearing aid features. We attempt to synthesize our current evidenced-based knowledge about hearing aids and the provision of hearing aid services with the goal of providing the reader a one-stop source. We again provide this information in a clinician-friendly step-by-step manner: Audiological pre-fitting testing; needs assessment and treatment planning; hearing aid hardware, software, and features; hearing aid selection, verification, orientation and counseling; post-fitting follow-up; and real-world validation. Of course, next year there will be another 200 or so hearing aid articles published, and maybe some changes in hearing aid features—but we hope this text will serve as a useful foundation going forward.

Putting forth the effort to develop an entire textbook is a rather daunting task, and we are all pretty busy. In teaching our hearing aid courses we were never satisfied, however, with what was available. None of the texts offered all of the material we wanted to include in a way that was accessible to audiology students. Also, we wanted to have a textbook that took a student through the entire hearing aid process from beginning to end in a logical and clinically applicable manner. So we set out to write a book that we would be able to use in its entirety in all of our hearing aid coursework, rather than needing different texts for different classes and picking a chapter here and a chapter there. We think we have achieved our goal and hope you also find it a good one-stop-shop for all clinical hearing aid courses. Of course we will be using articles from the research literature to supplement this text going forward, but all of the core material we talk about in our current classes is here. Given that many in our target audience are audiology students and busy clinicians, we also knew that we had to ensure the book's readability. We wanted to present our material in a manner that was a little unique but not distracting. Consequently, we followed a similar structure that we introduced previously and provided callouts where we could to add or emphasize a given point. Throughout the text, you will see short paragraphs that we have identified as Technical Tips, Things to Remember, Key Concept, and Points to Ponder. To keep the book manageable in size and weight, we have placed some related content on the PluralPlus companion website rather than include it in appendices. There you will find many of the forms and scoresheets needed to facilitate the pre- and post-fitting measures we describe in this text, as well as PowerPoint slides with all of the figures from the text arranged by chapter.

This is now the fourth book that the three of us have co-written. Fortunately, when it comes to hearing aid issues, we think pretty much the same, so when we say "we" we usually do really mean "we." Moreover, if you simply follow what has been carefully thought out and published in evidence-based best practice guidelines, the provision of hearing aid service is not as debatable as some people try to make it. That said, from new algorithms to new types of patient outcomes, discovery in the area of hearing aids marches on rapidly, and the evidence base remains limited for some of the newer techniques. As you might guess, the three of us are strong-willed, which often made for some fun debates in areas where research evidence is limited. Reaching consensus takes time—not as much time as generating content, but time nonetheless. As with a good scotch or wine, attentive blending and 12 years of aging (from concept to completion) was necessary to finish this work—we hope you enjoy every sip!

Acknowledgments

Regarding the contents of this book, it is important that we again acknowledge the tireless efforts of Elizabeth Stangl, AuD, from the Hearing Aid Lab at the University of Iowa. As was the case in our previous efforts, she is responsible for the construction of many of our figures, and she managed all the details regarding references, permissions, and overall organization of the book. Thanks, Elizabeth! Kade Schemahorn provided graphic design, and a number of other students in the Hearing Aid Lab at the University of Iowa were invaluable for their contributions: Curtis Hartling, Caitlin Sapp, Britany Barber, Kassie McLaughlin, Kelly Bailey, Erik Jorgenson, and Amy Carlson. In addition, Erin Picou, PhD, from Vanderbilt University, also provided a number of helpful suggestions and contributions. We also thank our families for putting up with years of hearing about "That Big @#$% Book"!

1
Evidence-Based Practice

The selection and fitting of hearing aids have always included components of both art and science. Although the field continues to push toward an increased evidence base, the ratio of art versus science favored art for a number of decades. Why? The science has not always kept up with the technological advances. With the current and forecasted health care reimbursement models, all clinicians must be prepared to offer true evidence of effectiveness, satisfaction, and/or benefit, if we want to be paid for our services! In this chapter we review the principles of evidence-based practice (EBP) and how we can apply them to our own practices.

Several studies have demonstrated the importance of EBP with regard to provision of hearing aid services. For starters, in the late 1990s, there was an overwhelming belief that "We have arrived!" with the first digital hearing aid release in the United States. Consumers and audiologists alike were yearning for hearing aids that provided better reproduction of sound, better hearing in noise, and better overall user satisfaction; many believed that these new digital products were the solution. An early, well-designed investigation of differences in outcomes over time, however, showed that we actually had *not* improved the likelihood of better hearing for the listener (Bentler & Duve, 2000) despite some pretty significant improvements in the technology. In that study, the 25 subjects were each fitted with hearing aids that spanned 100 years of practice, using the fitting approach appropriate to the era. A number of measures were taken with the hearing aids alone and with the hearing aids on the subjects.

The findings of the Bentler and Duve (2000) study were generally hard to swallow for many. Word recognition scores showed no significant difference across any of the conditions of testing, which included unaided, a nonelectronic ear trumpet, an old original body-style hearing aid, and the more recent analog and digital hearing aids used in the study. The only significantly different score was found with the 1930s body hearing aid, which was likely due to its inherent narrow bandwidth and high distortion. The ratings for sound clarity —assessed in the laboratory with cafeteria, office and traffic noise—did not differentiate the hearing aids in use from 1960 onward. Finally, the "real world" rating of ease of listening suggested that in difficult listening environments, such as a fast-food restaurant and a church service, none of these hearing aid processors worked better than the other. Although this all sounds negative for our efforts, the point to be made is: Newer is not always better. And if clinicians are to know what is better, we need to keep the evidence coming. A similarly eye-opening series of articles regarding today's technology recently was published by Cox et al. (2014, 2016)—more on that later.

Several studies have also shown that clinical intuition is often incorrect. Bias, either from the clinician or the hearing aid recipient, has been shown to cloud the true results. One study that clearly showed the strong biasing effects that are present by simply the labeling of hearing aids was completed more than a decade ago, and is often referred to as the "Bentler Hype Study" (Bentler, Niebuhr, Johnson, & Flamme, 2003). As part of this study, one group of hearing-impaired listeners had two one-month trials with hearing aids. For one month, participants wore the hearing aids labeled "state-of-the-art digital," and for the other month they wore hearing aids labeled "conventional." In reality the hearing aids were exactly the same hearing aids! It is important to note that digital hearing aids were still relatively new at the time of that study and were getting a lot of marketing press relative to their benefit over the older analog hearing aids. At the end of the first month-long trial, the participants completed a battery of speech recognition and self-report measures. After the testing was completed, the hearing aids were removed, the investigator left the room and came back, and participants were refitted with exactly the same hearing aids. Participants were then told they were wearing the opposite condition (conventional or digital) and sent out for another trial, after which the test battery was repeated. As expected there were no differences in speech recognition scores across the conditions; however, labeling clearly affected self-perception. The fitting labeled "digital" was scored significantly higher on some self-report subscales of the Abbreviated Profile of Hearing Aid Benefit (APHAB), and 33 of 40 participants expressed a preference for the fitting labeled "digital."

This type of placebo effect labeling bias was confirmed by a more recent study (Dawes, Hopkins, & Munro, 2013) during which 75% of participants expressed a preference for a hearing aid when it was labeled "new" over the same hearing aid model when it was labeled "conventional." Even though the effect was small (~4 percentage points), a striking additional finding was that the speech recognition performance was significantly better when the same hearing aids were labeled "new." This suggests that, in addition to differences in self-reported outcomes and preferences, the placebo effect can be so strong that patients may actually try harder (and consequently perform better) on objective outcome measures!

Although the presence of these biases is clear and must be considered in research design, their interactive effect on clinical perceptions may be less clear. A good example of the potential clinical implications is demonstrated by the findings of a study David Gnewikow completed as part of his dissertation at Vanderbilt University (Gnewikow, Ricketts, Bratt, & Mutchler, 2009). In this study, 90 patients were selected who all were fitted with the same model of omnidirectional hearing aid (old-HA) that were programmed to NAL-R targets prior to testing. A variety of outcome and preference measures were completed and compared to the same measures following another trial with a new hearing aid fitted exactly to exactly the same prescriptive gain targets (new-HA). The new-HA and old-HA were therefore identical in every way except that the new-HA could be programmed to use either fixed directional or fixed omnidirectional microphones (a trial with each of the microphone settings was completed). In addition, there was no labeling of "old" and "new"; however, participants were aware they were receiving new instruments. As expected, speech recognition in noise scores with noise sources surrounding the listener were identical for the new hearing aid and old hearing aid (both in omnidirectional mode) since they had essentially identical hearing aid responses. Somewhat surprisingly, however, there were no significant differences in subjective outcomes or preferences between the new-HA in directional and omnidirectional mode, but instead subjective outcomes were significantly higher for the new-HA over the old-HA (regardless of microphone type). These data demonstrate that the effect of bias can have a much greater effect on outcomes than a change of technology! Clinically, this same type of effect can happen. Is a new technology really better than an older one, or do patients report the new technology is better because we tell them it is? Although we can (and in our opinion should) let our patients know that we believe we have selected the best technologies for them, the actual effect size (ES) on outcomes must be based on evidence rather than our clinical intuition!

Are We Grounded in Evidence?

Evidence-based practice (EBP) has its roots in medicine. By definition, it is "the conscientious, explicit, and judicious use of current best evidence in making decisions about the care of individual patients . . . (by) integrating individual clinical expertise with the best available external clinical evidence from systematic research" (Sackett,

Rosenberg, Gray, Haynes, Richardson et al., 1996, p. 71). The literature is full of examples from medicine wherein practices deemed to be "best practice" at the time have turned out to be wrong or even harmful when scientific rigor was used to evaluate the effects. Examples include the ancient Greek practice of bloodletting for a variety of ailments, including hypertension. In the 19th century, opium was used to treat diabetes. In the 1940s, premature infants were "oxygenated" to prevent retrolental fibroplasia, a condition later found to be *caused*, not cured, by the treatment. The list goes on. The application of EBP principles in audiology has taken root in the past decade. Academic settings, clinicians, and manufacturers have important roles in the use of these principles for sound decision-making. Understanding our roles, as well as our roadblocks, is important for the successful move into everyday practice.

Concurrently, the field of audiology has witnessed an explosion in the availability of both technology and published literature. Clinicians have access to new diagnostic tools, measurement tools, processing schemes, and even style designs every few months. In addition, research publications have become increasingly abundant. A decade ago, it was reported that the number of papers published in the primary audiology journals had grown from 200 a year in 1960 to 1700 a year in 2003 (Thorne, 2003). At that rate, a clinician would need to read more than five papers a day for 365 days a year in order to keep up. If hearing science literature had been included, the total would increase to 4,350 papers per year and would require reading 12 papers per day. With today's online publishing and the increased number of professional journals, that number could easily exceed 10,000. In 2016, for example, more than 200 papers were published specifically related to hearing aid technology and fitting, in 17 different journals. The task of keeping up is daunting to any clinician. Yet, in this era of increased accountability (e.g., third party payers, legislation, and *ethics*), the clinician is often forced to make clinical management decisions without, in many cases, good available and supporting data.

In 2005, the American Speech-Language-Hearing Association (ASHA) first conducted a Knowledge-Attitude-Practices (KAP) survey on EBP among members. That survey was repeated in 2008, 2011, and 2014. Here are a few of the most recent findings (R. Mullen, personal communication, 2015):

- Most members could correctly define EBP and most members thought EBP was a good idea.
- "Insufficient time" was cited as a major or moderate barrier to EBP by more than 50% of audiology respondents (more than any other barrier).
- 59% of audiology faculty cited "lack of available evidence" more than any other barrier to the use of EBP.
- Respondents reported being "very likely" to use continuing education offerings (52%) and journals (56%) as sources of information to help make clinical decisions. These options followed "colleagues" (69%) by a considerable margin.
- It was often not clear to the clinician whether data provided from the hearing aid manufacturers are actual evidence or marketing copy.

All of these factors present significant roadblocks to the use of EBP principles. Nonetheless, we must consider that, if our profession is to survive, our practices must be based on data, and not educated guesswork. What may not be clear to the busy clinician is that the whole concept of EPB depends on three sources of information to inform clinical decision-making. Each can be considered one leg of a three-legged stool; all three must be functioning in order for the process (or stool) to work:

- Empirical evidence, or evidence from well-controlled research experiments;
- Clinical experience, or evidence gathered by repeated trials and tests with clinic patients;
- Patient characteristics, the specific needs and expectations of the patient for whom management plans are being considered.

Evidence-based practice is not viable without each of the three components outlined above. Often, audiologists "look to the research" for evidence that a particular signal processor should be used or that a new hearing aid feature is better than the previous one. Instead, all three sources of information should be considered in our daily work.

> **THINGS TO REMEMBER:**
> **"IF IT'S PUBLISHED, SHOULDN'T IT BE GOOD?"**
>
> Most new students—and some not-so-new clinicians—assume that if the information is published somewhere/anywhere, it must be true. We need to remember that there are many levels of "publication." Given the ease of desktop publishing and electronic dissemination, many things get published without much scientific scrutiny. Some things are published, but not subjected to peer review (i.e., a critical review by other scientists prior to acceptance for publication). On the other hand, a publication doesn't necessarily have to be peer-reviewed to be relevant to clinical decision making. And, even when something is peer-reviewed, the clinician must still take a critical look at what was done and its relevance to ongoing clinical decision making. The clinician needs to take responsibility for making this judgment, and that is more or less the main point of this chapter. In a hearing aid purchase, many would consider the patient to be the "consumer," but in fact, in most cases the consumer is really the clinician, as he or she will be making the important decisions for the patient—quite the responsibility.

What Is Good Evidence and How Do I Access It?

In most training programs, there is a course called *Introduction to Research* or the like. Although most clinicians do not pursue a career in research, all clinicians need to understand—or be able to differentiate—good research from not-so-good research. For example, good research has the following components:

- Study purpose
- Background literature
- Appropriate design including appropriate controls
- Sample size following power analysis
- Psychometrically sound outcomes used
- Intervention strategy explained
- Results, including dropouts
- Biases discussed
- Conclusions and clinical implications

As we discuss different types of evidence in this chapter, we will be referring to several different terms used in statistics and the critical review of research. We have summarized some of the terms in Table 1–1, adapted from Palmer et al. (2008).

Important Definitions

In the eyes of some, *research* and *evidence* might seem to be interchangeable terms. They are not. The different levels of the evidence that we draw from to help support our EBP don't always involve research. As shown in the well-known pyramid in Figure 1–1, evidence comes in many flavors; compelling evidence, however, comes from good and strong research. Let's review those EBP levels of evidence, starting with the lowest.

Expert Opinion

There are plenty of "experts" out there with opinions. Unfortunately, this is the lowest level of evidence that is considered in hearing aid research. Expert opinion can take the form of a workshop or lecture, an editorial in a journal, statements made in a book chapter (gulp), or even a manufacturer's trainer showing the newest design to a community of clinicians. In the world of EBP, there is little value placed on expert opinions without the supporting data. Expert opinion is a lot like clinical intuition: It is often unconsciously biased and introduces error into a process. For a very interesting discussion of these biases and their effects, consider Nobel Prize-winning Daniel Kahneman's excellent, *Thinking Fast and Slow*. While the focus of this book is examining

Table 1–1. Commonly Used Terms Used for Assessing Evidence

Sample Size	A sample is a subset of a population used to make inferences about the characteristics or behavior of the population. The size of the sample is the number of observations or measurements made. Typically, a larger sample size leads to more precise estimates of various population properties (see power).
Alpha	Probability level chosen by the researcher. Alpha = 0.05 means there is a 95% chance that a performance difference demonstrated between two sample study groups does truly exist in the general population.
Effect Size (ES)	The amount of difference the researcher is actually interested in detecting with a given study. For example, one study may be looking to detect a difference of 1.5 dB between groups (small ES), whereas another may be interested in only a 20 dB or greater difference between groups (large ES)
p value	The probability that a difference in sample group results would occur by chance even when there is no true difference in population groups (see alpha). Typical chosen as $p = 0.01$ or 0.05.
Power	The probability that study results will find a difference between sample group performance scores when a true difference between population scores does exist. Great power (≥ 0.80) is desirable in interpreting research results.
Statistical Significance	A finding considered to be statistically significant means that it is highly unlikely the finding would have occurred by chance, based on the chosen alpha level and ES.
Practical Significance	A finding can meet the requirements of statistical significance but not have practical value. For example, a study with a large enough sample size might find a statistically significant difference in scores of 5%, when a 5% difference has no real impact on a listener's overall function.

Note. Adapted from Palmer et al. (2008).

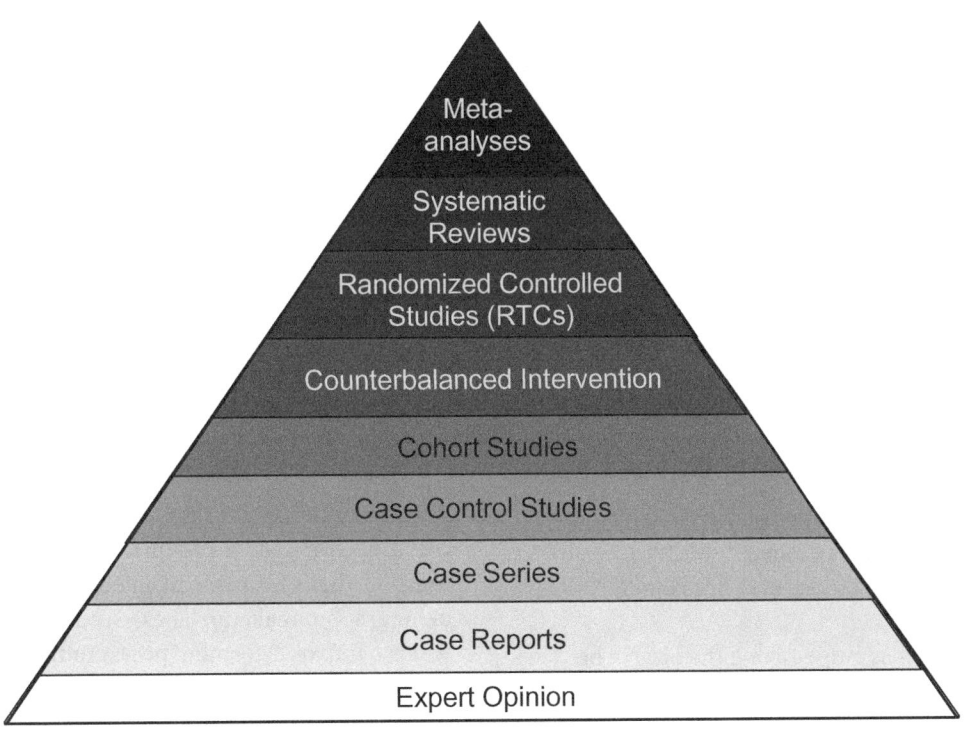

Figure 1–1. The pyramid of levels of evidence. Note that expert opinion is the lowest level of evidence, meanwhile meta-analysis offers the highest level of evidence.

how we make decisions, it provides many examples that demonstrate that expert opinion, on the average, is less accurate than a simple unbiased algorithm that includes expert opinion as just one equally weighted factor. In addition, many examples are given that demonstrate that clinical judgment is inherently biased by factors that are less important and more fluctuating than are the factors evidence shows to be the most important. A manufacturer who proclaims, "Two hearing aids should always be the goal in a fitting scheme," is really expressing an opinion favorable to company sales. The same would be true when a manufacturer recommends premier models (with a higher profit margin) over entry-level hearing aids. On the other hand, if that same "expert" were to produce data—of good quality—suggesting the same, the level of the evidence goes up significantly.

Case Reports or Case Series

Case reports or case series are also considered to be lower levels of evidence, but they are also often important to the development of the bigger questions of efficacy and effectiveness. A well-written case report will be clear about the importance of the observation; when multiple case reports show something similar, the next step might be a case-control study to determine if there is a relationship between the relevant variables. By themselves, case studies are nearly equivalent to testimonials.

Case studies include the following advantages:

- Can help in the identification of new trends in outcomes
- Can help detect new side effects and potential uses (adverse or beneficial)
- Are often educational—a way of sharing lessons learned
- Help identify unusual outcomes

Case studies include the following disadvantages:

- May not be generalizable
- Are not based on systematic studies
- Causes or associations may have other explanations
- Can be seen as emphasizing the bizarre or focusing on misleading elements

With respect to hearing aids, one of our favorite case studies of recent years was "The Case of the Missing Ping" (Mueller & Hawkins, 2006), which described the step-by-step procedure needed to determine why a golfer could hear the "ping" of his drive when he was not using his hearing aids, but could not hear the ping when they were inserted. Following sound-level meter measurements and extensive probe microphone testing with the patient, RECDs and RETSPLs, the "evidence" provided revealed that a low setting for the front-end AGCi limiting compressor of digital hearing aids can have a more fluctuating impact on real-world listening (see Chapter 10).

Case-Controlled Studies

A study that compares patients who have a disease or outcome of interest (cases) with patients who do not have the disease or outcome (controls) is known as a case-controlled study. Case-controlled studies are observational because no intervention is attempted and no attempt is made to alter the course of the outcome. Case-controlled studies can also be "retrospective studies" and "case-referent studies."

Advantages of case-controlled studies include the following:

- Require less time to conduct the study
- Can simultaneously look at multiple outcomes
- Are useful as initial studies to establish an association

Disadvantages of case-controlled studies include the following:

- May display more problems with data due to many uncontrolled variables (because these are often retrospective studies)
- Can be difficult to find a suitable control group

An example of a case-controlled study in our field could be comparing the quality of life of hearing aid users to that of non-hearing aid users with the same demographic makeup. These studies have shown that when compared to their peers, individuals who have treated their hearing loss with the use of hearing aids have better emotional stability, family relations, and sense of control over life events (Ciorba, Bianchini, Pelucchi, & Pastore, 2012; Swan et al., 2012).

Cohort Studies

A study design where one or more samples (called cohorts) are followed prospectively, and subsequent status evaluations with respect to a disease or outcome are conducted to determine which of the initial participants' exposure characteristics (risk factors) are associated with it, is a cohort study. As the study is conducted, outcomes from participants in each cohort are measured and relationships with specific characteristics determined.

Advantages of cohort studies include the following:

- Subjects in cohorts can be matched, which limits the influence of confounding variables
- Standardization of criteria/outcome is possible
- Easier and cheaper than a randomized controlled trial (RCT)

Disadvantages of cohort studies include the following:

- Cohorts can be difficult to identify due to confounding variables
- No randomization, which means that imbalances in patient characteristics could exist
- Blinding/masking is difficult
- Time required to obtained outcomes of interest can be considerable

An example of a cohort study related to hearing aids could involve research following groups of individuals with different technologies to determine adjustment timelines, preferred settings, and so on. One such study was conducted by Bentler and others in the early 1990s (Bentler, Niebuhr, Getta, & Anderson, 1993a and 1993b). In that study four groups of subjects using different analog "noise reduction" schemes were followed and tested over a period of one year to see if the benefit was different in some way across the groups. It was not.

Counterbalanced Intervention (CBI) Studies

One of the most common research questions is not whether a specific intervention works at all but, rather, which of multiple interventions works best. In this study design two or more intervention options are compared within a single group of participants. For example, do patients benefit more from one hearing aid or two? In order to offset timing and learning effects, the intervention (condition) the participant starts with and the order of conditions are counterbalanced across participants. For example, if we were comparing three interventions (A, B, and C), the number of participants that started with condition A would be equal to the number that started with condition B and the number that started with condition C. Furthermore, an equal number of participants would have conditions A, B, and C second and equal number would have conditions A, B and C third as well. Since this "within-subjects" design allows patients to serve as their own control group, these studies do not suffer from concerns that subject groups are not perfectly matched; therefore, group differences may be due to factors other than the specific intervention that are associated with some between-group studies. Due to the efficiency of having patients serve as their own control group, the CBI design is one of the most commonly used research designs found in the peer-reviewed literature of our field. Although there are some advantages to the CBI design, there are also several limitations that affect how we interpret the results of these studies.

Advantages of CBI studies include the following:

- Tight control over subject factors due to participants' serving as their own controls allows identification of fairly small differences.
- Not requiring a matched control group makes these studies much easier and quicker to complete, as well as more cost effective than the randomized controlled trials (RCTs) we describe in the next section.

Disadvantages of CBI studies include the following:

- Interpretation of longitudinal CBI studies is challenging, particularly in children, because the lack of control group does not allow the investigator to account for changes due to development and maturation. This limitation can greatly diminish the ability to make generalizations and the validity of the results.
- While offset by counter-balancing, learning effects can be present and contribute to variability. This can in turn weaken statistical power.

- If there is no control group we sometimes can't answer the question of whether the intervention works at all. That is, Intervention A could be better than B, but both could be worse than doing nothing at all.

Research of this type on hearing aids is often completed in a laboratory. The validity and applicability of the findings to clinical practice can be greatly strengthened, however, if the research is designed to have a real-world component. A recent example of this type of research is Cox Johnson & Xu, (2014) (more details are provided in Cox, Johnson and Xu, 2016; Johnson, Xu and Cox, 2017), in which outcomes with "premium" hearing aids and basic hearing aids are compared for speech understanding and quality of life. In that study, 25 participants, including both new and experienced hearing aid users, completed blinded, month-long trials with four pairs of hearing aids each: two basic and two premium. Their results indicated that all participants reacted very positively to the hearing aids (the good news); however, there were no statistically significant or clinically meaningful differences in improvement between the premium and basic-level hearing aids (the somewhat surprising news).

Randomized Controlled Trial (RCT)

Considered to be a very high level of evidence, RCTs are rare in hearing aid–related research. In this study design, participants are randomly assigned into an experimental group or a control group. The only expected difference between the control and experimental groups in a RCT is the outcome variable being studied. Commonly used in pharmaceutics research, an example might be investigation to determine whether a new drug has a different outcome than a sugar pill (*placebo*). Another type of RCT is comparison of an old intervention to a new intervention in two different groups. With this design however, it is often also important to include a third group (true control group) with either no intervention or a placebo to account for some of the weaknesses of the CBI designs described above. That said, there are many studies that use an RCT without a true control group. We think of this as sort of a hybrid design RCT—essentially a between-group version of the CBI design. This design can be quite appropriate, albeit depending on the experimental question, as demonstrated by the example study following. As with all experimental designs, RCTs have advantages and disadvantages.

Advantages of RCTs include the following:

- Randomization should eliminate population bias
- Statistical analyses can be clearly planned

Disadvantages of RCTs:

- Expensive to carry out in terms of time and money

**THINGS TO REMEMBER:
RESEARCH EVALUATING NEW TECHNOLOGY**

Robyn Cox (2005a) reminds us that there are some specific things that we should think about when we are evaluating research that addresses new technology. When you read about research evaluating new technology, ask yourself the following questions:

- How many subjects participated?
- How were they recruited?
- Are they representative of your patients?
- Is there a potential for bias in the way the study was conducted?
- Was there appropriate blinding of both subjects and data collectors?
- If the new technology was statistically better than the old, was the ES large enough to warrant the additional cost of this technology?

- Susceptible to volunteer bias; the subjects participating may not be representative of the population being studied
- No causal relationships can be made

Research of this type was conducted by Palmer (2012), who studied the starting point for using trainable hearing aids. Subjects (new hearing aid users) were randomly assigned to two different groups. The first group started hearing aid training on the day of the fitting; the second group used the hearing aids for a month (all fitted to NAL-NL1), and then started training. At the end of two months, the effects of the training, as measured by trained gain and patient preference, were assessed. Since this study was aimed at examining differences in technologies rather than technology benefit, there was no need for a true control group.

Systematic Reviews

A systematic review is a compilation of all relevant studies on a particular clinical or health-related topic/question. Cox (2005a) provides the flowchart of how a clinical recommendation can be derived from a systematic review in Figure 1–2. Fortunately, there are many search engines available today for assisting in a systematic review. Table 1–2 provides a review of some of the more popular ones. Google Scholar is another popular option; however, since results are ranked based on an algorithm that is not chronologically based, we find

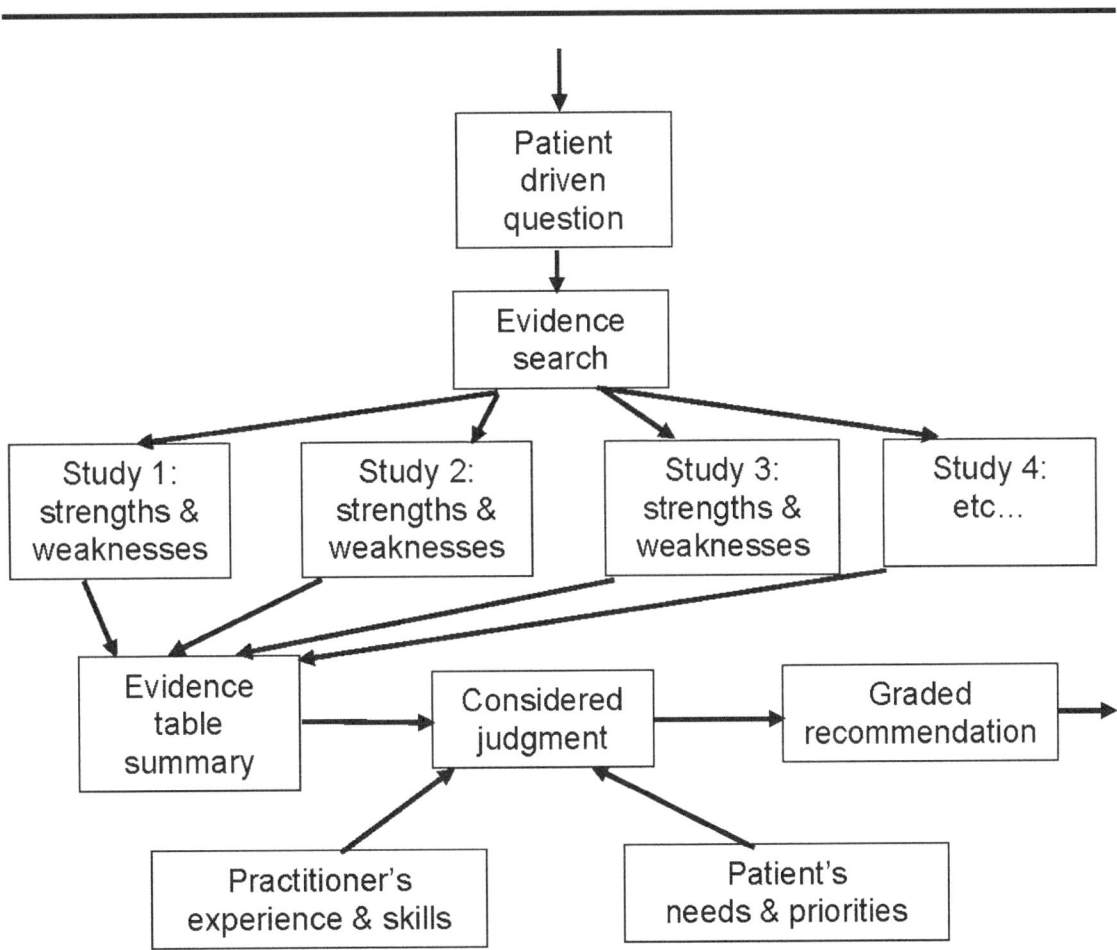

Figure 1–2. Schematic illustration of the application of the EBP method to generate a recommendation. This is consistent with a systematic or critical review, based on a given topic or clinical question. Adapted from Cox, 2005a, with permission.

Table 1–2. Example of the Various Search Engines Available for Systematic Reviews

Database and Website	Details
The Becker Library at the Washington University School of Medicine in St. Louis http://beckerguides.wustl.edu/audiology	Includes major databases, journals, and books, as well as other resources in the field of audiology and deaf education.
ComDisDome http://www.comdisdome.com	Includes more than 300,000 records in the communications disorders literature, dated back to 1911.
Cumulative Index to Nursing and Allied Health Literature (CINAHL) http://www.cinahl.com/	Includes journals, books, audiovisual, pamphlets, software, dissertations, and research instruments.
PubMed http://www.pubmed.gov	MEDLINE® is the largest module of PubMed. The biomedical journal citations and abstracts are created by the U.S. National Library of Medicine (NLM). MEDLINE® cites about 5400 journals, including journals in the area of audiological intervention that are published in more than 80 countries.
PsychINFO http://www.apa.org/pubs/databases/psycinfo/index.aspx	Covers the psychological literature since the 1800s. The database also includes some records from the 1600s and 1700s. Among the 42 million cited references, 80% are from journal articles, 8% are book chapters from authored and edited books, and 12% are dissertations and secondary sources.
Scopus http://www.scopus.com/	Contains multidisciplinary journal abstracts and citations, including physics, engineering, life and health sciences, psychology, social sciences and biological, etc. Nearly 18,000 titles are included, of which nearly 16,500 are peer-reviewed journals.
SumSearch http://www.ncbi.nlm.nih.gov/pmc/articles/PMC2000788/	Searches websites with evidence written by qualified experts, with the majority of links from the NLM, the Database of Abstracts of Reviews of Effectiveness (DARE) and the National Guideline Clearinghouse (NGC) and categorized as textbooks, review articles, practice guidelines, systematic reviews, and original research.
TRIP (Turning Research Into Practice) Database http://www.tripdatabase.com/	Searches more than 75 databases, including PubMed, the DARE and the NGC, and other evidence-based materials, such as systematic reviews, peer-reviewed journals, guidelines, e-textbooks, expert opinions, patient information.

Note. Adapted from Wong and Hickson (2012).

it more difficult to ensure a comprehensive list when using this tool.

Advantages of systematic reviews include the following:

- Exhaustive survey of the current literature
- Less costly to pull data from prior studies than to create a new study
- Less time required than conducting a new study
- Results can be generalized and extrapolated to the general population more broadly than can individual studies
- More reliable and accurate than individual studies
- Considered an evidence-based resource for clinicians

Disadvantages of systematic reviews include the following:

- Very time-consuming
- May not be easy to combine studies
- May be difficult to find studies that meet criteria of research question

In Chapter 5 for example, you will find that we frequently recommend the use of unaided frequency-specific loudness measures to determine the patient's loudness discomfort level (LDL). In part, this recommendation is based on the systematic review of Mueller and Bentler (2005). They asked the question: "Are the clinical measurements of LDL for adult patients predictive of aided acceptance and satisfaction of loudness for high inputs in the real world?" Nearly 200 articles were reviewed, and they reported that the evidence supported using unaided LDLs for selecting the maximum real-ear output of hearing aids (no recommendation could be made of aided LDLs—see associated Key Concept).

We are aware that many clinics do systematic reviews on various diagnostic and hearing aid issues; of course, this also is a common project for students in their research methods class or perhaps even a capstone project. These reviews often lead to modifications and improvements in the overall hearing aid fitting process.

Meta-Analysis

As was apparent in Figure 1–1, the highest level of evidence comes from the meta-analysis. In a meta-analysis, a number of studies are combined in order to develop a single conclusion that has greater statistical power. Such a conclusion is statistically stronger than the analysis of a single study, due to increased numbers of subjects, greater diversity among subjects, or accumulated effects and results. Meta-analysis would be used for the following purposes:

- To establish statistical significance with studies that have conflicting results
- To develop a more correct estimate of ES or magnitude
- To examine subgroups with individual numbers that are not statistically significant

KEY CONCEPT: MANY ARTICLES DO NOT MEET CRITERIA FOR REVIEW

As we mentioned, when conducting a systematic review, data from several articles can be used to reach evidence conclusions. Before conducting the review, it is important to formulate a very specific question, develop criteria, and only then use articles that meet these criteria. Although there are more than 200 articles published each year regarding hearing aid technology, selection, and fitting, location of articles that meet a given criteria is not always an easy task. An example of this was reported by Mueller and Bentler (2005). Intuitively, it would seem that assessing aided loudness discomfort behaviorally following the hearing aid fitting, and then making appropriate adjustments when necessary, would result in improved patient satisfaction. This has been recommended in best practice guidelines. But is there evidence to support this procedure? Mueller and Bentler (2005) report that, although they started with 187 articles related to loudness measures with hearing aids, after they eliminated those articles that did not meet the necessary level of evidence, did not assess behavior-aided loudness discomfort levels (LDLs), did not include real-world loudness outcomes, or did not directly compare real-world loudness outcome to clinical measures, no articles remained; hence, they could not reach a concluding recommendation on this seemingly important clinical measure. It is cases like this in which expert opinion may be the highest level of evidence available; if you care to think of us as experts, we've provided a step-by-step method for conducting this testing in Chapter 15.

> **TECHNICAL TIP: WHAT'S A "QUEASY" EXPERIMENT?**
>
> In our world of hearing aids, *quasi-experimental* studies are often encountered. A quasi-experimental design is one that looks a bit like an RCT except for one main difference: There is no random assignment of subjects to the control and experimental groups (RCT) nor to the experimental groups (cohort studies). Sometimes referred to as "queasy" experiments, they are considered to be less robust in terms of research design. With respect to internal validity, they often appear to be inferior to randomized experiments. But there is something compelling about these designs; taken as a group, they are more frequently implemented than their randomized cousins.

Advantages to meta-analysis include the following:

- Offers greater statistical power
- Provides confirmatory data analysis
- Has greater ability to extrapolate to the general population affected
- Considered an evidence-based resource

Disadvantages to meta-analysis include the following:

- Difficult and time consuming to identify appropriate studies
- Not all studies provide adequate data for inclusion and analysis
- Requires advanced statistical techniques

A meta-analysis published in 2015 by Akeroyd and Whitmer looked at the effects of hearing impairment and hearing aids on sound localization. Their findings indicated that hearing impaired listeners show poorer abilities than listeners with normal hearing in determining the spatial direction of sound from all directions, and especially so from the side. They also conclude that there is no experimental evidence that hearing aids improve the situation.

Levels of Evidence

Now that you are familiar with the designs in research, the levels shown in Figure 1–1 are more meaningful. Many clinicians, professors, and supervisors like to assign level-coding to the research design. You can see two different approaches in Tables 1–3 and 1–4. What is not always clear to students and clinicians when they first begin to study EBP is that levels and quality must go hand in hand. Even though a research team may decide to carry out an RCT, if they fail to meet certain quality markers, the research might not be included in a systematic review or a meta-analysis due to its poor quality, and in spite of its great design.

Table 1–3. Assignment of Level Coding to the Different Research Designs

Level	Description
Ia	Well-designed meta-analysis of more than one randomized controlled trial (RCT)
Ib	Well-designed RCT
IIa	Well-designed controlled study without randomization
IIb	Well-designed quasi-experimental study
III	Well-designed nonexperimental studies, i.e., correlational and case studies
IV	Expert committee report, consensus conference, clinical experience of respected authorities

Source: Robey (2004). Adapted with permission of the Agency for Healthcare Research and Quality.

Table 1–4. Another Example of Assignment of Level Coding to the Various Research Designs

Levels of Evidence	Description
1++	High-quality meta-analyses, systematic reviews of RCTs, or RCTs with very low risk of bias
1+	Well-conducted meta-analyses, systematic reviews of RCTs, or RCTs with low risk of bias
1	Meta-analyses, systematic reviews or RCTs, or RCTs with a high risk of bias
2++	High-quality systematic reviews of case-control or cohort studies *or* high quality case-control or cohort studies with a very low risk of confounding, bias, or chance and a high probability that the probability is causal
2+	Well-conducted case-control or cohort study studies with a low risk of confounding, bias, or chance and a moderate probability that the relationship is causal
2–	Case-control or cohort studies with a high risk of confounding, bias, or chance and a significant risk that the relationship is not causal
3	Nonanalytic studies, e.g., case reports, case series
4	Expert opinion

Source: Harbour & Miller (2001).

KEY CONCEPT: IS THE *POWER* SUFFICIENT?

For clinicians who look to the empirical evidence to guide clinical decision-making, knowing that a study was performed with an adequate number of subjects could instill additional confidence in the reported findings. Included in the list of quality markers discussed in this chapter is evidence of "sufficient power" to detect a true difference. In general, the more subjects the better, but that would introduce increased time and cost, without the real evidence that the investigator has enough subjects in the end. Sufficient power is tied to sample size in the following manner: Depending upon the ES that is considered to be clinically important, and the confidence the investigator wants relative to accuracy of the study in finding an effect (the p value), the sample size can be determined for various estimates of effect size, as shown in Figure 1-3. The good news for researchers is that there are many available software tools to help establish the sufficiency of the power for any design (Lau & Kuk, 2011).

A power analysis can be conducted prior to the start of the data collection (*a priori*) or after the data have been collected (*post hoc*). An increasing number of journal reviewers are asking for *a priori* power analyses to justify the sample size in a submitted paper, especially for those studies with a relatively small pool of subjects. What you will often see is that a power of .80 was used. What this means is that 80% of the time, if there really is a difference between two groups, we would obtain a statistically significant difference. This also means that 20% of the times that we conduct this experiment, we will not obtain a statistically significant effect between the two groups, even though there really is a difference.

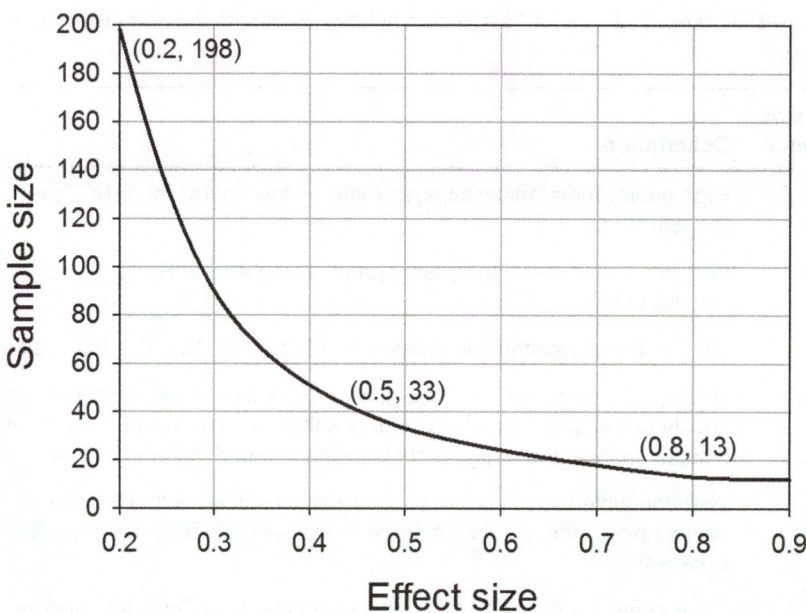

Figure 1–3. Relationship between the required sample size and the ES in a *t*-test with matched pairs for a significance criterion (α) of 0.05, and power of 0.8.

POINTS TO PONDER: HOW WAS SUBJECT SELECTION CONDUCTED?

We all have heard stories about how critical jury selection can be for an important criminal trial. Subject selection for hearing aid research can influence the results of a study in much the same way. We are aware of studies supporting various types of new technology where the results have been changed by simply repeating the study with a different set of subjects. For example, by screening subjects for cognitive function and using only those who pass, the end results could be significantly different. But do all of *your* patients have good cognitive function? The skeptical clinician will want to know many details about the subjects included in a study when determining if the findings are relevant to a given clinical situation. Some things to think about include the following (adapted from Palmer et al, 2008):

- How and from where were the subjects selected? Are they "professional subjects" as are used in many studies in a university setting?
- Did the subjects get paid?
- Do the subjects get to keep the "new" hearing aids? Or purchase them at a sizeable discount?
- What types of biases were built into the study (e.g., using the term "new" compared to "old" hearing aid)? Was the new technology in a more attractive case?
- What was the age range of the subjects?
- What was the level of education of the subjects (i.e., will this generalize to a larger population or to your patients)?

- What was the socioeconomic status of the participants (e.g., were they all college students, college graduates, retired professionals)?
- Were both men and women included?
- What types, degrees, and configurations of hearing loss were included?
- Was cognition level considered?
- Were these active individuals with high communication demands?
- Were the subjects blinded to the treatment condition?
- Was the researcher blinded to the treatment condition when measuring outcomes?

Quality Markers

As noted previously, the design alone does not warrant the level designated in Tables 1–3 and 1–4. Each discipline may develop the markers that designate *good* research. We choose to start with the "Jadad scale" in our assessment of study quality. The Jadad scale has been widely used to assess the quality of clinical trials (Jadad et al., 1996). The scale consists of five questions:

1. Is the study randomized?
2. Is the study double blinded?
3. Is there a description of withdrawals?
4. Is the randomization adequately described?
5. Is the blindness adequately described?

Originally, the scale was applied to trials describing pain treatment but has since been expanded to include other areas, including hearing aid trials (Taylor, Paisley, Davis, 2001). A Jadad score may not be calculated, but a summary similar to the one shown in Table 1–5 can be generated to show the quality of the chosen group of studies. In that systematic review (Bentler, 2006), it was difficult to find high quality studies among the studies

Table 1–5. Summary of Study Quality for Directional Microphone Review

Study	Randomization Procedures	Blinding	Follow-Up ≥80%	Power Calculation	Validated Outcomes
Boymans and Dreschler (2000)	X	S	✓	X	✓
Cord et al. (2002)	NA	NA	✓	X	✓
Gnewikow and Ricketts (2005)	NA	D	X	X	✓
Palmer et al. (2005)	NA	S	✓	✓	X
Preves et al. (1999)	✓	S	✓	X	✓
Ricketts et al. (2003)	✓	S	✓	X	✓
Surr et al. (2002)	✓	S	✓	X	✓
Walden et al. (2000)	NA	S	✓	X	X
Yueh et al. (2001)	**	X	✓	X	✓

Note. X = criterion not met; NA = not appropriate; S = single blinding; D = double blinding; checkmark indicates the quality marker was met.
**partial randomization (for two treatments only)
Source: Adapted from Bentler (2006) with permission.

chosen for inclusion (more to follow). Table 1–6 shows examples of a rating scheme that can go hand-in-hand with the final table.

Grading the Evidence

Assigning a level of evidence for a given study should be relatively straightforward, if the design is clear and the study itself is relatively free from limitations or weaknesses as determined by the quality markers. Unfortunately that is not always the case. Cox (2005a) suggests that the level be moderated by grading to account for variation in the quality of the studies considered. She suggests evidence levels should have associated grading as shown in Table 1–7, regardless of level.

Effect Size (ES)

Recently, studies have started to include ES analyses, and for good reason. If we consider that we are measuring the effect of our hearing aid intervention, then the ES becomes a meaningful concept because it really expresses the magnitude of a result. Consider that the more subjects enrolled in a study, the higher the likelihood of finding a significant finding, albeit often a very small one. The ES can be considered a standard score of the finding that considers how large the effect is regardless of the number of subjects tested. It can be calculated in several ways depending upon the type of data under analysis (see Hill & Thompson, 2004). A common approach is to compute ES as the standardized mean difference between the two groups, as shown in the following equation, commonly referred to as Cohen's d:

$$ES = \text{(mean of experimental group)} \; minus \; \text{(mean of the control group)} \; divided \; by \; \text{the pooled standard deviation.}$$

The formula is modified for a comparison of two groups as is often done in the quasi-experimental designs (such as crossover design) in hearing aid research. An ES of 0.2 is considered to be small; 0.5 is considered to be medium, and 0.8 is considered to be large. To give you an example of what these values mean, let's take a study that compared speech recognition performance for beamforming hearing aids to traditional directional ones, and the outcome was a Cohen's d of .80. What this means is that 79% of the treatment group (beamforming) will be above the mean of the control group (traditional directional), 69% of the two groups will overlap, and there is a 71% chance that a person picked at random from the treatment group will have a higher score than a person picked at random from the control group (probability of superiority). If 100 people go through the treatment (fitted with beamforming products), at least 28 to 30 more people will have a favorable outcome compared to their outcome had they received the control treatment (traditional directional). As you can see, this type of interpretation is helpful for taking the laboratory research findings into the clinic.

Another ES calculation that is commonly found in more recent publications, and is often associated with analysis of variance (ANOVA) techniques, is partial η^2 (pronounced partial eta squared). It generally follows similar underlying principles as Cohen's d, so similar ES rules apply. This is not true of all ES methods however. If you see a method you are not familiar with (e.g., omega squared), it may be informative to look up the accepted small, medium, and large values online (e.g., 0.01, 0.059, 0.138).

Table 1–6. System for Quality Rating of Individual Studies

Rating	Interpretation of Rating
++	Very low risk of bias. Any weaknesses that are present are very unlikely to alter the conclusions of the study.
+	Low risk of bias. Identified weaknesses or omitted information that probably would not alter the conclusions of the study.
−	High risk of bias. Identified weaknesses or omitted information that are likely or very likely to alter the conclusions of the study.

Source: Cox (2005a).

Table 1–7. An Example of Grading of the Evidence

A	Consistent level 1 studies
B	Consistent level 2 or 3 studies *or* extrapolations from level 1 studies
C	Level 4 studies *or* extrapolations from level 2 or 3 studies
D	Level 5 evidence *or* troublingly inconsistent or inconclusive studies of any level

> **KEY CONCEPT: DON'T LET YOUR EYES FOOL YOU!**
>
> In this chapter we talk about power analysis, statistical significance, effect size, and other factors that you must consider when determining whether a given finding is meaningful. Consider that in most of hearing aid research, when one technology is compared to another the differences will be small. Studies showing that "Hearing Aid A" is better than "Hearing Aid B" may be based on a Hearing In Noise Test (HINT) score difference of 2 dB or less, or no more than a 10 percentage point (e.g., 75% vs. 65%) improvement in speech recognition. What you might then see, especially in white papers and trade journal articles, are some creative graphics: Rather than a chart going from 0% to 100%, the chart may go from 60% to 80%, making that minimal 10 percentage point improvement look huge.

An example ES analysis is shown in Figure 1–4 (Cox, 2005a). The two pairs of plots (upper and lower boxes) depict hypothetical distributions of results for two experiments comparing a new hearing aid to an older model of hearing aid. The upper box (Study A) shows the same mean difference in scores of 17 points as is shown in the lower box (Study B). As can be seen in the figures, however, the subjects did not behave in a similar manner. In Study A, the standard deviation (SD) was four points, whereas in Study B, the SD was

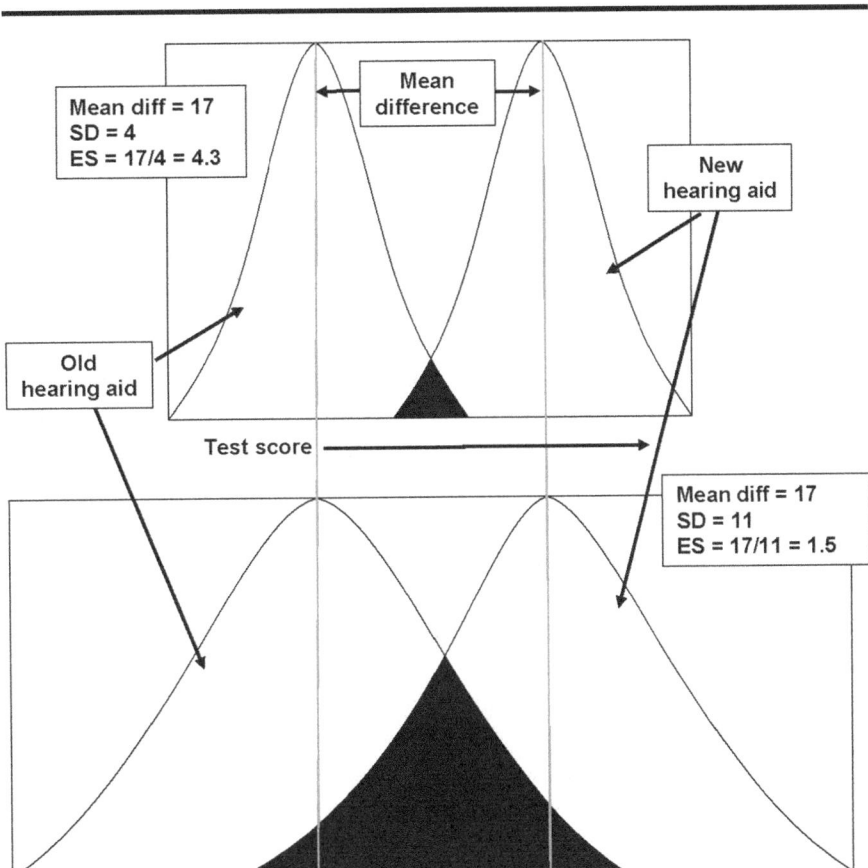

Figure 1–4. Example of two studies with same mean difference in hearing aid outcomes but differing ES (refer to text). Adapted from Cox, 2005a, with permission.

11 points, showing that there was significant overlap of the two groups in terms of their responses. By applying the formula for ES, we discover that Study A has an ES of 4.3, whereas Study B has an ES of 1.5. This means that most of the subjects in Study A had a better result with the new hearing aid, whereas in Study B several of the subjects had no real improvement from the new hearing aid.

Why is this important? If the clinician looks for significant findings, both studies indicate that to be the case. For Study B, however, the significance may not be *clinically* relevant. The ES can better direct us to accepting the findings and implementing them into our clinical practice. More to follow.

ES Plus Confidence Interval (CI)

When ES is combined with the CI, the results allow us to arrive at a more conclusive outcome. For example, in Figure 1–5A we see four studies comparing two hearing aids. For each study the ES is shown by the filled circle, along with its 95% CI. The 95% CI is the range of ESs you would expect to measure for 95 out of 100 replications of the study. If the CI intersects the bolded 0.0 line, the implication is that the results are not significant (the hearing aids were not deemed to have different outcomes). Based on the ES and 95% CI, each study provides us with a different conclusion:

- Study 1 produced an ES of 0.2, but the CI span was −0.2 to +0.6. This CI does intersect the 0 effect line, so the results are not significant. Because the CI is relatively wide, we cannot be confident that the ES of 0.2 will be seen again if the study is replicated.
- Study 2 produced the same ES of 0.2 as Study 1 but with a very narrow CI. This CI does not intersect the 0 line so we know the study did produce a significant finding (i.e., the new technology was superior to the older technology). In addition, since the CI is relatively small, we can be confident that this result is highly reproducible.
- Study 3 produced an ES of 0.5 with a CI from 0.75 to 0.25. This CI does not intersect the 0 line so we know that the study produced significant results. In addition, since the CI is relatively narrow, we are confident that the study result is highly reproducible.
- Study 4 produced the same ES as Study 3 but with a very wide CI. The CI does intersect the 0 line so we know that the results of the study were not significant.

Based on these interpretations, we can see that the value or importance of the ES is tied to the significance of the finding. In Study 2, the ES was small but the study produced a significant finding; that is, one hearing aid was significantly better than the other, albeit by a small amount. In Study 4, the ES was large, but so was the CI, resulting in a finding on "no significant difference between the hearing aids."

Combining Data

A final demonstration of the potential value of using ESs can be seen in Figure 1–5B. This figure illustrates the advantages of combining ESs across studies to increase power. In this case, Study 1 had an ES of 0.3 but the CI crossed the 0 line indicating that the results were not

---

KEY CONCEPT: "SHOW ME THE EVIDENCE"

The typical hard-working, fast-paced clinician is not likely to be involved in the calculation of significance and ES with any regularity. But to understand the terminology allows for better consumption of the relevant research. Without that understanding, we may fall prey to the common trap of mistaking marketing for evidence. Slick looking white papers from the manufacturer tend to look a lot like articles from refereed journals. Don't be afraid to ask: Was a power analysis conducted? What was the ES? Was the study blinded? Was it double-blinded? Was there a control group used? In other words, it's very reasonable to say, "Show me the evidence!" when offered a new product or a new feature.

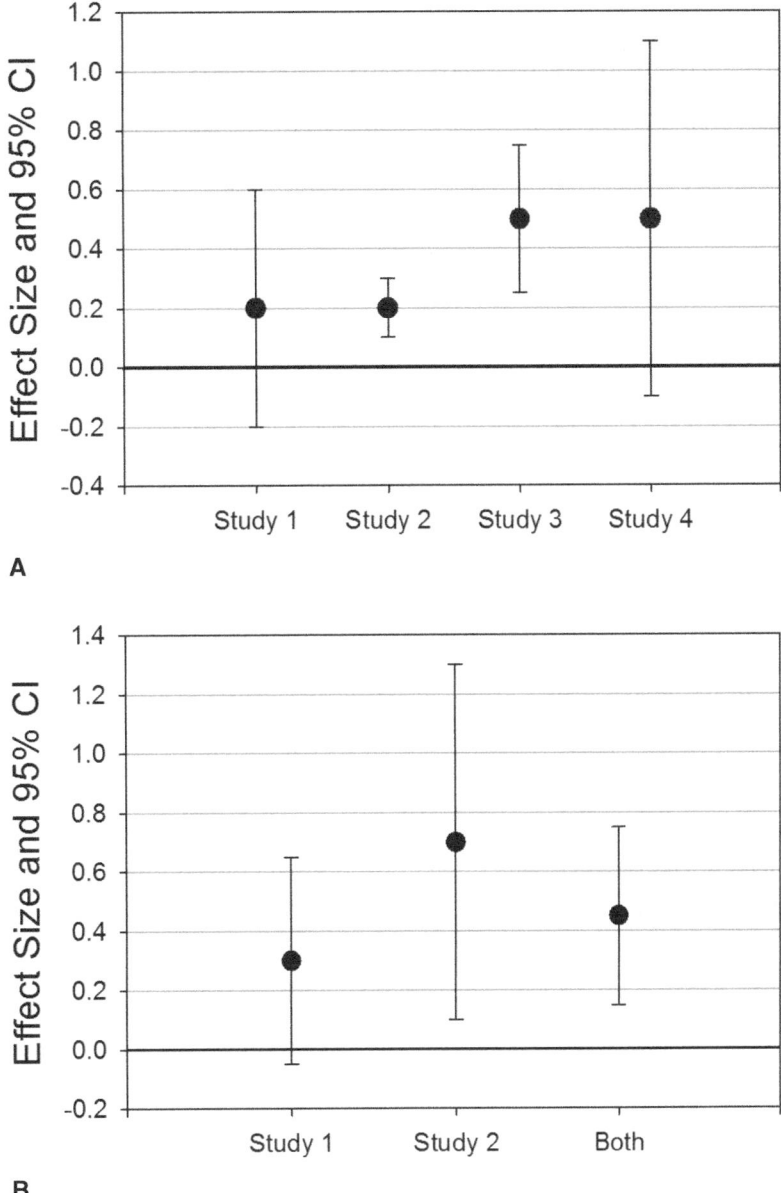

Figure 1–5. A. Example of smaller and larger ES and how the significance of the finding is related to the CI. **B.** Example of how combining data sets can show a significant outcome even when individual studies do not.

significant. In Study 2 there was a greater ES (0.7) but even wider CI, although the CI did not cross the 0 line. The interpretation of that study would be that the finding was significant, but the likelihood of a reproducible finding limited. By combining the two studies, we have an ES of 0.45 with a CI that does not cross the 0 line. Because we increased the number of subjects—and thus the power—we were able to show that the two technologies were significantly different, a finding that was less obvious when looking at the two studies independently.

> **THINGS TO REMEMBER: WHAT DOES THE EVIDENCE TELL US TO DATE ABOUT HEARING AIDS?**
>
> A few promising things. A long-time researcher in hearing aid effectiveness, Larry Humes, offers the following general findings, based on his systematic review of the evidence (Humes & Krull, 2012). Using the key words *hearing aid*, *outcome*, and *adults*, he initially searched through 783 articles to arrive at 33 appropriate studies of subjective and/or objective measures of hearing aid outcomes related to hearing aid benefit, satisfaction, and usage. This led him to several conclusions:
>
> - Although a fair number of good quality (Grade B) nonrandomized intervention studies (Level 3 evidence) have been completed in this area over the past two decades, only one randomized controlled trial (Level 2 evidence; Grade A) of hearing aid effectiveness (Yueh et al., 2001) is available. No studies have employed placebo groups as controls and the use of control groups has also been rare.
> - The overwhelming majority of nonrandomized intervention studies have made use of similar study samples: older adults with mild to severe sloping sensorineural hearing loss, fit bilaterally with hearing aids whose frequency response characteristics were verified via real-ear measurements. This facilitates pooling of the data and probably increases the likelihood for similar outcomes across studies, but does not aid in the generalization of findings to other groups of hearing-impaired adults or other protocols (e.g., unilateral amplification, failure to use real-ear measurements for verification).
> - Keeping the two conclusions noted above in mind, the following general observations were drawn from the analyses of the existing nonrandomized intervention studies conducted:
>   - Benefaction measures generally showed significant reductions in hearing handicap or the frequency of problems from unaided to aided conditions and generated typical responses of "helpful" and "satisfied."
>   - Usage measure typically showed self-reported usage of four to eight hours per day or "about three-quarters of the time."
>   - Speech understanding was significantly improved from unaided to aided test conditions, with the exception of high speech levels at low signal-to-noise ratios.

Evidence for Verification and Validation

To this point, most of our research examples have involved evidence for hearing aid technology, processing, or special features. This evidence is certainly important, but we are also interested in evidence for all the other components of the hearing aid fitting protocol. We have already mentioned some studies related to prefitting testing, but what about verification and validation methods? Does the evidence support our clinical practices?

In a Midwestern city of 50,000 people, next to the hospital, there is an audiology practice (Practice A) that sells hearing aids. At Practice A, all hearing aid patients have a needs assessment, complete a COSI, and receive a QuickSIN prior to the fitting. A validated prescriptive method is used, the fitting is verified with probe microphone measures, and adjustments are made to match targets for each input level. Aided loudness is then verified and the patient receives unaided and aided QuickSIN testing to demonstrate the benefits of amplification. A few weeks following the fitting, the patient returns and completes the COSI and the IOI-HA. Problems (if any) are discussed and other appropriate counseling conducted. Down the street from Practice A, located in a shopping complex next to the supermarket, is Practice B. Practice B sells the same brand of hearing aids for the same prices as Practice A. At Practice B, however, the only prefitting testing is a pure-tone audiogram and word recognition in quiet. The fitting itself consists of nothing more than a mouse click on the manufacturer's proprietary fitting algorithm icon. "Verification" is based on a single question: "How does that sound?" No outcome measures are conducted.

So what do you think? Do the people fitted at Practice A derive more benefit from their hearing aids? Are they more satisfied? Are the returns for credit higher for Practice B? Does Practice B have more patients with their hearing aids in the drawer? Is Practice A more profitable than Practice B? The answers to these questions are not as straightforward as you might think.

There is surprisingly little evidence regarding the value of hearing aid verification and validation, and what is available is often inferential. For example, in his 2005 article that was a systematic review of research with the NAL prescriptive fitting, Mueller reported that although the level of evidence was only moderate, there was evidence supporting the use of this prescriptive method (8 of the 11 studies that met criteria). As we discuss in Chapter 16, in a crossover design study conducted more recently by Abrams, Chisolm, McManus, and McArdle (2012), the NAL-N1 fitting was significantly superior to the manufacturers' default algorithm for real-world hearing aid benefit. Sanders, Stoody, Weber, and Mueller (2015) report that manufacturers' software-derived NAL-NL2 fittings do not meet NAL-NL2 targets in the real ear and adjustments of 10 dB or more typically are necessary in the higher frequencies. So if we then conclude that there is evidence for starting patients with the NAL fitting algorithm, and we know that this is possible only when ear canal SPL is measured, then there is indirect evidence for the practice of probe microphone verification for all patients.

Although not a high level of evidence (i.e., only Level 3), certainly the most extensive data regarding the value of verification and validation comes from the MarkeTrak VIII survey. We cannot derive a clear cause and effect from these data, but with a sampling from over 2000 patients, the findings certainly are compelling.

MarkeTrak VIII: Support for Verification and Validation

As the name indicates, MarkeTrak VIII was the eighth in a series of consumer satisfaction surveys (see Chapter 3). What makes MarkeTrak VIII unique, however, is that not only was patient satisfaction assessed but also considerable information was collected regarding how the hearing aids were fitted. The relationship between the fitting process and subsequent satisfaction has led to several articles discussing these data (e.g., Kochkin, 2010, Kochkin, 2011, Kochkin, 2014).

The Survey Process

The MarkeTrak VIII survey process has been explained in detail by Kochkin (2009), but a brief overview is as follows:

- A short screening survey was sent to 80,000 members of the National Family Organization households (balanced for age, income, location, etc.).
- This survey was completed by 46,843 individuals. Of this group, 14,623 stated that at least one family member had a hearing loss; 3,789 were owners of hearing aids.
- In 2009, a detailed seven-page survey was sent to the 3,789 hearing aid owners. There was a response rate of 84% (3,174).
- Narrowing this database to individuals who had hearing aids that were no older than four years resulted in 1,141 experienced users and 884 new users (total $n = 2,025$).
- The mean age (~71 years), gender (~55% male) and hearing aid age (~1.8 years) was similar for both groups (Note: *New users* identified individuals using their first pair of hearing aids, not *newly fitted* users).

As with most of the previous MarkeTrak surveys, satisfaction was assessed for several factors using a seven-point Likert scale. Using these data, overall success was measured using a statistical composite of the following factors:

- Hearing aid use
- Benefit and satisfaction
  - Satisfaction with hearing aids to "improve hearing"
  - Perception of problem resolution for 10 different listening situations (only ones that applied to them)
  - Satisfaction for different listening situations
- Patient purchase recommendations (e.g., recommend hearing aids for friends)

Important for our discussion here is that the respondents also reported on tests/services they received during the fitting process with a "yes or no" response. If they were "not sure," that also was provided as an optional response. Each of the items listed below was described in a manner that would be meaningful to the lay individual:

- Hearing tested in sound booth
- Loudness discomfort measurement
- Probe microphone measurement used for verification
- Measurement of objective benefit (e.g., pre–post measurement of speech understanding)
- Measurement of subjective benefit
- Outcome measure of patient benefit/satisfaction
- Auditory training software/therapy
- Enrollment in aural rehabilitation group
- Received self-help book/literature/video
- Referred to self-help group (e.g., Hearing Loss Association of America or HLAA).

As is probably obvious from the lists just presented, data analysis of these survey results could easily be used to examine whether there was a relationship between the verification and validation testing conducted, and patient success with hearing aids. Also, using other data from the survey, Kochkin was able the examine relationships between the testing conducted and repeat visits and patient loyalty. We will review each of these research questions.

Test Protocol and Patient Satisfaction

The findings of greatest interest to individuals fitting hearing aids from the MarkeTrak VIII survey was the relationship of patient satisfaction to the test protocol used in the fitting process. Does best practice pay off? To derive a total measure of success, a factor analysis was conducted on the outcome measures, resulting in a single index that was standardized to a mean of 5 and standard deviation of 2. In comparing above-average and below-average hearing aid user success, individuals who were at least one standard deviation below the mean ($n = 331$) on success and those who were at least one standard deviation above the mean on success ($n = 407$) were compared. Hearing aid users with above-average success were most likely to have received objective benefit measurements (+26%), subjective benefit measurements (+25%), loudness discomfort testing (+24%), probe microphone verification (+20%), and a patient satisfaction measurement (+17%).

We of course do not know if the increased satisfaction is a result of the test procedure itself (e.g., the maximum power output or MPO was changed when loudness testing was conducted) or simply that increased testing means that the patient spends more time with the audiologist, which probably gives the patient more confidence in the overall fitting process and a greater respect for the audiologist's professional credentials.

A different way to view these findings is shown in Figure 1–6. These data reflect the answer to the question: Does pre-fitting testing, verification and validation performed during the hearing aid fitting process have an additive or multiplicative impact on real-world success? The patients were ranked on the number of items (range 0–12) or protocol steps received during the hearing aid fitting process. The average total success scores are then derived by the number of protocol steps performed (see Figure 1–6). As is clearly shown, as additional steps are added—LDL + probe microphone + speech in noise testing + outcome measures—overall satisfaction rises steeply from below 2.0 (hearing test only) to nearly 6.0. (Note: Steps 8 and above reflect post-fitting rehabilitation and counseling).

If we consider that following best practice (Steps 1 to 7 in Figure 1–6) leads to improved satisfaction and success with hearing aids, then it's also important to consider other data from this research. The findings also revealed that 94% of the group in the

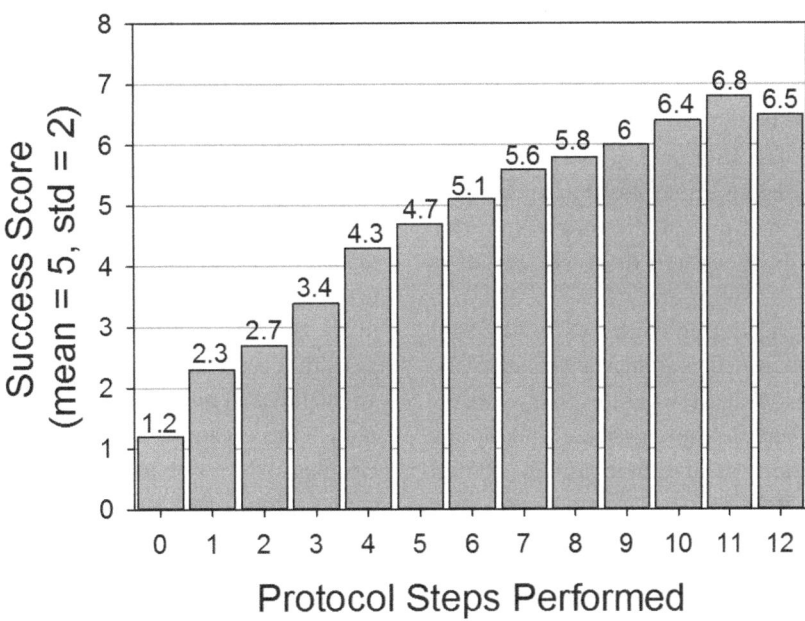

Figure 1–6. Success score as a function of number of protocol steps performed during the hearing aid fitting. Adapted from Kochkin et al., 2010.

POINTS TO PONDER: WHAT INFLUENCED SATISFACTION OUTCOME?

In the data we show in Figure 1–6, there certainly appears to be a strong relationship between the test protocol and success with hearing aids. What else could have influenced these findings? Kochkin et al. (2010) examined several possible variables. They report that age of the patient, gender, user sophistication (new vs. experienced), size of city (rural to metropolitan), price of hearing aid, style of hearing aid, and degree of hearing loss explained less than 1% of variance. In this study, 69% of hearing aids were fit by audiologists and 31% by hearing instrument specialists. The professional training of the hearing aid fitter explained less than one-half of 1% of the real-world success with respect to protocol used or hearing aid user. Yes, you just read that: *The professional training of the hearing aid fitter explained less than one-half of 1% of the real-world success with respect to protocol used or hearing aid user.* Why the small difference? We think this could also relate to evidenced-based practice procedures. While audiologists are typically trained to use best practice procedures, not all of them do. Data examining use of probe microphone verification suggest very similar percentages for audiologists and hearing instrument specialists. We suspect that similar percentages would also be found for a number of other best practice procedures as well. Being trained in best practices does not really help us if we don't apply them in our clinical practice, an observation that is reinforced in the following section.

---

top 15% of satisfaction would recommend their dispenser to others, whereas only 39% of the group with the bottom 15% of satisfaction would consider doing this.

Return Patient Visits

Unscheduled repeat visits during the fitting process can be considered an indirect measure of patient success.

For example, this was used by Shi et al. (2015) in a study of the value of LDL and QuickSIN testing. Kochkin (2011), using the MarkeTrak data, examined how the test protocol might influence repeat visits. To do this, he divided the patients into four groups (Figure 1–7), separating those that had both verification and validation from those that had one or the other. Note that 22% had neither (as in Practice B discussed earlier in this chapter).

The relationship to testing conducted at the time of the fitting and subsequent patient visits is also significant. The trend is what we would expect, with the big jump in visits present for those patients who did not receive any verification or validation measures (average of 2.4 visits vs. 3.6 visits).

Kochkin also provides the following data from this analysis:

- For patients with above average success, 76% were fitted in one or two visits compared to 40% of patients who experienced below average success.
- For patients with below-average success, 47% required four to six visits to fit their hearing aids compared to only 7% of patients who experienced above-average success.

Kochkin (2011) goes on to report that, in 2010, nearly 2.7 million hearing aids were fitted in the United States, representing over 1.5 million patients (e.g., estimating bilateral fitting rate of 75%). Assuming the same distribution of best practices as noted by patients in Figure 1–7 and the estimate that there is a reduction of 1.2 in the average number of patient visits, Kochkin suggests that the systematic utilization of both verification and validation procedures while fitting hearing aids will reduce unnecessary patient visits by a total of 521,779. He goes on to point out that this additional service consumes a lot of the audiologist's time (~400,000 hours/year) that could be better spent counseling others or fitting new patients with hearing aids. Moreover, and perhaps most importantly, he adds that these extra and unnecessary visits can be a huge inconvenience to the older patients, who often need a ride to the clinic and frequently have multiple disabilities that can include challenges with respect to mobility, danger from falls, and other potential problems. We agree.

Patient Loyalty

Most of us fitting hearing aids are pretty confident that the majority of patients leave our office with their new hearing aids with pretty positive thoughts about us and the fitting process. Based on this positive experience we probably also assume that these happy patients will steer their friends and relatives who need hearing aids our way. Furthermore, they will certainly be back to see us when they need replacement hearing aids. But how loyal are our patients? And how does our test protocol influence patient loyalty?

Patient loyalty and its relationship to the overall fitting process was yet another interesting area that could be examined by mining the MarkeTrak VIII data. Going back to 1986 and paraphrasing the classic book by W. Edwards Deming, *Out of the Crisis*, we've often heard that a happy customer (patient) who comes back is worth 10 new prospects. Happy customers spread their good news to eight other potential customers, but unhappy customers spread their bad news to 16 potential customers (and this was *before* the days of Facebook and Twitter!). The cost of acquiring a new customer is five times higher than keeping a customer satisfied. There has not been a lot of research in this area related

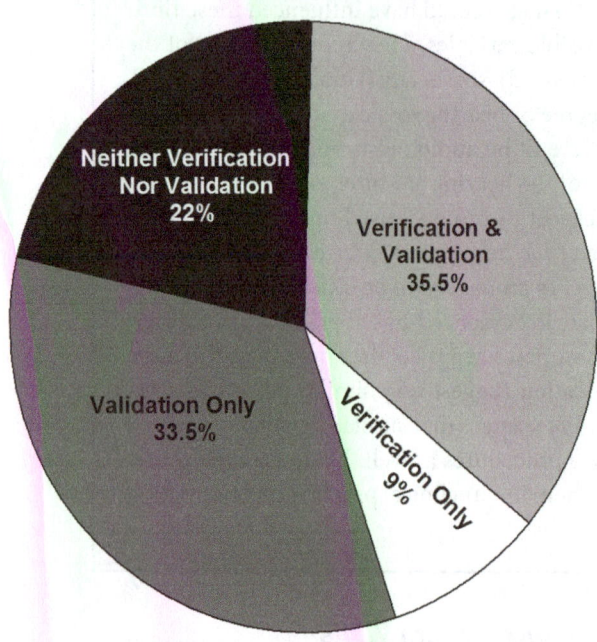

Figure 1–7. From Kochkin, 2011, the percent of survey respondents that had verification only (9%), validation only (33.5%), verification and validation (35.5%), and neither (22%).

to hearing aid sales but, to a large extent, a customer is a customer, whether the concern is repeat business for an airline, a coffee shop, or an audiologist's office.

In the MarkeTrak survey that we explained earlier, hearing aid users were asked to rate their dispenser (either audiologist or hearing instrument specialist) on seven factors using a seven-point Likert scale: "Very dissatisfied," "Dissatisfied," "Somewhat dissatisfied," "Neutral" (equally satisfied and dissatisfied), "Somewhat satisfied," "Satisfied," and "Very satisfied." They also then completed Likert scale ratings for the dispenser/audiologist on the following factors: (a) professionalism, (b) knowledge level, (c) explanation of hearing aid care, (d) explanation of hearing aid expectations, (e) quality of service during the hearing aid fitting, (f) quality of service post-fitting, and (g) level of empathy. For data analysis, an average of these last seven attributes was obtained to reflect a single dimension.

It is of course important to see how patient loyalty relates to the verification and validation procedures. Recall from our earlier discussion, an overall index of best practices was standardized to a Z-score with a mean of 5 and standard deviation of 2. For this analysis, scores were converted to percentile rankings and then grouped into 10 levels of best practices (BP) in deciles, where BP1 = minimal hearing aid fitting protocol – 10%, BP5 = average (50%) protocol, and BP10 = comprehensive (100%) protocol. Figure 1–8 shows the relationship between patient loyalty and the level of best practice provided by the dispenser. Observe that those with the highest level of best practices (BP10) have a 96% loyalty rating. Loyalty ratings rapidly decline to 34% for those using minimalist fitting protocols. In general, Kochkin reported an average loyalty rating of 57% for audiologists who do not conduct verification or validation, and an average loyalty rating of 84% for those audiologists who do.

To conclude this section on the MarkeTrak VIII verification and validation data, let's take those average patient loyalty findings, and go back to the Practice A and Practice B examples that we discussed earlier. To provide more background data, both practices have been in business for 10 years, and every year they each sell hearing aids to about 100 patients.

Approximately 80% of their fittings are bilateral, which then result in 180 hearing aids per year. After 10 years of practice, many of their patients should be returning to replace their hearing aids. But, about 20% have either died, moved away, or are not in a position to obtain new hearing aids, so we'll consider the potential annual return rate for both practices is 80% or 80 patients.

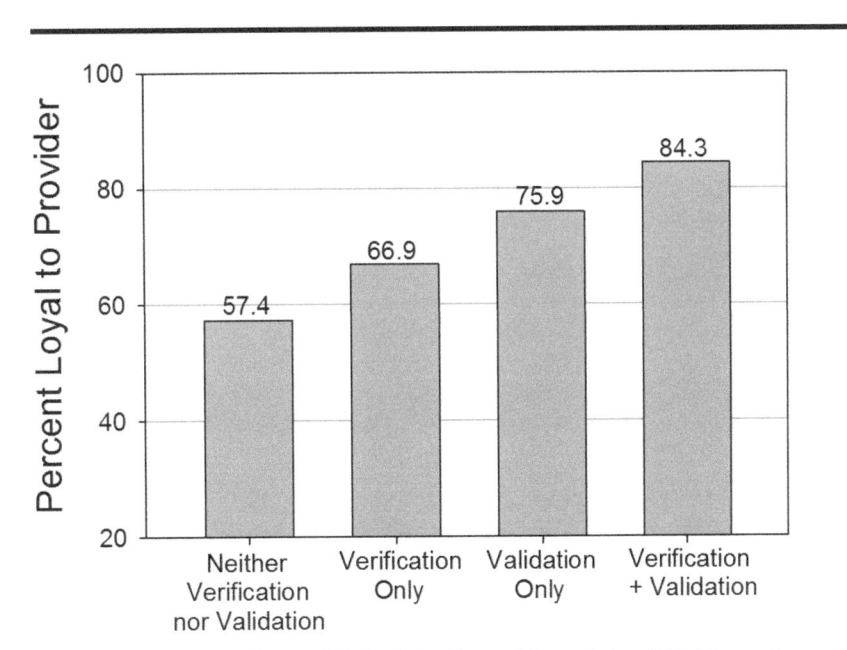

Figure 1–8. Relationship between patient loyalty and groupings as per best practice. Adapted from Kochkin, 2011.

Recall that Practice B did not conduct verification or validation, so we would predict their patient return rate to be 57%. To do the math: 57% of 80 (potential) × 1.8 (bilateral fittings) = 81 hearing aids sold to return patients. Now how about Practice A, where they work a little harder? Their patient return rate should be 84%. Again, to do the math: 84% of 80 (potential) × 1.8 (bilateral fittings) = 120 hearing aids—a 39 hearing aid difference, which we would predict to be present every year. So not only is best practice ethical practice, it is also good (and profitable) practice.

In Closing

It is unlikely that most clinicians will engage in high-level research endeavors such as the RCT. It is also unlikely that most clinicians will find the time in their busy practices to carry out a systematic review of relevant literature each time they have a hearing aid-related question. How do we resolve this dilemma of getting the evidence to the clinic? There are several options. All clinicians are required to maintain continuing education evidence (CEUs). Take advantage of those presentations that provide the evidence you are looking for. Bear in mind, however, that to best use these principles of EBP requires all three "legs" of information to provide the best management planning for our patients: empirical, clinician experience, and client characteristics. In this chapter we have helped sort through understanding of the empirical evidence and considered a number of published datasets relative to hearing aid effectiveness. Each practicing clinician brings a wealth of previous experience to the table each day that must be considered, as does each patient bring his or her needs and expectations. All three of the legs must be in place and balanced for the best outcome.

2
The Audiologist and Hearing Aid Provision

The selection and fitting of hearing aids has been associated with audiology since before audiology was called audiology. In fact, it is probable that the extensive work with hearing aids and aural rehabilitation by several individuals during World War II is what led to the coining of the words audiology and audiologist, but more on that later. In this chapter, we talk about how the profession of audiology is associated with the area of hearing aid fitting and dispensing, and discuss many of the overriding principles, guidelines, and regulations that have an impact on this relationship.

A Little History

Perhaps the first book to provide extensive guidance regarding the fitting of hearing aids was *Hearing Tests and Hearing Instrument,* written by Watson and Tolan, published in 1949. Neither Watson nor Tolan were audiologists, nor what we would now call audiologists. Thomas Tolan, a medical doctor, was the director of the Department of Otology at the Medical School of the University of Minnesota. Leland A. Watson was the president of the Maico Corporation, a company involved in the manufacture of audiometers and hearing aids. At the time this book was published, many viewed it as simply a promotion of Maico products (one reviewer commented "useful for salesmen"), and to some extent it was, but it also was the first organized publication of many hearing aid fitting concepts, some of which still apply today.

It was around this same time that the terms audiology and audiologist began to be commonly used. When exactly the term audiology was coined is debatable. According to research by Ken Berger, PhD (1976a), the term may have been used by a New York dentist in 1935 by two California hearing aid specialists (approximately 1939) or by individuals working for the Maico company in the late 1930s. Probably unrelated, but well documented, is that a song entitled "Audiology" was recorded around 1939. In the academic world, the first use of the term *audiology* usually is credited to either Hallowell Davis, Norton Canfield (prominent military otolaryngologist), or Raymond Carhart, all in the mid-1940s. Relating to what we now know as the profession of audiology, the first use of the word in print was in 1946, in publications in the *Journal of Speech Disorders* (in reference to the U.S. Naval Hospital in Philadelphia) and in the *Volta Review* (in a description of coursework offered at Northwestern University; Jerger, 2009).

Military Roots

Regardless of who actually coined the word audiology, there is little question that the advancement of the use of the term was linked directly to the establishment of rehabilitation centers during World War II. These sites were established to handle the large number of returning veterans suffering from hearing loss. Four major military regional sites were established: Hoff General Hospital (Santa Barbara, CA), Borden General Hospital (Chickasha, OK), Philadelphia Naval Hospital, and Deshon General Hospital (Butler, PA). Captain Raymond Carhart (Figure 2–1), a 1936 PhD graduate of Northwestern University (majoring in speech pathology, experimental phonetics, and psychology), was assigned to Deshon Hospital from 1944 to 1946. His work there has had a lasting effect on the field of audiology and, specifically, the selection and fitting of hearing aids. In 1946, Carhart published three articles describing the hearing aid selection and fitting procedures developed at Deshon (Carhart, 1946a, 1946b, 1946c). We talk more about the impact that Captain Carhart had on the clinical evaluation of hearing aids in Chapter 14.

Following World War II, there were several additional military audiology facilities established at major hospitals—Walter Reed Army Medical Center in Washington, DC, being the most notable. We also saw the emergence of several U.S. Department of Veterans Affairs (VA) audiology clinics. All of these facilities employed audiologists, both military and civilian, who conducted hearing aid evaluations and also dispensed hearing aids to veterans, active duty, and retired military personnel. Because of the ethical constraints placed on audiologists fitting hearing aids outside of the government—which we discuss shortly—these military and VA hospital clinics became known as excellent training sites for audiology students wanting to obtain hands-on experience with the selection and fitting of hearing aids.

It was also during this time that audiology training programs began to emerge. These early programs were in the Midwest, at locations such as Northwestern University, the University of Iowa, and Purdue University.

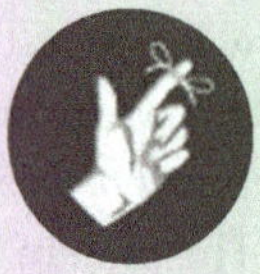

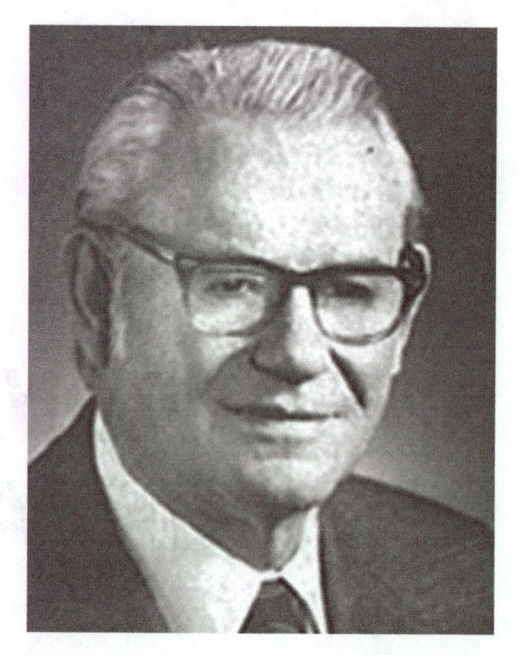

Figure 2–1. Raymond Carhart, PhD, often considered the father of audiology and at least partly responsible for coining the word audiology. Noted professor at Northwestern University until his death in 1975. He conducted pioneering work related to the selection and fitting of hearing aids while serving in the U.S. Army in the 1940s.

THINGS TO REMEMBER: WARTIME AUDIOLOGY

If you are interested in audiology history, you will enjoy the monograph written by Moe Bergman titled "American Wartime Military Audiology," a special issue of *Audiology Today* (2002). In it he writes: "It is important for every profession to document its origins. It should be of interest to today's practitioners of audiology to know how the American military 'aural rehabilitation' programs for hearing casualties in the twentieth-century world wars practiced what is now known as 'audiology.'" Even then, professionals were working to help rehabilitate individuals who suffered from hearing loss, many as a result of the unprecedentedly loud equipment and powerful explosives used in World Wars I and II.

The first PhD granted in audiology was from Northwestern in 1946 to John Keys, who went on to establish a noted audiology research and training program at the University of Oklahoma (Jerger, 2009).

Audiologists as the Middle Man

Although audiologists at military facilities enjoyed the benefits of directly dispensing hearing aids to their patients, in the civilian sector, until the 1980s, nearly all hearing aids were dispensed by hearing aid dealers (now referred to as hearing instrument specialists), not audiologists. As is true today, there were many storefront hearing aid sales facilities, many of them franchises.

Audiologists' clinical activities regarding hearing aid dispensing were influenced greatly by the American Speech and Hearing Association (ASHA), the primary professional organization for audiologists during this time frame. For arguably good reasons, the ASHA had the belief that it could be challenging to professional ethics if an audiologist were to evaluate a patient for a hearing aid, recommend a hearing aid, and then turn around and sell the patient the hearing aid he or she had just recommended. Selling hearing aids, therefore, was a violation of the ASHA ethical standards.

So it was that during this time frame, audiologists had a somewhat unusual role in the selection and fitting of hearing aids. During this era, although the majority of hearing aids were dispensed by a *dispenser* without the patient first going to an audiologist, there were situations when an audiologist was involved. When this happened, the general fitting process would go something like this:

- The patient would go to a university or hospital clinic to have his or her hearing tested and be evaluated for hearing aids. We say hearing aids, with an "s," although rarely did audiologists then recommend the use of two hearing aids. In fact, this often caused considerable friction between the hearing aid dealer and the audiologist, as dealers would more frequently fit people bilaterally ("Just a way to make more money," audiologists often would say).
- Audiologists of the time had a large stock selection of behind the ear (BTE) hearing aids on consignment from various manufacturers; it was not unusual to have 20 to 30 consigned aids. A common procedure then was to conduct aided sound field comparative speech testing, usually using monosyllables, with hearing aids from different companies. There usually was only time to test three hearing aids during a typical one-hour appointment; hence, this selection procedure became known as the *hang three* approach.
- Following the speech testing, the aided word recognition scores for each instrument were compared, and a winner was determined. In some cases, this might mean the patient only scored 2 to 4% higher with one of the instruments—but there had to be a winner. The audiologist would then *prescribe* this fitting (e.g., brand, model, settings of potentiometers).
- The patient was then referred directly to a given hearing aid dealer who sold that brand (most dealers only sold one or two brands) or, if the audiologist was concerned about the appearance of a conflict of interest, the patient was simply given a list of several dealers in the area, and the patient would then be on his or her own to find the product.
- The protocol for most facilities was that after the patient purchased the new hearing aids, he or she would return to the audiology clinic to obtain aided speech recognition testing with the new product. This was another situation rife with conflict, as in many cases the patient had purchased a hearing aid different from what the audiologist had recommended. The audiologist and dispenser often would disagree regarding what was best, and the patient was caught in the middle.

For a variety of reasons, the fitting and dispensing arrangement just described was less than ideal. Not only was the original comparative selection procedure flawed, but the audiologist was removed from the important post-fitting troubleshooting, tweaking, and counseling. As would be expected, the patients returned to the hearing aid dealer, not the audiologist, for these services. If only audiologists had been allowed to sell hearing aids, the process would have been so much more efficient.

Selling is Not a Bad Word (Anymore)

Regarding the ASHA code of ethics mentioned earlier, it is important to point out that in the 1960s and 1970s state licensure for audiology did not exist for most states. Clinical audiologists, therefore, valued their ASHA certification and did not want to jeopardize their standing as an ASHA member. And for the most part, audiologists not belonging to the ASHA were considered outsiders. Moreover, most audiologists, especially those in academia, tended to believe that selling hearing aids had a certain sleaze factor associated with it. There of course were audiologists who tested the system, and their expulsion from the ASHA was publicized. James Jerger devotes a couple of pages to *The Saga of Barry Elpern* in his book on the history of audiology (Jerger, 2009, pp. 48–49).

As time went on, however, more and more audiologists saw the benefits of providing complete services for their patients. In the early 1970s, we started to see audiologists going into a dispensing private practice—with little concern regarding the approval from the ASHA.

The movement to remove the violation for selling hearing aids from the ASHA code of ethics gathered steam in 1977 when a group of ASHA members formed the Academy of Dispensing Audiology (ADA). The name of the organization obviously was selected to make the point that selling hearing aids should be part of the audiologists' scope of practice (the name has since been changed to the Academy of Doctors of Audiology). Although one might think that this new organization was simply a handful of young maverick audiologists, it actually included several prominent members of the profession, most notably Leo Doerfler, PhD, who was not only the ADA's founding president, but also a former president of the ASHA.

While the internal pressure for change was resulting in many heated discussions at professional meetings, the event that probably triggered the change in ASHA policy was a 1978 U.S. Supreme Court ruling against the National Society of Professional Engineers, saying that their code of ethics could not be used to prohibit price interference for engineers' services. And so it was that selling hearing aids for profit became ethical. By the end of 1979, nearly 1,000 audiologists were selling hearing aids; that number grew to 5,000 by the end of the 1980s (Harford, 2000).

Audiologists in the Workplace

Things have changed considerably since the days when audiologists only dispensed hearing aids in government facilities. Today, there are approximately 16,000 licensed audiologists in the United States, and 60 to 70% of these dispense hearing aids. (Note, by comparison, there are approximately 8,000 licensed hearing instrument specialists.) Audiologists dispense from a variety of settings ranging from their own private practice, to an otolaryngologist's practice, to a university or hospital clinic, to an office owned by a manufacturer, or in more recent years, from a chain big box store (e.g., Costco, Sam's). Shown in Figure 2–2 are the most recent data from the American Academy of Audiology (AAA) summarizing typical work settings. Observe that the highest percent of audiologists are in privately owned audiology practices. Although this is the most common workplace, data from the AAA suggests that only 15 to 20% of audiology offices are owned and controlled by audiologists, much lower than for other similar professions (e.g., in optometry it's 75% and in dentistry, 93%). Private practice ownership among audiologists also has been decreasing significantly in recent years, as offices are being purchased by manufacturers and other buying groups.

Hearing Aid Distribution Channels

Indirectly and sometimes directly related to the workplaces in which we find audiologists dispensing hearing aids, is the overall hearing aid distribution system.

Manufacturers

We now have what is referred to as the *Big Six*, composed of Widex, Sivantos (Signia), Starkey, Great Nordic (GN) (ReSound), Sonova (Phonak), and William Demant (Oticon). Among them, these companies own or manage 15 to 20 other brands of hearing aids. In addition, there are probably another 25 to 30 lesser known hearing aid manufacturing companies. Most audiologists have one or two favorite companies and buy directly from these manufacturers, with over 90% of sales from the Big Six.

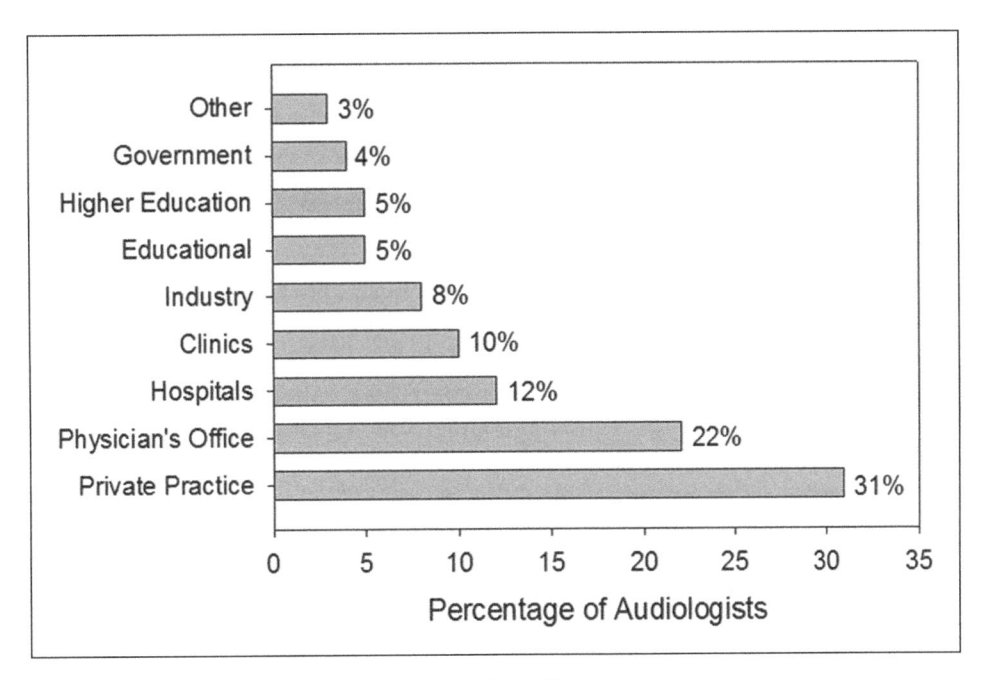

Figure 2–2. Workplace distribution for U.S. audiologists.

- Other: 3%
- Government: 4%
- Higher Education: 5%
- Educational: 5%
- Industry: 8%
- Clinics: 10%
- Hospitals: 12%
- Physician's Office: 22%
- Private Practice: 31%

Buying Groups

Some audiologists find it advantageous to work with a buying group. That is because, with the increased volume, the groups can demand discounts from the manufacturers and pass these savings on to members of the group. There are several different groups and different types of groups to choose from. Examples are Audigy, AuDNET, EarQ, AHAA, and Sonus. Many of the groups offer a range of practice assistance other than just hearing aid purchases. Some of the buying groups, however, more or less work exclusively with the brands of one or two manufacturers.

Retail Outlets

All of the Big Six have retail outlets, which may consist of established stores such as Beltone (owned by GN ReSound), companies with multicenter clinical sites such as Newport Audiology (Sonova) or HearUSA (Sivantos), or the manufacturer may be more subtly involved through corporate-owned, independent practices. Manufacturers also offer loans to audiologists, often used to purchase or expand a practice, which then ties the audiologist to that manufacturer's product. In addition to the Big Six, retail offices also are operated by Amplifon (Sonus and Miracle Ear), Costco, and Sam's Club (and probably several more since the writing of this chapter). All the retail outlets employ audiologists, although the audiologist or hearing instrument specialist mix varies considerably among sites.

Internet Sales

Consumers obtain much of their information about hearing loss and hearing aids from the Internet, so it is not surprising that they buy hearing aids through the Internet too. There are even sites that rate the Internet sales sites. An Internet purchase is possible by simply going to eBay or to Internet sites specializing in Internet sales (conduct an Internet search and you will see that there are several). Although most, if not all, manufacturers have issued a statement saying that they will not sell hearing aids to retailers who do not conduct an in-person fitting, this is difficult to control. For example, if a regular customer of a hearing aid manufacturer purchases 10 BTE hearing aids, how does the company know how and when they were sold? Internet sales also

> **POINTS TO PONDER: TO BUNDLE OR NOT?**
>
> Surveys indicate that 80 to 85% of audiologists who sell hearing aids use a *bundled* approach. That is, a single inclusive price that includes the audiologist's cost for the product, fitting fees, counseling, and follow-up visits (either through the life of the hearing aid or, in some cases, only during the warranty period). The patient is not informed what percent of the total cost is for the product nor what costs are for services, although our experiences suggest that the average patient believes the bulk of the cost is the product.
>
> Audiologists who use an *unbundled* approach break out the cost of the product, accessories, fitting fees, consulting, and follow-up services. This has the advantage of clearly showing the value of the fitting and counseling that goes along with dispensing hearing aids. Additionally, it eliminates the patient's concern that the audiologist is upselling when he or she recommends more features, as the fitting fee would likely stay the same (e.g., it does not require more time or counseling to fit a 20-channel product than a 4-channel product). Some audiologists, however, shy away from the unbundled approach because they believe that when the patient sees the true cost of the hearing aid, they will consider the audiologist's fees to be unreasonable (e.g., a $1,000 hearing aid—cost to audiologist—typically is sold for $2,000; in an unbundled scheme, keeping the total cost the same, this would suggest a $1,000 fitting/service fee). Also, audiologists fear that the patient may not return for the necessary follow-up visits because of the cost involved, and the end result will be dissatisfaction with amplification. Because of this, some audiologists use a partly unbundled approach.
>
> The reason we have included this topic as a "Points to Ponder" is because as Internet sales of hearing aids become more common, audiologists may have to think more about the value of their services, as patients will walk in the door already owning their hearing aids. Also, as over-the-counter (OTC) hearing aids/personal sound amplifiers (PSAPs) become more common, it will be more critical for audiologists to emphasize that they are providing a *service*, not a commodity. For a review of the pros and cons of bundling for hearing aid sales, see the *Audiology Today* article by Sjoblad and Warren (2011), and the comments of John Coverstone later in this chapter.

may be illegal in some states, but again enforcement is difficult; as you would expect, something of this nature has a low priority with enforcement officials.

The Ohio Hearing Aid Internet Work Group (September, 2011) compiled the chart shown in Table 2–1 regarding state laws related to Internet hearing aid sales. There have been some other states added and some revisions to these laws since that time. Currently this is a fast-moving target as you will see later in this chapter. We expect it will take a few more years before the dust settles, but there are currently large changes to hearing aid distribution systems that are already in progress.

In most cases, the hearing aid purchased through the Internet will need programming by an audiologist, not to mention that the patient will also need long-term follow-up rehabilitation care. How this is accomplished often becomes a sticky issue for dispensing audiologists. How are these patients handled when they show up for an appointment carrying their newly purchased hearing aids with them? Some Internet hearing aid sales sites like Hearing Planet (Sonova) have attempted to partner with dispensing audiologists—that is, the patient brings in the Internet-purchased hearing aids and the audiologist conducts the programming. In general, audiologists have not been receptive to this arrangement. Internet sales are not going to go away, however, so we expect that some type of arrangement will evolve so that this group of patients can receive effective benefit from their instruments.

Personal Sound Amplifier Product. We recognize that this is a product and not a distribution channel, but we explain the connection soon. When is a device a per-

Table 2–1. Examples of State Laws that Relate to the Internet Sale of Hearing Aids

State	Citation	Type of Restriction
California	CA BPC Code §3351.5	Catalog/direct mail sellers must be licensed HA dispensers in CA
Connecticut	CT Public Health Code §20-406-14 CT Public Health Code §20-406-1	Must be licensed by state to fit or dispense HA. Reference to "regular place of business" where licensee must be physically available to the public
Florida	FL Statute §484.054	Prohibition on sales or distribution of HA through the mail to the ultimate consumer
Maryland	MD Statute §391-2	Requires MD license for online dispensers; applies general commercial law to HA sales
Missouri	MO Statute §346.110	Fitting and testing must be done by Mo licensed HAD or AuD prior to mail order sale
Nevada	NV Statute §637A.243	Mail order sales require: proof of otoscopic exam; proof of audiometric exam; earmolds taken by NV licensee; attestation by consumer
Oregon	OR Statute §694.032	Fitting and sale of HA must be competed in state
Texas	TX Statue §402.451	Dispensing and fitting must be done by TX licensee
Washington	WA Statute §18.35.175	Requires face to face contact "to test or otherwise determine needs of purchaser"

sonal sound amplifier product (PSAP) and when is it a hearing aid? The distinction becomes more blurred each year. In March 2009, the Food and Drug Administration (FDA) issued guidance describing how hearing aids and PSAPs differ. This guidance defines a hearing aid as a sound-amplifying device intended to compensate for impaired hearing. PSAPs, the guidance states, are not intended to make up for impaired hearing. Instead, they are intended for non-hearing-impaired consumers to amplify sounds in the environment for a number of reasons, such as for recreational activities. You maybe have seen advertisements for such devices as "Game Ear" or "Hunter's Ear." Some PSAPs are more or less novelty items—see Figure 2–3. But today we also have advanced PSAPs advertised as having 14 bands and channels, digital noise reduction, feedback reduction, and a volume control wheel. Sounds a lot like a hearing aid to us, but such products are being sold over-the-counter at retail outlets.

In recent years, there has been considerable discussion regarding PSAPs and over-the-counter hearing aids. Because of the increasing similarity with hearing aids, the FDA issued a guidance document that specifically stated that PSAPs could not be used to treat hearing loss, nor could they be marketed as such (FDA, 2013). They further stated that the regulation of PSAPs was outside the purview of the FDA, but went on to say that the document was only guidance and not a rule. In 2015, the President's Council of Advisors on Science and Technology (PCAST) recommended that the FDA withdraw its guidance document on PSAPs (PCAST, 2015). In 2016, the Report by the Committee on Accessible and Affordable Hearing Health Care for Adults from the National Academies of Sciences, Engineering and Medicine (NASEM) suggested that the Food and Drug Administration should establish a new category of over-the-counter (OTC) wearable hearing devices. This device classification would be separate from "hearing

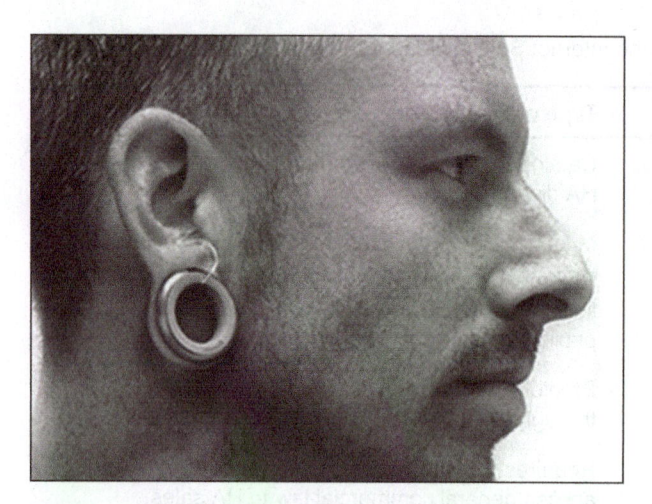

Figure 2–3. An example of a PSAP with a unique ear lobe placement. One of many styles developed to make PSAPs more interesting.

aids." They stated that OTC devices would be defined as wearable, OTC devices that can assist adults with mild to moderate hearing loss. In April of 2016, the FDA had a public workshop on "Streamlining Regulations for Good Manufacturing Practices for Hearing Aids." Following this workshop there were a number of comments from a variety of stakeholders. Several groups—including the American Academy of Audiology, American Speech-Language Hearing Association, and the Hearing Industries Association—generally advocated for continued regulation of hearing aids by the FDA because this was more likely to optimize patient outcomes. In opposition to this argument, several groups—including the Consumer Technology Association and the American Association of Retired Persons—argued that that accessibility and affordability were the most important factors (P and HLAA).

Early in 2017, Larry Humes and colleagues published an article that revealed that an OTC model could lead to outcomes which were similar to a more traditional hearing aid fitting model. Importantly, the OTC model included careful selection of appropriate patients with mild-to-moderate hearing loss through audiological assessment and also established normal cognitive status (screening). These participants were then asked to self-select a frequency response from one of three options which were all appropriate for listeners with mild-moderate hearing loss. Orientation in the OTC model included viewing a professionally developed video self-orientation in the laboratory and participants were encouraged to call with questions. Perhaps not surprisingly, this model revealed similar outcomes to participants that were individually fitted to NAL-NL prescriptions using the probe microphone techniques we describe in Chapter 17. Importantly, this study did not provide evidence that listeners can self-diagnose a mild-to-moderate hearing loss. Indeed, more that 40% of study respondents were not eligible to participate, many because their hearing thresholds fell outside the mild-to-moderate range. In addition, this study did not assess whether participants could self-fit, because only relatively appropriate frequency responses were available for selection. Importantly, 72% *did not* select the product programmed to the gain and output that would have been selected by an audiologist based on the NAL-NL2 fitting approach. As a result, the average aided SII, even for raised speech (65 dB SPL), was lower than what would have been obtained with an NAL-NL2 fitting (.60 vs. .65).

One study in 2017 also demonstrated that well-fitted advanced PSAP devices led to similar speech recognition for soft speech in noise to a well fitted hearing aid (Reed, Betz, Kendig, Korczak, & Lin, 2017). Conversely, a low-priced PSAP was found to *decrease* speech recognition in the same condition compared to wearing no device at all.

By August 2017, the Over-the-Counter Hearing Aid Act of 2017 had passed both houses of Congress and awaited expected presidential signature into law in the very near future. This bill amended the Federal Food, Drug, and Cosmetic Act to require the Food and Drug Administration (FDA) to create a category of OTC hearing aids for adult listeners (over 18 years) with mild to moderate hearing loss and issue regulations regarding those hearing aids. The act further specified that these regulations must: "(1) provide reasonable assurances of safety and efficacy; (2) establish output limits and labeling requirements; and (3) describe requirements for the sale of hearing aids in-person, by mail, or online, without a prescription." By the time you read this, we expect the law that establishes the category of OTC devices will be in place and multiple manufacturers (including both existing hearing aid companies and more general consumer electronics manufacturers) will have introduced, or will soon introduce OTC devices. AAA and other national organizations continue to work with the FDA to best address issues of patient safety and appro-

> ### SOAPBOX: WHAT ARE WE SELLING?
>
> We sometimes hear AuD students say in their first or second year, "I'm really not interested in hearing aids, as I don't want to have to *sell* something." Yes, there often is a financial transaction when working with hearing aids, but there are also charges involved for routine diagnostics, balance function testing, auditory processing disorder (APD) evaluations, and most all other audiologic services. Regarding hearing aids, the question really is, what are we selling? We know that properly fitted hearing aids and effective counseling will lead to long-term hearing aid use, benefit, and satisfaction. And, we know that effective hearing aid use is related not only to improved communication, but also increased earning power, emotional stability, improved family relationships, physical health, and increased social participation. So what we really are selling are our skills in addition to a product: our skills to educate the patient regarding the benefits of hearing aid use, our skills to provide the patient with the optimum fitting through verification and validation, and our counseling skills to handle any bumps in the road that might occur throughout the process. In most cases, a better quality of life for the patient is the result. Not a bad thing to *sell*.

priate labeling. In addition, considerable work still needs to be done to address the most appropriate OTC model relative to patient selection and delivery of any appropriate services. Regardless, it is clear that device delivery for some patients with mild-to-moderate hearing loss will likely look very different in two years than it did two years ago. If we get it right, however, that may be a good thing. We believe that provision of cost effective hearing health care for listeners with mild-to-moderate hearing loss, the vast majority of whom are not currently pursuing hearing aids, is a great goal for all. There are many exciting possibilities that are being proposed, some of which are expected to make hearing aids cost effective and accessible for more patients than ever before. Importantly, if we are careful, we may be able to accomplish this goal with no decrease in patient outcomes.

Laws, Regulations, Rules, and Guidelines Related to the Fitting of Hearing Aids

We know that it takes years of education and experience to be successful in the practice of fitting and dispensing hearing aids. The student of this area of audiology must know anatomy and physiology, hearing science, a variety of behavioral test procedures, hearing aid technology, fitting techniques, and a host of other things—superb counseling skills and a good bedside manner also are a must. Fortunately, these areas are all extremely interesting, and some might even say fun to learn. What often is thought of as not so much fun are all the rules and regulations that go along with the practice of dispensing hearing aids. Yet, they are just as critical for success. We briefly discuss some of them here.

Scope of Practice

A good starting point for this section is the scope of practice for audiology. Although we do not usually think of these as regulations or rules, they do serve as a foundation for the development of other documents. All major audiology organizations have a published scope of practice. For example, the AAA scope of practice (last updated January 2004) states as part of its purpose:

> This document outlines those activities that are within the expertise of members of the profession. This Scope of Practice statement is intended for use by audiologists, allied professionals, consumers of audiologic services, and the general public. It serves as a reference for issues of service delivery, third-party reimbursement, legislation, consumer education, regulatory action, state and professional licensure, and inter-professional relations.

Regarding the fitting of hearing aids, the document states:

> The audiologist is the professional who provides the full range of audiologic treatment services for persons with impairment of hearing and vestibular function. The audiologist is responsible for the evaluation, fitting, and verification of amplification devices, including assistive listening devices. The audiologist determines the appropriateness of amplification systems for persons with hearing impairment, evaluates benefit, and provides counseling and training regarding their use. Audiologists conduct otoscopic examinations; clean ear canals and remove cerumen; take ear canal impressions; and select, fit, evaluate, and dispense hearing aids and other amplification systems.

Licensure

Certainly, one of the most important concerns regarding the sale of hearing aids is obtaining appropriate licensure, which is controlled on a state-by-state basis. For audiologists, this could simply mean obtaining your *audiology license* for a given state; however, at this writing, in 13 states it also is necessary to obtain a second hearing aid dispensing license. For example, in the North Dakota state license for audiologists, it states that the board may refuse to issue or renew a license, or may suspend, revoke, or take other disciplinary action if the licensee has engaged in unprofessional conduct. Such *unprofessional conduct* includes the following:

> Receiving remuneration of any kind from the sale of any type of hearing aid, unless licensed under Chapter 43-33. (Note: Chapter 43-33 is the Hearing Aid Dealers license.)

As you might guess, the need for audiologists to hold this second license, and the associated requirements to pass a written and practical examination to obtain this license, has generated considerable angst among audiologists and their professional organizations over the years. In particular, the practical exam that often is required has been criticized; in some states, rumor has it that points can be deducted for using the wrong color pen for the right and left ear. Audiologists argue that, after completing the requirements of an AuD degree, the audiologist would have the necessary knowledge and skills needed for the evaluation and fitting of hearing aids. Moreover, to obtain the audiology license, the audiologist already has passed a national examination that includes questions regarding hearing aids and hearing aid dispensing. Not all laws are reasonable, however, and licensure for hearing aid dispensing has a longer history and is more established than that of audiology. These state laws do change fairly frequently, so we suggest that you check with the AAA or the ASHA to obtain the current status for specific states. In some states, even when the hearing aid dispensing license is not necessary, additional requirements to the standard audiology license do apply.

Board Certification

Board certification in audiology is available from both the AAA and the ASHA, although it is not necessary to belong to either organization to obtain and hold the certification. The AAA certification is granted by the American Board of Audiology; hence it often is referred to by the abbreviation ABA. The ASHA certification is the Clinical Certificate of Competence in Audiology, or CCC-A. Some audiologists have both, so when paging through the Yellow Pages you might see an audiologist listed as AuD, ABA, CCC-A.

Board certification is not required for dispensing hearing aids, and holding such certification, for the most part, is only indirectly related to the services provided. The written test required to obtain either certification often is the same as the test required to obtain state licensure. Board-certified individuals have mandatory continuing education unit (CEU) requirements, but mandatory CEUs also are required for licensure.

Hearing Aid Fitting Guidelines

As with other areas of clinical audiology, over the years various guidelines have been established regarding the selection and fitting of hearing aids. Typically, these guidelines are developed by a group of key experts and reflect what is considered good practice at the time of the writing. Whether these guidelines have had an impact on clinical practice is debatable. Portions of guidelines, however, have found their way into the body of state license documents, and some guidelines have been used by the ASHA when accrediting clinics and training programs. An example of the latter is the hearing aid fitting guidelines published in 1967, based on a 1966 Chicago meeting sponsored by the AHSA. The outcome was the 71-page ASHA Reports Number 2 1967). This document included not only recommended test procedures for adults and children but also minimal requirements for hearing programs.

In more recent years, there have been at least five different sets of guidelines written regarding the selection and fitting of hearing aids for adults:

- 1991: Vanderbilt/VA Hearing Aid Conference 1990 Consensus Statement: Recommended Components of a Hearing Aid Selection Procedure for Adults (Hawkins, Beck, Bratt, Fabry, Mueller, & Stelmachowicz (1991)
- 1997: The Independent Hearing Aid Fitting Forum (IHAFF) Protocol (Valente & Van Vliet, 1997)
- 1998: ASHA Ad Hoc Committee on Hearing Aid Selection and Fitting: Guidelines for Hearing Aid Fitting for Adults (http://www.asha.org)
- 2004: International Society of Audiology: Good Practice Guidance for Adult Hearing Aid Fittings and Services. Prepared by the Good Practice Working Group of the International Collegium of Rehabilitative Audiology (ICRA; http://www.isa-audiology.org)
- 2006: American Academy of Audiology: Guidelines for the Audiologic Management of Adult Hearing Impairment (http://www.audiology.org)

Best Practice

So far, we have talked about *guidelines* and *preferred practice*. The term *best practice* has been a popular buzzword used in industry and management for many years to describe a process of developing a standard way of doing things (a related example is ISO 9001 certification, a standard that has been attained by some hearing aid manufacturers). In more recent years, we have used this term for audiologic practice, with the general definition that best practice is a method or technique that has consistently shown results superior to those achieved with other means, and that this practice can be used as a benchmark. That is, it returns documented outcomes that can be replicated. Regarding the selection and fitting of hearing aids, we sometimes use the term *best practice guidelines* when referring to published hearing aid fitting guidelines. This may or may not be correct, as in some cases the guidelines may have been based more on expert opinion than on a critical grading of research evidence (see review in Chapter 1). When research evidence is used, the common term is *evidence-based practice*, which often is used interchangeably with best practice.

Because it usually takes considerable time for a given technique or treatment to be researched thoroughly and for this research to be published in peer-reviewed journals (and therefore qualify as a best practice), another term that has been used by the U.S. Department of Health and Human Services is *promising practice*. The definition is as follows:

> Promising Practice: At least preliminary evidence of effectiveness in small-scale interventions or for which there is potential for generating data that will be useful for making decisions about taking the intervention to scale and generalizing the results to diverse populations and settings.

THINGS TO REMEMBER: THIRD-PARTY REIMBURSEMENT

At one time, there was a requirement to hold the ASHA CCC-A to obtain certain types of third-party reimbursement. This was before the presence of audiology licensure in all states. We understand that this requirement has been lifted or can be successfully contested. Hence, both the CCC-A and the AAA ABA are optional board certifications.

> **KEY CONCEPT: ASHA PREFERRED PRACTICE PATTERNS**
>
> In 2006, the ASHA released a lengthy document titled "Preferred Practice Patterns for the Profession of Audiology," which has a section on the selection and fitting of hearing aids for adults. In the preamble, it was pointed out that the *preferred practice* patterns are neither a yardstick to measure acceptable conduct nor a set of aspirational principles. Rather, they reflect the standard of care relevant to a particular set of circumstances. How do preferred practice statements fit with documents labeled as guidelines? The ASHA document states that it is useful to regard these practice patterns within the conceptual framework of ASHA policy statements ranging in scope and specificity from broad to narrow. They are defined as follows:
>
> - Scope of Practice Statement: A list of professional activities that define the range of services offered within the profession of audiology.
> - Preferred Practice Patterns: Statements that define generally applicable characteristics of activities directed toward individual patients.
> - Position Statements: Statements that specify ASHA's policy and stance on a matter.
> - Practice Guidelines: A recommended set of procedures for a specific area of practice, based on research findings and current practice.
>
> American Speech-Language-Hearing Association. (2006). *Preferred Practice Patterns for the Profession of Audiology* [Preferred Practice Patterns]. Retrieved from http://www.asha.org

An example of a hearing aid feature that probably would fall into the promising practice category today would be frequency lowering. There appears to be some evidence that when children undergo training using this algorithm, there may be improved performance for the recognition and production of the /s/ and /sh/ sounds (see Chapter 12). At this point, the available evidence would be weak for best practice, but could be considered promising. A summary of these different terms is shown in Table 2–2.

Table 2–2. Different Levels of Best Practice

Research Validated Best Practice	A program, activity or strategy that has the highest degree of proven effectiveness. Supported by highly rated objective and comprehensive research and evaluation.
Field Tested Best Practice	A program, activity or strategy that has been shown to work effectively and produce successful outcomes and is supported to some degree by subjective and objective data.
Promising Practice	A program, activity or strategy that has worked within one organization and shows promise during its early stages for becoming a best practice with long term sustainable impact. A promising practice must have some objective basis for claiming effectiveness and must have the potential for replication.

Source: Adapted from the U.S. Department of Health and Human Services, Administration for Children and Families Program Announcement. (Federal Register, Vol. 68, No. 131, July 2003)

Evidence-Based Practice

Frank C. Wilson, MD, an authority in *evidence-based practice* once wrote:

> Neither unaudited experience nor logical thought can replace controlled clinical trials, so until documentation of a procedure's effectiveness can be demonstrated, it should be considered a false idol and worship withheld. (2009, p. 80)

Although the basic principles date back to the mid-1800s, evidence-based practice is relatively new to medicine, and even newer to audiology. Noted expert David L. Sackett, MD, describes it as "the conscientious, explicit, and judicious use of current best evidence in making decisions about the care of individual patients. The practice of evidence-based medicine [audiology] means integrating individual clinical expertise with the best available external clinical evidence from systematic research" (Sackett, Rosenberg, Gray, Haynes, & Richardson, 1996). We reviewed the issues surrounding evidence-based practice in Chapter 1.

The AAA Fitting Guidelines. We mentioned earlier that *fitting guidelines* are only best practice guidelines if they are constructed using the rules of evidence-based practice. The 2006 hearing aid fitting guidelines published by the AAA used this approach. For each recommendation, this guideline provides the level of evidence and a grade—see Table 2–3 for the grading system that was used. Table 2–4 is an example of six items taken from one of the Tables of Evidence. It includes some items on compression threshold (CT), compression limiting (CL), peak clipping (PC), and threshold of discomfort measures (TD). We selected a section from a table that had mostly Level 1 and Level 2 grades; however, this is not representative of the entire guideline. Michael Valente, chair of the committee who developed

Table 2–3. Grades of Recommendation

Grade	Criteria
A	Level 1–2 studies with consistent conclusions.
B	Level 3–4 studies with consistent findings or extrapolated evidence from Level 1–2 studies.
C	Level 5 studies or extrapolation from Level 3–4 studies.
D	Level 6 evidence; inconsistent or inconclusive studies of any level, any study having a high risk of bias.

Table 2–4. Sample Portion of a Table of Evidence Taken From the 2006 AAA Hearing Aid Fitting Guidelines

Treatment Decision	Level	Grade
Hearing aids with low CTs yield better outcomes when compared to linear PC. Patients prefer CL to at least one typical low CT instrument.	2	A
A wide range of CTs and time constants may be appropriate.	1	A
Speech recognition differences can be associated with increased number of compression channels.	1	D
Listeners with greater cognitive ability derive greater benefit from temporal structure in background noise when listening with faster time constants.	2	A
Quantification of a theoretical multichannel compression hearing aid, using intelligibility index And target-gain matching measures, indicate a seven-channel system would suffice for most audiograms in order to meet the strictest root-mean-square (RMS) error criterion evaluated.	2	B
Data support measurement of individual TD and setting of OSPL90 so it does not exceed TD in order to minimize chances of auditory discomfort in the real world.	3	B

these guidelines, provided a review of the recommendations and the procedures used for grading (Valente, 2006). He states that, overall, the combined Tables of Evidence contained 108 statements that were provided to support the 43 recommendations in the guideline. The following is the frequency with which the different levels of evidence were assigned for the 108 recommendations: Level 1: 4.6%, Level 2: 25.9%, Level 3: 14.8%, Level 4: 35.2%, Level 5: 4.6%, and Level 6: 14.8%. Note that less than one-third of the recommendations were judged as Level 1–2.

Efficacy, Effectiveness, and Efficiency

As we have discussed, the treatment of hearing loss using hearing aids falls into the category of a health care intervention, something that epidemiologists have been studying for many years. Simply stated, we need to ask three questions: Can it work? Does it work? And, is it worth it? British epidemiologist Archie Cochrane was one of the first to organize intervention research into three categories:

- Efficacy (Can it work?): This is the extent to which an intervention does more good than harm. This type of testing often is conducted under relatively ideal circumstances.
    Example: The directivity index of a new directional microphone algorithm is evaluated by the manufacturer in an anechoic chamber.
- Effectiveness (Does it work in the real world?): This evaluation assesses whether an intervention does more good than harm when used in a typical health care practice.
    Example: Patients are fitted with the new directional algorithm and compare this processing with omnidirectional processing in typical real-world listening situations.
- Efficiency (Is it worth it?): Is the effect of an intervention worth the additional cost that may be related to its use? Is the intervention cost-effective?
    Example: If the new directional algorithm provides an average 2 dB improvement in the patient's SNR (i.e., it is effective), but a pair of hearing aids with this algorithm cost the patient $500 more than other products, is the additional cost to the patient worth the benefit obtained?

In Robyn Cox's 2004 review of evidence-based practice, she offers the following additional explanation to assist us in differentiating efficacy from effectiveness:

- Efficacy: The *efficacy* of a treatment is how well it *can* work given the best possible scenario. This usually means the treatment is administered to highly motivated patients with uncomplicated problems, and the practitioners providing the treatment are extensively trained in the details of the treatment and have plenty of time to get things just right.
- Effectiveness: The *effectiveness* of a treatment is how well it *does* work in the real world where patients may not be very motivated or compliant, and they often lead complicated lives. Also, in the real world, practitioners have limited time and may not understand all the fine points of the treatment.

As an example, Cox (2004) discusses wide dynamic range compression (WDRC), a feature in nearly all hearing aids today that has been shown in research to improve audibility and speech recognition for soft speech; hence, it is *efficacious*. But, we know that some patients do not adapt well to this amount of gain for soft sounds: They may find it annoying and they may not want to go through the necessary adjustment period. It may even be that some patients never do adjust to this increased audibility. WDRC processing, therefore, is not always an effective treatment. Although efficacy is important, it is treatment effectiveness that drives our fitting practices.

FDA Regulations

As you might expect, there are government regulations relating to the manufacture, sale, and fitting of hearing aids. These issues are addressed by the U.S. Food and Drug Administration (FDA), Department of Health and Human Services, Medical Devices regulations (Subchapter H, Revised April 1, 2010). This regulation has definitions for both audiologist and dispenser.

Audiologist: Audiologist refers to any person qualified by training and experience to specialize in the evaluation and rehabilitation of individuals whose communication disorders center in whole or in part in the hearing function. In some states audiologists must satisfy specific requirements for licensure.

Dispenser: Dispenser refers to any person, partnership, corporation, or association engaged in the sale, lease, or rental of hearing aids to any member of the consuming public or any employee, agent, sales person, and/or representative of such a person, partnership, corporation, or association.

In general, the term dispenser is used in the regulation and, as shown in the definition above, this term would apply to audiologists involved in selling hearing aids.

FDA Red Flags

One of the things outlined in the FDA regulation are the eight *red flags* for referral (not to be confused with the *Red Flag Rules* issued by the Federal Trade Commission [FTC] in 2010). The regulation states that a dispenser should advise a prospective hearing aid user to consult a licensed physician (preferably an otolaryngologist) promptly if any of the following is observed through record review, case history, or testing:

1. Visible congenital or traumatic deformity of the ear.
2. History of active drainage from the ear within the previous 90 days
3. History of sudden or rapidly progressive hearing loss within the previous 90 days
4. Acute or chronic dizziness
5. Unilateral hearing loss of sudden or recent onset within the previous 90 days
6. Audiometric air-bone gap equal to or greater than 15 dB at 500 Hz, 1000 Hz, and 2000 Hz
7. Visible evidence of significant cerumen accumulation or a foreign body in the ear canal
8. Pain or discomfort in the ear

In general, even if these eight conditions were not present in the regulation, the prudent audiologist would probably refer the wearer if any of these conditions existed anyway. Depending on your definition of significant, one exception might be cerumen accumulation, which often does not require a medical referral and easily can be handled by most audiologists (assuming it is allowed by the state's licensure law).

FDA Medical Clearance

The FDA also regulates *condition for sale* of certain medical devices. Regarding hearing aids, one condition prior to December 2016 was medical clearance, which is summarized as follows (FDA Sec. 801.421 Hearing aid devices; conditions for sale):

- Prospective hearing aid users must obtain a medical clearance from a physician (preferably one who specializes in diseases of the ear) prior to being fit with amplification. The medical clearance must have occurred in the last six months. If the prospective user is over 18 years of age, they may waive this medical clearance and, instead, complete a medical waiver. The medical waiver must be in the language provided by the FDA.
- Prospective hearing aid users under the age of 18 years of age obtain a medical clearance from a physician (preferably one who specializes in diseases of the ear) prior to being fit with amplification. The medical clearance must have occurred in the last six months. Neither the child or their parent or guardian may waive this medical clearance requirement.

This rule for adults 18 and over changed suddenly on December 7, 2016. At a meeting of the NASEM, Eric Mann, Chief, Ear, Nose and Throat Devices Branch of the FDA announced that, effective immediately, the rule requiring a medical evaluation before obtaining most hearing aids would no longer be enforced. This was based on the assumption that most adults were simply signing the waiver. This was a critical step required for OTC legislation to move forward and eliminated decades long enforcement of this rule.

HIPAA

The Health Insurance Portability and Accountability Act (HIPAA) became law in 1996. The part of HIPAA that has the most impact on audiology practice is the Accountability or Administrative Simplification section. Contained in this section are rules regarding transactions and code sets, privacy, and security. There also are rules mandating that that the Employer Identification Number provided to the IRS be utilized when submitting claims to insurers and a rule that mandates the use of the National Provider Identifier (NPI) by audiologists when submitting claims to all insurers including Medicare and Medicaid. Each clinic or facility must also obtain a NPI.

The HIPAA guidelines regarding privacy and confidentially are extensive and complex; some even directly impact the fitting of hearing aids, such as the passwords for fitting software. A thorough description is beyond the scope of this chapter, but an excellent review is provided at the website of the AAA (http://www.audiology.org) and the ADA (http://www.audiologist.org).

Federal Trade Commission

The FTC has issued a set of regulations, effective in June 2010, known as the Red Flag Rules. These rules apply to any audiology practice that accepts and processes third-party payments or insurance, or acts as a creditor for its patients. This rule requires practices to create and implement written identity theft prevention, detection, and management policies and procedures in an attempt to protect their patients from identity theft. The Red Flag Rules can be considered an expansion of the HIPAA privacy rules. As with the HIPAA Privacy Policy, the audiology practice needs to create office policies and procedures that outline how the practice intends to identify, detect, and respond to identity theft red flags.

Laws and Statutes

There are several laws and statutes that have the possibility of relating directly to the sale of hearing aids. In particular, they apply when the audiologist or audiology practice is involved with reimbursement through Medicare or Medicaid.

Antikickback Statute

We are referring to the Medicare and Medicaid Patient Protection Act of 1987, as amended, 42 U.S.C. §1320a-7b. The section of the this statute that relates directly to the sale of hearing aids prohibits the offer or receipt of certain remuneration in return for referrals for, or recommending purchase of, supplies and services reimbursable under government health care programs. Violation of this statute is a felony; upon conviction the individual could be fined not more than $25,000 or imprisoned for not more than five years, or both. Specially, the statute states:

- Whoever knowingly and willfully solicits or receives any remuneration, including any kickback, bribe, or rebate (directly or indirectly, overtly or covertly, in cash or in-kind) in return for referring an individual to a person for the furnishing or arranging for the furnishing of any item or service for which payment may be made in whole or in part under [Medicare] or a state health care program;
- In return for purchasing, leasing, ordering, or arranging for or recommending purchasing, leasing, or ordering any good, facility, service, or item for which payment may be made in whole or in part under [Medicare] or a state health care program.

The antikickback statute requires intent, but considers that *remuneration* is anything of value, which could include gifts, points, free trips, or equipment that is linked to the purchase of hearing aids from a given manufacturer.

Stark Law

The federal statute dealing with physician self-referral is generally referred to as the *Stark Law*, although there have been modifications. Congress included a provision in the Omnibus Budget Reconciliation Act of 1989, which barred self-referrals for clinical laboratory services under the Medicare program, effective January 1, 1992. This provision is known as *Stark I*. Under this law, if a physician or a member of a physician's immediate family has a financial relationship with a health care entity, the physician may not make referrals to that entity for the furnishing of designated health services under the Medicare program. Generally, to determine whether the Stark statute applies to a particular arrangement, three questions must be answered: Does this arrangement involve a referral of a Medicare or

Medicaid patient by a physician or an immediate family member of a physician? Second, is the referral for a *designated health service*? Third, is there a financial relationship of any kind between the referring physician or family member and the entity to which the referral is being made? Violations of Stark can result in civil penalties: denial of payments for the services provided in violation of Stark; and exclusion from participation in Medicare, Medicaid, and/or any other federal health care program. The Stark statute does not require bad intent; a tainted financial relationship violates the Stark Law regardless of intentions.

False Claims Act

The False Claims Act (31 U.S.C. §§ 3729–3733, also called the *Lincoln Law* as it became law during Abraham Lincoln's administration) is a federal law that imposes liability on persons and companies who defraud governmental programs. As it relates to audiology, the False Claims Act deals with audiologists who submit claims for services that were not done or were not necessary. It applies to any federal health care program. Specifically, violation of this law would include:

- Knowingly submitting a false claim to a federal health care program;
- Submitting claims for services not performed, for medically unnecessary services, and for *upcoding* (i.e., coding at a higher level or for more services than were provided).

Gifts or Inducements to Beneficiaries

Gifts and inducements to beneficiaries are included under section 1128A(a)(5) of the Social Security Act (the Act), enacted as part of HIPAA. Specifically the law states:

> It is unlawful to knowingly offer or give remuneration to Medicare or Medicaid beneficiaries to influence their choice of provider for any item or service covered by Medicare or a state health care program.

You might wonder what this has to do with the sale of hearing aids? Exactly what remuneration would audiologists be giving away? The answer is free hearing testing, which usually is termed *free hearing screening*. It is not unusual to see a newspaper ad offering a special "This week only! Come in for your free hearing screening!" There is some debate about whether screening might be okay and threshold testing might not, but it is no secret that the purpose of the ad is to increase office traffic, and hopefully hearing aid sales. But is it legal? Bryan Liang, who is an MD, PhD, and JD, has spoken on this topic at numerous audiology meetings. Here is the opinion he voiced in 2000:

> This is a very, very difficult and important issue and audiologists are justified in being concerned about it . . . At the outset, let me emphasize that free hearing screenings are not *per se* a violation of fraud and abuse laws; it is just that they might be. One thing

---

TECHNICAL TIP: CODING

In our discussion of the false claims act, we list *upcoding* as an example of a violation. If you are new to the profession, that term might not have much meaning, so we provide a brief explanation. Current Procedural Terminology, which simply is referred to by the abbreviation CPT, are codes containing a set of five numbers assigned to most tasks and services provided by an audiologist. They are used by insurers to determine the amount of reimbursement. All audiologists use the same set of CPT codes. Within health care, thousands of codes are in use, and they are updated annually. Development and maintenance of these codes is overseen by the American Medical Association. Relative to upcoding, if an audiologist only conducted air conduction thresholds for a given patient, that would be CPT Code 92552. If the audiologist entered 92557, which is the Code for *comprehensive audiometry threshold evaluation and speech recognition*, a higher reimbursement rate, that would be considered upcoding. These codes often change—for clinical practice you will need to obtain an updated listing, available from the AAA, ADA or the ASHA, as well as other sources.

I think is clear, however: if it is a public health situation where you are not trying to induce referrals to yourself, and if Medicare, Medicaid and other federal health programs are not involved, you are probably okay. If the free screenings become tied to or eventually involve Medicaid or Medicare or the VA program, there may be a problem. (Grayson & Liang, 2000)

Guidance from the ASHA is not as vague. Provisions state: "Providing free hearing tests when you are a Medicare provider appears to be a clear violation of Medicare rules and regulations. Medicare prohibits offering free services such as hearing testing as an inducement to generate other services such as diagnostic audiologic services."

Billing and Reimbursement

Although this text focuses mostly on the selection and fitting of hearing aids, we cannot lose sight of the fact that there is a business side to audiology. Any successful practitioner knows the rules of reimbursement, the specifics of proper coding, and the legalities of billing and financial relationships. To cover all these topics appropriately, we would need several book chapters, or maybe even an entire book, such as the one by Glaser & Traynor (2013). Billing and coding change frequently, and staying current is critical—it's not something we'll go into here. Rather, we recommend that you monitor the articles and workshops of audiology experts such as Debbie Abel, Kim Cavitt, and Bob Fifer, which provide excellent up-to-date information.

More on Bundling and Unbundling

We brought up the topic of bundling and unbundling earlier in this chapter under "Points to Ponder." While the majority of audiologists appear to be in favor of bundling, there are a few who speak out in favor of unbundling. One of them is audiologist John Coverstone, and here are what he considers to be the advantages of unbundling for the audiologist, taken from one of his recent articles (2012):

- Unbundling requires conducting a cost analysis. Performing a cost analysis can provide you with a completely different perspective on how your business operates. It can also provide you with a lot more confidence in your fees when you eventually use this information to set them.
- You can ensure that you are paid for the services that you provide. An unbundled

---

POINTS TO PONDER: VIOLATION OR NO VIOLATION?

Example #1: A private practice audiologist notes that a new otolaryngologist opened a practice down the street. The otolaryngologist does not employ an audiologist. The audiologist takes the otolaryngologist out to a nice dinner. They discuss the services the audiologist offers, including the dispensing of hearing aids. Violation of Antikickback Law?

Example #2: An otolaryngologist employs an audiologist who dispenses hearing aids. The otolaryngologist refers all patients needing hearing aids to this audiologist. The audiologist earns a handsome salary, which is based almost entirely on commissions from the hearing aids sold. The percent of the commission escalates as a function of the number of units sold each month. Violation of Stark Law?

Example #3: An audiologist sells a large number of hearing aids that are reimbursed through a government agency. The reimbursement rate is very low and to help him or her out a manufacturer provides a 25% discount on the Level 1 hearing aids purchased for this population. The invoice sent to the audiologist, however, states the single-unit price, not the discounted price. The audiologist submits this invoice to the government agency for reimbursement, as this is the *true* price of the hearing aid. Violation of False Claims Law?

model focuses on fees that are appropriate for the time and resources that you dedicate to caring for your patients.
- You have something to promote. There is a good possibility that you will be the first in your area to adopt this fee structure.
- Many audiologists enjoy the intangible benefits of unbundling more than the business ones. Unbundling promotes an image of a professional rather than one of a sales person.
- There is an additional increase in confidence among patients when they know that the recommendations you are making are not tied to how much you will make from the sale. Unbundling removes the burden of tying the income you receive to the product you recommend.
- Unbundling makes it much easier to practice in the modern hearing aid dispensing world:
  - Insurance companies are used to a medical model. Unbundling allows you to fit into that model very easily—and probably bill out more of what you are doing in the process.
  - If you currently bundle and then bill insurance when you can, there is a very good chance that you are in violation of your contract and possibly federal law (if you accept federal insurance). Medicare, in particular, does not allow you to bill anyone else less than you bill Medicare. If you include evaluations in the price of a hearing aid, as many people do, you cannot then charge Medicare for the same service.
  - Direct hearing aid sales are not going away. Wherever patients purchase the device, unbundling makes it easy for you to provide the services that are so essential for successful hearing aid use.

Ethics

As with all areas of clinical audiology, ethical guidelines relate to several different aspects of dispensing hearing aids. Are the patients treated properly? Do the fitting and verification procedures assure that the patients obtained what is best for them? Are there outside incentives that influence clinical decisions? Ethical guidelines related to hearing aid fitting can also originate from several sources: professional organizations, state licensure documents, hearing aid manufacturers, and health care organizations.

Code of Ethics of Professional Organizations

When we think of codes of ethics, we usually first associate them with professional organizations. You might even know someone who was removed from an audiology organization because of a violation of a given organization's standards. The ethical guidelines for both the AAA and the ASHA can be found at their respective websites.

The code of ethics for an organization typically covers a wide range of activities, including such areas as maintaining high standards of professional competence, maintaining patient confidentiality, providing appropriate services and products, making accurate public statements, avoiding commercial interests that could impact patient care, and abstaining from dishonesty or illegal conduct that could adversely affect the profession.

Ethics Related to Hearing Aid Fitting Procedures. One area of the code of ethics that is often overlooked (or simply not remembered) includes statements involving clinical practice. That is, if an audiologist is not performing a given audiologic task appropriately, is that then unethical behavior? For example, we know that preferred practice guidelines say that word recognition testing should be conducted using standardized *recorded* speech material. What if an audiologist used monitored live voice? Some do, we hear. Is this an ethical violation?

This area of ethics was brought to light in a 2009 article by Catherine Palmer, PhD, in which she related these guidelines specifically to the fitting of hearing aids. Let us say that there are data available that show that certain hearing aid verification and validation methods improve benefit and satisfaction. What if an audiologist does not utilize these measures in the fitting of hearing aids? Is this unethical behavior?

Palmer draws our attention to the following statement from Principle 2 of the AAA *Code of Ethics*, which states: "Members shall maintain high standards of professional competence in rendering services . . . " Principle 4 of the same ethics code states: "Members shall provide only services and products that are in the best interest of those served." She also mentions Principle of Ethics II from the ASHA *Code of Ethics*, which states: "Individuals shall honor their responsibility to achieve and maintain the highest level of professional competence." Palmer adds that all of these statements point to the assumption that an ethical practitioner will follow the best practices supported by evidence and published by his or her professional organizations.

So is failing to comply with best practice guidelines unethical and justification for removal from an organization? Some might say that this is taking the ethical practice guidelines a bit too far. But the point we are making is that ethical practice is not just about keeping your nose clean and staying out of jail—it is about being a good audiologist, which includes appropriate clinical practice.

Specific Guidelines Regarding Incentives from Manufacturers. In 2003, the AAA added some ethical guidelines regarding financial incentives from hearing aid manufacturers. These guidelines are titled, "Ethical Practice Guidelines on Financial Incentives from Hearing Instrument Manufacturers." There did not appear to be a particular event or series of events that prompted this document, although it was at about this time that the Office of the Inspector General issued guidelines for gift-giving for the pharmaceutical industry. Perhaps the thought was that a proactive approach would be best, as some of these ethical concerns also could be construed as illegal. Here are some examples of what was considered *okay* or *not okay* in the AAA document.

Things that are *probably okay*:

- Gifts that primarily benefit the patient and are related to the audiologist's work that do not exceed $100 in value.
- The cost of reasonable travel expenses to attend a legitimate educational program.
- Meals and social functions that are part of a legitimate educational program.
- Co-op advertising if there are no strings attached.
- Modest meals from a manufacturer's rep when business related.
- Discount programs as long as they do not compromise professional judgment. (*Authors'*

Note: This becomes less of a problem each year as the array of products from each manufacturer expands.)
- Obtaining a loan from a hearing aid manufacturer is sort of okay; see exact wording in document.
- Consulting for a company, or owning stock is okay, but it must be disclosed to the patient if you fit the patient with that product.

Things that are *probably not okay*:

- Accepting invitations to private convention parties or paid tickets for golfing, sporting events, opera, theater, and so forth.
- Any expenses related to a spouse or significant other attending an educational meeting (e.g., meals, travel, lodging, entertainment).
- Accepting gifts that are over $100 or that do not relate to patient care.
- Incentives or credit toward product purchases (including audiologic or hearing aid related equipment) that are tied to hearing aid purchases.

Hawkins, Hamill, Van Vliet, and Freeman (2002) conducted a survey of audiologists regarding many of the potential conflicts of interest we mention here. Sixteen different scenarios were rated as either *nothing wrong; may not be in patient's best interest, but comfortable with it; highly suspect; borders on unethical;* or *clearly unethical*. In addition, they included the ratings provided by hearing impaired patients for the same items—a reasonable factor to sample, as the *perception of unethical* can be considered unethical.

Hawkins, Hamill, and Kukula (2006) repeated the survey four years later (for audiologists only) to determine if the increased focus on potential ethical violations by professional organizations had an impact on audiologists' perceptions. We have included a summary of the data from both surveys in Table 2–5. For this summary, we combined the ratings of *borders on unethical* and *clearly unethical*. Observe that over the four-year interval, audiologists appeared to become more vigilant concerning what activities might be unethical. Also note that for some items there is a considerable gap between the views of audiologists and those of consumers.

So far, we have discussed the ethical guidelines of a professional organization. One might ask: What about

Table 2–5. Summary of possible unethical behavior as rated by audiologists and consumers

Possibly Unethical Behavior	Percent who believe action to be unethical		
	Audiologists (year 2002)	Audiologists (year 2006)	Consumers
Earning credits from companies per hearing aid purchased, redeemable for gifts or cruises	38	70	71
Receiving professional development money from companies for each hearing aid purchased	19	31	85
Receiving equipment from company in exchange for agreeing to purchase a number of aids during the year	30	51	85
Receiving $100 traveler's check for each high-end instrument purchased from company	43	69	85
Receiving visits from sales representatives to discuss company's products	0	1	2
Receiving pens and notebooks with names of company's new products	4	4	7
Sales rep bringing lunch to office while company's new products are discussed	6	8	22
Sales rep taking Audiologist and spouse out to dinner to discuss company's new products	22	48	41
Attending an open party given by manufacturer at a convention regardless of whether they use the company's product	2	3	12
Attending an invitation only party at a convention given by a company	7	16	24
Attending a company sponsored, state approved CEU workshop in town	2	2	10
Attending a company sponsored, state approved CEU workshop in town, with breakfast and lunch provided	3	4	17
Attending CEU workshop in another city; company pays audiologist's expenses to attend	17	32	38
Attending CEU workshop in another city; company pays audiologist's and spouse's expenses to attend	45	74	69
Using Brand X almost exclusively because Aud thinks it is a good product and receives 20% volume discount	7	16	21
Purchasing a franchise and using the product line almost exclusively	9	15	28
Receiving salary plus a commission based on number of instruments sold while working in a clinic	12	19	26

Source: Hawkins et al., 2006.

all the audiologists who do not belong to a professional organization? Would it seem that they would then be exempt from these codes of ethics? Just let your membership in the AAA expire, and then you can take free trips from manufacturers? Well, it is not quite that simple, as state licensure also has ethical guidelines.

Ethics Related to Licensure

In addition to the ethical guidelines of professional organizations, state licensure laws also have ethical guidelines, and failure to comply could result in losing your license—something most audiologists would view as worse than being kicked out of their favorite professional organization. The wording usually is something like this regarding the suspension or revocation of the license: "Engaging in unprofessional conduct, as defined by the rules established by the board, or violating the code of ethics adopted and published by the board."

Most of these licensure ethical violations, of course, involve fairly serious acts such as misrepresentation, violation of patient confidentiality, discrimination statutes, fraud, deceit, and so forth. There are some items that are more in the gray area, however, and do relate to the selling of hearing aids. An example follows:

> Participating in activities that constitute a conflict of professional interest and adversely affect the licensee's ability to provide appropriate audiology services.

The key here is that it not only must be a conflict of interest but also must adversely affect audiology services. In most cases, even when a potential conflict of interest exists, hearing aid services are not negatively affected. But what about the following examples? (1) You work at a dispensing practice owned by one of the Big Six hearing aid manufacturers or (2) you have a huge loan from one of these major manufacturers. Both situations are a common occurrence nowadays. You are audited each month to assure that you are selling a high percentage of their product (e.g., 80%, 90%, or whatever is required). What if you have several patients who require a special feature that is implemented much more effectively by another manufacturer, but you continue to sell the products of your parent company to meet your monthly quota? Is this appropriate audiologic service?

Hearing aid licensure laws also have ethical standards. These ethics tend to be more directly related to the sale of hearing aids. Here are some examples taken from the North Dakota Hearing Aid Dealers' license, a license required for all dispensing audiologists in the state. Two of the items listed are fairly straightforward—the patient needs to have been tested properly and the patient has to have a need for amplification. Ethical violations include the following:

- Sale of a hearing instrument to a person without adequate and proper audiometric testing.
- Sale of a hearing instrument to a person when the need for a hearing instrument has not been established after adequate and proper audiometric testing.

POINTS TO PONDER: OKAY TO HAVE A FAVORITE MANUFACTURER?

Many audiologists purchase 80% or more of their hearing aids from a single manufacturer. (See Johnson, Mueller and Ricketts, 2009, for a review of audiologists purchasing trends.) Although some might frown on this, we certainly do not consider this unethical, as long as the amplification needs of each patient are being met. There are many advantages of using a primary manufacturer. The most significant is the greater familiarity with the products and the fitting software. Fine tuning hearing aids quickly on a busy day can be quite challenging for even the seasoned audiologist if several different manufacturers are used. Not only does manufacturer software differ greatly in how changes are made to different hearing aid features, but those features probably will be given different names. In addition, controls with the same name (e.g., gain for soft) may have different effects on compression parameters depending on the specific manufacturer. Another advantage of only using one or two manufacturers is the increased familiarity with the manufacturer's support staff, which can help solve fitting, ordering, repair, and administrative problems. If enough hearing aids are purchased each month, there also will likely be a reduction in the cost of the products, which can be passed along to the patient.

At this point, we could have a lengthy discussion of what really is *adequate* testing and how do you really know when hearing aids will *not* benefit a patient? But, we save that discussion for later chapters of this book. Below, we have listed four other ethical violations from the same licensure law. The examples included are from us, not the statute, but do represent actual potential violations that we are aware of from other states:

- Using, or causing, or promoting the use of any advertising matter, promotional literature, testimonial, guarantee, warranty, label, brand, insignia, or any other representation, however disseminated or published, which is misleading, deceptive, or untruthful.
  Example: An audiologist sends out a direct mail piece saying: "Having trouble understanding in background noise? With the advanced NoiseStopper algorithm from MagicTone, you'll notice a remarkable improvement in understanding conversations in background noise."
- Advertising a particular model or type of hearing instrument for sale when purchasers or prospective purchasers responding to the advertisement cannot purchase the advertised model or type, if it is established that the purpose of the advertisement is to obtain prospects for the sale of a model or type other than that advertised.
  Example: Audiologist places a full-page newspaper ad that says: "Thousands of hearing impaired people are now using the totally invisible Phantom II deep-canal hearing aids from MagicTone [very tiny aid shown on the finger tip in the photo]. Stop in today to place your order during a special discount offer." (Note that the audiologist knows that because of the very small size, the fit-rate for the Phantom II is only about 5% of patients; the audiologist nearly always fits the Phantom I, a much larger, more visible completely in-the-canal (CIC) style).
- Advertising a manufacturer's product or using a manufacturer's name or trademark that implies a relationship with the manufacturer that does not exist.
  Example: The dispenser has a newspaper ad that reads: "Be the first to experience the new neural digital technology from MagicTone. Our center has been selected as a MagicTone research site. Enroll in the latest MagicTone research study for new hearing aid users by calling 701-223-XXXX. (Note: This dispenser does sell MagicTone's products, but there is no MagicTone research study.)
- To directly or indirectly give or offer to give, or permit, or cause to be given money or anything of value to any person who advises another in a professional capacity as an inducement to influence them or have them influence others to purchase or contract to purchase products sold or offered for sale by a licensee, or to influence persons to refrain from dealing in the products of competitors.
  Example: A dispenser says to a patient: "What? You're going to go check prices at Bob's Hearing Aids? I've seen some of his patients, and none of them were fit correctly. He doesn't even do probe-mic testing!"

More Ethical Guidelines

It is not just professional organizations and licensure laws that have ethical guidelines. Manufacturers, organizations, medical centers, and other entities sometimes have guidelines that are more rigid than those of the AAA or the ASHA.

Hearing Aid Manufacturers. Although you might think that it is the hearing aid manufacturers that are encouraging audiologists to stray from the straight and narrow (which indeed sometimes has been true in the past), some manufacturers have guidelines more rigid than those of the professional organizations. We know of one company, for example, that has a strict policy regarding issues that are relatively minor, such as who gets a free lunch. If a sales rep takes out an audiology customer for a business lunch, and the audiologist's spouse joins them, the spouse pays for his or her own food. A rep who generously pays the entire bill would most likely receive a letter of reprimand. The same rep takes a group of Chicago audiology customers to a Cubs game? That just might cost the rep his or her job with this company.

Veterans Affairs (VA). The VA employs about 1,000 audiologists, most of whom dispense hearing aids and, therefore, work closely with hearing aid manufacturers. About 15% to 20% of all hearing aids sold in the United States are to VA clinics. Nearly all major manufacturers have products approved by the VA and, as part of this, the manufacturers provide off-site product training, usually at a major city (e.g., an East Coast VA audiologist might go to Las Vegas for training). Again, the VA has guidelines that are at least as rigid as those of professional organizations. For example, food and lodging can be no more than 150% of the government per diem. This means that if the government per diem for meals for a given city were $56 (e.g., San Antonio, TX), the manufacturer could spend no more than $84/person (150% of $56) for meals and beverages for the day of training. If you consider that the attendees would be served three meals plus snacks, and that a bowl of potato chips or pretzels may cost $25 from hotel catering, you can quickly calculate that the manufacturer will not be serving an expensive wine with dinner Actually, they would not be serving any wine at dinner, as providing alcoholic beverages also is prohibited. The manufacturer could be removed from the VA contract for noncompliance. The VA guidelines also state the following:

> Excluded expenses or extras include transportation to and from home/airport, car rental, mileage (gas), baggage fees, entertainment of any kind, cruises, tours, or tickets to any form of entertainment. Contractors will not pay expenses for spouses or partners of government employees.

Medical Centers. And, finally, if your dispensing practice is part of a medical center, conflict of interest guidelines may be even more rigid. Recall that the AAA guidelines state that it is okay to accept small gifts (under $100 in value) from manufacturers, as long as the gift relates to your practice or patient care. Certainly a $50 pen would fit into that category—we all need to write something now and then at work, right? Well, that pen had better not have "Starkey" or "Signia" printed on it, or you could be in trouble. Several medical centers, including our own Vanderbilt, do not allow the use of any gift item that displays the name or logo of a product that potentially could be recommended or sold at the Center.

KEY CONCEPT: IS A GIFT EVER JUST A GIFT?

Most of the data regarding the acceptance of gifts and how they might influence the behavior of the medical professional relate to gifts from pharmaceutical companies to physicians. If we assume that the impact would be similar for hearing aid manufacturers and audiologists, here are some things to remember:

- Companies work harder to influence you than you work to resist their efforts.
- You probably believe that your professional colleagues will be influenced, but that you will not.
- You are probably more influenced than you think.
- Small gifts pack about the same punch as larger ones.

Again, if we use the data from previous studies related to pharmaceuticals and apply the findings to gifts to dispensing audiologists, here are some potentially negative outcomes:

- Dispensing more of a given brand without complete consideration of options.
- Dispensing a higher tier product (more channels, features, etc.) than is needed for certain patients.
- Inability to recognize false claims from the favorite brand.
- Developing a close relationship with the manufacturer's rep.

Now, you might be saying, isn't that going a bit too far? Why would the pen I use have any bearing on what brand of hearing aids I sell to my patients? If you are asking that question, especially if you are an audiology student, you might be interested in the intriguing study regarding free pens published by Grande, Frosch, Perkins, Barbara, and Kahn (2009). This was a randomized controlled study of 352 third- and fourth-year medical students at two different medical schools: the University of Miami and the University of Pennsylvania. At the time, these two schools had different policies regarding pharmaceutical marketing items; a more restrictive policy and more negative, school-level attitude toward marketing was in place at the University of Pennsylvania. The medical students were given small marketing items (pens and notepads) promoting Lipitor. There was an exposed and control group at both universities and attitudes were measured pre and post gifts for both Lipitor and Zocor using the Implicit Association Test.

What did they find? The small gifts had no effect on the third-year students at either university, but fourth-year students at the University of Miami formed a more favorable attitude toward Lipitor (the drug that was marketed). It is interesting to note that the free gifts had a reverse effect at the University of Pennsylvania, where a more restrictive policy was in place. So free pens do matter. Which leads us to ask: In the marketing world, is a gift ever just a gift?

In Closing

As we have discussed, there is a long history between audiology and the fitting of hearing aids. There is a long and storied history regarding audiology and hearing aid dispensing too. Consider that as recently as the late 1970s, it was considered unethical for audiologists to sell hearing aids, compared with today, when a large portion of hearing aids sold in the United States are by audiologists who own and operate their own private practice.

Regarding the distribution and manufacturing of hearing aids, we now have the Big Six companies, which include over 90% of the hearing aids sold. But, as you might expect, the landscape is constantly changing. Two of the Big Six companies have been put up for sale in just the last few years. Nobody is too sure what the impact will be from increased Internet sales or the proliferation of PSAPs. And, what about the increasing number of private practices owned by manufacturers? Are we going back to the days of mostly *franchise offices*?

For the audiologist interested in dispensing hearing aids, we have reviewed many of the related background issues that need to be considered: licensure, certification, guidelines, regulations, laws, reimbursement, and ethics. These topics are maybe not as intriguing as directional beamforming, new noise reduction algorithms, or Bluetooth connectivity, but they are vitally important, nonetheless.

3
Understanding the Hearing Aid Candidate

Data from surveys conducted by the National Family Opinion (NFO) panel from over 80,000 households suggest that approximately 30 million, or about 10% of the U.S. population of approximately 320 million, have some degree of hearing loss. It is usually estimated that around 95% of hearing impaired individuals can be helped with hearing aids, at least for some listening conditions. For the current U.S. population, that would be about approximately 30.5 million. Yet, we know from other surveys that only 20% to 25% of those who report having a significant hearing loss use hearing aids, suggesting that there may be 20 million or more individuals in the United States in need of treatment.

As reviewed by Mueller and Johnson (2013), some industry leaders believe that the untapped market is not as large as 20 million, due to an overestimation of the pool of potential hearing aid consumers. This is based on the notion that just because a person has an admitted hearing loss does not mean he believes that he needs hearing aids or is interested is using hearing aids. Data show that only about one-third of the people with admitted hearing loss perceive themselves as having significant need for hearing aids. The real untapped potential market for hearing aids, therefore, may be closer to about 10 million today, considering the latest estimate of people in the United States who have a hearing impairment (NIDCD, 2016).

According to recent data from the Hearing Industry Association (HIA), more than 3.3 million hearing aids are sold each year in the United States. Since about 80% of hearing aids are sold in pairs (for bilateral fittings), however, only about 1.62 million people actually purchase hearing aids each year; 1.3 million people purchase two hearing aids and the remaining 6,600,000 purchase one hearing aid. The unit volume of hearing aid sales has been slow to increase over time, considering that one million hearing aids were sold for the first time back in 1983. In 2004, the unit volume of hearing aid sales reached two million, indicating only an average of 4.7% increase in sales per year over the 21-year period from 1983. These relatively low sales numbers become even more significant today, given the improvements in hearing aid technology and the "aging of America." Sales have increased more rapidly in recent years however (5–7%), due mostly to increased purchases by the VA and big box retailers (Costco's market share is around 12%).

Not surprisingly, the prevalence of hearing loss increases with increasing age: approximately 314 in 1,000 people over age 65 have hearing loss, and 40% to 50% of people 75 and older have a hearing loss. Although we know that decreased hearing sensitivity is part of the aging process, the majority (65%) of the 30 million people with hearing loss are under the age of 65, shown in

Figure 3–1. Hearing aid use within this younger majority is significantly less than the already disturbing low 20 to 25% figure mentioned earlier—more details on these demographics shortly. Here are some general summary data from http://www.betterhearing.org regarding the incidence of hearing loss:

- Three in 10 people over age 60 have hearing loss.
- One in six baby boomers (ages 41 to 59), or 14.6%, have a hearing problem.
- One in 14 Generation Xers (ages 29 to 40), or 7.4%, already have hearing loss.
- At least 1.4 million children (18 or younger) have hearing problems.
- It is estimated that 3 in 1,000 infants are born with serious to profound hearing loss.

We of course know that individuals with hearing loss have problems understanding speech. But in addition to this obvious difficulty, we also know that hearing loss is associated with other serious negative consequences such as academic difficulties, various problems in the workplace, and psychosocial problems such as social isolation, depression, anxiety, loneliness, lessened self-efficacy, and mastery (e.g., Abrams & Doyle, 2000; Newman, Jacobson, Hug, & Sandridge, 1997).

MarkeTrak

As mentioned in our introduction, market penetration regarding the use of hearing aids is poor, and the reasons that people do not use hearing aids are complex. This has been a topic of considerable study over the past two decades. In 1984 the Hearing Industry Association (HIA) published a landmark survey of the U.S. hearing aid market. Following an initial large-scale NFO screening survey to identify individuals with hearing loss, a comprehensive 120-question survey was sent to 1,050 hearing aid non-owners and 550 owners of hearing aids.

Percentage of U.S. Citizens with Hearing Loss by Age

- 65-74, 17.1%
- 75-84, 15.2%
- 85+, 4.5%
- <18, 4.5%
- 18-34, 8.1%
- 35-44, 11.4%
- 45-54, 19.1%
- 55-64, 20.1%

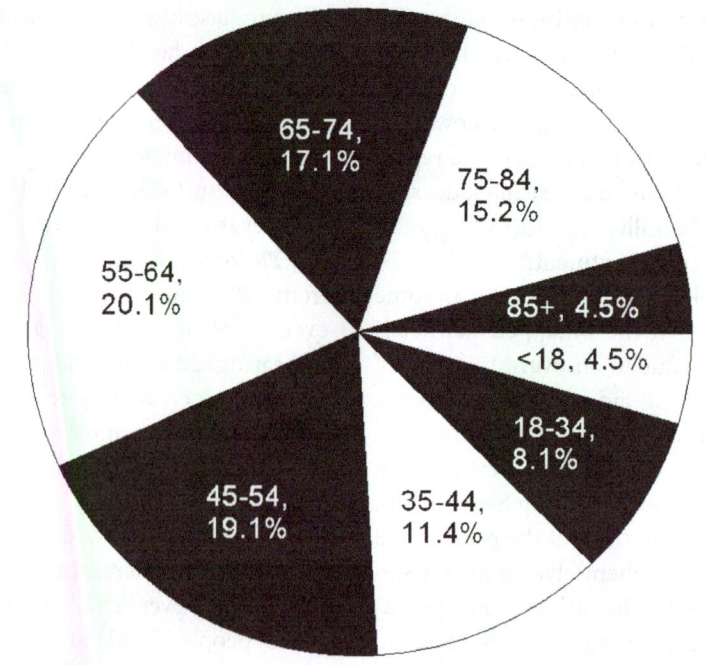

Total number of Americans with hearing loss is about 31.5 million

Figure 3–1. Distribution of U.S. citizens with hearing loss as a function of age.

> **THINGS TO REMEMBER: NEGATIVE CONSEQUENCES**
>
> Data from MarkeTrak9 (Abrams and Kihm, 2015) reveal that individuals who recently purchased hearing aids had known that they had a hearing loss for an average of 13 years. This delay in taking action is important to consider when we view the negative consequences of untreated hearing loss:
>
> - Irritability, negativism, and anger
> - Fatigue, tension, stress, and depression
> - Avoidance or withdrawal from social situations
> - Social rejection and loneliness
> - Reduced alertness and increased risk to personal safety
> - Impaired memory and ability to learn new tasks
> - Reduced job performance and earning power
> - Diminished psychological and overall health
>
> *Source:* Better Hearing Institute, Washington, DC

The results provided the first-ever systematic look at the hearing aid market. Given that several decades have passed since this survey was conducted, it is interesting to consider some of the major findings from this landmark survey. How much has really changed?

- Consumers knew where to go for help with their hearing, but 40% of non-owners had never discussed their hearing loss with a physician or an audiologist.
- There was a preference to obtain the hearing aids from the ear, nose, and throat (ENT) doctor and have the hearing aids prescribed.
- Physician recommendations for hearing aids were biased toward the older patients.
- A significant number of non-owners (17%) were told that a hearing aid would not help them (53% by otolaryngologists; 22% by audiologists)
- It is surprising to note that background noise, the price of hearing aids, or cosmetics was not considered a major problem in converting non-owners.
- And finally, nearly 14% of hearing aid owners did not use their hearing aids.

As you can see, some of the findings from 1984 have not changed significantly today. Unfortunately, one of them is the percentage of *in-the-drawer* (ITD) hearing aids. Throughout all the MarkeTrak surveys over the years, this percentage has remained disturbingly high, although dropping to only 3% for MarkeTrak9, compared to 12% for MarkeTrak VIII. One area that has changed since 1984 is that otolaryngologists are now much more likely to recommend hearing aids—this, of course, is largely because hearing aids are sold in most otolaryngologists' offices, usually by audiologists working for the otolaryngologist, although some otolaryngologists are also licensed dispensers.

The results of this HIA (1984) survey led to many initiatives and recommendations, one of which was to launch a family physician education program, based on the importance that survey respondents placed on a family doctor's recommendation. An in-depth review and further analysis of many of the HIA (1984) survey findings was reported in a 1990 *Hearing Instruments* article by Sergei Kochkin entitled, "One more time . . . What did the 1984 HIA market survey say?" At the time, Kochkin had been recently hired by Knowles Electronics as Director of Strategic Planning, with the main responsibility of "developing and market-testing programs to impartially grow the market for hearing instruments." It was in May, 1990, in a *Hearing Journal* publication, that Kochkin introduced MarkeTrak (a consumer-oriented tracking survey of the hearing instrument market), and in this article, he published initial findings from two surveys conducted in 1989. Since this first MarkeTrak report, now referred to as MarkeTrak I, Kochkin and

Knowles Electronics teamed to conduct five more surveys of the U.S. hearing loss population, MarkeTrak II through MarkeTrak VI. MarkeTrak VII and MarkeTrak VIII were conducted and published by the Better Hearing Institute (BHI), with Knowles Electronics sponsorship, and also were reported by Kochkin. MarkeTrak9 was conducted by the Hearing Industries Association (HIA) and completed in 2014. Much of the data we report in this chapter originate from one or more of the MarkeTrak surveys.

While our focus is on the U.S. MarkeTrak surveys, it is important to mention that since 2009 similar surveys have been conducted in Europe, sponsored by the European Hearing Instrument Manufacturers Association (EHIMA). EHIMA was founded in 1985 and represents the six major European hearing instrument manufacturers, producing up to 90% of the hearing aids made in Europe. The European survey is referred to as EuroTrak; the most recent EuroTrak 2015 included data from Germany, France, UK, Italy, and Switzerland. The EuroTrak survey methods are similar to MarkeTrak9, and the findings from these surveys, therefore, have been directly compared (e.g., see Hougaard, Ruf, Egger, and Abrams, 2016).

Willingness to Use Hearing Aids

As we discussed earlier, market penetration regarding hearing aid use is poor. Why is this? As part of MarkeTrak VII, Kochkin examined some of the obstacles to hearing aid use for adults. One area that emerged as significant was the effects of age—that is, there is a perception that the use of hearing aids is probably okay for older people, but not okay for younger people. This is summarized nicely in Figure 3–2. For this analysis, Kochkin (2007) separated degree of hearing loss into 10 hearing loss deciles (#1 = mild, #10 = severe/profound), and then shows hearing aid use as a function for five different hearing loss categories. As expected, the use of hearing aids increases with the degree of loss for all age groups; overall adoption percentages range from 1.9% for decile #1, to 15.5% for decile #5, to 59.9% for decile #10. But, observe that age has a strong influence. For example, for decile #5 (moderate hearing loss), the use rate is over 60% for individuals over 75 years of age but only around 20% for hearing impaired people in the 55 to 64 age range. The 55 to 64 age range group would have to fall in decile #10 before their hearing aid adoption would exceed 60%.

There are many other interwoven reasons for which hearing impaired people are reluctant to use hearing aids. Many of these reasons are summarized in Figure 3–3, which is taken only from deciles #6 through #10 (more significant losses). Note that the leading reason is type of hearing loss. Kochkin (2007) explains that this means that the person believes there is something unique about his or her hearing loss, suggesting that hearing aids will not be beneficial. In many cases, they believe that their hearing loss is not severe enough to

---

THINGS TO REMEMBER: MARKETRAK9—A NEW BASELINE?

As we discuss in this chapter, there have been several MarkeTrak surveys dating back to 1984. HIA's latest MarkeTrak survey completed at the end of 2014, MarkeTrak9, is a significant departure from the eight preceding surveys in terms of the strategies and techniques used to collect consumer information. For this reason, some have suggested that it be considered a new baseline rather than used as a direct comparison to the other MarkeTrak surveys. One notable difference was that the previous eight MarkeTrak surveys used the National Family Opinion (NFO) mail panel, using paper-and-pencil surveys distributed though the United States Postal Service. In contrast, MarkeTrak9 employed an online survey technique, which could have influenced the characteristics of the respondents (e.g., younger, more tech savvy). For example, the average age at which the respondents reported purchasing their first hearing aid was 63.3 years (vs. 68.9 years for MarkeTrak VIII), and compared to MarkeTrak VIII, there was a higher percentage identifying themselves as first-time buyers (57% vs. 37%).

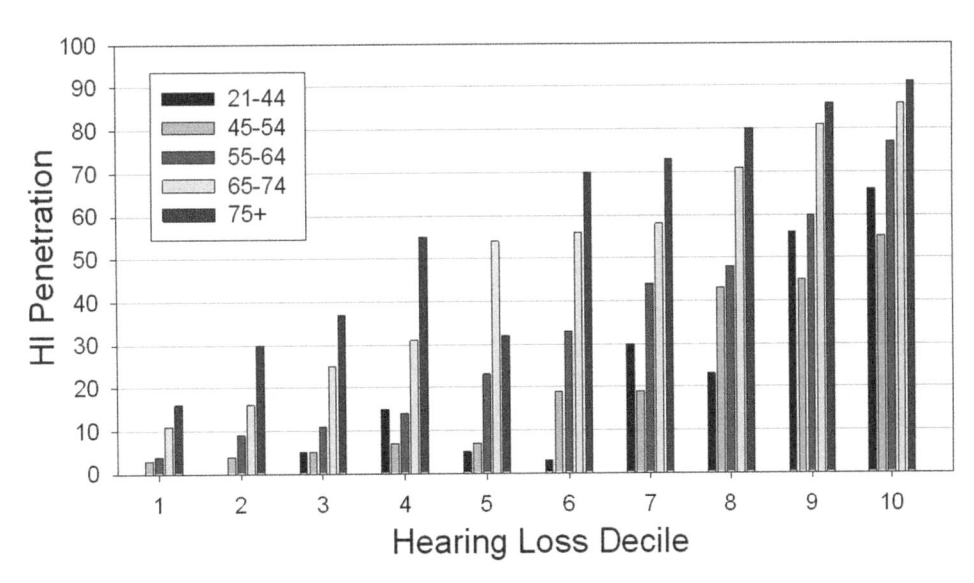

Figure 3–2. Degree of hearing loss categorized into 10 deciles (1 = mild, 10 = severe/profound), showing the percent of hearing aid use for five different hearing loss categories. (Adapted from Kochkin, 2007.)

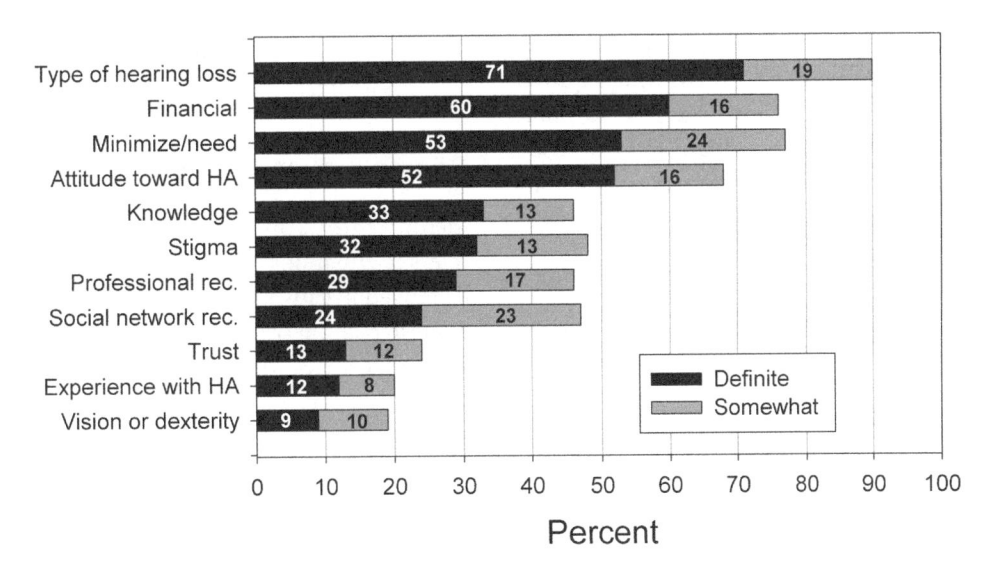

Figure 3–3. Leading reasons for not using hearings aids reported by individuals with hearing loss. (Adapted from Kochkin, 2007.)

warrant the use of hearing aids. The second leading factor is financial. To examine the integrity of this response, Kochkin compared the incomes for this group (controlling for age) with those nonusers who said they could afford hearing aids. For three of the five age groups, there was close to a $40,000 difference in mean household income, suggesting that indeed, the *can't afford* group is probably being truthful. Indeed, this concern was cited heavily as justification for the OTC hearing aid bill discussed in Chapter 2. Another significant factor, probably related to age differences shown in Figure 3–2, was the social stigma associated with the use of hearing aids. This is an interesting area, which we discuss in some detail in the next section.

Effects of Stigma

Despite considerable marketing effects to the contrary, in most Western cultures like the United States, people with hearing loss are often thought of as old, less able, and maybe even cognitively impaired. This belief is held not only by society in general, but also by the people who have hearing loss (self-stigmatization). This can have a profound effect regarding the initial adoption of amplification as well as the use and acceptance of hearing aids. Because hearing loss is not visible, to avoid stigmatization, some individuals may try to deny or hide their hearing loss. As described by Gagné, Southall, and Jennings (2009), a variety of strategies might be used.

For example, they will isolate and insulate themselves from the world around them. In this way, they will not need to use communication strategies (e.g., asking someone to repeat) that will reveal that they have a hearing loss. The efforts expended to conceal the hearing require emotional and cognitive resources, which then can lead to an overall decrease in quality of life.

In 1996, Hétu proposed two models related to the stigmatization that occurs for individuals with acquired hearing loss: the *stigmatization process* and the *normalization process*. The work of Hétu (1996) was discussed by Gagné et al. (2009), and the following is a brief summary taken from their review:

Stigmatization Process
- Stigmatization occurs because of *shame* related to their hearing impairment. Shame refers to an emotion that accompanies threats to one's sense of social belonging.
- The shame is related to communication breakdowns that occur when people with hearing loss interact with people who have normal hearing. The person may feel guilt about themselves related to the hearing loss.
- As a result of the feelings of incompetency that might develop, the person's self-esteem and social identity are diminished.
- This may lead the person to attempt to conceal the hearing loss or withdraw from social activities.

Normalization Process (Step 1)
- The normalization process is to help the person who is stigmatized by the hearing loss regain a more normal social identity.
- The individual begins by meeting and interacting with other people who have hearing loss. This creates an environment where they can share their feelings and discuss their unsuccessful social interactions.
- They realize that they are not alone, and that many other people have the same feelings of being denigrated or ashamed.
- They begin to realize that the feelings they have are normal.

Normalization Process (Step 2)
- The person with hearing loss needs to meet and interact with family and friends who do not have hearing loss.
- The hearing impaired person is encouraged to tell family and friends that they have a hearing issue.
- The use of effective communication strategies will help restore a more factorable social identity; the person with hearing loss will gain more confidence; and as a result, they will be more likely to participate in social situations.

Stigma-Induced Identity Threat

Identity threat, often referred to as stereotype threat, refers to situations in which individuals feel they might be judged negatively because of a stereotype. The threat refers to being at risk of confirming, as self-characteristic, a negative stereotype about one's group. Identity threat can lead to self-handicapping strategies and a reduced sense of belonging to the stereotyped domain or their value of the domain in question. Studies in this area often have been focused toward minority or gender issues, but identity threat is also something that may need to be considered with hearing aid candidates. We have already discussed one example.

As reviewed by Gagné et al. (2009), stigma related to hearing loss and hearing aid use can put a person at risk for identity threat. This may occur when the patient judges the demands imposed by a stigma-relevant event as potentially harmful to his or her social identity, and when the stress induced exceeds the patient's ability to cope with the demands of the situation. We have already discussed one example. Recall from Figure 3–2 that hearing aid use rate is more than 60% for individuals with moderate hearing loss who are over 75 years of age, but the use rate is only 20% for the same hearing

Table 3–1. Components of an Audiologic Counseling Strategy Designed to Address Identity Threat for the Hearing Aid Candidate

1. Describe and discuss the stigma-induced identity threat, and explain to the patient the cause, consequences and the potential costs of the stress related to identify threat.
2. Establish a hierarchy of situations in which identity threat occurs.
3. Discuss the effectiveness of the patient's typical coping strategies. Introduce new adaptive strategies when necessary.
4. Implement a problem-solving approach to address a situation of stigma-inducing identity threat identified by the patient.
5. Train and encourage the patient to apply the selected coping strategies in a secure environment (may be practiced during the counseling session).
6. Meet with the patient to discuss the process of implementing and the consequences of applying the strategies discussed.
7. Attempt a similar experience in a slightly more threatening situation.
8. Increase the number of situations in which the patient discloses his or her hearing loss and applies appropriate coping strategies.

Source: Adapted from Gagne et al., 2009.

loss group in the 55 to 64 age range. It is reasonable to assume that the use of hearing aids is an identity threat to the younger group. In Table 3–1, Gagné et al. (2009) provide a set of guidelines to help the audiologist counsel the patient with identity threat.

The Benefits of Hearing Aid Use

As shown in the preceding section, MarkeTrak studies have examined the reasons why people delay their decision to purchase hearing aids. Certainly one reason is that they simply are unaware of the fact that receiving early treatment for hearing loss has the potential to literally transform their lives (e.g., my hearing loss is too mild to benefit from hearing aids). Research by the National Council on the Aging on more than two thousand people with hearing loss, as well as their significant others, demonstrated that hearing aids clearly are associated with substantial improvements in the social, emotional, psychological, and physical well-being of people with hearing loss in all hearing loss categories from mild to severe. Specifically, hearing aid usage is positively related to the following quality of life issues. Hearing loss treatment (use of hearing aids) was shown to improve:

- Earning power
- Communication in relationships
- Intimacy and warmth in family relationships
- Ease in communication
- Emotional stability
- Sense of control over life events
- Perception of mental functioning
- Physical health
- Group social participation

As part of this research, significant others were asked to rate changes they observed in several different areas of their life that they believed were due to the respondent using hearing aids. These findings are shown in Figure 3–4. In general, for nearly all quality of life areas assessed, the observed improvements were

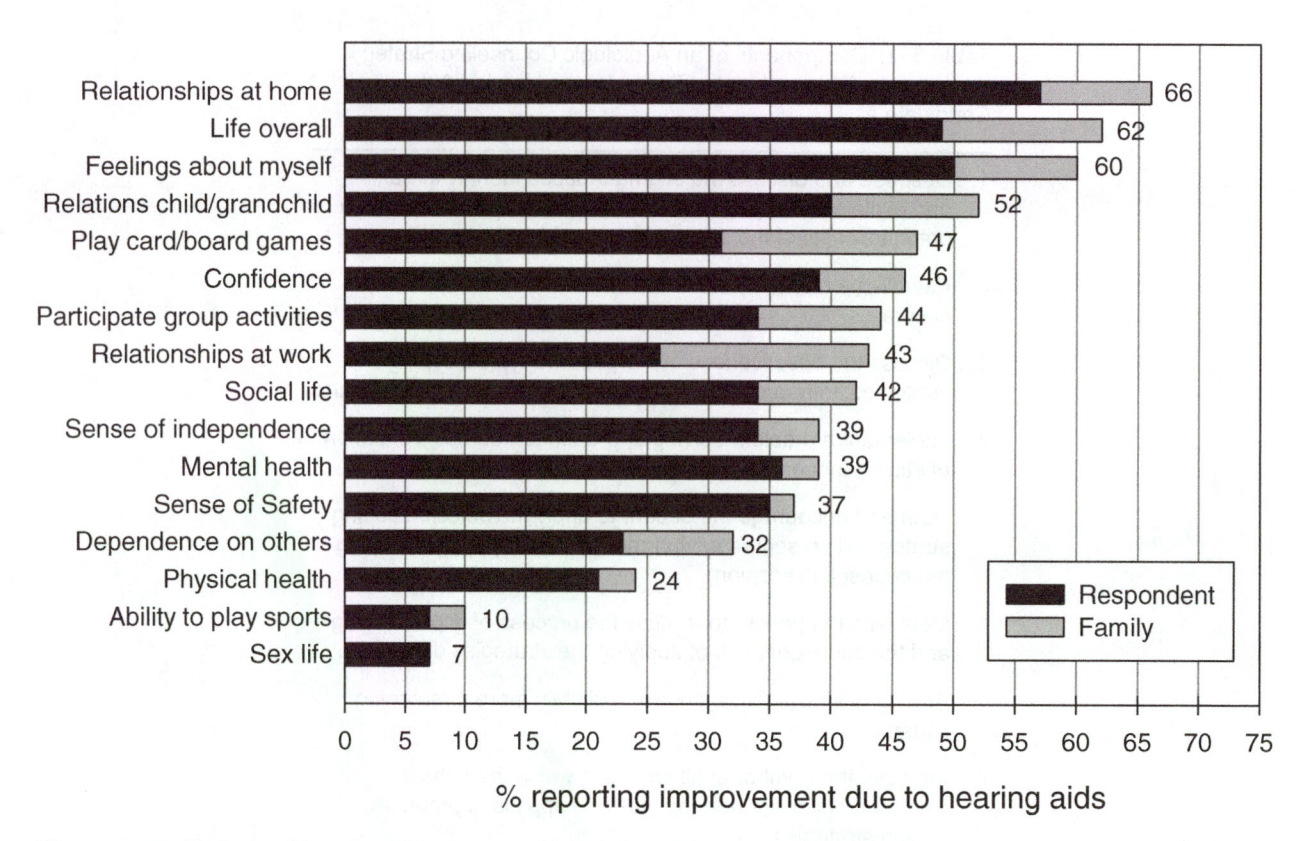

Figure 3–4. Percent of hearing aid owners and their family members reporting improvement in their quality of life in 16 different areas due to the use of hearing aids. Note that in nearly all cases, the family members report that the hearing aid user is experiencing more benefit than the user reports.

positively related to the degree of hearing loss. Family members in nearly every comparison observed greater improvements than the respondent. The top three areas of observed improvement for both respondents and family members were *relationships at home, feelings about self,* and *life overall.* As might be expected, the most substantial improvements were observed for the individuals with more severe hearing loss.

Perhaps just as important, this research found that hearing loss treatment was shown to reduce:

- Discrimination toward the person with the hearing loss
- Hearing loss compensation behaviors (i.e., pretending you hear)
- Anger and frustration in relationships
- Depression and depressive symptoms
- Feelings of paranoia
- Anxiety
- Social phobias
- Self-criticism

Given all the factors that can be improved with the use of hearing aids, it is somewhat difficult to explain the large percent of nonusers. Indeed, it could be that they are not aware of the potential advantages. But what about the ITDs—the people who have purchased hearing aids, did not return them during the trial period, but are not using them? Why didn't these patients receive benefit? Why they were not satisfied? This also has been studied, and the reasons are quite variable and include aspects of the patient, the hearing aid, and the environment (see "Things to Remember" on this topic). To combat nonuse, it is important to consider these factors and the potential for them to affect individual patients during the process of establishing candidacy, selecting and fitting the hearing aid, and providing counseling. In this way, future nonuse can be reduced.

> **POINTS TO PONDER:
> A LINK BETWEEN HEARING LOSS AND DEMENTIA?**
>
> In recent years, there has been considerable discussion regarding the potential link between untreated hearing loss and early dementia. It's an "attention-getting" topic that has been popular in the lay press and the focus of many television news shows. Much of the data on this topic is from the Johns Hopkins research laboratory and the Baltimore Longitudinal Study on Aging; Frank Lin, MD, is the primary spokesman. One compelling finding was for individuals who underwent yearly magnetic resonance imaging (MRI) to track brain changes for up to 10 years. At the starting point, 75 had normal hearing and 51 had impaired hearing. After analyzing their MRIs over the following years, those participants whose hearing was already impaired at the start of the study had accelerated rates of brain atrophy compared to those with normal hearing, losing more than an additional cubic centimeter of brain tissue each year. Those with impaired hearing had significantly more shrinkage in particular regions, including the superior, middle and inferior temporal gyri.
>
> Other research has shown a relationship between hearing impairment and the incidence of dementia and cognitive decline in older adults—suggesting a 30 to 40% greater risk of cognitive decline if hearing loss is present. It is difficult to say if this is because of the hearing loss per se or the withdrawal from communication and social isolation that often accompanies hearing loss. Although it is tempting to conclude that this could be prevented by the early use of hearing aids, this has yet to be shown in well-controlled clinical trials.

Satisfaction with Amplification

We have talked about some reasons why individuals do not use their hearing aids, but fortunately most patients do, and most of these individuals are reasonably satisfied. Satisfaction with amplification is something that has been tracked by MarkeTrak over the years, with several surveys examining specific aspects of hearing aid fittings (e.g., bilateral versus unilateral, directional versus omnidirectional, custom instruments versus BTE). These surveys are archived (http://www.betterhearing.org). For the satisfaction ratings, the MarkeTrak surveys have used a five-point Likert scale: very dissatisfied, dissatisfied, neutral, satisfied, and very satisfied. The satisfied and very satisfied categories are then often combined for a single satisfaction measure. Results from surveys over the past 12 years have revealed satisfaction levels significantly higher than when the first survey was conducted, going from 60% in 1989 to 74% for MarkeTrak VIII in 2008. MarkeTrak9 shows a substantial increase to 81%, but recall that this was a different sampling procedure. Interestingly, there was a drop in satisfaction in the mid-1990s. Our best guess is that this relates to the heavy promotion of digital technology during this period, which brought in new users, was significantly more expensive, raised expectations, but may not have delivered value. But that's just a guess.

In addition to overall satisfaction, it is important to consider satisfaction for different listening situations. This is shown for MarkeTrak VIII in Figure 3–5. Note that satisfaction is very high for one-on-one communication (92%) and even conversations in small groups (85%). As noise and/or reverberation is added, satisfaction predictably goes down. For common listening situations where background noise is present, such as a restaurant or large group, satisfaction is 68 to 75%. Although these later numbers are not as high as we would like, it is important to point out that as recently as 1995 (e.g., MarkeTrak IV), satisfaction for use in restaurants was only 52% (23% poorer) and the satisfaction for listening in large groups was below 40% (20% poorer). We suspect that the significant increase we have seen in recent years is some combination of today's advanced algorithms, better fitting procedures (more audibility), and probably better counseling.

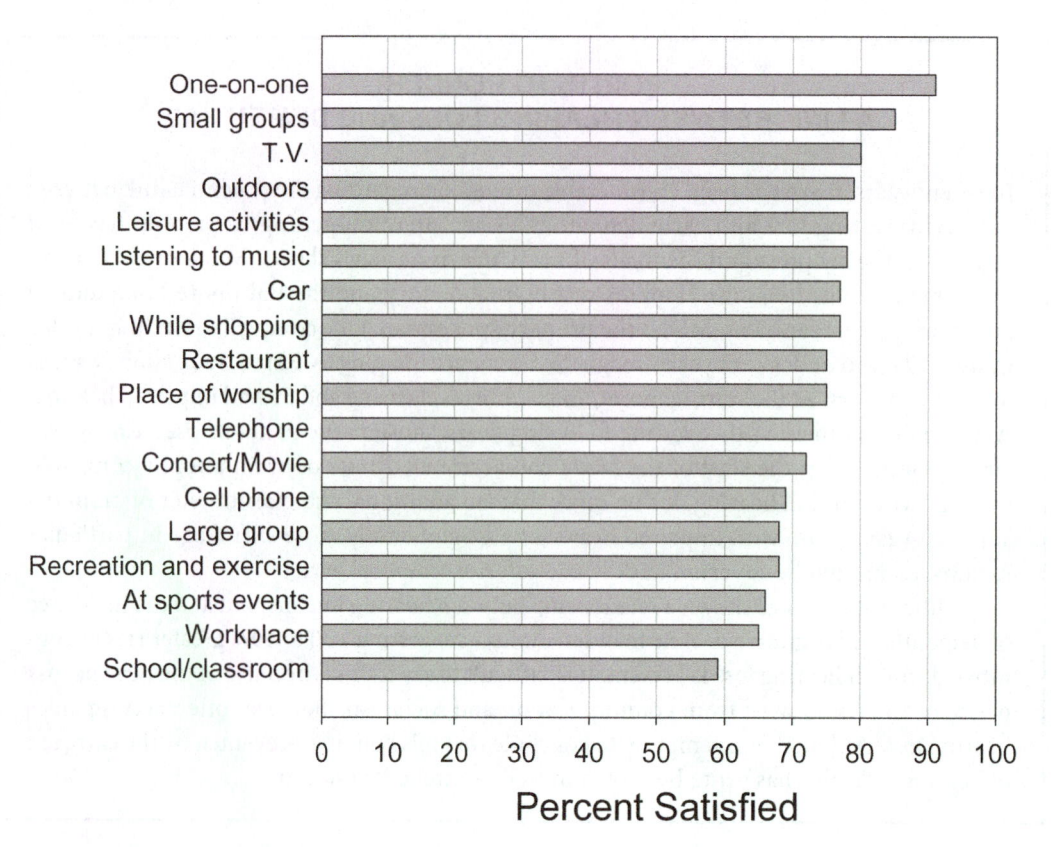

Figure 3–5. Data from MarkeTrak VIII showing satisfaction rates for 18 different listening conditions. (Adapted from Kochkin, 2010.)

THINGS TO REMEMBER: OFTEN CITED FACTORS FOR HEARING AID NONUSE

Earlier in this chapter, we examined the reasons why people with hearing loss do not use hearing aids. These data were primarily for individuals who never had tried hearing aids. But what about the people who own hearing aids and do not use them? The main reasons (according to MarketTrack surveys rank ordering) are listed below. As we read through the different reasons, we can speculate that perhaps some patients simply have unrealistic expectations, but we also have to wonder whether some of these factors could have been reduced or eliminated with improved verification, validation, and counseling.

- Lack of benefit
- Lack of benefit in noise
- Poor cosmetics
- Disbelief that they need help
- Inability to insert the earmold
- Poor fit and/or comfort
- Negative side effects
- Poor sound quality for own voice
- Poor sound quality for external sounds
- Feedback
- Broken hearing aid

Another area of satisfaction that can be studied is related to sound quality and the sounds of potentially annoying aspects of hearing aid use (e.g., wind noise, sound of own voice). These data from MarkeTrak VIII are shown in Figure 3–6. Again, the satisfaction values are not as high as we would like, but nearly all of them are 10 to 15% better than those in the surveys from the 1990s. For example, the *use in noisy situations* satisfaction rating of 62% is substantially higher, by 25%, than that recorded in MarkeTrak IV.

Understanding the Patient

A patient is not defined only by his or her hearing loss or communication needs but by a variety of factors. This understanding and respect for individuality must begin the moment a patient walks in the door and continue throughout the entire professional relationship with him or her. As clinicians, we must also recognize the strengths and limitations of our own personality and

---

**POINTS TO PONDER:
WHAT IS A GOOD SATISFACTION RATING?**

We have seen an upward trend in overall satisfaction with hearing aids in the past 20 years, and we are now at 81%. We do not expect to ever have 100% satisfaction, but what is good? How does 81% compare with other services and products? The good news is that it is about 15% higher than network TV, the IRS, and McDonald's. It is approximately the same as satisfaction levels for banks, hotels, and waste disposal. Coming in somewhat higher are beer and utility companies. BMW owners have an 84% satisfaction rate, and topping the list at 86% is that for processed food (e.g., Heinz® Ketchup) at 86%. As of this writing, satisfaction with the U.S. Congress is at 18% and has been at historically low levels for some time now!

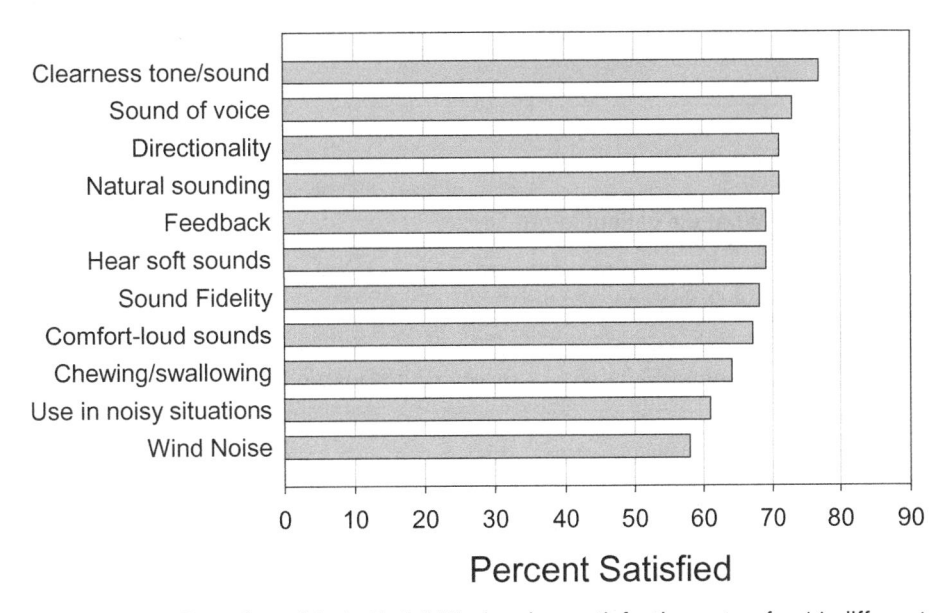

Figure 3–6. Data from MarkeTrak VIII showing satisfaction rates for 11 different conditions related to hearing aid use. (Adapted from Kochkin, 2010.)

how that might interact with the patients. In this way, we can optimize rapport with each patient and maximize our chances at the most positive outcome possible.

Stages of Grief

As reviewed by Taylor and Mueller (2011), it is a commonly held belief that adults with acquired hearing go through Kübler-Ross's five stages of grief: denial, anger, bargaining, depression, and acceptance. It is helpful when initiating the opening counseling and conducting our case history if we have a general understanding of which stage each patient falls into. Whenever possible, it is useful to involve family members and other significant others, as this will help identify the patient's stage. Their assistance also will be helpful as you guide the patient through the first four stages in preparation for using hearing aids—stage five. The time it takes a patient to travel through the five stages is extremely variable; for some patients, it seems to happen in a single afternoon, whereas for others it may take years. Not everyone goes through all of the stages or goes through them in linear fashion. Some stages may not be experienced at all. Because hearing loss usually is a slow and gradual process, it is very common to experience a patient in denial. On the other hand, because it is gradual and not life-threatening, the stages of anger and depression are not observed as often as they might be with other pathologies. We do see these stages more commonly in sudden hearing loss, however.

With the typical patient considering the use of hearing aids, the denial stage is so common that it is almost expected. We all have seen a patient in our office who had tried hearing aids four or five years earlier, and returned them for credit because they "did not provide the expected benefit," and who is now back to try hearing aids again. Our testing reveals that the hearing loss and speech recognition has not really changed in five years, but this time the patient reports that hearing aids provide significant benefit and becomes a satisfied user. Was this because of the changes in hearing aid technology over the years? Maybe, but it is more probable that the fitting is now successful simply because the patient now is accepting of the hearing loss and ready to seek assistance. Insights into how the five stages of grieving can influence patient behavior can be helpful in counseling the new hearing aid user. Examples for each stage are provided in Table 3–2.

Identifying the Hearing Aid Candidate

With all of the problems associated with hearing loss, it is important to discuss what makes someone a hearing aid candidate. Although this question has been debated for decades, it is clear that the answer is much more complex than simply the presence of a certain degree

Table 3–2. The Elisabeth Kubler Ross Five Psychological Stages of Grieving, Applied to Hearing Loss

Stage	What the patient might say:
Denial	"I don't have a hearing problem, other people mumble." "I hear everything I need to hear."
Anger	To their friends—"Are you purposely talking behind my back?" To the professional: "Are you sure you did the testing correctly?"
Bargaining	"Okay, maybe I just wasn't listening, I'll pay more attention." "Let's see if I'm still having problems next year, maybe my hearing will get better."
Depression	"It seems like my family avoids me because of my hearing loss." "There are things I'll probably never hear again." "I'm getting old."
Acceptance	"Wearing hearing aids is really no big deal." "My quality of life will probably improve with the use of hearing aids." "A lot of people my age have worse health problems than hearing loss."

Source: Adapted from Taylor and Mueller, 2011.

of hearing loss. In fact, success with hearing aids can be more affected by a patient's motivation than the exact degree of hearing loss. Factors such as difficulty hearing sounds, communication difficulty, motivation for improved hearing, financial constraints, expectations related to hearing aids (both positive and negative), and a host of other factors affect candidacy. Before establishing candidacy, the patient must make some effort to be evaluated. Specifically, the patient, sometimes under the direction (or strong encouragement) of a spouse or significant other, must seek help for his or her hearing problem.

Making the decision to seek help is obviously a complex one as is shown by the survey data we have discussed. One factor is the magnitude of hearing loss. Specifically, more than 85% of nonusers fall in the range of mild-to-moderate hearing loss and data from Flamme et al. (2005) reveal that fewer than 6% of individuals with mild-to-moderate hearing loss pursue amplification. It is tempting to conclude that these individuals with mild-to-moderate hearing loss may simply not encounter hearing-related communication difficulties, although this contradicts everything we know about the importance of audibility and speech understanding. In agreement, Newman, Jacobson, Hug, and Sandridge (1997) reported that even younger adults with mild hearing loss report a variety of psychosocial problems affecting everyday life.

Concerns about lack of benefit, concerns about how they might look wearing hearing aids (cosmetics), negative reports from friends and others about hearing aids, and high cost can also keep patients from pursuing amplification. Although it is tempting to think that cosmetic and cost concerns might dominate the worries related to hearing aid use and lead to a patient's avoidance of seeking help, they are clearly not the only factors. Surprisingly, one survey reported that only 35% of individuals who self-report having a hearing loss, but currently do not have a hearing aid, would wear an instrument even if it was free and invisible (Kochkin, 2001). Recent data suggests that number has gone up to 55% (Kochkin, 2012)—a sign of the economy perhaps? Obviously, as we discussed earlier, concerns such as expected lack of benefit, negative consequences, and other issues also are being considered by prospective patients.

Once an individual seeks help, it is important to determine if she or he is an appropriate candidate. At the simplest level, candidacy for adults can be described by a combination of the presence of hearing loss to a degree that obstructs communication (or other reported hearing difficulties) and the motivation to improve hearing. Although these criteria are likely the most important to keep in mind when considering candidacy, a few specific question areas should usually be explored when considering candidacy. Whereas we as clinicians must sometimes gently encourage patients to try amplification, we must also be willing to halt the entire process if the patient is not ready. The answers to a few specific questions can help frame future questions and help us as clinicians decide how much counseling needs to be done prior to thinking about hearing aid selection. Depending on whether there is a red flag or not, the answers to these specific questions might lead to (1) some counseling during the hearing aid selection stage, (2) the potential need for significant further counseling, or (3) possibly the conclusion that the patient is not an appropriate candidate at this time. Examples of typical and red flag answers are shown in Table 3–3. These are all answers that we actually have heard in the clinic on more than one occasion.

Although it may seem quite surprising on the surface, many adults who seek assessment of their hearing difficulties reject recommendations for remediation of hearing loss. Therefore, in addition to recognizing how the lack of treatment may impact a given individual considering amplification, it is also relevant to determine if and how other nonauditory factors might affect the prognosis for amplification, and whether these factors should be formally assessed. Nonauditory, contextual factors can be internally or externally based.

- Internal (i.e., personal contextual) factors impacting communication include cognitive decline, personality characteristics (expectations, motivation, willingness to take a risk, assertiveness), additional sensory impairments (manual dexterity, visual acuity), prior experience with amplification, general health, and other otologic conditions (e.g., tinnitus).
- External (i.e., environmental contextual) factors include environmental characteristics (such as occupational demands and recreational habits) and patient support systems.

Questions asked during the case history should be tailored to address these issues and not just focus on

Table 3–3. Questions and Answers That Can Help Frame the Counseling Process

Q1. Why are you here?
- Expected Answer: I have been having some problems hearing (or understanding), especially in background noise.
- Red Flag: **My wife thinks I can't hear.**

Q2. Whose idea was it to come in? (usually indirectly asked)
- Expected Answer: My daughter suggested that I should come in, and I guess she is right. I've been putting if off for years.
- Red Flag: **My husband says he thinks I have a problem, but I really don't.**

Q3. What is your biggest concern?
- Expected Answer: That I won't be able to use a hearing aid correctly.
- Red Flag: **That we really can't afford the hearing aid and my wife will find out we have financial problems.**

Q4. Do you believe you can be helped by the use of hearing aids?
- Typical Answer: I think so. I certainly hope the hearing aids will help me.
- Red Flag: **I really don't have much of hearing problem, so I really don't need help.**

---

hearing. There is no strong evidence to suggest that any one or a combination of these nonauditory issues can be used to reliably predict success or failure with hearing aids (Valente, 2006). Nevertheless, identifying these factors should be addressed in counseling and in establishing realistic expectations with the patient. In Chapter 6, we review several self-assessment scales that can assist in obtaining important information (which often is not part of the case history) and categorizing candidacy.

Motivational Interviewing

Based on the patient's answers during the case history and their personality, a number of different counseling approaches might be necessary when talking to a patient about hearing aid candidacy. It is beyond the scope of this book to address many of these approaches in detail; however, there are many other textbooks that directly address counseling techniques. One counseling philosophy is motivational interviewing, described by Miller and Rollnick (2002; for more information visit http://www.motivationalinterview.org). Motivational interviewing is a directive, client-centered counseling style for eliciting behavior change by helping our patients explore and resolve ambivalence. This counseling approach, which evolved from treatment of substance abusers, points out the futility of confrontational approaches ("See, you have a hearing loss just like your wife said, now what are you going to do about it?"). Instead, the fact that the patient may experience ambivalence about treatment (a feeling of uncertainty about something due to a mental conflict) that must be explored and resolved is highlighted. Although interested readers are referred elsewhere for detailed techniques, it is worthwhile to at least attempt to capture the spirit of motivational interviewing (see "Technical Tip" on this topic).

In their counseling textbook, Clark and English (2003) describe similar themes that are more directly related to hearing loss including the importance of getting patients to take ownership of their hearing problem. They describe techniques that can be used for children and adults related to identification of specific problems or difficulties related to hearing and discussing how best to counteract those problems. This type of counseling requires that the clinician switch roles during their time spent with a patient. Specifically, the clinician must relinquish his or her role as the expert who is determining what is best for the patient until after the patient makes the decision to be willing to accept help and pursue amplification.

In addition to the patient, we must also be honest with ourselves as clinicians. This not only includes

> **TECHNICAL TIP: THE SPIRIT OF MOTIVATIONAL INTERVIEWING**
>
> - Motivation to change is elicited from the patient and not imposed from without.
> - It is the patient's task, not the audiologist's, to articulate and resolve his or her ambivalence.
> - Direct persuasion is not an effective method for resolving ambivalence.
> - The counseling style is generally a quiet and eliciting one.
> - The audiologist is directive in helping the patient to examine and resolve ambivalence.
> - Readiness to change is not a patient trait, but a fluctuating product of interpersonal interaction.
> - The therapeutic relationship is more like a partnership or companionship than expert/recipient roles.
>
> (Adapted from http://www.motivationalinterview.org.)

recognizing when we may be stressed or have external pressures that may affect our performance but also recognizing our own personality and how it might interact with that of our patients. Some clinicians have naturally warm and friendly styles; others are more businesslike and direct in their approach. Both of these approaches can be successful, although they will likely have the greatest appeal to different patient personalities. Regardless of personality, a caring professional approach and a genuine interest in addressing each individual patient's communication needs is critical for establishing patient trust and building rapport. Without this rapport, many patients will be much less likely to trust your recommendations. The unfortunate consequence of this lack of trust may be reduced satisfaction with hearing aids or even failure to pursue further help for a period of time.

The Patient's Story

Erdman (2009) discusses the importance of an empathetic practitioner-patient relationship, which can facilitate engagement of the patient and which in turn may improve their management of the treatment and their adherence to the treatment regimen. The understanding is based on the accurate perspective of the patient experience and appropriate emotional reactivity.

Part of this biopsychosocial counseling approach is the patient's story. Listening to a patient's story will facilitate the counseling process, and the patients are there to tell their story. It is why they made the appointment. You just need to help them a little. Erdman (2009) provides some guidance in this area:

- Use open-ended statements: "What brought you here today?"
- If at all possible, sit with the patient in a private area face to face. Make eye contact and show that you are sincerely listening.
- Allow the patient to answer. Wait. He or she may not respond immediately. If the patient does not respond in 10 to 20 seconds, rephrase the question and try again.
- Listen to the story and develop a shared understanding of what the experience of hearing loss means to the patient. This will help you engage the patient and facilitate achieving the treatment goals.

The Four Habits Model

In the final section of this chapter, we take some of the things that we have discussed so far and put them into a model that you can use with your patients. The model that we prefer is from Frankel and Stein (1999) from their article, "Getting the Most Out of the Clinical Encounter: The Four Habits Model." As pointed out by these authors, our bedside manner has a direct influence on the outcome of the treatment; research has shown that patients probably are more concerned about how much we care than how much we know. Four intentions support the Four Habits:

- To establish rapport and build trust rapidly
- To facilitate the effective exchange of information
- To demonstrate caring and concern
- To increase the likelihood of treatment adherence and positive health outcomes

Habit 1: Invest in the Beginning

It is recommended that three tasks are accomplished at the beginning of the patient encounter, as is exemplified in Table 3–4.

Creating Rapport Quickly

The first few moments of the encounter are important for establishing a trusting relationship. Actions such as the following are suggested:

- At the initial introduction, to obtain trust and respect, it is helpful if the patient is addressed at the same level of authority. That is, if you are Dr. Smith, then the patient would be Mr. Jones.
- A handshake during the introduction initiates touch.
- Assure name of patient and correct pronunciation; include names of others if family members or significant others are present.
- Adapt voice tone and language level to the patient.
- If possible, review the chart before the initial introduction and inform the patient of this.
- If the patient is not seen on time, acknowledge this with something like: "I'm sorry for keeping you waiting."

Eliciting Patient Concerns

The second task is to determine the reason(s) for the appointment. Regarding the fitting of hearing aids, this often will help assist in determining if the patient is ready for amplification. Frankel and Stein (1999) recommend two different strategies:

- Draw out the patient's concerns with open-ended questions, for example, "I understand you're having some problems with your hearing?" "Can you tell me about that?"
- Use *continuers*. Once the patient begins to describe the hearing and communication

Table 3–4. Habit #1: Invest in the Beginning

Create rapport quickly	• Introduce yourself to everyone in room.
	• Acknowledge wait if patient not seen on time.
	• Convey your knowledge of patient's history.
	• Make social comment or ask a non-medical question to put the patient at ease.
	• Adapt own language and the pace of the conversation to that of the patient.
Elicit patient's concerns	• Use open ended questions: "What prompted this visit?" "What can I help you with today?" "I understand that you are here because of _____, tell me more about that." "What else would you like to discuss?"
Plan the visit with the patient	• Repeat patient's concerns back to them to check understanding.
	• Describe course of action. Let the patient know what to expect.
	• Prioritize course of action if necessary. "I know you'd like to talk to someone about your dizziness and the soreness in your right ear, but let's start with conducting the hearing evaluation."

problems, this then includes vocalizations such as "Uh huh," "Go on," and "Tell me more," and nonverbal behaviors such as silence, head nodding, and an engaged listening posture.

Once you have heard the concerns of the patient, it is time to plan the visit. You could use a summary statement as follows: "So it sounds as though you're having some trouble understanding speech, especially when background noise is present. What I'd like to do is conduct some testing, so I can tell you what is going on, and then we'll develop a plan together if treatment is needed."

Typically, a patient who is being seen by an audiologist for the potential use of hearing aids has a fairly straightforward problem. It is not like a patient who may have a list of five or six problems going in to see his or her general practice physician, In some situations, however, the patient might present ear-related issues that need attention that are not directly related to the fitting of hearing aids (e.g., external or middle ear pathology, balance function problems, tinnitus). Two strategies are suggested for handling this:

> Prioritization: Inform the patient about what can be accomplished during the office visit. "In the time we have today, I want to first make sure we obtain a good measure of how you're hearing and conduct a few tests to identify what might be causing your hearing problems." If time is running short, use *I wish* statements. "I wish I had more time today to talk about the ringing in your ears, but . . ."

> Time-framing: Patients usually know the time of their appointment, but are not aware of the time that was allotted for them. It is therefore helpful to provide them information such as: "Mr. Smith, you were scheduled for a 30-minute appointment today. We can take care of your other concerns in a follow-up appointment."

Habit 2: Elicit the Patient's Perspective

The purpose of this habit is to assess the patient's point of view concerning the hearing problem and what treatment he or she is seeking. Eliciting the patient's perspective consists of three skills: assessing patient attribution, identifying patient requests for care, and exploring the impact of symptoms (as reviewed in Table 3–5).

Assessing Patient Attribution

This consists of determining the patient's perspective about what caused the hearing loss. It is important to ask open-ended questions and to allow the patient to express his or her concerns. This may help you provide reassurance when the testing is finished—a patient who believes that his or her hearing loss is due to a brain tumor will be relieved to know that the hearing loss is consistent with presbycusis. Because most hearing losses are from similar causes, as audiologists it is tempting to help out the patient with the case history: "Oh, you like to hunt; your hearing loss probably is from noise exposure." Although this may be true, it is important to know what the patient thinks. It has been shown that patients who understand and who are able to explain

Table 3–5. Habit #2: Elicit the Patient's Perspective

Ask for patient's ideas	• Assess the patient's point of view regarding their hearing problems: "Why do you think that you have a hearing loss?" "What worries you about this problem?"
	• Ask the patient's friends and family their opinion.
Elicit specific requests	• Determine the patient's goals or desired outcome: "What are you hoping that I can help you with regarding your hearing problems?"
Explore the impact the hearing loss is having on the patient's life	• How has this hearing loss affected your social life? Work? Relations with family members?
	• Ask the patient's friends and family the same questions.

> **THINGS TO REMEMBER: TIME MANAGEMENT CAN BE TRICKY**
>
> The Four Habits Model discusses the use of prioritization and time-framing when working with patients. This is based on a busy medical practice in which patient visits might be scheduled every 15 minutes. Some audiology clinics only allow 30 minutes for a diagnostic appointment, which doesn't leave much time for discussion treatment strategies. When seeing patients who are hearing aid candidates, the audiologist needs to exercise some clinical judgment when a time crunch exists. There is something to the old adage "strike while the iron is hot." If after testing and your follow-up counseling a patient appears to be ready to order hearing aids, we suggest that you somehow find time to follow through with this at that patient visit. Often, the patient will be willing to simply wait an hour or so until you have a break, rather than come back on another day—which may not happen for years!

the problem (e.g., I've worked as a carpenter for the past 20 years, and I'm pretty sure I got my hearing loss from all that saw noise) are able to recall more of the information that we provide them, and are more responsive to treatment (Tuckett, Boulton, Olson, & Williams, 1985).

Identifying Patient Requests

In general, when the patient arrives at your clinic, he or she brings along not only a set of problems, but also expectations regarding the recommendations and treatment that you will provide. This could be related to past experiences, stories from friends, or information acquired from the media. We all have seen the patient who believes that hearing loss could be cured by a simple operation. It is helpful to ask a question such as, "How were you hoping that I could help you with your hearing loss today?" It is interesting to note that Eisenthal and Lazare (1977) found that patients whose requests were fully listened to were more satisfied with their care, regardless of whether the requests were granted.

Exploring the Impact

The final skill in Habit 2 is determining the impact of the patient's hearing loss on their daily activities, work, and family relations. This is best accomplished by using a structured self-assessment scale designed for this purpose. One example is the Hearing Handicap for the Elderly or Adult (HHIE or HHIA). This scale, described in detail in Chapter 6, examines the social and emotional handicap caused by the hearing loss. Another helpful scale, also described in Chapter 6, is the Client Oriented Scale of Improvement, or COSI. Because the COSI relies on communication situations generated by the patient, this often uncovers specific areas regarding work and family where the hearing loss is causing problems.

Habit 3: Demonstrate Empathy

It is of course important to build rapport and show empathy throughout the patient visit, but perhaps the most important time is while you are establishing the patient's concern(s). A review of how this can be accomplished is shown in Table 3–6.

Being Open to the Patient's Emotions

As we have already discussed, clinical practice can be busy, and many times we just want to get down to business—get the patient in the booth, do the testing, order the hearing aids. When do we have time to experience empathy? Frankel and Stein (1999) explain that one strategy is to look for brief windows of opportunity for responding to patients' emotions, a skill noted in outstanding clinicians. And, it may not take as long as you think. Research at the University of Western Ontario by Stewart, Brown, and Weston (1989) shows that medical professionals who are sensitive to and explore patients' emotional concerns take on the average only one minute longer to complete a patient visit compared with

Table 3–6. Habit #3: Demonstrate Empathy

Be open to patient's emotions	• Assess changes in body language and voice.
	• Look for opportunities to use brief empathic comments or gestures.
Make at least one empathic statement	• Name a probable emotion: "That sounds really upsetting."
	• Compliment the patient on efforts to address the problem.
Convey empathy nonverbally	• Pause; use body language.
Be aware of your own emotions	• Use your feeling as a clue to what the patient might be feeling.
	• Take a break if necessary.

those who do not. It is also important to identify hints of emotion that patients might use as a trial balloon. The comment, "I'm thinking about retirement," seems simple enough, unless one considers that communication problems at work could be driving the decision.

Frankel and Stein (1999) suggest that there are two general options available when responding to a potential empathic opportunity:

- The audiologist can avoid the opportunity by changing the topic, ignoring the statement, or by offering premature reassurance. This is the easiest approach and, unfortunately, often the one employed.
- The audiologist can encourage the expression of the emotion by using open-ended continuers like "Please go on . . . ," "Tell me more," and so forth. Some empathetic responses suggested by Bird and Cohen-Cole (1990) include:
    - Reflection—"I can see that you are . . . "
    - Legitimation—"I can understand why you feel . . . "
    - Support—"I want to help."
    - Partnership—"Let's work together . . . "
    - Respect—"You're doing great."

Habit 4: Invest in the End

This habit is more about delivering information than collecting it. It relates to tasks that occur at the end of the patient visit: delivering diagnostic information, encouraging patients to participate in decision making, and negotiating treatment plans (e.g., the fitting of hearing aids). Table 3–7 reviews some of the key skills related to this habit.

Delivering Diagnostic Information

Frankel and Stein (1999) suggest that the most important principle regarding the delivery of diagnostic information is to use the patient's original statement of concerns to frame information to be shared. "Well Bob, you mentioned that you might have a hearing loss because of all that noise exposure during construction work? Well, it looks like you were right." "Well Mrs. Smith, you mentioned that you were having trouble understanding your grandchildren. This testing clearly explains why you have that problem."

Informational Counseling. When we sit down with our patients following the initial audiologic testing, we typically explain the test results. This is something that

---

KEY CONCEPT: ABOUT PATIENT CARE

Dr. Francis Peabody was a well-known pioneer in the area of internal medicine. At the age of 45, he became seriously and incurably ill. His final talk was titled "Care of the Patient," in which he stated the now famous dictum, "the secret of the care of the patient is in caring for the patient."

Table 3–7. Habit #4: Invest in the End

Deliver diagnostic information	• Describe the test results in a way that relate back to the patient's concerns: "You were right, you do have problems understanding speech when background noise is present."
	• Test to determine if patient is understanding your comments.
Provide education	• Explain why you did each test.
	• Explain prognosis: "This is a permanent hearing loss and it is unlikely it will improve." "Your hearing loss will likely gradually become worse due to the natural aging process."
	• Provide written materials of support.
Involve patient in making decisions	• Discuss treatment goals: "I believe you will receive significant benefit from the use of hearing aids. We can start the process today if you like."
	• Listen to the patient's preference.
	• Set limits respectively. "It's certainly possible that your friend's hearing was helped by surgery, but you don't have that type of hearing loss. The use of hearing aids is the only treatment."
	• Assess the patient's ability and motivation to carry out the treatment plan.
Complete the visit	• Ask the patient for additional questions?
	• Assess satisfaction: "Is there anything more about your hearing loss or the use of hearing aids that you would like to know?"
	• Reassure the patient of follow-up care.

in general audiologists enjoy doing, almost to a fault. This process is referred to as *informational counseling*. Bob Margolis (2004b) has written on this topic, and here are some tips that he provides:

- Present the most important information first.
- Patients are best at remembering the first thing you tell them.
- Give advice in the form of concrete instructions.
- Use easy-to-understand language such as short words and sentences.
- Repeat the most important information.
- Stress the importance of recommendations or other information that you want the patient to remember.
- Ask for questions and confirm the patient understands before moving on to the next category.
- Don't present too much information.
- Present only the information that is important for the patient to remember.
- Supplement verbal information with written, graphic, and pictorial materials that the patient can take home.
- Plan on going slower and spending more time with older individuals who may have cognitive problems.
- Again, repeat the most important information.

Involving Patients in Decision Making

Patient involvement in the decision-making process is important for all types of treatment, including the fitting of hearing aids. As we discuss in the preceding section, it is first important that the patient understands your explanation of the problem. With a typical patient with a presbycusic-type hearing loss, it is counterproductive to rush into the ordering of hearing aids only to have the patient call you the next day to ask about what surgery options are available. Checking comprehension of your informational counseling is important. Once this has been established, proceed with presenting the treatment plan. The model of Frankel and Stein is primarily geared

> **POINTS TO PONDER: WHAT IS REALLY REMEMBERED?**
>
> We all have sat down with a patient and provided a detailed description of our test findings, how this relates to ear anatomy and real-world speech communication, and what treatment strategies are needed, such as the use of hearing aids. At the end of our little spiel, we maybe even pat ourselves on the back for doing such a thorough job. Here are a few points to ponder (from Margolis, 2004a):
>
> - About 50% of the information presented to a patient is forgotten immediately.
> - About 50% of the information that the patient *does* remember, is incorrect.
> - One large study reported that 68% of the patients could not remember the diagnoses that were told to them.
> - In another study, the patient and their physician agreed on what needed follow-up only 45% of the time.

toward medical treatment plans, and we recognize that some modifications may need to be made when the sale of hearing aids is involved (see our earlier discussion regarding the barriers to obtaining hearing aids). The basic principles of the model that they outline still apply, however:

- Provide a clear rationale. Let the patient know why the fitting of hearing aids is the best option. Explain why other treatment options do not apply to them. Use graphics to help explain your plan (see Chapter 5) and take-home, written material to supplement your statements and help them remember.
- Explore potential barriers to implementation. After providing a clear rationale for the plan, check with the patient to determine what barriers might exist. You could ask a question such as: "What might prevent you from purchasing hearing aids?"
- Provide support. Explain to the patient the complete fitting process, pointing out that the two of you will work as a team to assure that optimum benefit is achieved. Acknowledge that this is an important decision, but also remind the patient of the potential benefits of amplification discussed earlier in this chapter. Investing in the end ensures the patient that a partnership exists.

As summarized by Frankel and Stein (1999), the Four Habits Model blends the logic of clinical decision making with the logic of social interaction. With hope, this leads to successful relationships with your patients, which often determines the successfulness of the treatment—in our case, obtaining benefit with and satisfaction from the use of hearing aids. It often has been stated that the fitting of hearing aids is both an art and a science. In the following chapters, we focus mostly on the science, but you'll find the science works much better by understanding and implementing the concepts discussed here.

In Closing

As we have reviewed, understanding the hearing aid candidate goes far beyond evaluating his or her pure-tone thresholds and speech recognition scores. We know that the majority of individuals who need hearing aids do not obtain them. And sadly, 5 to 10% of people who own hearing aids never use them. Why is this? Certainly the stigmatization of hearing loss and hearing aid use is one reason. Younger individuals must have a much greater hearing loss than older individuals before they will adopt hearing aid use. And, surveys have shown that, even with the new technology available, many of the expected benefits with amplification are not present.

On the positive side, satisfaction with hearing aids continues to increase. Most notably, there has been a 20% increase in the number of patients who are satisfied with their hearing aid's performance while listening in background noise. Recent surveys also have shown that the use of hearing aids significantly improves many quality of life issues, with 50% of wearers reporting improvement for *feelings about myself* and *life overall*.

We must recognize that the patient brings many concerns and feelings to the prefitting appointment. How we deal with this can impact the overall fitting process. By listening to the patient's story, using motivational interviewing, and following some of the guidelines of the Four Habits Model, we can better understand our patients and prepare them for the use of hearing aids. It is then our job to select the right technology, fit it correctly, and conduct appropriate postfitting follow-up and counseling—all things we address in future chapters.

4
Speech Acoustics

As we discussed in the preceding chapter, there are a large number of factors that are important when assessing and understanding the patient and hearing aid candidacy. As we describe in the following chapters, there also are a series of audiologic tests, both behavioral and self-assessment, that play an important role in the overall fitting protocol. The most common reason patients seek help, however, is because of difficulties in hearing and recognizing speech. There are many variables to consider for speech recognition, but as stated eloquently by Pascoe (1980), detecting sound is the first imperative:

> Although it is true that the mere detection of sound does not insure its recognition, it is even more true that without detection the probabilities of recognition are greatly diminished.

Given the importance of speech recognition to patients and the importance of audibility to speech recognition, it is not surprising that improving speech audibility is the core goal of most hearing aid fittings. One characteristic that is shared by all hearing aids is that they are able to increase sound level. Modern hearing aids affect sound level in sophisticated ways, however. That is, they can provide more amplification at some input levels than at others, provide less amplification for some types of sounds than others (like noise), and provide this variable amplification differently for different frequency bands. Given the importance of speech recognition and the potential complexity of modern amplification schemes, it is important to examine how audibility and speech recognition are related. For example, do all parts of the speech signal have to be audible for maximum speech recognition? Are all speech frequencies equally important to speech recognition?

To lay the foundation for examining the potential effect hearing aid amplification processing can have, which we do later in this book, we spend considerable space in this chapter defining speech in terms of its level and the frequency regions of importance. Then, the impact of the environments in which speech is produced on speech recognition is discussed. With the information presented in this chapter as a foundation, one can then form a better understanding about how hearing aid processing might interact with audibility and room acoustics, giving us a good chance of forming realistic expectations related to hearing aid benefit for current, as well as future, processing strategies. As you will see in later chapters, we introduce tests to illustrate how individual patients handle speech communication both in quiet and in background noise.

Long-Term Speech Acoustics

Before considering speech audibility and importance functions, it is first relevant to quantify speech acoustically. Most often speech is described in static terms (overall level, overall frequency shape, etc.). By static we mean that a single number representing an average value over time is used rather than representing the signal moment by moment. For example, even though the level of speech naturally fluctuates over time, it is common to examine the level across frequency (spectrum of speech) after averaging over some predefined segment (e.g., an entire passage). Graphic plots of these data are referred to as a Long-Term Average Speech Spectrum (LTASS). The LTASS representation is particularly useful because it can be used to quantify the relationship between speech levels and hearing thresholds, giving us a specific indication of audibility for a given patient. By comparing audibility with and without a hearing aid, we can directly demonstrate the degree that a specific hearing aid fitting changes audibility for an individual listener. An LTASS is usually defined by the vocal effort required for its production rather than being based on the perceived sound level (Pavlovic, 1989; Pearsons, Bennett, & Fidell, 1977). That is, rather than asking listeners to turn the level of a recorded talker up and down until the speech signal is rated "soft," talkers are asked to speak softly, and the level is measured at a predefined distance, typically one meter.

The specific test conditions and instructions matter as well. For example, a talker may be asked to speak at a conversational level, and their vocal output is measured at a distance of one meter. Work that is often referenced in this area is that of Pearsons et al. (1977). Table 4–1 is a summary of their mean speech levels in A-weighed decibels (dBA) for casual, normal, raised, and shouted speech for males, females, and children.

The listener also has an effect on the LTASS, presumably because people talk louder if they know a listener has a hearing loss. For instance, estimates place the overall level of normal conversational speech measured at one meter at 70 dB SPL when the listener has impaired hearing; however, when the listener has normal hearing,

> **TECHNICAL TIP: THREE FACTORS FOR QUANTIFYING SPEECH ACOUSTICS**
>
> - Level at each frequency and overall level for various vocal effort levels (e.g., soft, casual, raised, shouted)
> - Dynamic range for a single vocal effort level (i.e., range of levels from lowest to highest portions of speech at specified frequencies, often referred to as the "banana")
> - Level change over time (sometimes described by how quickly level changes from segment to segment—amplitude modulation rate—and how much level change occurs—amplitude modulation depth).

Table 4–1. Mean speech levels in dBA and unweighted sound pressure levels for casual, normal, raised, loud, and shouted speech by males, females, and children in an anechoic chamber. Unweighted sound pressure levels in [ ]. Standard deviations in ( ).

	Casual	Normal	Raised	Loud	Shouted
Females	50[54] (4)	55[58] (4)	63[65] (4)	71[72] (6)	82[82] (7)
Males	52[56] (4)	58[61] (4)	65[68] (5)	76[77] (6)	89[89] (7)
Children	53[56] (5)	58[61] (5)	65[67] (7)	74[75] (9)	82[82] (9)

Note. All values are rounded to the nearest dB.
Source: From Table 1 and Figure 16, 17, and 18 in Pearsons et al. (1977).

> ## THINGS TO REMEMBER: SPEECH LEVELS
>
> - Soft vocal effort results in speech that has an overall level of approximately 53 dB SPL.
> - Conversational vocal effort results in speech that has an overall level of approximately 62 dB SPL.
> - Shouted vocal effort results in speech that has an overall level of approximately 83 dB SPL.
> - There is a lot of variability across talkers. Shouted speech might be 72 dB SPL for one talker and 85 dB SPL for another. On average, there are also gender differences; the intensity levels produced by males are about 7 dB higher than those of females.
> - Note that these all are *SPL values*. They correspond to approximately 40, 50, and 70 dB HL, for soft, conversational, and shouted levels when presented through headphones from an audiometer.

> ## KEY CONCEPT: PROBE MICROPHONE TESTING
>
> Let us go back to the clinic for a moment. The importance of the speech spectrum becomes clear in our probe microphone verification of hearing aid fittings—a technique often referred to as *speech mapping*, which we discuss in Chapters 16 and 17. This testing approach has increased the awareness of the LTASS and the effects of LTASS amplification among clinicians. Hearing aid verification methods have long used test signals that are intended to mimic some of the properties of speech. Early probe microphone systems used swept pure tones or noise that was shaped (filtered) to mimic an LTASS. In more recent probe microphone testing systems, however, we have seen the introduction of test signals that are generated to include both the spectral and temporal modulation properties of speech. Such samples include International Collegium of Rehabilitative Audiology (ICRA) signals, samples of real speech, samples of real speech signals that are shaped to some agreed-upon standard LTASS, and a real speech signal that is spliced together from a variety of speech signals that differ in terms of talker and language, such as the International Speech Test Signal (ISTS).

the overall level decreased to approximately 63 dB SPL (Stelmachowicz, Mace, Kopun, & Carney, 1993).

As implied, a typical LTASS is an average of many spectra. Although some LTASS can reflect an average of many similar talkers, those applied in some hearing aid test equipment also reflect gender, age, and other conditions. Figure 4–1 shows the effect of talker gender and age on the LTASS at a single vocal effort level. Other factors, such as the inclusion of one or many languages and the type of speech material, are also important when defining an LTASS (Pavlovic, 1989, Byrne et al, 1994). One choice relates to whether speech material is chosen that is phonemically balanced (uses all phonemes in a language equally) or, more commonly, phonetically balanced (the phonemes in a language are represented using the same proportion for which they occur in usual speech). There are many common phonetically balanced passages in use. The most commonly

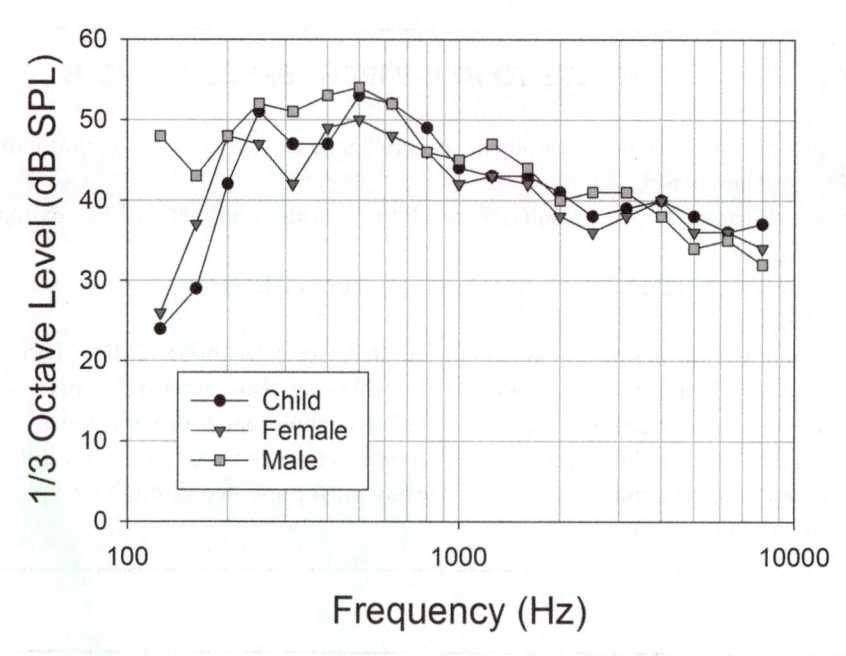

Figure 4–1. Example of LTASS measured for adult male, adult female, and child talkers speaking with average vocal effort. (Adapted from Pearsons et al., 1977.)

referred to being the *Rainbow Passage* and the shortest recognized passage is about a shoe bench. (See related Points-to-Ponder.)

Differences Across LTASS

Different LTASS will be measured depending on the conditions chosen. That is, there is not just one LTASS, even for the same vocal effort level. On the surface, it might appear that this fact would make it difficult to measure speech recognition clinically. Fortunately, standards organizations work to reach a consensus on measurement procedures and on which measurements will be accepted. Two common such organizations are the American National Standards Institute (ANSI), which was initially formed in 1907, although it was not reorganized into its current form until 1969, and the International Electrotechnical Commission (IEC), which was formed in 1904.

Even though there are many LTASS samples, the spectra across studies and over a wide range of different populations do have some similarities. The characteristic pattern for average vocal effort reveals a peak around 500 Hz and a spectral slope (drop in level across frequency) of about 9 dB per octave (e.g., ANSI S3.5-1997; Dreschler, Verschuure, Ludvigsen, & Westerman, 2001; Pavlovic, 1989; Pavlovic & Studebaker, 1984). It is assumed that the spectral peak corresponds to approximately the frequency of the first formants. The shape is also affected by vocal effort; the spectral slope is slightly steeper for soft speech and becomes flatter as speech level increases as shown in Figure 4–2 (see the Key Concept on this topic for description of why this figure is different from Figure 4–1). The frequency of the spectral peak also is higher for shouted speech than lower vocal effort levels. In fact, if you record shouted speech and play it at the same level as soft speech, one of the most striking (and perhaps surprising) features is that the shouted speech has a higher apparent pitch. Finally, the shape of the LTASS can be affected by the language spoken (Byrne et al., 1994), although those frequency and intensity differences have been deemed fairly insignificant in the fitting of hearing aids.

The spectral levels in Figure 4–2 are based on ANSI S3.5-1997 (average and shouted vocal efforts) and Pearsons et al. (1977; Soft speech).

> **POINTS TO PONDER: RAINBOW PASSAGE AND THE SHORTEST PHONETICALLY BALANCED PASSAGE**
>
> ■ **Rainbow Passage:** When the sunlight strikes raindrops in the air, they act as a prism and form a rainbow. The rainbow is a division of white light into many beautiful colors. These take the shape of a long round arch, with its path high above, and its two ends apparently beyond the horizon. There is, according to legend, a boiling pot of gold at one end. People look, but no one ever finds it. When a man looks for something beyond his reach, his friends say he is looking for the pot of gold at the end of the rainbow. Throughout the centuries, people have explained the rainbow in various ways. Some have accepted it as a miracle without physical explanation. To the Hebrews, it was a token that there would be no more universal floods. The Greeks used to imagine that it was a sign from the gods to foretell war or heavy rain. The Norsemen considered the rainbow as a bridge over which the gods passed from earth to their home in the sky. Others have tried to explain the phenomenon physically. Aristotle thought that the rainbow was caused by reflection of the sun's rays by the rain. Since then, physicists have found that it is not reflection, but refraction by the raindrops which causes the rainbows. Many complicated ideas about the rainbow have been formed. The difference in the rainbow depends considerably on the size of the drops, and the width of the colored band increases as the size of the drops increases. The actual primary rainbow observed is said to be the effect of superimposition of a number of bows. If the red of the second bow falls upon the green of the first, the result is to give a bow with an abnormally wide yellow band, since red and green light, when mixed, form yellow. This is a very common type of bow, one showing mainly red and yellow, with little or no green or blue.
> ■ **Shortest Balanced Passage:** "Joe took father's shoe bench out; she was waiting at my lawn."

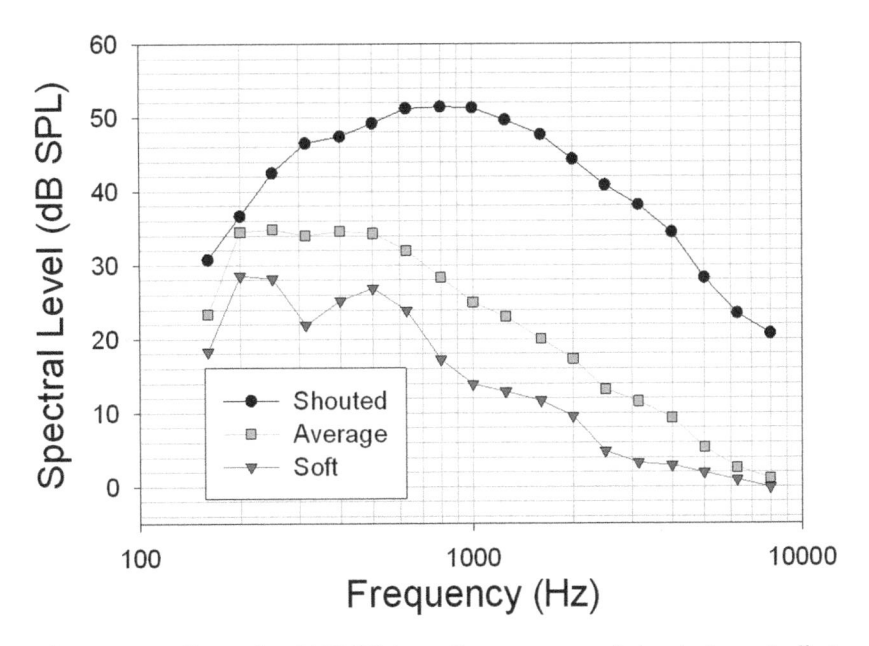

Figure 4–2. Example of LTASS for soft, average, and shouted vocal effort levels. (Adapted from Pearsons et al., 1977 and ANSI S3.5-1997.)

> ### TECHNICAL TIP: THE LTASS AND PRESCRIPTIVE FITTING APPROACHES
>
> Although similar, there are several different speech spectra used in clinical audiology and the fitting of hearing aids. One example relates to the development and verification of prescriptive fitting algorithms, which we discuss in detail in Chapter 14. Currently there are two primary fitting algorithms in use: the National Acoustic Laboratories Non-Linear version 2 (NAL-NL2) and the Desired Sensation Level version 5.0a (DSL v5.0a).
>
> - NAL-NL2: The development of the NAL-NL1 and NL2 algorithms has been based on the assumed input signal represented by the one-third-octave levels of the International Long-Term Average Speech Spectrum (ILTASS) published by Byrne et al. (1994).
> - DSL v5.0a: The evolution of the DSL fitting scheme has focused on placement of third octave speech levels at a desired sensation level for a given hearing loss. The actual values for that speech are an average of male/female/child recordings of speech obtained 30 cm in front of the talker and recordings taken at ear level of the child.

Dynamics of Speech

Directly related to the LTASS is the dynamic range of speech. The dynamic range of speech at any frequency refers to the difference between the lowest level (speech minima) and highest level (speech maxima). Typically, instead of actually defining the dynamic range with regard to the absolute highest and lowest level segments, some percentage of total energy is often used. For example, the maxima might be defined as the level at which 90% of the speech energy falls below and the minima might be defined as the level for which 10% of energy falls below (i.e., the 10% to 90% dynamic range). Differences between reported values for the dynamic range of speech in the research literature also reflect differences in experimental variables like frequency range and the length of sampling interval (e.g., Pavlovic, 1987, 1989). Specifically, the shorter the sampling interval, the larger the dynamic range. If we average the intensity level of speech over 500 ms blocks of time, there will be a significantly narrower range than if we average over 1ms blocks of time. This is because averaging acts to smooth out some of the very short-term peaks and valleys in the speech signal.

Why a 30 dB Dynamic Range?

Choosing the appropriate interval duration is not straightforward because it is of interest to reflect a segment length that is perceptually relevant. That is, the dynamic range of speech is not quantified for purely acoustic reasons; rather, we want to define a range that represents what a listener perceives so that we can estimate audibility.

Most commonly, a dynamic range of 30 dB is advocated for making predictions of speech recognition, although more recent data suggest a dynamic range of greater than 30 dB must be available to optimize speech recognition for all listeners across all conditions. Therefore, we believe that 30 dB should be considered a somewhat conservative estimate of the dynamic range of speech. Data also suggest that the 30 dB dynamic range is not symmetric around the LTASS; rather, it may be best represented as LTASS +12 and −18 dB for the speech maxima and minima, respectively (Pavlovic, 1989). These issues are primarily still research considerations, however, and it is common to assume a dynamic range of 30 dB that is symmetric around the LTASS. Although perhaps not 100% accurate, this

> **KEY CONCEPT: BAND-LEVEL ACOUSTICS**
>
> - You may remember from acoustics that, although the level of a signal is most commonly expressed in total level (that is considering all frequencies present and often referred to as *overall* level), we can also describe the sound level of the same signal in a more frequency-specific manner. That is, we can describe the level measured within a particular bandwidth.
> - In the specific cases of Figures 4–1 and 4–2, the level in each one-third-octave wide band and one-hertz wide band (spectral level) are given, respectively. This is why the two figures appear at first glance to be so different in level. The relative effect that measurement bandwidth has on level values is demonstrated in Table 4–2.
> - It is very common to use one-third-octave band level representations of speech when verifying hearing aid targets, particularly when using "speech mapping" techniques, as we describe in Chapters 16 and 17. This is in part due to the fact that calculations of output targets for the modern prescriptive methods described in Chapter 14 are based on one-third-octave speech level inputs.
> - The following two formulas can be used to move between the levels of relatively narrow and wide measurement bandwidths:
>
> Level of Wider Bandwidth (dB SPL) = Level of Narrower Bandwidth + 10 log [Wider Bandwidth (Hz)/Narrower Bandwidth (Hz)]
>
> Level of Narrower Bandwidth (dB SPL) = Level of Wider Bandwidth − 10 log [Wider Bandwidth (Hz)/Narrower Bandwidth (Hz)]

> **TECHNICAL TIP: CONSIDERING A PERPETUALLY RELEVANT DYNAMIC RANGE**
>
> - Let us assume that the acoustic dynamic range of speech for a single talker is measured to be 50 dB using a very small time averaging window.
> - If listeners only require 30 dB of this range (e.g., the 40 to 90% dynamic range) to optimize speech recognition, no matter what the listening condition, one could argue that the remaining 20 dB of this range (which is composed of very short-term maxima and lower level and short-term minima in the speech signal) is not perceptually relevant.

simpler explanation is considered accurate enough for most uses. Clinically however, the 30 dB dynamic range really only encompasses a single vocal effort; if we want to consider the dynamic range across a full range of vocal efforts, the range is much larger as we discuss in the next section. This is why we use a range of input levels in the hearing aid verification process (see Chapter 17).

Table 4–2. The LTASS level at octave frequencies for various vocal efforts as measured using spectral, 1/3 octave, and octave measurement bandwidths

Frequency	Bandwidth	Vocal Effort				
		Soft	Normal	Raised	Loud	Shouted
250	S. Level	—	34.75	38.98	41.55	42.50
	1/3 octave	48.00	52.38	56.61	59.18	60.13
	Octave	—	57.25	61.48	64.05	65.00
500	S. Level	—	34.27	40.15	44.85	49.24
	1/3 octave	50.00	54.88	60.76	65.46	69.85
	Octave	—	59.77	65.65	70.35	74.74
1000	S. Level	—	25.01	33.86	42.16	51.31
	1/3 octave	42.00	48.65	57.50	65.80	74.95
	Octave	—	53.52	62.37	70.67	79.82
2000	S. Level	—	17.32	25.32	34.39	44.32
	1/3 octave	40.00	43.96	51.96	61.03	70.96
	Octave	—	48.84	56.84	65.91	75.84
3000	S. Level	—	11.55	20.15	28.21	38.13
	1/3 octave	33.00	40.18	48.78	56.84	66.76
	Octave	—	—	—	—	—
4000	S. Level	—	9.33	16.78	25.41	34.41
	1/3 octave	32.50	38.96	46.41	55.04	64.04
	Octave	—	43.86	51.31	59.94	68.94

Source: Adapted from ANSI S3.5, 1997

Audibility and Speech Recognition

Although there is a movement to switch to an SPL representation of both hearing loss and the speech spectrum level when discussing hearing aids, it is still common to describe the patient's thresholds in dB HL (decibels hearing level) in the clinic. Because this is so common, the dynamic range of speech for the average vocal effort LTASS shown in Figure 4–2 often has been replotted in dB HL (see Figure 4–3 for example). This dynamic range is shown along with an example hearing loss to demonstrate how hearing loss can impact audibility of speech that was produced at an average vocal effort. When plotted in this way, which is similar to an audiogram, speech that falls below the hearing threshold (*above* the threshold line in this figure) is not audible; speech below the plotted audiogram is audible. In this example, showing speech produced with average vocal effort, no speech sounds above 1500 Hz would be audible to the patient. In Chapter 5, we provide several other examples of using the LTASS and the audiogram, and discuss how this association can be used for patient counseling and illustration of the benefits of amplification.

As we mentioned earlier, the commonly used 30 dB dynamic range of speech shown in Figure 4–3 only applies to a single vocal effort level. To provide you with an idea of the *total dynamic range* of speech for a wide range of vocal efforts, the dynamic range from the minima for soft speech to the maxima for shouted speech, expressed in HL, are shown in Figure 4–4. These data suggest that a reasonable clinical estimate of the

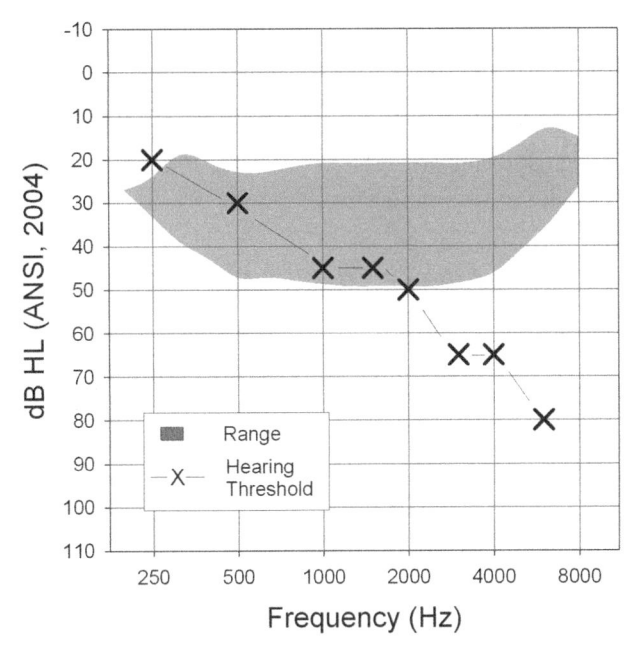

Figure 4–3. An example of speech audibility for the average vocal effort levels in a patient with a sloping hearing loss configuration.

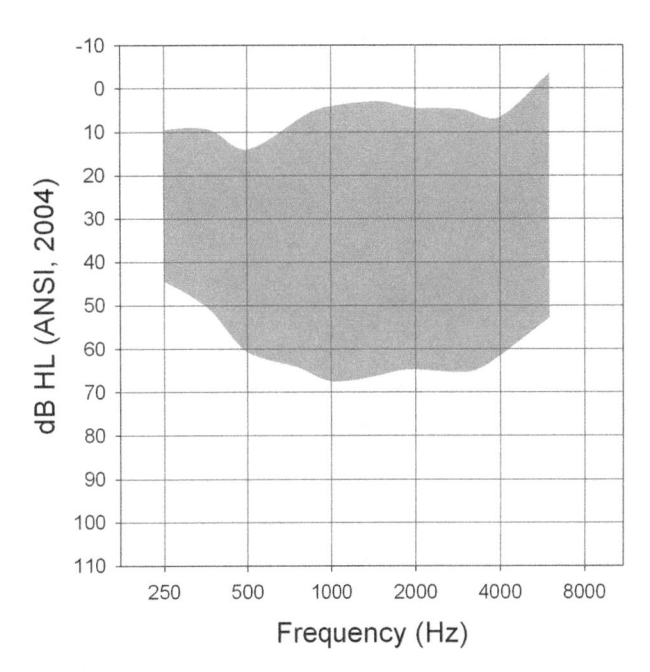

Figure 4–4. Conservative estimate of the full dynamic range of speech across a range of vocal efforts encompassing from the soft speech minima to the shouted speech maxima.

total dynamic range of speech is at least 60 dB. When accounting for individual differences in talkers, however, this range is likely more than 70 dB.

The Articulation Index/Audibility Index

Because speech levels and dynamic range have been quantified in so many studies, it is possible to calculate the audibility of speech under conditions of hearing loss and/or masking by a noise signal with a fairly high degree of accuracy. To do this as accurately as possible, we need frequency-specific hearing thresholds, thresholds of discomfort, any background noise levels, and the maxima and minima of the exact speech signal of interest. With this information, the audibility of speech at each frequency can be displayed as shown in Figure 4–3; however, rather than just knowing audibility, it is of interest to know how frequency-specific audibility translates into importance for speech recognition performance. Calculation of not just audibility, but importance-weighted audibility as well, is the explicit goal of what is referred to as the Articulation Index, or simply AI. These procedures, in one way or another, have been employed since the early 1900s, with the first detailed approach published by Fletcher and Galt (1950). Refer to Figure 4–5. ANSI standards have been developed regarding this measurement, including the current ANSI standard method, which is called the Speech Intelligibility Index (SII; ANSI S3.5-1997 [R2007]).

To examine how AI calculations might be conducted, let us start with an experiment in which we divide the entire dynamic range of speech into blocks. In this experiment, we decide to make the blocks 5 dB high and one-third octave wide. We could then present different combinations of these blocks by masking out other blocks with background noise and look at the corresponding speech recognition scores. Sounds like a really fun experiment does it not? Although such experiments might prove tedious for participants, they are a way to precisely quantify the relative importance of the speech signal in each frequency band (importance weightings) and can be plotted as Frequency Importance Functions (FIFs) or Band Importance Functions (BIFs).

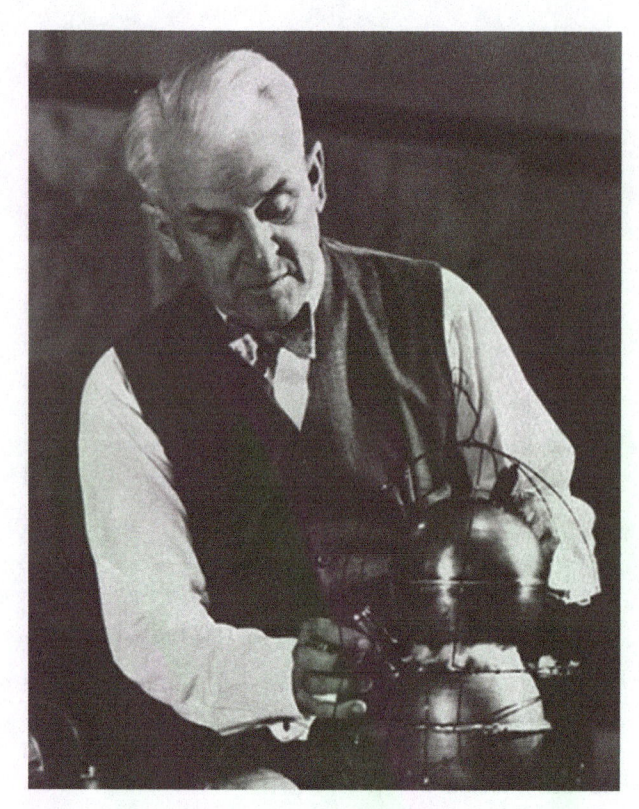

Figure 4–5. The individual most credited with developing the articulation index is Harvey Fletcher, based on his research at Bell Labs conducted over three decades, with the finely tuned version finally published in 1950. Dr. Fletcher is also known for his research relating to loudness scaling, equal loudness contours, loudness summation, and critical band theory. Dr. Fletcher was elected an honorary fellow of the Acoustical Society of America in 1949, the second person to receive this honor after Thomas Edison.

BIFs are usually plotted so that the total importance for all bands adds up to 1.00 (i.e., 100%). An example is shown in Figure 4–6. If we were to add up the frequency importance values on any one line in this figure, the total would always be 1.00 (that is, 100% of available speech deemed important).

Band Importance Functions

Band Importance Functions differ in shape depending on the exact speech material evaluated. However, there are some general patterns based on how much contextual information is present. When there is little context, as is the case with nonsense syllables (e.g., /ba/, /da/, and /ga/), the BIF usually peaks in the higher frequencies (around 2000 Hz to 3000 Hz). This is not that surprising when we consider what is needed for correct identification of nonsense syllables. To distinguish /si/ (see) from /ʃi/ (she), a listener must actually hear the difference in the high frequency consonant signals. Increasing the amount of context (i.e., moving from nonsense syllables to running speech) leads to a shift of importance toward the lower frequencies, as shown in Figure 4–6. This shift can be explained by the positive effect that context has on filling in missing information. For example, try reading aloud this target sentence:

"The children _oveled _and on the beach."

Most listeners can fill in the missing two speech sounds and realize the intention was, "The children shoveled sand on the beach." Actually *hearing* the soft high

---

TECHNICAL TIP: AI AND SII—SAME OR DIFFERENT?

One thing you may have noticed is that we have referred to AI as both the Articulation Index and Audibility Index, and referred to the ANSI standard method of the SII. Why are there so many terms? Articulation Index was the original term for these calculations but, as several authors have pointed out, these calculations are really based on audibility, even though they do use audibility importance weighted by frequency. We go into a more detailed explanation of this issue later in this chapter. To make a long story short, AI and SII have both been used to refer to general and specific procedures, whereas the SII is the current standard. Although there is certainly not complete consensus on the issue, we have chosen to use AI as a general term encompassing all procedures of this type and SII to refer to the current specific ANSI standard procedure.

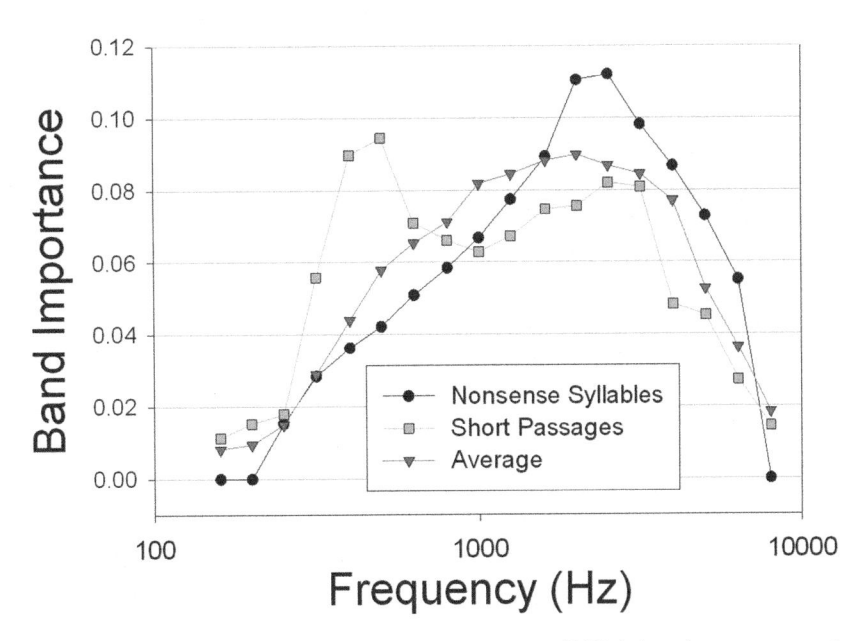

Figure 4–6. The band importance functions (BIFs) for three types of speech, which vary by the amount of contextual information. (Adapted from ANSI S3.5-1997.)

KEY CONCEPT: CALCULATING BAND IMPORTANCE FUNCTIONS

Let's take a very simple example and just divide speech into two parts or bands, frequencies above 3000 Hz and frequencies below 3000 Hz. That is, we will take a masking noise and cover up all speech energy above 3000 Hz (3000 down) and then cover up all speech energy below 3000 Hz (3000 up) and test speech recognition.

- Depending on the speech material, we would expect that speech recognition scores might be about 100% for the 3000 down condition and about 40% for the 3000 up condition.
- By doing more testing and a little math, we might conclude (in this example) that 80% of speech importance falls below 3000 Hz and about 20% falls above 3000 Hz. This corresponds to BIF weightings of 0.8 and 0.2 for our two tested frequency bands.
- Note that you cannot simply add up the scores from the two conditions because the entire speech signal does not need to be present to obtain 100% correct because of context and redundancy. Listeners with normal hearing only need to have about 40% of the total available weighted important speech energy to obtain 100% correct when listening to sentences.
- This type of work first started in Bell Labs in the 1920s and 1930s (as described, for example, by French & Steinberg, 1947, and Fletcher & Galt, 1950). The Bell laboratory work identified the bandwidth of 300 Hz to 3000 Hz as providing enough speech information for listeners to generally understand all words, and this bandwidth is still used today in many telecommunication systems.

frequency consonants is therefore less important when you have context to help fill in the blanks.

For calculation of an AI, the audibility of each of the BIFs is examined in order to derive a single number that reflects importance weighted audibility. Specifically, once the importance of various frequency bands for speech (BIFs) is known, the band audibility (BA), or how much of each of these frequency bands is audible, can be calculated based on the 30 dB speech dynamic range. To keep things simple, audibility is also calculated as a portion of the whole. In other words, if 100% of speech is audible in a frequency band (the full 30 dB dynamic range), audibility in that band is 1.00.

If masking noise and/or a hearing loss is present, the full 30 dB dynamic range may not be audible. For example, if only 20 dB of the full 30 dB dynamic range is audible, then the BA would be calculated as: 20/30 = 0.66. Once audibility is measured and band audibility is calculated in each frequency band, the BA is multiplied by that frequency band's BIF, and the resulting product in each band is summed over all the bands. This is described mathematically in the following formula:

$$AI = \sum_{i=0}^{n} (BIF \times BA)$$

Frequency Bands for AI

The number of frequency bands used in the calculation of AI depends on the procedure and the chosen bandwidth (ANSI S3.5-1997; Mueller & Killion, 1990; Pavlovic, 1984; Pavlovic & Studebaker, 1984). Specifically, common procedures currently divide up the frequency range of speech using from 4 to 21 bands. The smaller the bandwidth and larger the number of bands, the greater the calculation accuracy, but obviously the calculation and measurement become more time-consuming as more bands are added. For this reason, some procedures have sacrificed precise accuracy (approximately 2 to 3%) to provide a procedure that is easy to use and understand and is clinically friendly (Mueller & Killion, 1990; Pavlovic, 1991). We discuss this clinical application later and in more detail in Chapter 5.

The narrowest bandwidth used is termed the *critical bandwidth*. The critical bandwidth refers to the assumed bandwidth of the human auditory filters. That is, the total level of any and all signals within the critical bandwidth are integrated over the entire bandwidth and perceived as a single level. Therefore, it is usually assumed that bandwidths smaller than the critical bandwidth are not perceptually relevant because,

---

KEY CONCEPT: IMPORTANT AI CONSIDERATIONS

There are many AI derivations that are not perfectly equivalent across test conditions. We explain some of those factors here.

- The AI is not a direct predictor of speech recognition. To improve prediction accuracy, the appropriate band importance function derived specifically for the speech material of interest must be used, and a second formula (specific AI/SII to percent correct transfer function) must also be applied. A commonly used chart for this purpose is based on data from Davis and Silverman (1960) and displayed in Figure 4–7. Even when these steps are taken, prediction of speech recognition performance will only be accurate on average. Clinically, however, these measures can be used to predict expected changes in scores due to amplification, noise, or other changes in audibility within an individual listener.
- The AI was developed for listeners with normal hearing. That said, it is often effectively applied to those with hearing loss. To improve accuracy for groups of listeners with hearing impairment, hearing loss desensitization (HLD) and level distortion (LD) factors are sometimes applied.
- HLDs are applied because of evidence that speech recognition decreases with increasing hearing loss, even when audibility is accounted for. Originally it was called the *Speech Desensitization* factor (Pavlovic, Studebaker, & Sherbecoe, 1986), and was a single

multiplier based on averaged thresholds and then applied to the total AI value. Although HLDs assume that performance decrements are directly related to the magnitude of loss, they do not specify what factors are responsible for the deficit (sort of a catch-all correction based on degree of loss). There currently is disagreement with respect to how HLDs should be applied and whether frequency specific corrections may be needed (Ching, Dillon, & Byrne, 1998; Ching, Dillon, Katsch, & Byrne, 2001; Hornsby and Ricketts, 2003, 2006; Humes, 2002). Accuracy can also be improved for all AIs by applying corrections for age and for language proficiency.

- LD factors are applied because data clearly demonstrate that speech recognition performance decreases when speech is presented at very high levels, especially near the threshold of discomfort. In the SII standard, the LD factor is a simple multiplier based on the speech level in each frequency band.
- Instead of using simple band audibility to estimate audibility when calculating an SII, modulation transfer function techniques (described later in this chapter when discussing the Speech Transmission Index) can be used to estimate signal-to-noise ratio to better account for the effects of room acoustics on speech recognition.

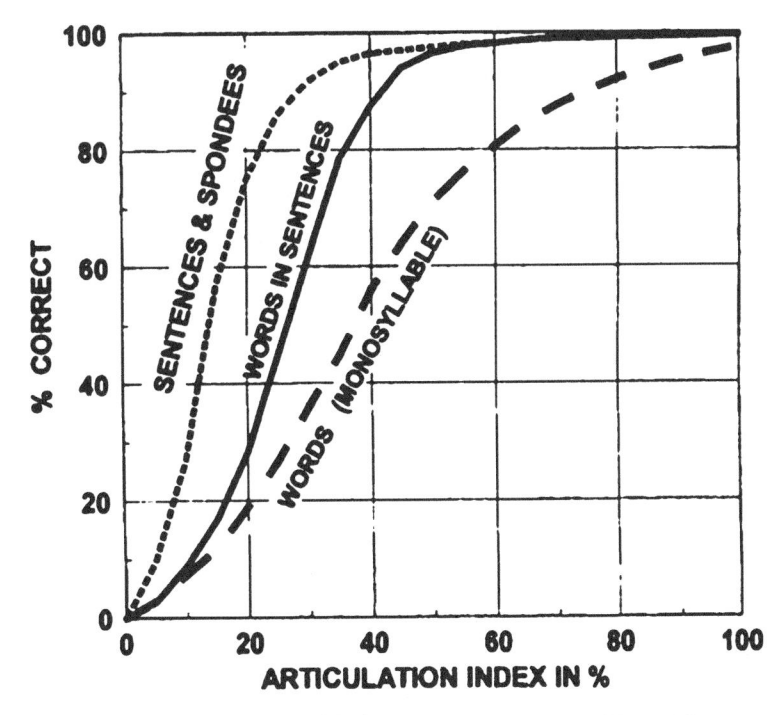

Figure 4–7. The relationship between an *average* AI and the percent correct for a variety of speech materials. (Adapted from data presented by Davis and Silverman, 1960.)

perceptually, sounds within the critical bandwidth are grouped together. Although a complete description of all of the factors affecting AI calculation are well beyond the scope of this chapter, AI can be of clinical utility provided that we keep several considerations in mind.

Short-Term Speech Acoustics

Although it is important to discuss the LTASS when considering speech audibility, it is clearly the case that speech level fluctuates over time. We can easily see this by looking at a plot of instantaneous speech amplitude as a function of time as shown in Figure 4–8. In case you are not familiar with this type of display (called a *time waveform*), we provide some background information that will help the interpretation.

Figure 4–8 is the time waveform of one sentence spoken by a male talker. A quick glance at this figure shows that there are segments of speech produced at fairly high levels (at the peak of 0.5 in this example) and other segments produced at much lower levels. Recall

---

TECHNICAL TIP: INTERPRETING TIME WAVEFORMS

- Figure 4–8 shows a common way to display sound using commercially available, computer-based, analysis software; the axis along the bottom (*x*-axis) displays time. In this case, time is shown in seconds, and observe that the entire sample is a little more than three seconds long.
- The axis along the side (*y*-axis) is relative amplitude. In this case, the scale is just in relative numbers, but in some software it is shown in relative dB. Relative amplitude measures like these start in the middle. That is, lower and higher signal levels will appear on the *y*-axis as having smaller and larger excursions, respectively. This is denoted by the brackets marked Lower Level and Higher Level.
- The highest level signal that can be displayed (0.5/−0.5 for a peak-to-peak amplitude of 1 in this example), commonly corresponds to the highest level that can be output by the computers sound card before physical limiting (clipping).
- The dynamic range of the computer sound card, that is the range from the lowest to highest level signals that can be output, will depend on the physical limitations of the sound card and theoretical limitations imposed by the number of bits used when sampling. The theoretical limit is 6 dB per bit, so a 16-bit sample will have a theoretical dynamic range of ($16 \times 6 = 96$ dB).

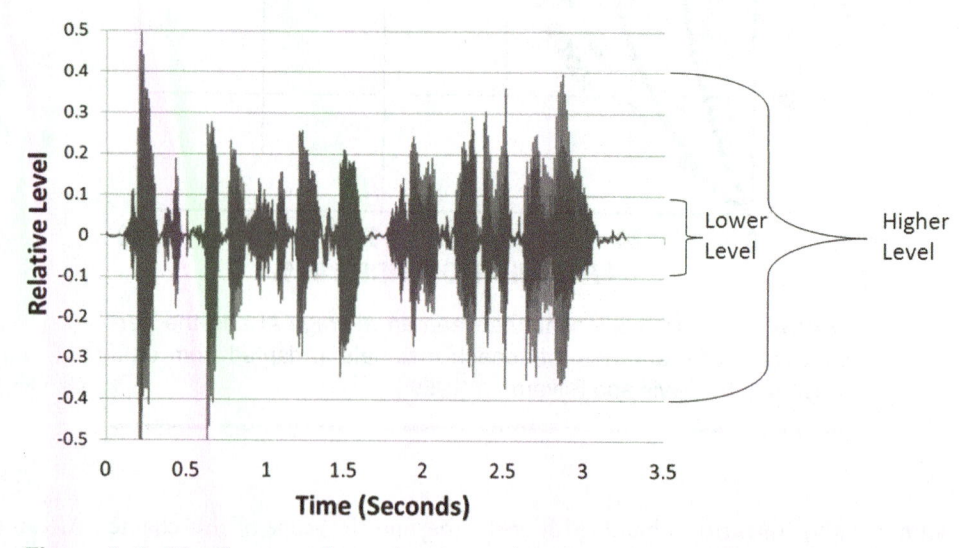

Figure 4–8. The time waveform of an approximately 3.2-second speech sample.

that we described this previously as the dynamic range of speech for a single talker at one vocal effort, which we said was around 30 dB. We can see from this recording that the simple explanation of a 30 dB dynamic range of speech is a little misleading, however, because not all levels are present at the same time. This is true even when we examine all frequencies at the same time as we are doing in this figure. If we look at this figure closely, we can see that the amplitude changes occur over different periods of time.

Looking at the Envelope

It is possible to visualize each syllable in Figure 4–8 by highlighting its general outline, commonly referred to as the syllable amplitude *envelope*, by using a bolded black line for the two-second speech sample. This is shown in Figure 4–9. By doing this, we can see a change in the level that corresponds to each syllable that occurs every 125 to 250 ms (0.125 to 0.25 seconds in Figure 4–9). In contrast, we could look as a much smaller time segment of speech. In Figure 4–10, we show a single word *she* that has a total duration of about 275 ms (0.275 seconds). In this case, we can see amplitude changes corresponding to individual phonemes that are much shorter, ranging from approximately 50 ms to 150 ms.

We can look at a variety of speech segments in this way and see a large range in duration both across and within each type of segment. Figure 4–11, adapted from data presented by Plomp (1986), gives an indication of the range of average durations associated with the amplitude changes within various segments of speech. It is important to note that the x-axis of this figure is on a logarithmic scale. With scaling in mind, we can see the duration of these amplitude changes ranges from about 33 ms, for the shortest phoneme transitions, to more than a few of seconds for sentences.

Instead of discussing the duration associated with amplitude changes within various speech segments, it is more typical to refer to these changes in level over time as amplitude modulations. For example, instead of describing level changes due to the duration of consonants as 50 ms in length, we describe the amplitude modulation associated with these consonant as occurring 20 times a second or, more simply, a modulation rate of 20 Hz (1000 ms [duration of 1 second]/50 ms [duration of level change associated with this consonant]). Using this convention, we can describe speech as having amplitude modulations ranging from about 30 Hz (e.g., 33.3 ms duration) for the shortest phonemes to less than 0.5 Hz (e.g., two-second duration) for some sentences.

In addition to the modulation rate, we can also describe speech in terms of its modulation depth; that

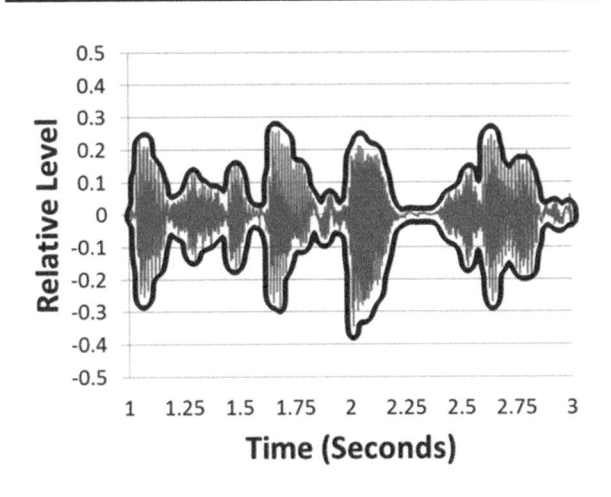

Figure 4–9. The time waveform of a 2-second speech sample. In this example, a bold black line is used to highlight the general amplitude envelope of individual syllables.

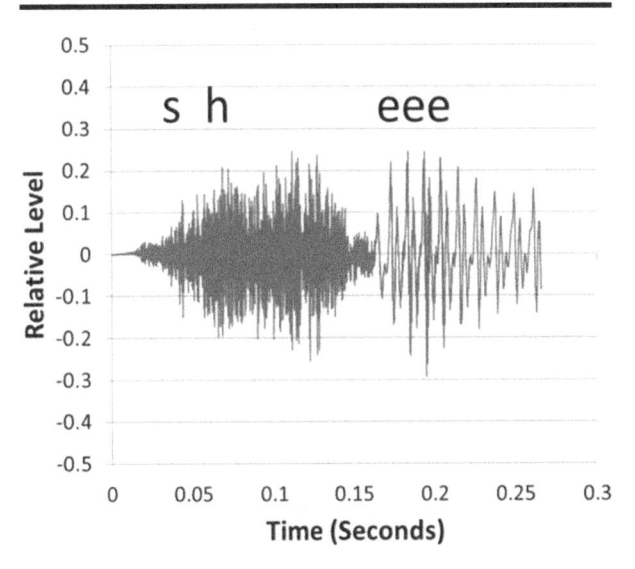

Figure 4–10. The time waveform of the spoken speech sample /shi/, *she*.

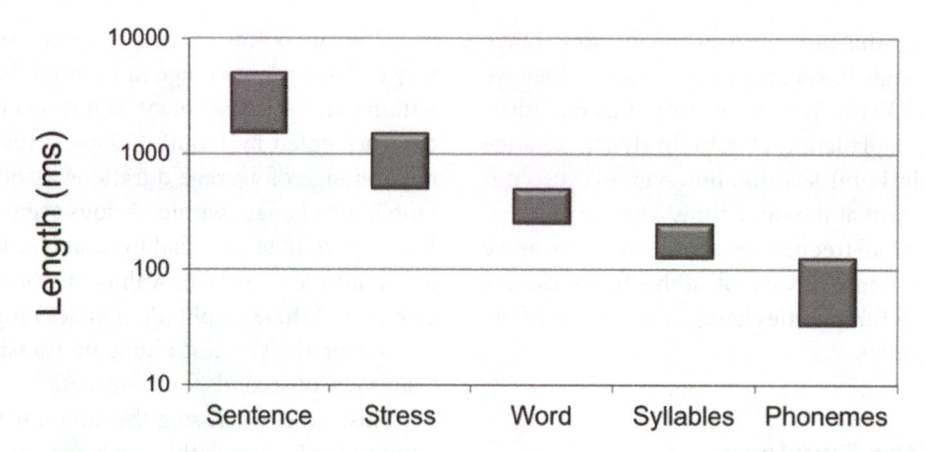

Figure 4–11. The range of average durations of various speech segments. These durations are associated with the amplitude changes within the segments of each type. (Adapted from Plomp, 1986.)

is, how large of a change in amplitude there is from the maxima of the signal to its minima. We have already discussed the assumption that the dynamic range of speech for a single vocal effort level is approximately 30 dB; therefore, this same value can be assigned to the modulation depth of speech. Putting all this information together, we can describe the majority of speech signals as amplitude modulated from approximately 0.5 Hz to more than 20 Hz with a modulation depth at each of those modulation frequencies of about 30 dB.

Practical Applications

You might be wondering why we are spending so much time discussing speech acoustics in a hearing aid textbook. Let us discuss a couple of specific examples of why this information is so important.

First, amplitude modulation information can be useful in hearing aid signal processing when attempting to identify speech. Today's hearing aids utilize a *signal classification system* in which an attempt is made to classify a signal as speech in quiet, speech in noise, broadband noise, music, and so forth. The results of this classification can then be used in controlling features such as digital noise reduction, directional technology, automatic compression learning, and so forth. Specifically, if the incoming signal is not amplitude modulated, or has a modulation rate higher than 30 Hz or so, we can be confident that it is *not* speech. Unfortunately, however, we are not assured that the signal is speech, just because it has a modulation rate in the range common to speech signals, but usually the classification system is correct if it is speech-in-quiet. We discuss other factors that are used when attempting to differentiate speech from other signals in Chapter 11.

A second, even more important reason for understanding the speech signal, relates to how the listening environment and hearing aid processing affect acoustics. For example, several factors related to hearing aid processing and the listening environment can affect the modulation depth of speech. What happens to the modulation depth when noise is added? Let us first look at this schematically. In Figure 4–12, an unmodulated noise that has a level that is well below that of speech has been added to the same speech signal displayed in Figure 4–8. We can see that the noise fills in the modulation valleys, so the lowest level portions of speech are masked by the noise. We can also see that this decrease in modulation depth occurs equally for all modulation rates. That is, there is not greater masking for high modulation rates than for low rates.

Effects of Reverberation

What about environmental factors other than noise? How might reverberation affect the modulation depth of speech? We can examine this question by playing the speech shown in Figure 4–8 in a reverberant room. The

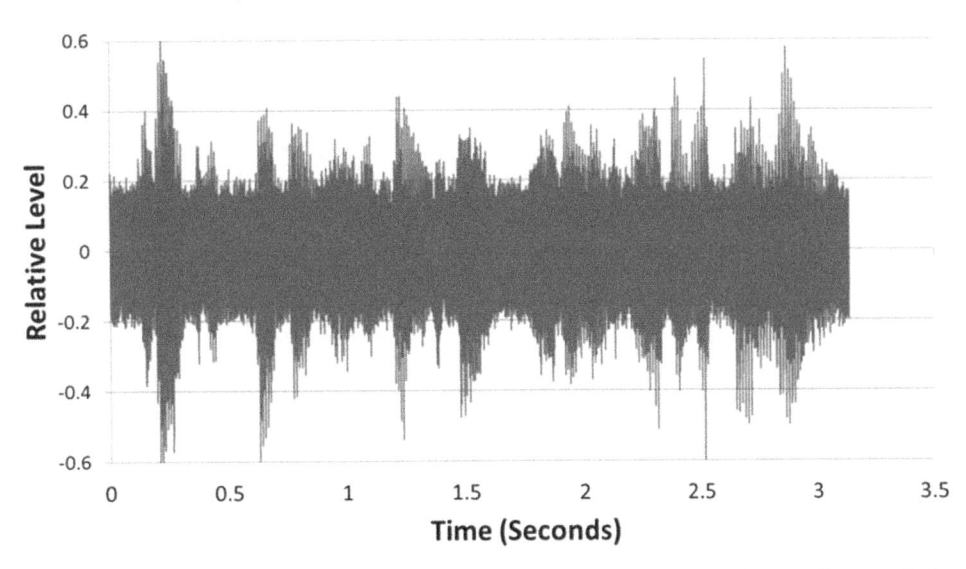

Figure 4–12. The time waveform of an approximately 3.2-second speech sample in background noise. The SNR is +3 dB.

KEY CONCEPT: SOME POINTS ON REVERBERATION

For the most part, we have been talking about speech signals delivered in ideal surroundings. We know, however, that our hearing aid patients will be out in reverberant conditions. In fact, it often is the poor understanding of speech in these difficult conditions that prompt the patient to obtain hearing aids. How does reverberation impact the speech signal?

- One of the most common measures of a room's effect on sound propagation is reverberation time. Commonly, reverberation time is defined as the time required for a signal to decrease in level by 60 dB after its offset (ANSI S1.1-1994).
- Reverberation occurs because sound generated from any source inside a room will be reflected (bounced) off room surfaces. Due to these reflections, there will be multiple angles of arrival for sound energy other than the angle of origin. That is, there will be a direct sound pathway (D) and several reflected sound pathways (R), which in combination are referred to as the reflective or reverberant sound field (Figure 4–13).
- There are usually many more reflected sound pathways than shown here, and some sound pathways may never reach the listener before they decay away (become so low level they are not heard).
- As the distance from the sound source increases, the level of the direct sound will decrease. According to the inverse square law, every doubling of distance will halve the intensity. In contrast, the reverberant sound level remains approximately constant (although this changes with proximity to reflective surfaces—for example, the reverberant level might go up near a wall). In consequence, as a sound source and a listener are separated in space, there is an increase in the reverberant to direct sound ratio. The distance at which the level of the direct signal is equal to that of the reverberant signal is referred to as the critical distance (Egan, 1988; Peutz, 1971). An example demonstrating direct sound, reverberant sound, and a combination of the two as a function of distance, is shown in Figure 4–14.

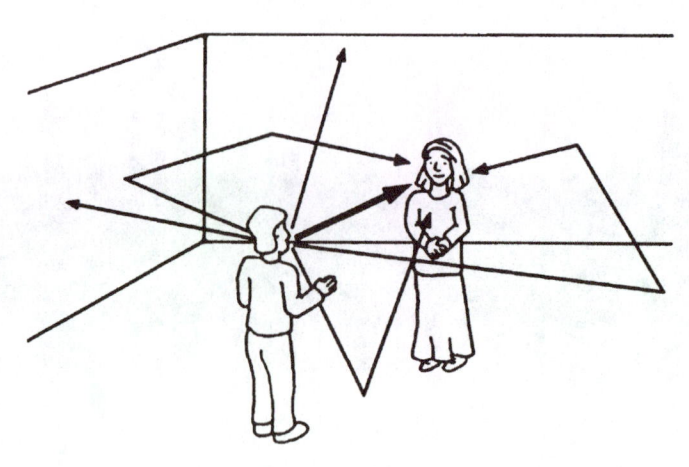

Figure 4–13. A representation of direct (*bold arrow*) and reflected (*thin arrows*) sound pathways, produced by a talker (illustrated by Wilder Boule).

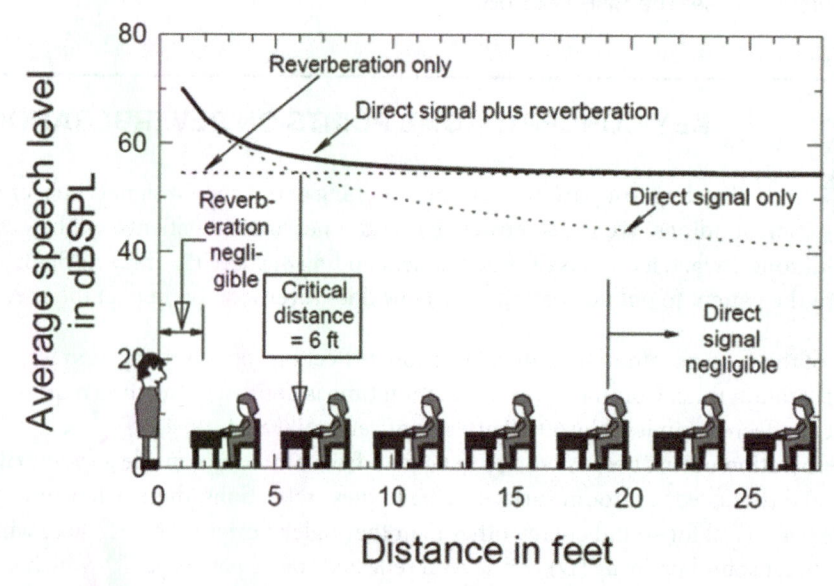

Figure 4–14. Predicted long-term average speech level as a function of the distance from the talker in a room measuring 30 × 20 × 9 feet with a reverberation time of 500 ms.

recording of this signal in a room with a high amount of reverberation (average reverberation time approximately four seconds) is shown in Figure 4–15. We can see that reverberation acts to fill in modulation depth somewhat similarly to noise as was shown in Figure 4–12. Further, the longer the reverberation time, the more the modulation depth is filled in. The effect is a little different from noise, however, because this masking is occurring because echoes from early portions of speech act to mask later portions (overlap masking) or echoes from a speech segment act to mask that same speech segment (speech self-masking). In consequence, shorter reverberation times or earlier reflections mainly fill in the modulation depth when the modulation rate is high. For lower modulation rates, the echoes may not last long enough to fill in the gaps. Therefore, we must exam-

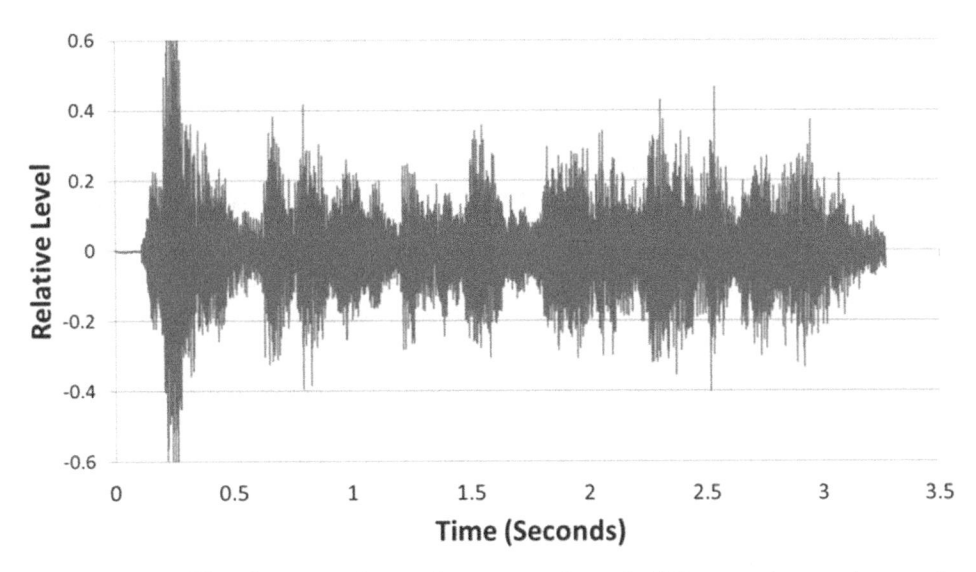

Figure 4–15. The time waveform of an approximately 3.2-second speech sample recorded in a reverberant room.

ine modulation depth over a range of realistic modulation rates for speech to obtain a complete picture of how an environment might affect speech modulations (Houtgast, 1981; Houtgast & Steeneken, 1985; Houtgast, Steeneken, & Plomp, 1980). A graphical representation of how an environment, noise, or any change affects the modulation depth across modulation frequencies of speech is commonly referred to as a modulation transfer function (MTF).

Signal-to-Noise Ratio

Because speech is such a dynamic signal, it might be expected that environmental (e.g., noise, reverberation, distance) and processing factors that affect the MTF might also affect speech recognition. For example, it has been suggested that individuals with normal hearing require a signal-to-noise ratio (SNR) of at least +6 dB for satisfactory communication (e.g., Moore, 1989). SNR refers to the level of the speech in comparison with the level of the noise. Specifically, positive SNR values indicate that, on average, the speech is a higher level than the noise, whereas negative SNRs indicate the noise is at a higher level than the speech. Although poor SNRs are a problem for all listeners, data overwhelmingly support the contention that individuals with sensorineural hearing loss generally require a significantly greater SNR to obtain speech recognition performance equivalent to listeners with normal hearing (Carhart & Tillman, 1970; Cooper & Cutts, 1971; Dirks, Morgan, & Dubno, 1982; Groen, 1969; Killion, 1997; Plomp, 1976; Schum, 1996; Sutter, 1985).

From a patient counseling standpoint, it is also important to remember that, although we increase our vocal effort as a function of the level of the background noise, there is not a one-to-one relationship. That is, the more intense the background noise, the less favorable the SNR despite the increase in vocal effort. This is illustrated in Figure 4–16 (adapted from Pearsons et al., 1977), which shows the level of speech on the y-axis and the level of the background noise on the x-axis. To help your interpretation of this chart, some specific examples are shown in Table 4–3. As you see from Figure 4–16, as noise levels exceed 75 dB SPL, the SNR continues to become more adverse. If you consider that many large group social events and restaurants have background noise levels greater than 75 dB SPL, it is easy to understand the problems faced by the hearing impaired listener.

We discuss different speech-in-noise tests that can be used in the clinic that consider various factors including audibility and the effects of noise in Chapter 6. Some of them apply a fixed SNR for testing, whereas others

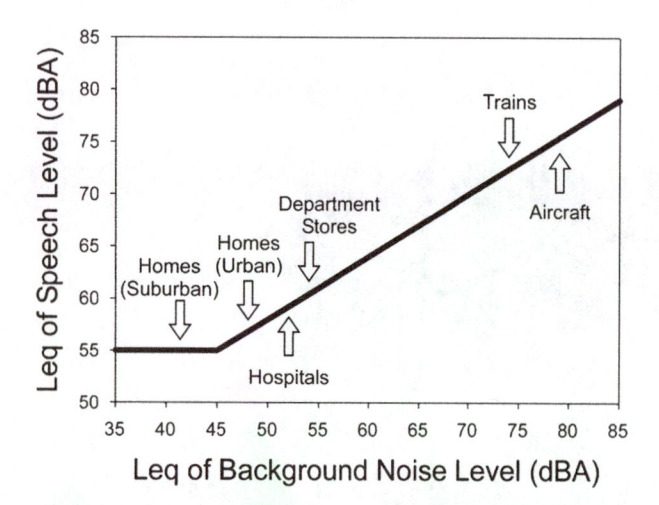

Figure 4–16. The change in SNR as a function of background noise level. (Adapted from Pearsons et al., 1977.)

Table 4–3. SNR as a Function of Background Noise.

If background noise is:	Speech is:	SNR
45 dBA	55 dBA	+10 dB
55 dBA	61 dBA	+6 dB
65 dBA	67 dBA	+2 dB
75 dBA	73 dBA	−2 dB

use an adaptive approach, with either the target speech signal or the background competing signal changing in intensity. In addition to the effects of noise and audibility, data also clearly show decreases in speech recognition with increasing reverberation (Bistafa & Bradley, 2000; Bradley, Reich, & Norcross, 1999; Crandell & Smaldino, 2000; Moncur & Dirks, 1967). The negative effect of reverberation is also clearly increased with a greater talker-to-listener distance.

The STI

Quantifying the effect of environmental factors such as reverberation on speech recognition is the impetus behind the Speech Transmission Index (STI; Houtgast & Steeneken, 1971, 1973; Steeneken & Houtgast, 1980; IEC 60268-16). The STI shares some general similarities with AI calculations, but there is a considerable difference related to how background noise is represented. Both procedures require summing the product of an estimate of speech importance: the band importance function and another factor of importance calculated across several bands. Instead of calculating simple audibility within each band (BA) as in the case of traditional AI procedures, however, a type of SNR is estimated in each band by calculating or measuring modulation MTFs for modulation rates that are similar to speech. The typical STI procedure examines or calculates MTFs for modulation frequencies ranging from 0.63 Hz to 12.5 Hz within each of seven octave bands centered at 125, 250, 500, 1000, 2000, 4000, and 8000 Hz. If the modulation depth approaches the case of being completely filled in across modulation frequencies (e.g., by noise and/or due to the effects of reverberation), the SNR function approaches 0. If there is little change in the modulation depth, the SNR function approaches 1:

$$AI = \sum_{i=0}^{n} \left(BIF \times \frac{SNR + 15}{30} \right)$$

The standard STI differs from AI in a few more subtle ways as well. For example, the STI is typically calculated using no more than seven octave bands. In addition, the assumed band importance function is much flatter for the STI than assumed for most AI procedures, although some authors have proposed corrective modifications (e.g., Humes, Dirks, Bell, Ahlstrom, & Kincaid, 1986). The flatter band importance function assumed by the STI generally makes it less sensitive to filtering effects, however, than the ANSI standard AI procedure, the SII. That is, noise that drops in level precipitously as a function of frequency provides much less masking than noise that has a more gradual drop in level. These effects are generally not well represented in the standard STI due to the flatter band importance function. Still, the STI is much more adept at demonstrating the effect of room acoustics on speech recognition than the original SII. To try to improve accuracy and consider room effects, the SII standard also describes an alternative method for measuring or calculating SNR using procedures similar to those used in the STI.

One way STI has been used is to calculate Percentage Articulation Loss of Consonants (%ALcons). The calculation of %ALcons is used to estimate how much recognition of consonants is degraded based on STI measures. For example, 2% ALcons would indicate a small degradation, whereas 20% ALcons would indicate a much larger and significant degradation. The %ALCONS measures are often reported by acoustical consultants when describing room effects and are often calculated based on specific measurement equipment. One of the most common formulas used to derive ALcons from STI is: *ALcons = 10(1−STI/0.46)*; however, empirical formulas, such as: *ALcons = 170.5405 (e−5.419 × STI*, are also sometimes used. Because STI is computationally intensive, it presented a challenge for earlier portable test equipment. As a consequence, a simplified STI referred to as the Rapid/Room Acoustics STI (RASTI) is sometimes used. With continued advancements in modern test equipment, however, the STI is often advocated over the RASTI due to its greater accuracy.

Mini-Summary

That was a lot of information presented over the last few pages. Before we discuss some clinical applications, here is a mini-summary.

- There are many LTASS. The average shape and overall level of the LTASS depends on factors such as vocal effort, language, and talker characteristics. Speech produced using average vocal effort has an overall level of approximately 62 dB SPL and has a dynamic range of approximately 30 dB. The dynamic range of all speech at all effort levels is greater than 60 dB.
- There are many different AI procedures. In general, these procedures calculate a single value that provides a general indication of the importance-weighted magnitude of speech audibility. AI accuracy can be improved by using actual measured speech and noise levels and the correct band importance function. AI accuracy can further be improved by using hearing loss desensitization, language proficiency, and presentation level factors. Speech can be described as an amplitude modulated signal with a modulation depth of 30 dB and modulation rates ranging from approximately 0.5 to 20 Hz.
- The STI is a measure that can be used to examine how room acoustics (e.g., reverberation and distance) and noise can affect the transmission of speech information. It is based on measuring or calculating MTFs.
- Room effects such as reverberation can also be accounted for in the SII by using an alternative method for calculating or measuring SNR based on the MTF.

Clinical Use of the AI and the STI

All of the technical aspects of AI and STI may be interesting from a research standpoint, and understanding the effects of audibility and room acoustics on speech recognition performance is clearly important theoretically so that we can really understand how much difficulty a patient might be having and how much benefit a particular hearing aid or processing algorithm may provide. As audiologists, however, we must ask how useful the actual AI and STI measures are in the clinic. We certainly do not have time to measure and calculate the standard SII for all the environments our patients might be in. So, is it of interest to know if there are clinically applicable procedures and, more importantly, really opportunities for their use?

With regard to AI/SII, aided and unaided calculations increasingly are showing up on commercial probe microphone equipment and in hearing aid fitting software. Is there a good reason to use these measures clinically? We certainly argue there is; however, there are several potential pitfalls in clinical use.

Despite some apparent limitations, the AI can be used clinically as a measure of importance-weighted audibility. When used in this way it can help when counseling patients and caregivers of children with hearing impairment regarding what to expect in terms of speech audibility and benefit from a hearing aid. For example, you might use an AI to confirm to a patient, spouse, caregiver, or parent that the hearing loss in question leads to the loss of a significant amount of speech sounds. When using AI procedures for patient counseling, it is sometimes useful to display the findings graphically (see examples in Chapter 5). We believe that AI calculations are likely not needed for many clinical situations, but they can provide a useful starting point for some patients

> **TECHNICAL TIP: CLINICAL AI CONSIDERATIONS**
>
> - AI provides an indication of relative changes in audibility but is not useful for precise prediction of an individual patient's speech recognition score.
> - It is important to remember that there is not a one-to-one relationship between the AI and speech understanding—for example, a 70% AI does *not* equal a 70% speech recognition score.
> - For an average patient (cochlear hearing loss, no cognitive deficit), the AI can be used to predict speech recognition for different speech material when an appropriate *transfer function* is applied (see Figure 4–7).
> - It is important to remember that the prediction will be for *average-level speech*, and therefore, their speech recognition might be higher or lower for other input levels.
> - The predicted score is based on the AI in quiet and does not consider the masking effects of background noise (although this can be simulated).
> - As seen in later chapters (and detailed in Chapter 17), the highest AI does not typically lead to the best hearing aid fitting. (If it did, we could just give 100 dB of gain to everyone.) The goal of a hearing aid fitting is never just to maximize AI without also considering listening comfort, sound quality, and loudness perceptions. Making all speech at all levels audible (maximum AI) will typically lead to most signals being too loud for patient comfort.
> - For some patients, increases in audibility in some frequency regions may not lead to increases in speech recognition (see our discussion of effective audibility and cochlear *dead regions* in Chapter 5). In general, use of the AI may lead to an overestimation of the increase in speech recognition expected from an increase in audibility after fitting a hearing aid if cochlear dead regions and/or HLD factors are not considered. It is also important to note that the AI is quite accurate for prediction of relative changes in speech recognition performance, however, even without considering HLDs, for listeners with hearing thresholds better than approximately 65 to 70 dB HL.
> - We must also remember to consider *level* effects. As speech peaks approach the listener's threshold of discomfort, the magnitude of speech recognition improvement will be less than predicted from AI if a level desensitization factor is not considered.

when talking about the degree of communication deficit, potential hearing aid benefit, or hearing assistive technology (HAT) candidacy and/ or expectations.

On the following pages, we provide an introduction to clinical AI procedures that are easy to use. There are many clinical procedures available, but rather than overwhelm you, we focus on the detail of only a few of our favorites.

Before we start, let's get a better idea of the expected average relationship between speech recognition and AI. To make things simple enough for clinical use, we will assume an average AI procedure that in turn assumes an average band importance function and does not include corrections for hearing loss, level, age, or any other factor. We can obtain a rough idea about this relationship by going back to Figure 4–7. As we mentioned earlier, these data provide a graphical representation of the AI-to-speech-recognition transfer functions. In Figure 4–7, the x-axis is the SII, and the y-axis is the predicted percent correct score for a given speech material.

Imagine a person who has a downward sloping hearing loss going from 20 dB at 500 Hz to 60 dB at 6000 Hz. Approximately half the speech cues will be available to this listener, and the AI would equal about 0.5. The relationship between AI and intelligibility is not linear, however (see Figure 4–7). We can see that the most linear function between AI and the percent correct scores is for single words. This is important because it suggests that higher AI values are especially important when there are fewer speech context cues available.

The effect of context can be demonstrated clearly by our example of the listener with hearing loss and an AI of 0.5. Even though this listener misses 50% of the speech cues, he or she will miss only about 30% of the words in a NU-6 monosyllabic word list and only 5% of sentences. The dramatic difference is a result of the brain's remarkable ability to use context to fill in missing information.

One important example of limited context occurs in children who are first learning speech. In this case, the context might be available in the speech source, but the child may not yet know how to use it. As a result, he or she may not be as able to fill in the blanks as well as an adult when the child misses certain words or sounds. As we pointed out previously, another surprising thing we can see from Figure 4–7 is that for sentence materials, the AI only needs to be about 0.4 for adult listeners with normal hearing to approach 100% correct identification. This of course is for sentences in quiet—performance may be much different in background noise.

Clinical AI Procedures

As we have discussed, formal AI procedures can involve considerable mathematical calculations. Even with the computer scoring methods that are available today, use of these procedures has been overwhelming or too time-consuming for most clinicians. Recognizing this, Chas Pavlovic designed a simplified method referred to as A_0 (pronounced A-zero), which was published in 1989. One of the advantages for the A_0 was that no form was required and the procedure could be applied to any audiogram. The calculation is based on only four frequencies (500, 1000, 2000, and 4000 Hz), each having the potential of 30 audible dB. Consider the speech box or *speech block* shown in Figure 4–17 that represents a rough estimate of the dynamic range of speech from the minima at 20 dB HL to the maxima at 50 dB HL. The procedure is equally weighted, so we have four frequencies with 30 dB at each frequency for a total of 120 potential audible dB. To illustrate how this might be used, let us take an individual with a downward sloping hearing loss of 30 dB at 500 Hz, 45 dB at 1000 Hz, 50 dB at 2000 Hz, and 65 dB at 4000 Hz. Applying this to the

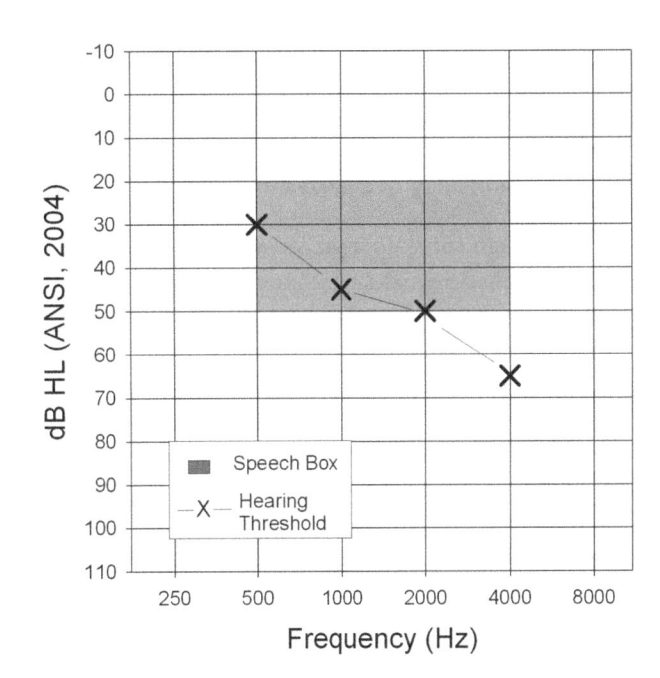

Figure 4–17. An example of the A0 procedure applied to an audiogram.

speech block shown in Figure 4–17, we see that this patient would have 20 audible dB at 500 Hz, 5 dB at 1000 Hz, 0 dB at 2000 Hz, and 0 dB at 4000 Hz. If we add the audible dB together (20 + 5 + 0 + 0) we find that 25 of the possible 120 dB are audible, for an AI of 0.21 (25 / 120). Pretty simple, huh?

Well, not simple enough for some because dividing anything by 120 in a speedy manner might require a calculator or pencil and paper. As a consequence, the 1988 publication of Pavlovic led to several other simplified AI procedures:

- Mueller and Killion (1990) develop a procedure that has 100 dots representing the speech spectrum, commonly called the *count-the-dots audiogram*.
- Humes (1991) develops a similar count-the-dots audiogram, although he only uses 33 dots (and they are bigger).
- Pavlovic (1991) develops a *count-the-squares* procedure, using 100 squares with a somewhat different speech spectrum than Mueller and Killion or Humes.
- Lundeen (1996) publishes a 100-dot version modeled after the 100-square work of Pavlovic.

- Kringlebotn (1999) develops an audiogram form with 100 points for SII calculation.
- In 2010, Killion and Mueller revise their 100-dot audiogram to more closely align it to the SII (more high frequency dots).

Although these approaches are all slightly different, the similarities are such that any of them could be applied for routine clinical use. That is, it is unlikely that your clinical decision making will be changed based on an AI difference of 5% or less, which is probably the biggest difference you will see among methods. In addition, when fitting hearing aids, you will more likely use the automatic calculations of the probe microphone equipment, which may also be different, depending on what speech spectrum or AI method is being used by a given manufacturer. The popular Audioscan Verifit, for example, uses a speech spectrum slightly raised from the 20 to 50 dB HL range of Killion and Mueller (2010) and, therefore, a higher (better) unaided AI will result.

In the next chapter, we illustrate how these count-the-dot audiograms can be used in patient counseling and for making decisions related to hearing aid candidacy. In Chapter 15 we show how the AI (or SII) can be applied during the verification process.

Situational Hearing Aid Response Profile

Another and somewhat different, clinically useful AI-based procedure that we want to mention is the Situational Hearing Aid Response Profile (SHARP), which was developed by Patricia Stelmachowicz and colleagues (Stelmachowicz, Mace, Kopun, & Carney, 1993) and recently revised. The SHARP is a computer program that provides a graphical representation of speech audibility for 16 typical listening conditions commonly experienced by children. This program also calculates unaided and aided SII for each of the listening conditions it includes. Aided audibility can also be visualized after applying nonlinear frequency compression. Because this tool was developed for pediatric hearing aid fittings, it is not surprising that long-term average speech spectra representations include important situations for children. These include a teacher speaking at various distances, the hearing aid wearer's own voice, a child in a cradle position, and a number of other situations. An example of the SHARP graphical output is shown in Figure 4–18. The shaded areas in this figure give a clear indication of the area of audible speech. Similar figures are now available on many probe microphone systems; however, they usually only include aver-

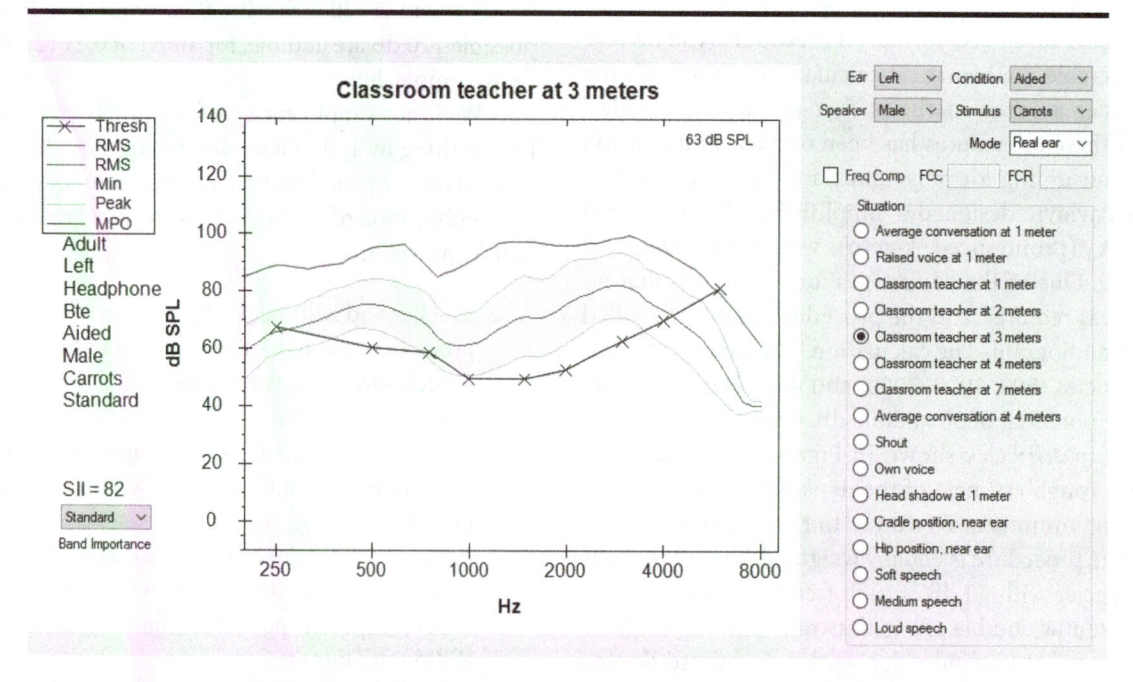

Figure 4–18. An example of aided audibility for a theoretical child in one listening situation calculated using the SHARP.

> **POINTS TO PONDER: "A" IS FOR ARTICULATION OR AUDIBILITY?**
>
> As we have discussed, the abbreviation AI is commonly used for the *Articulation Index*, but the word articulation makes it sound like the calculation has more to do with how we speak than how we hear. For the most part, what we are measuring is the audibility of speech cues, so wouldn't *Audibility Index* be a better term? We could still keep the "A." In 1993, Mead Killion, Gus Mueller, Chas Pavlovic, and Larry Humes, who had all independently designed a simplified AI procedure, published the article "A Is for Audibility," in support of the switch from the word articulation. Twenty-five years have passed and articulation still seems to be the word of choice. Perhaps this is only fitting, as this is the term that Harvey Fletcher used over 80 years ago, and his work has certainly withstood the test of time.

age speech spectrum shapes, even when multiple signal levels are possible. The SHARP is a nice tool for those fitting hearing aids on children and can be used with any hearing aid prescription. In addition to the school setting application, the inclusion of long-term average speech spectra corresponding to the very close listening positions that are experienced by infants and toddlers are especially helpful for counseling purposes. Copies of SHARP can be obtained by e-mailing audiosharp@boystown.org.

Clinical STI Procedures

Given that estimation of the STI requires measurements in a room and/or complex calculations, rather than just the readily available clinical information, it is reasonable to question whether there are clinical applications for the STI. Although perhaps not convenient in routine clinical hearing aid practice, the STI can be useful when considering the impact of room acoustics, acoustic room treatments, or hearing assistive technology. A complete discussion of this topic is well beyond the scope of this textbook; however, clinicians who routinely do this type of work often choose to obtain a sound level meter and/or computer program that is able to measure and calculate STI or one of its simplified versions such as the Rapid Speech Transmission Index, or RASTI. More recently rough measurements and calculations of the STI for public address systems have even been introduced as smartphone applications.

We should mention that it is also possible to obtain free STI software that can be used in conjunction with an existing personal computer, loudspeaker, and microphone. For example, Harry Levitt has developed a program that can be used to make such measures and is available free of charge from Gallaudet University (search the Internet for http://www.hearingresearch.org and LexSTI). This small, easy-to-use program can be quite useful (for example) for clinicians in a school setting arguing for acoustic treatment of a room or hearing assistive technology. In addition, a number of other versions are available for free that include MatLab script versions. A note of caution is also warranted, however. The STI should generally not be used after measuring the modulation transfer function at the output of modern hearing aids. This limitation is due to the fact that some types of commonly used signal processing, such as amplitude compression, are known to affect STI values without producing a concomitant effect on speech recognition.

Mini-Summary

- The calculation of the AI can be helpful for patient counseling and making decisions regarding amplification.
- Maximizing the AI is clearly not the only consideration when assigning hearing aid gain and is expected to lead to excessive and undesirable loudness in many cases. In addition, hearing loss desensitization and level effects must also be considered when interpreting clinical AI values.
- There are several clinically friendly AI approaches available. In general, they

produce similar and comparable clinical AI values. Clinical application of aided audibility for a variety of different long-term average speech spectra, as is possible with the SHARP instrument, can be useful for examining speech audibility across a range of environments in children.

In Closing

Understanding the acoustics of the speech signal is paramount to managing the most common desire of potential hearing aid candidates: understanding speech better. Without a basic understanding of the factors that impact the LTASS (such as vocal effort, talker variables, and measurement techniques), it is not possible to alter or adjust the hearing aid processing in a meaningful or effective manner. Knowing the interactions between speech dynamics and the hearing aid's classification system leads to a better understanding of the function of automatic hearing aid algorithms. Quantifying the resultant audibility after a hearing aid fitting allows both the clinician and patient to better understand the potential success of the effort. Adding the effect of noise and reverberation to that audibility calculation provides a better real-world indication of the potential for success.

5

Pre-Fitting Tests Using Frequency-Specific Measures

In the next few chapters, we discuss some of the pre-fitting tools that we use to assess the patient, the patient's hearing handicap, and their communication needs to begin making decisions regarding hearing aid candidacy and selection. Assessing communication needs for the purpose of hearing aid selection requires knowledge in several areas. Given the time limitations in a typical clinic setting, it is necessary that an appropriately small number of measures are selected that provide the most important information for each specific patient in an efficient manner. Because every patient is different and there is not sufficient time to gather exhaustive clinical data, this handful of assessment tools must be selected individually for each patient's situation out of the large group of possible assessment measures available. This is often an iterative process during which the clinician uses information gathered earlier (e.g., general case history, type and degree of hearing loss, general patient goals, and problems) to determine what additional information is most critical to gather for the individual patient via additional assessments. In the next three chapters we provide you with a variety of tools, ranging from tests using pure-tone stimuli, speech recognition in quiet, speech in background noise, and several self-assessment measures.

To select the best assessment measures and interpret their results to assist in selecting the optimal hearing aid model, style, and processing for a given patient, it is important to know how hearing aids work and the various features available. For example, loudness discomfort measures go hand-in-hand with setting the maximum output of the hearing aid; the patient's QuickSIN score might influence the recommendation of wireless streaming technologies, and so forth. Because the hearing aid selection process requires knowledge in so many areas, we sometimes describe assessment tools and techniques without first providing a clear indication of exactly when and how the test results should be applied and interpreted. It is our philosophy that the cookbook method of learning about hearing aids is of little use in the long run, so subsequent chapters provide information about the philosophy underlying the use of these techniques so that future techniques can also be appropriately applied.

Although it is easy to get caught up in learning how to conduct and score all the test procedures and then trying to understand when and how to best implement them, we must remember that each patient is an individual. One of the most challenging and interesting aspects of hearing aid selection and fitting is recognizing this individuality and appropriately modifying the process for each patient. Protocols are a wonderful starting place and an excellent mechanism for helping ensure quality control in our practice. A protocol should only serve as a point of reference, however, and the personality, desire, and needs of the individual patient must drive clinical decision making from beginning to end.

Using the Audiogram for Counseling and Predicting Audibility

In the previous chapter, we provided a detailed description of the speech signal and explained the importance of understanding the components of this signal as they relate to the fitting of hearing aids. As we describe, a big part of the success of the overall fitting relates to making speech audible, with the caveat that it also must have the appropriate loudness, minimal distortion, and a reasonable sound quality. It is helpful during the prefitting appointment to assure that the patient understands the fitting goals. For the new hearing aid user who still might be questioning the need for hearing aids, it might be necessary to illustrate how much of the average speech signal is *not* audible. For the experienced hearing aid user obtaining a new pair of hearing aids, it might be helpful to explain why the new hearing aids will sound different from the old ones. For example, if more high frequency gain is being added, an explanation of the importance of these speech cues might encourage the user to be more accepting to this new amplification strategy. These visual demonstrations also can be very helpful for family members who might be wondering why Mom can "hear but not understand."

The history of audiology is linked to the audiogram. (See Mueller, Ricketts, and Bentler, 2014, Appendix H, for an interesting hearing loss timeline dating back to Hippocrates in 377 BC.) There are several methods of using the patient's pure-tone audiogram for prefitting counseling. Some are more detailed than others, and the method selected often relates to the sophistication of the patient, the level of interest in learning about hearing loss, and how the loss might impact speech understanding.

Using the Speech Banana with Symbols

As was discussed in the previous chapter, when we plot the LTASS range on the HL scale, it more or less resembles a banana—so much so that even many lay people know what the *speech banana* is. This is commonly used for counseling patients regarding their hearing loss. Some audiologists only have the banana shaded on the audiogram, other forms have symbols for common environmental sounds or have the various speech consonants or vowels printed on the audiogram—this is a common option in the software of computer-based audiometers. Usually this is not the audiogram placed in the patient's records or sent out to referral sources but rather simply something unofficial that can be used for counseling and that the patient can take home for review.

Many audiologists have the speech banana on their standard clinical audiogram, as it provides an immediate reference for the speech range. Figure 5–1 is an audiogram that does not have a banana per se, but shows the individual speech sounds that are contained within the banana. Several environmental sounds also

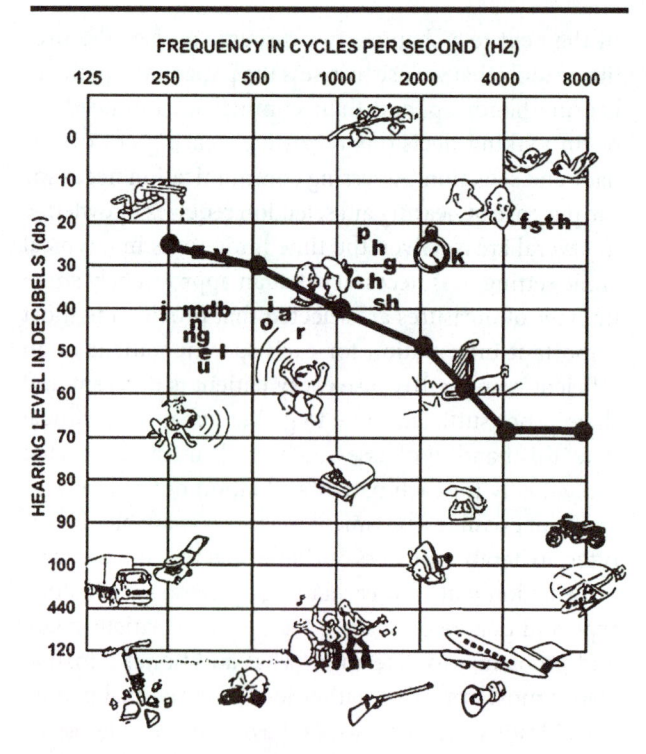

Figure 5–1. Typical downward sloping hearing loss plotted on an audiogram displaying common speech and environmental sounds.

are displayed. This is not an audiogram that you would use in a medical record, but it is helpful for patient counseling. After plotting the hearing thresholds, you could then talk about the portion of the banana that was not audible, the speech sounds that are not audible, and also point out specific environmental sounds that might not be heard or not perceived as readily as for people with normal hearing. This latter form is a bit extreme, as most audiologists would not want all these symbols for environmental sounds—personally, we probably wouldn't include the whispering chimpanzees on our form. The point is, many forms of this type are available and can serve as useful counseling tools.

Using the Speech Banana With Dots

In the previous chapter, we introduced you to the AI and the SII, and discussed some simplified clinical methods for making these calculations. Of the several methods we reviewed we like the count-the-dots procedure for busy clinicians because the frequencies often important in hearing aid fittings, 1500 and 3000 Hz, are now also included, and the calculation of AI only involves counting dots—no addition, subtraction, or division required. In case it is not obvious, you would count the dots below the hearing thresholds. If you want to venture into the world of math and it is a mild hearing loss, you might want to count the dots above the hearing thresholds and subtract this number from 100.

The 1990 Mueller-Killion audiogram was based on a 200-dot SPL chart that was used in industrial acoustics in the 1960s (Cavanaugh, Farrell, Hirtle, & Waters, 1962). The density of the dots changes as a function of frequency to represent the importance function of speech. We have found the count-the-dot audiogram to be particularly helpful when counseling patients who are in denial regarding the degree of handicap that they might have. Using a percentage to make the point is something that everyone can relate to. Showing someone graphically that they are missing 60% of average speech, although they have just said they hear everything, can

---

SOAPBOX: PICK YOUR BANANA CAREFULLY!

As we have mentioned, it is common to place the speech banana (average LTASS) on the audiogram and use this for counseling. There have been several studies of average speech over the years, and LTASS findings do vary somewhat from study to study, but they are more or less in pretty good general agreement. So why is it then, that if we would do a Google image search on *Speech Banana* today, we find audiograms (apparently used in offices and clinics somewhere) with the 1000 to 2000 Hz frequency region of the LTASS ranging anywhere from 15 to 45 dB for the upper boundary and 40 to 70 dB for the lower boundary, with everything in between also used? A 25 dB difference! This is a pretty fundamental concept of audiology: Wouldn't it be nice if we all could get it right? Imagine if you took your three-year-old son in for testing and the audiometric results revealed that he had a 35 dB loss (or is it really a loss?). If he were tested at Clinic A, where they use the 15 to 45 dB banana, you would be told that your son was missing about two-thirds of the important sounds of average speech. On the other hand, if he were tested at Clinic B, where the audiologists use the 40 to 70 dB speech banana, you would be told that all is well—he is hearing 100% of average speech. In our opinion, this borders on malpractice, as a child suffering from middle ear effusion (which often results in a hearing loss of 30 to 35 dB) might go untreated for months or years, simply because the parents were given the wrong counseling based on the wrong banana.

Refer back to Chapter 4 for more details on the correct LTASS. In general, we recommend using a spectrum that has the soft components for the mid-frequencies around 20 to 25 dB, with the loud components of the LTASS at 50 to 55 dB (see Figure 5–1).

> **KEY CONCEPT: HEARING, NOT UNDERSTANDING**
>
> Although we believe that using *percent audibility* of average speech can be effective for patient counseling, we do need to mention a fine point that often needs to be clarified. It is important to clearly state that this is the percent of speech that the patient *hears*, not the percent of speech that he or she *understands*. Patients sometimes want to think of it as percent understanding or even percent hearing loss. As we discussed in Chapter 4, it is possible to make a rough conversion from the audibility index to speech recognition using the chart shown in Figure 4–7. As illustrated in this chart, a person who is only hearing 50% of average speech could be understanding nearly 100% of sentence material if listening in quiet.

be a convincing message. As we discussed in Chapter 3, patients often forget much of what we tell them during the pre-fitting counseling process, but they usually remember the percentage of dots they could hear.

The dots also can be useful in educating referral sources, as it soon becomes clear that an individual with a high frequency, noise-induced hearing loss really does not have normal hearing for the *speech range*, as this patient often is missing over 40% of average speech. Or, the dots also work effectively for illustrating the audibility deficit a child with middle ear effusion might suffer. In 2010, Mueller and Killion modified their 1990 count-the-dot procedure (Killion & Mueller, 2010). The authors state that the form was changed to reflect the research behind the new ANSI standard S3.5-1997 (R2007), "Methods for Calculation of Speech Intelligibility Index," which produced a new SII importance function that gives more weight to higher frequencies. The new version, therefore, slightly redistributes the 100 dots and includes weightings for 6000 and 8000 Hz. The revised 2010 audiogram is shown in Figure 5–2. Note that the audible dots for this patient are roughly 20%. Killion and Mueller (2010) reviewed the basic differences between the newer and older forms:

- The new audiogram has 11 dots above 4000 Hz, whereas only six dots were above 4000 Hz in the older version. There is also an additional dot at 4000 Hz in the new version. Because there are only 100 dots to work with, these extra high-frequency dots were carefully lifted from the frequencies below 4000 Hz.
- Because a few dots from the mid-frequencies were removed, the typical patient with a gradually downward sloping hearing loss might have an AI score 2 to 3% lower with the new SII version than with the older one.

One thing that did not change in the new Killion Mueller count-the-dot audiogram is the overall speech spectrum, which is based on a 60 dB SPL equivalence. As we have discussed earlier, there are several different speech bananas in clinical use. Killion and Mueller (2010) state that their selection of this spectrum was based on the work of Margo Skinner, who recommended that all conversational speech tests be conducted at 60 dB SPL, 5 dB softer than the generally accepted average

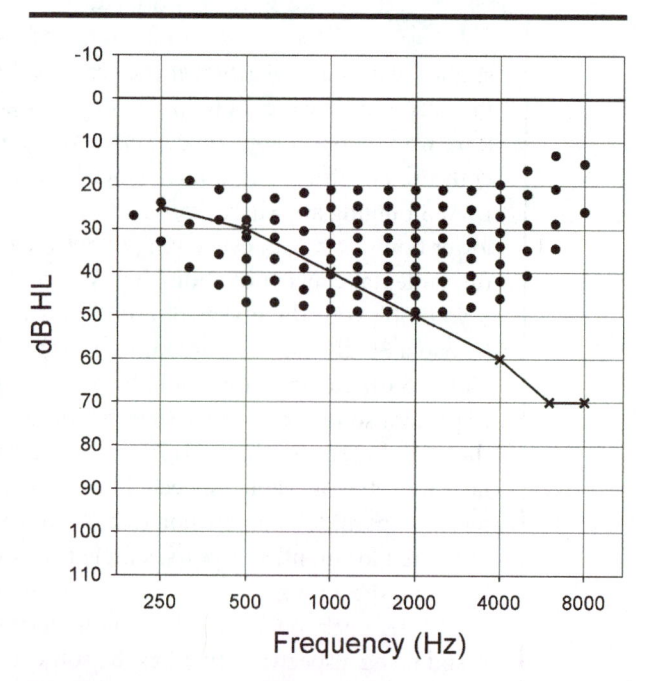

Figure 5–2. Typical downward sloping hearing loss plotted on an audiogram displaying the 2010 Killion and Mueller count-the-dots SII speech spectrum.

for conversational speech, as this level is a better measure of the listener's ability in everyday life (Skinner, Holden, Holden, Demorest, & Fourakis, 1997).

Although the audibility calculations that we have been discussing can be computerized easily (and they have been), there is something to be said about using the paper-and-pencil version. Sitting at a desk with a patient, plotting the audiogram, having the patient help you count the audible dots, showing what happens when the low-frequency dots are covered up because they are masked by noise, all tends to have a memorable counseling impact. The patient takes the sheets home with him or her, and in general, the patient seems to get it. But computer automation is a good thing too, so we discuss how the illustration of audibility also can be used with your fitting software and probe microphone equipment.

Using Fitting Software or Probe Microphone Equipment

Most hearing aid fitting software also provides a counseling module, which often includes a method to relate the hearing loss to average speech. We have observed that some of these do not use the correct level for the banana, so proceed with caution if you choose to use this approach. An easy and more accurate way to illustrate how the patient's hearing loss relates to an average speech signal is to use your probe microphone equipment. The advantage of this is that we now have converted everything to ear canal SPL, and we are using an SPL-O-gram, a display method where loud sounds actually fall appropriately above soft sounds, unlike the standard audiogram. One way to use this display is to plot the patient's hearing threshold and use the average speech spectrum that is stored for screen display. This is shown in Figure 5–3. In general, this is more intuitive for patient counseling than the standard audiogram, as we see that what is *not* audible falls below the patient's thresholds, and what is audible falls above. This display does not involve any extra testing; the probe microphone equipment monitor is simply used to facilitate the counseling.

It is possible to add a bit more face validity into the pre-fitting counseling and actually measure an average speech spectrum in the patient's ear canal while comparing the speech levels to hearing thresholds. This is displayed in Figure 5–4. What you see here are

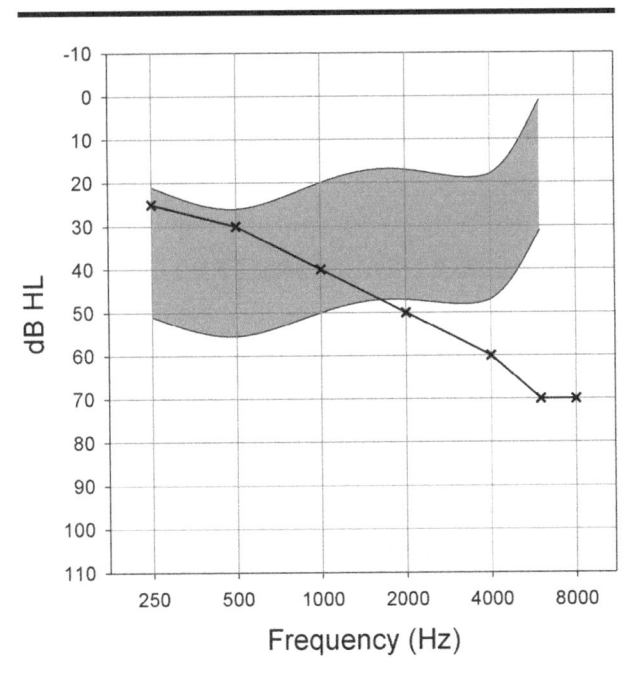

Figure 5–3. Typical downward sloping hearing loss plotted on an audiogram displaying the average speech spectrum.

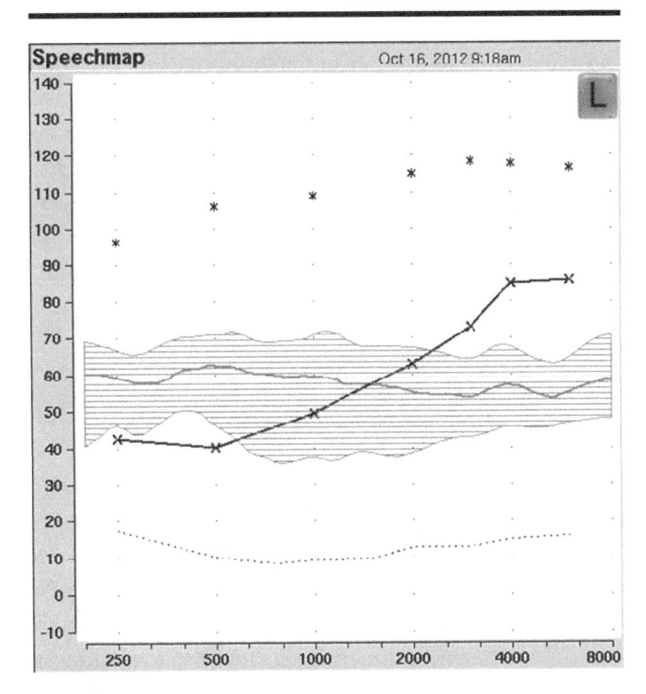

Figure 5–4. Typical downward sloping hearing loss (same as used in Figures 5–1 to 5–3) plotted in the SPL-O-Gram format (reference = ear canal SPL). Rather than displaying the average speech spectrum, the spectrum shown was obtained from a real-speech signal (65 dB SPL) delivered to the patient's open ear with the probe microphone tip at the patient's eardrum.

the same hearing thresholds as before, compared with the measured real-ear output of the calibrated LTASS (*carrot passage—male talker*) of the Audioscan Verifit probe microphone equipment (i.e., the measurement is conducted with the test probe at the patient's eardrum). This equipment automatically calculates the SII, which in this case was 41%. This is considerably better than the 20% that we calculated for Figure 5–2, but recall that the Killion-Mueller spectrum was based on a 60 dB SPL overall level, rather than the approximately 62 dB SPL level used by the SII. The patient's free-field-to-eardrum transfer function also will impact these measures (see Chapter 16). Depending on the time that is available, this counseling and demonstration can be expanded by presenting speech of different input levels (soft, average, loud), or even using live speech of family members to illustrate to the patient what he or she is missing.

What Does It All Mean?

What we have shown in this section is that there are many ways that the pure-tone audiogram can be used to help patients understand their hearing handicap and how it relates to speech understanding. For the most part, it is pretty simple. But, we need to focus on the fact that the goal in this case is not perfect scientific accuracy—we don't care if one SII estimate is 2% different from another. The overall purpose is simply to show patients the impact that hearing loss potentially could have for understanding speech so that they can make informed decisions regarding the use of hearing aids.

Loudness Discomfort Level Testing

The most critical aspect of the hearing aid verification process is ensuring that both the gain and the maximum output are adjusted correctly for a given patient. Although these two adjustments are not totally independent (one could not achieve high gain levels for average inputs without a moderately high output setting), for the average patient it is usually possible to vary the gain by 40 dB to 50 dB and the MPO (for maximum power output) by at least 20 dB. Gain prescriptions are typically based on audiometric thresholds, but how do we determine the best MPO setting? The logical approach, which also has been specified in best practice guidelines for the past 25 years, is to conduct frequency-specific loudness discomfort level (LDL) measures, and use these values to set the hearing aid MPO (often by manipulating the output compression limiting kneepoint) so that loud sounds are loud, but not too loud. These frequency-specific LDL measures should be a routine part of the pre-fitting hearing aid battery.

Background

The loudness growth function for both normal hearing and hearing impaired individuals, at some point, reaches a level where the sound is uncomfortable. This is referred to as the uncomfortable loudness level, threshold of discomfort, or the term we use throughout this book, the loudness discomfort level (LDL).

POINTS TO PONDER: DOES THE TERMINOLOGY REALLY MATTER?

As we explain in Table 5–1, there are many terms used to denote the point at which loud sounds become uncomfortable: UL, UCL, ULL, TD, LDL, and so forth. Does it matter what term we use? This topic has been discussed several times over the years in the Mueller and Bentler "How Loud Is Allowed" trilogy (Mueller & Bentler, 1994, 2002, 2008). Dr. Bentler points out (supported by research; Warner & Bentler, 2002) that TD is the most appropriate term, as dimensions other than the loudness of a perceptually abusive sound play a part in what is considered uncomfortable—it is not determined by the RMS level of the signal alone. Factors that tend to cause LDLs to be rated lower include annoyance, peakiness, high-frequency content, and the subjective perception of tinniness. These factors are particularly important during the aided verification process (see chapter 15). For this book, however, despite Dr. Bentler's fondness for the TD descriptor, we use LDL to describe this loudness perception.

Table 5–1. Terminology Associated with the Measurement of Loudness Discomfort

- Uncomfortable Loudness (UCL). This is perhaps the most commonly used term among clinicians to describe the point at which loud sounds become uncomfortable. The common use of the letter "C" in the abbreviation is somewhat puzzling, and indeed, some simply use the abbreviation UL. The abbreviation ULL also is used, with the final "L" referring to *level*.
- Loudness Discomfort Level (LDL). The term that we prefer and what we will use throughout this chapter. It is used interchangeably with UCL/ULL.
- Threshold of Discomfort (TD). Another term for the same measure. For the most part (see Point to Ponder on this topic), it can be used interchangeably with LDL, UCL and ULL.
- Upper Level of Comfort (ULC). The category of loudness falling just below the LDL. When using the 7-point Cox Contour Anchors we discuss later, this is the #6 Loud, But Okay rating. In general, we want the output of the hearing aid to fall at this level; the DSL prescriptive software has used ULC values for this purpose.
- Highest Comfortable Level (HCL). The same as the ULC.
- OSPL90: The broadest most powerful output of a hearing aid with the gain control "full on" measured in a 2-cc coupler using 90 dB swept pure tones. A component of ANSI standard S3.22 and used for hearing aid specification, documentation, and quality control.
- Maximum Power Output (MPO). In some cases, the term MPO is used synonymously with OSPL90. More commonly, however, in the clinic, MPO refers to the maximum output of the hearing aid when specific settings have been made (e.g., settings of gain, input and output compression), and not the *potential* maximum output of the instrument (the OSPL90). The MPO, therefore, cannot be higher than the OSPL90, and often it is significantly lower. For example, lowering the AGCo compression kneepoint for a given patient would lower the hearing aid's MPO.
- Real-ear saturation response (RESR). This is an MPO measure obtained with the hearing aid fitted to the patient's ear rather than in a 2-cc coupler. Typically, this measure is made with the hearing aid's gain and compression parameters set to approximate use conditions using an 85 to 90 dB swept pure tone.
- Real-ear coupler difference (RECD). This is a measure which compares the output of a hearing aid in the real ear to the output in a 2-cc coupler with identical settings. If the RECD is known, it can be added to the hearing aid coupler MPO (*not* the OSPL90) to predict the maximum output in the ear canal.
- Reference equivalent thresholds in SPL (RETSPL). Difference between HL dial setting and output in a 2-cc or 6-cc coupler. Because insert earphones (which are calibrated in a 2-cc coupler), are typically used for HL LDL testing, RETSPL values can be used to convert HL LDLs to 2-cc coupler values (so you can speak the same language as your fitting software).
- Real-ear dial difference (REDD). This is the addition of the RETSPL and the RECD (or it can be measured directly); using this you can convert from HL LDL to ear canal SPL. This provides the RESR output targets you see on the probe-mic fitting screen.
- Automatic Gain Control-input (AGCi): Input compression, typically having a low activation kneepoint (in which case it is referred to as WDRC). It can be used to control the hearing aids' MPO if kneepoints are low enough and the ratios are big enough. Note: Amplitude compression processing will be discussed in much greater detail in Book Two and is purposefully oversimplified here.
- Automatic Gain Control-output (AGCo): Output compression, typically having a high activation kneepoint and high compression ratios (in which case it is referred to as compression limiting)—the most common method to control the MPO.

A long-standing component of the fitting process is to assure that the MPO of the hearing is appropriate for the patient. Carhart's procedure from the 1940s (1946a) included a "determination of instrument efficiency," which included "transmitting loud sounds without undue discomfort."

Although intuitively it seems likely that the maximum output of the hearing aid could influence use, benefit, and satisfaction, one might question if there are data to suggest that this is a problem. There are. In 2003, in a large survey of audiologists, Jenstad, Van Tasell, and Ewert (2003) reported that "aids too loud" was the most common complaint audiologists received from patients fitted with hearing aids. "Satisfaction with loudness" also has been a common question on the MarkeTrak surveys. Although overall satisfaction with hearing aids has gone from a low of 53% (1994) to a high of 81% (2015), as recently as 2008 the MarkeTrak VIII survey revealed that satisfaction for "comfort with loud sounds" was only 67%, which had a .60 correlation with overall satisfaction (Kochkin, 2010). It is also important to mention that the comfort for loud sounds category only had 42% satisfaction as recently as 2002 (Kochkin, 2002).

In a related finding from MarkeTrak VIII, Kochkin et al. (2010) reported that highly satisfied users from the sample were more apt to have undergone loudness testing during the fitting process than individuals who were not satisfied. For the weighted protocol, these differences were substantial: For the bottom 15% of satisfaction ($n = 275$), only 40% received the testing versus 98% for the top 15% of satisfied hearing aid users ($n = 276$). The study did not differentiate between loudness testing conducted pre-fitting under earphones or aided during the fitting process.

The research surrounding the clinical measure of LDLs was addressed in an evidence-based review by Mueller and Bentler (2005). Because of the limited number of studies that met their criteria ($n = 3$), the level of evidence, and the statistical power of the studies, they were unable to make a strong recommendation concerning the clinical use of LDL measures. One prospective study published since the Mueller and Bentler (2005) review compared two different fitting protocols: One included LDL measures and the other did not (Shi, Doherty, Kordas, & Pellegrino, 2007). The aided Abbreviated Profile of Hearing Aid Benefit (APHAB) and Satisfaction of Amplification in Daily Life (SADL) findings for the two groups were not significantly different following hearing aid use. When the authors examined patient-driven adjustments in the first 45 days following the fittings, however, there were nearly twice as many adjustments made to the group who were fitted without the LDL measures (mean = 2.7 versus 1.5 adjustments). The authors speculate this was because of the alterations of the output based on the LDL values.

Measures of LDL Variability

An important question regarding the pre-fitting measurement of LDLs relates to the variability of loudness discomfort among individuals. Are the LDLs of the hearing impaired about the same as people with normal hearing? Do individuals with the same hearing loss more or less have the same LDLs? If for example, most all patients with a 50 dB cochlear hearing loss have LDLs within a 10 dB window, then it probably would not be worth the time investment to conduct LDL testing during the pre-fitting process. We would simply predict it from the audiogram.

Perhaps the most extensive study of LDLs was reported by Bentler and Cooley (2001). They compiled LDLs for a total of 433 subjects (710 ears) with presumed cochlear pathologies. They obtained LDLs using an ascending method of limits similar to our recommendations in the next section. Their data (averaged for five test frequencies) is displayed in Figure 5–5. Several important teaching points are evident:

1. From 20 to 60 dB hearing loss, there is no average change in LDLs.
2. Above 60 dB, average LDLs go up roughly 5 dB for each 10 dB increase in hearing loss.
3. The range of LDLs for different individuals with the same hearing loss is 40 to 50 dB or greater for most hearing loss levels.

Other findings from the 2001 Bentler and Cooley study have clinical importance (multiple regression analysis

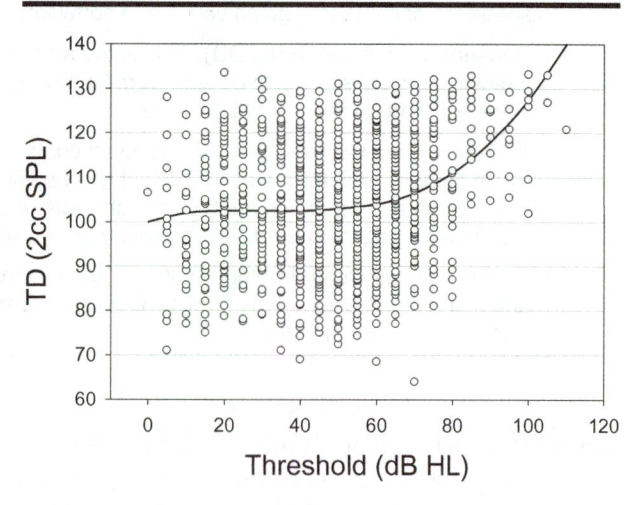

Figure 5–5. Display of LDLs (TDs) referenced to a 2-cc coupler as a function of hearing loss obtained from 710 individual ears. Data points averaged for frequencies 500 to 4000 Hz. (Adapted from Bentler and Cooley, 2001.)

using almost 2,000 LDLs; subjects ranging in age from 11 to 97 years):

1. LDLs did not vary as a function of the frequency tested (when hearing loss was matched).
2. There were no gender differences.
3. There were no age differences.

As mentioned above and readily observed in Figure 5–5, the variability of LDLs for individuals with the same degree of hearing loss is very large. For example, if we take a common 50 dB hearing loss, we see that values ranged from the mid-70s to more than 130 dB—nearly a 60 dB range. Perhaps more important than the range per se is that there were not just one or two outliers but a fairly even distribution between the lower and upper values. If we were to use average values to predict the correct MPO setting, in this example, the value would be around 102 dB (re: 2-cc coupler; see regression line). Bentler and Cooley (2001), however, report that only 32% of measured LDLs fell within ±5 dB of this average. Assuming that we would not want an MPO mistake of greater than 5 dB, this clearly points out the problems that can exist when average values are used.

Dillon and Storey (1998) also reported LDL findings for a large group of subjects, showing average values similar to that of Bentler and Cooley (2001). The range of variability for their subject group was smaller, however, at around 40 dB, primarily because they did not observe LDLs less than approximately 90 dB once the hearing loss was 50 dB or greater. But even with this somewhat smaller range, predicting from the audiogram could be risky.

If It Is Not Right?

So what happens if we fit a hearing aid and the MPO is not right? Perhaps the biggest problem would be to select an output that is too high, exceeding the patient's LDL. Some probable adverse outcomes are as follows:

- Because there is not a control for MPO, the patient will turn down gain (and will then not have appropriate audibility for soft and average inputs).
- The patient will only use the hearing aids when knowing that no loud sounds will be present (missing out on appropriate amplification for the majority of listening situations).
- The patient will have some initial negative experiences and will simply stop using the hearing aids.

So what if the MPO is set unnecessarily lower than it needs to be? Unlike setting the output too high, this probably will not result in rejection of amplification, but there are several potential negative consequences:

- Speech may sound somewhat distorted, as the peaks often will be limited by the MPO of the hearing aid (typically an AGCo algorithm).
- Speech may not have the necessary amplitude dynamics, as the peaks will be limited or clipped. Music may sound dull.
- The range of loudness perceptions will be limited—average and loud inputs may only differ by a few decibels following processing.

POINTS TO PONDER: *BEST* PRACTICE VERSUS *REAL* PRACTICE

Starting with the Vanderbilt Report of 1991, all subsequent best practice guidelines have included the recommendation of conducting frequency-specific LDLs as part of the pre-fitting of hearing aids. So is this a common practice? Mueller (2003a) conducted a survey of more than 500 audiologists and Hearing Instrument Specialists who were actively fitting hearing aids and found that 61% routinely conducted pre-fitting LDL measures. Only 27% of these respondents, however, used frequency-specific test signals (speech stimuli was by far the most popular). If we do the math (27 of 61%), we find that only 16% of audiologists or dispensers were conducting pre-fitting LDL testing according to established protocols. That of course was in 2003. Maybe things are different today?

- For some speech-in-noise listening situations (those with a slightly positive SNR), unnecessary MPO limiting could make the SNR more adverse.

Let the Fitting Software Do the Work?

In the next few pages, we present a clinical protocol that easily can be used to measure the frequency-specific LDL, and then these values can be used to set the MPO of the hearing aid for individual patients. Before we do that, however, it is relevant to discuss what is the most common pre-fitting clinical method of deciding the hearing aid's MPO: It is using the decision making function of the manufacturer's software. Depending on the audiologist and the manufacturer, there are several options regarding how this could be handled:

- No LDLs entered into the software; the software selects MPO values based on the average for the patient's hearing thresholds using algorithms from validated prescriptive fitting methods. The two most popular methods are the NAL-NL2 (for National Acoustics Laboratory–Nonlinear 2) and the Desired Sensation Level Version 5 (DSL5.0)—see Chapter 14.
- No LDLs entered into the software; the software selects MPO values based on the average for patient's hearing thresholds using the manufacturer's correction values.
- LDLs entered into the software; the software selects MPO values based on HL to 2-cc corrections using data from validated fitting methods (e.g., DSL5.0). *Note:* The NAL-NL2 does not use measured LDLs for MPO calculations, although it is possible that a given manufacturer could use its own correction factors for setting the MPO in conjunction with the NAL-NL2 algorithm.
- LDLs entered into the software; the software selects MPO values based on the manufacturer's HL to 2-cc coupler corrections.

Could these different approaches result in different MPO settings? Most certainly. When LDLs are not entered, the DSL prescribes different output values than the NAL-NL2. Moreover, it is reported that some manufacturers use the 1988 data of Pascoe, which are nearly 10 dB higher than the average values from Bentler and Cooley (2001) for common hearing losses in the 50 to 60 dB range. Even when LDLs are entered, not all manufacturers have the same philosophy regarding how the MPO should relate to the measured LDL. Should MPO be set exactly at the LDL? Above? Below?

A Comparative Study of MPO. To examine some of these differences, Mueller, Bentler, and Wu (2008) conducted electroacoustic measures (MPO for a 90 dB SPL swept tone) for the premier hearing aid of each of the top six manufacturers. The hearing aids were programmed based on the manufacturers' default settings for a flat 50 dB HL hearing loss. The authors first conducted the fitting without entering LDLs—they found an approximate 20 dB difference in the MPO among instruments.

The authors then entered a 90 dB HL LDL for all test frequencies and reprogrammed the instruments. Again, they found a range of about 20 dB, although the ordering among manufacturers has changed. Some dropped the MPO by 10 dB, but for others no change was present (that is, the entered LDLs were ignored). Given the variability of the MPO selected by the different manufacturers, even when LDLs are entered, it seems reasonable that the prudent audiologist would want to select the MPO themselves, which is what we discuss in the next section.

Administration and Scoring

Although measuring LDLs is usually considered a fairly simple task and can be conducted effectively by a technician, there are two important procedural conditions that, if not followed correctly, will significantly reduce the validity and reliability of the task: the use of loudness anchors and appropriate instructions. In fact, we suspect that when audiologists state, "I don't do LDL testing because the results are just too unreliable," it is probably because these critical components have not been implemented into the test protocol.

Loudness Anchors

Loudness anchors are used to give the patient a reference for the loudness perceptions that he or she will be experiencing. They indicate boundaries and intermediate steps, which facilitate the understanding of the task and improved reliability; the patient has words to attach to a perception. The loudness anchors that we recommend, shown in Figure 5–6, are from Robyn Cox (1995) and were used in the development of the Cox Contour Test, which became part of the hearing aid fitting protocol of the IHAFF (Independent Hearing Aid Fitting Forum; Cox, 1995; Mueller, 1994b). These anchors are an abbreviated form of those used by David Hawkins in much of his LDL research (e.g., Hawkins, Walden, Montgomery, & Prosek, 1987).

Prior to the testing, the patients are familiarized with the loudness anchors and are provided the chart to use during testing. They can respond either by stating the loudness category or by simply giving the number. We prefer to have the chart quite large (e.g., 2′ × 3′), mounted on cardboard, which patients can hold in their lap during testing. They then have the option of pointing to the category rather than calling out the term or the number. (Savvy clinicians have learned to associate the certainty of the judgment with different pointing techniques—a true #7 hits the board with a little more force than an uncertain one.) The pointing technique of course only works if you have the patient positioned in the booth so that you can observe the response. Many audiologists simply have the chart printed on standard size paper and hand it to the patient or have the chart mounted on the test booth wall. However you do it, our main point is—*use the anchors!*

Instructions

Going hand-in-hand with the anchors are the instructions. The measured LDL can vary by 15 to 20 dB simply based on the instructions that are used. Given that we are using the loudness anchors of Cox (1995), it is appropriate to use the instructions that were developed in association with these anchors also. They are provided in Figure 5–7. We have modified Cox's instructions slightly by adding the sentence, "It is okay to repeat a loudness category, and it is okay to skip a category," as we've found that patients sometimes have problems regarding these issues. For example, they give a #6 rating when it really is a #7 because they think they have to say #6 at least once or they immediately go from #4 to #5 because the tone got louder, and they already had said #4 once. Perhaps the most important statement of the instructions is at the end, "... louder than you would ever choose on your radio no matter what mood you are in." What we are looking for is when the sound is *first* uncomfortable. Audiologists who are somewhat haphazard in delivering LDL instructions often say something like, "we want to see what you can tolerate." The difference between uncomfortable and tolerable can be 10 to 20 dB for some patients. We can assure you that when new hearing aid users experience an environmental noise that exceeds their LDL, they do not sit back and say, "Gee, I wonder if I could tolerate that?" Rather, they turn down gain as quickly as possible, which often makes soft speech inaudible. Alternatively, in cases where there is no volume control, the patient may reject the hearing aids completely.

We find it convenient to paste the written instructions on the back of the board that has the loudness anchors on the front. This way you can be reading (yes, reading) the instructions while the patient is looking at the anchors. We cannot overstate the importance of using precise and consistent instructions when the goal is a reliable and valid measure.

Test Procedures

Typically, LDL testing is conducted in the test booth, as that is where the equipment is located, and the patient is already seated and hooked up to earphones for the

---

Loudness Anchors

#7. Uncomfortably Loud

#6. Loud, But Okay

#5. Comfortable, But Slightly Loud

#4. Comfortable

#3. Comfortable, But Slightly Soft

#2. Soft

#1. Very Soft

Figure 5–6. Loudness anchors used for LDL testing. Anchors adapted from those used for the Cox Contour Test (Cox, 1995).

> **LDL Instructions**
>
> THE PURPOSE OF THIS TEST IS TO FIND YOUR JUDGMENTS OF THE LOUDNESS OF DIFFERENT SOUNDS.
>
> YOU WILL HEAR SOUNDS THAT INCREASE AND DECREASE IN VOLUME. YOU MUST MAKE A JUDGMENT ABOUT HOW LOUD THE SOUNDS ARE. PRETEND YOU ARE LISTENING TO THE RADIO AT THAT VOLUME. HOW LOUD WOULD IT BE?
>
> AFTER EACH SOUND, TELL ME WHICH OF THESE CATEGORIES BEST DESCRIBES THE LOUDNESS. IT IS OKAY TO REPEAT A LOUDNESS CATEGORY, AND IT IS OKAY TO SKIP A CATEGORY.
>
> KEEP IN MIND THAT AN UNCOMFORTABLY LOUD SOUND IS LOUDER THAN YOU WOULD EVER CHOOSE ON YOUR RADIO NO MATTER WHAT MOOD YOU ARE IN.

Figure 5–7. Instructions that are read to the patient prior to administering LDL measures. (Modified from Cox, 1995).

diagnostic testing. If the equipment is available in a hearing aid fitting room, there is no reason that earphone LDL testing could not be conducted there instead, as ambient room noise is not an issue. Once the patient is seated, the earphones have been inserted properly (deep fit of foam tip), the patient has the loudness anchors and the instructions have been given, we recommend the following protocol:

- Use pulsed pure tones as test signal and select frequency.
- First, conduct practice run.
- Begin testing at or near the patient's MCL (e.g., 60 to 70 dB HL).
- Present signal and obtain rating (will probably be #4).
- Use ascending approach in 5 dB steps and obtain loudness rating for each subsequent level.
- Stop run at the level that results in the first #7 rating.
- Following the practice run, repeat procedure.
- After again establishing the #7 rating, conduct a second run.
- If the #7 rating of the second run is within 5 dB of the first, average the two and record this as the LDL. If the difference is larger than 5 dB, conduct a third run and average the last two.
- Repeat the procedure for other selected frequencies (practice run no longer necessary).
- Repeat the procedure for the other ear.

An example of calculating LDL is shown in Figure 5–8. In this case, we are using the worksheet from Robyn Cox, which is available at her website (http://www.memphis.edu/csd/harl/index.htm). For this patient, testing started at 500 Hz in the right ear. The first run produced a #7 rating of 90 dB HL. Notice that the #7 rating for the second run was 100 dB, 10 dB above the first, so a third run was conducted. The average of the second and third runs resulted in an average LDL of 98 dB (100 + 95 / 2, and rounded up). For 3000 Hz, the first and second runs resulted in the same value, so it was not necessary to conduct a third run. For the left ear, observe that the lower frequency selected was 1000 Hz rather than 500 Hz—this was because the patient had normal hearing for 500 Hz. (No hearing loss, no gain, no MPO problem.) For both frequencies tested in this ear, the #7 values fell within 5 dB for the two runs.

Notice that on the form shown in Figure 5–8, we have the loudness rating for each presentation level. Although it is interesting to see the loudness growth

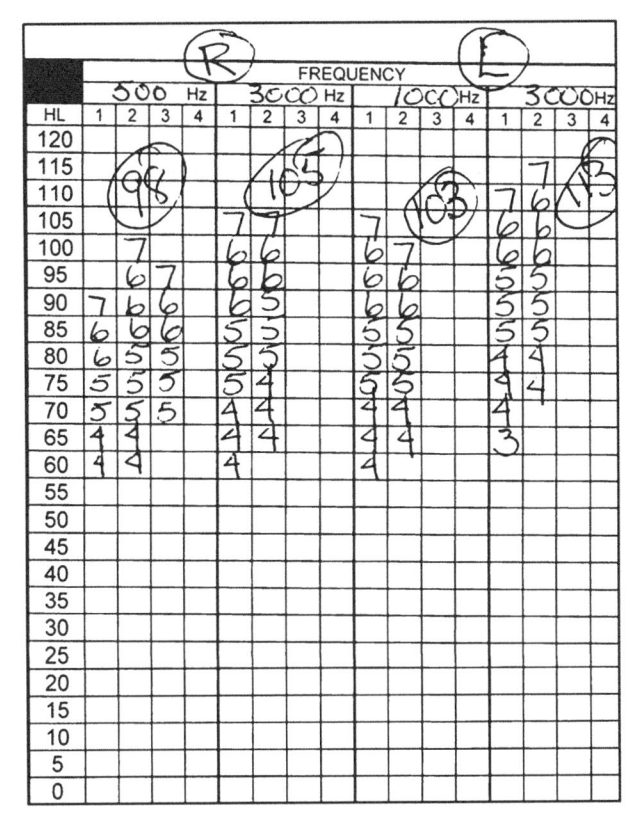

Figure 5–8. Sample score sheet completed by an audiologist while administering LDL measures for 500 and 3000 Hz for the right, and 1000 and 3000 Hz for the left. The numbers that are circled at the top represent average values for the different runs. These average values are then used for setting the hearing aid MPO. The score sheet itself is from the Cox Contour Test.

pattern, you really do not have to record the ratings for anything but #7. Most of us can remember the #7 value of the first run, so all you have to record is the average of the two. If that is all you are going to record, the worksheet is a bit of overkill—you could just record the #7 values on the audiogram, scratch paper, or even a bar napkin, if you like.

So, now that the LDLs are measured and recorded, what happens next? Will this extra effort and time (five minutes or so) result in a better fitting? That comes next.

Clinical Applications

As we discussed earlier, when programming the hearing aids, one option is to enter the measured LDLs into the fitting software. And, as we also discuss, the impact this has on the setting of the hearing aid MPO varies considerably among manufacturers. If you fit most of your patients with hearing aids from a single manufacturer (85% of audiologists do), then it might be worth taking some time and entering different LDLs into the software (e.g., all 80s, all 90s, all 100s) and observe how this influences the MPO settings. Do they change? Do the settings agree with your beliefs? It is possible that the manufacturer(s) that you use will do these calculations correctly. If not, we recommend the procedure outlined below.

> ### TECHNICAL TIP: BILATERAL LDLS FOR BILATERAL FITTINGS?
>
> A common question regarding LDL measures is if it is necessary to conduct bilateral LDLs for a bilateral fitting. On the surface, it would seem that this might be necessary, as we know that usually there are binaural summation effects that can be 6 dB or more at suprathreshold levels. But it is not that simple. First, the binaural loudness summation that can impact listening through hearing aids may not be the same as that experienced with earphone testing or unaided soundfield measures. A partial explanation is that full summation can occur only when the inputs are the same at both ears (and eardrums). That rarely occurs, especially across the frequency range. Second, it seems that summation may be present when the task is a loudness matching paradigm, but when it is couched in loudness discomfort terms, the summation is not observed. This could be related to the improved sound quality of bilateral listening, which may counteract the summation effects that are present (see Mueller and Bright [1994] and Mueller and Hornsby [2002], for review). The fact that bilateral LDLs are essentially the same as unilateral ones is a good thing for both the patient and the audiologist. For the patient, it means that the ceiling of their dynamic range was not reduced, so with bilateral summation effects the overall dynamic range should be expanded. For audiologists, it means that each ear can be treated independently without making alterations when the patient uses bilateral amplification.

Converting to 2-cc Coupler

A continual disconnect in the fitting of hearing aids is that we conduct testing in HL; manufacturers commonly provide hearing aid software referenced to 2-cc coupler levels in SPL, and we verify hearing aids in ear canal SPL. As a result, we are continually converting among the three references. If that makes you feel like you are going in a circle, you might enjoy Larry Revit's article, "Circle of Decibels" (Revit, 1997), which nicely illustrates these relationships (see chapter 16). So for our task at hand, we have LDLs in HL, but we want to program hearing aid MPO for specific frequencies, which are defined in the fitting software in 2-cc coupler SPL. How do we get from HL to the 2-cc coupler levels? Fortunately, this is more common of a correction than you might think, and we have an ANSI standard (S3.6-2004) for making these corrections. These values are referred to as *RETSPLs*. This is an acronym for the Reference Equivalent Threshold in SPL and is pronounced *Rhet-Spull*, in case you are curious. It is the difference between HL and the output in a 2-cc or 6-cc coupler. The reason that this is commonly used is that audiometers are calibrated using RETSPL values. For our discussion here, things work out conveniently because insert earphones, which you used for conducting the LDL measures, are calibrated in a 2-cc coupler, just like hearing aids. If we convert HL values using the RETSPL, it makes it easy to talk to the fitting software, which also is in the language of 2-cc SPL, when adjustments are needed.

As mentioned, RETSPL values for insert earphones are contained in ANSI Standard S3.6-2010, and these values are shown in Table 5–2. Note that the values are somewhat different for the two types of 2-cc couplers commonly used with hearing aids (HA1 and HA2) although except for 4000 Hz and 6000 Hz, these differences are small. For our example here, we will use the HA1 coupler values (the coupler type commonly used with custom hearing aids such as ITEs). These are mostly positive numbers, which means that they are added to the HL values to convert to 2-cc. Refer back to our LDL testing shown in Figure 5–8. Note that the LDL for 500 Hz was 98 dB, and the LDL for 3000 Hz was 105. Using the corresponding RETSPLs from Table 5–2, we would then do the following corrections:

For 500 Hz: 98 + 6.0 = 104 dB (re: 2-cc coupler)

For 3000 Hz: 105 + 2.5 = 107.5 (108) dB (re: 2-cc coupler)

This little bit of simple math gives us the values that we need to go into the fitting software and make the necessary adjustments for this patient.

Software Adjustments

All manufacturers have methods to adjust the MPO in their fitting software; in most cases this can be accomplished relatively independently of gain for soft, aver-

---

TECHNICAL TIP: THINKING ABOUT THE RETSPL

One of our favorite quiz questions for audiology students or interns is to ask them to describe the expected differences in the RETSPL for infants versus adults. We have had some interesting answers over the years. The point of course, is that RETSPLs are *device* specific, not *people* specific. You use the same RETSPL corrections for big ears and tiny ears. In contrast, Real-Ear Coupler Differences (RECDs) are *ear* specific.

Table 5–2. Reference Equivalent Threshold values in SPL (RETSPL) for Insert Earphones from ANSI S3.6-2004

	250	500	1K	1.5K	2K	3K	4K	6K
3A/5A insert (HA-1)	14.5	6.0	0.0	0.0	2.5	2.5	0.0	−2.5
3A/5A insert (HA-2)	14.0	5.5	0.0	2.0	3.0	3.5	5.5	2.0

age, and loud(er) input levels. As a consequence, it is preferable to adjust the gain and low threshold compression parameters so that loud speech is loud but okay, and then use the MPO adjustment to assure that loud environmental noises do not exceed the LDL. Rather than having default controls for gain and compression parameters, most modern hearing aids have separate handles (sometimes within each compression channel) to control gain for soft, average, and loud input levels, in addition to MPO control and sometimes control of gain for even more input levels. That is, there are different controls for different purposes. These controls attempt to directly affect gain and output as a function of input, but the exact gain, compression, and limiting algorithms manipulated to do this are often kept out of view. When AGCo compression is used to limit the hearing aid output, the compression ratios are usually 10:1 or greater, so the AGCo kneepoint and the MPO value tend to be essentially the same. It is also possible to implement lower threshold compression using smaller compression ratios and then use peak clipping to limit the output, but that approach is seldom used.

We encourage you to work through this MPO adjustment process with the software from your favorite manufacturer, but we have given you an example here. One thing that fortunately has changed in recent years is that we now have the capability of setting the MPO independently for many different channels. It was not too long ago that the MPO was adjusted in hearing aids using a single-channel output limiter, commonly implemented using AGCo, meaning that you had to pick one value, which usually was driven by the real-ear peak of the response, set the MPO to this value, and then let the MPOs at all the other frequencies fall where they may. Single channel limiting, in an effort to set the MPO low enough for one specific frequency, often meant unnecessarily reducing headroom for many others. By comparison, in the example that we have here, this product has 16 adjustment possibilities for 16 channels of AGCo—enough MPO software adjustment capability to satisfy even the most fastidious audiologist.

Figure 5–9 illustrates the MPO adjustment screen from one manufacturer. Note that there are 16 channels and the bottom values in the chart represent the MPO settings. In the software, this display is accompanied by a graph of the output, which we are not showing due to space limitations. Going back to our earlier calculations, we would simply go to the 500 Hz tab and set the MPO, currently set at 105 dB, to 104 dB—for 1 dB it may not be worth the effort. In some low-power instruments, the output at 500 Hz might not go to 104 dB, which in this case we would simply set it as high as it goes. We would then go to 3000 Hz and set this MPO (currently set at 116 dB) to 108 dB. Then, using basic interpolation, we would set all the other intermediate channels to correspond to these values accordingly (e.g., increasing gradually from 104 to 113 dB).

Although these types of adjustments might seem a little confusing the first few times, they quickly become routine. And we have to believe that you and your patient will be in a better place than if you had randomly picked a value within a range of 50 to 60 dB (shown in Figure 5–5).

FAQs about LDL Measures

Once audiologists begin conducting LDLs routinely, there tend to be a lot of clinical questions, so we thought we'd end this section with some FAQs.

200	500	1K	1.5	2K	2.5	3K	3.5	4K	4.5	5K	5.5	6K	6.5	7K	7.5	ALL
-7	-7	2	2	7	12	14	12	10	8	8	2	-1	-3	-4	-6	Loud
3	3	12	12	17	21	23	22	20	18	16	10	7	4	0	-4	Moderate
13	13	20	20	24	30	32	30	27	24	22	16	13	9	5	1	Soft
98	105	111	111	114	114	116	116	112	109	107	103	101	100	99	98	MPO

Figure 5–9. Screenshot from the software of a major manufacturer illustrating the selection of frequency-specific MPO across several channels. MPO values are displayed in the bottom row.

How Many Frequencies to Test?

Although the "more is better" adage usually applies, we do need to be practical: How much information is really needed to make a good clinical judgment? There is no reason to waste time in a busy clinic conducting LDLs at unnecessary frequencies when that time could be spent conducting other pre-fitting measures or patient counseling. Two frequencies per ear usually are enough, although for some configurations, three probably work a little better. Fortunately, most hearing aids today have multichannel MPO control, but if you are fitting a hearing aid with only single-channel control of output, then one frequency is probably enough. It is hoped you pick the right one—as you will not be able to shape the output signal anyway.

What Are the Best Frequencies to Test?

It would be nice if we could simply give you two frequencies to test and that was all you had to remember. It is not that simple, as the best LDL frequencies change from patient to patient. Here are some general rules to remember:

- If the patient has a relatively flat or gradually downward sloping hearing loss across all frequencies, we recommend conducting LDL measures at 500 or 1000 Hz and 3000 Hz (and Bentler & Nelson, 2001, showed 750 Hz and 3000 Hz to be most predictive of broadband/real-world LDLs). If the hearing loss is not changing significantly frequency to frequency, we certainly would not expect that the LDLs would either. Hence, if you have one value at 500 Hz and one at 3000 Hz, you could set the MPO at the intermediate frequencies by interpolation.
- Many patients have normal hearing in the lower frequencies. If it is obvious that you will not be applying gain for 500 Hz, or applying very little gain, then there is no reason to conduct LDLs for this frequency, as the MPO setting will not impact the fitting. If the patient has normal hearing at 1000 Hz? Then the same logic applies for this frequency.
- As we discuss in a later section of this chapter relating to cochlear dead regions, some patients have downward sloping hearing losses where the extent of the loss makes it very unlikely that we can obtain aided audibility using traditional amplification (e.g., loss of approximately 90 dB or greater). In this case, we might decide to give up on chasing this frequency and even roll off gain to help prevent feedback. So again, if we are not planning to apply gain, then there is no reason to conduct LDLs at this frequency.
- To summarize our points, although we often will conduct LDLs for the two frequencies of 500 and 3000 Hz to obtain loudness anchors for the corners of the fitting range, let's take a patient with normal hearing through 1000 Hz, dropping to a 30 dB loss at 1500 Hz, down to 60 dB at 2000 Hz, and then 90 dB thresholds at 3000 and 4000 Hz. Although not a common audiogram for a hearing aid fitting (fortunately), we do see audiograms like this. So what are the LDL testing rules for this patient? Well, if the lows are normal and we are not going to chase the highs, then in this case we would do LDL testing at 1500 and 2000 Hz, as this is the frequency region where a correct setting of the MPO will most probably determine the success of the fitting.

Several Audiologists Use Speech Signals, Such as Spondee Words to Obtain LDLs: Is This an Acceptable Substitute for Pulsed Tones?

In a word, no. The reason for conducting earphone LDLs is to determine the values for setting *frequency-specific* MPO values—the level at which output is limited. Consider this example—your Monday morning patient being fitted for hearing aids has a gradually downward sloping hearing loss ranging from 30 dB in the lows to 75 dB at 4000 Hz. You do speech LDLs and obtain values of 95 dB bilaterally? How do you convert this HL value to 2-cc coupler so you can talk to the software? How do you use this number to set the AGCo kneepoint at 1000 Hz? At 3000 Hz? At any frequency? We are aware that there are some state dispensing laws that specify that speech material be used for LDL measures. We have no explanation for why this would be the preferred method.

For Patient Flow Purposes, When Is the Best Time to Conduct LDLs?

If you have worked in a busy clinic, you know that what is time-consuming for most audiometric testing is often not the test itself, it is things like finding a booth that is free, getting the patient back to the booth, listening to the patient's stories about their grandchildren, getting the inserts to fit deeply enough, and so on. For this reason, we recommend conducting LDL testing at the same time that the routine audiogram is conducted. The patient is already seated, they just had some practice listening to pulsed tones, and now all you have to do is go in the room, hand them the loudness chart, and explain the test procedure. Granted, at this point you do not know if the patient will decide to purchase hearing aids and you indeed will end up conducting testing for many patients who do not, but it still will increase your efficiency in the long run. Moreover, even if the patient does not return for hearing aids for a year or so, if a check of audiometric thresholds at that time reveals that thresholds have not changed, there is a good chance LDLs are the same too and your testing will already be completed.

Why Use Pure Tones for Testing? The Patients Do Not Hear Pure Tones in the Real World

We partially already answered this earlier when we explained that we somehow have to talk the language of the fitting software, which uses values based on 2-cc coupler, pure-tone measures. It is true that listeners do not normally hear pure tones in their daily environment, but they do hear narrowband signals that drive the output of the hearing to a level nearly as high (shrill dog bark, baby crying, clattering of dishes). Our goal is to prepare the patient for a worst case situation. Moreover, recall that we recommend setting the hearing aid to the #7 rating, which in fact is uncomfortable. We could use #6, which is typically 3 to 5 dB lower, but because the hearing aid is seldom driven to the output produced by a pure tone, we have a cushion of a few dB—and the #7 rating from pure-tone testing seems to work pretty well in the real world. This was supported by the work of Bratt, Rosenfeld, Poek, Kang, Williams, and Larson (2002) and Munro and Patel (1998). And of course, before the patient ever leaves the clinic, we will conduct aided LDL testing using loud speech and obnoxious environmental noises (see Chapter 15), so we should always be okay.

Is It Okay to Use a Warble Tone or Narrowband Noise as the Stimulus?

This is a common question and the short answer is that it probably does not matter. But, we wonder, why you would want to use these stimuli? Given that pulsed pure tones work well for audiometric thresholds and that the patient has just had practice listening to these signals during the audiometric threshold measurements, it seems logical to use these signals for LDL testing too. Why introduce a new signal that could possibly confuse the patient?

Are the Results of LDL Testing Reliable?

The reliability certainly is adequate for clinical measures. This has been studied quite extensively with similar findings among researchers—test/retest variability is around 3 to 4 dB, not much worse than for pure-tone thresholds (Hawkins, Walden, Montgomery, & Prosek, 1987; Ricketts & Bentler, 1996). The variability will be somewhat influenced by the test procedure employed. Palmer and Lindley (1998) used a LDL test protocol very similar to what we recommended earlier (an ascending method using the Cox Seven-Point Contour Anchors and Cox instructions). They reported a mean test-retest difference of 2.6 dB across five test frequencies for the #7 (uncomfortably loud) anchor rating; 94% of the test-retest differences were less than 10 dB. Related to this question, we might mention that there also does not appear to be a learning effect for the task—repeat measures days or weeks after the initial testing have not shown large differences (Cox, Alexander, Taylor, & Gray, 1997; Palmer & Lindley, 1998).

What if the Patient's LDLs Are Above the Limits of the Audiometer?

With TDH earphones the upper limit of most audiometers is 120 dB HL, which is probably loud enough (although Bentler and Cooley, 2001, appear to have gone to 130 dB in their data collection.) But with insert earphones the maximum output usually drops to 110 dB or even lower. Assuming that most audiologists are using insert phones, this can be somewhat of a problem. First, however, if the patient's LDL is greater than 110 dB HL, then you already know that this is not a "sound sensitive" individual, so the exact hearing aid MPO setting is probably not as critical as for someone who is. If you are getting #6 ratings (Cox Anchors) for 110 dB, then it's fairly safe to assume that the LDL is around 115 dB; usually we see a 5 dB or so difference between the #6 rating and the patient's LDL (#7 rating). Or as an alternative, for these patients you could use the predictive algorithm for MPO from your prescriptive fitting method (e.g. the NAL-NL2). And of course, you will still have your aided verification ahead of you to do the final tweaking of the AGCo kneepoints.

Does the Patient's LDL Go Up After Hearing Aid Use?

This is a reasonable question because, if it did, it would be necessary to reassess LDLs periodically after the hearing aid fitting and then readjust the MPO settings accordingly. At one time (e.g., 1940s), researchers actually suggested *tolerance training* to expand the useable dynamic range. Tolerance training is not part of our fitting practices today—at least it is not conducted intentionally.

Research that has examined LDLs after hearing aid use has sometimes noted a slight increase, but there does not seem to be a significant change in loudness perceptions (e.g., Bentler, Niebuhr, Getta, & Anderson, 1993b; Hamilton & Munro, 2010; Lindley, Palmer, Durrant, & Pratt, 2000). These studies, however, did not purposely expose patients to outputs above their LDLs but rather initially fit the hearing aids with output corresponding with the patient's unaided loudness ratings. Similarly, Bratt et al. (2002) followed potential changes in LDLs over a nine-month period following the fitting of hearing aids for 360 patients and noted an average increase of the LDL of only 1 to 3 dB across the five frequencies observed (500, 1000, 2000, 3000, and 4000 Hz).

An interesting exception to all this regarding plasticity for loudness discomfort was reported by Hamilton and Munro (2010). They compared LDLs for individuals fitted bilaterally with those of patients who were fitted unilaterally; both groups had similar symmetric hearing losses. The LDLs for the group aided bilaterally were symmetrical. They found that for the patients fitted unilaterally, there was a significant interaural asymmetry of 3 to 5 dB, with higher LDLs in the fitted ear and lower LDLs in the not-fitted ear. They suggest that changes in the LDL may be a feature of asymmetric sensory input and are consistent with a central gain mechanism.

If the Patient Has a Conductive Loss, or a Large Air-Bone Gap, Is It Still Necessary to Conduct LDL Testing?

In general, we would expect that LDLs would be elevated at about a 1:1 factor of the conductive component. Known to be precise, Harvey Dillon suggests it is actually 87.5% of the conductive component. This means that if the patient has a 60 dB loss with a 30 dB conductive component, and we use average LDL values for cochlear pathology, it is probable that the LDL is 125 dB or greater—beyond the limits of the earphones. So, in many cases testing probably is not necessary. However, (see Figure 5–5) note that some patients with a 60 dB cochlear loss have LDLs around 90 dB. If again we add the effects of the conductive component (90 + [.875 × 30]), we will have a desired MPO of around 117 dB. For this patient, you will want to adjust the hearing aid output accordingly. Given the minimal time it takes to conduct a quick LDL check, it might be worthwhile even when a conductive loss or conductive component is present.

For Open-Canal Fittings, Do the Same Rules Apply for Setting the MPO?

Good question. We talk about that in Chapter 17, but it is good to discuss it here too. It gets a little complicated, but stick with us (see Mueller & Ricketts, 2006, for detailed review). The technique we provided earlier for converting LDLs to 2-cc coupler and then adjusting the MPO is based on the assumption that the patient has an average real-ear coupler difference (RECD). If your patient truly has an open fitting, the RECD is much smaller (remember Boyle's Law), which will *reduce* the ear canal SPL. But, on the other hand, the patient may retain all or most of the open ear resonances, which will *increase* the ear canal SPL. For patients who have average or larger-than-average resonances, this will outweigh the RECD reduction; the net effect is that the real-ear MPO will be greater with an open fitting (in the 2000 to 4000 Hz range) than with a closed fitting. You may have to set the hearing aid MPO *lower* for this frequency range for an open fitting. It is also possible that the sound going through the open canal and striking the ear drum directly will be greater than the output of the hearing aid. This of course is why we also check aided loudness during the verification process.

Why Is It Necessary to Conduct Pre-Fitting LDLs if Aided LDLs Are Assessed at the Time of the Fitting?

We certainly recommended aided loudness verification; we discuss a protocol for this in Chapters 15 and 17. And it is true that a good verification protocol could take care of many fitting mistakes that result when pre-fitting LDL testing is not conducted. There is one factor, however, that must be considered. With some fitting algorithms, such as the DSL 5.0, the LDL that is entered into the software is not just used for selecting the maximum output. It also is used in the calculations of desired gain for soft, average, and loud speech inputs. Here is a simple example to make this point. Consider a patient with a 50 dB loss who has LDLs of 110 dB—a fairly common finding. This patient has a 60 dB dynamic range. Now, what if this patient with a 50 dB hearing loss had LDLs of 90 dB—also a common finding? A 40 dB dynamic range. In general, for patients with the same hearing loss, when the dynamic range becomes smaller, the patient's preferred listening level for average speech falls at a less intense level. Some fitting algorithms, therefore, provide different fitting targets for the same hearing loss for a 40 dB versus a 60 dB dynamic range. If you wait until the verification stage, and then find out that the patient's LDLs are not what you had predicted, you may not only have to change the maximum output, but also may need to go back and change the gain for soft and average. This is why it makes sense to us to include the patient's LDLs up front so that these values can be used in the initial programming prior to verification.

It Seems That Older People Are More Bothered by Loud Noise; Isn't This Related to Lower LDLs for This Group?

First, we already mentioned earlier that Bentler and Cooley (2001) found no effect of age in their large sample of nearly 2000 LDLs. However, *bothered by loud noise* is somewhat different from the perception of uncomfortably loud. We can, however, look at the aversiveness scale of the APHAB (described in detail in Chapter 7). The norms for this scale include aversiveness results for both young normal hearing and elderly with few or no hearing problems. If we examine the percentage of problems for the two groups, the percentile distributions are very similar. If anything, the elderly are less bothered by loud noises—the 50th percentile for the young listeners is 20% problems, whereas for elderly listeners the 50th percentile is 10%. These were people, however, with normal or near-normal hearing. But in general, data to date does not support setting the hearing aid MPO any differently for the elderly than for younger adults when both groups have the same LDLs.

What if Some Patients Simply Don't Understand the Task?

This does happen on occasion. The tip-off usually is when you raise the intensity of the tone by 5 dB, and the patient calls out a number lower than what they had rated the previous softer signal. We usually try reinstructing and give it one more shot. If problems still occur, we then just predict the MPO from the pure tones using an approach such as that used by the NAL-NL2. In a typical clinic, we'd estimate that 90 to 95% of the patients understand the LDL task well enough to provide valid and reliable responses.

At What Point Do Low LDLs Mean the Patient Has Hyperacusis?

There has been a lot of talk about *hyperacusis* in recent years and, indeed, individuals suffering from this under-researched condition do have lower-than-average LDLs. You've probably also heard terms related to hyperacusis such as phonophobia, misophonia, and selective sound sensitivity syndrome, known as 4S (see Hall, 2013 for review). Given that it's sometimes difficult to differentiate these disorders, we'll refer to the general condition as "decreased sound tolerance" (DST).

For the most part, the patient with DST is a different type of patient from those we have been talking about here. DST is not related to cochlear disorders; in fact, the typical patient with this disorder has normal hearing. In some instances, the term hyperacusis has been inappropriately applied; a patient who simply has LDLs somewhat lower than average is labeled hyperacusic. A comprehensive review of this pathology was provided by Baguley (2003), and in this review he gives the following definition for hyperacusis:

Hyperacusis has been defined as "unusual tolerance to ordinary environmental sounds" and, more pejoratively, as "consistently exaggerated or inappropriate responses to sounds that are neither threatening nor uncomfortably loud to a typical person." (p. 582)

These are patients that often will not leave the house because of the fear that a loud sound may occur. These are not the typical patients you see for hearing aid fittings who happen to have LDLs 10 to 20 dB or so below average.

A Final Message

At some point in the fitting process, we have to get the MPO set correctly. You probably have heard the old adage, "There's never enough time to do it right, but there is always enough time to do it again."

We believe that taking a few minutes to conduct earphone LDLs will pay off in streamlining the adjustments on the day of the fitting. True, we also recommend aided loudness verification and, yes, one could wait until then to set the MPO, but the process will be much simpler if the hearing aids already are at or near the desired levels. Moreover, for some fitting algorithms, the patient's LDL impacts gain for soft, average, and loud, so if you do not have it right from the beginning, you are more or less starting over with all the hearing aid programming.

Real-Ear Coupler Difference (RECD)

Many of you already have heard of how the RECD applies to the fitting of hearing aids for children, and certainly that is the primary application. There are some compelling reasons, however, why we might want to consider greater use of the RECD when fitting hearing aids to adults.

1662: It Was a Very Good Year

We start this section with a word about Robert Boyle (1627–1691), a 17th-century philosopher, chemist, and physicist. In the world of audiology, he is best known for describing what is now referred to as Boyle's Law, which was published in 1662.

Boyle's Law: This principle states that the absolute pressure and volume of a given mass of confined gas (air) are inversely proportional, if the temperature remains unchanged within a closed system. That is, if the volume of the closed space becomes smaller, the pressure (i.e., SPL) becomes proportionally greater; if the volume becomes larger, the pressure becomes smaller.

If we now relate this to the residual volume of the ear canal when an earphone tip, earmold, or hearing aid is in place, consider that if we reduce the volume by one-half—the tip is placed deeper in the ear canal, or the patient's ear canal is only one-half as large as average—then the sound pressure within this volume will double. A doubling of sound pressure corresponds to an increase of 6 dB.

Here is one example of the application: A couple in their seventies went to the audiology clinic to have their hearing tested. Bob was a big burly guy with large ear canals. His wife Mary was petite with small ear canals. When the testing was completed, it showed that they both had bilateral downward sloping losses, and the audiologist observed that both Bob and Mary had a 50 dB loss at 2000 Hz in their right ear. Because Bob had a large ear canal residual volume following the placement of the insert earphone tip, when the audiometer dial read 50 dB HL the output at his eardrum (what he *heard*) was 55 dB SPL. Because Mary had a small ear canal and a small ear canal residual volume, the output at her eardrum when the dial was set to 50 dB was 65 dB SPL. So Mary's hearing really was 10 dB worse than Bob's at 2000 Hz. But when Bob and Mary are fitted with hearing aids, will this 10 dB be taken into account or will the audiologist simply enter 50 dB into the fitting software for both of them? Should it be taken into account?

Background

Few clinicians measure an adult patient's RECD in clinical practice. But, it actually could improve the fitting by providing a more accurate estimate of hearing threshold for calculation of real ear gain and output targets. As the name suggests, the RECD is the difference between the output of a signal in the real ear versus the output of the same signal in a 2-cc coupler. Because the residual volume of the real ear with an insert earphone or hearing aid/earmold in place is nearly always less than 2 cc, the RECD value is usually a positive number (i.e., output in the ear canal exceeds the output in the coupler). As would then be expected, infants and children have larger RECDs than adults, as the residual volume is even more different than 2 cc. Because the RECDs for infants and children are less predictable, reliable Real-Ear Aided Response (REAR) measures used in hearing aid fittings are more difficult to obtain in children, and because these patients are not able to provide extensive subjective reports regarding the hearing aid fitting, RECDs are an important part of the fitting process with this population. Several studies have collected RECD data from individuals of different ages, and provided average findings. Table 5–3 shows one example taken from the DSL5.0 (based on foam-tip inserts and the HA2 coupler). Importantl,y however, these data pre-date the current standard RECD method that we describe below.

The primary clinical application of the RECD in children and difficult to assess adults is to use this value to predict ear canal output, which may be difficult to measure, based on the hearing aid's 2-cc coupler output, which is easy to measure. For example, if we know that a hearing aid has a maximum output of 112 dB SPL in the 2-cc coupler at 2000 Hz and the patient's RECD is 8 dB at 2000 Hz, then we would predict that the MPO in the ear canal would be 120 dB SPL (112 dB + 8 dB). Or, if you knew you wanted the output in the ear canal to be any given value, then the RECD can be applied (in this case, subtracted from the 2-cc coupler), so that the hearing aid is programmed to the corresponding desired values. This application can be used for setting both the input level-specific gain and the maximum power output (e.g., AGCo kneepoints). In other words, if RECD values are known, the hearing aid can be accurately fitted to real-ear target values in the 2-cc coupler test box.

RECD Applications for Adults

As we have mentioned, the RECD is commonly used with infants and toddlers to predict real-ear SPL when conventional probe microphone measures for verification are not feasible. But why have we included the RECD as a pre-fitting test for adults? We talked about the RETSPL in the previous LDL section, but to help explain why the *individual* (rather than average) RECD might be useful for fitting adult patients, it is necessary to introduce another term, the REDD.

REDD: This acronym is the Real-Ear Dial Difference. As the name indicates, it is the difference between the intensity setting in HL on the audiometer dial and the output in the ear canal. It is composed of the RETSPL, which takes us from the audiometer HL to the 2-cc coupler, and the RECD, which takes us from the 2-cc coupler to the real ear. If you like formulas: REDD = RECD + RETSPL. The REDD also can be assessed directly by using probe microphone

Table 5–3. A Sampling of Age-Related Foam-Tip HA-2 RECD Values

Age/Freq	250	500	750	1000	1500	2000	3000	4000	6000
1 month	3	8	9	12	15	15	16	20	23
12 months	3	6	8	10	10	11	11	15	17
24 months	3	5	7	9	9	10	10	14	15
36 months	3	5	7	9	8	9	9	13	14
60 months	3	5	7	9	7	8	8	13	13
8 yrs–Adult	3	4	6	8	7	7	8	13	13

Note. Values are from DSL 5.0 but differ from DSL in that values from 119 months have been used for ages>119 months. DSL 5.0 RECDs differ from DSL 4.1 RECDs.

Source: Adapted from Audioscan Verifit User Manual.

equipment to measure the ear canal SPL when a pure tone is presented from the audiometer. The primary use of this correction factor is related to the probe microphone verification of hearing aid performance. For example, if we know a patient's HL threshold is 50 dB at 3000 Hz, the RETSPL for 3000 Hz is 3 dB, and the patient's RECD is 8 dB at 3000 Hz (which would then give us an REDD of 11 dB), then we would calculate that the patient's threshold in ear canal SPL would be 61 dB for 3000 Hz (50 + 11 dB).

When we conduct REAR measures such as *speech mapping* with our probe microphone equipment, the patient's thresholds and the LDLs are converted to ear canal SPL from the HL values using the REDD. It is common to use the average REDD for this conversion, which includes the average RECD—recall that RETSPLs are not patient specific. The converted thresholds shown on the screen are then often used to determine whether soft sounds have been made audible, and if average speech is matching prescriptive targets, which have been derived from these average values. The converted LDLs are used to determine whether the MPO of the hearing aid falls into the appropriate region. Consider, however, that if the patient's RECD differs significantly from average, the on-screen ear canal SPL plots will not be correct and, potentially, what might appear as a good fitting might not be as good as it appears.

RECD Variability

It is important to consider what variability might exist in adult RECDs and how this variability might affect hearing aid fittings. One of the first studies on this topic was published by Valente, Potts, Valente, Vass, and Goebel (1994). Part of the design of the study was to compare supra-aural (TDH39) earphones with insert earphones (ER3A). Given that today insert earphones are routinely used, we only refer to these results, displayed in Table 5–4. These data are from 50 adult ears; a 90 dB HL pure-tone signal at the frequencies shown was the input stimulus. The mean values are the resulting output ear canal SPLs that were measured (top line on Table 5–4); the difference between these values and 90 dB would be the mean REDD. For the present discussion, however, our interest is not so much with the absolute REDD but rather in the variability, shown by the standard deviations and the range for each frequency. Notice that for the key frequencies of 2000 to 4000 Hz, standard deviations are 4.0 to 5.6 dB, with ranges of 20 to 29 dB. If we look at 3000 Hz, where the range is the largest at 29 dB, in practical terms this means that for two different patients with the same hearing loss expressed in HL, their true hearing loss may differ by this amount. Obviously, this could affect prescribed gain and output. Also, consider that this was a research study where the earphone foam tip was carefully placed at a controlled depth. Everyday clinical differences could be even larger.

The largest database for adult RECDs was reported by Saunders and Morgan (2003). Their work included 1,814 ears of 904 subjects; 69% were male. They report RECD standard deviations of 3.1 dB for 1000 Hz, 3.5 dB for 2000 Hz, and 5.4 dB for 4000 Hz. The range between the 5th and 95th percentiles was roughly 10 to 17 dB between 1000 and 4000 Hz, increasing as a function of the frequency tested. Mueller, Ricketts and Bentler (2014) review how these differences could influence fitting to prescriptive target.

Table 5–4. Mean and Output Range of 90 dB HL Input Signal Measured in the Ear Canal of 50 Adults

	ER-3A Earphones					
Frequency	500 Hz	1000 Hz	1500 Hz	2000 Hz	3000 Hz	4000 Hz
Mean	88.9	92.9	96.3	99.5	92.6	88.7
SD	5.8	2.9	4.3	5.6	4.0	5.6
Range	23.0	12.0	21.0	29.0	20.0	25.0

Note. Real-ear SPL values shown were obtained using 90 db HL input signal. Mean REDDs can be calculated by subtracting 90 dB from the mean output values shown in the top line.

Source: Adapted from Valente et al., 1994.

> ### KEY CONCEPT: AUDIOGRAM INTERPRETATION FOR YOUNG CHILDREN
>
> Our discussion here has centered on the effects that ear canal acoustics can have on interpreting the standard audiogram with adults. It is also important to remember this concept when viewing serial audiograms for young children that have been obtained over several years. Consider a child whose true hearing thresholds have not changed. As the young child's ear canal becomes larger when they grow, the residual ear canal cavity for the insert earphone also will become larger. This means that it will require more SPL to reach the child's threshold. This in turn will result in a higher HL value, which when recorded on the audiogram will give the appearance that hearing thresholds have become worse, when in fact they have not.

Methods to Measure the RECD

As we have stated, calculating the RECD involves two measurements: the output of a test signal in a 2-cc coupler and in the real ear. Although this sounds rather straightforward, there are many variations possible for this measurement, which can lead to different RECDs. These differences could be as large as 10 dB or more between certain test protocols. In Chapters 16 and 17, we provide some step-by-step guidelines regarding the measurement of the RECD, but some of the issues to consider follow:

- Not only is the RECD dependent on the individual ear residual volume, it also is dependent on the acoustic impedance of the sound source, the coupling system, and the coupler that is used.
- The transducer for the RECD can be an insert earphone attached to an audiometer or a probe microphone system, or a special-purpose transducer developed for RECD measures.
- Some have suggested that a hearing aid be used for the transducer (e.g., Munro & Millward, 2006), but the settings of compression and other algorithms of this hearing aid then introduce a new set of variables.
- The transducer used for the RECD measurement can be coupled to the ear using a special-purpose eartip, a foam eartip, or the patient's own custom earmold.
- Both the HA1 and the HA2 coupler have been used as the 2-cc reference, which also introduces differences. Measurements are referenced to the HA-1 coupler in the current standard, however, and the effect of the acoustics of the coupling system has been removed.
- Although traditionally the real-ear output is measured using conventional probe microphone measures, in recent years two hearing aid manufacturers have introduced a hearing aid equipped with a probe tube that can then generate the test signal *and* measure it in the real ear, eliminating the need for probe microphone equipment (assuming these measures are reliable and valid). This in situ testing is discussed in more detail later in this chapter.

As illustrated from the above review, the measurement of the RECD is not a simple straightforward matter. This is why you will see different RECD values published and why it has been difficult to settle on a standard for RECD measures. The latest ANSI standard for real ear measurement (S3.46-2013) is the first in North America to standardize the RECD. This standard states that the coupler must be the HA1, the test signal must come from a high-impedance source transducer, and the same earpiece (either a foam tip or an earmold) must be used for both the ear measurement and the coupler measurement. We will go into details on this in Chapter 16—also see Scollie (2016) for review.

Clinical Applications

As we have discussed, RECDs often are used to predict real-ear hearing aid output when traditional probe microphone measures are not feasible. When this is the purpose of the RECD, all the measurement variables we just mentioned must be carefully considered. Presently, however, we only are concerned with using the RECD for making appropriate corrections of the audiogram and the LDLs when going from HL to ear canal SPL. The measurement of the RECD requires probe microphone equipment, and each manufacturer has some equipment-specific procedures. We suggest you follow their user's manual: Each manufacturer provides an easy-to-follow, step-by-step protocol, which we will discuss in more detail in Chapter 17.

An example of the probe microphone (probe-mic) RECD measure using an insert earphone is displayed in Figure 5–10. What we see at the top of the screen is the real-ear output with the coupler response below it. This particular equipment then automatically subtracts these two values and what you see on the bottom of the screen is the resulting RECD. The average RECD also is displayed, indicating that this patient's RECD is 3 to 5 dB larger than average. The RECD shown here has the general appearance of what you would expect to see, but an RECD doesn't always look this "predictable." There are a couple of things to troubleshoot when things don't look quite right:

- A negative RECD in the lower frequencies often means a poor seal.
- A negative RECD in the higher frequency suggests a plugged or poorly placed probe tip.

Applying the Measured RECD

Once the RECD has been measured, it now can be applied as a correction in fitting software and in your probe-mic equipment. To illustrate specifically how this can affect a fitting, we conducted probe-mic speech mapping with a hearing aid programmed to provide appropriate audibility for soft speech. Shown in Figure 5–11, Panel A, is the aided soft speech output (55 dB SPL input; LTASS for the male talker of Audioscan Verifit). This display is based on average RECD values for this patient. Observe that the average of soft speech (the dark line in the speech spectrum) falls about 5 dB above the patient's threshold. This patient, however, had a RECD somewhat larger than average, fairly similar to that shown in Figure 5–10, so we entered these values into the probe microphone software to recalculate the REDD, which in turn changes the ear canal SPL plotting of the audiogram and the LDLs. The results of this adjustment are displayed in Figure 5–11, Panel B. We need to emphasize that the output of the hearing aid is the same, but now the average of the soft speech signal is barely above the hearing thresholds.

The data shown in Figure 5–11 provide just one illustration of how these RECD measures can improve the accuracy of the fitting. This is a pretest that probably is best accomplished on the day of the fitting, just before probe microphone verification begins. Recall that the objective here is to provide a more precise evaluation regarding the patient's thresholds and the ear canal SPL generated by the hearing aid. In Chapter 17, we discuss

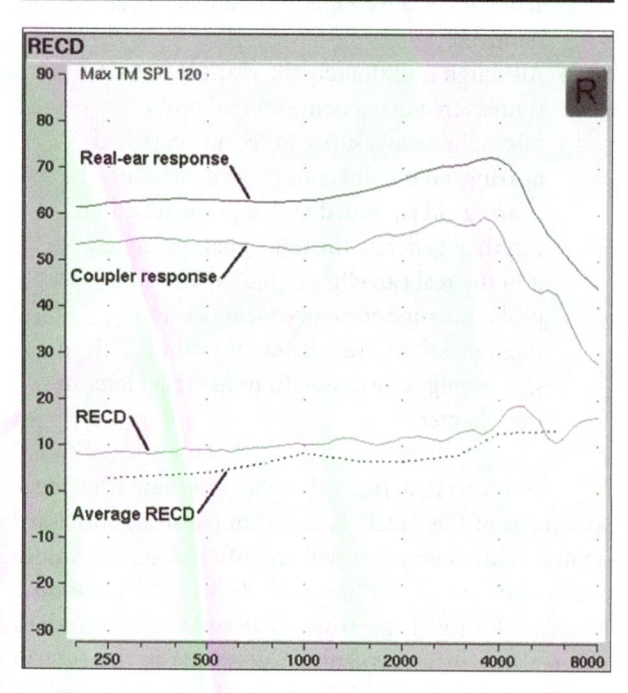

Figure 5–10. Upper portion of the chart shows the absolute values for the input signal measured in a 2-cc coupler compared with the real ear. The lower part of the chart shows the calculated difference between the two upper curves—the patient's RECD—compared with the average RECD.

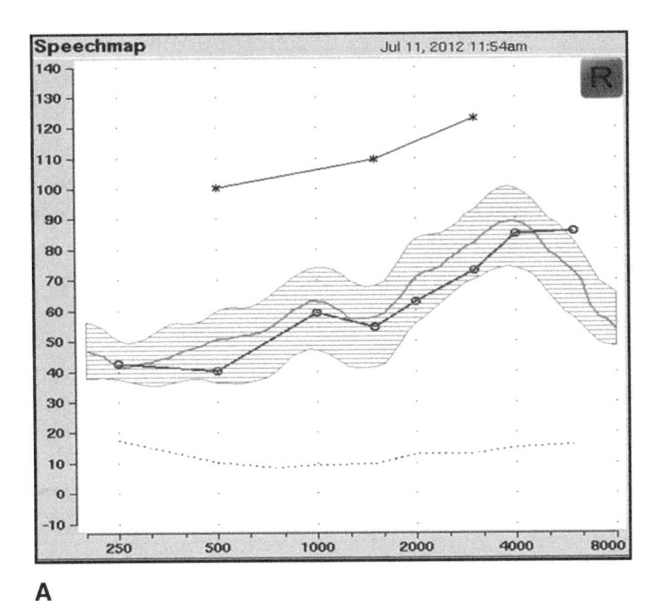

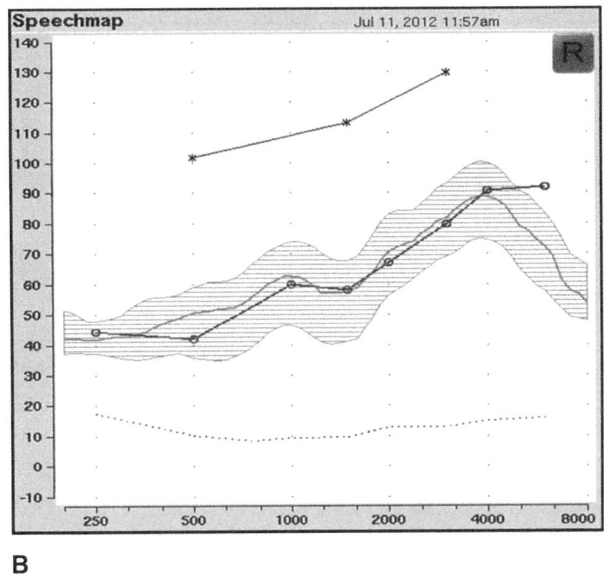

Figure 5–11. SPL-O-Gram plot of the patient's thresholds (*dark line, connected circles*) converted to ear canal SPL. Hatched area represents the amplified real speech signal from the hearing aid. **Panel A:** Hearing thresholds plotted using average correction. Note that the majority of the amplified signal appears audible (above the threshold plot) for the 2000 to 3000 Hz region. **Panel B:** Hearing thresholds plotted using the patient's measured RECD. Note that now only about 50% of the speech signal is audible for the 2000 to 3000 Hz region.

TECHNICAL TIP: USE OF THE INDIVIDUAL RECD FOR FITTINGS

As we discuss in this section, the measured RECD can be used to individualize the fitting process with respect to the assessment of audibility (see Figure 5–11). But, as we mentioned, it is also possible to enter an individual RECD into some prescriptive algorithms and manufacturers' fitting software. One potential problem, however, is to use the individual RECD with an algorithm to which the average RECD already has been added. Care should be taken to assure that only one RECD is used or significant errors will result.

---

the use of the ANSI standard method for measurement of RECD, how this measures can be used for verification, and various sources of error.

In Situ Testing

Another pre-fitting measure that can be conducted which could potentially enhance the fitting process is in situ testing. What we are referring to is audiometric thresholds or loudness judgments that are conducted using the hearing aid to transmit the test signal. In situ is a Latin term meaning "in place." Related to audiology, there is sometimes confusion regarding what is meant by in situ testing, as historically, probe microphone measures also have been referred to as in situ—that is, testing conducted in place at the ear rather than in a 2-cc coupler. There doesn't seem to be a better term to use, however, than in situ when the hearing aid is used to deliver signals, so that's what we'll use here.

When in situ testing is implemented, the testing itself is driven by the fitting software of the manufacturer. The hearing aid is fitted to the ear and the signals are then delivered. The response from the patient (e.g., threshold, MCL, or LDL) is recorded in the software, much the same as with computerized audiometry. These digital values can then be converted to traditional HL values or used internally by the software to alter the hearing aid fitting.

Background

In the previous section, we discussed how the RECD can be used to account for individual ear canal differences, which has the potential of improving the preciseness of the fitting. In situ audiometry can play much the same role. With the hearing aid serving as the transducer, pure tones, continuous or pulsed, are played directly into the ear for threshold testing. By doing so, many of the same ear canal acoustic properties are taken into consideration as we discussed with RECD measures. It has been suggested that determining an unaided threshold response with the hearing aid/earmold in situ can increase the precision of the hearing aid fitting (Kuk, 2003). With the hearing aid coupled to the ear in the same manner as the user would wear it in everyday listening situations, considerations such as residual volume of the ear canal or the effects of venting—intended or slit-leak—are accounted for in the initial stages of fitting the device. Other purported advantages include time saved in the fitting process and space saved in the office.

One possible source of concern involves the reliability of threshold measurements taken in situ. There seems to be little evidence, however, that hearing aid in situ measures are less reliable than those obtained using standard TDH or insert earphones (Smith-Olinde, Nicholson, Chivers, Highley, & Williams, 2006; O'Brien, Keidser, Yeend, Hartley, & Dillon, 2010), although this has not been examined with all devices currently available.

Administration

Obtaining in situ thresholds is similar to obtaining thresholds in a more traditional manner. The patient is seated near the computer used for programming of the hearing aid. The patient's earmold or an appropriate dome tips (depending on the manufacturer and the model of hearing aid chosen) are inserted into the ear. Several of the systems also allow for an evaluation of the environment to determine if the ambient noise level is acceptable. The patient is instructed to indicate (by raising a hand or finger) when he or she hears the tone in the test ear. Depending upon the hearing in the non-test ear, it is advisable to plug that ear to avoid any false positive responses. The thresholds are obtained in the manner of choice (e.g., down 10, up 5) by the examiner with the computer functioning very much like current computer-based audiometers, with the keyboard or the mouse tracking the frequencies and intensities.

KEY CONCEPT: POTENTIAL USES OF HEARING AID IN SITU MEASURES

Most of the major manufacturers offer the capability of using the hearing aid to conduct in situ measures. In general, we see three major areas of utilization:

- To conduct audiometric testing when standard audiometry is not available to allow for a "first fit" of a hearing aid.
- To make corrections to standard audiometry for alteration of the fitting algorithm. This can involve changes relative to the residual ear canal volume with the hearing aid in place (as we discussed with RECD measures) or the effects of venting. Applications need to be considered for open canal fittings (Keidser, Yeend, O'Brien, & Hartley, 2011).
- For hearing aid verification of gain and output when traditional probe microphone measures are not available.

Currently, there are at least six manufacturers of hearing aids that provide in situ testing capabilities in their software. Table 5–5 shows some of the similarities and differences across these options. It is obvious that the frequency ranges, intensities, and even graphic presentation can vary. The manner in which the collected data are used, also will vary.

A Comparative Study

As we mentioned earlier, research has shown that the reliability of hearing aid in situ testing is good. Many audiologists use this as a replacement or addition to conventional pure-tone thresholds when hearing aids are fitted. This seems to be particularly true when a manufacturer's proprietary fitting algorithm is utilized.

Given that there are now a number of manufacturers who have in situ testing available, we questioned if the same thresholds would be obtained for a given patient with the different systems. This of course is a different question from one of test reliability. To do this, we used the right ear of a 64-year-old male patient with a confirmed cochlear hearing loss. We used the premier mini-BTE RIC product for each manufacturer and its "closed" fitting tip. In general, the tightness of the different domes was similar among manufacturers. Testing was conducted in a quiet hearing aid fitting room.

In Figure 5–12, the results of in situ testing are shown for the hearing aid patient. The circles indicate the measures obtained using a calibrated audiometer and insert earphones. Each of the other symbols represents the thresholds obtained using the six in situ options. There is a noticeable difference observed in the low frequencies: All in situ thresholds are lower than earphone, some as much as 20 to 30 dB. This is no doubt a reflection of the leakage from the fitting tip when compared to the tight fitting foam of the insert earphone. Even in the high frequencies we see some relatively large differences among manufactures—20 dB at 4000 Hz and 6000 Hz. Interestingly, at 3000 Hz, all thresholds were remarkably similar.

Table 5–5. Comparison of In Situ Audiometry Measurement Parameters

Manufacturer	Frequency Range	Intensity Range	Overlays	Measurement of TDs	Mouse or Keyboard Control	Stimuli
Oticon	250–8000 Hz	20/40 to 65/110 dB HL*	None	Can be measured but not stored	Both	Continuous or Pulsed Pure Tone
Phonak	250–6000 Hz	20/25 to 80/100 dB HL*	None	Yes	Both	Continuous Pure Tone
ReSound	250–6000 Hz	20 to 80/100 dB HL*	Audiogram, Speech Banana, Phonemes, and Familiar Sounds	Can be measured but not stored	Both	Continuous or Pulsed Pure Tone or Warble
Signia	250–6000 Hz	10 to 40/95 dB HL*	Audiogram	No	Both	Continuous Pure Tone
Starkey	250–4000 Hz	30 to 100/120 dB HL*	Speech Spectrum and Familiar Sounds	Yes	Both	Continuous or Pulsed Pure Tone
Widex	250–8000 Hz	0 to 80/120 dB HL*	None	No	Both	Pulsed Chirp

*Intensity and frequency range depends on frequency and instrument model.

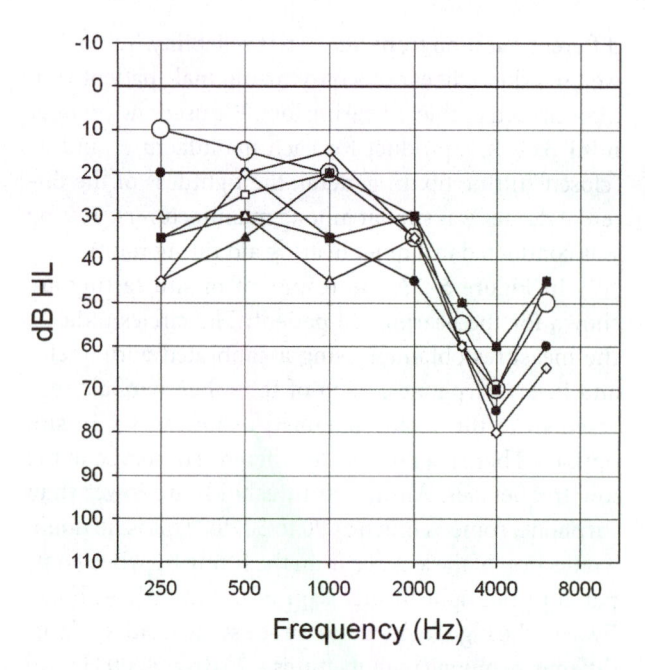

Figure 5–12. In situ thresholds obtained using the software and hearing aids (mini-BTEs) from six major manufacturers and the manufacturers' stock closed fitting tips. Earphone thresholds are shown for comparison (*larger open circles*).

The purpose of this testing was not to determine what method or device was best. Although the earphone threshold is included as a reference, it's certainly possible that any one of the in situ thresholds might be "best" for the fitting of this product—depending on how these data are used in the software. Perhaps a more interesting question would be what real-ear gain is present for each instrument when these in situ data are applied? Research with one of these products revealed that the RECDs obtained differed substantially from those obtained using traditional RECD methods (DiGiovanni and Pratt, 2010). These RECDs, when applied to the output, would then lead to less-than-desirable gain values. The results from Scollie, Bagatto, Moodie, and Crukley (2011) were somewhat more encouraging, as they found predictive accuracy for the REAR to be within 5 dB between 500 and 4000 Hz for 14 out of 15 ears tested. In general, however, until more definitive research is available, we don't see in situ measurements as a clearly accurate replacement for verification using probe microphone speech mapping.

Threshold-Equalizing Noise Test

Another test utilizing pure tones (and noise) that can be used in the pre-fitting assessment is the threshold-equalizing noise (TEN) test. This test is designed to detect regions of the cochlea where the inner hair cells are not functional. These areas are commonly referred to as *dead zones* or *dead regions*.

Background

As you probably recall from your ear physiology studies, the basilar membrane is tuned. That is, each place on the membrane is tuned to respond best to sounds of a narrow frequency range—high frequencies toward the base and low frequencies toward the apex. The frequency that induces the maximum vibration for a given region is termed the *characteristic frequency*. The role of various cells is quite complex with a variety of interactions and sharing of information. A very simplified explanation of the role of various cells is that the outer hair cells sharpen the frequency-specific tuning and amplify the signal, whereas the inner hair cells detect the signal and transmit it to the cranial nerve VIII.

The majority of acquired cochlear hearing losses begin with damage to the outer hair cells. The likelihood that there will also be damage to the inner hair cells typically increases with greater hearing loss. Audiometric, damage to the inner hair cells is usually present for hearing losses of 55 to 60 dB HL and greater. In some cases, particularly with more severe hearing loss, there may be regions where the inner hair cells become nonfunctional, the aforementioned dead regions. These regions are difficult to detect with traditional pure-tone testing as a high intensity signal in the area of a dead region will produce enough basilar membrane vibration that there will be a response (the patient hears a tone) at a different region where the inner hair cells are healthy, even though that region is not specifically tuned to the test frequency. This is most notable in steeply sloping hearing losses (either downward or upward). For example, a person with a downward sloping hearing loss with a threshold of 40 dB at 2000 Hz and a dead region at 4000 Hz, may present with a threshold of 80 to 90 dB at 4000 Hz simply because the 4000 Hz tone is being detected by neurons tuned to lower frequencies at which hearing is more normal.

Why is this important for the selection and fitting of hearing aids? Research has shown that providing audibility for a frequency range within a dead region is less useful (or maybe not useful at all) than when dead regions are not present. If the clinician is fairly certain that a dead region is present, he or she might try various mitigation approaches:

- Not be as aggressive in trying to provide audibility for this frequency range, which might help eliminate acoustic feedback issues;
- Provide the patient with alternative programs with and without gain for the dead regions for real-world comparison;
- Be more likely to consider hearing aid technology that provides frequency lowering. (This only applies to high-frequency dead regions; see "Key Concept" comments;)
- Provide the patient specific counseling regarding the realistic benefits of high-frequency amplification.

Historically, the assessment of the tuning capabilities of the damaged cochlea was assessed by measuring tuning curves—a procedure reserved for auditory research laboratories. In 2000, Moore, Huss, Vickers, Glasberg, and Alcántara (2000) introduced the TEN test, a procedure that was relatively easy and quick to administer by clinicians. A few years later, a second version of the TEN test was developed, called the TEN(HL) test (Moore, Glasberg, & Stone, 2004). The basic concept of the TEN test is as follows:

- The *threshold equalizing noise* is spectrally shaped so that, for normal hearing individuals, it gives equal masked thresholds for pure-tone signals at all frequencies within the test range.
- When a patient has hearing loss and there are surviving inner hair cells corresponding to the specific test region with elevated audiometric thresholds, the test signal in that frequency region is detected by hair cells with characteristic frequencies close to that region. When this is true, the masked threshold in the equivalent noise will be similar to that for normal hearing listeners (provided that the noise intensity is sufficient to produce significant masking).
- When the inner hair cells for the test frequency are nonfunctional, however, the signal will be detected by inner hair cells with different characteristic frequencies than the signal frequency. In such a case, it will require a higher equivalent noise level to mask these thresholds, a level significantly higher than normal.

KEY CONCEPT: FREQUENCY-LOWERING TECHNOLOGY

- As we discuss extensively in Chapter 12, all major manufacturers provide the option of frequency-lowering technology in their products. As the name suggests, when a severe-to-profound, high-frequency hearing loss exists, this algorithm is designed to transfer important speech sounds from the higher frequencies (e.g., 3000 Hz to 6000 Hz) where they are presumed to be inaudible to lower frequencies where there is less hearing loss and the probabilities of audibility are greater.
- The signal transfer can be conducted using frequency compression, transposition, or duplication and lowering—different approaches are used by different manufacturers.
- If continued research reveals that this technology provides significant benefit and the magnitude of benefit equals or exceeds that provided by simply providing high-frequency amplification, then TEN test results could help determine when to apply frequency lowering. The TEN test perhaps could even be delivered by the hearing aid itself.

Since its introduction, the TEN test has been used in numerous studies to assess the prevalence of dead regions and examine the effects these dead regions might have on speech processing and amplification requirements. Although we often think of dead regions occurring in patients who have severe-to-profound, steeply downward-sloping hearing losses, Hornsby and Dundas (2009) report that it is not quite this straightforward. Some of their findings are summarized in Figure 5–13. Observe in the center panel of Figure 5–13, that when the TEN finding was "no dead region (DR)," there was a clear association with hearing loss. Nearly all ears (>80%) with a hearing loss of 40 dB or less had negative findings, whereas very few ears with a hearing loss >80 dB had negative findings. If we look at the top panel of Figure 5–13, we see that when a positive finding for dead regions was obtained, however, there was little difference in dead region prevalence/hearing loss level once the hearing loss reached 50 dB.

Hornsby and Dundas (2009) also examined positive versus negative dead region findings as a function of hearing loss slope (i.e., steep, gradually sloping, flat). The majority of the inconclusive findings (approximately 60%) were for subjects with a steep slope and only 10% of the negative dead region findings were for this group. For conclusive positive dead region findings, however, the prevalence (approximately 30%) was the same for the flat slope audiograms as for the steep slope.

Clinically, when we consider utilizing frequency lowering algorithms, we usually are interested in the presence of dead regions in the 3000 to 4000 Hz region. Specifically studying the prevalence of dead regions at 4000 Hz using the TEN test (98 ears; hearing loss ranging from 60 dB HL to 85 dB HL), Aazh and Moore (2007) report the prevalence of dead regions at 4000 Hz increased with increasing hearing loss and exceeded 50% for hearing losses greater than 70 dB. Using 70 dB HL as the cutoff criteria resulted in a sensitivity of 62% and a specificity of 63%. In agreement with Hornsby and Dundas (2009), they did not find a significant relationship between the presence of the dead region and the slope of the audiogram for the frequency region below 4000 Hz.

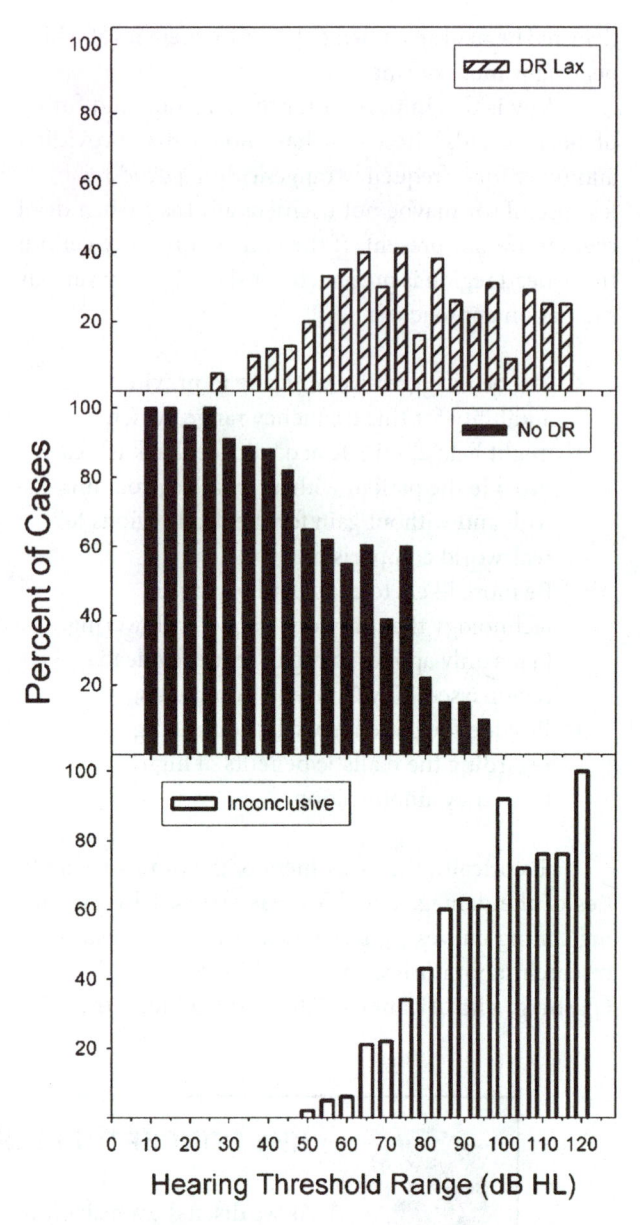

Figure 5–13. Distribution (percent of subjects) of the cochlear dead regions categorized for three classifications. *Top Panel:* Positive for the dead region using lax criteria. *Middle Panel:* Negative for the dead region. *Bottom Panel:* Inconclusive, unable to interpret due to test limitations. (Adapted from Hornsby and Dundas, 2009.)

Administration and Scoring

Until recently, the TEN(HL) test could only be conducted by use of a CD player connected to an audiometer. In the past few years, the test has been implemented within a few PC-based audiometers. For the CD version, the tones are recorded on one channel and the equalizing noise on the other. All calibrations are in dB

HL, therefore audiometric thresholds can be measured either using the tones generated by the audiometer or by using the test tones from the CD; the results should be very similar.

Administration

The test procedure for detecting a test signal in the TEN is determined using the same method as would be used for traditional audiometry except that a 2 dB step size is used when the tone is in the region of the detection threshold; larger steps can be used initially to find the approximate threshold. Moore (2010) provides general guidelines for administering the test:

- For frequencies at which the hearing loss is less than or equal to 60 dB HL, set the TEN level to 70 dB HL.
- When the hearing loss is 70 dB HL or more at a given frequency, set the TEN level 10 dB above the audiometric threshold at that frequency.
- If the TEN is found to be unpleasantly loud or if the maximum TEN level of 90 dB HL is reached, then the TEN level can be set equal to the audiometric threshold.
- It may be difficult or impossible to apply the TEN(HL) test when the hearing loss at the test frequency is 90 dB HL or more—although it is quite likely that a dead region would be present with such a severe hearing loss and this might be apparent from the audiometric configuration.

Scoring the TEN Test

The test is scored as either a positive or negative indicator of a dead region for each ear-specific frequency tested. The following are general guidelines regarding the scoring of the TEN test (from Moore, 2010):

- For a person with normal hearing, the threshold of the test tone in the TEN is typically equal to the TEN level. For example, if the TEN level is set to 70 dB HL, the threshold for detecting the test tone is about 70 dB HL for any frequency from 500 to 4000 Hz.
- If a patient has a cochlear hearing loss but does not have a dead region at the test frequency, then the threshold of the test tone in the TEN is typically a few dB above the TEN level. For example, if the TEN level is set to 70 dB HL, the threshold for detecting the test tone might be around 73 dB HL. The difference between the reference level and the threshold detection level is referred to as the SNR(T).
- When the test tone frequency falls in a dead region, the threshold for detecting the test tone in the TEN is typically well above the TEN level. The criteria for diagnosing a dead region at a specific frequency are:
  1. The threshold of the test tone in the TEN is 10 dB or more above the TEN level.
  2. The threshold of the test tone in the TEN is 10 dB or more above the audiometric (absolute) threshold.
  3. If the TEN level is selected as we described earlier, then criterion #2 automatically will be satisfied when criterion #1 is satisfied.

Clinical Application

The clinical applications of TEN test results are based on the assumption that people with cochlear dead regions will not benefit from amplification well inside that frequency region. It is important to explain what we mean by the term *well inside*. Again, we refer to the work of Brian Moore (see summary from Moore, 2010). The recommendations of Moore and his colleagues are that for a high frequency, downward sloping hearing loss, we would only apply amplification up to about 1.7 times the *edge* (beginning) of the dead region (Baer, Moore, & Kluk, 2002). For example, let's take a patient with a very steeply downward sloping hearing loss going from 30 dB at 1000 Hz, 70 dB at 1500 Hz, and 80 dB or worse above 1500 Hz. TEN test results are normal for 1000 Hz but indicate dead regions for 1500 Hz and above—in this example, 1500 Hz would be considered the edge frequency. We would then attempt to restore audibility for frequencies up to about 2500 Hz (1500 × 1.7 = 2550 Hz), but not higher.

The audiogram example that we just used is not very common of course. More common is the audiogram where the severity of the loss does not approach dead region territory until 3000 Hz. If this were the case, according to Moore's recommendations, we then would provide amplification up to 5000 Hz (3000 × 1.7 = 5100 Hz). For the most part, this is no different from what we would do if we did not know the patient had dead regions. If the edge is at 2000 Hz, Moore's guidelines suggest providing amplification up until 3400 Hz, which would be somewhat of an alteration to the typical fitting. For this reason, Vinay and Moore (2007) suggest that for hearing aid fittings for downward sloping losses, we would conduct the TEN for the frequencies of 2000 Hz and below when the hearing loss reaches the level where dead regions may be present (e.g., approximately 60 dB).

These guidelines, however, are loosely interpreted in clinical practice. Many audiologists withhold amplification at the *suspected edge* of the dead region. We say suspected because this decision usually is made by examining the pure-tone audiogram and not by conducting the TEN test. There are data to suggest that withholding amplification near the edge of the dead region is a mistake, and we address that at the end of this section.

Although we normally encounter high-frequency dead regions, and this is what most research has been concerned with, there also are patients with low-frequency dead regions. Although not as common, the actual impact on the hearing aid fitting might be greater for this population. For low-frequency dead regions, the guidance from research is to only amplify to 0.57 dB below the edge (Vinay & Moore, 2007; Vinay, Moore, & Baer, 2008). Consider a patient with Ménières disease with a severe loss in the lows rising to only a mild loss at 2000 Hz and above. If this patient had dead regions at 250, 500, and 1000 Hz, we then would only amplify down to 570 Hz in the lower frequencies. In this case, amplifying at and *above* the dead region is probably helpful.

Dead regions also are present in other less common audiometric configurations, such as the cookie bite, *V-shaped*, or *inverted V-shaped*. It is difficult to provide amplification rules to these configurations and it often is helpful to utilize clinical speech testing at different sensation levels to assess the benefits of audibility (see review by Halpin, 2002). This is, of course, helpful for all configurations.

TEN Test Findings and Hearing Aid Adjustment

Let's talk about how we might use the TEN test results for fitting hearing aids for the typical patient. That is, not the patient with a 50 dB/octave drop in their audiogram with thresholds of >90 dB at 3000 Hz and above, but rather, people with more gently sloping audiograms with losses in the 70 dB to 90 dB range in the higher frequencies—the kind of hearing loss we more frequently encounter. This has been researched in several studies using real hearing aids in real-world environments (e.g., Cox, Johnson, & Alexander, 2012; Mackersie, Crocker, & Davis, 2004; Preminger, Carpenter, & Ziegler, 2005). In a nicely designed study, Cox and colleagues (2012) used 18 matched pairs to examine the effects of providing prescribed amplification (i.e., NAL-NL1 fitting algorithm) versus rolling off high frequency gain (low-pass) for people with dead regions identified by the TEN test, compared with their matched pair who did not have dead regions (DR). Cox and colleagues (2012) concluded that "they did not observe any situation in

---

POINTS TO PONDER: SENSITIVITY AND SPECIFICITY OF THE TEN

Sensitivity and specificity calculations for a given test usually involve a comparative *gold standard*. For the TEN test, the standard commonly used is psychophysical tuning curves (PTC). Summers, Molis, Müsch, Walden, Surr, and Cord (2003) compared these two measures and found agreement (presence or absence) for only 10 of 18 cases (56%). The disagreement was because the TEN results suggested the presence of dead regions whereas the PTC results did not, suggesting poor specificity. More recently, Warnaar and Dreschler (2012), using a modified PTC procedure and the TEN(HL) test ($n = 24$), found an agreement between these measures of around 75% when frequency-specific agreement for each test ear was studied. If the comparison was simply the presence or absence of dead regions, then the agreement was quite good: 88% (21 of 24 ears).

which typical hearing aid patients with DRs were penalized by the provision of high frequency gain similar to the NAL prescription: either they benefited from more high frequency gain or they performed no worse with it."

Because some earlier work had used subjects with dead regions at several consecutive frequencies, it is important to point out that only 17% of the Cox et al. (2012) patients had dead regions below 2000 Hz, 61% only had a dead region at one frequency, and 33% only had dead regions at 4000 Hz. But again, these were typical hearing aid patients and, in their data analysis, the authors did not observe any interactions with these factors.

Our General Recommendations. Our general recommendations, therefore, for using TEN testing to assist in programming hearing aids are as follows:

Probably not too helpful for—

- Downward-sloping audiometric configuration when the high frequency hearing loss (e.g., 3000 to 4000 Hz) is such that it is not probable that average speech can be made audible (approximately 90 dB or greater). The amplification decision based on the audiogram alone—to give up on these frequencies—will probably be no different from when known dead regions are present.
- Downward-sloping audiometric configuration when the high frequencies are aidable (e.g., approximately 65 to 85 dB). In this case, it would be reasonable to apply prescriptive gain whether or not dead regions are present.
- Determining when to use frequency-lowering algorithms. This would most probably be determined by the degree of high frequency hearing loss and not TEN test results (for the reasons cited in the first two examples).

May be helpful for—

- Upward sloping or flat configurations when the potential exists for low-frequency dead regions or that dead regions exist for several consecutive frequencies.
- Cookie-bite or V-shaped audiometric configurations when a severe loss exists in the mid-frequencies.

For counseling purposes, we would expect the TEN test findings to be helpful for a greater range of patients, as most research suggests that these patients do not experience the same benefit from audibility as their counterparts without dead regions. Preminger et al. (2005), for example, showed aided APHAB scores that were considerably worse than expected (based on degree of hearing loss) for a group of individuals with dead regions. Although this chapter's focus is *pre-testing*, it might be useful to conduct TEN testing *post-fitting* for select patients who do not have the expected benefits for understanding speech when using hearing aids.

In Closing

It might sometimes seem tempting to skip pre-fitting testing in the name of clinical time pressures. Considerable data have shown, however, that a simple pure-tone audiogram is a poor indicator of patients' individual communication abilities and listening needs. Furthermore, there is considerable variability across patients with similar hearing thresholds. Some of the most critical individual patient differences relate to speech recognition and self-reported factors such as motivation, hearing handicap, noise tolerance and other factors we will discuss in the next two chapters. With respect to the current chapter, however, ignoring individual LDL measures in any patient can lead to a hearing aid fitting with too much or too little output, which in turn can result in a patient rejecting hearing aids completely. Also, using audibility to help counsel patients can really help when discussing hearing aid expectations and general listening strategies. Depending on the patient, RECD measures and assessment of low frequency dead regions may help improve fitting accuracy or guide appropriate gain modifications respectively. Given realistic clinical time pressures, it is of course important that we carefully select the most important pre-fitting measures for each patient. Doing so is a worthwhile exercise since it can eliminate some of the post-fitting problems that will come up without this information. We expect that patients who experience fewer problems during the fitting process will likely be happier with the entire experience and with the professional services received.

6
Pre-Fitting Testing Using Speech Material

In the previous chapter, we reviewed how pure-tone and narrowband signals can be used to obtain useful information prior to the fitting of hearing aids. And in Chapter 7, we review how pre-fitting self-assessment inventories also assist in treatment planning and counseling. Although both areas certainly are important, it is commonly recognized that the cornerstone of pre-fitting testing lies with speech audiometry. Not only is speech testing part of the routine diagnostic battery, but there are many speech tests available that have direct use for the fitting of hearing aids.

Prior to the fitting, what is it that we would like to know? How the patient understands speech in quiet? Or the patient's recognition of speech in background noise? What is his or her annoyance level with respect to background noise when attempting to understand speech? How do patients assess their ability to understand speech in background noise—does this agree with their *true* ability? And what about their central auditory processing capabilities for speech signals? Or cognitive issues related to speech communication?

In this chapter, we review the different areas of pre-fitting speech testing and provide samples of appropriate tests to use depending on the pre-fitting question that is being asked. Some of the speech tests reviewed also can be used for aided verification (see Chapter 15), hence an application of the pre-fitting test findings will be establishing a baseline for post-fitting comparisons.

But, there also are many other uses. To get us started, we review some general clinical considerations when conducting these tests.

General Considerations

The basic speech test conducted by most audiologists is monosyllable word recognition in quiet using phonetically or phonemically balanced (PB) word lists—often simply referred to as *word-rec* testing or *PB-testing*. We discuss this in the next section, mostly because the test is so popular for basic diagnostics, not because we believe it is a very useful hearing aid pre-fitting measure. Unfortunately, in some offices and clinics it is the only speech test conducted, so we believe it is important to provide guidelines on the administration and interpretation of this test. The rest of the chapter relates to speech testing in the presence of a competing signal.

Speech-in-Noise Testing

It is common for best practice guidelines related to the fitting of hearing aids to recommend *speech recognition in noise* as a routine measure prior to the hearing aid fitting, and we certainly agree. There are several reasons, including those that follow, for why these tests are important, aside from the fact that the speech recognition score in quiet is a poor predictor of a patient's speech-in-noise performance:

- To address the patient's complaints. It is very likely that problems understanding speech in background noise are the primary reason why the patient is seeking assistance. Conducting this testing conveys to the patient that you understand, and are interested in learning about, his or her problem.
- To select and adjust the best technology. The results of these tests can impact your selection of the fitting arrangement (e.g., unilateral versus bilateral), the hearing aid style, how you set features aimed at reducing noise, and/or the need for special features such as remote microphones.
- To establish a baseline. The information collected during this testing can be used as a baseline for measuring aided benefit.
- To monitor performance over time. A patient's ability to understand in background noise may become significantly poorer without an associated change in hearing thresholds or speech understanding in quiet.
- To assist with counseling. How does the patient's score compare with individuals with normal hearing or other individuals with the same degree of hearing loss? As we discuss in detail in Chapter 7, part of the fitting process is to maintain realistic expectations for the patient. The results of speech-in-noise testing will assist in identifying real-world situations where the patient may or may not do well.
- To help a patient make a decision. Many times, a patient may be on the fence regarding the use of hearing aids and maybe has heard that hearing aids do not work. An aided versus unaided speech test during the initial visit provides an example of potential benefit (see example later in this chapter) and often provides encouragement for the patient to move forward.

Words or Sentences?

When conducting speech-in-noise tests, we have the option of using tools that require the recognition of single words, key words embedded in sentences, or entire sentences. There does not seem to be a consensus around what is best, as there are pros and cons of using either words or sentences. As reviewed by Wilson and McArdle (2008), there are advantages to using sentence materials:

- Better face validity; similar to what the patient experiences in everyday listening.
- Perhaps better approximation of how a person understands conversational speech; monosyllables have a lack of lexical, semantic, and syntactic redundancies and dynamic phonotactic cues.

On the other hand, monosyllables may be preferred due to the following disadvantages of using sentences (Wilson & McArdle, 2008):

- With sentence material, context contributes heavily to intelligibility and makes basic auditory function difficult to determine.
- The syntactic and semantic structures of sentence-length stimuli can influence performance.
- Sentences involve more complex cognitive skills; more working memory effort is required; these demands could differentially affect older versus younger patients.

Competing Noises

There are several different types of competing noises used with popular speech tests. The different noises have different characteristics, which can impact the performance for a given test. Most importantly, using the wrong noise can affect list equivalency, resulting in a clinician drawing the wrong conclusion about measured differences between test conditions (e.g., performance for the right versus left ear). It is important, therefore, to use the type of competing noise with each speech test that was used in its development when normative data were collected. Commonly used competing noises include the following:

- Speech noise (speech shaped noise): As the name indicates, this is a broadband, typically non-modulated, noise that usually has been shaped to be consistent with the LTASS. An advantage of this type of competition is that the lack of modulation typically leads to more reliable results for small segments of speech since the SNR is typically more precisely controlled. An example would be the Hearing In Noise Test (HINT), where an effort was made to shape the speech noise specifically so that it was very similar to the LTASS of the HINT sentences.

- Multitalkers: In this instance, the competing signal is competing talkers. We separate this category from our next category, multitalker *babble*, as the conventional definition of speech babble is that none of the background conversations are intelligible. With fewer talkers, however, it is possible to detect meaningful words or strings of words if the patient tunes in to the competing signal. This increases the informational masking (versus energetic masking), which can impact performance. Furthermore, because speech is amplitude modulated, this type of background noise allows listeners who are able, to *listen in the gaps* between competing speech segments improving face validity. Examples of this type of competing signal are the Quick Speech In Noise (QuickSIN) and the Bamford-Kowal-Bench Sentences in Noise (BKB-SIN), which have a four-talker background competition (one male, three females).
- Multitalker babble: With a multitalker babble, individual words from the talker are not recognizable, making it a true babble. This is accomplished by using more talkers, recorded from more loudspeakers and/or recorded in an uncorrelated manner. For example, the multitalker babble available from Auditec of St. Louis contains 20 talkers. There is some research to suggest that multitalker babble provides more separation between listeners with hearing loss and those with normal hearing than a competition of speech noise. Examples of tests that use a multitalker babble for a competing signal are the Words In Noise (WIN) and the Revised Speech-In-Noise (R-SPIN).
- Cocktail party/cafeteria noise: A background that is sometimes used as competition for speech testing is cafeteria or cocktail party noise. These noises are similar to multitalker babble, but usually have greater spectral bandwidth and contain transients as they typically have the clinking of glasses and dishes as well as multiple talkers. These background noises are usually recorded at a party or cafeteria, and then overdubbed with

> **KEY CONCEPT: ENERGETIC OR INFORMATIONAL MASKING?**
>
> When we conduct speech-in-noise testing, there is a masking effect from the background signal. There are different kinds of masking effects, however. As described by Jerger (2006), energetic masking occurs when the neural excitation evoked by the competing signal (speech or noise or both) exceeds the excitation produced by the target speech—for the most part, the masking effect is the energies and the synchrony of the energies of the two signals. There is a second type of masking that can cause an additional interference, or interference independent of energetic masking, which also serves to reduce speech recognition. This is referred to as informational masking (also perceptual or central masking). As the name suggests, this refers to the informational content of the masking signal. To relate these two masking effects to clinical testing, the background signal of the HINT and the WIN are strictly energetic, whereas the background signal of the QuickSIN and BKB-SIN also have an informational component. In laboratory studies, Hornsby, Ricketts, and Johnson (2006) found that hearing aid benefit is poorest when the background signal contains both energetic and informational masking. Unfortunately, this is the type of background noise experienced by most listeners in the real world.

- time offsets to provide a more unified signal and to reduce amplitude fluctuations.
- Speech: When the goal of the testing is to assess higher level auditory processing, it often is desirable to use single-talker speech as the competition. An early example of this was the Synthetic Sentence Identification Test (SSI), in which the competing signal for the synthetic sentences was James Jerger reading a story about Davy Crockett. When dichotic testing is conducted, unless a directed response is used (the patient is instructed to focus on one ear), there is not a defined *competing* signal, as the signal presented to each ear is competing against the other. Two examples of this are the tests that we discuss later in this chapter, the Dichotic Digit Test (DDT; two digits presented simultaneously to each ear) and the Dichotic Sentence Identification (DSI) test (synthetic sentences presented simultaneously to each ear).

Adaptive Versus Fixed SNR

In the clinic, speech-in-noise testing can be conducted by using an adaptive or a fixed SNR. With adaptive testing, either the speech or the noise level is fixed, and the other signal level is then varied. The variance of the adaptive signal can be at predetermined intervals with a wide range of SNRs tested (e.g., WIN, BKB-SIN, Quick-SIN). Alternatively, the adaptive signal can be varied as a function of the individual's performance on the previous item. An example of this is the HINT, in which the target sentence material is raised or lowered in 2-dB steps for each sentence, whereas the background noise is fixed. In either case, the purpose of the testing typically is to determine the SNR where the patient is obtaining a score at or near 50% correct. This is referred to as the speech reception threshold (SRT) in noise (often denoted as SNR-50 or SRT50), or in the case of the HINT, it is dubbed the Reception Threshold for Speech (RTS). The QuickSIN and the BKB-SIN compare the patient's 50% correct score with that of individuals with normal hearing, and the score is reported as *SNR loss* (i.e., deviation from normal-hearing norms). Although these SNR loss values are easy to interpret, there are some factors that affect the SNR loss. These factors may include:

- Age. Patients who are older are more likely to have more SNR loss (Walden & Walden, 2004).
- Test ear. Even with similar hearing in both ears, on average, patients have less SNR loss in their right ear than left ear (Walden & Walden, 2005).
- Presence of cochlear dead regions. Patients who have dead regions are more likely to have more SNR loss (Preminger, Carpenter, & Ziegler, 2005).
- Working memory capacity. Patients who have larger working memory capacity may have less SNR loss (Parbery-Clark, Strait, Anderson, Hittner, & Kraus, 2011).
- Musical training. Patients who are professional musicians may have less SNR loss (Parbery-Clark et al., 2011).

An alternative method of conducting speech-in-noise testing would be to use a test that has a fixed SNR. That is, the SNR is not adjusted for the individual patient but is presented at the same level for all. Speech tests that use a fixed SNR are the R-SPIN (+8 dB) and the Speech Recognition In Noise Test (SPRINT; +9 dB). The Connected Speech Test (CST) also is a fixed-level test, although the background multitalker babble can be adjusted to different SNRs. For example, for the CST:

- We commonly choose speech presentation levels of approximately 53 dB SPL (soft speech vocal effort) when we have the goal of determining the patient's ability to recognize soft speech or when demonstrating to the patient that hearing aids work.
- We use levels associated with speech produced with average vocal effort (62 dB SPL) or higher when we are demonstrating directional microphone capabilities. In this case, we present the speech from the front and the noise from behind.
- Based on the guidance provided by the research of Pearsons et al. (1977), we typically use fairly positive SNRs (e.g., +10 dB) for lower speech presentation levels and poorer SNRs (e.g., +3 dB) for higher speech presentation levels to reflect what commonly occurs in the real word.

There are clinical advantages to both the adaptive and fixed SNR methods of measuring speech recognition in background noise. First, some advantages of the adaptive model:

- Eliminate floor and ceiling effects (i.e., scoring nearly all correct or all incorrect), a common problem when a fixed SNR is used.
- The 50% correct point for most patients can be obtained more reliably and efficiently than a lengthy word list.
- Better able to determine significant differences between patients or between the right and left ears of the same patient.

But, there also are some disadvantages of measuring the reception threshold for speech compared with using a fixed SNR approach:

- Difficult to explain test results to the patient—telling a patient his or her speech reception threshold (SRT) in noise is 10 dB is not very meaningful.
- Difficult for patients to relate their performance to the real world. Because of the way the test is designed, two individuals with very different speech recognition ability would both report that they got about one-half of the words correct.
- Difficult to relate findings to third parties and referral sources. Even audiologists are not always certain if a SNR-50 score of +4 dB is good or bad. And, the SNR-50 score that is good for one speech test might just be okay for another (e.g., see norms for BKB-SIN versus WIN).
- Administration and scoring may be somewhat more cumbersome.

Presentation Level

An important consideration when conducting speech-in-noise testing is to select an appropriate presentation signal. The level selected is directly related to the question being asked and the overall purpose of the testing. Here are some examples:

- Choice #1: Conduct testing at the level at which the norms were collected. This is the most reasonable choice, as it allows for comparison with the norms and should ensure the best inter-list reliability.
- Choice #2: Conduct testing at the level at which the best performance is predicted. This should provide the best indication of true recognition ability and best predict potential performance with amplification.
- Choice #3: Conduct testing at the average real-world levels, which should provide the best prediction of how the patient performs in the real world. (Note: We say *best* not *accurate*—clinical testing is not too good at predicting real-world performance.)
- Choice #4: Conduct testing at the specific level that relates to a patient complaint; a patient with a mild hearing loss whose primary complaint is understanding soft speech might be tested at the level of soft speech.

For some individuals and some speech tests, the four considerations above may result in fairly similar presentation levels. In other cases, there may be large differences. Let's take two of the most commonly used speech-in-noise sentence tests, the QuickSIN and the HINT. With the HINT, it is recommended that the background noise be set at 65 dB (A) SPL. For the QuickSIN, it is recommend that the sentences are presented at 70 dB HL if the pure-tone average (PTA) is 45 dB or less, and at the patient's *loud but okay* loudness rating if the PTA is greater than 50 dB—this rating would probably occur at 85 to 90 dB HL for someone with this degree of hearing loss. Some quick HL to SPL conversions tell us that if standard protocols are followed, the QuickSIN will be presented at a considerably higher levels (e.g., 10–20 dB) than the HINT, which could impact the resulting SRT-50.

What may be most important as a clinician is to understand what question really is being answered when the test is conducted, which means we have to know the question being asked or the question that needs to be asked. If the question is, "What's this patient's optimum speech recognition performance in background noise?" and the patient has a downward sloping hearing loss, knowing that audibility for the high frequencies is a concern, a relatively high presentation level should be selected (e.g., testing at the "loud but okay" loudness level). On the other hand, if the purpose of the testing is to establish a baseline for aided verification measures, a lower presentation level should be used (e.g., 40–50 dB HL range). If a high presentation level is used in this instance, it is very possible that aided measures will be no better than unaided, suggesting to the patient that the hearing aids provide no benefit for understanding speech in background noise.

Earphones or Sound Field?

As with presentation level, the use of earphones versus sound field testing depends somewhat on the purpose of the test and how the test was normed. In general, there are compelling reasons to conduct the testing using earphones:

- Calibration/standardization is much easier.
- Ability to obtain individual ear information.
- Ease in masking non-test ear when necessary.
- Not constrained by upper output limits of sound field speakers.
- Accommodation for the many audiologists fitting hearing aids who do not have appropriate sound field systems.

Despite these advantages for earphones, there may be some times when sound field testing is the best choice or required by the test protocol. There are also different ways to do earphone testing. So essentially, we have three options for sound delivery:

- Earphone testing (unilateral): Even people with symmetric hearing loss may have different word recognition (in noise) ability for the right and left ears. Knowledge of this can be helpful during the fitting process (e.g., recommending what ear to use on the telephone) and during post-fitting counseling (e.g., helping explain why the patient notices an ear difference in a bilateral fitting). In most cases, ear-specific testing is recommended.
- Earphone testing (bilateral): This should provide the best indication of optimum recognition ability—although the results will probably not be much better than best ear performance from unilateral testing. The design of some speech tests require bilateral presentation (e.g., dichotic material), and at least one test, the SPRINT, is normed for bilateral earphone presentation. The Acceptable Noise Level Test (ANLT) does not tend to be ear-specific, and although it is normally conducted in the sound field, bilateral earphone testing should work okay.
- Sound field testing: Some speech tests used with fitting hearing aids were normed in the sound field. Also, if the only purpose of the testing is to serve as a baseline for aided verification, if pre-fitting is conducted in the sound field, it is then possible to conduct aided testing using the same test paradigm. We do not recommend attempting ear-specific testing in the sound field, as it is difficult to eliminate the non-test ear, even when using well-fitted earplugs. Unrelated to the fitting of hearing aids, some government agencies, for reasons we do not quite understand, require unaided sound field measures of speech recognition. Obviously, good calibration of the sound field system is critical—something we talk about next.

Sound Field Calibration

As we mentioned, some speech-in-noise tests that we discuss later in this chapter are designed to be conducted in the sound field. It is important to calibrate every signal from every audiometer channel from every loudspeaker position you will use. For example, if you present the competing noise track for a given test from both the front and back loudspeaker, it is important to calibrate the noise track from each one of the two loudspeakers separately. Also, it is important to remember that what is in the test room affects calibration. That is, all equipment and furniture that is typically present should remain in the test room during calibration.

Although not precisely accurate, we find that even cheap sound level meters such as those found online for less than $100 are good enough for these purposes and are typically accurate within a decibel or two—and more importantly, give a repeatable measure. A smartphone application can work, but it is important to first verifying accuracy. Many sound meter apps allow for calibration and can be reasonable accurate, but it is worthwhile to double check in your actual test environment because the smartphone microphone may not be equally sensitive at all distances, levels, and angles.

We have given you several considerations in this section to think about. We encourage you to keep these in mind as you review the many speech tests we have outlined.

Speech Recognition in Quiet

As we mentioned in the introduction, monosyllable word recognition in quiet is probably our least favorite speech test for the fitting of hearing aids, but the fact remains, unfortunately, that it sometimes is the only speech test conducted. There are several monosyllabic word tests available and we have selected two of them for discussion here. The first is the Northwestern University Test #6 (NU#6; Auditec version)—this choice was easy; it is clearly the most researched and clinically applied speech test of the past several decades. If you are still a fan of the W-22s, consider switching.

The second test we discuss is the Maryland CNCs. Although not as popular as the NU#6, this is the test used by the VA clinics, a group of audiologists who happen to fit 20% of all hearing aids each year in the United States. Moreover, many audiologists not directly affiliated with the VA see veterans on a contract basis, and this test is then also sometimes required.

Northwestern University Test #6

The primary monosyllabic word list that we recommend is the NU#6. As the name indicates, this list was developed at Northwestern University in the 1960s. Research at the time was conducted with several lists, all given different numerical designators. Original monosyllabic research was with List #4, which was then expanded to four 50-word lists, categorized as List #6.

Background

Because of the known limitations of the then popular PAL-50 and CID W-22 word lists, Tillman, Carhart, and Wilber (1963) worked to develop a new monosyllabic test. At the time, Lehiste and Peterson (1959) had promoted the notion that monosyllabic word lists should have phonemic rather than phonetic balance. Tillman et al. (1963), therefore, used the word list of Lehiste and Peterson partially for this reason, but also because these were words that had been selected on the basis of a high degree of familiarity, and they were all consonant-nucleus-consonant.

The early recordings (reel-to-reel tape) of the NU#6 lists that were used clinically had Tom Tillman as the talker, but these were soon replaced by the Auditec recording, released in the early 1970s. One of the first laboratory studies of the Auditec material was by Wilson, Coley, Haenel, and Browning (1976), who conducted testing for a group of listeners with normal hearing and a second group with sensorineural hearing loss. Their results demonstrated good inter-list equivalence for the Auditec version for both groups. They also conducted comparative intelligibility functions for the Auditec and the original Northwestern versions of the NU#6. They did find a slight difference between the two recordings, but they concluded that for clinical purposes the two versions could be considered equivalent.

There are different versions of the NU#6 recording available. By far, the Auditec recording is the most commonly used among clinicians.

It is important to point out the purpose of conducting traditional monosyllabic testing when used as a hearing aid pre-fitting test. First, we mention three things that this testing is *not* intended to do:

- We are not conducting the testing to determine how this person performs in the real world—monosyllables, under earphones, in quiet, in a test booth are a far cry from the real world (see related "Key Concept").
- Second, this test is also not useful for assessing whether a patient is a good candidate for hearing aids or for making decisions about what types of signal processing or features the hearing aid should have.
- Finally, we are not conducting the testing to determine how this person performs for *average-level* speech. This approach possibly could be used as a hearing aid verification test (see Chapter 15), but it is not an important pre-fitting question to answer.

> **KEY CONCEPT:**
> **POOR PREDICTOR OF BENEFIT AND SATISFACTION**
>
> As we have mentioned, we are not encouraging the use of monosyllabic testing in quiet for the purpose of predicting hearing aid benefit or satisfaction. Taylor (2007) conducted an evidence-based review regarding the use of earphone word recognition testing to predict real-world success with hearing aids. He states that out of the 11 studies that met his criteria, only four indicated a weak correlation, and none of the 11 revealed a strong predictive relationship between word recognition scores (in quiet) and success with amplification. Much of the research in this area has been conducted by Larry Humes, PhD, of Indiana University. For review, see his 2003 article on modeling and predicting hearing aid outcomes.

So why are we doing this testing? There are two things that we would like to know: What is the maximum performance possible for this patient? And, is there a significant difference between ears? That is, when we deliver the words at the optimum presentation level—enough, but not too much audibility—what score is obtained? This measure is termed *PB-Max*. We would expect that, if fitted properly, the aided performance will equal or maybe even exceed this value. The task then is to use a test protocol that best assures that the scores we obtain are a close approximation to PB-Max. That is what we discuss in the next section.

Administration and Scoring

Given that clinical monosyllabic word testing has been around for over 70 years and that it is one of the most routine and fundamental tests conducted by audiologists, one might think that a universal test protocol existed. It may exist somewhere in best practice guidelines, but unfortunately audiologists seem to be fond of modifications and shortcuts. This often makes it nearly impossible to compare results conducted at two different clinics, or even compare results for testing conducted at two different times at *the same clinic*.

Although the testing is conducted in many different ways, audiologists do at least agree that the testing is conducted with earphones and that individual ear results are desirable. The scoring is also standard: The patient scores 2% for each word repeated correctly using a 50-word list. An exception to this is when the 10-word or 25-word screening test is used, which we discuss shortly. Most critical for obtaining valid and reliable scores are the presentation level and the presentation format.

Presentation Level. As we mentioned earlier, the goal of this testing is to find PB-Max. In a research lab, this would consist of conducting a performance/intensity (PI) function in small steps (2 or 4 dB), with levels ranging from just above the threshold to the patient's loudness discomfort level. In a busy clinic, the audiologist usually will only conduct testing at one level. How do you know what level is best? First, we list three methods that are still sometimes used, which we know are *not* best:

- A fixed SL (30 or 40 dB) added to the patient's SRT.
- A fixed SL (30 or 40 dB) added to the patient's pure-tone average.
- The patient's most comfortable level (MCL) for speech.

There is no single level or procedure that will work the best for finding PB-Max for *all* patients (other than a PI/PB function using small steps). But if we choose to use a single presentation level, we must then pick one that gives us the best chance of being right most of the time. Fortunately, we have some research data to help us make that decision.

In general, the presentation goal relates to audibility of the speech signal, especially the important high frequency signals needed to identify PB words (e.g.,

> **POINTS TO PONDER: THE HISTORY OF PBs**
>
> Throughout this section we may sometimes refer to monosyllabic word recognition testing as *PB testing*. We also talk about an important test concept, referred to as *PB-Max*. If you are new to audiology, you might question the history of PB and why it is commonly used (at least by older audiologists). When monosyllabic word lists were first introduced, it was considered to be important that each 50-word list was *phonetically balanced*, abbreviated PB. Since the 1960s, we have used the NU#6 lists, which actually are not phonetically balanced, but phonemically balanced. But, because we maintained the *P*, the terms *PB list*, *PB testing*, and *PB score* have more or less survived.

2000 to 3000 Hz region). This is why in many cases, for patients with a downward sloping hearing loss, using a 30 to 40 dB fixed SL approach is not effective. Although maximizing audibility is good, the presentation level also has to be below the patient's LDL (for loudness discomfort level). In 1983, Kamm, Morgan, and Dirks found that, for downward sloping hearing losses, PB-Max most commonly occurred around 95 dB SPL (for average hearing losses of 50 dB or less). This translates to approximately 75 dB HL (earphones), and many clinics that only use one presentation level have selected either 75 or 80 dB HL for routine use.

Research by Guthrie and Mackersie (2009) revealed two other approaches, which also seem to work quite well, and in fact in their study these methods were slightly better than the fixed 75 to 80 dB HL method. The first of these two approaches is to measure the patient's LDL for speech and then conduct testing 5 dB below this level. This should accomplish the two goals we stated earlier: maximizing audibility without infringing on the LDL. As we discuss later in this chapter, it has been recommended to conduct some other tests such as the QuickSIN at the "Loud, But Okay" loudness level, which for many patients is indeed 5 dB below their LDL. The downside of this approach of Guthrie and Mackersie (2009), however, is that an extra speech test is required—we normally would not conduct an earphone speech LDL (see Chapter 5).

A second approach suggested by Guthrie and Mackersie (2009), the one that we prefer and that was essentially as effective as the LDL minus 5 dB method, is to use a variable sensation level (SL) based on the 2000-Hz threshold. The SL becomes smaller as the threshold becomes worse. The values they recommend are shown in Table 6–1.

It is possible that when using this approach, the speech signal will be "Uncomfortably Loud" for some patients. When this happens, simply reduce the intensity in small steps until the speech signal is judged "Loud, But Okay." We do need to point out that when you first start delivering speech to patients at 75 to 80 dB HL, it is very common for them to act a little startled and say something like, "That's really loud." At this point, it is important to have the patient make the distinction between "Really Loud" and "Uncomfortably Loud." You might say something like, "I realize the speech is loud, but we need to have it loud to obtain the best test results. Is it truly uncomfortable, or just louder than you would like?" In most cases, after some thought, the patient will decide that it's really okay. We suggest using live voice and talking to the patient at the proposed test level intensity to assure that all is well before initiating the actual recorded-speech testing.

Table 6–1. Recommended Presentation Levels for Monosyllabic Word Recognition Testing

The SL values shown below are added to the 2000 Hz threshold to obtain presentation levels:	
2000 Hz Threshold	<50 dB HL: 25 dB SL
2000 Hz Threshold	50–55 dB HL: 20 dB SL
2000 Hz Threshold	60–65 dB HL: 15 dB SL
2000 Hz Threshold	70–75 dB HL: 10 dB SL

Source: Guthrie and Mackerzie, 2009.

List Length. As we mentioned, research has shown that the Auditec recording of the NU#6 lists has a good list equivalency (Wilson et al., 1976). This of course was for the full 50-word lists. This does not necessarily hold true for the first or second half of any given list (e.g., the use of a 25-word list)—we have heard that in some clinics, the use of *half lists* is common practice. Consider the following example using the NU#6 List—we limit our discussion to List 1A, as that is the most commonly used. Research by Hurley and Sells (2003) identified the 10 most difficult words for each NU#6 list (actually, all 50 words are rank-ordered for difficulty). For List 1A, it just happens that eight of those words are in the first half and two are in the second half. So let's say a given patient simply misses the 10 hardest words. If a full 50-word list had been used, the score would be 80%. If someone were to use a half list and the right ear was tested first, however, the patient's scores would be 68% for the right ear and 92% for the left. Some otolaryngologists would order an MRI when presented with this degree (24%) of asymmetry for word recognition. If the patient needed hearing aids, and stated that he only wanted to purchase one, some audiologists might fit the left ear because it was the "best," when, in fact, the left ear probably was the same as the right—it just got lucky and got the easy half of the list!

In addition to the validity issue, another reason to use the full 50-word lists is that when the test has more items, critical differences become smaller. We talk about that in detail shortly, but here is a preview. At the .05 level of confidence, for a 50-word list, if a patient has a score of 72% for the right ear, the score for the left ear must be poorer than 54% or better than 86% before the left ear can be considered significantly different from the right. If only 25 words are delivered, then the left ear score must be worse than 48% or better than 92%—the range of *non-significance* grows to 44%, and expands by 12 percentage points. This of course is clinically important, as one of the reasons we are doing the test is to determine if there is a significant difference between ears (the same issue exists when determining if speech recognition has changed over time).

We are not certain of all the reasons why some audiologists choose to use a half list, but one thing that is commonly mentioned is time—it does not take as long. We could point out that a *one-word list* is even faster! If an extra minute or two is really that critical, there is a way to speed up testing and still use 50 words. The NU#6 recording has a standard interstimulus interval (ISI), however, the recorded list also is available with a shortened ISI. For many, if not most patients, the shortened ISI works fine. If not, it is always possible to pause the test. Specifically, if ordering from Auditec of St. Louis, the CD that you want is: *NU-6 Ordered by Difficulty, Version II, Short Interval*. We explain the "ordered by difficulty" aspect of this title in the next section. With the increasingly common computer-based audiometers, the audiologist can present each word at a pace consistent with the patient's response, which sometimes is even faster than the shortened ISI.

Ten Best (Worse) Words. After just telling you that it is risky practice to only use 25 words, we are now going to say that it is sometimes okay to only use 10—if you use the *right* 10! Some patients with mild losses, but who are still hearing aid candidates, might understand monosyllables in quiet very well and have scores of 96 to 100%. It is possible to identify these patients quickly, and save some valuable clinic time that could be used for counseling, by presenting the 10 most difficult words of a given NU#6 list first.

Research by Hurley and Sells (2003) identified the 10 most difficult words of the four NU#6 lists (Auditec recording). Their research revealed that if a patients correctly recognizes 9 or 10 of the first 10 words (which are ordered by difficulty), you can then predict (.05 level of confidence) that their true score using a full 50-word list would be 96 to 100%. Given this high probability, there would be little reason to continue with the other 40 words of the list.

If the patient misses four or more words from the first 10, then conduct the entire 50-word list. If, however, the patient only misses two or three words of the first 10, then compute the score again at the end of 25 words—the next 15 words also are ordered by level of difficulty. If after 25 items, the patient still has only missed two or three words, you can then stop testing, with the prediction (.05 level of confidence) that the true score is 94 to 96%. The NU#6 lists ordered by difficulty can be obtained from Auditec of St. Louis—they even provide an additional 10-second delay after the 10th and 25th words while you are thinking about whether you will go on or stop the test. We advocate always using this version of the NU#6, as the worst case is that you'll present all 50 words, which is what you would have done anyway. This word-difficulty ordering only applies to the Auditec recording of the words.

SOAPBOX: SRT + 40 DB—JUST SAY *NO*

A little story about a patient evaluated at a large, ear-nose-throat audiology center. The patient, a 55-year-old male, was self-referred, with the complaint of reduced hearing in both ears and some tinnitus. He had a history of noise exposure (hunting without hearing protection since a teenager); his primary reason for the visit was to see if hearing aids would help. His pure-tone thresholds were quite symmetric, with normal hearing in the low frequencies, dropping to a 60 to 75 dB loss in the 3000 to 6000 Hz range. There was a difference between ears, however, at 2000 Hz, where the right ear threshold was 40 dB, and the left ear dropped to 60 dB. The patient had SRTs of 10 dB in both ears, agreeing with his low-frequency thresholds. When the audiologist conducted word recognition testing, she used the *SRT +40* approach (resulting in a 50 dB HL presentation level for both ears) and obtained word recognition scores of 96% for the right ear and 80% for the left—a 16% difference between ears. The patient was then seen for his ear-nose-throat exam, and because of the word recognition asymmetry, an MRI was ordered to rule out a space-occupying lesion.

Does anything about this bother you? We certainly could question why a 16% interaural difference should trigger an MRI, or for that matter, why any monosyllabic recognition finding should trigger an MRI. But, the fact is that these are the guidelines from the American Academy of Otolaryngology (AAO), which are shown in this chart:

Recommendations for Screening MRI for Asymmetric Sensorineural Hearing Loss SNHL

PTA	Speech Discrimination
Mean PTA ≤30 dB, then asymmetry of >15 dB at two contiguous frequencies	A difference in speech discrimination scores of greater that 15%
Mean PTA >30 dB, then asymmetry of >20 dB at two contiguous frequencies	

So, the otolaryngologist was simply following the guidelines from the parent organization. But, does anyone really think those guidelines were intended for word recognition scores obtained from patients who were tested at a presentation level that was 10 dB below their 2000 Hz threshold? On the other hand, shouldn't we be able to assume that values placed in someone's medical records are *correct*?

Testing of this patient a year later at a different facility, using 80 dB HL presentation levels in both ears revealed a 94% score for the right ear and 92% for the left. Our soapbox is directly related to the often cited quote of David Pascoe (1980):

> Although it is true that mere detection of a sound does not ensure its recognition . . . it's even more true that without detection, the probabilities of correct identification are greatly diminished.

This unfortunate case begs the question—why would anyone conducting a diagnostic speech test purposely present the speech at a level that would nearly guarantee invalid test results and potentially lead to additional (expensive) testing, not to mention the undue stress to the patient? Selecting the correct presentation level for word recognition testing is not rocket science—let's do it right!

Presentation Mode. Just as we do not attempt to whistle the pure tones from 250 to 8000 Hz when we conduct air-conduction threshold testing, we also do not use monitored live voice when we conduct word recognition testing. The speaker can have a significant impact on the word recognition score (WRS). Substantial research has been conducted with the Auditec of St. Louis recording of the NU#6, and using this recording has become the standard presentation format. The words are presented from CD or with some computer-based audiometers from an internal wave file. Using this standard test format allows for the patient's performance to be compared with clinical norms, and for comparisons to be made from clinic to clinic and from visit to visit in the same clinic.

The test is the *recorded* version. Using a haphazard personal modification and then placing these scores into medical records would be considered unethical by many—and certainly could have serious medical-legal consequences.

Clinical Significance: Binomial Model. Once the WRS has been obtained for both ears, we want to decide if the results will influence our decision making regarding amplification. Is the patient's right ear score different from the left? Did the scores change since the patient's last visit? Did the scores change since the patient started using hearing aids? The question then becomes: What percent difference is truly a difference?

In what has become a classic article, Thornton and Raffin (1978) modeled the performance on clinical tests of speech recognition as a binomial variable. This binomial model was tested against data from 4,120 speech recognition scores. They developed tables for determining significant deviations between scores. One of these tables (.05 level of confidence) is shown as Table 6–2 for a 50-word list. As we mentioned earlier, the number of items used is important because variability in scores is inversely related to the number of items in the test. Also inherent in the model is that the variability of the scores is the greatest in the middle of the range (e.g., 50%) and is lowest at the extreme ranges (0% and 100%).

The Thornton and Raffin tables have more or less withstood the test of time, and are commonly used in clinical practice and in the interpretation of research findings. If this sort of thing interests you, however, you might enjoy reading Harvey Dillon's critique of the Thornton and Raffin (1982) model in an *Ear and Hearing* paper and the letters to the editor from both Thornton and Raffin, and from Dillon, which followed in a later 1982 issue. Carney and Schlauch (2007) examined a critical difference table for monosyllables using a computer simulation and compared these findings with the Thornton and Raffin table. They did find some small differences, but none greater than the score that would result from missing one word. Close enough for us.

If the critical differences shown in Table 6–2 are new to you, we will walk you through an example. Let's say you have a patient with a symmetric hearing loss who has been using a hearing aid in the right ear for several years. The patient is in your office today and tells you that he thinks his left ear (the unaided ear) has been getting worse. The patient particularly notices it on the telephone. You see that when he was tested three years ago, the word recognition score for the left ear was 78%. Today it was 62%. So did his speech understanding get (significantly) worse? To use the chart, first pick one of the two numbers—it does not matter which one—so we will take the higher score of 78%. Locate 78% on the chart and you will see that the critical range (the

---

KEY CONCEPT: THE WORDS ARE *NOT* THE TEST

We've already been "On The Soapbox" once the past few pages, so we'll do this one from ground level. Repeat after us: The words are not the test. The recorded version is the test. This point was made nicely by Fred Bess, in his 1983 book chapter on speech audiometry. He compared four different *recorded versions* of the same NU#6 lists and found that, at some sensation levels, average performance varied by as much as 60% for hearing impaired listeners among the different recordings.

Table 6–2. Thornton and Raffin (1978) Binomial Model Critical Differences at the .05 Confidence Level

Score %	N = 50	N = 25	Score %	N = 50	N = 25
0	0–4	0–8	52	34–70	28–76
2	0–10		54	36–72	
4	0–14	0–20	56	38–74	32–80
6	2–18		58	40–76	
8	2–22	0–28	60	42–78	36–84
10	2–24		62	44–78	
12	4–26	4–32	64	46–80	40–64
14	4–30		66	48–82	
16	6–32	4–40	68	50–84	44–88
18	6–34		70	52–86	
20	8–36	4–44	72	54–86	48–92
22	8–40		74	56–88	
24	10–42	8–48	76	58–90	52–92
26	12–44		78	60–92	
28	14–46	8–52	80	64–92	56–96
30	14–48		82	66–94	
32	16–50	12–56	84	68–94	60–96
34	18–52		86	70–96	
36	20–54	16–60	88	74–96	68–96
38	22–56		90	76–98	
40	22–58	16–64	92	78–98	72–100
42	24–60		94	82–98	
44	26–62	20–68	96	86–100	80–100
46	28–64		98	90–100	
48	30–66	24–72	100	96–100	92–100
50	32–68				

range where the score is *not* significantly different) is 60 to 92%. Because 62% (the new test score) falls within this range, you would conclude that today's score is not significantly poorer than the score of three years ago. Notice that if you had first picked 62%, the score of the poorer ear, the range would have been 44 to 78% and you would have reached the same conclusion.

We encourage you to use the Thornton and Raffin—or similarly derived—tables whenever comparing word recognition scores. In fact, many audiologists find it is difficult to write a report without it. Some audiologists have expressed concern that the .05 level is too rigid for clinical use—there is a .10 level chart available, if that is more to your liking.

Clinical Significance: Comparison to Pure-Tone Average. Another area where clinical significance is an issue relates to a patient's word recognition score compared to the degree of hearing loss. That is, we often look at a word recognition score, then look at the degree of hearing loss and form an opinion somewhere between "Yeah, that's about what I expected" and "That just doesn't look right." We do have data, however, to help us make this judgment more precisely. Using the Auditec recordings of the NU#6 word lists and testing over 400 adults with cochlear hearing loss, Dubno, Lee, Klein, Matthius, and Lam (1995) compared PB-Max with the patient's pure-tone average. They then used a best fit regression to provide a 95% confidence limit for these measures. We can then use these data to determine if our patients' word recognition scores are "appropriate" for their hearing loss.

We have audiologist Linda Thibodeau to thank for taking the Dubno et al., 1995, data and putting it into an easy-to-use chart. In fact, you get double-your-pleasure with this chart, as she combined the Dubno data with the Thornton and Raffin chart that we discussed earlier. The chart we are referring to is shown in Figure 6–1; it's dubbed the SPRINT, for speech recognition interpretation (Thibodeau, 2007). What we are showing in Figure 6–1 is the version for when a 50-word list is used; there also is a version for 25 words. The Dubno data are the same for both charts, whereas the range for the critical differences for the Thornton and Raffin model of course becomes larger for the 25-word chart.

Let's go back to the patient that we discussed earlier. Recall that he originally had a word recognition score of 78%, which had now dropped to 62%. We concluded that the difference between these two scores was *not significant* (50-word list). Not surprisingly, we reach this same conclusion when we compare the two scores using the SPRINT (the intersection of 78% found on the bottom abscissa and 62% found on the right ordinate column, which falls within the vertical arrow signifying *non-significance*).

To determine if these word recognition scores agree with the patient's pure-tone hearing loss, we need to use his pure-tone average (500, 1000, and 2000 Hz). The PTA at the time of the first test was 33 dB, and at the time of the second test it had dropped slightly to 36 dB. We now look at the intersection of the first word recognition score (78%) found on the lower "*x*-axis," and the PTA of 33 dB found on the left "*y*-axis." Note that the intersection does not fall in the shaded area—the PTA would have to be 24 dB or better for a score of 78% to be disproportionately low. If we now look at this patient's second word recognition score of 62%, and determine the intersection with the second PTA of 36 dB, we see that this indeed does fall into the edge of the shaded area. This could mean that we failed to obtain PB-Max, or perhaps that there is some other factor contributing to his poorer word recognition performance (e.g., auditory processing, reduced cognition). As you can see the SPRINT chart can be a helpful companion when making day-to-day decisions regarding word recognition performance and counseling patients.

Clinical Applications

As we mentioned earlier, earphone monosyllabic word recognition scores in quiet are poor predictors of who is a candidate for hearing aids and who will benefit from the use of hearing aids. There are some clinical applications, however, where these scores may be helpful in clinical decision making.

Bilateral versus unilateral versus BiCROS fitting: In general, we would consider everyone with a bilateral hearing loss a candidate for two hearing aids (see Chapter 8 for review). But what if a person has a relatively symmetrical bilateral hearing loss (e.g., poorer ear falling 10 to 15 dB below the better ear), but the WRSs were approximately 80% in the good ear and approximately 40% in the bad ear? Not a common finding, but it does happen. Is this person still a candidate for bilateral hearing aids? Probably, but if after trying hearing aids, this person reported to us that the bad side just did not seem to be getting much benefit from the hearing aid, our counseling might be different than if both ears had had WRSs around 80%. There are other cases, in which pure-tone symmetry may be somewhat greater, and we see the bad ear as low as 10 to 20%—this may be an indication for a trial with a BiCROS fitting.

Selecting an ear to fit: Although we might encourage most all of our patients with bilateral hearing losses to use two hearing aids, for a variety of reasons, some patients will chose to use only one. When the pure-tone hearing loss is symmetric, which ear do you fit? In some instances, the patient may have specific listening situations that will help you make the decision (e.g., frequently travel as a passenger in the car and need to hear the driver), but in other cases they do not. People

SPRINT CHART for 50-WORD LISTS

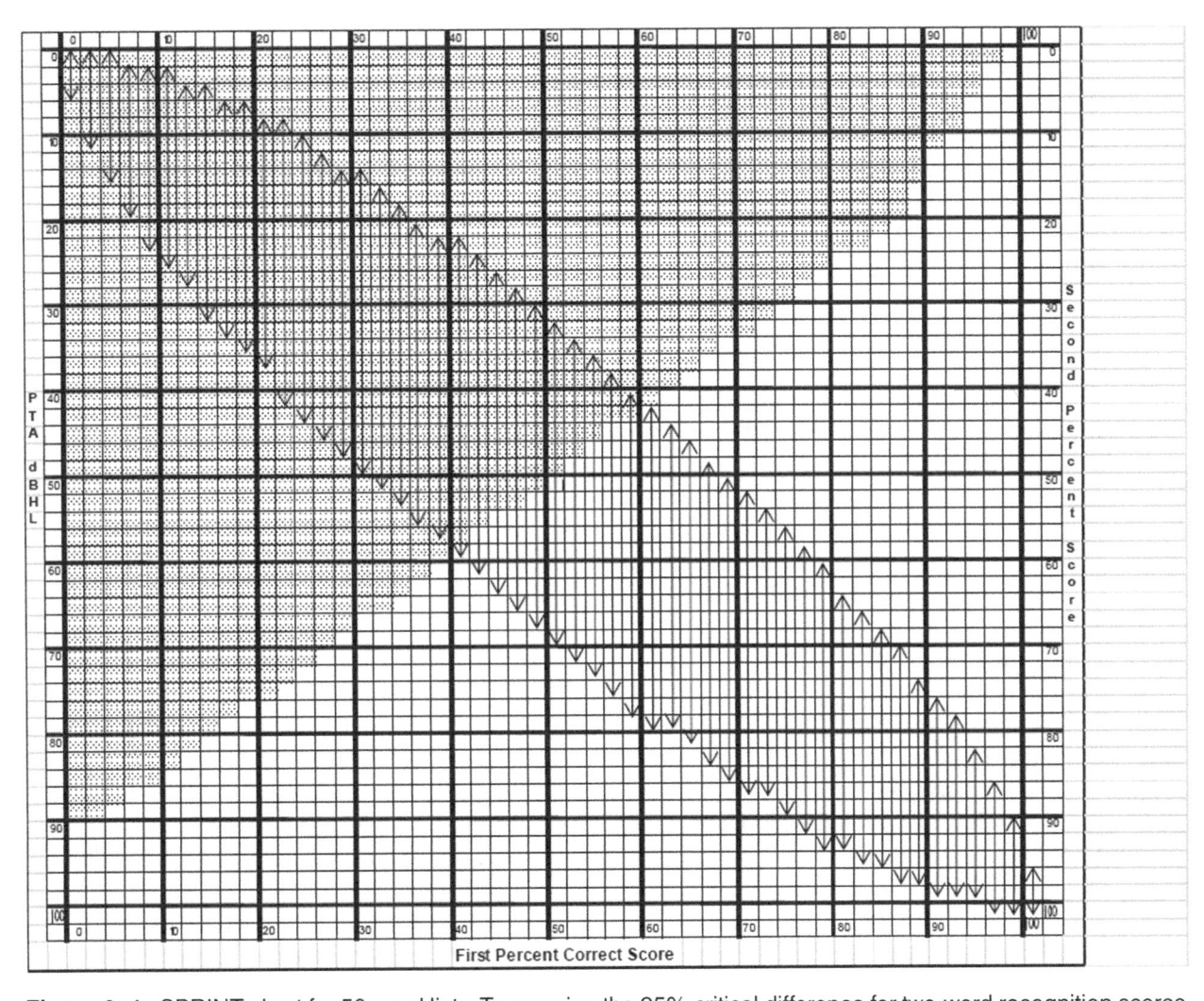

Figure 6–1. SPRINT chart for 50-word lists. To examine the 95% critical difference for two-word recognition scores, determine the intersection of the first (bottom x-axis) and the second (right y-axis) score. If the intersection point falls within one of the vertical arrows, the two scores *are not* significantly different from each other (based on the work of Thornton and Raffin, 1978). To examine the 95% confidence limit for PB-Max on the Auditec NU#6 list, determine the intersection of the word recognition score on the bottom x-axis, and the patient's PTA on the left y-axis. If the intersection of these two values falls within the shaded area, the word recognition score is considered disproportionately low (based on the work of Dubno et al., 1995). The SPRINT chart is reproduced here with permission from its developer, Linda Thibodeau, PhD (Thibodeau, 2007).

typically have similar WRSs in both ears if their hearing loss is symmetrical, but it is possible that you will see a significant ear difference. In this case, you might want to fit the better ear. This of course only applies if the difference between ears is truly a difference (see Table 6–2).

Change over time: An elderly patient of yours, whom you fit bilaterally with hearing aids five years ago, arrives at your office with the complaint that the right hearing aid is not working correctly. You check out the aid and it seems to be fine, so you decide to evaluate the

> **KEY CONCEPT: ONLY USE STANDARDIZED TESTS**
>
> Although we are not sure why, given all the well-developed speech recognition in noise tests, some clinicians continue to use standard monosyllable word materials for testing in the presence of background noise. That is, speech noise, white noise, or some other background noise is added to the standard word lists. We urge caution in doing this as several studies have shown that the standard lists are not equivalent when presented in noise. Moreover, as we mentioned, there are several speech tests that have been designed to be used with background noise—we review most of them later in this chapter.

patient's hearing. There has been no significant change in pure-tone thresholds, but the WRS for the right ear has dropped from 84 to 56%—the patient later tells you she had a mild stroke a few months ago. In this case, the results of word recognition testing will make you a better counselor. It is probably obvious, but we say it anyway—comparisons of this type only can be conducted if you follow the test protocol we discussed earlier.

Test Availability

There are several versions of the NU#6, but we recommend using the Auditec of St. Louis recording. As discussed earlier, it makes good sense to routinely use the list ordered by difficulty with the shortened interstimulus interval.

Maryland CNCs

Although this section on speech recognition in quiet focuses on the NU#6, we believe it is also important to briefly discuss a second monosyllabic test—the Maryland CNCs. The primary reason is that this is the standard word recognition measure conducted at all VA hospitals and clinics, where about 20% of hearing aids in the United States are fitted. Also this is the test used for the Compensation and Pension Evaluation Guidelines established by the VA (Speech Recognition and Identification Materials, Disc 2.0, produced in 1998). It is common that clinical audiologists who are not employed by the VA also may be requested to conduct this testing for select patients. The test is very similar to the NU#6, and, therefore, all the factors we discussed in the previous section regarding use for the fitting of hearing aids apply to the Maryland CNCs as well.

Background

We assume that the name *Maryland* comes from the location of the Biocommunications Research Laboratory, where Don Causey, PhD, of the VA conducted much of his research. This laboratory was located at the University of Maryland, not far from the VA audiology headquarters in Washington, DC. Causey was the primary researcher in the development of the Maryland word lists. Like the NU#6, the Maryland CNCs rely heavily on the revised CNC lists of Peterson and Lehiste (1962). Causey, Hood, Hermanson, and Bowling (1984) mention some of the goals in the development of the Maryland word lists:

- Uniform distribution of word familiarity
- Phonetic and/or phonemic balance
- Maximum inter-list equivalence and high test-retest reliability
- More equivalent lists than from the NU#6
- Better differentiation among word recognition abilities of individuals with normal hearing versus those with sensorineural hearing loss
- Better accounting for the effects of consonant-vowel and vowel-consonant transitions. To accomplish this, each key word was embedded in the phrase, "Say the word _____ again." Other monosyllable tests had used either, "You will say _____." or "Say the word _____."

In early research, Causey et al. (1984) studied the performance-intensity function of the Maryland CNCs

> **THINGS TO REMEMBER:
> ALWAYS, ALWAYS, ALWAYS, AND NEVER**
>
> If you simply skimmed this section on monosyllabic testing or did not read it at all, at least take a look at our four procedural rules:
>
> 1. Always use presentation levels that optimize audibility (see the 2000 Hz threshold + SL approach).
> 2. Always use a 50-word list, unless the patient passes 10-word or 25-word screening.
> 3. Always use critical differences for decision making when comparing scores between ears or sessions.
> 4. Never use live-voice presentation.

and examined the equivalency of the 10 original lists (24-year-old male talker) and test-retest reliability. They found a 2.1% per dB increase in word recognition in the linear portion of the performance-intensity function for normal listeners and a 1.3% per dB increase for hearing impaired listeners. Six of the ten lists were judged to be equivalent (Lists 1, 3, 6, 7, 9, and 10), and good test-retest reliability was reported. Over the years, the original lists have been made available through the work of Richard Wilson, PhD, and colleagues of the VA.

Administration and Scoring

If the Maryland CNCs are simply used as a replacement for the NU#6 list for the pre-fitting of hearing aids, we refer you to the administration and scoring guidelines from the previous section. If the lists are used specifically for a veteran for compensation or pension, however, then the procedures of the VA handbook for compensation and pension exams should be followed.

Clinical Applications

The Maryland CNCs are commonly used for compensation and pension evaluations for veterans, but the findings certainly would apply to the fitting of hearing aids, in the same manner as we discussed for the NU#6. In fact, if the performance-intensity protocol recommended by the VA is used, the resulting scores may be more representative of the patient's true performance than if testing was only conducted at a single level, which usually is the case with the NU#6. In general, the clinical applications of these results would be the same as we discussed for the NU#6.

Obtaining the Maryland CNC Test

The Maryland CNC test is available on the Departments of Defense and Veterans Affairs Audiology Materials, Disc 1.0, and also Speech Recognition and Identification Materials, Disc 4.0. Frye Electronics also has a CD available containing these lists (http://www.Frye.com).

Speech Recognition in Noise

As we described in the introduction to this chapter, when speech testing is conducted for the purposes of fitting hearing aids, we nearly always want to use a speech-in-noise test rather than a speech-in-quiet test. The speech-in-noise tests tend to fall into two general categories: speech recognition measures with a fixed SNR that result in a percent correct score or the use of a variable speech/noise signal that results in a SNR-50 score. This section reviews three tests that fall in the first of these two categories.

Speech Perception in Noise (SPIN) and R-SPIN

The Speech Perception in Noise Test (SPIN) was developed under contract from the National Institute of

Neurological Disorders and Stroke to assess the degree of impairment in auditory reception and/or utilization of context (Kalikow, Stevens, & Elliott, 1977). As we have mentioned before, the problem with traditional tests of speech perception is that they are not good estimates of real-world performance. Considering that the purpose is to assess a person's ability to understand speech in everyday situations, the need for a better test was clear at the time of the development of the SPIN. Instead of examining primarily acoustic-phonetic processing, the authors sought to investigate the *cognitive* aspects such as working memory and receptive language skills (Kalikow et al., 1977).

Background

In the development process, Kalikow and colleagues began with 285 key words placed each in high-probability (PH) and low-probability (PL) sentences, and then culled the list based on phonetic balance, predictability in the PH condition, and word familiarity. The result was ten 25-sentence list pairs for which only the final word is scored. Initial testing was performed to compare the intelligibility of the low-probability sentences with traditional, neutral context words in noise. The results showed comparable intelligibility scores (Kalikow et al., 1977).

A study from Hutcherson, Dirks, and Morgan (1979) assessed score differences between PH and PL sentences with a range of SNRs. The authors found that for SNRs between −2 and +2, "the difference between the PH and PL score is approximately 40%." They also found that ceiling and floor effects resulted in smaller differences outside of that SNR range. The slopes of the PI functions from this study showed a steeper function for the high-context items, which is evidence for context as a significant contributing factor to speech recognition.

The Revised SPIN. Bilger, Neutzel, Rabinowitz, and Rzeczkowski (1984) set out to standardize the SPIN and

---

TECHNICAL TIP: IS THE SPIN FOR KIDS?

Elliott (1979) conducted a study with children of different ages to identify the age at which children begin to perform at the same level as adults. Results of tests on four different age levels revealed that children younger than 15 to 17 years of age perform significantly poorer than adults on the SPIN. She recommended that the SPIN should not be used in the pediatric population. In related research, Fallon, Trehub, and Schneider (2000) sought to explore the idea that noise affects children's speech understanding more than it does for adults, and they found that children age 11 and younger required more favorable SNRs than adults did, particularly with low-context materials.

KEY CONCEPT: IS THE SPIN A COGNITIVE TEST?

Recall that earlier we mentioned that a design characteristic of the SPIN was to assess cognitive status as well as word recognition. Owen (1981) examined this by using a battery of non-audiometric cognitive tests to evaluate whether the SPIN test difference score (the difference between low and high predictive sentences) is truly a measure of the listener's use of context. His analysis revealed that the difference score is actually more closely related to audibility, as opposed to contextual cues. Owen (1981), however, suggested that it may be possible to use the low-predictability sentences to evaluate more central auditory processing skills such as auditory closure—the ability to decode a whole word after hearing only part of it.

posited that normal hearing subjects would not provide a good estimate of the SPIN's reliability. As a consequence, they tested a variety of subjects with hearing loss at a level well above the threshold, with a +8 dB SNR, based on the work of Pearsons, Bennett, and Fidell (1977), who suggested that this was a common SNR encountered in everyday environments. The +8 dB SNR has since become the standard—and basis for normative data—and what typically is used today.

In that study, Bilger et al. (1984) also called attention to the fact that the lists did not meet the qualifications for equivalency. In addition, they stated that "performance reflects two skills that may be largely uncorrelated: ability to listen in noise and to use context." They then revised the test based on the analysis of each test item and removed 31 key words and their corresponding sentences. This resulted in a total of four 50-item list pairs. Today you see this revised version referred to as the R-SPIN or the SPIN-R (Bilger, 1984). Examples of sentences (using the same key words) from the R-SPIN are as follows:

High Predictability
- The baby slept in his crib.
- The farmer baled the hay.

Low Predictability
- He can't consider the crib.
- Tom discussed the hay.

We mentioned earlier that the R-SPIN is a fixed SNR test; however, Wilson, McArdle, Watts, and Smith (2012) demonstrated that this test can be configured into a multiple SNR paradigm to estimate SNR-50, but that additional research will need to be conducted to develop distinct lists from each of the 200 key words that would be reliable across listeners of representative age and hearing loss.

Administration and Scoring. The SPIN and the R-SPIN take approximately 10 minutes to administer and require a verbal or written response of the last word in each sentence. Both tests are designed for adults but may be used with teenagers as young as 15 years old.

Patient instructions should include the following:

- Listen carefully to each of the following 50 sentences and write down or repeat only the last word. If you are writing your answers down, be sure to put each answer in its corresponding blank space.
- You will have plenty of time, so write legibly and check your spelling.
- The last word will be a common word that you have heard many times before, but some may be easier to understand than others.
- Take a guess if you are unsure. You will not be penalized for wrong answers.

To set up the test, calibrate using the 1000 Hz calibration tone, and then set one channel to the signal and the other to the babble, and present both to the same ear. Present the sentences with plenty of time in between each item for the patient to respond.

The recommended procedures for selecting the presentation level are as follows:

- Once the babble has been appropriately calibrated, determine the patient's threshold for the babble.
- Set the speech signal to 50 dB above the speech babble threshold.
- Set the babble to 8 dB below the speech signal (SNR = +8 dB).

The R-SPIN score is reported as a percentage. Sum the number of correct high-probability words and the number of correct low-probability words separately. Then, using the scoring nomograph, shown in Figure 6–2, find the corresponding number in the high probability axis and read over to the corresponding number for low probability. That number is called "the percentage hearing for speech" and should fall within the normal region (the outlined area). If the score does not fall within that area, it could be underestimating the patient's hearing for speech. Numbers that are crossed out indicate invalid test results or that the patient may have additional contributing factors that determine the test score. Specifically, as we discussed earlier, non-auditory factors that may contribute to test scores include cognitive declines, difficulty using context, and so forth.

This scoring and interpretation is quite different from most other speech tests, so to be clear, we include the actual wording of this concept from the R-SPIN manual:

Scores based on the administration of the R-SPIN test are valid estimates of percent hearing for speech if, and only if, the patient's scores in the high- and

Number Correct – Low Context

	0	1	2	3	4	5	6	7	8	9	10	11	12	13	14	15	16	17	18
25	50.0	65.9	72.2	75.8	78.5	80.8	82.4	84.1	85.3	86.6	87.7	88.7	89.6	90.5	91.3	92.1	92.9	93.6	94.3
24	34.1	50.0	56.8	61.4	64.8	67.4	69.9	71.9	73.9	75.8	77.3	78.8	80.2	81.6	82.9	84.1	85.3	86.7	87.9
23	27.8	43.2	50.0	54.8	58.3	61.0	63.7	65.9	68.1	69.9	71.9	73.6	75.2	76.7	78.2	79.7	81.1	82.6	83.9
22	24.2	38.6	45.2	50.0	53.6	56.8	59.1	61.8	63.7	65.9	67.7	69.2	71.2	72.9	74.5	76.1	77.9	79.4	81.1
21	21.5	35.2	41.7	46.4	50.0	53.2	55.6	58.3	60.3	62.6	64.4	66.3	68.1	69.9	71.6	73.2	75.2	76.7	78.5
20	19.2	32.6	39.0	43.2	46.8	50.0	52.8	55.2	57.5	59.5	61.4	63.7	65.5	67.4	69.2	70.9	72.6	74.2	76.1
19	17.6	30.1	36.3	40.9	44.4	47.2	50.0	52.4	54.8	56.8	59.1	61.0	62.9	64.8	66.6	68.4	70.2	72.2	73.9
18	15.9	28.1	34.1	39.2	41.7	44.8	47.6	50.0	52.4	54.4	56.4	58.7	60.6	62.6	64.4	66.3	68.1	70.2	
17	14.7	26.1	31.9	36.3	39.7	42.5	45.2	47.6	50.0	52.0	54.4	56.4	58.3	60.3	62.2	64.1	65.9		
16	13.4	24.2	30.1	34.1	37.4	40.5	43.2	45.6	48.0	50.0	52.0	54.0	56.0	57.9	59.9	62.2			
15	12.3	22.7	28.1	32.3	35.6	38.6	40.9	43.6	45.6	48.0	50.0	52.0	54.0	56.0	57.9				
14	11.3	21.2	26.4	30.8	33.7	36.3	39.0	41.3	43.6	46.0	48.0	50.0	52.0	54.0					
13	10.4	19.8	24.8	28.8	31.9	34.5	37.1	39.4	41.7	44.0	46.0	48.0	50.0						
12	09.5	18.4	23.3	27.1	30.1	32.6	35.2	37.4	39.7	42.1	44.0	46.0							
11	08.7	17.1	21.8	25.5	28.4	30.8	33.4	35.6	37.8	40.1	42.1								
10	07.9	15.9	20.3	23.9	26.8	29.1	31.6	33.4	35.9	37.8									
9	07.1	14.7	18.9	22.1	24.8	27.4	29.8	31.9	34.1										
8	06.4	13.3	17.4	20.6	23.3	25.8	27.8	29.8											
7	05.7	12.1	16.1	18.9	21.5	23.9	26.1												
6	05.0	10.9	14.5	17.4	19.8	22.1													
5	04.4	09.7	13.1	16.9	17.9														
4	03.8	08.5	11.5	14.0															
3	03.0	07.2	09.8																
2	02.3	05.7																	
1	01.5	00.4																	
0	0.0	02.3																	

(Number Correct – High Context is the y-axis)

Low Context

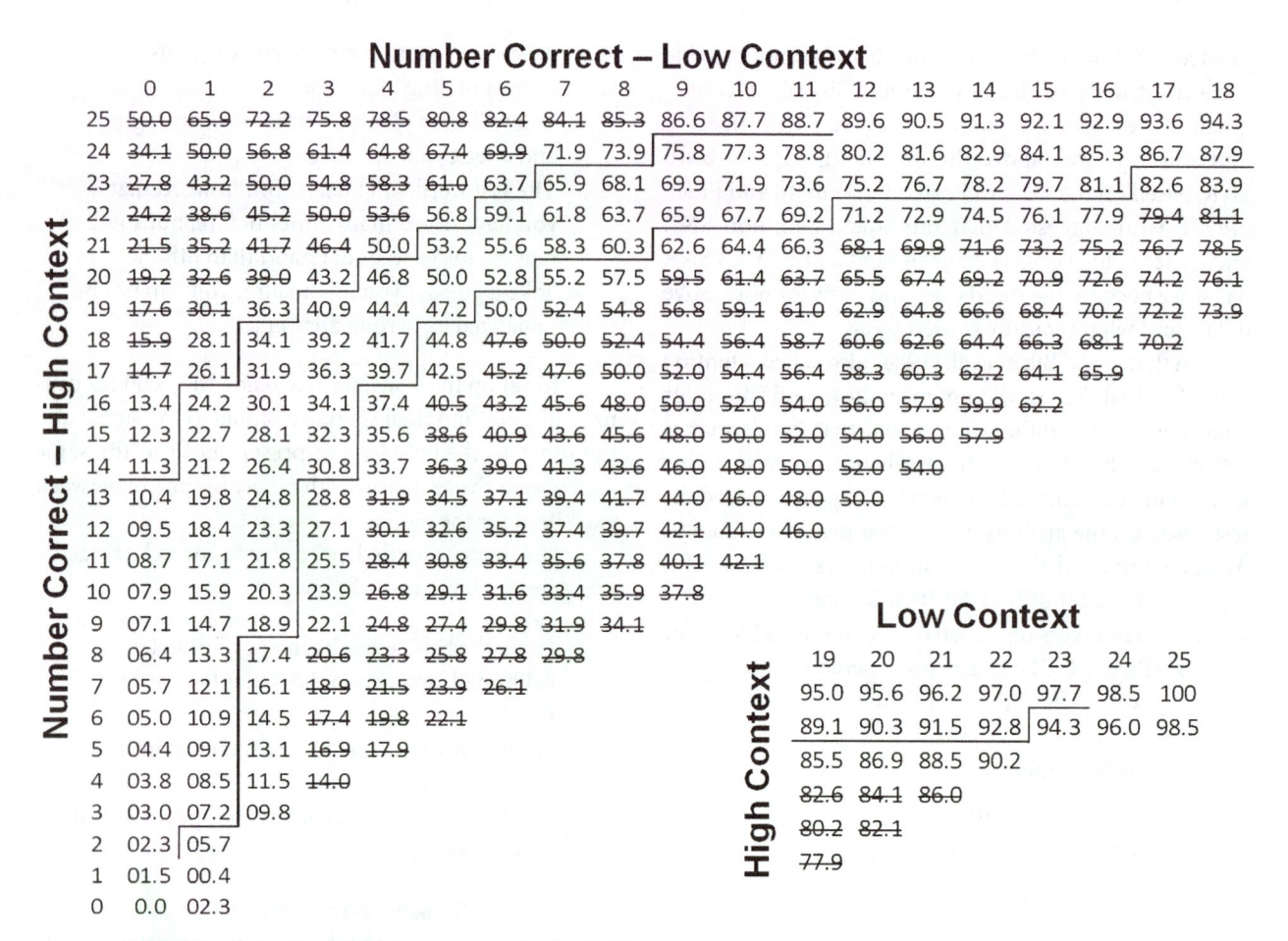

High Context	19	20	21	22	23	24	25
	95.0	95.6	96.2	97.0	97.7	98.5	100
	89.1	90.3	91.5	92.8	94.3	96.0	98.5
	85.5	86.9	88.5	90.2			
	82.6	84.1	86.0				
	80.2	82.1					
	77.9						

Figure 6–2. Nomograph used for scoring the R-SPIN. The chart is used to determine the intersection of the number of correct items of the low-probability and high-probability words (Adapted from *Manual for the Clinical Use of the Revised SPIN Test* by R. C. Bilger, 1984. Champaign, IL: University of Illinois Press.)

low-predictability subtests place her/him in the acceptance region of the scoring nomograph. Scores that fall outside the acceptance region underestimate the patient's ability to hear speech and probably reflect non-auditory factors.

Using the nomograph shown in Figure 6–2, let's take a patient who scored 23/25 for the high-context items (*y*-axis) and 13/25 for the low-context items (*x*-axis). The R-SPIN *percent hearing* score would be 76.7 (where the two scores meet on the chart). Note that if the high-context scores were only 15/25, the percent hearing would drop to 56.0%, and observe that this score has been lined out, suggesting that the high-low difference is greater than normal and that there may be contributing factors to the R-SPIN score.

Clinical Applications. There are several potential applications of the R-SPIN related to the selection and fitting of hearing aids:

- To evaluate the degree of handicap for speech recognition in background noise for patients with hearing loss.
- To evaluate whether or not a patient is able to make use of the contextual information to which they have access (difference between low- and high-predictability scores).

> **TECHNICAL TIP: AGE EFFECTS AND THE R-SPIN**
>
> In a large study of speech recognition using different materials, Dubno, Lee, Matthews, and Mills (1997) conducted the R-SPIN for 129 subjects (256 ears) divided into three age groups: 55 to 64 years, 65 to 74 years, and 75 to 84 years. They found that after the effect of average hearing loss on maximum scores was accounted for, 11.6% of the remaining variance in scores for males can be explained by age, whereas the corresponding value for females was 0.3%. For the R-SPIN, statistically significant decreases in scores for males were observed for words in high-context sentences; a declining trend with age was also observed for words in low-context sentences, but this was not significant. These results suggest that, for male patients, you may expect to see an effect of aging, in addition to auditory effects of hearing loss.

- To predict hearing aid benefit. Kalikow et al. (1977) suggest that the comparison of high- and low-predictability scores "has the potential of predicting the ability of a hearing-impaired listener to perform in everyday communicative situations, and thus may help estimate the benefit that the individual is likely to gain from a hearing aid."
- To evaluate ear-to-ear differences or differences over time, if using a complementary list pair.

Unfortunately, the R-SPIN only contains 25 items of each type per list and, therefore, is not sensitive to small changes and is vulnerable to variability. In addition, it tests only monosyllabic nouns, and the test is relatively time-consuming compared with other available tests of speech perception. The R-SPIN has been used in considerable research related to hearing aid verification, often using different SNRs from the standard +8 dB, and, because of ceiling effects, only the low-predictability sentences.

Obtaining the R-SPIN. The R-SPIN can be obtained for a nominal charge through the Department of Speech and Hearing Science, University of Illinois, Champaign, IL 61820.

Connected Speech Test (CST)

Developed in the Hearing Aid Research Laboratory at the University of Memphis, the CST is a sentence recognition test designed to approximate everyday conversations in which contextual cues are usually available and includes both audio-only and audiovisual versions (Cox, Alexander, & Gilmore, 1987; Cox, Alexander, Gilmore, & Pusakulich, 1988). That is, the CST can be administered with or without the talker's face being visible.

Background

The CST consists of 24 equivalent pairs of passages of speech. Each passage has 9 or 10 sentences about a familiar topic, such as windows, an umbrella, grass, and so forth. These sentences, spoken by a female talker, were constructed to be syntactically and semantically simple. The topics and vocabulary were based on children's reading materials. The CST also includes 8 practice passages and 16 learning passages. An example of a CST passage about a woodpecker is shown in Figure 6–3.

The CST was designed to be used primarily as a criterion measure for research studies of hearing aid benefit. Because the test has a high number of equivalent lists, good test-retest variability, and high content validity, it has been used extensively in hearing aid research (e.g., Arehart, Kates, & Anderson, 2010; Boike & Souza, 2000; Picou & Ricketts, 2011; Wu & Bentler, 2010) and has been recommended to be an integral part of a standardized research test battery (Walden, 1997).

Administration and Scoring

The CST is a sentence recognition test during which a patient hears a sentence and repeats that sentence as precisely as possible. The clinician scores the patient's response based on standardized key words in each

> The woodpecker is a bird with a **STRONG BEAK**.
> It bores **HOLES** in **TREES** looking for **INSECTS**.
> Woodpeckers **LIVE** in all parts of the world.
> The **TOES** of woodpeckers **ARE VERY UNUSUAL**.
> Two **POINT FORWARD** and two face **BACKWARD**.
> This allows the **BIRD** to cling to **TREES**.
> The **TAIL FEATHERS** of a woodpecker are **STIFF**.
> **THEY** can **USE** their tails as a **SUPPORT**.
> They also use their tails to grasp **TREES**.
> Woodpeckers **HAVE** long **TONGUES** with pointed **TIPS**.

Figure 6–3. This is a sample CST passage. The general topic of the passage is woodpeckers (the patient is informed of this) and the key words are in bold. Note that the passage contains 25 key words. (Adapted from the Hearing Aid Research Lab, University of Memphis, Memphis, TN).

sentence. There are 25 key words in each passage; standard administration is to use two passages at a time, yielding 50 key words. Whether presenting the materials as audio-only or audiovisual, it is important that the patient be told the passage topic before presentation of every list. Note that in Figure 6–3, the key words are bolded in caps for ease of scoring.

The speech sentences and background noise are on separate tracks on the disc, which allows for presentation in quiet or in any SNR the clinician chooses. The selection of the speech level and SNR for this test should be based on your clinical goal, as we discussed earlier in this chapter.

The two-channel calibration noise contains steady state noise in both channels. Importantly, the noises in each channel are not the same, as one matches the spectrum of the CST babble and the other matches the spectrum of the speech. Following the most up-to-date test manual when calibrating any speech test is always encouraged. The CST provides an example of why this is so important as this test has the somewhat unusual calibration instructions of adjusting the VU meter to –5 dB for the noise channel and –4 dB for the speech channel.

Manual scoring is accomplished by counting the number of key words the listener misses out of 50 for each passage pair. We simply make tick marks for every word missed on a piece of scrap paper. Alternatively, one could print out copies of the passage pair text and mark out the actual words missed. The recordings contain pauses after each sentence presentation, so that the patient has time to repeat the sentence and to facilitate scoring. As a consequence, test administration and scoring after calibration simply consists of telling the patient the passage topic, pressing play, and keeping track of the number of key words that are not correctly repeated.

The speech track of the CST can be routed to one earphone or to a loudspeaker, and the noise track can be routed to the same earphone or loudspeaker to evaluate speech recognition in noise without spatial separation, or to another loudspeaker (e.g., behind the patient) to evaluate speech recognition in noise with spatial separation—for example, to evaluate directional benefit for counseling purposes. The video track of the DVD can then be routed from the DVD player to either a television or other video monitor using the appropriate video cord (e.g., S-video, DVI, HDMI). A sound level meter will be required to calibrate the level at the position of the listener's head for loudspeaker presentation.

Obtaining Speech Intelligibility Ratings

As an alternative to use as an objective speech recognition measure, the CST materials can also be used to estimate subjective perception of performance. Although the same corpus of sentences is used, a male talker is used instead, the instructions are different, and the test is referred to SIR (for Speech Intelligibility Ratings; Cox & McDaniel, 1989). In this test, listeners rate the intel-

> **THINGS TO REMEMBER:
> THE HARL AT THE UNIVERSITY OF MEMPHIS**
>
> As we mention here, both the CST and the Speech Intelligibility Ratings (SIR) are available from the Hearing Aid Research Laboratory (HARL) at the University of Memphis. Both tests can be ordered from its website, which is a treasure trove for audiologists needing tests and self-assessment scales related to hearing aid selection and fitting; most of the material is from the research of long-time HARL director Robyn Cox. In addition to the tests we just mentioned, this is also where you find other fitting applications such as VIOLA and the Contour Test (Chapter 5), as well as pre-fitting measures that we discuss in Chapter 7 such as the APHAB and ECHO, and also popular outcome measures like the SADL, IOI-HA, and DOSO, which we discuss in Chapter 19. All in all, it is a very useful website to visit.

ligibility of test passages on an equal-appearing interval scale from 0 to 100. A rating of 0 should reflect a situation in which none of the words is understood and a score of 100 would represent a situation in which all of the words are understood.

Asking participants to estimate the percentage of words they understood yields very similar results as objective speech recognition scores. Although listeners with hearing loss generally underestimate their performance, they do so consistently. Therefore, to estimate objective hearing aid benefit, one could gather subjective data on the perception of intelligibility in both aided and unaided conditions. Listeners who underestimate their performance unaided will also underestimate their performance aided, giving similar estimates of hearing aid benefit (Cox, Alexander, & Rivera, 1991). Similar results have been reported with the SIR (Cox & McDaniel, 1989) test and the Revised SIR (Cienkowski & Speaks, 2000). In total, these results suggest that subjective impression of perceived intelligibility may be a useful measure for evaluating the effects of hearing aids on speech recognition. Therefore, one may choose to use the SIR instead of the CST if interested in the performance with a male instead of a female talker.

Clinical Applications

The CST was designed for, and is used most often in, hearing aid research studies. Although we find it is a bit long for routine clinical use, there are some specific clinical situations where the CST is useful. Many speech recognition in noise measures are limited in the context they provide, which in turn limits their face validity relative to the continuous discourse that is often present during typical conversations. Even more striking, the vast majority of speech recognition measures are presented without the visual cues that are commonly available during typical communication. One reason for this limitation is there are more logistical challenges and greater costs associated with presenting audiovisual materials than just the audio.

Despite these challenges, it is sometimes of interest to determine either the benefit to speech recognition from visual cues or, more likely, the performance advantage provided by a hearing aid with visual cues present. This latter question may be of interest especially in listeners with very poor speech recognition (typically severe-to-profound loss) who are unable to understand speech without visual cues. For example, for counseling purposes, during the pre-fitting visit, you may be interested in showing a patient with profound hearing loss that a directional hearing aid might be able to provide benefit. Unfortunately, this patient is unable to accurately repeat any words in noise without having visual cues. With the audiovisual presentation of the CST and presentation of the noise from behind the listener, you can demonstrate how the directional microphone can make things easier to understand when the talker's face is visible. Repeating this testing at a very challenging SNR also can help you demonstrate how an FM system or remote microphone may be needed instead in difficult listening situations. Such demonstrations can provide a useful starting point when counseling patients on the use of different microphone technologies.

> **TECHNICAL TIP: CRITICAL DIFFERENCES FOR THE CST**
>
> If you are conducting the CST using earphones for ear-specific findings, you might want to know if there is a significant difference between ears. If you conducted this pre-fitting testing as a baseline for later amplification, you might want to know if aided findings are better than unaided. When is a difference really a difference? Cox et al. (1988) reported that the 95% critical difference for scores based on mean performance across two pair of passages (100 key words) per condition is 14 rau (rationalized arcsine units, a measure similar to percent correct). For adults with hearing impairment, the critical difference is 15.5 rau. This means that, for a hearing aid to have a significant effect for a listener, the difference between aided and unaided speech recognition should be approximately 15% or more. This difference of course will need to be larger if only one passage pair per condition is used.
>
> You might have noticed we use the term rau. What is a *rau* you might ask? For starters, it is the abbreviation for rationalized arcsine unit. Arcsine transformations are used to transform proportions to make them more suitable for statistical analysis. These arcsines, however, sometimes do not have an obvious relationship to the original proportions. The *rationalized* arcsine provides values that are numerically close to the original percentage values over most of the percentage range. They still, however, retain the desirable statistical properties of the arcsine transform. See Studebaker (1985) for review.

> **THINGS TO REMEMBER:
> HOW CHANGING SNR AFFECTS PERFORMANCE**
>
> Cox et al. (1988) reported that, for normal hearing listeners, the slope of the performance-intensity function of the CST is 12 rau per dB. For listeners with hearing loss, the slope of the function was 8.5 rau per dB. This means that, for every change in dB, we might expect approximately a 10 % change in speech recognition. This information can be used to adjust the SNR and avoid floor and ceiling effects.

Obtaining the CST

The audio-only version of the CST and the SIR Test are included on the HARL Speech Intelligibility Tests audio CD. The audiovisual version of the CST is available on DVD and organized into six-passage, audiovisual-equivalent sets as discussed in Cox & McDaniel (1989). Both versions can be obtained from the HARL website at the University of Memphis (http://www.memphis.edu/csd/harl/cstest.htm). Also available is an automated scoring system for the audio-only CST.

Speech Recognition in Noise Test (SPRINT)

For many years, the SPRINT was considered a test that only was of interest to military audiologists, as it was developed by U.S. Army audiologist researchers to assist in determining fitness for duty. In recent years, however, this test has found its way into civilian audiology clinics, and therefore, we believe it is important to include a summary of the test in this chapter. The reason that some civilian audiology clinics have started using the test is that they find themselves testing military personnel, particularly reservists and National Guard members, through contractual arrangements. It can also be used for any patient to simply examine more thoroughly the effects of high frequency hearing loss on speech recognition. The test is lengthy (200 words), however, so the time commitment could be a deal breaker for some clinics.

Background

As mentioned, the SPRINT was developed at Walter Reed Army Medical Center for use in the U.S. Army. To understand the reason for its development, it is first necessary to briefly review the fitness for duty requirements. Soldiers in the army are profiled in six different categories, referred to as PULHES:

- P = Physical capacity
- U = Upper extremities
- L = Lower extremities
- H = Hearing-ears
- E = Vision-eyes
- S = Psychiatric

In each of these categories, a numerical rating of 1, 2, 3, or 4 is assigned. An H-1 profile indicates normal function, while an H-4 profile indicates *"unfit for duty."* Clearly, these profiles have a huge impact on a soldier's career.

Individuals need to meet the H-2 profile guidelines to be inducted. Retention standards are not as rigid. Primarily because of the occurrence of noise-induced hearing loss in the military, it is common for soldiers who enter active duty having an H-1 or H-2 profile, to suffer high-frequency hearing loss and, as a consequence, have thresholds exceeding H-2 levels at 3000 and/or 4000 Hz. This bumps them into the H-3 category. In most cases, their SRT will be ≤30 dB without hearing aids and nearly always with hearing aids, so it is unlikely that soldiers with noise-induced, high-frequency hearing loss will be classified as H-4.

As reviewed by Cord, Walden, and Atack (1992), soldiers with H-3 profiles may be required to go before a Military Medical Retention Board (MMRB) that makes a determination to retain, reclassify, or separate the soldier from active duty. This is based on the soldier's ability to perform his or her duties. As a result, the H-3 profile generates the most discussion and was the motivation for developing the SPRINT.

The SPRINT consists of the 200 monosyllabic words from Form C of the NU#6 lists. The words are prerecorded in a background of multitalker babble noise, with a +9 dB speech-to-babble ratio. Cord et al. (1992) explains that this level was chosen so that normal hearing soldiers score 95 to 100% on the test. The goal of this word recognition in noise test is to provide information to the MMRBs for fitness of duty and also to allow for the comparative evaluation of different people holding the H-3 profile.

Normative Data. In early research with the SPRINT, 319 soldiers with H-3 profiles were evaluated. The mean score for the group was 163 items correct (81.5%) with a range of 65 (32.5%) to 196 (98%). Outside of the military, there has not been much research with the SPRINT. One exception is the work of Wilson and Cates (2008), which compared the SPRINT with the WIN test (a test that determines SNR-50, reviewed later in this chapter) for normal hearing and hearing impaired subjects. They report that listeners with normal hearing obtained 92.5% correct on the SPRINT with a WIN-50 score of 2.7 dB SNR. The listeners with hearing loss obtained 65.3% correct on the SPRINT and a WIN-50 at 12.0 dB SNR. The SPRINT and WIN were significantly correlated ($r = -0.81$), indicating that the SPRINT had good concurrent validity. As expected, these authors also report that the high-frequency, pure-tone average (1000, 2000, 4000 Hz) had higher correlations with the SPRINT and WIN than did the traditional three-frequency, pure-tone average (500, 1000, 2000 Hz).

Administration and Scoring

Some general guidelines for administering the SPRINT are as follows:

- The test is delivered using standard audiometric equipment via earphones, using standard calibration procedures. (Note: Given the purpose of this test and the relatively low presentation level, correct calibration of the signal is essential.)
- The monosyllabic words and the multitalker babble are prerecorded at the +9 dB speech-to-babble ratio on the same track of the CD; therefore, only one channel is needed.

- The test is conducted using a *bilateral presentation* (i.e., separate ear scores are *not* obtained).
- The presentation level is 50 dB HL.
- The complete 200-word test must be administered for this test to be valid.

The recommended instructions for the test are as follows:

> You will be hearing a recording of a man's voice saying some words. In the background, there will be the sound of several people talking at once. I want you to repeat back the words that the man is saying. Some of the words may be difficult for you to hear. If you're not sure what the word is, take a guess. There are four lists containing 50 words each for a total of 200 words. This will take about 20 minutes. You will be hearing the words and the background talkers in both ears.

The patient's SPRINT score is simply the number of monosyllabic words that were correctly identified (i.e., 0 to 200). To compare the score with the standardization sample, it is necessary to convert the score to a percentile ranking within the frequency distribution depicted in Table 6–3. For example, if the patient only correctly identifies 133 of the 200 monosyllabic words, the patient would then fall in the 10th percentile, and therefore, we would predict that 90% of all patients with similar hearing losses will score higher than he or she on the SPRINT. When used for military personnel, other

Table 6–3. Conversion Table for the SPRINT*

Score	Percentile	Score	Percentile
0–75	1	162	37
76–100	2	163	40
101–107	3	164	42
108–116	4	165	45
117–122	5	166	48
123–124	6	167	49
125–126	7	168	51
127–128	8	169	53
129–130	9	170	55
131–135	10	171	57
136–138	11	172	59
139–140	12	173	62
141	13	174	64
142	14	175	67
143–144	16	176	70
145	17	177	72
146	18	178	74
147	19	179	76
148	21	180	78
149–150	22	181	80
151–152	23	182	83
153	24	183	86
154	26	184	89
155–156	28	185	92
157	29	186–187	95
158	30	188	96
159	32	189	97
160	34	190	98
161	35	191	99

*Using this table, the item correct score is converted to a percentile.
Source: Adapted from Cord, Walden, & Atack, 1992.

TECHNICAL TIP: PRACTICE EFFECT FOR THE SPRINT?

Although performance for all 200 words of the NU#6 list is used for scoring the SPRINT, Wilson and Cates (2008) examined scores for each 50-word list independently. They found that for the normal hearing group, the scores for Lists 1 to 4 were: 89.0, 93.7, 92.8, and 94.4%. The respective scores for the hearing loss group were: 62.1, 66.8, 67.3, and 65.2%. In both cases, there appears to be about 4% poorer performance for List 1, reflecting a possible learning effect for the speech-in-noise task. An alternative explanation would be poor inter-list equivalency; however, Wilson et al. (1976) showed good inter-list equivalency for these Auditec NU#6 recordings.

charts and considerations are considered to determine fitness for duty (see SPRINT manual).

Clinical Applications

As we mentioned in the introduction, the SPRINT was designed to provide additional information regarding fitness for duty for army personnel. In the military, it is usually administered to all active duty soldiers who are identified as having a permanent H-3 profile and retested when soldiers with an H-3 profile demonstrate a significant, permanent threshold shift.

When making fitting decisions based on the results of speech tests, we normally are looking at results from testing conducted at a relatively high presentation level—we discussed why this is important earlier in this chapter. The SPRINT is delivered at 50 dB HL (around the level of average conversation speech), considerably softer than we would normally use for other pre-fitting speech tests. There would be one benefit, however, of using this lower level. Although we are not aware of real-world validation, we would expect that patients with a significantly poorer SPRINT score are having more difficulty in their everyday communication than the patients with the higher SPRINT scores. This difference, in fact, likely would be greater for the SPRINT than for other tests administered at higher presentation levels. Recall, however, that the SNR for the SPRINT is +9 dB. Individuals with a high SPRINT score, therefore, could be having significant problems in more adverse listening situations—a high SPRINT score does not necessarily mean the patient is not a candidate for hearing aids.

The 200 items of the SPRINT makes it one of the longer speech tests, so it is unlikely an audiologist would adopt this for routine testing when fitting hearing aids. But, if the testing is already being conducted for military reasons, then it seems worthwhile to consider the patient's performance on the SPRINT along with other pre-fitting measures.

Obtaining the SPRINT

The SPRINT can be obtained from Auditec of St. Louis. If using the test for military purposes, we suggest obtaining the test guidelines (militaryaudiology.org/site/2009/01/sprint-test/).

Reception Thresholds for Speech-in-Noise

In the preceding section, we discussed speech-in-noise tests that were designed to use a fixed SNR. These tests answer the clinical question regarding how a patient performs for a given listening situation. These tests, however, often are not good at differentiating patients, primarily because of floor and ceiling effects. Consider two different patients, both with similar high frequency hearing losses. One of these patients does very well in background noise and does not start to have problems until the SNR reaches 1 to 2 dB. The other patient starts to have problems when the SNR is around 6 to 7 dB. These two patients, with the same hearing losses and fitted with the same hearing aids, might have different real-world outcomes affecting hearing aid satisfaction. But, if the speech-in-noise test selected had a fixed SNR, and that SNR was relatively good (such as the R-SPIN at +8 dB), these two patients might appear more similar than they really are due to ceiling effects.

TECHNICAL TIP: TEST-RETEST RELIABILITY

Cord et al. (1992) report test-retest data for 30 normal hearing listeners. The mean score for the initial administration of the SPRINT was 164.6 words correct ($SD = 15.46$), and the mean score for the retest was 166.8 words correct ($SD = 14.21$). The authors found a correlation coefficient of .93 ($p < .01$), suggesting good test-retest agreement. The slightly better (approximately 2%) mean performance for the second administration could be related to the apparent learning effect reported by Wilson and Cates (2008), which they observed following the first 50 words.

Adaptive speech tests, as the name indicates, vary either the speech or the background noise level for each patient. Rather than a percent correct, the test is scored at the SNR where the patient obtained 50% correct. As mentioned previously, this is referred to as the speech reception threshold (SRT) in noise (often denoted as SNR-50 or SRT50); or in the case of the HINT, it is dubbed the reception threshold for speech (RTS). We describe four of these tests in this section.

Finally, it is important to point out that it is risky to generalize the 50% correct for speech-in-noise performance for a given patient without referring back to the test itself and performance for that test for individuals with both normal hearing and hearing loss. Fortunately for our discussion in this chapter, Wilson, McArdle, and Smith (2007) just happened to compare the four SNR-50 speech tests that we describe. They found that for a group of individuals with hearing loss, the mean SNR-50 results for the four different tests were as follows:

BKB-SIN	SNR-50 = 5.0 dB
HINT	RTS = 8.9 dB
QuickSIN	SNR-50 = 12.3 dB
WIN	SNR-50 = 14.0 dB

The above mean values are from the same patients, so that if we only knew that a given patient from this group had an SNR-50 of 8 dB, it would not tell us much. That performance would be considerably better than average for the WIN but worse than average for the BKB-SIN. As you might expect, these scores from hearing impaired individuals differed significantly from people with normal hearing, but the degree of difference also varied for the different tests. The difference was as low as 4.2 and 5.6 dB for the BKB-SIN and the HINT (which have more context in the material) compared with 7.9 and 10.1 dB for the QuickSIN and the WIN.

Hearing in Noise Test (HINT)

For audiologists working with hearing aids, the HINT is one of the most well-known speech-in-noise tests, because for the past 20+ years, it has been the favorite test of researchers when comparative hearing aid performance is conducted. Hence, audiologists are accustomed to thinking about things like the benefit from directional technology in terms of HINT scores—manufacturers often use these scores in promotional literature. The test is favored by researchers of course; because of the adaptive nature of the HINT, floor and ceiling effects are avoided. Moreover, using the SNR-50 approach, which zeros in on the steepest portion of the performance-intensity function, it is more probable that small differences in true performance will be observed.

Although most audiologists know about the HINT, it is not commonly used in the routine hearing aid fitting protocols for adults. This is probably because of several reasons including administration and scoring

---

TECHNICAL TIP: VARY THE SPEECH LEVEL OR THE NOISE LEVEL?

In this section, we discuss adaptive procedures for determining the speech reception threshold in noise (i.e., SNR for 50% correct). For some tests, the noise is fixed and speech varies (e.g., the HINT), and in others the speech is fixed and the noise varies (e.g., BKB-SIN). In most real-world listening situations, it is the noise that is fixed, so that approach would seem to have to the most face validity. But, there also are certain advantages of having a fixed speech signal. One might ask if the test outcome differs depending on which of the two is the variable signal? Wilson and McArdle (2012) did ask this question using modified versions of the R-SPIN, and they found, at least for this test, that it *does not* matter. The mean 50% points were slightly lower (better) on the speech-variable, babble-fixed condition, but the small differences (0.1 to 0.4 dB) are not clinically significant. Larger differences might be expected, however, if lower presentation levels are used and there is an interaction with the audibility of the speech signal.

of the original CD versions that are more cumbersome than most other tests, the results are in SNR rather than percent correct, and availability of the test has been spotty. Nevertheless, it is one of the most researched speech tests and certainly could be adopted for routine clinical use. Conversely, the version for children (Pediatric HINT) is used more commonly, likely because it was more readily available (previously available as the HINT-C CD).

Background

The HINT was originally developed for testing related to the evaluation of bilateral versus unilateral hearing aid fittings. Prior to the HINT, one of the only adaptive speech reception threshold tests reported was the Dutch test developed by Plomp and Mimpen (1979)—which influenced the development of the HINT. The now-classic article describing the development of the HINT at the House Ear Institute of Los Angeles was published by Nilsson, Soli, and Sullivan (1994). The following are some details regarding the development of this test (Nilsson et al., 1994; Vermiglio, 2008):

- The HINT material was derived from the BKB (for Bamford-Kowal-Bench) sentences, which were from British children. The language level is approximately a first-grade reading level.
- The 336 BKB sentences were revised, roughly equated for sentence length, rated for naturalness by native speakers of American English, and were rescaled to obtain equal intelligibility. Following these measures, 252 of the 336 sentences remained; Figure 6–4 shows the sample sentences.
- The current American English version of the HINT for adults has 25 lists of 10 sentences. It is common (and recommended) to use two lists/test (20 sentences). Each list is phonemically balanced and the twelve 20-sentence lists are equivalent.
- The HINT masking noise is a speech spectrum noise that was spectrally matched to the long-term average spectrum of the stimulus sentences.

As we have discussed, there are several adaptive speech tests available from which an audiologist can

1. (A/the) **boy fell from** (A/the) **window**
2. (A/the) **wife helped her husband**
3. **Big dogs can be dangerous**
4. **Her shoes** (are/were) **very dirty**
5. (A/the) **player lost** (a/the) **shoe**
6. **Somebody stole** the **money**
7. (A/the) **fire** (is/was) **very hot**
8. **She's drinking from her own cup**
9. (A/the) **picture came from** (a/the) **book**
10. (A/the) car (is/was) **going too fast**

Figure 6–4. Sample of a 10-item list from the HINT. (Adapted from *HINT Manual Two*, House Ear Institute).

choose. Are these tests all pretty much the same? Mueller, Johnson, and Weber (2010) tested a group of adults with mild-moderate downward sloping hearing loss using both the HINT and the QuickSIN. They found a relatively strong 0.75 correlation between these two measures. Wilson et al. (2007) sought to determine which adaptive speech test would be the best for separating hearing impaired listeners from individuals with normal hearing using four different adaptive speech tests: HINT, QuickSIN, BKB-SIN, and the WIN—the latter three tests are discussed in detail later in this chapter. They concluded that separation between groups was greater for the QuickSIN and the WIN (8 to 10 dB), compared with the HINT and the BKB-SIN (4 to 6 dB). These results suggest that, although there is a strong correlation between these adaptive tests, the QuickSIN and the WIN may be most sensitive to the effects of hearing loss.

Administration and Scoring

The recommended instructions from the HINT manual are as follows:

> This is test of your ability to hear soft speech in a noisy situation. First you will hear background noise. Then you will hear a man reading a sentence. The

> **THINGS TO REMEMBER: THE HINT GOES INTERNATIONAL**
>
> There is little question that the HINT is the most internationally used speech test. In a special issue of the *International Journal of Audiology* (2008), there were summaries of research and norms published for the HINT for the following different languages: Latin American Spanish, Brazilian Portuguese, Turkish, Castilian Spanish, Bulgarian, French, Korean, Norwegian, Malay, Japanese, Canadian French, Cantonese, Taiwanese Mandarin, and Mainland Mandarin. The HINT software currently includes presentation in 22 languages in the adult version and five languages in the pediatric version. Consequently, if your practice setting includes serving patients in languages other than English, this test may allow you to complete speech in noise testing on a greater percentage of your population.

loudness of the man's voice will change during the test. Sometimes it will be very faint. Please repeat anything you hear, even if it is only part of the sentence. I will stop after each sentence to allow you to repeat what you heard. It is all right to guess.

Once the patient is ready to take the test, follow the recommended process:

- Set the noise channel to the HL dial reading that was determined to deliver 65 dB SPL.
- The first sentence is presented at a level which is 5 dB below the noise.
- This first sentence is played and repeated, increasing the level in 4-dB increments until the patient responds correctly. Record this level on the score sheet.
- Begin testing at this level with Sentence #1. An adaptive approach is applied for the intensity of the sentences—the intensity is increased when the patient does not provide a correct response and decreased when the response is correct.
- 4-dB steps are used for Sentences #1 to #4.
- 2-dB adaptive steps are used for Sentences #5 to #20.

Scoring the HINT. The HINT is no longer available on CD; however, if you work at a clinic that still has an old CD copy, the process of administering and scoring the HINT requires a bit more attention than for most recognition measures. First, you will need to listen carefully to the patient's response and determine if the patient got all the key words of the sentence correct. All words must be correct for the sentence to be scored correct. If correct, a "+" is placed on the score sheet; if not correct, "−" is recorded. Then quickly, the intensity level must be lowered or raised, so that the next sentence is presented at the correct level. To help illustrate this method, we have a completed score sheet shown in Figure 6–5. This paper-to-dial visual task—and remembering that for "plus" turn the dial down and for "minus" turn the dial up activity—is not the kind of speech recognition scoring that allows you to simultaneously sip coffee, read text messages, or even daydream. The current HINT that is available in either software or internet versions automate much of this process, but we still feel it is important that we understand what is going on behind the scenes.

Details regarding the scoring (20-sentence list) for HINT are specified below:

- The score placed for Column 21 is based on the patient's performance for Sentence #20. If the patient got Sentence #20 correct, the score for Column 21 is 2 dB lower than what was recorded in Column 20. If the patient missed Sentence #20, then the score placed in Column 21 is 2 dB higher.
- The presentation levels for Columns 5–21 are then summed and divided by 17 to obtain an average. For example, we see in Figure 6–5 that the total of the 17 presentations was 1,164.5; divided by 17 we have an average value of 68.5 dB.
- To obtain the RTS, we need to subtract the HL reference level that was used for the 65 dB SPL calibration. In this case, that value was 60 dB HL, and therefore our RTS is 68.5 dB minus 60 dB or 8.5 dB.

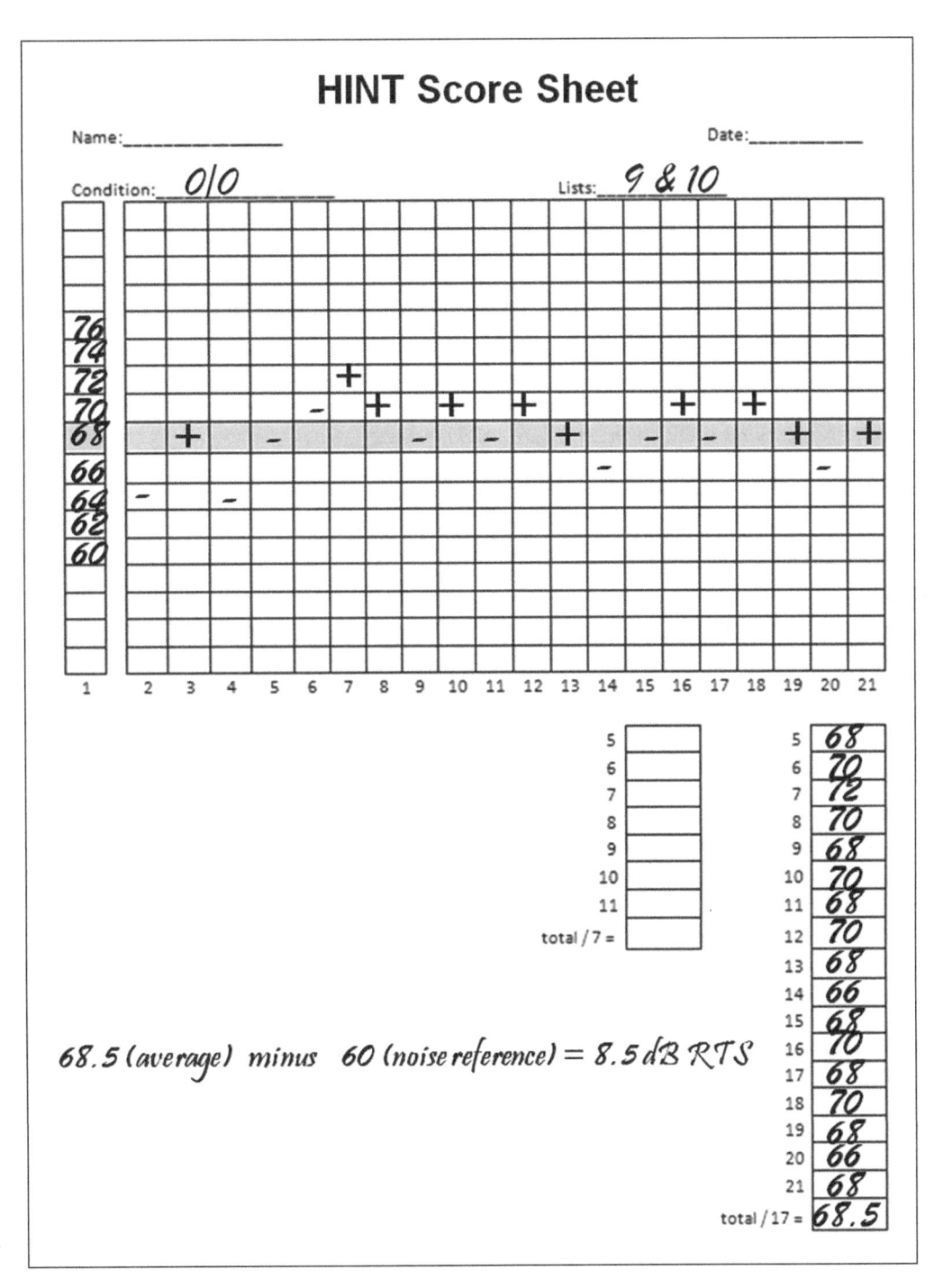

Figure 6–5. Sample of a completed score sheet from the HINT. The "+" and "–" markings indicate when the patient had a correct or incorrect response for a sentence for a given presentation level. The RTS value shown was calculated by subtracting the level of the background noise (60 dB HL) from the average of the last 17 presentations levels (68.5).

> ### POINTS TO PONDER: WHEN IS THE HINT NO LONGER THE HINT?
>
> In various published research studies related to the evaluation of hearing aids and hearing aid candidates, we have observed numerous modifications of the HINT. Often, in these studies it is reported that the HINT was used as the speech material, although we question if it is really the HINT if the test is not administered and scored as originally intended. Some modifications we have observed include the following:
>
> - Presentation levels of the fixed noise signal are lower or higher than the recommended 65 dB SPL.
> - Multitalker babble, cocktail party noise, ISTS (for International Speech Test Signal), the HINT sentences themselves, and other noise signals are used as competition instead of the standard HINT noise.
> - The silent gap between the sentences is filled in with noise.
> - An introductory phrase is used for each sentence.
> - Rather than an adaptive presentation, the background noise is presented at a fixed SNR or in quiet. This is a common procedure for patients with cochlear implants.
> - Rather than scoring each sentence as all or nothing, each word of each sentence is scored.
>
> What really gets confusing is that we have even heard mention of using the HINT with no background noise, which would then seem to make it the HIQT rather than the HINT. When administered using these nonstandard manners it is important that the normative data no longer apply and you cannot even assume the lists are equivalent. Concern over nonstandard clinical use led to the cessation of distribution of the HINT on CD.

> ### TECHNICAL TIP: PERFORMANCE-INTENSITY FUNCTION OF THE HINT
>
> When using the HINT, it is sometimes desirable to think of different HINT RTS scores in terms of predicted intelligibility change. That is, if a person experienced a 3-dB reduction in his HINT RTS, how could we express that as a percent of reduced speech recognition? To obtain an estimate, we can look at performance as a function of the SNR. Nilsson and Soli (1994) reported a slope of 9.5%/dB between 10 and 90% of the range. Eisenberg, Dirks, Takayanagi, and Martinez (1998) reported the slope of the PI function as 11.8% between 20 and 80%. Roughly then, 10 to 12%/dB SNR for the midrange of the function would be a reasonable estimate to remember.

Clinical Applications

One of the clinical applications of the HINT is to determine how a given patient's score differs from people with normal hearing. Shown in Table 6–4 are norms from the HINT manual for sound field testing with both the signal and noise presented from a 0 degree azimuth. Shown in Table 6–5 are HINT norms for bilateral earphone testing (Vermiglio, 2008). Also included in Table 6–5 is the expected intelligibility change from

Table 6–4. HINT Norms for Sound-Field Testing with Both Sentences and HINT Noise Delivered from a Loudspeaker at 0° Azimuth

Percentile	Hint RTS
90th	−4.2
70th	−3.4
50th	−2.8
30th	−2.3
10th	−1.5

Source: Adapted from Koch, Nilsson, & Soli, 2004.

Table 6–5. HINT Earphone Norms For Bilateral Presentation, Noise Front Condition

Percentile	Hint RTS	Intelligibility Change
90th	−3.9	14%
70th	−3.3	7%
50th	−2.6	0%
30th	−1.9	7%
10th	−1.3	14%

Note. Also shown is the expected intelligibility change from the mean (50th percentile).
Source: Adapted from Vermiglio, 2008.

the mean (50th percentile). Note that these two different sets of norms are very similar, within 0.2 to 0.3 for the 90th, 50th, and 10th percentiles.

If we look at the norms for normal hearing individuals, we then have an estimate of where our patient falls. For example, if the HINT RTS is 7 dB, we would then assume that the patient would need the speech turned up or the noise turned down about 9 to 10 dB compared with normal hearing individuals (see 50th percentile for Tables 6–4 and 6–5). This is similar to the SNR loss designator that is used for the QuickSIN, which we explain in the next section. The degree of this SNR loss can be used in pre-fitting counseling. We also know that a patient with an RTS of 2 dB may require different counseling than one with a 10 dB RTS. The same would apply to large ear differences for the HINT. A second application of the HINT is related to spatial separation. The HINT remains one of the few speech in noise tests that includes normative data for conditions in which the speech and noise are presented from the same loudspeaker or earphone (colocated) and when the speech is presented from directly in front and the noise is presented from the side (spatial separation). This allows us to measure spatial release from masking for speech, potentially indicating how important it is to maintain localization cues in individual patients. This has implications for the selection of hearing aid technologies that distort interaural cues such as bilateral beamforming technologies (see Chapter 11).

There are no norms per se for people with sensorineural hearing loss, primarily because there is such variance in the hearing losses studied. Also, many of the studies have modified the HINT, using different background noises, loudspeaker arrangements, and presentation levels. It is common, however, with typical downward sloping hearing losses, to see scores in the +3 to +12 dB RTS range; in the research we mentioned earlier from Mueller et al. (2010), who used the standard HINT format, they reported the mean RTS was 6.4 dB with a range of 0.4 to 16.3 dB.

In addition to providing useful information for counseling, pre-fitting HINT measures can serve as a baseline for later hearing aid verification. Because of the adaptive nature and the 2-dB steps, the sensitivity of the HINT is better than many speech tests for detecting differences in hearing aid performance, for example, the benefits of directional technology. We should mention that if the patient only has a mild-to-moderate hearing loss and the HINT was conducted at a fairly high presentation level, it is very possible that the aided HINT RTS will be no better than the unaided—more on this in Chapter 15.

Obtaining the HINT

The original HINT CD and HINT for children CD (HINT-C) are no longer available. Currently, the HINT is available through software, standalone (hardware and software), and web-based versions. The software enables HINT administration using loudspeakers or headphones. Both the sound field and headphone protocols include conditions with spatial separation of the speech and noise sources. The headphone protocol uses head-related transfer functions (HRTFs) to simulate the spatial locations of the speech and noise sources. This simulation has been validated a number of times with different HINT languages. The HINT software is PC-based and exists in several forms. The standalone and full software versions of the HINT include both fixed and adaptive test protocols using the adult sentence lists for any of the 22 languages and the pediatric sentence lists in five languages (including American English). The standalone HINT can also be used with cochlear implant (CI) recipients by directly connecting the output of an interface box to the auxiliary input on the implant. Special versions of the adaptive protocols can be selected for CI testing. Individuals with one or two CIs can be tested in this manner, as well as individuals with a CI in one ear and acoustic hearing in the other ear.

In 2012, Hearing Test System, LLC, (HTS) obtained the exclusive license to commercialize the HINT technology from the House Research Institute. Both the standalone and web-based versions of HINT are available from HTS (http://hearingtestsystems.net/). Unrelated to hearing aid fitting, a web-based version of the HINT for use in occupational hearing screening is also available. This application is primarily with government agencies that have public safety and law enforcement staff. Federal, state (provincial), and local agencies in the United States and Canada are using the HINT for this purpose.

Quick Speech in Noise (QuickSIN) Test

As we have discussed, understanding speech in background noise is not predictable from a patient's pure-tone thresholds (Dirks et al., 1982; Killion & Niquette, 2000; Lyregaard, 1982; Walden & Walden, 2004). Some early attempts to create clinical tests such as the Speech in Noise test (SIN; Killion & Villchur, 1993) and the R-SPIN (Bilger et al., 1984) turned out to be less than ideal because they were lengthy, and in some cases the lists were not equivalent or they were too difficult for some patients (Bentler, 2000). The QuickSIN was developed to overcome some of these limitations (Killion, Niquette, Gudmundsen, Revit, & Banerjee, 2004).

Background

The QuickSIN was designed to be short enough for routine clinical use but yet provide a quick and reliable way to measure a listener's speech understanding ability in noise. The test certainly is quick, as a single list only requires about a minute to administer after instructions. When introduced, the QuickSIN joined the HINT as a measure that tests multiple SNRs by design. As a result, a threshold SNR, for which approximately 50% of the material is correctly repeated, is determined (commonly referred to as an SNR-50), and the difficulty of choosing a single, correct SNR that avoids floor and ceiling effects is eliminated.

There are a total of 18 lists (plus three practice lists), although in the original design it was pointed out that only 12 lists could be used as single lists (the other six could be used in three pairs). Research since that time has revealed that not all of these 12 lists are equivalent, (see "Things to Remember" passage in this section), so only eight of the lists should be used for routine clinical testing. Sentences are spoken by a female talker who is reading sentences from the speech corpus of the IEEE (1969). The IEEE sentences were designed to be syntactically appropriate and meaningful but still provide limited contextual information. For example, one practice sentence is copied below:

"One step more and the board will collapse."

The QuickSIN sentences are presented in a multitalker background at six predetermined SNRs, which become progressively more difficult with each sentence in 5-dB steps. That is, the first sentence is presented at a +25 dB SNR and the second sentence is presented at a +20 dB SNR. The final sentence is the most difficult and is presented at a 0 dB SNR. The presentation level of the speech is fixed, and the level of the multitalker background varies when SNR is adjusted. The competing signal is somewhat unique because it is not a true babble as used with some of the other tests we describe. It is only four talkers and one of the talkers, a female, is the same talker who is reading the target sentences. At the adverse SNRs (when the multitalkers become louder) many patients report that they have a tendency to try to follow the woman in the competing noise. We discussed information masking earlier in this chapter, and of course, this type of background noise is not unlike what many of our hearing aid patients frequently experience.

The standard QuickSIN lists are available in both a mixed version (target sentences and competing talkers on same track) for standard testing through a headphone or single loudspeaker and a "separated" version where the noise and speech are on separate tracks so they can be routed to separate loudspeakers. The mixed version is helpful as you do not have to be concerned with the calibration of two different channels to maintain the correct SNR.

The standard QuickSIN lists were also modified to generate High Frequency Emphasis (HFE) and High Frequency Emphasis-Low Pass (HFE-LP) lists. These lists are designed to be used in combination to assess the importance of maximizing high-frequency gain for patients with steeply sloping high frequency hearing loss (see "Clinical Applications"). Both HFE lists are the standard lists with approximately 30 dB of high frequency gain applied to simulate the hearing aid gain that might be applied for a listener with 60 to 70 dB of hearing loss. To generate the HFE-LP lists, a low-pass filter was applied with a cut-off frequency of 3,000 Hz to simulate a hearing aid that provides high frequency gain but only through approximately 3000 Hz.

Administration and Scoring

The traditional method of administering the QuickSIN is using the commercially available CD in a CD player routed to a clinical audiometer. The QuickSIN manual describes specific calibration and scoring methods:

- For standard measurement of the SNR-50, the presentation level should be 70 dB HL (83 dB SPL) for patients with pure-tone averages 45 dB or less and should be set to "loud but okay" (just below the patient's LDL) for patients with more hearing loss.
- The test can be administered under headphones (bilaterally or unilaterally) or in the sound field, depending on the desired use (see "Clinical Applications").
- The patient's task is to repeat the sentence spoken by the female talker. Each sentence consists of five key words, and patients receive credit for each key word correctly repeated; unlike the HINT, which we discussed earlier, they do not need to get the entire sentence correct.
- The test is easily scored (with minor math applications) using the standard score sheet, copies of which are available online. The clinician simply marks the number of key words correctly repeated for each sentence and then sums these numbers to calculate a total score, shown in Figure 6–6.

The QuickSIN is scored as SNR loss, rather than SRT-50, because the score is adjusted based on average performance for normal hearing individuals. That is, the number of correctly repeated key words is subtracted from 25.5 (SNR loss = 25.5 – Correct Key Words). This

---

TRACK 21

Practice List A   Score

1. The <u>lake</u> <u>sparkled</u> in the <u>red</u> <u>hot</u> <u>sun</u>.   S/N 25   _____
2. <u>Tend</u> the <u>sheep</u> <u>while</u> the <u>dog</u> <u>wanders</u>.   S/N 20   _____
3. <u>Take</u> <u>two</u> <u>shares</u> as a <u>fair</u> <u>profit</u>.   S/N 15   _____
4. <u>North</u> <u>winds</u> <u>bring</u> <u>colds</u> and <u>fevers</u>.   S/N 10   _____
5. A <u>sash</u> of <u>gold</u> <u>silk</u> will <u>trim</u> her <u>dress</u>. S/N 5   _____
6. <u>Fake</u> <u>stones</u> <u>shine</u> but <u>cost</u> <u>little</u>.   S/N 0   _____
                                                                TOTAL _____

Figure 6–6. Sample list from the QuickSIN. (Adapted from the *QuickSIN User Manual*, Etymotic, Inc.).

number reflects the SNR at which a patient correctly repeats approximately 50% of the key words, with the normal hearing correction (Killion et al., 2004). For example, let's say a patient repeated all the words correctly for the first four sentences (a total of 20 words; 5 key words/sentence), and was not able to get any of the words correct for the last two more difficult sentence presentations (presented at an SNR of +5 dB and 0 dB). We would then subtract 20 (words correct) from 25.5, and this patient would have an SNR loss of 5.5 dB.

Critical difference values for the QuickSIN are shown in Figure 6–7. You can see that these values drop pretty rapidly as the number of lists per condition increases from one to three. Given the very fast test time of giving one list, we believe it is worthwhile to present at least two lists per condition when comparing conditions (e.g., HFE versus HFE-LP or right ear versus left ear). In this case, the time investment is still less than five minutes and critical differences approach 2 dB with 90% confidence. For a single condition (e.g., measuring the patient's SNR loss), it is probably worth your time to present three lists to gain a more accurate and reliable measure. When using more than one list, score each list individually, and then average the SNR loss scores.

Clinical Applications

There are several ways that the QuickSIN findings can be used to assist in hearing aid selection and patient counseling (See the clinical case studies of Mueller, 2016). We review a few of them here.

Hearing Aid Selection. One of the most obvious clinical uses for the QuickSIN may be as a pre-fitting

---

> **KEY CONCEPT: BACKGROUND FOR SCORING THE QUICKSIN**
>
> Audiologists often ask why is it that for scoring the QuickSIN, we use the number 25.5? Why not subtract the missed words from 30, as this is the number of items. Let us explain. This calculation was modeled after the Tillman and Olsen (1973) spondee threshold method. The math is kept simple by using five words per step and a 5-dB step size—in other words, one word per dB. In this case, one-half of the step size (2.5 dB) is added to the starting SNR (+25 dB) and then 2 dB is subtracted from this value because normal hearing listeners score +2 dB SNR on the average. As the authors explain, "if someone repeats all the words correctly down to 15 dB SNR and then misses everything beyond that point, they gave 15 correct responses (five each at 25, 20, and 15 dB SNR). Because they scored 100% correct at 15 dB SNR and 0% correct at 10 dB SNR, their SNR-50 would be about 12.5 dB, halfway between 15 and 10."

Lists per Condition	1	2	3	4	5	6	7	8	9
95% C.D. +/-, in dB	3.9	2.7	2.2	1.9	1.7	1.6	1.5	1.4	1.3
90% C.D. +/-, in dB	3.2	2.2	1.8	1.6	1.4	1.3	1.2	1.1	1.1
80% C.D. +/-, in dB	2.5	1.8	1.5	1.3	1.1	1.0	1.0	0.9	0.8

Figure 6–7. Critical differences for the QuickSIN for different number of lists used. (Adapted from the *QuickSIN User Manual*, Etymotic, Inc.).

> **THINGS TO REMEMBER:
> DO NOT USE THESE QUICKSIN LISTS**
>
> For a standard administration, the QuickSIN is a quick and reliable method of estimating a patient's ability to understand speech in noise. As we have mentioned, you will want to use two or three lists per ear when conducting your testing. It is important, therefore, that all lists are equivalent. Research by McArdle and Wilson (2006) suggests that they may not be. In studying individuals with hearing loss, they found that the range among lists was 10.0 to 14.3 dB SNR. The data from their study indicated that for purposes of homogeneity of test results, for individuals with hearing loss, lists 4, 5, 13, and 16 *should not* be used.

measure to aid in hearing aid selection and counseling decisions. Once a clinician has determined the SNR loss, this information can be combined with knowledge of the patient's communication needs to provide evidenced-based recommendations to the patient regarding hearing aid features, in particular, microphone technology. For example, let's assume a patient has the communication goal of better speech understanding in a noisy mall, for which you estimate the SNR to be +4 dB. If the patient has a QuickSIN score indicating the SNR at which they can repeat 50% of words in sentences (SNR-50) of +6, they might expect to obtain important benefits from directional technology. Conversely, if the patient has a goal of communicating in a noisy club in which you estimate the SNR to be +1 dB and their QuickSIN SNR-50 is +15 dB, we would predict that he or she would not obtain any benefit from directional technology, and an FM system or remote microphone may need to be considered—and you may have some counseling about realistic expectations to do as well.

We find that information regarding SNR loss as it relates to goals and realistic expectations for counseling purposes is one of the best uses for the QuickSIN—this counseling then ties into the pre-fitting completion of the Client Oriented Scale of Improvement (COSI) that we discuss in the next chapter. There also is some evidence that unaided SNR loss may be a significant predictor of amplification success in everyday living. That is, people who have more SNR loss may report less success with hearing aids (Walden & Walden, 2004).

High Frequency Gain. An additional clinical use of the QuickSIN capitalizes on the HFE (for high frequency emphasis) lists (Tracks 36 to 47) and HFE-LP (for high frequency emphasis-low predictability) lists (Tracks 52 to 63). As we discussed in Chapter 5, there is some question as to whether or not people with steeply sloping high frequency hearing loss, particularly those with cochlear dead regions, can benefit from high frequency amplification. Although data suggests that, on average, benefit is expected, it does not occur for all listeners; it appears that the degree to which a patient can make use of high frequency cues depends on the individual. For some patients, providing high frequency amplification may actually impair speech recognition, and for others, high frequency amplification provides additional speech cues, improving speech recognition (Hornsby, Johnson, & Picou, 2011; Rankovic, 1991; Turner & Cummings, 1999). Therefore, a clinician could use the HFE and HFE-LP QuickSIN lists to determine if an individual patient would benefit from high frequency gain, or if that patient would be better served to not have the prescription gain and instead have less high frequency gain. The advantages to not providing high frequency gain for a patient, who would not benefit from it, are that providing high frequency gain may actually impair speech recognition for some patients, especially with steeply sloping high frequency hearing loss. Feedback is generally easier to manage if maximizing high frequency gain is not essential. Therefore, using a couple of QuickSIN lists to determine the usefulness of maximizing high frequency gain could potentially save a clinician (and the patient) considerable time and energy, if high frequency gain proves to be not helpful.

Unilateral Versus Bilateral. The QuickSIN may also be helpful in determining whether to fit unilateral or bilateral amplification. For some patients, especially those that are older, it is possible that using only one hearing aid allows them to understand speech better than with two hearing aids (Walden & Walden, 2005). Whether or not a patient will benefit from two hearing aids is not necessarily predictable from his or her audiogram. That is, even patients with symmetric hearing losses and symmetrical word recognition in quiet may perform better with only one hearing aid in background noise. Therefore, using the QuickSIN under headphones to evaluate SNR loss in each ear and also a bilateral SNR loss could help guide clinical recommendations for hearing aid selection. For example, if a patient has an SNR loss of 4 dB in the right ear, 9 dB in the left ear, and 12 dB bilaterally, the best clinical recommendation may be to encourage the patient to try only the right hearing aid, and then switch to using both hearing aids for specific difficult listening situations during their hearing aid trial period. Depending on patient feedback, this patient may prefer keeping only the right hearing aid (although some patients with this pattern of QuickSIN results may still prefer keeping both instruments for other reasons). Because the SNR loss in the left ear is worse than the right ear and because the bilateral SNR loss is worse than either ear alone, the right ear is a prime candidate for amplification. Dichotic speech testing also will be helpful in making this decision—see our discussion later in the chapter. Of course, the patient's listening needs must be considered when these decisions are made. If the patient rarely is in background noise, it is probably not wise to withhold the benefits of bilateral hearing aids just because of this one factor.

Obtaining the QuickSIN

The QuickSIN CD is available from Etymotic Research (http://www.etymotic.com/pro/) and also from Auditec of St. Louis (https://auditecincorporated.wordpress.com/).

Bamford-Kowal-Bench Sentences in Noise (BKB-SIN)

The BKB-SIN (Etymotic Research, 2005) is another speech-in-noise test that uses the SNR-50 approach. Like its cousin the QuickSIN, it was developed to quickly and accurately assess speech recognition performance in background noise during a routine clinic visit.

Background

The BKB-SIN consists of sentences from the Bamford Kowal-Bench corpus spoken by a male talker with a multalker babble background noise (the same four-talker background that is used for the QuickSIN). The sentences are appropriate for use with pediatric populations because the sentences were derived from language samples taken from young children (Bench, Kowal, & Bamford, 1979) and are at approximately a first-grade reading level (Nilsson & Soli, 1994). Recog-

---

THINGS TO REMEMBER: RELIABILITY OF THE QUICKSIN

For HFE and HFE-LP administration, it may be necessary to test a patient with eight lists—four HFE lists and four HFE-LP lists. By using eight lists, the 95% confidence interval is 1.9 dB. In other words, if the average difference between the HFE and HFE-LP scores is 2 dB or greater, you can assume that the difference is real. So, if a patient achieves a score that is more than 2 dB better with the HFE lists than with the HFE-LP lists, you can conclude that this patient is likely helped by high-frequency gain and you should strive to provide the recommended high-frequency gain for this patient. The research of Johnson and Cox (2009) revealed Lists 1, 4, 5 and 10 of the HFE and HFE-LP lists were the most sensitive to reduction of high-frequencies and should give the most valid information regarding about benefit from high-frequency cues. Therefore an alternative procedure would be to only use these four lists (two per condition) when the QuickSIN is used for this purpose.

nition of the words in the sentences in each list progressively becomes more difficult by increasing the noise +3 dB for each sentence. That is, the SNR progressively changes in 3 dB steps from +9 to −6 dB (List Pairs 1 to 8) and from +21 to 0 dB (List Pairs 9 to 18). Each list pair consists of two lists, each with 8 to 10 sentences. A sample list is displayed in Figure 6–8.

Although not quite as quick as the QuickSIN, it is still quite fast. In addition, the BKB-SIN holds several other advantages including better reliability, better list equivalency, and more normative data including norms for cochlear implant users and children. For these reasons, we favor the BKB-SIN over the QuickSIN for most of the clinical applications we described earlier for the QuickSIN. There are two caveats to this recommendation. First, there are currently no HFE or HFE-LP lists available for the BKB-SIN, so the QuickSIN still must be used for assessing benefits for high-frequency amplification. Second, and perhaps more importantly, the Quick-SIN results in larger differences between normal and hearing impaired listeners, likely due to differences in talker gender and sentence complexity, and is therefore more sensitive to difficulties with understanding speech in noise.

Administration and Scoring

Administration and scoring is nearly identical to the QuickSIN, which we detailed in the previous section. In brief, the easiest method of administering the BKB-SIN is using the commercially available CD in a CD player routed to a clinical audiometer. The BKB-SIN manual describes specific calibration and scoring methods. For determining an SNR loss and comparison with normative data, the presentation level should be 70 dB HL for patients with three-frequency pure-tone averages 45 dB or less and should be set to "loud but okay" for patients with more hearing loss. The test can be administered under headphones (bilaterally or unilaterally) or in the sound field, depending on the desired use (see "Clinical Applications"). The patient's task is to repeat the sentence spoken by a male talker. The instructions are as follows:

> Imagine you are at a party. There will be a man talking and several other talkers in the background. The man will say, "Ready," and then will say a sentence. Repeat the sentence the man says. The man's voice is easy to hear at first because his voice is louder than the others. The background talkers will gradually

List 9A	Key Words	# Correct	SNR
1. The football player lost a shoe.	4	_____	+21 dB
2. The painter used a brush.	3	_____	+18 dB
3. The lady sat on her chair.	3	_____	+15 dB
4. The milkman brought the cream.	3	_____	+12 dB
5. The dog chased the cat.	3	_____	+9 dB
6. Mother shut the window.	3	_____	+6 dB
7. The apple pie was good.	3	_____	+3 dB
8. Rain falls from the clouds.	3	_____	0 dB
	Total Key Words Correct	_____	
	SNR − 50 = (23.5) − (# correct)	_____	

Figure 6–8. Sample list from the BKB-SIN.™ (Adapted from the *BKB-SIN™ User Manual*, Etymotic, Inc.).

become louder, making it difficult to understand the man's voice, but please guess and repeat as much of each sentence as possible.

The BKB-SIN contains 18 equivalent list pairs, but both lists in the pairs must be administered and included in the score to retain maximum reliability and equivalency. Each sentence consists of three or four key words—the first sentence has four, the rest have three—and patients receive credit for each key word correctly repeated. The number of key words correct is subtracted from 23.5 to determine the SNR-50, or the SNR at which a patient understands 50% of the words (SNR loss = 23.5 − Correct Key Words). Calculate an SNR-50 for each list and then average the values for both lists in a list pair to calculate an overall SNR-50. This number reflects the SNR at which a patient correctly identifies approximately 50% of the key words.

Once the SNR-50 is obtained, the BKB-SIN manual contains normative values that can be used to calculate an SNR loss, which is analogous to the SNR loss derived using the QuickSIN. SNR loss is calculated by subtracting the average SNR-50 for a population from the patient's SNR-50 (SNR loss = Patient's SNR-50 − Normative Data SNR-50). These normative values are found in the BKB-SIN manual and are displayed in Table 6–6. For example, if you tested an adult hearing aid candidate and calculated the SNR-50 to be 10 dB, you could then calculate the SNR loss (SNR loss = 10 dB − (−2.5 dB) = 12.5 dB). The same data interpretation can be used for the BKB-SIN as the QuickSIN (see Table 6–6). That is, for this patient, you have discovered a moderate SNR loss, relative to adult listeners with normal hearing.

There are some important points to note relative to these data interpretations. First, these normative values are only applicable when using the CD, a calibrated audiometer, List Pairs 1 to 8, and moderate-to-loud presentation levels. These data are not to be used if testing was completed with a system that has not been calibrated, soft presentation levels (35 to 40 dB HL), or the Split Track tests. The Split Track CD contains recordings with the speech and noise on separate channels and is useful for sound field testing.

Clinical Applications

Like the QuickSIN, the BKB-SIN can be used to estimate SNR loss to assist in hearing aid selection, to guide realistic expectations counseling, to demonstrate the benefits of amplification, and to evaluate directional microphones. There are some notable differences between the BKB-SIN and the QuickSIN. First, the BKB-SIN takes approximately three minutes to complete, whereas the QuickSIN is only one minute per list. In addition, recent evidence suggests that the BKB-SIN is easier than the QuickSIN (Wilson et al., 2007). Because it is easier, the BKB-SIN may be more appropriate than the QuickSIN for use with patient populations who would otherwise struggle with speech-in-noise testing like children, patients with severe hearing losses, or patients with cochlear implants. Although the BKB-SIN contains normative data for a variety of ages, the interpretation of the results is more difficult for children. Speech, language, and academic skills and experience can play a role in susceptibility to background noise and learning in children. Therefore, poorer performance may be attributed, at least in part, to developmental and other factors unrelated to SNR loss.

Similar to the QuickSIN, the BKB-SIN may be related to other self-reported outcomes. More specifically, some investigators have reported that higher SNR losses, as measured with the BKB-SIN, are significantly related to self-perceived communication difficulties for adults who use cochlear implants. That is, people who

Table 6–6. BKB-SIN Test Norms (List Pairs 1–8)

	Adults		Children		
	Normal Hearing	CI Users	Ages 5–6	Ages 7–10	Ages 11–14
Mean SNR-50	−2.5	*	3.5	0.8	−0.9
St. Dev.	0.8	1.6	2.0	1.2	1.1

Source: Adapted from Etymotic Research, 2005.

> **THINGS TO REMEMBER: RELIABILITY OF THE BKB-SIN**
>
> Because one use for the BKB-SIN is to compare performance with one ear versus the other, it is important to consider how different scores need to be to be considered reliably different. This minimum difference score varies based on patient population. Figure 6–9 displays the critical differences for the BKB-SIN for each patient population and for each confidence interval. The confidence interval indicates how certain you can be that the difference you have found is real. If the difference between two lists is larger than the 95% confidence interval, you can assume that there is only a 5% chance that the difference between the lists is not real. For example, let's say you test a hearing aid candidate and find a score of 10 dB SNR-50 for the right ear and a score of 7 dB for the left ear. Using the table shown in Figure 6–9, you can see that there is better than a 95% chance that the difference between the two ears is real. To obtain meaningful differences that are smaller than the values listed, a clinician would need to use more than one list pair per condition.

have more significant SNR loss, are more likely to report difficulties communicating in daily life, even with a cochlear implant (Donaldson et al., 2009). This information can be used to help guide expectations counseling for both hearing aid and cochlear implant users.

Obtaining the BKB-SIN

The BKB-SIN is available from Etymotic Research (http://www.etymotic.com/pro/) and also Auditec of St. Louis (https://auditecincorporated.wordpress.com/).

	Number of Lists =	1	2	3	4	5	6	7	8	9	
Adults	95% C.D. Test +/-	2.2	1.6	1.3	1.1	1.0	0.9	0.8	0.8	0.7	dB
	80% C.D. Test +/-	1.8	1.3	1.0	0.9	0.8	0.7	0.7	0.6	0.6	dB
Adult CI Users	95% C.D. Test +/-	4.4	3.1	2.6	2.2	2.0	1.8	1.7	1.6	1.5	dB
	80% C.D. Test +/-	3.6	2.6	2.1	1.8	1.6	1.5	1.4	1.3	1.2	dB
Children by Age											
5-6	95% C.D. Test +/-	5.4	3.9	3.1	2.7	2.4	2.2	2.1	1.9	1.8	dB
	80% C.D. Test +/-	4.4	3.1	2.6	2.2	2.0	1.8	1.7	1.6	1.5	dB
7-10	95% C.D. Test +/-	3.5	2.5	2.0	1.8	1.6	1.4	1.3	1.2	1.2	dB
	80% C.D. Test +/-	2.9	2.0	1.7	1.4	1.3	1.2	1.1	1.0	1.0	dB
11-14	95% C.D. Test +/-	3.2	2.3	1.9	1.6	1.5	1.3	1.2	1.1	1.1	dB
	80% C.D. Test +/-	2.6	1.9	1.5	1.3	1.2	1.1	1.0	0.9	0.9	dB

Figure 6–9. Critical differences for the BKB-SIN™ for the different number of lists used. (Adapted from the *BKB-SIN™ User Manual*, Etymotic, Inc.).

> **THINGS TO REMEMBER: THE BKB-SIN FOR KIDS?**
>
> The focus of this chapter is testing for adults, but as we mentioned above, there is also BKB-SIN normative data for children provided in the user manual. This research found that the BKB-SIN test can be used for children as young as five years old. Reliability is considerably lower for children under 7 years old, however. Still, of the speech-in-noise tests using sentence materials mentioned in this chapter, the BKB-SIN is probably the best suited for the pediatric population.

Words in Noise (WIN) Test

So far in this section, we have discussed three different SNR-50 tests that easily could be used for hearing aid pre-fitting testing. The HINT is a sentence test (all words in the sentence must be correct for the sentence to be correct); the QuickSIN and the BKB-SIN also use sentences, although the scoring is for individual key words within each sentence. The final test in this category is the WIN (for Words in Noise), which uses the NU#6 monosyllables. Recall that in the beginning of this chapter, we reviewed some benefits of using sentences material for speech-in-noise testing, but there also are associated limitations:

- With sentence material, context contributes heavily to intelligibility and makes basic auditory function difficult to determine.
- Sentences involve more complex cognitive skills; more working memory effort is required. These demands could differentially affect older versus younger patients.

These factors could lead us to select a monosyllable test for speech-in-noise testing. If so, the WIN seems to be the most carefully researched tool available.

Background

Wilson (2003) describes that several factors entered into the development of the WIN test including a test that would use traditional word stimuli, that would fit a clinical protocol, that would evaluate recognition performance at multiple SNRs, and that would generate a performance metric that was easy to compute and easy to interpret. The WIN then evolved with the following characteristics (Wilson, 2003):

- The NU#6 monosyllabic materials recorded by a female speaker were selected. This test was already in widespread use in VA clinics and, therefore, familiar to clinicians. This word list also was selected because of its sensitivity to the variety of word-recognition performances in quiet exhibited by individuals with hearing loss. This enables word-recognition data to be obtained in quiet and in the background noise using the same speaker, speaking the same words.
- The justification for selecting multitalker babble as the competing background noise was based on evidence that multitalker babble is the most common environmental noise encountered by listeners in everyday life (Plomp, 1978). The multitalker babble used with the WIN test was recorded by audiologist Donald Causey and consists of three female and three male speakers talking about various topics (Sperry, Wiley, & Chial, 1997).
- The level of the multitalker babble is fixed relative to the varied level of the speech signal. This is designed to mimic the real world, in which background noises are maintained at fairly constant levels for given listening situations. To reduce test variability, the words were time-locked to a unique segment of babble for reduced variability.
- To be efficient, the test was designed to use multiple speech presentation levels in which

10 words were presented at each of seven levels (a total of 70 words).
- Finally, the WIN test design was amenable to quantification in terms of percent correct at each signal-to-babble ratio, of the overall percent correct, and of the 50% correct point of the signal-to-babble function.

The above provides some of the original goals, and the clinical WIN test of today is mostly the same. It has been shortened to 35 monosyllables (see Wilson & Burks, 2005), which are presented in seven groups of five with a fixed babble level; the level of the words change in 4-dB steps equating to SNRs ranging from 24 to 0 dB, see score sheet shown in Figure 6–10.

In 2011, Wilson published a summary of WIN test results for a rather impressive number of test subjects—3,430. In this study, he compares the WIN findings with age, degree of hearing loss, and performance on the NU#6 test in quiet. One of the major findings supports our statements at the beginning of this chapter—it is very difficult to predict a patient's speech understanding in noise from his or her speech recognition in quiet. Wilson reports that 70% of the participants had recognition performances in quiet (NU#6) that were good or excellent, but only 6.9% of these same patients had normal performance for the WIN. For the 222 participants who had normal performance for the WIN, 218 (98.2%) also had excellent word recognition in quiet (92% correct or better). And perhaps most important, 1,383 (46.1%) of the 3,000 participants with abnormal performances on the WIN had excellent performances on the NU#6 in quiet (92% or better). In other words, normal performance on the WIN pretty much assures normal performance for speech in quiet, but the opposite is not true. The general relationship between word recognition in quiet and the WIN is shown in Figure 6–11. As expected, WIN performance also became poorer when the hearing loss became greater. This relationship is shown in Figure 6–12 for both the 500, 1000, and 2000 Hz pure-tone average and the high-frequency average (1000, 2000, and 4000 Hz).

Administration and Scoring

The WIN test protocol that we describe here is that developed by Richard Wilson, PhD, and is available from the VA CD, Speech Recognition and Identification Materials, Disc 4.0. The mixed speech in noise is in one channel and only the test stimuli are on the other channel, which is not used for testing. This second channel can instead be used by the clinician to hear the words clearly for monitoring and scoring purposes. Test administration is about six minutes.

- With the pure tone calibrated to 0 VU (0 dB), the babble is 20 dB below the level of the calibration tone indicated on the monitoring meter.
- The words-in-noise testing is completed under headphones. The words-in-noise are on the left channel, and the words-in-quiet at a constant level are on the right channel (for monitoring purposes only). Therefore, the left channel should be routed to whichever ear is being tested.

KEY CONCEPT: PRESENTATION LEVEL EFFECTS

Wilson (2003) examined the effects of presentation level of the WIN for two different levels (70 versus 90 dB SPL) for groups of normal hearing and hearing impaired individuals. He found that for the listeners with normal hearing, 20% of the performances were better for 70 dB SPL than for 90 dB SPL; 32% were better for 90 dB SPL than for 70 dB SPL; and 48% of the performances were equal at the two presentation levels. The same analysis for the listeners with hearing loss revealed 33% of the performances were better for 70 dB SPL than for 90 dB SPL; 30% were better for 90 dB SPL than for 70 dB SPL; and 36% of the performances were equal at the two presentation levels. Overall, there was a fairly even distribution for both presentation levels with no clear winner.

Words-in-Noise (WIN)

Name_____SS#_____Age_____

Date_____By_____Ear_____Level_____

Track 25, List 1, Random 1

24-dB S/B		12-dB S/B		0-dB S/B	
1	pain	16	hate	31	gaze
2	youth	17	shack	32	life
3	wheat	18	tool	33	get
4	dodge	19	voice	34	read
5	cool	20	rush	35	bath
20-dB S/B		**8-dB S/B**			
6	ditch	21	turn		
7	ring	22	young	# Correct	
8	kick	23	bite	Threshold (50%)	
9	chair	24	pick	dB S/B	
10	luck	25	half		
16-dB S/B		**4-dB S/B**			
11	base	26	far		
12	wire	27	learn		
13	red	28	mood		
14	time	29	talk		
15	judge	30	note		

Ear_____Level_____

Track 25, List 2, Random 1

24-dB S/B		12-dB S/B		0-dB S/B	
1	food	16	good	31	back
2	road	17	search	32	dab
3	juice	18	pass	33	kill
4	late	19	witch	34	nice
5	hire	20	chief	35	calm
20-dB S/B		**8-dB S/B**			
6	tire	21	sour		
7	such	22	doll	# Correct	
8	shawl	23	deep	Threshold (50%)	
9	haze	24	soap	dB S/B	
10	gun	25	make		
16-dB S/B		**4-dB S/B**			
11	live	26	beg		
12	date	27	mess		
13	gas	28	long		
14	have	29	mouse		
15	dog	30	sheep		

	# Correct	Threshold
	1	25.2
	2	24.4
	3	23.6
PROFOUND	4	22.8
	5	22.0
	6	21.2
	7	20.4
	8	19.6
	9	18.8
	10	18.0
SEVERE	11	17.2
	12	16.4
	13	15.6
	14	14.8
	15	14.0
MODERATE	16	13.2
	17	12.4
	18	11.6
	19	10.8
	20	10.0
	21	9.2
MILD	22	8.4
	23	7.6
	24	6.8
	25	6.0
	26	5.2
	27	4.4
	28	3.6
	29	2.8
NORMAL	30	2.0
	31	1.2
	32	0.4
	33	-0.4
	34	-1.2
	35	-2.0

Figure 6–10. Example of score sheet used for the WIN test. (Adapted from the Clinical Protocol for Speech Testing, Eastern Tennessee State University, Johnson City, TN).

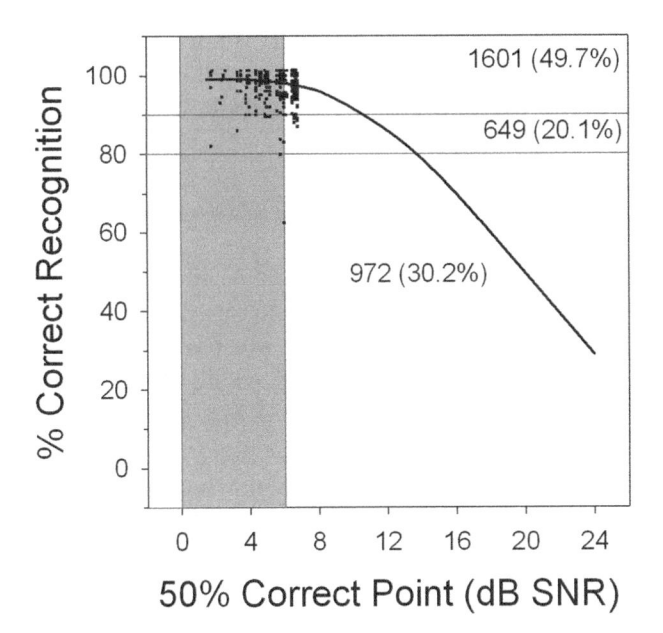

Figure 6–11. Bivariate plot of WIN test performance as it relates to word recognition scores in quiet. (Adapted from Wilson, 2011).

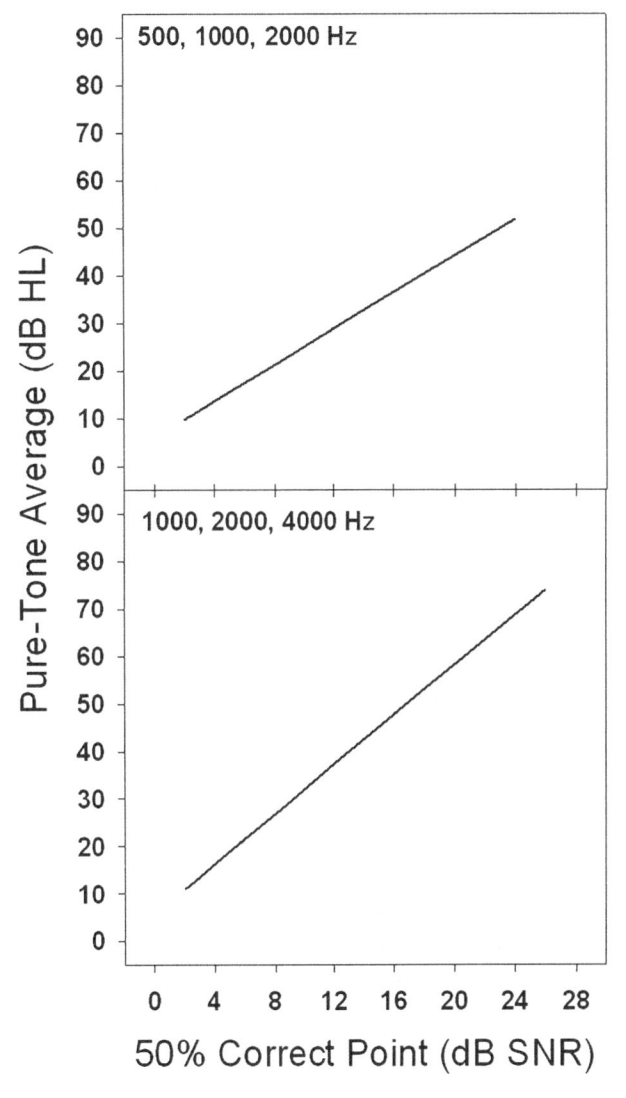

Figure 6–12. Bivariate plot of WIN test performance as it relates to hearing loss for both standard pure-tone average (500, 1000, and 2000 Hz) and for the high frequency average (1000, 2000, and 4000 Hz).

- The score sheet selected determines the tracks that are presented (i.e., if the next score sheet is for Tracks 3 and 4, then those tracks are presented to the patient).
- The presentation level for the WIN is determined from the following:
  - Pure-tone average ≤40 dB HL: the HL is set to 80 dB. This puts the babble at 80 dB SPL (60 dB HL) with the words ranging from 104 dB SPL (84 dB HL) to 80 dB SPL (60 dB HL).
  - Pure-tone average >40 dB HL to 59 dB HL: the HL is set to 90 dB. This puts the babble at 90 dB SPL (70 dB HL) with the words ranging from 114 dB SPL (94 dB HL) to 90 dB SPL (70 dB HL).
  - Pure-tone average ≥60 dB HL: The ETSU protocol recommends not conducting the WIN when hearing loss reaches this level, as background data are not available.

To score the WIN, the number of words repeated correctly is counted for each signal-to-babble ratio (five possible for each of seven levels). Some audiologists also plot the number of correct responses on the WIN normative chart; the shaded region represents the 90th percentile for people with normal hearing, shown in Figure 6–13. This graphic representation can be helpful for patient counseling. The scores for each level are then added to determine the total correct and the SNR-50 (SNR for 50% correct) is then obtained from the chart on the right hand side of the score sheet (see Figure 6–10). These thresholds correspond to the descriptors used

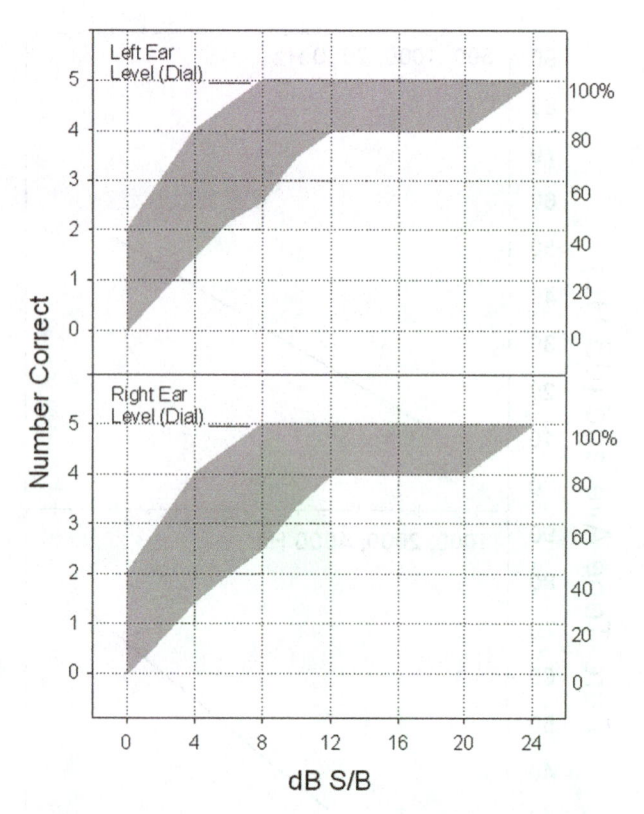

Figure 6–13. Chart for plotting the results of the WIN. The shaded area represents the 90th percentile cutoff. (Adapted from the Clinical Protocol for Speech Testing, Eastern Tennessee State University, Johnson City, TN).

in the threshold chart on the score sheet (e.g., normal, mild, moderate, severe, or profound), and these terms can be used to describe the patient's performance.

If the look-up SNR-50 chart is not available or if you just enjoy doing a little math, the following equation can be used to calculate the WIN SNR-50 based on the raw score:

WIN Score = 26 − (80% of total correct words)

Thus, the best WIN score that can be attained (35 correct) is −2.0 dB SNR-50 (80% of 35 = 28; subtracted from 26 = −2 dB SNR), and the worst WIN score possible (0 correct) is an SNR-50 of 26.0 dB (80% of 0 = 0; subtracted from 26 = 26 dB SNR). Lower WIN scores, therefore, are indicative of better performance on this test, as is also the case for other measures of SNR-50, such as the BKB-SIN, QuickSIN, and HINT.

Clinical Applications

As we mentioned in the introduction of this chapter, SNR-50 scores for a given patient must be interpreted relative to the test that was used. The following are the general WIN test interpretation guidelines provided by Wilson and Burks (2005):

- Normal: ≤6.0 dB.
- Mild: 6.8 to 10.0 dB.
- Moderate: 10.8 to 14.8 dB.
- Severe: 15.6 to 19.6 dB.
- Profound: >20 dB.

Armed with the chart above and with the average data from the large sample of patients displayed in Figures 6–11 and 6–12, the patient's WIN test findings can

---

THINGS TO REMEMBER: LIST 3 FOR PRACTICE ONLY

Presently there are two 35-word WIN lists for a total of 70 words. When the WIN test was developed, researchers originally had identified 150 words from the NU#6 list that potentially would be appropriate. Wilson and Watts (2012) examined the possibility of constructing a third list of 35 words for the WIN test from the 80 that were left over. There are times, both in the clinic and in research, when a third list would be useful. In their research, the authors found that the 90th percentiles for Lists 1 and 2 for the listeners with normal hearing were both 6.0 dB SNR, which is exactly the 90th percentile established with the original WIN (Wilson, Abrams, & Pillion, 2003). In contrast, the 90th percentile for List 3 was 10.6 dB SNR. A large difference also was present on List 3 for individuals with hearing loss. The authors recommend, therefore, that List 3 could be used as a practice list but should not be used for clinical testing.

be used to assist in making fitting decisions and providing appropriate counseling. For clinical purposes, we usually consider a difference of 3 dB significant for the WIN test. Here are some examples of how WIN test results might be used:

- The patient's WIN scores are 6 to 8 dB in both ears. The speech-in-noise recognition is at or near that of people with normal hearing. We would expect the patient to do quite well in background noise with the hearing aids if we provide appropriate audibility.
- The patient's WIN scores are 16 to 18 dB in both ears. We would expect this patient to have significant problems in background noise even with properly fitted hearing aids. They should be counseled accordingly and strongly encouraged to use FM, remote microphones, or other assistive listening technology.
- The patient's high frequency pure-tone average is 30 dB and the bilateral WIN score is 17 dB. A patient with a high frequency average of only 30 dB typically has a WIN score around 10 dB. The 17 dB score, therefore, suggests that this patient may have cognitive and/or auditory processing difficulties that impact the ability to understand in background noise.
- The patient has relatively symmetrical hearing and word recognition in quiet, but the WIN score is 8 dB for the right ear and 14 dB for the left. If this patient has a strong preference to only purchase one hearing aid, consider aiding the right ear. If this patient is fitted with bilateral amplification, consider that the hearing aid for the left ear may not be helpful for listening in background noise.

Obtaining the WIN

The VA Auditory and Vestibular Research Laboratory have three audio compact discs available. The WIN is included on Disc 4.0, Speech Recognition and Identification Materials.

KEY CONCEPT: WIN AND QUICKSIN—SAME OR DIFFERENT

Earlier in this chapter, we talked about another SNR-50 test, the QuickSIN, which is a sentence recognition task. McArdle, Wilson, and Burks (2005) compared the recognition performances of 36 listeners with normal hearing and 72 listeners with sensorineural hearing loss on the WIN test and the QuickSIN. Two different lists were used for each test. The listeners with hearing loss had mean SNR-50s for both tests that were 7 to 8 dB higher than those of the listeners with normal hearing. The mean SNR-50 performance for the WIN for the two lists was 12.3 and 12.4 dB; for the QuickSIN 10.1 and 13.3 dB. The difference between the WIN and QuickSIN performances was not significant, suggesting that at least for these two tests, words and sentences in multitalker babble provide the same differentiation between performances by listeners with normal hearing and listeners with hearing loss. Therefore, both the WIN and QuickSIN would seem to be equally sensitive to the effects of hearing loss.

THINGS TO REMEMBER: THE WIN TEST FOR KIDS?

The focus of this chapter is testing for adults, but it is worth mentioning that the WIN test also has been normed for children (see Wilson, Farmer, Gandhi, Shelburne, & Weaver, 2010). This research found that the WIN test can be used for children as young as six years old. Suggested upper cutoffs for each of the seven age groups ranged from 13.2 dB SNR-50 (6-year-olds) to 8.4 dB SNR-50 (9- to 12-year-olds).

Further information, score sheets and contact information and instructions for ordering these materials can be found online (http://www.avreap.research.va.gov/AVREAPRESEARCH/Resources/CliniciansResearchers/Speech_Recogition_Test_Materials.asp).

Speech-Based Subjective Ratings

To this point, we have discussed several tests that are objective measures of speech recognition in noise—some use sentence material and others use monosyllables. Some have a fixed SNR, whereas others use an SNR-50 approach. What these tests all have in common, however, is that they require a response from the patient that is then objectively scored by the audiologist. In this upcoming section, we discuss two speech-in-noise tests that are somewhat different. Both of these tests utilize a subjective response from the patient. In one case, the patients relate at what point they are bothered by background noise; in the other instance, the patients report how well they believe they are understanding speech.

Acceptable Noise Level (ANL)

It is possible to combine speech and noise and have the patient make judgments regarding the signal. One such measure is the *acceptability* of the level of the background noise while listening to speech. This is the design of the acceptable noise level (ANL) test. Although the ANL is a relatively new *clinical* procedure, it has been used in research for over 20 years. The development of the ANL is credited to the research of Anna Nabelek at the University of Tennessee. The ANL just might be the most researched speech-in-noise test in the past decade or so. In 2014, Olsen and Brännström published a review article, revealing that there had been 45 peer-reviewed articles on the ANL since 2004.

Background

The first publication describing the ANL procedure was by Nabelek, Tucker, and Letowski in 1991. At that time, the test was called the *tolerated SNR*. And, speaking of names, it is important to point out that the term ANL is somewhat of a misnomer, as the test score is a *difference value*, not a *level* per se. More precise, it is an SNR, as indicated by its original name. The test consists of two measures and a calculation:

- Measurement #1: Most Comfort Level (MCL). The patient first adjusts running speech in quiet, using a bracketing procedure, until the MCL has been determined.
- Measurement #2: Background Noise Level (BNL). Leaving the running speech set at the patient's MCL, multitalker babble is introduced. Again, a bracketing procedure is used, and the listener adjusts the babble to the maximum level that is deemed acceptable and that still enables the listener to follow the speech passage *without becoming tense or tired*. This determines the BNL.
- Calculation: Acceptable Noise Level (ANL). The BNL is subtracted from the MCL, which provides the ANL. For example, if the patient's MCL is 72 dB HL and the BNL is 64 dB HL, then the ANL would be 8 dB.

As apparent from the procedure just described, small ANLs (e.g., 5 dB or less) are normally considered good, as this means that the patient is willing to put up with a considerable amount of noise while listening to speech. On the other hand, big ANLs (e.g., >15 dB) are not so good, as it means that the patient is easily bothered by background noise. As reported by Plyler (2009), data from years of ANL research at the University of Tennessee laboratory show ANL values ranging from −2 to 38 dB for listeners with normal hearing and from −2 to 29 dB for listeners with hearing impairment. Plyler (2009) reports that their most common ANL value is around 10 dB for both groups of listeners, and both groups have similar ANL distributions.

An interesting factor associated with the ANL test is that the patient's ANL seems to be unaffected by many test variables that sometimes do affect objective speech recognition measures. For example, research has shown that there are several things that do not appear to affect ANL scores—see Freyaldenhoven (2007) and Plyler (2009) for a complete review. The following variables have been shown *not* to affect the ANL:

Age, gender, primary language, degree of hearing loss, acoustic reflex thresholds, otoacoustic emissions contralateral suppression, type of speech material, type of background noise, patient's speech recognition in quiet or in background noise, whether the testing is aided or unaided, and experience using hearing aids.

We talk about some of these factors in more detail shortly. Given the list above, at this point you might be asking, what *does* affect the ANL or what is related to the ANL? Limited research suggests association could exist with the following (Freyaldenhoven, 2007; Plyler, 2009):

- Presentation Level: ANLs tend to be larger (worse) as the presentation level of the speech signal becomes higher (although ANL growth patterns are the same for normal hearing and hearing impaired individuals).
- One study revealed a 4-dB increase in speech presentation level yielded a 1-dB increase in ANL. Given that the MCLs for individuals being fitted for hearing aids usually fall in relative small range (e.g., 20 dB or so), this factor should not have a large impact on ANL clinical interpretation.
- Plyler (2015) reports that the addition of visual cues improved ANL values for normal hearing listeners; however, visual cues only improved ANL values for listeners with impaired hearing when they were using their hearing aids. Interestingly, the effect of visual cues on the ANL was larger for listeners with poor ANL values than for those with good ANL values; however, it was not related to speech reading ability. These results are consistent with previous studies examining the role of visual cues on the ANL in normal hearing listeners (Wu, Stangel, Pang, & Zhang, 2014).
- One study revealed that normal hearing listeners classified as Type B personality had significantly smaller ANL values than listeners classified as Type A personality. That is, people who are more "high strung," prefer a higher level of control, and are more detail oriented (Type A personality) tend to have larger ANL values—are more easily bothered by background noise.
- Research with patients diagnosed with ADHD/ADD found that ANLs improved while the patients were on stimulant medication.

A point we make in this chapter and others regarding pre-fitting testing is that it is not feasible to do all the tests, so when you select your test battery you will want to use tests that provide *different* information. Because of this, it has been common to compare ANL findings with more commonly administered objective speech recognition measures. The results of these studies have been in agreement, showing that the patients' ANL was not significantly related to their performance on the SPIN (Nabelek, Tampas, & Burchfield, 2004), the HINT

THINGS TO REMEMBER: HEARING AND TECHNOLOGY AND THE ANL

Given that we usually think of small ANLs as good, it is reasonable to question whether hearing aid technology can improve the ANL. Freyaldenhoven et al. (2005) showed that directional microphone technology resulted in an average 3 dB improvement (lowering) of the measured ANL. Note, the patient's ANL is not really changing; the SNR in the ear canal is. Regardless, we would expect that the patient would now accept 3 dB more of background noise. Mueller, Weber, and Hornsby (2006) reported similar findings for digital noise reduction (DNR); an approximate 4 dB improvement. These DNR findings should be interpreted with caution, however, as the noise was the competing speech-shaped broadband signal of the HINT. The magnitude of the benefit would likely be smaller if a more speech-like noise were present.

(Mueller et al., 2006), or the QuickSIN (Mueller et al., 2010). Although it may seem that a patient with hearing loss who has an excellent aided score on the QuickSIN (e.g., SNR loss around 2 dB) would also have a small aided ANL, this relationship does not exist consistently. This suggests that, at least for some individuals in a controlled clinical setting, the desire to perform well on a speech recognition test trumps the annoyance of the noise. In real-world listening, however, the patient may avoid those situations, develop stress or fatigue in those situations, or not use the hearing aids. Therefore, the inclusion of the ANL into a clinical test battery may give a clinician additional valuable information.

Administration and Scoring

Research suggests that the speech signal and the type of background noise that is used for the ANL measurement does not matter too much; however, given the large body of research conducted with the *standard material*, we recommend that you obtain this CD if you are going to use this test. The primary speech signal is a male talker reading a travelogue about Arizona and the background noise is a multitalker speech babble; specifically, the babble is from the revised SPIN test we discussed earlier in this chapter.

Given that the calculation of the ANL only requires two measurements and some first-grade math skills, a standard test form or score sheet is not really necessary. Most clinics do develop their own worksheet, however. This is helpful for repeat testing, as then you also will know the measured MCL and BNL. The test commonly is presented sound field, although using earphones (bilateral presentation) is okay too. Because the ANL is not affected by the degree of hearing loss or speech recognition ability, there usually are not ear differences, and you can save a little time by conducting the test bilaterally. In the case of a unilateral fitting, you might want to test each ear just to confirm that there are not significant ANL differences. For example, if all other audiometric results are symmetrical and if there were an interaural ANL difference, you might consider fitting the ear with the lower ANL score. When conducted in the typical sound field manner, the test will take no longer than two or three minutes to conduct. The instructions for the MCL portion of the test are as follows:

> You will listen to a man reading a story through the loudspeaker. After a few moments, select the loudness of the story that is most comfortable for you as if you were listening to a radio. I will adjust the loudness for you—just signal to me if you want it turned up or down. But first, I'd like you to have me turn the loudness up until it is too loud and then down until it is too soft. Then, have me turn the loudness up and down until we find the loudness level that is the most comfortable for you.

We suggest starting the test at around 30 to 40 dB HL and initially using 5-dB steps to establish the general upper and lower limits. Then switch to 2-dB (or 2.5-dB) steps for more precise final bracketing. Once this value is obtained, provide the instructions for the BNL procedure, which are as follows:

> Now you will listen to the same story as before, except there now will be background noise of several people talking at the same time. After you have

---

TECHNICAL TIP: HOW GOOD IS TOO GOOD

As we have described, the task for the patient when setting the noise level is to adjust it to "the most you would be willing to accept or put up with without becoming tense and tired while following the story." The key point here is that the patient must still be able to follow the story. We have found that some patients are focusing so intently regarding what they can put up with that they forget this other important part of the instructions. The result will be unusually low ANL scores, maybe even a negative ANL score. Consider that few people will be able to follow the story when the noise is equal to the signal. If you see scores that seem unusually low, we suggest reinstruction and repeating the test. If you continually see small ANLs—check out your calibration, especially if you do not commonly conduct two-channel speech testing.

> **THINGS TO REMEMBER: RELIABILITY OF THE ANL MEASURE**
>
> Given that the BNL portion of the ANL procedure is a somewhat unique measure (e.g., most patients are not accustomed to assessing what level of noise they can put up with), Mueller et al. (2006) examined the test-retest of this component of the ANL calculation (during a single test session). In all, the BNL was repeated three times for each of three different test conditions for 22 hearing-impaired subjects, a total of 66 BNLs. They found that in 15% of the cases, the BNL did not change at all; in 61%, the largest difference among the three measures per person was 2 dB (2-dB steps were used in the research); and in 13%, the BNLs differed by 4 dB. The largest test-retest difference observed was 6 dB, present for 11% of the 66 ANLs calculated.
>
> The findings of Mueller et al. (2006) suggest that the BNL is a relatively reliable measure, although these researchers did not address the variability of the MCL, which has the potential to be unreliable in that, for most patients, it is a *range* and not a single dB value. Considering the minimal time it takes to conduct the MCL and BNL (and calculate an ANL), we would suggest repeating both measures and taking an average of the two ANLs.

listened to this for a few moments, select the level of background noise that is the MOST you would be willing to accept or "put-up-with" without becoming tense and tired while following the story. First, have me turn the noise up until it is too loud and then down until the noise is soft and the story becomes very clear. Finally, adjust the noise (up and down) to the maximum noise level that you would be willing to put up with for a long time while still following the story.

Clinical Applications

For starters, the thing to remember is that small ANLs are good; large ANLs, are not so good. Good for what, you might ask? And what constitutes a good ANL? The cutoffs that generally are used, based on studies from the University of Tennessee that we discussed previously are:

- Low: 7 dB or less
- Midrange: 8 to 12 dB
- High: 13 dB or higher

Intuitively, it would seem that someone who is not bothered much by background noise would be a more successful hearing aid user. That may be true. A large-scale study ($N = 191$) on this topic was reported by Nabelek, Freyaldenhoven, Tampas, Burchfield, and Muenchen (2006). Unaided ANLs were compared for individuals who had been fitted with hearing aids. Based on a questionnaire regarding hearing aid use, the subjects were divided into three groups: full-time users ($n = 69$), part-time users ($n = 69$), or nonusers ($n = 59$). The authors found that full-time users had significantly smaller ANLs than the other two groups (mean ANL of 7.7 dB); however, there was little difference in mean ANLs between the part-time users and nonusers (13.5 and 14.4, respectively).

Freyaldenhoven, Nabelek, and Tampas (2008) examined the relationship between ANLs and the APHAB. They found that there was *not* a significant relationship between the unaided or aided ANLs and aided benefit scores and any APHAB subscale. Taylor (2008) used the International Outcome Inventory for Hearing Aids (IOI-HA) questionnaire and found a weak but significant correlation with the ANL. More specifically, the high ANL group (ANLs >12 dB; $n = 4$) had poorer overall IOI-HA scores, primarily due to lower scores for the Factor 1 questions (which does include a question regarding hearing aid use).

The work of Schwartz and Cox (2011, 2012) has been less encouraging regarding the clinical utility of the ANL. Although they do report that it was significantly correlated to the aversiveness scale of the APHAB—people with large ANLs are more bothered by loud noises—it was not significantly correlated to the other outcomes of the APHAB or findings from the HHIE or the SADL. Looking at several domains, such as benefit, satisfaction, quality of life, and so forth, they found the prediction accuracy to range from 52% to 64%, with the highest accuracy for hearing aid use (64%).

So what is the practical take-home message from these ANL studies? First, given that there is not a consensus, it appears that more research is needed before we make a strong recommendation. But for the moment, let us assume that there is at least a weak relationship between the ANL and hearing aid use. Going back to the Nabelek et al. (2006) data, if someone has an ANL of 20 dB do you simply tell them that they'll probably never use their hearing aids, so they might as well save their money? Of course not, but you might put a "Red X" by their name and target them for more intense counseling and post-fitting audiologic rehabilitation. It would be reasonable to consider them at risk for not being successful with amplification. If they tell you that loud noises are bothering them, that would be a predictable outcome. If you normally only have your new hearing aid patients come back for follow-up visits once or twice during the first month after the fitting, you might consider seeing the high ANL patients more frequently.

Finally, you might ask if a patient's ANL score would alter the hearing aid technology that you will select or the way special features will be adjusted. The answer is not yet clear. Although we would agree that someone with a large ANL probably needs directional technology and DNR, we are going to fit this technology to someone with a small ANL too. Adjust the DNR to maximum strength rather than medium? Maybe, but there is no evidence to suggest that this will make a difference. Remote microphone technology, of course, would be beneficial, especially if they are avoiding noisy listening situations. Some preliminary data from the Vanderbilt University research, however, suggests that moving to more aggressive sound cleaning technologies (e.g., using a remote microphone instead of directional microphone) may be more likely to be preferred by those with poor ANLs.

Given the significant relationship between large ANLs and real-world annoyance from loud sounds (Schwartz & Cox, 2011), if your patient's ANL is significantly larger than average, you might spend more time than usual during the fitting process assuring that environmental sounds are not "Uncomfortably Loud" (see recommended procedures in Chapter 15).

Obtaining the ANL Test

The standard CD with the travelogue and the R-SPIN competing noise is available from Frye Electronics (http://www.frye.com).

Performance-Perceptual Test (PPT)

As the name suggests, the Performance-Perceptual Test (PPT) also requires the patient to make a subjective judgment. In this case, however, the *perceptual* part is a judgment regarding speech recognition. That is, the patients self-score their performance. The measure of most interest is not the perceptual score itself, but how the perceptual score differs from the true performance score; this difference is referred to as the performance-perceptual discrepancy or PPDIS.

Background

Saunders (2009) explains that the PPT originally was developed to study individuals with obscure auditory dysfunction (OAD). Persons with OAD report difficulties hearing speech in noise, yet have clinically normal hearing. In her early research, Saunders found that people with OAD tended to underestimate their hearing ability. This led to the notion that the misjudgment of speech understanding ability also could be related to hearing aid satisfaction.

The speech test that is the basis for measuring the patient's perceptions of word recognition and calculating the PPDIS is the HINT, which we discussed earlier in this chapter. The performance score of the PPT, therefore, is obtained using the standard HINT protocol; that is, the background noise is constant and the intensity level of the sentences are adaptively raised or lowered depending on the patient's response for the preceding sentence. The patient repeats back what he or she hears, and the audiologist determines whether all words of the sentence are correct. For the perceptual portion of the PPT, the intensity of the sentences is altered based on whether patients think that they correctly recognized all the words of the sentence. Rather than repeat back the sentence, the patient simply responds with a *Yes* or *No*.

We discuss the norms later but, in general, the average patient tends to have similar scores for the performance and perceptual administration of the HINT. What we are interested in are those who do not, and for that reason we calculate the PPDIS. This defines the extent to which the patient misjudges his or her hearing ability. If the perceptual HINT RTS is more adverse (a more difficult SNR) than the performance RTS, it suggests that patients overestimate their speech recognition ability. If, on the other hand, the perceptual RTS is less adverse (an easier SNR) than the performance RTS, this indicates patients who underestimate their speech recognition ability. Ideally, we want patients who have a PPDIS around 0 dB, as there could be problems associated with both significantly positive and negative PPDIS scores.

You might wonder how this unique speech test correlates with patient characteristics or other hearing aid pre-fitting measures that might be conducted. Here is a brief summary of some related findings:

- PPDIS is not related to age or degree of hearing loss (Saunders & Forsline, 2006).
- PPDIS is not significantly related to other pre-fitting tests, such as the ANL or QuickSIN (Mueller et al., 2010).
- PPDIS is related to self-perceived hearing handicap. Saunders, Forsline, and Fausti (2004) examined the relationship between unaided HHIE/A scores (see Chapter 6 for description) and the PPT. They found a significant relationship, in that people whose HHIE/A scores were worse than what would be expected from their hearing loss tended to have PPT scores that underestimated their speech recognition ability.
- PPDIS may be related to hearing aid dissatisfaction. Saunders (2009) reports that negative PPDIS scores (underestimators) tend to associated with more hearing aid dissatisfaction.

Although at this point we are talking about using the PPT for pre-fitting testing, it of course also can be a valuable outcome measure. Of interest, Saunders and Forsline (2006) reported that when the unaided PPDIS was compared with the aided PPDIS, the aided score had less variance. The mean unaided and aided PPDIS did not differ significantly. That is, although the patient's absolute scores may have changed, the use of hearing aids did not influence the relationship between his or her measured and perceptual judgments.

Administration and Scoring

As we mentioned, the PPDIS consists of using the standard HINT material. Refer back to the HINT section of this chapter for the recommended test procedure. The PPT is administered in the sound field, although bilateral earphone administration would probably yield similar results. The scoring of the PPT, using 20-sentence HINT lists, is as described earlier in this chapter for the HINT and illustrated in Figure 6–5. The perceptual portion is always administered first. The reason for this, as described by Saunders, is that if you do the performance portion first, the patient will know that you already have scored them on the same test and are probably trying to catch them out (this is somewhat true), which could influence their perceptual judgments (see Mueller, 2010, for review).

To calculate the PPDIS, we want to know the difference between the two HINT scores. The basic rules for calculation and interpretation are as follows:

PPDIS = HINT *Performance* RTS minus HINT *Perceptual* RTS

Positive PPDIS = Patient *overestimates* speech recognition ability

Negative PPDIS = Patient *underestimates* speech recognition ability.

Clinical Applications

It is first important to consider how the average patient performs regarding his or her PPDIS. It appears that, on average, the perceptual and performance scores are fairly similar, with a mean unaided PPDIS of −1.4 dB, indicating a slight trend for individuals to underestimate their speech recognition ability. These data are similar to those reported by Saunders et al. (2004); these authors offer the following interpretation guidelines:

- Underestimation: PPDIS <33rd percentile of normative data (value ≤ −3)
- Accurate: PPDIS between 33rd and 66th percentile of normative data (value > −3 and < +0.2)

- Overestimation: PPDIS >66th percentile of normative data (value of ≥ +0.2)

Mueller et al. (2010), however, reported mean values that were 2 to 3 dB higher than shown above—their subjects had a slight tendency to overestimate their speech recognition ability. The authors speculate that this may be because their subject sample only included hearing aid users who were satisfied with their hearing aids; recall that dissatisfaction with amplification is associated with negative PPDIS scores. In general, your primary counseling efforts will be directed toward patients who fall significantly outside of these normative values (e.g., PPDIS more negative than −3 dB or more positive than +3 dB).

It is unlikely that a patient's PPDIS score will be helpful for selecting fitting arrangements or different technology; however, there are certainly counseling insights that can be gained. Particularly for the new hearing aid users who either overestimate or underestimate their speech recognition ability, the PPDIS score can provide general areas for discussion regarding their adjustment to amplification. For example, if you know that someone is an under-estimator, before they leave your office with their hearing aids you might encourage them to try guessing when they do not understand or assume they understand when they are uncertain. Saunders (2009) and Mueller et al. (2014) provide a summary of how PPDIS scores can be used in patient counseling including recommended solutions. Because we know that negative PPDIS scores are associated with hearing aid dissatisfaction, special attention should be paid to this group.

A somewhat different pre-fitting use of the PPDIS would be for those individuals with significant communication problems who believe that they do not really need hearing aids. In many cases, these people are overestimators. By conducting the PPT, it is possible to show the patient the difference between the true score and perceptual score, which might be helpful in initiating the trial of hearing aids.

In a 2009 article, Dr. Saunders was asked why it was that some people judge their speech understanding different from what it really is. Her response is as follows:

> I don't have a definitive answer for that, and most likely the reasons vary from person to person. The explanation might be related to personality (being perfectionist, anxious, or lacking self-confidence) or to past experiences. Or it might be associated with expectations about hearing. It might be specific to hearing or it might not be.
>
> From a practical perspective, I suggest that being aware that not everyone has an accurate perception of their own ability to understand speech is more important than figuring out why—unless, of course, the reason why can be used to fix the problem. If misjudgment is personality-based, changing that trait is going to be difficult. Therefore, I propose that we address the implications of misjudgment of hearing, not its causes. That's why PPT-based counseling focuses on behavioral changes—not explanations.

Obtaining the PPT

All the normative data to date for the PPT have been with the HINT; see our comments regarding obtaining this test in that earlier section of this chapter. It is possible that a different speech test, such as the QuickSIN, could be used, although norms would need to be established.

TECHNICAL TIP: TEST-RETEST RELIABILITY OF PPT

Saunders et al. (2004) report good test-retest reliability for the PPT. The authors reported reliability data for the perceptual ($r = 0.95$), the performance ($r = 0.97$), and the PPDIS ($r = 0.88$), all in unaided listening conditions. As mentioned by the authors, it is somewhat surprising that patients are as reliable with the perceptual task as they are with performance, as we usually do not think of subjective measures as being as reliable as objective ones. The reliability of the PPDIS is of course somewhat lower, as it is derived from the two other measures, each with their own variability, but it still is considered excellent for a test like this.

Dichotic Speech Tests

The 1960s was an exciting time for diagnostic audiology. We were moving beyond simple air and bone conduction threshold testing and beginning to construct diagnostic tests that would allow us to identify pathologies of nerve VIII, the brain stem, and yes . . . even the brain. In James Jerger's now classic 1969 book, *Modern Developments in Audiology*, there was an intriguing review chapter on central auditory processing by Italians Bocca and Calearo. It was there that many audiologists first read about the cognitive theory of the *redundancy principle*—extrinsic, the linguistic redundancy of the test stimuli, versus intrinsic, the multiplicity of auditory processing pathways. Simply stated, when conducting clinical speech testing, the principle reminds us that the more subtle the auditory disorder, the more the redundancy of the test stimuli needs to be reduced for the speech test to be sensitive. Certainly, one way to reduce redundancy is to present different speech stimuli to the two ears simultaneously, which we refer to as dichotic testing. It was more than 50 years ago—in 1961—when Doreen Kimura published two articles describing how dichotic digit testing could be used to help describe central auditory processing. Her explanation of the crossed auditory pathways, ipsilateral suppression, and the *right ear effect* has withstood the test of time, and laid the groundwork for the design and interpretation of many audiologic speech tests that followed. We review a revised version of her dichotic digit test later in this section.

So what does all this have to do with hearing aid selection and fitting? Although dichotic speech tests can be used to help identify a specific auditory pathology or disorder, the results of this testing also can be used in a more general framework to gauge a patient's overall processing ability. In many cases, especially with older adults, cognitive factors contribute to the poor performance on dichotic tests. When used in conjunction with fitting hearing aids, there are two primary results that might impact the fitting and/or patient counseling:

- Performance for both ears is significantly reduced, more so than expected based on pure-tone thresholds and other monaural speech-in-noise tests. When this finding occurs, the patient would be counseled regarding realistic expectations for hearing aid benefit in background noise or when multiple talkers are present, and FM technology or other wireless assistive listening devices would be strongly encouraged.
- Performance for one ear is significantly worse than the other, more so than predicted by pure-tone thresholds or other monaural speech tests. This patient would be considered

---

TECHNICAL TIP: TERMINOLOGY

When describing the presentation mode for auditory processing tests, specific terminology usually is used, which is somewhat different from what is used for other speech testing.

- Monotic: The signal or signals (e.g., speech and competition) are presented to only one ear. This essentially is the same as a unilateral or monaural presentation. Tests such as the QuickSIN or WIN are presented unilaterally for hearing aid prefitting testing.
- Diotic: The same signal is presented to both ears. The SPRINT, which we discussed earlier, is presented diotically. The QuickSIN and BKBSIN can also be presented diotically via headphones.
- Dichotic: Two different competing speech signals are presented to each ear simultaneously (often carefully timed to have the same onset). The task is to identify both signals or, in some cases, the signal for a pre-cued ear. The two tests that we discuss in this chapter, the DSI and the DDT, are examples of clinical dichotic tests.

at risk for optimum benefit with bilateral amplification. This finding would probably not negate a bilateral fitting because of the potential advantages unrelated to dichotic speech understanding, but these results do alert the audiologist to pay close attention to patient comments in this regard on post-fitting visits and to perhaps have some specific suggestions for hearing aid use (e.g., only use one hearing aid for parties). Moreover, if the patient only desires to purchase one hearing aid, it would be reasonable to fit the ear with the best dichotic speech score (assuming the between ear difference was significant).

Free-Recall Versus Direct-Recall

There have been two different types of recall patterns used when dichotic speech testing has been conducted:

- Free recall: In the free-recall condition, the patient has to attend to and report the speech signal(s) heard in both ears. The ear-order of report is not cued (for difficult dichotic tasks, most patients do tend to report the right ear signal first).
- Directed recall: For this response mode, the patient is instructed to only report the signal for one ear. He or she hears the speech signals presented to each ear but can focus on the signal heard in the cued ear while disregarding the signal presented to the non-cued ear. This results in a reduced demand on cognitive processing.

Clearly, the free-recall condition places greater stress on attentional resources than the directed-recall condition. When recognition performance is below normal in the free-recall condition but improves substantially in the directed-recall condition, then we assume the problem is primarily in the cognitive domain because memory and attention abilities are insufficient for successful performance when both ears must be monitored simultaneously.

When performance is below normal in both the free- and directed-recall conditions, then the problem is interpreted to be primarily in the auditory domain because performance does not improve by reducing cognitive demands (Jerger, Stach, Johnson, Loiselle, & Jerger, 1990).

Effects of Peripheral Hearing Loss

One concern in the clinical interpretation of all auditory processing tests is the influence of a concurrent peripheral hearing loss. That is, how is one certain that results showing an ear difference or reduced overall performance are related to higher processing function, rather than simply due to lower-level peripheral pathology? In the general population this is not so much an issue, as often the patient suspected of having an auditory processing disorder has normal hearing. When these tests are used as part of the hearing aid pre-fitting battery, however, it is always something that must be considered in test interpretation. Although it is very difficult to eliminate the influence of a peripheral hearing loss when using these speech tests, we have selected two tests to discuss in this section that appear to be the most resilient to hearing loss and, therefore, the best choice for use in the hearing aid selection process.

The Dichotic Sentence Identification Test

As we have mentioned throughout this chapter, the purpose of adding speech tests to the pre-fitting battery is to obtain unique information about the patient. In the case of the Dichotic Sentence Identification Test (DSI), the new information that might be gathered, particularly for older adults, is the presence of a more central processing deficit rather than what might be detected using tests such as the QuickSIN or the WIN. Research has shown that the DSI may be successful in making this identification.

Background

The DSI was introduced by Fifer, Jerger, Berlin, Tobey, and Campbell (1983). The test used the 10 sentences of the well-established Synthetic Sentence Identification (SSI) test. These 10 sentences were paired with each other and presented dichotically (one sentence to each ear). To make the sentences more appropriate for dichotic pairing, the items were edited and equalized for overall intensity. Also, to enhance timing alignment, the duration of each sentence was adjusted to equal two seconds by editing out or expanding the vowel segments of the sentences. The authors stated that one of the goals was to design a dichotic test that was relatively resistant to the effects of peripheral hearing loss. In this early work, the authors report that the DSI indeed was resistant to the influence of hearing loss until the pure-tone average (average of 500, 1000, and 2000 Hz) exceeded approximately 50 dB HL. In a later study (Jerger, Chmiel, Allen, & Wilson, 1994), DSI testing was conducted on individuals with PTA asymmetry as great as 30 dB. Even with this lax criterion of symmetry, analysis showed that only 5% of variance in the DSI ear differences could be accounted for by the PTA average.

Shortly after the introductory report by Fifer et al. (1983), a shortened clinical version of the DSI was developed, which only included six of the original 10 sentences of the SSI. These sentences are shown in Figure 6–14. Each sentence is delivered five times to each ear and paired accordingly with each of the other five sentences, resulting in a total of 30 test items.

Because of its relative resistance to hearing loss, the DSI has been used to study processing in older individuals. Chmiel and Jerger (1996), for example, evaluated 115 elderly subjects over the age of 60 with high frequency sensorineural hearing loss. Using the free- and directed-recall conditions for the DSI test, they found that 29% of the subjects were categorized as having an auditory-specific processing deficit. In an earlier study using a similar DSI procedure, Jerger et al. (1990) administered this dichotic test to 172 elderly hearing impaired subjects (60 to 90 years). In this study, 58% showed below-normal performance in one ear in the free-recall condition with a significant improvement in the directed-recall condition, suggesting a cognitive-based disorder. Another 23% showed a deficit in both response modes. Only 19% of this sample showed no deficit in either ear for either DSI condition.

In DSI research from 1994, Jerger et al. confirmed a progressively larger right ear advantage or left ear deficit with increasing age. This effect was shown for both the free-recall and directed-recall test modes. These authors also report a gender difference in the effect of age on the left ear deficit. Males showed a larger effect than females for both modes of test administration.

The 60- to 90-year age group studied in the Jerger et al. (1990) study is fairly representative of the individuals we fit with hearing aids. If it is true that 80% of these individuals have a cognitive or auditory specific deficit that is preventing them from processing speech effectively, how do we account for that during the hearing aid fitting process?

Administration and Scoring

In general, the DSI can be given to individuals with a pure-tone average (500, 1000, and 2000 Hz) of 50 dB HL or less. General test procedures are as follows:

- The test is conducted under earphones.
- The patient is given the card with the six sentences printed on them (large bold print should be used).
- The patient is then instructed to listen for two different sentences presented to both ears simultaneously, find the two sentences from among the six on the printed list, and call out the corresponding numbers of the sentences heard.
- The test items are delivered at 50 dB SL relative to the pure-tone average (500, 1000, and 2000 Hz) for the respective ears. If this level exceeds the patient's LDL, lower the intensity to the "loud but okay" loudness rating of the patient.
- With the intensity set at desired levels for both channels/ears, talk to the patient (bilateral presentation) to assure a relative loudness match between ears is present. Your voice

---

1. Agree with him only to find out.
2. Down by the time is real enough.
3. Go change your car color is red.
4. Women view men with green paper should.
5. Built the government with the force almost.
6. Small boat with a picture has become.

Figure 6–14. The six sentences used for DSI testing. Sentences were taken from the original sentences of the SSI test.

should be localized to the center of the head. Adjust intensity if necessary.

We typically deliver the test using free-recall. If the findings are abnormal, the test certainly could be repeated using directed-recall to gather additional information—although it probably will not alter your counseling to a great degree. As we mentioned, the DSI consists of 30 sentence pairs and scoring for each ear is reported in the percent correct (each correct item is multiplied by 3.3%). Given that there are only six sentences, one might think that the patients would guess a lot, given the probability of a correct guess. It is surprising that this does not happen very often. When they do not get it, they simply do not respond. It is true, of course, that they really only need to identify one key word of the sentence, and this is okay.

The chart shown in Figure 6–15 can be used to assist in test interpretation. Because we know that the results will be affected by hearing loss, this is accounted for in this chart. For example, note that for PTA up to 25 dB, DSI scores of 75% or better are considered normal—we would expect younger patients to fall closer to the top of this range. As the PTA increases, the cutoff for normal decreases. Notice that a 50% score would be in the normal range for someone with a PTA of 40 dB. If the hearing loss is relatively symmetric, we would expect DSI scores to be within 16 to 20% between ears.

An exception might be patients older than 80 years, in whom we would expect a left ear deficit.

Clinical Applications

As we discussed in the introduction portion of this section, there is a general belief that dichotic speech tests, such as the DSI, can be used to help predict who might show the greatest benefit from amplification. Chmiel and Jerger (1996), for example, used the HHIE outcome measure (see Chapter 7) to examine the reduction of handicap for new hearing aid users after six weeks of first-time hearing aid use. They compared the improvement for the HHIE to the patients' pre-fitting DSI performance and found that there was a significant improvement in average HHIE scores but only for the DSI-normal category. In the subgroup with dichotic deficits (DSI-abnormal group), average HHIE scores did not change significantly after hearing aid use.

In their 1994 article, Jerger et al. suggest that a patient's score for a particular ear for the DSI is the linear contribution of four different factors:

- Speech Recognition: The patient's ability to recognize a target sentence in the presence of contralateral competition by a difference

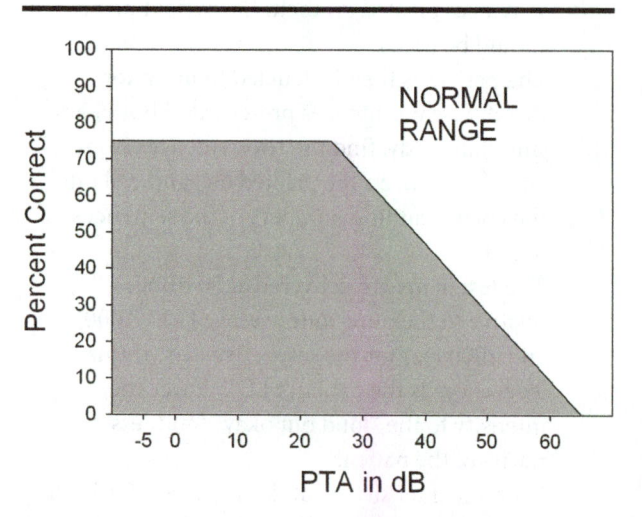

Figure 6–15. Normative data as a function of hearing loss for interpreting DSI findings. (Adapted from Auditec of St. Louis).

TECHNICAL TIP: SCORING OF DOUBLE CORRECTS

We often see that patients who are having trouble with the DSI will attempt different listening strategies. One of these is to self-impose a directed-ear response. That is, they will focus on the right ear for a period of time, and you will notice that they are getting all the right ear sentences correct. Then, they will switch their focus to the left ear, and they will get all the left ear sentences correct. But, they never (or seldom) get both correct. For this reason, we find it useful to also score *double corrects*: that is, the percentage of time that the patient gave the correct response for both ears. We suspect that a patient who scores 50% in both ears with 50% double correct responses is different from the patient who scores 50% in both ears with no double correct responses.

sentence. This factor is assumed to be equivalent for right and left ears.
- Left Ear Deficit: This is a performance difference favoring input to the right ear due to left hemisphere dominance for speech signals. This factor favors the right ear score over the left ear score and operates in both the free-recall and directed-recall modes.
- Task Deficit: A deficit in performance resulting from the cognitive demands of the instructional set. This is associated with the demands on memory and speed of mental processing inherent in the behavioral response in the dichotic paradigm. It is assumed to be equivalent for right and left ear scores but operates primarily in the free-recall mode.
- Interaction Effect: An additional task deficit resulting from the interaction between the patient's report bias and the task deficit. If, for example, the patient is biased toward responding first to the right ear input, then the left ear score might be more affected by the task deficit factor than the right ear score. This is primarily a factor in the free-recall mode.

Although understanding why reduced DSI scores are present is important, the clinician will want to know how a given score influences the fitting process. It is certainly possible that a patient could score well on tests like the QuickSIN or the WIN, yet have an abnormal DSI score. For this information, refer back to the beginning of this section, where we outlined some of the potential practical uses of dichotic speech results.

Obtaining the DSI

The DSI can be obtained from Auditec of St. Louis. It also can be found on Audiology VA CD, Disc 2 (http://www.etsu.edu/crhs/aslp/audiology/resources/Aud_VA_CD_Disc_2.aspx).

The Dichotic Digit Test (DDT)

As we discussed with the DSI test, there may be instances during the pre-fitting process when a dichotic test is needed to assess the cognitive and/or central auditory processing integrity of the patient. The Dichotic Digit Test (DDT) is an easily administered auditory processing test that can be used for this purpose. In general, the test is similar to the DSI, and similar results would be expected. It is unlikely that you would administer both the DSI and the DDT to a given patient.

Background

As we mentioned in the introduction of this section, much of the early work with dichotic listening, dating back to the early 1960s, utilized dichotic digits. The test was seldom used in clinical audiology, however, until the 1980s. The rediscovery of this processing test among clinicians was due in large part to an article by Frank Musiek (1983). In this article, he presented his version of a DDT, norms for both normal hearing and individuals with mild to moderate cochlear hearing loss, and also 21 subjects with intracranial lesions. Unlike some of the earlier dichotic digit tests, which used three digits per ear, Musiek's version only used two digits per ear. The digits from 1 to 10, excluding the number seven (the only two-syllable digit in this range) were paired to form 20 test items, 40 for each ear.

To establish cutoff values for clinical differential testing, Musiek (1983) used the means and two standard deviations (with some rounding to obtain easy-to-use numbers) for the normal hearing and cochlear hearing loss group. Although it is known that a right ear advantage is sometimes observed for dichotic speech testing, this effect was very small for the normative data and, therefore, no ear-specific norms are necessary. The following normative values were reported:

- Normal hearing: 90% or better
- Hearing loss: 80% or better.

For clinical use today, there are three different dichotic digits tests to choose from: the Musiek version we just discussed, an Auditec of St. Louis version, and a version developed by Richard Wilson and colleagues of the VA system. The VA version has one, two, and three digit pairs available. Table 6–7 shows the mean values reported by Strouse and Wilson (1999) for the two-pair dichotic digit presentations (similar to Musiek DDT) for different age groups for the free-recall paradigm.

Notice that for these mean values, there is an age-related decrease in performance, especially for the left

Table 6–7. Mean Values for the Two-Pair Dichotic Digit Presentations for Different Age Groups for the Free-Recall Paradigm

Age Group	Right Ear	Left Ear
20–29	97.6	96.9
30–39	95.1	86.5
40–49	94.3	88.3
50–59	90.7	78.4
60–69	91.9	83.8
70–79	90.6	74.3

Source: Adapted from Strouse & Wilson, 1999.

ear. Strouse and Wilson (1999) also tested these same subjects using a directed-recall mode. As expected, the results were considerably better. The poorest performance was again for the oldest group, but the mean values were 95.7% for the right ear and 90.7% for the left. One might question whether the reduced performance shown in Table 6–7 for the older groups was simply because these subjects had greater hearing loss. They did indeed have greater hearing loss, but Strouse and Wilson (1999) addressed this issue and provided three convincing reasons why this probably was not related to the poorer performance for the dichotic digits: (1) reduced performance was not observed for the one-digit dichotic presentation, (2) reduced performance was not observed for the directed response, and (3) scores for monosyllabic word testing, delivered at the same HL (70 dB), were not reduced.

As we discussed earlier, from a clinical standpoint, it is meaningful to have a general idea of what percentage of our older patients have some sort of processing deficit. Recall that one study (Jerger et al., 1990) suggested it may be as high as 80%. To examine this for their sample, Strouse and Wilson (1999) looked at a subsample of their population, the subjects in the 60- to 79-year age range (*n* = 60). They report that within this group, 48% had a deficit in at least one ear for free-recall condition, and 7% of these subjects also showed the deficit for the directed recall. Although the free-recall versus direct-recall differences are academically interesting, when we relate the test results to hearing aid fittings, they become less important, as our fitting and counseling strategies will be very similar for both a cognitive-based and an auditory-based cause.

Administration and Scoring

The administration of the DDT is similar to our previous discussion for the DSI. As mentioned, there are different dichotic digit tests available—we base our review here on the Musiek Auditec version, which seems to be the most commonly used (for further information regarding administration of this test, see Guenette, 2006):

- A two-channel audiometer is required, and the test is presented from a CD. It is important that the audiologist is certain about which channel is going to each ear (confer with the patient if necessary) and that each channel is calibrated.
- In most cases, a presentation level of 50 dB above the SRT is appropriate. If the SRT was not conducted, use 50 dB above the pure-tone average (500, 1000, and 2000 Hz). Exceptions to this include the following:
    - If the patient has normal hearing in the low frequencies (resulting in an SRT of approximately 10 dB) and a sharply falling hearing loss (e.g., resulting in >50 dB for 2000 Hz and above), 50 dB SL may not result in a high enough setting.
    - In a relatively moderate flat hearing loss (SRT approximately 40 to 45 dB), using a 50 dB SL may place the test signals at or above the patient's LDL.
- For both of the above situations, we recommend using a presentation level of 75 to 80 dB HL or the patient's "Loud, But Okay" loudness rating for speech, which should be about 5 dB below their speech LDL.
- With the intensity set at desired levels for both channels/ears, talk to the patient (bilateral presentation) to assure a relative loudness match between ears is present. Your voice should be localized to the center of the patient's head. If the patient reports that one ear is louder than the other, raise the intensity of the softer ear to match the loudness of the louder ear.

- Deliver the three pairs of practice items. Repeat if the patient seems to have trouble understanding the task.
- Deliver the 20 test items.
- Give the patient ample time to respond, even though this probably will require pausing the CD occasionally (the norms were established to allow patients as much time as they wish to respond).
- If a patient cannot respond orally, he or she can write the digits or point to them on a large response board.

The following are sample instructions:

You will be hearing two numbers in each of your ears. Listen carefully in both ears and repeat all the numbers you hear. The order that you repeat them doesn't matter. If you are unsure of the numbers, please guess. The first few items will be for practice. At this point the audiologist might also want to give the following example: "You might hear the numbers 3 and 9 in your right ear, and the numbers 4 and 8 in your left ear. What you then would repeat back to me is all four numbers—3, 9, 4, and 8. Any questions?"

The DDT is scored by percent correct. The Musiek version has 20 pairs or 40 items, so the patient is given 2.5% for each correct digit per ear.

Clinical Applications

The DDT is similar to the DSI, and we would expect similar results. Hence, the clinical applications are essentially the same as we discussed in the DSI section. As with the DSI, the DDT can be conducted in both a free-recall and a directed-ear mode. In some cases, we see large improvement for one ear in the directed-ear condition but not for the other. This finding may give some indication of which ear to fit for patients who are purchasing only one hearing aid.

In general, bilaterally reduced DDT scores are a red flag that additional counseling may be needed. Included would be guidelines for effective listening and encouragement to use assistive listening devices. As with the DSI, a significantly low DDT score in one ear only may influence decisions and counseling regarding bilateral amplification.

Obtaining the DDT

There are two different versions of the DDT available from Auditec of St. Louis. A third version of the DDT is available from Audiology VA CD Disc 2 (http://www.etsu.edu/crhs/aslp/audiology/resources/Aud_VA_CD_Disc_2.asp).

In Closing

In this chapter we have attempted to give you a review of the most commonly used speech-in-noise tests and a few pointers on testing speech in quiet as a bonus. It should now be obvious why all hearing aid best practice guidelines recommend the use of speech-in-noise measures.

One More Just for Fun

And just when you thought we had covered all the speech tests that could be used with hearing aid fitting, we have one more to mention. Not everyone is using it clinically in hearing aid users, but it has been used a lot in cochlear implant and bimodal stimulation research.

AzBio Sentences

The AzBio sentences are perhaps the newest member of our ever growing list of speech-in-noise tests. These sentences are commonly used with cochlear implant patients. The AzBio sentences were first described by Spahr and Dorman (2004) and were developed in the Department of Speech and Hearing Science at Arizona State University. The development of these sentence materials was enabled by a grant from the Arizona Biomedical Institute at ASU (currently known as the Biodesign Institute), and, in appreciation, the resulting speech materials were dubbed the AzBio sentences (see Spahr et al., 2012 for review).

The AzBio sentence materials are available on an audio CD designed specifically for use with a clinical audiometer and consist of 15 lists of 20 sentences each. There is a 10-talker babble on the second track of the CD. Unlike some other sentence tests we have discussed, the AzBio sentences differ considerably in length. For example, for List 1, three sentences only have five words and three contain 10 words. Some lists have sentences of four or 11 words, but most are seven to nine words. The total words possible for each 20-sentence list then also varies and ranges from 133 to 154.

Schafer, Pogue, and Milrany (2012) examined the equivalency of the 15 AzBio Sentence Test lists on the commercially available CD at two SNRs. They tested participants with normal hearing and a second group with cochlear implants. These authors concluded that when the AzBio Sentence Test is used with the background noise for clinical or research purposes, only Lists 2, 3, 4, 5, 8, 9, 10, 11, 13, and 15 are recommended.

The AzBio test is increasingly used much with the typical hearing aid patient, so consider it if your goal is to select a sentence test with a fixed SNR. The AzBio is available from http://www.auditorypotential.com.

Cognitive Measures

We certainly all would agree that the patient's cognitive function will affect the hearing aid fitting process and will influence our counseling during the pre-fitting testing. Some might even suggest that cognitive function can be used to help determine the best signal processing as we discuss in Chapter 10. It seems reasonable, therefore, to perhaps include a cognitive test in our pre-fitting battery. We did not specifically include any cognitive speech tests here. You may recall, however, that comparing free recall versus directed recall for dichotic speech tests, such as the DSI, may provide insight into cognitive function.

There are other speech tests available that are designed to assess cognitive function. One recommended by Pam Souza (2012) for clinical use is the Reading Span Test (although it sometimes is given as a reading test first so that the results are not contaminated by reduced speech recognition). This test was designed to measure simultaneous storage and processing capacity. The patient is asked to determine if a particular sentence makes sense and then, after several sentences have been presented, the patient is asked to recall the first or last words of those sentences. The number of sentences presented prior to recall increase during the test, and the final score is the percentage of correctly recalled words (Souza, 2012). This is just one example of cognitive testing that one day may be fairly routine in hearing aid pre-fitting testing.

In Closing (Again)

So there you have it. Quite a buffet of speech tests to choose from. We reviewed two speech tests that are given in quiet, four that use a fixed SNR, four more that use an adaptive SNR-50 approach, a couple of tests that require a subjective response, two dichotic speech tests, and a few bonus tests at the end. You certainly have several to choose from—we have our favorites and hope you will find yours.

7
Self-Assessment Scales for Pre-Fitting Testing

To this point, we have discussed objective pure-tone, narrowband, and speech recognition tests that can be used during the assessment prior to the fitting of hearing aids. We recommend also using self-assessment inventories to complement the objective findings. That is, some type of formal questionnaire completed by the patient that relates to their hearing difficulty, communication needs, the use of hearing aids, or their candidacy in general should be included in this pre-fitting battery.

In some ways, these scales are not much more than an extended case history, but they allow the clinician to collect information in an organized manner; in most cases, the patient's responses can be compared with average data from large samples. The information collected using these inventories can significantly influence pre-fitting counseling and in some instances alter fitting decisions. In some cases, the scores collected before the fitting serve as a baseline, as they may be compared with results measured after a patient wears hearing aids for a period of time to quantify directly subjective hearing aid benefit, reduction in hearing handicap, or other outcomes of interest—we talk about this extensively in Chapter 19.

As we reviewed in the previous chapter, there are many speech recognition tests to choose from, and the notion is that we select a specific test to answer a specific question we might have about the patient (e.g., How much are they bothered by background noise? How well do they understand speech in background noise?). The same is true regarding self-assessment inventories. There are some pre-fitting inventories that are geared toward determining communication difficulty, whereas others are geared toward examining the patient's expectations. Others may be focused toward perceived handicap, how the patient judges loudness, or their motivation to use hearing aids. Once the audiologist determines the types of questions that need to be answered, inventories that address these specific issues can be selected. Of course clinical time is quite limited, and we need to be as efficient as possible. If we already know something about the patient, it is typically not worth our limited time to use a formal inventory for the sole purpose of confirming this same information. Consequently, narrowing down the type of information needed to enhance development of our treatment plan and selecting the appropriate tools to obtain that information is part of the art of our profession and requires time to effectively master.

Reasons to Use Pre-Fitting Self-Assessment Scales

To get us started, we first list a few areas where self-assessment pre-fitting tests might be helpful for the overall hearing aid fitting process. Our examples include names of specific tests. You might not be familiar with these tests just yet, but all are explained in detail later in the chapter. Here are seven general uses for standardized scales as part of the pre-fitting process:

- Assist in determining if a patient is a candidate for hearing aids.

    Example: A patient has a very mild hearing loss; normal hearing through 2000 Hz, dropping down to a 40 dB loss in the 3000 to 6000 Hz range. The Hearing Handicap for the Elderly (HHIE) or Abbreviated Profile of Hearing Aid Benefit (APHAB) scores, however, show significant handicap and considerable communication problems. This might lead us to make a different decision regarding amplification than if the HHIE or APHAB scores were consistent with someone with normal hearing.

- Assist in determining if a patient is ready to be helped.

    Example 1: A patient has a bilateral downward sloping hearing loss ranging from 30 dB in the lows to 70 dB in the highs. The Audibility Index (AI) is 38% for the right ear and 32% for the left. The scores for the HHIE and the APHAB, however, are consistent with someone with normal hearing. If this person denies these communication problems, will he or she accept the use of hearing aids? Is counseling needed before even attempting to move forward?

    Example 2: A patient with a mild hearing loss scores in the 10th percentile for the motivation subscale of the Hearing Aid Selection Profile (HASP). Is this patient ready to accept and use hearing aids, or is the patient a *return for credit* waiting to happen? Why did the patient make the appointment for the hearing aid evaluation? Or did someone else make the appointment?

- Assist in establishing realistic expectations.

    Example: A patient with a moderately severe bilateral hearing loss is being fit with hearing aids for the first time. The results of the ECHO show that the patient believes that the use of hearing aids will resolve 100% of the communication problems including understanding speech in adverse background noise situations. It is probably best to readjust the patient's expectations before he or she begins to use hearing aids.

- Assist in establishing a baseline.

    Example: The patient's results for the aversiveness scale of the APHAB reveal a low tolerance for loud sounds (e.g., using the Cox anchors, the patient judges sounds to be Uncomfortably Loud when most individuals consider these sounds to be Loud, But Okay). This information might be helpful in setting the AGCo kneepoints at the time of the fitting and will be useful in interpreting the post-fitting ratings on these scales (e.g., the patient may complain that sounds are too loud despite seemingly appropriate hearing aid output settings).

- Assist in establishing goals to select and prioritize technology as well as providing topics that may require further counseling.

    Example: A patient lists specific goals related to telephone use and listening in noisy restaurants on the COSI. This information is combined with the patient's speech recognition in noise performance and threshold information to make decisions related to prioritizing hearing aid features, appropriate expectations counseling, and appropriate telephone listening technologies. Establishment of specific hearing aid goals is critical for developing an intervention plan that targets each individual patient's listening needs and leads to increased patient satisfaction and use.

- Quality Assurance Management

    Example: An audiology private practice has three different clinics in a large metropolitan area. The HASP is administered to all potential hearing aid candidates over a six-month period. The results from each clinic are analyzed to determine if the patient population is different for categories such as motivation, physical limitations, or cost. These findings could be used to change staff, test protocols or office procedures, or could

> **TECHNICAL TIP: A GOOD "QUICK SIX"**
>
> Although we recommend the use of validated self-assessment scales, there will be times, for one reason or another, when administration will not be possible. Here are six open-ended questions that can be used to obtain information quickly that is similar to that obtained with related scales (adapted from Taylor & Mueller, 2017). It is actually reasonable to use these questions with all patients, as using them will help establish your concern for the patient's problems and supplement the pre-fitting information gathered from other more formal measures. Remember, as we discussed in Chapter 3, once you have asked the question, you will need to sit back, quietly listen to the response, and make sure that you really hear the individual patient's answers without leading them to the most common answer.
>
> 1. Tell me what brought you into the office.
> 2. How long have you been noticing difficulty with communication?
> 3. Do other people notice you are having difficulty with communication?
> 4. Tell me about the areas you are having difficulty with communication.
> 5. Would you be willing to accept help or assistance with the difficulties you are having?
> 6. On a scale of 1 to 10, with 1 being "I don't need help" and 10 being "I need help right away," how would you rate your ability to communicate?

be helpful in explaining different dispensing patterns among offices.

In this chapter, we review several different self-assessment scales that can be used in the pre-fitting process. Clinically, it is common to use only one or two of these with any given patient, although that is often related more to time constraints than the clinical value of the scales themselves; some scales might only be used for special cases. Nonetheless, it is important to be familiar with as many as possible because all the measures we describe can provide unique and important information for at least a small number of patients.

Some clinicians comment that it would be nice to use pre-fitting scales more routinely, but they just don't have the time. Given how much information these scales can provide, however, we find that spending the time on appropriate pre-fitting measures up front can in fact save time by helping in the selection process and providing a focus on the most important counseling issues. In addition, there are many ways to facilitate administration to make the process as streamlined as possible. These include mailing the scale to the patient so they can complete it at home before arriving at the clinic or having them complete the scale in the waiting room, with assistance from support personnel if needed. Although having the patient complete the scale on his or her own is certainly preferable to skipping the scale altogether, we have to be aware that data clearly show this leads to significantly less reliable answers than when questions are given to patients in interview form. Another way to increase efficiency is to administer a scale orally as part of the case history.

Regardless of the administration method, we highly recommend the use of modern computer technology to automate scoring. Without this, there may simply not be enough time to score the scale in an efficient enough manner to easily use the data during the selection appointment to facilitate selection and counseling. As the average patient becomes more computer savvy, this technology can also be used to facilitate administration—that is, the patient can simply complete a couple of scales using a tablet (e.g., iPad), which is then handed to you when you begin your initial pre-fitting counseling. In some cases, a tablet can be used to complete the scale through an interactive interface that would be expected to improve reliability when compared with old-fashioned pen and paper administration.

> **SOAPBOX:**
> **SOME THINGS YOU JUST HAVE TO MAKE TIME FOR!**
>
> We have all heard the old saying, "You can't judge a book by its cover." A saying that is maybe not as well-known, but is even truer is, "You can't judge a hearing aid candidate by his audiogram." Patients and their individual listening needs differ in so many ways that are not displayed in Xs and Os or word recognitions scores. There is an excellent battery of validated preselection self-assessment inventories available. They are easy to administer and score. The results of these scales will shape the fitting process, assist in technology decisions, and are invaluable for developing counseling strategies and a relationship with the patient along the way. The routine use of these scales is not only a good thing to do, it is the right thing to do.

A One Question Assessment?

It is even possible to obtain useful information from a pre-fitting questionnaire containing only one question. An example of this was reported by Palmer, Solodar, Hurley, Byrne, and Williams (2009). In a retrospective study of more than 800 adults aged 18 to 95 years, these authors examined the relationship between the patient's rating of his or her hearing ability and their subsequent decision to purchase hearing aids. The patients were asked the following question:

"On a scale from 1 to 10, with 1 being the worst and 10 being the best, how would you rate your overall hearing ability?"

The answer to the above question was then compared with whether the patient purchased hearing aids. Table 7–1 is a probability chart that resulted from the data analysis. Note that the results showed that there appear to be two distinct groups: those who are very likely to purchase hearing aids (ratings #1 to #5) and those who are likely *not* to purchase hearing aids (ratings #8 to #10). Palmer and colleagues suggest that these initial ratings can be used to determine the best counseling approach for a potential hearing aid user.

A Preview of the Assessment Scales

A large number of inventories have been introduced over the years. Rather than reviewing every measure

Table 7–1. The Relationship Between the Patient's Self-Rating of Hearing Ability and Probability of Purchasing Hearing Aids

Patient Rating of Hearing Ability (#1 = Worst, #10 = Best)	Predicted Probability of Hearing Aid Purchase
1	98%
2	96%
3	92%
4	83%
5	73%
6	58%
7	37%
8	20%
9	10%
10	6%

Source: From Palmer et al., 2009.

here, we have selected a subset of measures that we believe are useful, each of which provides unique information. More specifically, we have selected six different self-assessment inventories that can be used in the pre-fitting process. There are several other excellent self-assessment inventories and new ones which meet our criteria of being brief enough for clinical use, but data are still limited regarding validity and reliability.

> **KEY CONCEPT:**
> **SPOUSES, RELATIVES, AND FRIENDS WANTED!**
>
> In most cases, the pre-fitting self-assessment scales are completed during the pre-fitting appointment. We know that it is important to have the patient who is seeing you for the first time to bring a companion. The companion is someone who can make the consultative appointment more comfortable for the patient. In fact, subjective pre-fitting measures have been developed that are specifically targeted to significant others such as the HHIE-SP, described later in this chapter. Some reasons why we recommend having a significant other present during the pre-fitting appointment:
>
> 1. Provide details about the general health of the patient.
> 2. Give a second opinion about how the patient is communicating in daily living.
> 3. Facilitate discussion during the needs assessment and testing phase of the appointment.
> 4. Help the patient remember what was said during the evaluation.
> 5. Assist in making treatment and purchasing decisions.

Validation studies are time consuming, but in our opinion, critical, prior to routine clinical use. We also should point out there are a number of other self-assessment inventories that we will not review here, that can be quite useful when the patient has a very specific complaint. The Tinnitus Handicap Inventory (THI) is one good example (Newman, Jacobson and Spitzer, 1996). Here is a brief summary of the measures we will review:

- Hearing Handicap Inventory for the Elderly/Adult (HHIE/A). Measures the degree of handicap for emotional and social issues related to hearing loss.
- Abbreviated Profile of Hearing Aid Benefit (APHAB). Provides the percentage of problems the patient has for three different listening conditions involving speech understanding (in quiet, in background noise, and in reverberation) and for problems related to annoyance with environmental sounds (aversiveness scale).
- Expected Consequences of Hearing Aid Ownership (ECHO). Measures the patient's expectations for four different areas: positive effect, service and cost, negative features, and personal image.
- Client Oriented Scale of Improvement (COSI). Requires patients to identify three to five very specific listening goals/communication needs for amplification. Can then be used to measure patients' expectations related to these specific goals.
- Hearing Aid Selection Profile (HASP). Assesses eight patient factors related to the use of hearing aids: motivation, expectations, appearance, cost, technology, physical needs, communication needs, and lifestyle.
- Characteristics of Amplification Tool (COAT). Nine questions designed to determine the patient's communication needs, motivation, expectations, cosmetics, and cost concerns.

Hearing Handicap for the Elderly/Adult (HHIE/A)

Perhaps the oldest and most well-known self-assessment scale related to the pre-fitting of hearing aids is the HHIE. As the name suggests, this scale assesses handicap—specifically related to the emotional and social aspects of having a hearing loss.

Background

There have been some modifications to the HHIE scale over the years, so to get started, here is a brief summary:

- HHIE: The original 25-item questionnaire (Ventry & Weinstein, 1982), designed for the elderly—people 65 and older.
- HHIE-S: (*Note:* S = Screening.) A modification of the HHIE containing only 10 items (Weinstein, 1986).
- HHIA: (*Note:* A = Adult.). A 25-item of the HHIE for individuals younger than 65 years (Newman, Weinstein, Jacobson, & Hug, 1990).
- HHIA-S: (*Note:* S = Screening.) A modification of the HHIA containing only 10 items (Newman, Weinstein, Jacobson, & Hug, 1991).

Research has shown the shortened versions have comparable reliability and validity compared to the longer 25-item version, with an adequate internal consistency and high test-retest reliability (Newman et al., 1991; Ventry & Weinstein, 1983). For clinical use, therefore, we recommend the 10-item versions of both the HHIE and the HHIA. If we look at the 10-item versions, there are only two items that are different between the elderly and adult scales:

Question #3

- HHIE: Do you have difficulty understanding when someone speaks in a whisper?
- HHIA: Does a hearing problem cause you difficulty hearing/understanding coworkers, clients, or customers?

Question #6

- HHIE: Does a hearing problem cause you to attend religious services less often than you would like?
- HHIA: Does a hearing problem cause you problems in the movies or theater?

As you can see from the comparative questions, the adult version is geared more to someone who is still employed. If your 70-year-old patient is indeed still actively employed, there are no rules (that we know of) that say you cannot give him the HHIA-S rather than the HHIE-S. One might even question if the age cutoff is the same today as it was when the scales were developed: Is age 65 "elderly?"

The HHIE was designed to have questions that fall into two general areas: emotional and social/situational. These questions are sometimes designated by an "E" or an "S" on the form; there are five of each category on the HHIE-S and HHIA-S. The emotional scale examines the patient's attitudes and emotional feelings related to their hearing loss:

"Does a hearing problem cause you to feel embarrassed when you meet new people?"

The social/situation scale measures the perceived effects of hearing loss for a variety of communication situations:

"Does a hearing problem cause you difficulty when in a restaurant with relatives or friends?"

Many of the self-assessment scales that we describe in this chapter are designed to provide additional information to assist in hearing aid selection and counseling for the candidate. The HHIE, on the other hand, often has been used to determine whether or not the patient is a candidate. For example, the HHIE-S is recommended by the ASHA (1997) as a screening tool for hearing disability in older adults. In some instances, the HHIE even is used in marketing in an attempt to convince a potential hearing aid user that they have communication problems. For example, you might see the HHIE as part of a full-page hearing aid promotional ad in the Sunday newspaper. The readers are encouraged to answer the questions, score themselves, and rate their handicap.

Considerable research has been conducted comparing HHIE scores with the patient's audiogram. For example, Lichtenstein, Bess, and Logan (1988) validated the HHIE-S against pure-tone audiometry for 178 patients over age 65. They report that an HHIE-S score from 0 to 8 resulted in a likelihood ratio of 0.36 and a 13% probability of hearing loss (95% confidence interval, 0.19 to 0.68); a score of 26 or more yielded a likelihood ratio of 12.00, and a 84% probability of hearing loss (95% confidence interval, 2.62 to 55.00).

In one of the largest studies of this type, Wiley, Cruickshanks, Nondahl, and Tweed (2000) used the HHIE-S in the study of 3,471 adults (1,963 women,

> **TECHNICAL TIP: AN HHIE SCALE FOR THE SPOUSE TOO!**
>
> In addition to the HHIE and the HHIA and their screening companions, there is also the HHIE-SP, described by Newman and Weinstein (1986). The HHIE-SP is identical to the HHIE except for the substitution of "your spouse" for "you" in each question. This then provides an indication of how the spouse views the hearing problem. Newman and Weinstein (1986) report the husband's score (they used all male subjects in the study) were significantly higher (worse) than the wives for both the social and emotional scale (31 versus 24 points for the 25-item, 100-point version). Correlations between the HHIE and the HHIE-SP reveal a stronger relationship for the social/situational scale than for the emotional scale—probably because the hearing impaired person's handicap in social situations is often observable, whereas his or her thoughts about the situation might not be as obvious. It is important to remember that differences in the perceptions of hearing handicap between the patient and his or her spouse do not indicate that either party is right or wrong. It can be useful, however, to examine areas of discrepancy or agreement and use these emotional or social situations to shape counseling objectives.

1,508 men), as part of a large epidemiologic study of hearing disorders in older adults. Participants were divided into four groups based on age, which ranged from 48 to 92 years. Figure 7–1 illustrates the percentage of significant hearing handicap (HHIE-S >8) as a function of the degree of hearing loss. Although you might assume that as people age their hearing handicap will become worse, the authors report that, after accounting for the degree of hearing loss in men and women, self-reported hearing handicap was *lower* for older age

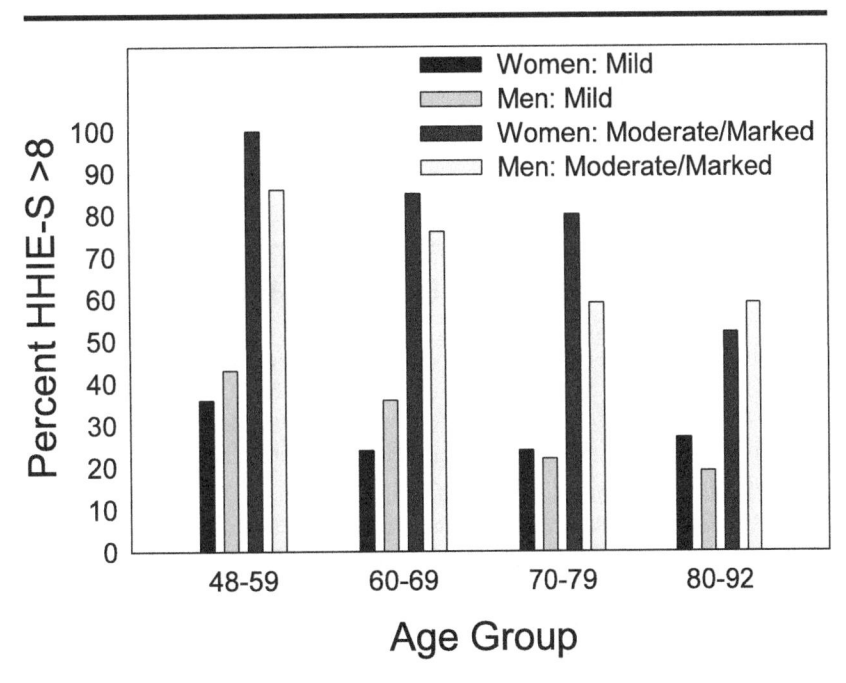

Figure 7–1. Illustration of the percentage of significant hearing handicap (HHIE -S>8) as a function of the degree of hearing loss, separated for men and women. (Adapted from Wiley et al., 2000.)

groups. After adjusting for the degree of hearing loss, handicap declined 24% for every five-year advancement in age. There are several possible reasons for this:

- Elderly individuals may minimize or ignore health problems.
- The older population is simply less bothered by problems such as hearing loss and may cope more successfully. Some may simply accept hearing loss as a natural part of aging.
- The generation of older individuals studied may have experienced greater hardships during their life, which led to lower expectations and stronger tolerance.
- The younger individuals are more active and place greater demands on their communication skills.
- The younger individuals are not as accepting of having a hearing loss.

Another large-scale study that utilized the HHIE was the Blue Mountains Hearing Study, conducted in a representative, older Australian community during the years 1997 to 1999 (Sindhusake et al., 2001). The study included 1,817 individuals who had both audiometric threshold testing and completed all questions on the HHIE-S (scores >8 were considered indicative of hearing handicap). Using the audiogram as the gold standard, a receiver operating characteristic (ROC) curve for HHIE-S score for mild, moderate, and marked hearing impairment was computed, as shown in Figure 7–2.

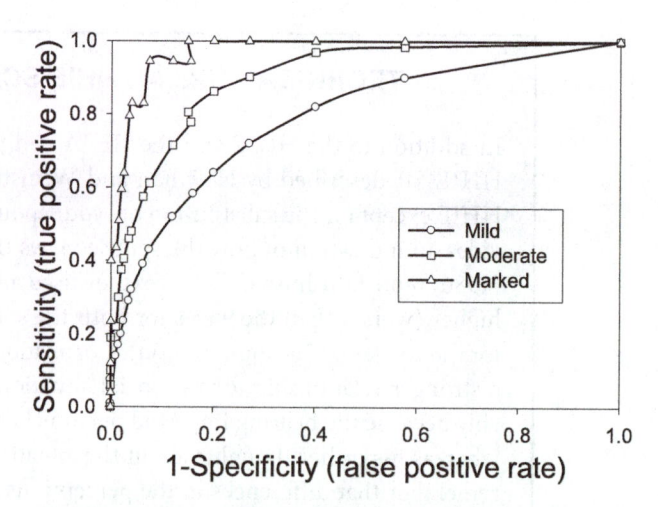

Figure 7–2. Illustration of the receiver operating characteristic curve (ROC) for HHIE-S scores (scores >8 were considered indicative of hearing handicap) for mild, moderate, and marked hearing impairment. Based on data from 1,817 individuals who had both audiometric threshold testing and who completed all questions on the HHIE-S. (Adapted from Sindhusake et al., 2001.)

The authors of the study consider that the ROC curves shown in Figure 7–2 confirm the usefulness of an HHIE-S score >8 in identifying moderate hearing loss but suggest that a lower HHIE-S cut-point score (e.g., >6) might be more useful in screening for mild hearing loss and a higher cut point score (e.g., >14), for marked hearing loss. It is interesting to note that the HHIE-S performed best in younger male subjects. The overall

---

TECHNICAL TIP: ROC CURVES

We mention the study using the HHIE-S findings and the audiogram to construct ROC curves. Here is a little information to help interpret Figure 7–2.

- Sensitivity: The percentage of time that a positive test finding will result for people who have the disease/pathology in question.
- Specificity: The percentage of time that a negative test finding will result for people who *do not* have the disease/pathology in question.

In signal detection theory, a receiver operating characteristic (ROC), or simply ROC curve, is a graphical plot of the sensitivity, or true positive rate, versus the false positive rate (1-specificity). These curves then allow for comparison of the trade-off between sensitivity (hit rate) and 1-specificity (false positive rate) as the pass or fail criteria of the test are manipulated. In this case, we are looking at the sensitivity of the HHIE to detect hearing loss.

prevalence of hearing loss in the study was 39.4%. The prevalence was lower, however, for the moderate and marked hearing loss groups, and therefore, the HHIE-S had higher negative predictive rates and lower positive predictive rates for these subject samples.

The HHIE-S also was used in the ongoing hearing study of the Framingham Heart Study cohort. The gold standard used in this study was an audiogram showing a pure-tone threshold of 40 dB HL or poorer at 1 and 2 kHz in one ear or at 1 or 2 kHz in both ears. Gates, Murphy, Rees, and Fraher (2003) reported that the HHIE-S (cutoff score >8) had a sensitivity of 35% and a specificity of 94% for detecting the criterion hearing loss.

Given the significant correlations that have been shown between HHIE score and degree of hearing loss, it is reasonable to assume that the HHIE score also is correlated with the decision to use hearing aids. As part of MarkeTrak IV, Kochkin (1997) included the HHIE-S in a survey of 3,000 hearing aid owners and 3,500 hearing impaired nonowners (response rate approximately 80% for each group). The relationship between hearing aid ownership (percent penetration) and the HHIE-S score is shown in Figure 7–3. As illustrated, there is a systematic (and significant) relationship between the HHIE-S score and the decision to own hearing aids. Note that even when HHIE scores are 30 or greater, however, approximately 50% of this group did not own hearing aids.

Administration and Scoring

One feature of the HHIE that has contributed to its popularity is that it is very easy to administer and score. It is recommended that the HHIE be delivered face-to-face to help prevent patients from skipping a question because of the belief it is not applicable to them. In this

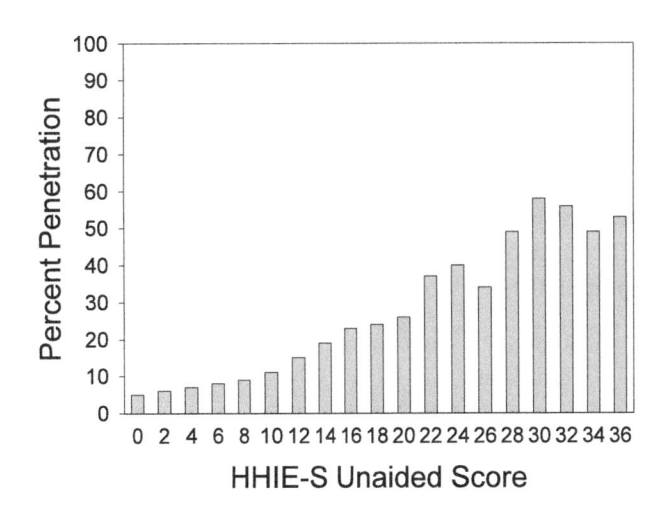

Figure 7–3. Data from MarkeTrak IV that show how unaided average HHIE scores relate to hearing aid ownership for individuals who state they have hearing loss. (Adapted from Kochkin, 1997.) As expected, hearing aid ownership increases as HHIE scores become worse, although even when HHIE scores are 30 or more, ownership is only around 50%.

regard, the instructions also state, "Do not skip a question if you avoid a situation because of your hearing loss." For each of the 10 questions of the HHIE/A-S, the patient has the choice of three answers:

- Yes (scored 4 points)
- Sometimes (scored 2 points)
- No (scored 0 points)

We have seen forms where these answers have been changed to Always, Sometimes, and Never. The MarkeTrak IV survey we discussed earlier, Kochkin (1997) used Frequently, Sometimes, and Never.

KEY CONCEPT: THE IMPORTANCE OF CONSISTENT INSTRUCTIONS

Clinicians should keep in mind that different instruction sets should not be used interchangeably. There are a large number of studies that clearly have shown that the specific instructions and response scale used can greatly affect the measured results of subjective questionnaires. Therefore, if the goal is to compare your patient to normative data, the specific instructions and response scale used when collecting the normative data must be used. It's very likely that using "Frequently" versus "Always" versus "Yes" for the 4-point HHIE response might all result in different scores for the same patient.

Once completed, the scores for the 10 items are simply added, with 40 representing the highest (worst) score, a significant handicap. A separate score can be calculated for each of the two different subscales (emotional and social), although typically just the overall score is used (especially for the screening version).

The following general guidelines are used for interpreting the results:

- 0 to 8: No significant perception of a hearing handicap
- 10 to 22: Mild to moderate perception of a hearing handicap
- >22: Perception of a severe handicap

Clinical Application

As with some of the other scales we will discuss, the unaided HHIE often is used as a baseline for measuring hearing aid benefit following the fitting of hearing aids. One hopes that, with the use of hearing aids, we will observe the scores improve from the unaided findings. The HHIE also is a very useful tool for pre-fitting counseling. Assume our patient is a 74-year-old male who is semi-retired. He has a history of noise exposure and a bilaterally symmetrical downward sloping hearing loss, with near-normal hearing in the lows that drops to 50 dB at 2000 Hz and 70 dB in the 3000 to 4000 Hz range. His HHIE-S scores are 16 for social/situational and 4 for emotional, giving him a total score of 20. The total score of 20 places him in the moderate perception of handicap category. The 16 score for the social subscale indicates that he is having problems in several different communication settings. It would be worthwhile to discuss these problems more as they might make good items for the COSI. It is a little unusual that his emotional score is as low as it is, given the 16 score for social. It could indeed be that, although he is having considerable difficulty, it really does not bother him or his family. On the other hand, he simply may be denying that he is frustrated and embarrassed, or he maybe has not really accepted his hearing loss. This too would warrant discussion prior to the fitting.

What if a patient with this same hearing loss had an overall HHIE-S score of 36? It seems unlikely that this degree of hearing loss would cause that much handicap. Could it be that this patient is purposely exaggerating his or her handicap for some other reason? Why did the patient make the appointment? Other health problems? This takes us back to many of the issues we discussed in Chapter 3—except you are now armed with HHIE findings to assist in the counseling process.

Obtaining the HHIE/A

The HHIE/A is not copyrighted. Because most clinicians use the screening versions and because it is only 10 questions, clinics or individuals often design their own template of the questionnaire.

Abbreviated Profile of Hearing Aid Benefit (APHAB)

In the previous pages, we discussed the HHIE, perhaps the most utilized hearing aid fitting pretest over the past few decades. We would guess that the second most popular, and gaining ground, is the APHAB, a scale developed by Robyn Cox and colleagues at the University of Memphis.

POINTS TO PONDER: ARE HHIE-HHIA MERGING?

If you have used the HHIE/A in a busy clinic, you know that it is somewhat of a pain to use the two different forms and make sure the patient receives the correct form based on their age or employment status (or whether they attend religious services). Help is on the way. Barbara Weinstein tells us that a single, merged screening form for the HHIE/A is now available and is being used in at least one research project. Forms and normative data will be available soon, although the data undoubtedly will be very similar to what we have been using, given that most questions are the same and the scoring has not changed. Be on the lookout for this new form!

Background

Although normally thought of as an outcome measure, the APHAB also is a popular pre-fitting tool for one main reason: To calculate benefit with hearing aids, we need an unaided baseline. As we discuss shortly, there are several good reasons why the APHAB should be used as a measure prior to the hearing aid fitting other than simply obtaining baseline unaided information.

As you might predict from the word *abbreviated*, the origins of the APHAB are from other more extensive self-assessment scales, also developed at the University of Memphis. The first of these was a scale designed to assess hearing aid users' opinions about the helpfulness of their hearing aids. This scale was the Profile of Hearing Aid Performance (PHAP; Cox & Gilmore, 1990). This questionnaire consisted of 66 items distributed among seven subscales. Five subscales addressed the problems people have communicating in daily life, and two subscales related to the unpleasantness of everyday sounds. The PHAP was then modified so that the questions could also be answered by the unaided listener, making it possible to assess opinions regarding the benefit of using hearing aids. This revision of the PHAP was dubbed the Profile of Hearing Aid Benefit (PHAB; Cox, Gilmore, & Alexander, 1991). It was comprised of the same items and the same subscales as the PHAP. The PHAP and the PHAB were developed as research tools; the 66 questions and scoring for seven subscales were not generally considered *clinically friendly*. This led to the development of the shortened (or abbreviated) version of the PHAB, the 24-item, four-subscale APHAB (Cox & Alexander, 1995).

The APHAB is composed of 24 items that are scored in four subscales (six questions each). The subscales are:

- Ease of Communication (EC): The strain of communicating under relatively favorable conditions. (e.g., "I have difficulty hearing a conversation when I'm with one of my family members at home.")
- Reverberation (RV): Communication in reverberant rooms such as classrooms. (e.g., "When I am talking with someone across a large empty room, I understand the words.")
- Background Noise (BN): Communication in settings with high background noise levels. (e.g., "When I am listening to the news on the car radio and family members are talking, I have trouble hearing the news.")
- Aversiveness (AV): The unpleasantness of environmental sounds. (e.g., "The sounds of running water, such as a toilet flushing or a shower running, are uncomfortably loud.")

Cox, Alexander, and Gray (2003) compared unaided APHAB scores with four different audiometric variables: pure-tone hearing loss and three speech recognition tests—speech reception thresholds, monosyllables in quiet, and the revised Speech-In-Noise (R-SPIN) test. They report that for EC and RV subscales, 4 to 5% of additional variance was accounted for by combining a second variable with the one most strongly related to the subscale. For these subscales, the combined audiologic variables accounted for 45% (EC) and 51% (RV) of the variance in APHAB scores. For the BN subscale

---

THINGS TO REMEMBER: THE APHAB AND THE IHAFF

In the early 1990s, a group of 12 audiologists banded together to form what was dubbed the Independent Hearing Aid Fitting Forum (IHAFF). The goal was to develop a better way to fit hearing aids and provide a step-by-step protocol that could be adopted by audiologists across the United States (and maybe the world). Critics (or perhaps they were realists) suggested that the complete name should have been: "IHAFF-A-DREAM." Regardless, in 1994, after a couple of years of meetings, the IHAFF group indeed did emerge with a complete fitting protocol (Mueller, 1994b). Robyn Cox was a member of the IHAFF, and her APHAB, launched as part of this protocol, was a key component to the overall IHAFF fitting philosophy. Today, the IHAFF is mostly forgotten, but the APHAB is still going strong.

scores, however, combining audiometric variables did not improve their ability to predict APHAB scores. And it is interesting to note that it was not the R-SPIN, but rather monosyllabic word recognition in quiet that was the most closely related to the BN score. Differences in word recognition accounted for 26% of the differences in BN scores. As we might expect, scores for the AV subscale were not significantly associated with any audiometric variable.

The authors remind us, however, that although there was a modest correlation between audiometric findings and the EC and RV subscales, it is still risky to attempt to predict communication problems from audiometric data on an individual basis. This is clearly shown in Figure 7–4. If there were a close relationship, all data points would be clustered along the diagonal regression line. Instead, as shown, it was common for the true APHAB score to differ by 30% or more from the predicted. For example, if we observe the results for an unaided predicted score in the 50 to 60% range (a common clinical finding), note that true APHAB scores range from 20 to over 80%. Differences such as this one are precisely why we believe that in addition to objective tests, subjective tests such as this are an essential component of the hearing aid fitting process.

As part of MarkeTrak IV, Kochkin (1997) questioned if the unaided APHAB was related to hearing aid ownership. For this analysis, he averaged the three subscales—EC, RV, and BN—and referred to the result as *percent disability*. The APHAB was completed by 5,954 individuals with self-admitted hearing loss. The results showed a strong relationship between ownership and the unaided score, as illustrated in Figure 7–5. These data suggest that average unaided APHAB scores would need to exceed 65% before hearing aid ownership reaches 50% of individuals admitting to having a hearing loss. We can compare this with the norms for satisfied users of hearing aids (Johnson, Cox, & Alexander, 2010). These data show the 50th percentile average for the combined EC-AV-BN scales is 69%.

Administration and Scoring

The APHAB can be administered as a paper and pencil test or as a computer software version (e.g., the APHAB is included in the Questionnaire Module of the NOAH software). The 24 items of the APHAB are scored on a seven-point scale. A percent value, shown on the form, is designated for each letter answer:

- A: Always (99%)
- B: Almost Always (87%)
- C: Generally (75%)
- D: Half-the-time (50%)
- E: Occasionally (25%)
- F: Seldom (12%)
- G: Never (1%)

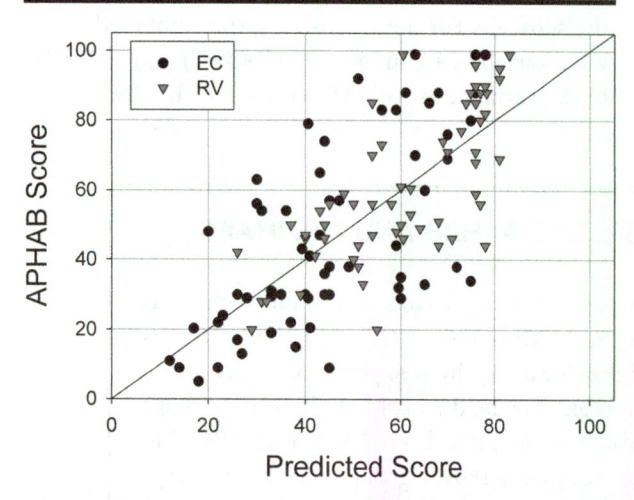

Figure 7–4. The APHAB score for the EC and BN subscales, predicted from audiometric measures, compared with the patient's true APHAB score for the same two subscales. (Adapted from Cox et al., 2003.)

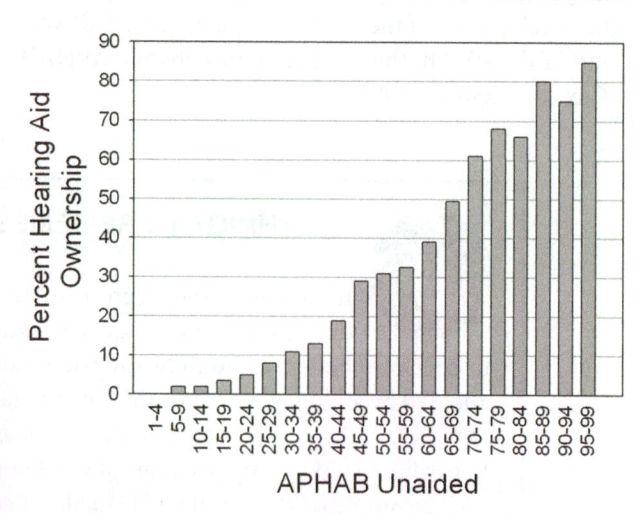

Figure 7–5. The relationship between the unaided APHAB score (percentage of problems) and hearing aid ownership. (Adapted from Kochkin, 1997.)

If a computer version of the APHAB is used, scoring is automatic and the results are displayed with comparative normative data. It is a little tedious and you might need a calculator, but it is relatively easy to score the APHAB by hand. Guidance for this can be found at the Hearing Aid Research Lab (HARL) website. If you plan to administer this test during the hearing aid selection visit, however, computer scoring is highly recommended so that the information can quickly and efficiently be used to aid in selection.

The instructions for completing the APHAB are as follows:

Please circle the answers that come closest to your everyday experience. Notice that each choice includes a percentage. You can use this to help you decide on your answer. For example, if a statement is true about 75% of the time, circle 'C' for that item. If you have not experienced the situation we describe, try to think of a similar situation that you have been

> **TECHNICAL TIP: ADMINISTERING THE APHAB**
>
> In her 1997 article describing the administration of the APHAB, Cox provides tips regarding two potential problems that could arise.
>
> - Patients sometimes have difficulty responding to a particular item because they do not experience the specific situation described in their daily life. She states that, in this case, we should attempt to help them identify a similar situation in preference to leaving the item blank. If we must leave items blank, Cox states that we probably should not give much weight to subscale scores derived from fewer than four responses.
> - A second important point is to tell the patient that each item must be read carefully because sometimes a response of *always* means a lot of problems, and sometimes it means few or no problems. Cox reports that the items were written this way to make sure that patients pay close attention to their content, and not simply read the first one or two and then give the same answer to all the rest. She states that if we tell the patients about this feature of the questionnaire and perhaps even show them some items that demonstrate the point, the great majority of people will complete the questionnaire successfully.
>
> Clearly these issues suggest that the reliability and validity of the APHAB can be enhanced by face-to-face administration or, at the least, by reviewing the answers with the patient.

> **KEY CONCEPT: LOOKING AT PREVIOUS ANSWERS IS OKAY!**
>
> As with some of the other pre-fitting scales we discuss, one of the primary uses of the pre-fitting APHAB is to serve as a baseline for the *aided* APHAB that will be conducted following the fitting. Be sure to use the same form for both; as Cox (1997) states, to maximize the validity and reliability, the patient should be allowed to see his or her responses to the Without Hearing Aid portion while he or she is completing the With Hearing Aid part. Cox further states that the patient should be encouraged to review the earlier responses, and they are allowed to change responses to the Without Hearing Aid part retrospectively. Seeing the unaided answers tends to recalibrate the patient and improves the quality of the With Hearing Aid answers.

in and respond for that situation. If you have no idea, leave that item blank.

Clinical Application

Cox (1997) states that there are four potential clinical uses of the APHAB:

1. To predict success from unaided scores
2. To compare results with different hearing aids
3. To evaluate fittings in an absolute sense
4. To measure benefit from the fitting

Both the first and fourth of these clinical uses apply to this chapter. We discuss the fourth one first. The most common use of the APHAB is to calculate the benefit with amplification. To do this, one must first have the unaided baseline for comparison. This is best obtained before the patient begins to use the instruments. We question if the patient really remembers accurately how they were doing without hearing aids after a month of hearing aid use. Before actually using the unaided APHAB for pre-fitting patient counseling, it is helpful to compare these scores with other tests of the pre-fitting test battery that you might have conducted. Here are a few examples:

- Do the EC subscale problems agree with the pure-tone audiogram or the AI scores from the count-the-dots calculations (see Chapter 5)?
- Does the BN subscale score agree with the WIN or the BKB-SIN SNR Loss (see Chapter 6 for review of these tests)?
- Do the patient's problem areas identified on the APHAB (e.g., lectures, grocery store, in car) agree with the items nominated on the COSI?

When using the APHAB for pre-fitting counseling, it is helpful to examine the scores for each one of the four subscales. Below are the results for a 74-year-old man with a mild-to-moderate downward sloping hearing loss (the same patient whom we discussed in the previous HHIE section). He still works part-time in his office supply business, which involves frequent meeting with clients. His average APHAB percent of problems for each subscale are:

- EC: 27%
- BN: 58%
- RV: 62%
- AV: 19%

Once these scores have been obtained, you will then want to compare them with normative data (norms). One counseling approach is to compare the patient to individuals with normal hearing. We prefer to plot the findings on one of the charts provided by Cox when the APHAB was first introduced (Cox, 1997); they are also part of the APHAB module included with the NOAH software.

This type of plot is shown in Figure 7–6, with our patient's scores included. Our patient is 74 years old, which some consider elderly, so we are using these norms for this patient as well as those for young people with normal hearing for comparison. As shown in Figure 7–6 (left panel), this patient's problems for both the BN and RV subscale exceed the 95th percentile of

---

THINGS TO REMEMBER: USING PERCENTILES FOR POST-FITTING COUNSELING

Although we are focusing on the use of the APHAB for pre-fitting testing, it is important to point out that the chart shown in Figure 7–6 can be very helpful for post-fitting counseling (see Chapter 19). The patient's aided APHAB can be plotted just as we plotted the unaided scores. It often is pleasing to see how closely our patients are performing compared with people with normal hearing, which we eagerly share with the patient. The graph also is a helpful reminder that a patient who still has 20% problems in background noise following hearing aid use is actually experiencing only slightly more problems than the 50th percentile of young normal listeners.

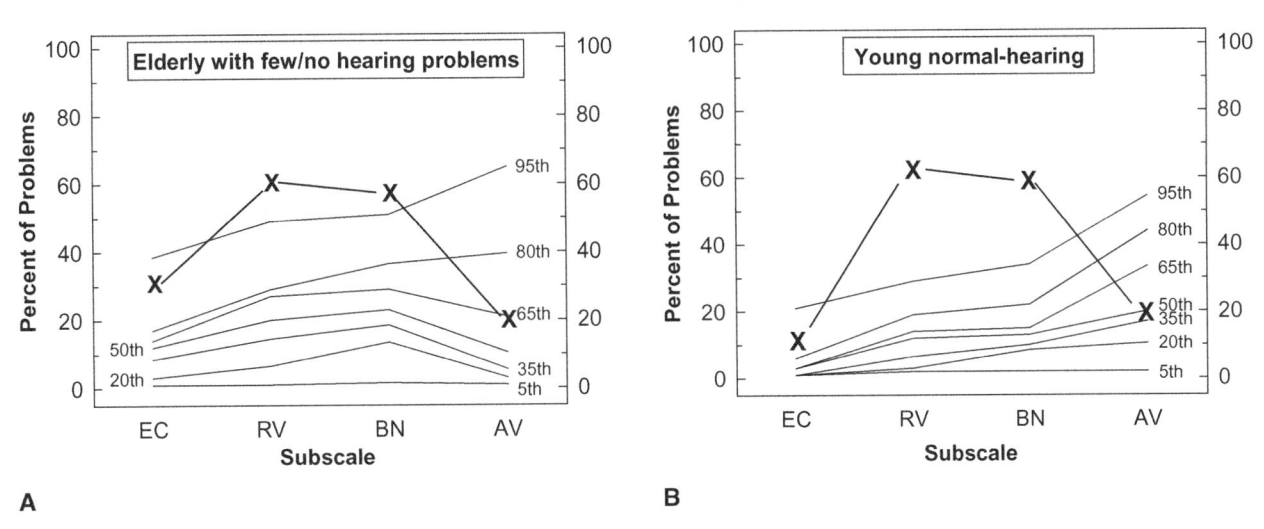

Figure 7–6. The plotting of the unaided APHAB scores for an individual patient for two different set of norms: elderly with few or no hearing problems (*Panel A*) and young normal hearing individuals (*Panel B*).

elderly people with normal hearing—that is, more than 95% of elderly people with normal (or near-normal) hearing do not have this large a number of problems.

Another way to view this patient's unaided APHAB scores is to compare them with norms of successful hearing aid users. This can be done by using a table available from Robyn Cox's HARL website and displayed in Figure 7–7 (adapted from Johnson et al., 2010). Using this table, we see that our patient falls around the 5th percentile for the EC subscale, 30th percentile for RV, 20th for BN, and 60th for AV. In general, while the patient's problems worse than his peers with normal hearing, they are not as severe as the average hearing aid user.

Obtaining the APHAB

Complete APHAB information can be obtained from Robyn Cox's website (http://www.memphis.edu/ausp/harl/). APHAB scoring software also is available. Some

---

TECHNICAL TIP: PERMISSIONS FOR USING THE APHAB

Many audiologists like to post the APHAB (and other self-assessment scales) on their website. Here is the word regarding APHAB permissions straight from the developer, Robyn Cox, PhD:

You do not need permission to post the APHAB on your website for use by your patients as long as you follow certain procedures. The APHAB is under copyright, which means that no one but the authors can legally copy, distribute or adapt the questionnaire without permission. We make the questionnaire freely available on HARL's website (http://www.memphis.edu/ausp/harl/). This means that we have given you permission to download it and use it. However, you cannot change it, sell it, or claim to have created it. I suggest that you download the "Form A-New Format" version to post to your website because it has a few additional instructions that would help patients complete the questionnaire correctly before their appointment.

Thank you, Robyn!

Percentile	EC	RV	BN	AV
95	99	99	99	70
80	83	87	89	35
65	75	81	81	21
50	63	71	75	14
35	56	65	67	9
20	46	58	58	3
5	26	47	41	1

Figure 7–7. Percentiles of unaided APHAB scores for successful hearing aid users. (Adapted from Johnson et al., 2010.)

hearing aid manufacturers have included the APHAB as part of their software, and the APHAB is part of the Questionnaire Module of NOAH, a free add-on for registered NOAH users that is available for download (http://www.himsa.com).

Expected Consequences of Hearing Aid Ownership (ECHO)

As the name indicates, the Expected Consequences of Hearing Aid Ownership (ECHO) is all about *expectations*. It is generally believed that expectations can influence satisfaction. Overly high expectations can lead to disappointment. And on the other hand, it seems reasonable that a person with low expectations may be more apt to be satisfied. We are reminded of Benjamin Franklin's often repeated statement: "Blessed is he who expects nothing, for he shall never be disappointed." Anecdotal reports suggest that most audiologists would prefer to have a patient with relatively low or, at the least, moderate expectations and some audiologists might even attempt to lower the patient's expectations if they appear to be too high. The ideal would seem to be realistic expectations as we discuss below. But unless we measure expectations and compare our findings to realistic

---

POINTS TO PONDER: ARE HIGH OR LOW EXPECTATIONS GOOD?

We probably all have had the experience of going into an unknown seedy restaurant only to walk out incredibly satisfied with our dinner. But if we had had the same meal at Ruth's Chris or the Palm, our satisfaction might have been considerably lower. When it comes to dining at restaurants, it is reasonable to conclude that it is more likely to be satisfying if our expectations are low. But does this also apply to obtaining hearing aids? Many clinicians are concerned that if their patients' expectations are too high (e.g., my new hearing aids will help me do better in all listening situations), amplification may not meet the expectations, and the patient will not be satisfied. This seems reasonable. On the other hand, some people are simply optimistic. They may have high expectations, but their attitude toward the use of hearing aids (and life in general) is such that they will make good things happen. If they believe that a positive outcome will result, it probably will. Limited research shows that the latter example might be especially true for hearing aid fittings. For example, Schum (1999), in his work developing the Hearing Aid Needs Assessment (HANA), found that patients who expected more help in noisy situations reported that they received more help in this listening condition. And relative to our discussion here of the ECHO, Cox and Alexander (2000) report that for the *Positive Effect* subscale, there was a significant positive correlation between higher expectations and greater satisfaction. (The other subscales were not significantly correlated in either direction.) This is not necessarily a cause and effect finding, however, and could likely be related to a third variable such as optimism. In related research, Cox, Alexander, and Gray (1999) found that extroverted individuals tended to report more hearing aid benefits in all types of listening settings. The bottom line is: If your patient believes that the new hearing aids are going to work well, that is probably okay (as long as expectations are within reason).

norms, it may be difficult to know what counseling on this topic is needed.

Background

The ECHO was introduced by Cox and Alexander in 2000. It was designed to be a companion scale for the Satisfaction of Amplification in Daily Life (SADL; Cox et al., 1999). The SADL is an outcome measure of satisfaction, designed to be used following the hearing aid fitting (see Chapter 19). The questions used on the ECHO are essentially the same as those of the SADL, only slightly reworded. The items on the SADL are questions, whereas for the ECHO, the sentence is transformed into a statement of expectation. Here is an example:

- SADL: How natural is the sound from your hearing aid?
- ECHO: My hearing aid will have a natural sound.

The ECHO consists of 15 items that are divided among four subscales. A description of the subscales is as follows (Cox & Alexander, 2000):

Positive Effect: This subscale comprises six items addressing the domain of improved performance and function. Two items concern acoustic benefit, one is about sound quality, and three address psychological dividends accompanying hearing aid use (e.g., "getting hearing aids is in my best interest"). Cox and Alexander (2000) report that this domain appears to be the largest single contributor to the variance in overall post-fitting satisfaction with amplification.

Service and Cost: This subscale includes two items about service and one item on cost. If the individual is not paying for the hearing aids, the cost item is omitted.

Negative Features: Each of the three items in this subscale addresses a different potentially negative aspect of hearing aid use. All three were often identified by hearing aid users as relatively unsatisfactory. This subscale provides an estimate of the status of matters that can often detract from an otherwise highly satisfactory fitting.

Personal Image: The fourth subscale, also with three items, addresses the domain of self-image and hearing aid stigma. The image or stigma content area has been implicated repeatedly over time as highly influential in the decision to try amplification and in ultimate hearing aid satisfaction.

The background research in the development of the ECHO consisted of four separate experiments. The following are some general observations and conclusions taken from the Cox and Alexander (2000) paper:

- The data gathered regarding expectations only represent a small portion of *potential* hearing aids candidates; that is, the ECHO data are from individuals who decided to seek help and who probably have different attitudes toward their hearing loss and toward the psychosocial impact of using hearing aids than those who do not.
- The typical novice hearing aid user does not have a realistic view of the hearing aid's strengths and weaknesses.
- Expectations differ significantly among patients.
- Informational counseling is warranted for individuals who do not understand the potential negative features of hearing aids or have unrealistic expectations related to personal image.
- A high score for the Positive Effect subscale was significantly correlated with increased satisfaction. Cox and Alexander caution, however, that this does not mean you should try to raise expectations, as we do not really know that it was these higher expectations that caused the better outcome. They support the common thought that unusually favorable opinions about the anticipated benefit from hearing aids might predispose the patient to disappointment.

Administration and Scoring

There are 15 questions, and each question is scored on a seven-point scale indicating the extent that the patient agrees with the statement. The subject simply circles the best answer for each question. The seven answers for each item are as follows (points assigned are 1 through 7 for answers A through G, respectively):

A: Not At All
B: A Little
C: Somewhat
D: Medium
E: Considerably
F: Greatly
G: Tremendously

The appropriate subscale for each question and scoring guidelines are available at Robyn Cox's HARL website. For each subscale, the values of the three or six answers (for the Positive Effect subscale) are then averaged. For example, if for the three items of the Service and Cost subscale, the patient answered Considerably (5 points), Greatly (6 points), and Considerably (5 points), the score for this subscale would be 5.3 (5 + 6 + 5 = 16; 16/3 = 5.3). Four of the 15 items of the ECHO are *reversed scored*, meaning that an answer of Not At All would receive 7 points rather than 1 point. An overall *Global Score* (average of the four subscales) also is calculated, although for clinical use, you will probably want to focus more on each individual subscale to know where to focus your counseling. The ECHO easily can be scored by hand, and scoring software also is available. Again, the use of scoring software is highly recommended if the ECHO is to be administered during the selection appointment.

Once the answers have been scored, the average values are plotted on the ECHO Reality Norms form shown in Figure 7–8. *Reality Norms* meaning that this is what you might expect from the average patient seeking amplification. The black circles on the form for each category represent the mean, and the gray bars illustrate the 20th to 80th percentile scores.

Clinical Application

It is reasonable to believe that that when pre-fitting counseling is targeted toward specific attitudes of the patient, post-fitting use and satisfaction will follow. The ECHO questionnaire is an excellent tool to target specific issues that need to be addressed. The Reality Norms provide a convenient way to compare your patient's expectations with the average. In general, low scores are more problematic than high scores, but if unusually high ratings

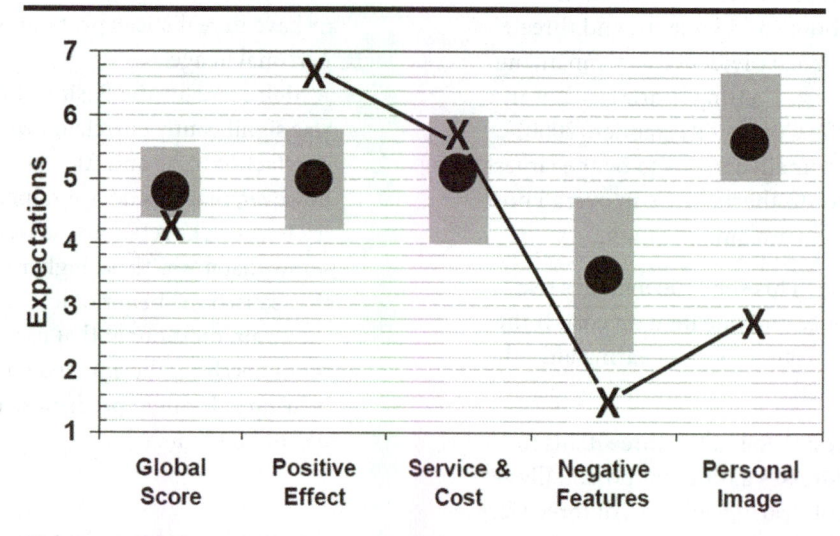

Figure 7–8. Score sheet for the ECHO. Black dots represent mean performance for average individuals with hearing loss (Reality Norms). The gray bars represent the 20th to 80th percentile score. The "Xs" on the chart are the scores for a given patient.

> **TECHNICAL TIP: WHAT DO HIGH ECHO SCORES MEAN?**
>
> We have found that when clinicians first start using the ECHO and see the patient's scores plotted on the Reality Norms form, it is not always intuitive to interpret what a deviation from the norm is telling them. It is easy to interpret the Positive Effects scale: A high score means that the person has high expectations regarding the performance of hearing aids and the benefits of amplification. This makes sense. But what about the Personal Image scale? Do high scores mean that the person has high expectations regarding the appearance of hearing aids (e.g., that he or she thinks the hearing aids will be invisible?) That might be a difficult individual to work with. But look at a question from that subscale: "I will be content with the appearance of my hearing aids." If the person answers Greatly or Tremendously, a high ECHO score will result and that is the answer most clinicians would like to hear. So, a high score is *good*. Likewise, with the Negative Features scale, a high score does *not* mean that the patient highly expects negative things to occur, but rather, they do not believe that there are negative features (which is not always good either if their beliefs are unreasonable).

are based on erroneous information or beliefs, this may require additional counseling as well.

A sample case is plotted on Figure 7–8. First, observe that the patient has a fairly average Global Score, although ratings are *not average* for three of the four subscales. Recall that the gray bars represent the 20th to 80th percentiles. The patient has a very optimistic approach toward the potential benefits of amplification (Positive Effects), which is probably okay, and the score for Service and Cost is average. The very low score for negative features indicates that the patient has either experienced or heard several negative things regarding hearing aids. This is a topic that should be explored further before fitting. For example, many of the past negative concerns regarding acoustic feedback no longer apply, given the sophisticated feedback reduction circuitry now routinely available. The extremely low score for personal image is also a concern, as it indicates the patient rated all three questions low. This means that the patient believes that people will notice the hearing loss more when wearing the hearing aids, that the patient will not be happy with the appearance of the hearing aids, and that using hearing aids will make the patient appear less capable. These attitudes easily could sabotage the fitting, as they might outweigh the patient's positive attitude regarding hearing aid benefit. This is clearly something that needs to be discussed with the patient.

Obtaining the ECHO

The forms for the ECHO can be obtained at HARL's website (http://www.memphis.edu/ausp/harl/). Software scoring also is available, and can be purchased from the AUSP Software Group (http://www.memphis.edu/csd/research/software.htm) at the School of Communication Sciences and Disorders at the University of Memphis.

Client Oriented Scale of Improvement (COSI)

The COSI is probably the most commonly used *outcome* measure among clinicians. It is also very useful for formalizing the specific listening goals a patient has for hearing aids, which is why we've included it here as a pre-fitting assessment tool. As we discuss in this section, the specificity of these goals can be particularly important as we prioritize hearing aid features and consider hearing assistive technology (HAT). In addition, we have found that this scale is useful for assessing expectations. Because it already is being used for outcome assessment, expectations easily can be assessed without introducing a new scale to the patient.

Background

One issue related to almost all standardized self-assessment scales is that the item must be relevant for the hearing aid user. Asking about his or her ability to understand speech at church or in a noisy restaurant is not useful if the patient does not go to either. To some extent, scales have tried to account for this by adding shortened versions—the APHAB is a shortened version of the PHAB; the HHIE-S is a shortened version of the HHIE—or by having somewhat different scales for different groups (e.g., the HHIE and the HHIA). This somewhat reduces irrelevance, but not completely, as patients still often omit items. Stuart Gatehouse (1994) weighed in on this issue. He suggested that, when assessing unaided disability, we should consider such factors as how often the patient is in a given situation and how much trouble he or she has communicating in this situation. The COSI was designed to accomplish these goals as well as eliminate irrelevancy. Furthermore, it allows patients to identify and rank order listening goals that are most important to them as an individual. For example, two patients may both have the goals of understanding speech in a noisy restaurant and understanding small children speaking. The importance of these two goals, and which one is most important, however, may be very different for the two patients.

The COSI was introduced in an article by Dillon, James, and Ginis in 1997. In short, the COSI allows patients to design their own questionnaires. The patients provide specific listening situations that are important for them. Making situations very specific is useful because it allows patients to easily remember and pay attention to situations when asked about hearing outcomes. From a hearing aid selection and counseling standpoint, however, it can also be quite useful as demonstrated in the clinical example we present later. After providing three to five specific situations, they are then rank ordered for importance. Recall that the COSI was designed for measuring outcomes, but the rationale for relevancy and situation importance also applies to selection and expectation ratings. Dillon et al. (1997) cite four goals related to the development of the COSI: (1) acceptable reliability (test-retest stability); (2) acceptable validity (correlations to other scales believed to be valid); (3) convenient to use; and (4) capable of improving, as well as measuring, rehabilitation outcomes.

If you have worked with the COSI but never used it for measuring expectations, you might be curious about how perceptions of benefit after hearing aid use compares with the patient's initial expectations. Palmer and Mueller (2000) provide some insight in this area in their study of 50 individuals (25 experienced users and 25 new users) who were fitted bilaterally with hearing aids as part of a larger study. Each subject completed a Patient Expectations Worksheet (PEW; a scale developed at the University of Pittsburgh that is very similar to the COSI) and listed five different communication situations in which they would like to obtain improvement (a total of 250 items). Their expectations were obtained using the five-point scale of the COSI, in which they identified the percentage of time that they believed they would be successful in a given situation following the use of hearing aids: Hardly Ever, Occasionally, Half the Time, Most of the Time, or Almost Always. Following a month of hearing aid use, the subjects rated their benefit for each situation using the same rating scale.

The results from Palmer and Mueller (2000) are shown in Figure 7–9. Note that expectations were met for a large percentage of the items (slightly greater for the previous user group, who may have had more realistic expectations), and moreover, expectations were exceeded for approximately 20% of the items. If we combine the Met and Exceeded categories, we have about

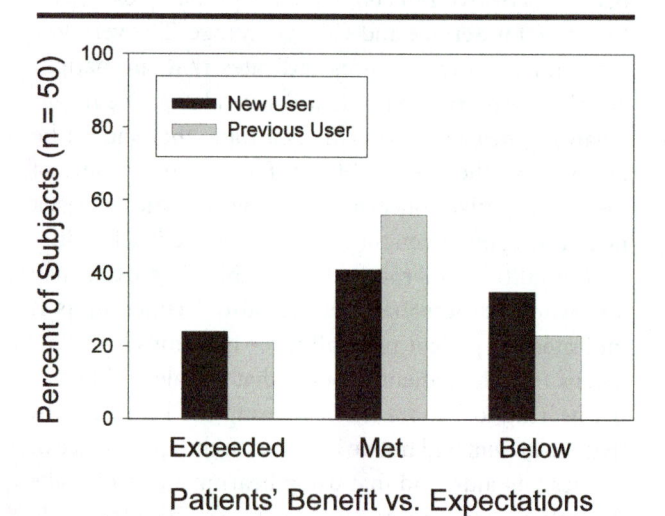

Figure 7–9. The degree that new and previous users exceeded, met, or fell below expectations when a COSI-like scale was used as a pre-fitting expectations tool.

a 70% success rate for all the items. That research was conducted quite a while ago, so we might expect even better results with today's technology.

Administration and Scoring

Unlike any other scale, the COSI starts off as a blank sheet. It is certainly possible that, after seeing hundreds of patients, no two COSIs will look the same. The process begins by having the patient identify up to five specific listening situations in which he or she would like to hear better. It is important to stress these are *listening situations* and not necessarily just communication. For some patients, the listening goals may all focus on communication, but for other listeners (e.g., a patient with a severe hearing loss), the goal may be to better hear when someone knocks at the door. Some patients will happily list six or seven, but for other patients, it is a struggle to come up with three. We suggest having at least three whenever possible. We find some patients are simply not talkative and are somewhat unresponsive in the interview process. For these individuals, it may be more productive to administer a more closed set questionnaire such as the APHAB or HHIE in lieu of the COSI.

It is important to make each item as specific as possible. "Hearing in background noise" would not be specific enough. After some questioning, this could be narrowed to, "Hearing my friends while playing cribbage at the bar at the Elks Club." Once one situation is identified, you then move on and establish other situations. After all situations have been identified, it is then helpful to go back, review all situations, and rank order them. Simply place a #1 for most important, #2 for the second most important, and so on in the box to the left of the item. Often, the item that the patient mentions first is something that just happened recently and is not the most important.

Shown in Figure 7–10 is the completed "expectations" COSI form for a 68-year-old male patient with a moderate downward sloping bilateral hearing who was being fitted with his first set of hearing aids. With some prodding, he nominated four different items, listed in the order that he provided them (he had just been out playing pool the night before). We then went back and prioritized the items, as is reflected by the numbers in the box to the left of each item.

Once the items are identified and prioritized, we normally then make a photocopy of the page. This is so we will have a clean sheet to use when he (the patient in Figure 7–10) comes back and rates his benefit with the hearing aids. We would prefer that he not see his expectations when he does the benefit rating—this is different from comparing unaided with aided, where we usually *do* want the patients to see their pre-fitting ratings. If that does not matter to you, then you have saved some time and you are ready to move ahead. We usually just have the patient rate expectations for the Degree of Change section.

Observe that this patient's expectations were *Better* for three of the four items and *Much Better* for hearing his friends at the pub. The *Better* ratings are quite reasonable, and we have a good chance of meeting his expectations for these. The benefit might even be *Much Better* for the TV listening situation. His expectations

---

THINGS TO REMEMBER: NUMBER OF COSI ITEMS

As discussed, we usually have the patient nominate as many as five COSI items. It is important to have the patient then rank order the items and, in particular, identify the two most important. Why is this? Research by Elaine Mormer and Catherine Palmer (2001) revealed that when people were asked again to nominate items two to three weeks later, 96% identified two of the same, but only 64% named three of the same. None of the individuals who initially listed four items named the same four items on retest. It appears that there probably is a recency bias for items of lesser importance, but at least two items remain constant.

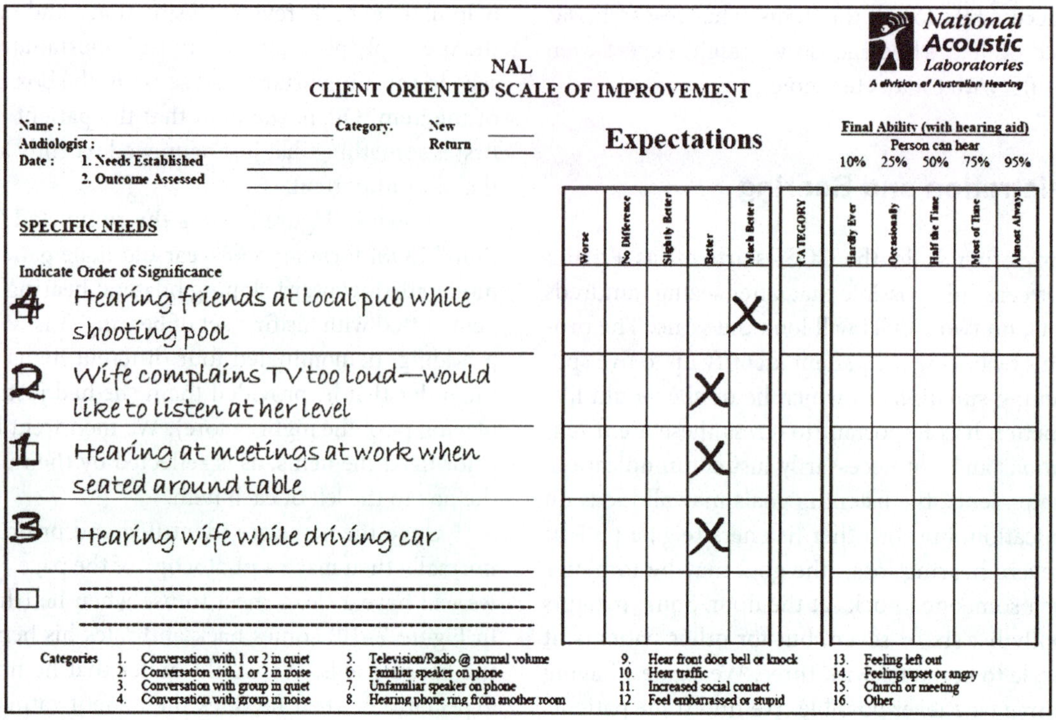

Figure 7–10. Completed pre-fitting COSI form showing the four nominated items by the patient, the patient's 1 to 4 ratings for the importance of these items, and the patient's expectations of how much benefit will be obtained when the patient starts using hearing aids ("X" markings in rating boxes). The "Expectations" heading is our modification of the standard COSI form.

TECHNICAL TIP: NOMINATING COSI ITEMS

As discussed, the items for the COSI are obtained by having a discussion with the patient, and having him or her nominate situations in which the patient has problems and would like improvement. On occasion, a patient will seem to only focus on the most difficult situations, often situations where normal hearing individuals have difficulty. This can be a problem for three reasons: (1) these situations possibly are not really the most important; (2) these situations probably occur infrequently; and (3) it will be difficult to meet expectations as these are the very situations where we expect the least benefit from amplification. Often, a quick glance at the audiogram tells us that the patient must be having trouble in other listening situations—like hearing conversations involving soft speech—even though the patient is not mentioning this. One way to *calibrate* the nomination process is to have the patient account for time. You might say: "Bob, you have named four different situations involving listening in background noise. In any given week (month), about how much time do you spend in these situations?" It is not unusual for Bob to answer, after some thought, that it is only four hours per week. Your next question then is: "So Bob, what do you do the other 96% of your waking hours?" This may uncover some other real and perhaps even more important listening situations in which Bob has difficulty.

for the pub, however, are a little concerning. We have been to the Blarney Stone; it has a cement floor and exposed brick walls, and the evening noise levels are nearly always 80 dBA or greater. If you look back at our discussion of communication in background noise in Chapter 4, you see that with this noise level it is unlikely to experience a positive SNR for an average conversation. This patient's QuickSIN score was 8 dB SNR loss. This expectation, therefore, is something we will want to talk to him about before he leaves the office with his new hearing aids. It may also lead us to discuss additional assistive technology that may allow him to communicate in this situation.

Obtaining the COSI

The form for the COSI can be downloaded (http://www.nal.gov.au/pdf/COSI-Question naire.pdf).

Hearing Aid Selection Profile (HASP)

The Three-Clinic HASP was developed by researchers (clinicians) at the Henry Ford Hospital in Detroit, MI; the Cleveland Clinic Foundation in Cleveland, OH; and the Mayo Clinic in Rochester, MN (Jacobson, Newman, Fabry, & Sandridge, 2001). Although many pre-fitting scales focus directly on communication problems and the effects of having a hearing loss, we know that there also are many *non-auditory* factors that can impact the benefit from and satisfaction with hearing aids. That's what the HASP is all about.

Background

The purpose of the HASP is to include patients' self-perceptions in many areas related to the core beliefs and attitudes that might impact the successful selection and fitting of amplification. The notion is that the results of the HASP improve overall hearing aid satisfaction by choosing the right amplification options for a given patient. Although probably too long for routine clinical use in many clinics, the HASP has clinical utility for specific situations as discussed later in this chapter. For a similar tool that is more efficient, readers are referred to the Characteristics of Amplification Tool (COAT), which is described in the next section.

The HASP is a 40-item self-report measure containing eight subscales, each consisting of five items. The response format is a five-point Likert scale with anchors of *Strongly Agree* and *Strongly Disagree,* that yield a maximum score of 20 points per subscale. The following is adapted from the Sandridge and Newman (2006) review regarding the construction of the HASP, in which three of the eight subscales address issues directly related to hearing aids:

- Motivation to wear hearing aids (e.g., "I want to wear a hearing aid even if I have difficulty in some situations.")
- Expectations regarding hearing aid performance (e.g., "A hearing aid will restore my hearing to normal just as eyeglasses restore vision to normal.")
- General communication needs (e.g., "It is very important for me to hear conversations when I am in a larger group, for example, at a party.")

The remaining five subscales contain items that assess a patient's perceptions and attitudes about issues not directly related to the use of hearing aids:

- Importance of physical appearance to others (e.g., "There is nothing wrong with using plastic surgery to improve one's appearance"; this subscale is reversed scored.)
- Attitude toward cost of commercial goods and services (e.g., "I don't think that I need the best money can buy"; this subscale is reversed scored.)
- Attitude toward technology (e.g., "I feel that new technology has improved our lives.")
- Physical functioning and manual dexterity (e.g., "It is easy for me to use small objects such as paper clips, coins, small buttons, and/or zippers.")
- Lifestyle (e.g., "I consider myself to be an active, busy, on-the-go kind of person.")

Mueller, Ricketts and Bentler, et al. (2014) review how different patient factors are related to HASP scores. Jacobson, Newman, Sandridge, and McCaslin (2002) used the HASP to study retrospectively the characteristics of individuals who rejected hearing aid use and returned their hearing aids for credit. There were three significant findings:

- The return-for-credit group fell at the 20th percentile for the Motivation subscale.
- The return-for-credit group demonstrated greater problems with manual dexterity, scoring between the 20th and 50th percentile for the Physical Functioning subscale.
- The return-for-credit group also had reduced listening needs, where scores also fell between the 20th and 50th percentile for the Communicative Needs subscale.

Administration and Scoring

As with many other pre-fitting tests, the HASP usually is administered (paper and pencil test) before discussing the use of hearing aids with the patient. As mentioned, there are 40 total items on the HASP, and each item is answered on a five-point scale ranging from Strongly Agree (4 points) to Strongly Disagree (0 points). There are eight subscales with five questions each; therefore, the total potential score for each subscale is 20 points. The questions for each subscale are randomized within the questionnaire; an identifying letter by the number of the question signifies the relevant subscale. Table 7–2 is an example of how the scoring would work for the five questions of the Motivation subscale. If you total the points for the five questions (far right column), we see that this patient has a score of 15 for this subscale. A simple pencil and paper score sheet like that in Table 7–2 easily could be used for each subscale. We recommend, however, using the Excel spreadsheet that is available through http://www.audiologyonline.com (see specifics at the end of this section).

Once the score for a given subscale has been determined, you would then compare this score with the HASP norms. These are shown in Figure 7–11, along with all the subscale scores for our patient (see open circles). Notice that the subscale score we calculated in Table 7–2 (15 points) places this patient exactly at the 50th percentile for Motivation. For clinical use, you could have a copy of these norms printed, and then each subscale score could be marked by hand on this chart. As mentioned earlier, however, we would recommend the use of a spreadsheet and electronic graphing and printing for efficient clinical use.

It is important to point out that the Appearance and Cost subscales are *reversed scored*. That is, the total points from the five subscale questions are *subtracted* from 20: The questions are worded so that Strongly Disagree is the answer most consistent with good hearing aid candidacy. In this way greater diversions from the 0 baseline will always have positive connotations regarding hearing aid candidacy for all eight subscales.

Clinical Application

In general, the HASP was designed to provide the audiologist with a wide range of information that could be useful in the hearing aid selection process. As obvious from the names of the subscales, this could involve such

Table 7–2. Sample of Questions and Scoring for the Motivation Subscale of the HASP

Q#	Question	Answer	Points
16	I want to wear a hearing aid even if I still have difficulty hearing is some situations.	Neutral	2
20	I know that a hearing aid will help me.	Agree	3
29	I am prepared to do what it takes to improve my hearing.	Strongly Agree	4
34	I am certain that I want a hearing aid	Agree	3
35	I am having a significant problem understanding speech.	Agree	3

Hearing Aid Selection Profile

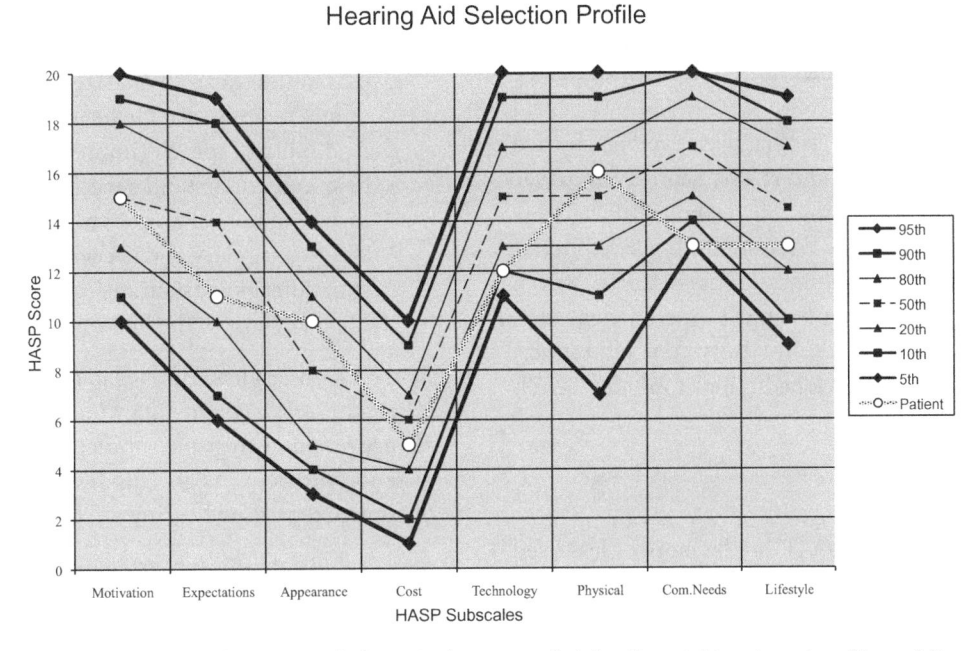

Figure 7–11. HASP norms (5th to 95th percentile) for the eight subscales. The white circles represent performance for a given individual.

things as listening needs, dexterity problems, concern with cost of the instruments, or cosmetics issues. Certainly, some of these factors could affect the selection of hearing aid style or special hearing aid features.

The results of the HASP also could be used as a predictor of who is at risk for unsuccessful use of hearing aids. For example, we know from the research of Jacobson et al. (2002) that people who returned their hearing aids for credit tend to have below average HASP subscale scores for Motivation, Physical (hand and finger dexterity), and Communication Needs. If this is known before the patient leaves with the hearing aids, counseling can be focused on these areas and the patient can be targeted for more attention during the first few weeks of hearing aid use. In general, almost all subscale scores that fall significantly below the 50th percentile need to be addressed. See Mueller et al. (2014) for other specific uses of HASP scores.

Let us return to Figure 7–11 and discuss how we might use this person's HASP scores in counseling or hearing aid selection. One way to approach it is to ask: How is this patient different from average (deviation from the 50th percentile)? That is, how will you differ from your average counseling and average selection procedure? Note that for Motivation, Expectations, Cost, and Physical, the patient is fairly close to the 50th percentile (white circles on chart above). The patient is somewhat less than average regarding concerns about appearance—this is good, as it allows you to offer a wide range of styles. The patient is at the 10th percentile for technology, significantly below average. This suggests that simple might be better. This probably is not someone who will be comfortable with five memories, a remote control for training the hearing aid, and extensive wireless connections. The Communication Needs are minimal (5th percentile), which agrees with the patient's lower Lifestyle scores. As these pieces fall together, it is much easier to determine the best fitting options.

Obtaining the HASP

The HASP form and the Excel spreadsheet for scoring and graphing are available at http://www.audiology online.com (askexpert/display_question.asp?question_id=815).

Characteristics of Amplification Tool (COAT)

The COAT is a pre-fitting test that was developed by two of the four developers of the HASP, Sharon Sandridge and Craig Newman of the Cleveland Clinic. These authors recognized the documented psychometric adequacy and clinical usefulness of the HASP; however, they mention that it is not the most time-efficient tool, which limits its application in a busy clinical practice. For this reason, they developed a new tool, the COAT.

Background

For time efficiency, the COAT can be more or less used as a replacement for the HASP. The COAT consists of nine items. Sandridge and Newman describe the rationale for including each item (Sandridge & Newman, 2006):

Item 1: Please list the top three situations where you would most like to hear better. This item is similar to the COSI. When patients are allowed to indicate specific areas of desired improvement, they play a more active role in the fitting process and in selecting the hearing aids that will meet their individual needs.

Item 2: How important is it for you to hear better? This item assesses the patient's global priority for hearing. For example, the retired individual whose primary activity is reading may not place as much importance on hearing as the individual involved in a variety of social activities.

Item 3: How motivated are you to wear and use hearing aids? A patient without motivation to use hearing aids sets the stage for failure; therefore, it is critical to assess motivation levels.

Item 4: How well do you think hearing aids will improve your hearing? Unrealistically high or low expectations regarding the use of hearing aids may lead to poor outcomes. Unrealistic expectations can result in decreased satisfaction with, or complete rejection of, the devices.

Item 5: What is your most important consideration regarding hearing aids? Four important considerations when selecting hearing aids are rank ordered by the patient:
- Cosmetics (hearing aid size and the ability of others not to see the hearing aids)
- Audibility of speech (improved ability to hear and understand speech)
- Listening in background noise (improved ability to understand speech in noisy situations like restaurants/parties)
- Finance (cost of the hearing aids)

Item 6: Do you prefer hearing aids that are totally automatic, allow you to adjust the volume and change listening programs, or no preference? This question provides insight into the patient's locus of control regarding hearing aid functionality.

Item 7: Indicate which hearing aid style(s) you would not *be willing to use.* Pictures illustrating six styles of hearing aids are displayed. The six styles include: traditional BTE, mini BTE with open ear tubing, full-shell ITE, half-shell ITE, ITC, and CIC. The patient is asked to indicate which style(s) of hearing aids is *not* acceptable.

Item 8: How confident are you that you will be a successful hearing aid user? The degree of self-efficacy (i.e., domain-specific belief that one can successfully complete a task) can be a predictor of successful hearing aid use. If a patient indicates low self-efficacy (i.e., lack of confidence), the audiologist can explore what concerns the patient has regarding hearing aid use.

Item 9: Select the cost category that represents the maximum amount you are willing to spend. This last item focuses on the patient's willingness to pay, guiding the clinician to select a level of technology consistent with the patient's desired financial investment.

Clinical Application

The items on the COAT cover a large range of pre-fitting areas including patient-specific listening needs, motivation, expectations, financial concerns, and cosmetics. The audiologist can easily use this form to focus on areas that need to be discussed or use the response to narrow the pool of products that are appropriate.

In the 2006 original article describing the COAT, authors Sandridge and Newman present a case study that nicely describes how the COAT can be used clinically to assist in the hearing aid selection. We have modified the original case slightly and present it here:

The case study is a 59-year-old male who is being seen for a Hearing Needs Assessment appointment. His audiometric results indicate a mild-to-moderate sensorineural hearing loss, bilaterally. He scored +12 dB SNR-50 on the Quick-SIN, consistent with poor speech recognition in noise. Upon review of his responses on the COAT, the following is noted:

- Wants to hear his customers in restaurants, his grandchildren at family gatherings, and coworkers at company social functions (Item 1).
- Hearing better is very important to him (Item 2); he is very motivated to use hearing aids (Item 3); and he expects that they will greatly improve his hearing (Item 4).
- Rates hearing aid size as the most important consideration followed by cost, understanding in background noise, and improved ability to hear speech (Item 5).
- Prefers hearing aids that are automatic (Item 6).
- Is unwilling to use any style of hearing aids except CICs (Item 7).
- Indicates high level of confidence for successful hearing aid use (Item 8).
- Did not complete the cost item (Item 9).

Combining all factors (age, hearing loss, responses on the COAT), a mini-BTE would be recommended with open ear fitting. He is initially uncomfortable with this recommendation because he is very concerned about cosmetics. The advantages and disadvantages of an open-ear fitting over the CIC are discussed, the excellent cosmetics of the open mini-BTE style are demonstrated on the ear, and he agrees to try them. The level of technology is discussed. He needs devices that have directional beamforming technology and noise-reduction processing that also addresses impulse sounds (dishes clinking) to provide him better speech recognition and more relaxed listening in restaurants and social events. This increases the level of technology needed and hence the device cost. He is not willing to commit to the higher recommended level of technology. Mid-Level devices are then chosen with the understanding that his hearing in background noise may be compromised to a certain degree and he may notice the clatter of dishes more in his restaurant. He understands that and wishes to proceed with the devices that fall within his budget.

Obtaining the COAT

The COAT is available for general use and the form can be downloaded from a link contained in the original 2006 COAT publication (http://www.audiologyonline.com/articles/article_detail.asp?article_id=1541).

In Closing

We have reviewed several different self-assessment scales, all of which measure somewhat different aspects regarding the potential use of hearing aids. We recognize that it is not feasible, or even necessary, to conduct all of them for a single patient; you will need to develop a battery that works the best for your situation, or different batteries for different patients. And how many scales really are enough? In part that depends on what we want to measure, how well we want to do it, and how much time we are willing to invest. The most important take-home point from this chapter is that there are many aspects of a patient's communication needs that cannot be predicted by routine audiometric measures. It is important to allow the patient to tell his or her story, and one effective way to do this is through the use of pre-fitting self-assessment scales.

8
Hearing Aid Styles and Fitting Applications

In the preceding chapters we have discussed the general attributes of the hearing aid candidate, the importance of speech information and how it interacts with the environment, several objective tests that we can use to assess the candidates' ability to process speech, and additional tests to refine our fitting. We have also reviewed the self-assessment scales that further define the patient's problems and listening needs, and also provide insight regarding the patient's handicap, motivation, and expectations. We are now ready to sit down with the patient and start making collaborative decisions. The first of these is selecting the best hearing aid style. Although the signal processing of the hearing aid is often of utmost concern, packaging this processing in an unacceptable style can lead to rejection of the amplification device.

Although the most obvious differences in hearing aid styles are cosmetic (size and shape), it is important to understand that style choices also can affect hearing aid acoustics, comfort, and ease of use. There are several benefits and limitations that are tied to hearing aid style that are unrelated to cosmetics. It often is the audiologist's job to strike a reasonable balance between *form* and *function*. We start by considering the look and physical characteristics of different hearing aids styles. Then, we continue by discussing bilateral versus unilateral fittings, and reviewing fittings aimed at specific special populations and applications.

Despite differences in style, hearing aids share several commonalities. At their most basic levels, all hearing aids include three stages that can be generally described as follows:

- The sound pick-up stage usually consists of a microphone or telecoil.
- The sound processing and amplification stage is where the bulk of the signal processing work is done to change the signal into the desired level and form.
- The sound delivery stage is primarily made up of a tiny loudspeaker (along with supporting processing) referred to as a receiver. Instead of a receiver, the output stage may include a vibrating oscillator that stimulates the cochlea through bone conduction or a variety of other specialized transducers, including those associated with middle ear implants.

Although there may be multiple goals, which we detail in Chapter 10, the primary function of the electronic components and sound processing is to work together to increase the amplitude in a frequency-specific manner. The frequency-specific increase in sound level for a signal at the output of a hearing aid, in comparison with the sound level at the input, is referred to as *gain*. Gain is really just the opposite of attenuation (a decrease in frequency-specific level, commonly expressed in dB). In fact, gain can be thought of as negative attenuation, whereas attenuation can be thought of as negative gain. This is an important concept to understand because some styles of hearing aids seal into the ear canal very well and, although they provide positive gain for a wide range of frequencies, negative gain (attenuation) may also occur in some frequency regions—more on that later in this chapter.

Unilateral Versus Bilateral Amplification

At some point in the hearing aid selection process, a joint decision must be made between the clinician and the patient regarding whether one or two hearing aids will be fitted. This sometimes is dictated by the audiogram (hearing in one ear is either too good or too bad for hearing aid use), but the majority of patients (i.e., 85 to 90%) are at least potential candidates for bilateral amplification. Although the intuitive notion that two ears are better than one is usually true, not all patients benefit from bilateral amplification, and not all patients who do benefit want to wear two hearing aids.

It might be surprising to some of you that bilateral fittings have not always been embraced by audiologists. As recent as the early 1970s, it was common for audiologists to tell patients that a single hearing aid was adequate and in some cases, when the patient returned from a dispenser (hearing instrument specialist) wearing two hearing aids, the audiologist accused the dispenser of simply trying to double the profit. Contributing to the *unilateral-is-okay* belief was a 1975 ruling by the Federal Trade Commission regarding the hearing aid industry that stated:

> No seller shall prepare, approve, fund, disseminate, or cause the dissemination of any advertisement which makes any representation that the use of two hearing aids, one in each ear, will be beneficial to persons with a hearing loss in both ears, unless it is clearly and conspicuously disclosed that many persons with a hearing loss in both ears will not receive greater benefits from the use of two aids, one in each ear, than the use of one hearing aid.

The importance for children to be fitted bilaterally, however, was beginning to be widely accepted about this time, and the general understanding of bilateral fittings then gradually transferred to adults. This move to consider bilateral the *routine* fitting probably was also fueled by the large number of audiologists who began direct dispensing in the late 1970s (see Chapter 2 for details). It was not until the 1990s, however, that the majority of people in the United States were fitted bilaterally. Current estimates are that about 80% of the U.S. fittings are bilateral (slightly less for first-time users), and about 90% of those with bilateral hearing loss are fitted bilaterally. This of course does not mean that they are *using* two hearing aids—or even using one hearing aid.

Potential Advantages of Bilateral Amplification

There are several benefits of *binaural hearing* and many of these benefits will be experienced with *bilateral fittings*. These benefits are assuming that you have selected an individual who is a reasonable bilateral candidate from an audiometric standpoint. That is, there must be

> **KEY CONCEPT: BILATERAL VERSUS BINAURAL**
>
> You may have noticed that in our discussion here and in other chapters that both the words bilateral and binaural have been used in reference to hearing with two ears. There is an important difference, however, between these two terms. When we refer to the auditory system, we use the terms binaural hearing and monaural hearing. The concepts of binaural hearing and the related advantages are mostly based on research with normal hearing individuals. When we are talking about hearing aids, we use the terms bilateral fittings and unilateral fittings. For example, if you presented the same speech signal to both ears (referred to as a diotic presentation), your patient would have *bilateral* processing but not the same phase and amplitude differences observed in *binaural* processing. In general, you can presume a *bilateral fitting* improves *binaural hearing*, but this is not always the case, which is why we have this differentiation.

aidable hearing in both ears, adequate speech recognition and central processing ability, and not too much asymmetry. How much is too much asymmetry? A rule of thumb is that we would like to have the *aided* speech signals within 15 dB of each other (see our "Technical Tip" on this topic). We would expect the greatest bilateral benefit when the amplified signals are relatively equal. With that in mind, we review the primary bilateral benefits here. It is important to have a basic understanding of each of the advantages because in many cases you will want to explain them to your patients and provide real-world examples. Some audiologists even use take-home handouts.

Elimination of the Head-Shadow Effect

High-frequency sounds arriving from one side of the head are attenuated by 10 to 15 dB for reception in the opposite ear. In the case of a unilateral fitting, patients may then still lack important audibility if they are not able to turn their head to face the talker when the origin is from their unaided ear. This is illustrated nicely in Figure 8–1, which shows the attenuation effects for different key frequencies as a function of the presentation angle. Assuming a relatively symmetrical hearing loss,

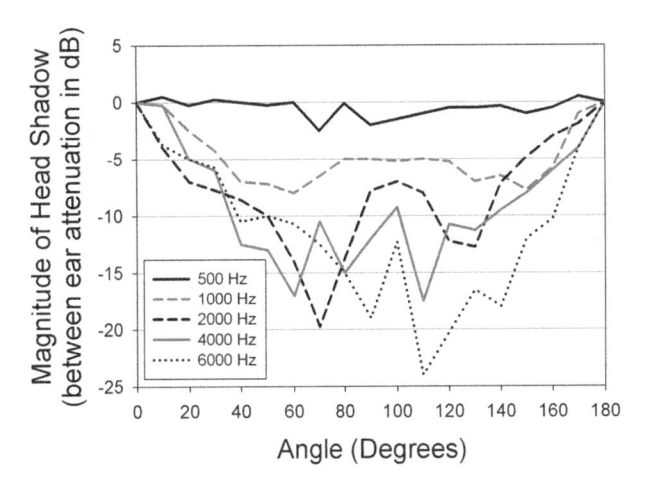

Figure 8–1. Effects of head shadow as a function of frequency. Attenuation shown for signals presented from 0 to 180 degrees.

**KEY CONCEPT:
HEARING AID VERSUS HEARING AIDS (WITH AN "S")**

As we discuss in this section, there indeed are some patients with a bilateral hearing loss where a single hearing aid is the best solution. The majority of patients, however, are best served with a bilateral fitting. Many of these patients will come to you with the belief that they need only one hearing aid. Following a diagnostic procedure, it is not uncommon for a patient to ask: "So do you think I need a hearing aid?" Only rarely does a patient ask: "Do you think I need a pair of hearing aids?" Why is this? Perhaps they have a friend who only uses one. Perhaps they have a mild loss and think two hearing aids are only for people with severe loss. Maybe it is simply wishful thinking (one hearing aid is less hassle, less money, etc.). We have found, however, that a common reason is that the patient has been told at one time or other that they only need a single hearing aid. Maybe not directly, but they have heard the word *aid* used in the singular rather than the plural form. For example, the family physician may have said, "Your hearing is getting worse; I think you probably need a hearing *aid*." Or the clinic receptionist may have said, "We have you scheduled for a hearing *aid* evaluation." For some individuals, when they arrive at their appointment and hear that two hearing aids are recommended when they were expecting to be fitted with only one, this new concept requires some time to digest (see the review of effective pre-fitting counseling in Chapter 3). So what is our point? As with most things that come in pairs (e.g., eyeglasses, shoes, chopsticks, and turtle doves), using the plural term *hearing aids* or *pair of hearing aids* early on in your discussions with patients might reduce the need for extended counseling down the road.

a bilateral fitting will eliminate the head-shadow effect. This will have an impact on speech understanding, as the patient no longer has a bad side.

Loudness Summation

This refers to the auditory system's ability to integrate and fuse sounds from each ear. That is, the sound level has to be reduced to produce the same loudness when listening with two ears in comparison to listening with one. Much of the research on this topic has been conducted with people with normal hearing, but the results for individuals with cochlear hearing loss appear to be similar. In general, summation effects become greater as a function of the degree that the signal occurs above the person's threshold. At threshold, summation effects are 2 to 3 dB, but summation may be 6 to 8 dB, or even higher at suprathreshold levels (depending on symmetry, individual variances, listening paradigm, and input level). If the expected practical advantage for the hearing aid user is that less amplifier gain is needed to reach the preferred loudness level, then the hearing aids are less prone to feedback. If lower gain levels are used, there also would be less likelihood of loud sounds exceeding the patient's LDL. And, for some patients with severe hearing loss, the extra loudness might be the only way to achieve the desired overall loudness level.

Improved Auditory Localization

We discuss auditory localization later in this chapter. In brief, localization requires the comparison of phase and amplitude differences between the two ears to determine the location of a sound. Research has clearly shown that this is accomplished more effectively in a bilateral fitting than in a unilateral one (see Simon, 2005, for review). In fact, a person with a mild-moderate symmetrical hearing loss could have worse localization after being *aided unilaterally* than when he or she was unaided, especially when first fitted. There is evidence to show that it is possible that patients fitted bilaterally may have localization ability rivaling that of those with normal hearing (Drennan, Gatehouse, Howell, Van Tasell, & Lund, 2005).

Improved Speech Understanding in Noise

Bilateral amplification and binaural processing allows for an improvement in speech understanding in background noise. We expect this advantage to be a 2 to 3 dB improvement in the SNR. There are two factors that account for this:

- Binaural redundancy: There is an advantage to hearing the same signal in both ears. The brain essentially has two chances of extracting the correct information, as illustrated by the *diotic* condition in Figure 8–2. For high input levels, this bilateral advantage may not be present, as the signal might be heard in the unaided ear for a unilateral fitting.
- Binaural squelch: Through central auditory processing, the brain can compare two individual speech-in-noise signals, and the result will be a fused signal with a better SNR than either of the two. As pointed out by Dillon (2001), the squelch effect will already be present if the low-frequency components of both the speech and noise are above thresholds in both ears for a unilateral fitting.

Although there has been a general belief for the past 30 years or more that bilateral amplification is superior to unilateral for understanding speech in background noise, there has not been much study of this topic recently. An exception is the publication of McArdle, Killion, Mennite, and Chilsolm (2012). These find-

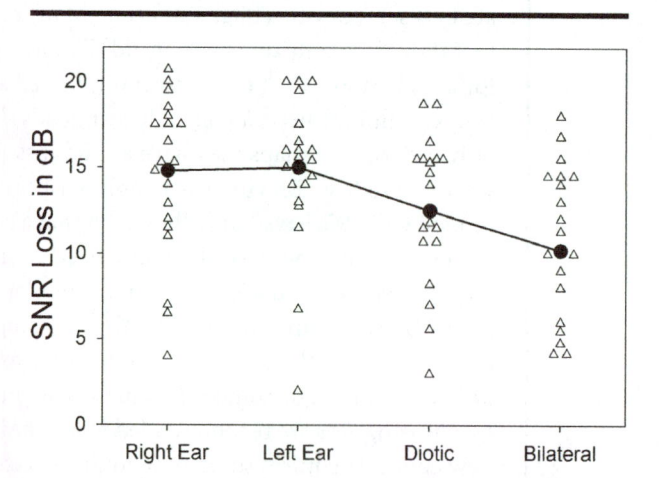

Figure 8–2. Average performance (SNR loss) for four different conditions: right ear, left ear, diotic (same signal to both ears), and bilateral (separately recorded signal to each ear). (Adapted from McArdle et al., 2012).

ing are summarized in Figure 8–2. This figure shows speech recognition in background noise (uncorrelated) for a group of hearing impaired listeners. The signal was recorded from the Knowles Electronics Manikin for Acoustic Research (KEMAR) and played to the subjects via earphones. Both the redundancy and squelch effects are apparent. Note that for the diotic presentation (signal recorded from a single ear but presented to both ears), there is an approximate 2 dB advantage, compared with either the right or left ear. We expect this advantage due to redundancy. When the subjects listened to the speech and noise signals that were recorded bilaterally (reflecting phase and amplitude differences), and these two different recordings were played to the two different ears, another 2 dB improvement was observed, for a combined 4 dB advantage when compared with the independent performance of the right or left ears. (Note that the measure is SNR loss, so lower numbers indicate an SNR improvement.)

Improved Sound Quality and Better Spatial Balance

If you have ever compared one versus two earphones while listening to your iPod, we do not have to tell you that bilateral listening provides better sound qual-

---

SOAPBOX: CLINICAL SPEECH MEASURES FOR BILATERAL FITTINGS

Some audiologists conduct earphone bilateral speech testing following the standard unilateral testing to determine if the patient will benefit from two hearing aids. Clinicians also are sometimes tempted to conduct aided speech testing in the clinic to demonstrate to the patient why two hearing aids are better than one. There are several reasons why we do not recommend these practices:

- We would only expect to see the bilateral advantage when noise is present and the listening task is difficult. For an earphone test such as monosyllables in quiet, we would expect the outcome to be no better than that of the best ear, taking into consideration the Thornton-Raffin critical differences (see Table 6–2), unless PB-Max was not correctly obtained during the initial unilateral testing.
- Regarding aided testing, we would only expect the bilateral benefit to be obtained if the person was in a distributed noise field and the noise was uncorrelated (e.g., a typical real-world environment). Most clinics do not have the sound field loudspeaker arrangement or recorded speech and noise material to conduct this type of testing.
- The aided bilateral benefit we are observing is small, and may be smaller than the test-retest and critical differences of the speech material used (again, see the critical differences discussed in Chapter 6).
- The speech-in-noise advantage only will be noticeable with clinical speech testing when an SNR improvement of 3 dB has an impact on a given patient's speech recognition—that is, when testing is conducted around his or her 50% intelligibility point. If the clinical test condition is too difficult or too easy (and this will vary from patient-to-patient), the benefit will not be observed. A variable or adaptive SNR test as described in Chapter 6 is required.
- Even though a substantial portion of patients may choose unilateral amplification after a bilateral trial, it does not appear that clinical tools are sensitive enough to predict which individuals these will be. Moreover, the decision to use only one hearing aid often is related to factors other than speech recognition.

ity than unilateral. There is sense of fullness, and the sound seems in your head rather than at the ear. This also applies to the hearing impaired and hearing aids, and has been substantiated by research (e.g., Balfour & Hawkins, 1992).

It is difficult to measure *spatial balance* in the clinic, but what we mean by this is the general sense of being in sync with your surroundings. We frequently hear from bilateral hearing aid users who had to be without one hearing aid because of a repair issue that they felt *unbalanced* by only wearing one hearing aid. Cox, Schwartz, Noe, and Alexander (2011) report that when individuals compared wearing two versus one hearing aid in the real world, *balance* was the leading reason for preferring the bilateral fitting.

Avoidance of the Unaided Ear Effect

We recall hearing stories from the 1970s of unscrupulous hearing aid dealers telling potential customers that they needed to buy two hearing aids because, if they only used one, the other ear would become lazy and their hearing in that ear would get worse. Once viewed as merely a sales tactic, science now tells us that there was some truth to what these salesmen were saying. An article published by Silman, Gelfand, and Silverman (1984) garnered attention when these authors reported that a sizeable percentage of people, who once had a symmetrical hearing loss and word recognition scores, suffered a reduction in word recognition in the unaided ear after being aided unilaterally for several years (with no significant change in pure-tone thresholds). In a retrospective study, Hurley (1999) reported that this effect was present for about 25% of unilateral hearing aid users.

This often has been referred to as auditory deprivation or late onset auditory deprivation, although we prefer the term *unaided ear effect*. The reason for the use of this term is that it does not seem to happen unless the opposite ear is aided. Specifically, people with a bilateral hearing loss who are not fitted with a hearing aid do not experience *deprivation*, even though their hearing loss is the same as the unaided ear of the people who were fitted unilaterally. Why is this? Part of it indeed may be due to deprivation. When people start wearing a hearing aid on one ear, their world generally becomes softer

---

TECHNICAL TIP: THE UNAIDED EAR EFFECT (AUDITORY DEPRIVATION)

The unaided ear effect is an intriguing topic that is still in need of considerable research. Much of what we know is from retrospective reports or illustrative cases, not controlled studies. Here is a brief summary, however, of what we believe to be true:

- The unaided ear effect will occur in about one-quarter to one-third of the people with symmetrical hearing loss fitted unilaterally.
- A significant effect (decrease in word recognition) may be noticed as soon as within one year or may occur more gradually over three to five years. (Is this possibly related to daily hearing aid use? Amount of daily communication? Degree of hearing loss in unaided ear?).
- At some point, the effect seems to plateau and no further reduction in speech recognition occurs.
- When the unaided ear is fitted with amplification after the effect has occurred, recovery in word recognition occurs for some individuals but not others—possibly related to the age of the patient (brain plasticity) and/or duration of the effect.
- This effect is also commonly observed in cochlear implant users; however, the negative effects appear to be even larger, suggesting those with greater hearing loss are likely more susceptible to the effect.

(people do not have to talk to them as loud, the TV is softer, etc.). Hence, there probably is less audibility for the unaided ear than if they were not wearing a hearing aid. But also, the use of amplification in one ear leads to a mismatch centrally, with the aided ear having the stronger signal. Over time, the brain may become more dominant for the stronger signal and pays less attention to the signal from the weaker ear. Recall that we talked about a similar effect in Chapter 5 regarding loudness discomfort measures. Regardless of the cause, the effect rarely occurs in bilateral fittings (Hurley, 1999), which is why this is often considered a compelling reason to use two hearing aids.

Potential Contraindications for Bilateral Amplification

Although there certainly are many reasons to think of the routine fitting as bilateral, there also are some reasons why a unilateral fitting might be the best choice. We have listed the most common.

Degree of Hearing Loss

Simply put, to be a candidate for bilateral hearing aid amplification, the hearing for each ear cannot be too good or too bad. Regarding minimal hearing loss, there

---

TECHNICAL TIP: COMMON FITTING DILEMMA

Regarding bilateral fittings, a common dilemma is when a patient has one ear with a 30 to 40 dB loss (PB-Max around 85 to 90%), and the other ear has a loss of 60 to 70 dB (PB-Max around 50 to 60%). You could decide to give up on the poorer ear and give the patient one close-to-normal ear by fitting only the better ear. Or, you could decide to give the patient pretty good symmetry and fit only the bad ear. Or, you could fit the patient bilaterally. Our default choice would be a bilateral fitting for a couple of reasons. First, the patient probably thinks that the good ear is normal. If you only aid the better ear, the patient will always wonder why you did not aid the ear with the hearing loss. Given that the good ear has a 30 to 40 dB hearing loss, if only the bad ear is aided the patient would still be lacking audibility for soft speech; it would be tough to achieve enough gain to make soft speech audible in the bad ear—which then leaves us with a bilateral fitting.

Although this patient probably will not experience all of the desired binaural benefits, we would expect improved localization simply because many sounds are now audible in the poorer ear. It is true that the decision would be easier if word recognition were better for the poorer ear. But we do know that, in general, patients will achieve an aided bilateral word recognition score equal to the better ear. In other words, you do not have to be concerned that amplification of the poorer ear will *pull down* overall speech understanding (unless this patient falls into the 5 to 10% of people with binaural interference). In fact, the brain might be able to use loudness from the poorer ear, combined with speech clarity from the better ear, to provide the patient with overall benefit, especially when people are talking from the bad side and the patient cannot turn his or her head (such as while driving or riding in a car). And also you might find that, when aided, the word recognition score for the poorer ear is better than what you obtained with earphones.

Another alternative we have not mentioned is a BiCROS, which we discuss in a later section. But for a patient like this, we would always try a bilateral fitting first. We would put our chances of success at fifty-fifty or better, which makes it worth the effort. The success will depend somewhat on the resulting aided symmetry for speech. If the aided asymmetry is too great, the patient will simply perceive all sounds in the good ear and consider the hearing aid in the poorer ear a useless nuisance.

are no rules regarding how much hearing loss is necessary to justify hearing aid use—we would expect, however, that the patient would have some hearing loss (>20–30 dB) in the speech range. It is relatively common today to fit hearing aids to someone with normal hearing through 2000 Hz if he or she is experiencing communication difficulty. Individuals with open fittings and normal low frequency hearing may be able to use unaided audible low frequencies to provide adequate localization, binaural squelch, and binaural redundancy, even when fitted unilaterally. Consequently, their remaining bilateral benefit will be more limited and mostly related to head shadow and a sense of balance for high-frequency sounds. Conversely, one of the causes for rejection of bilateral amplification, increased occlusion effect, will not be present in the open fittings so many of these patients will still be excellent candidates for bilateral amplification (see the section on open fittings later in this chapter for more details).

Regarding severe hearing losses in cases with a large asymmetry between the ears, sophisticated feedback reduction systems allow us to provide more feedback-free gain than ever before, and with smaller instruments. This allows us to fit the poorer ear in the vast majority of cases. The optimal intervention, however, for this population keep changing as advancements occur with cochlear implants and hybrid fittings.

Cost

Hearing aids are expensive. The patient's income level affects hearing aid adoption in general and also influences the purchase of one versus two hearing aids. In many clinics, the cost of two entry level products is about the same as one premier product. Given that the standard features on most entry-level products are quite satisfactory, if the patient only has a fixed amount of funds, we would recommend two lower priced instruments rather than one super instrument. But, even two entry-level hearing aids might be more than some people can afford.

Convenience

Some patients have considerable trouble putting the hearing aids in and taking them out, changing batteries, and making adjustments. Some consider the wearing of a hearing aid uncomfortable or annoying. A bilateral fitting doubles the problems. Wireless connectivity helps somewhat with this—a single button adjusts the volume or changes programs on both instruments. Remote controls and rechargeable batteries also can be helpful. But the patient will still have the other issues of dealing with two instruments.

Binaural Interference

There is a small portion of the population (approximately 5 to 10%) who have a *reduction* in speech recognition when they experience bilateral amplification. Believed to be due to a central auditory processing deficit, this is referred to as binaural interference. This would not necessarily be a contradiction for a bilateral fitting, however; the patient simply would only use one hearing aid when listening in background noise or competing signals. We would expect this person to obtain all the other benefits of bilateral amplification for other listening environments; the average user spends the majority of their time in situations without significant background noise. However, appropriate counselling needs to be provided and the potential limitations should be discussed with the patient so an appropriate decision to keep one or both hearing aids can be made during the trial period.

Perceived Benefit

Earlier, we described several real and potential benefits of bilateral amplification. One might think, therefore, that if we selected people with symmetric hearing losses, who audiometrically were candidates, who were able to easily handle two hearing aids, and allowed them to experience using one versus two hearing aids in the real world, there would be a large preference for bilateral amplification. However, it is simply not true. Cox et al. (2011) reported that after three months of real-world use of bilateral versus unilateral amplification, only 54% ($n = 94$) of individuals selected bilateral amplification. The research included assessing potential predictors of bilateral versus unilateral preference such as demographic, audiometric, auditory lifestyle, personality, and binaural processing variables. The authors concluded, however, that at this time, there is no accurate method that will predict which patients will prefer one hearing aid rather than two. Because preference cannot be predicted and hearing aid returns are possible, many clini-

> **TECHNICAL TIP: SCREENING FOR BINAURAL INTERFERENCE**
>
> As we mentioned, research suggests that as many as 10% or so of patients may have binaural interference when using two hearing aids. This is not something that likely would be detected prior to the fitting, as it often is not reflected in the pure-tone audiogram or routine speech recognition testing. As we discussed in Chapter 6, possible screening tests for binaural interference are the DSI and the dichotic digits. It seems reasonable to expect that significant ear asymmetry observed with these earphone dichotic tests also could influence a bilateral hearing aid fitting. Unfortunately, these are not tests conducted routinely in the hearing aid fitting process. Nevertheless, this would be something that could be implemented in post-fitting visits when a patient has an otherwise unexplained negative experience understanding speech in background noise when using two hearing aids. We also described in Chapter 6 the use of sound field presentation of speech recognition measures such as the Quick-SIN or BKB-SIN as a method to screen for binaural interference at the selection appointment. The measures can also be used to measure the presence of binaural interference after the fitting by comparing unilateral and bilateral performance.

cians will select bilateral amplification as the default and then return one of the instruments if the patient indicates unilateral amplification is preferred. Appropriate counseling at the time of the fitting and during the first few weeks of hearing aid use is also necessary to help ensure every patient ends up with the optimal fitting (i.e., unilateral or bilateral).

Two Important Factors Influencing Hearing Aid Style Selection

Several style related factors affect hearing aid acoustics including position of the microphone, position of the receiver, separation of the receiver and microphone, type of coupling to the ear, and so forth. Two considerations, however, that cut across all hearing styles are acoustic feedback and the occlusion effect. Before reviewing specific styles, we review some of the problems associated with feedback and the occlusion effect, and offer a few solutions.

Acoustic Feedback

Acoustic feedback occurs when amplified sound from the receiver finds a pathway back to the microphone and is re-amplified by the hearing aid repetitively in a feedback loop. The transfer function measured when comparing the sound input with the sound output is referred to as the *closed loop* response. It is differentiated from an *open loop* response that is measured when the receiver and microphone are acoustically isolated from each other. With typical hearing aid fittings, acoustic feedback is almost always present; however, the level is usually not high enough to result in the oscillation that produces *audible* feedback. That is, acoustic feedback is not a problem if the amount the signal level is reduced (attenuated) when it travels the feedback pathway (from the receiver to the microphone) is greater than the amount of amplification provided by the hearing aid. Instead, feedback will become a problem when the output of the receiver that reaches the microphone exceeds the original input level, as we describe in more detail soon. It is important to note that a feedback loop can occur regardless of the level of the original sound in the environment (even ambient noise). For many hearing aid fittings, the microphone is somewhat isolated from the receiver, providing attenuation to this looped signal that helps to reduce the likelihood of feedback.

In many fittings, including the common open fittings described later in this chapter, the feedback path does not provide enough attenuation to offset the hearing aid gain, and there is the potential for the signal to become larger (amplified) on every loop. This amplification will only occur, however, if the re-amplified sound adds in phase with the original sound. That is, for the signals to add in phase the duration of the entire loop must be equal to, or an integer multiple of, the period of the signal. If this *in-phase* addition occurs, it can generate an audible oscillation commonly described by the patient as squealing, howling, or whistling. A hearing aid will generate audible feedback at any frequency that has a period that is an integer multiple of the travel time required for sound to travel the entire feedback and gain loop (the duration of the closed loop response) if hearing aid gain amplification is greater than the feedback loop attenuation (unity gain exceeds 0 dB). In Figures 8–3 and 8–4, we walk you through two examples of how acoustic feedback might occur. Although in both cases, the input signal is the same, note that in Figure 8–3, we have more amplifier gain and less attenuation, and as a result, we have feedback.

Critical Gain Measures

In the past few years, it has become common practice for audiologists to conduct *open loop gain* or *critical gain* measures with the hearing aid fitted to their patient. It

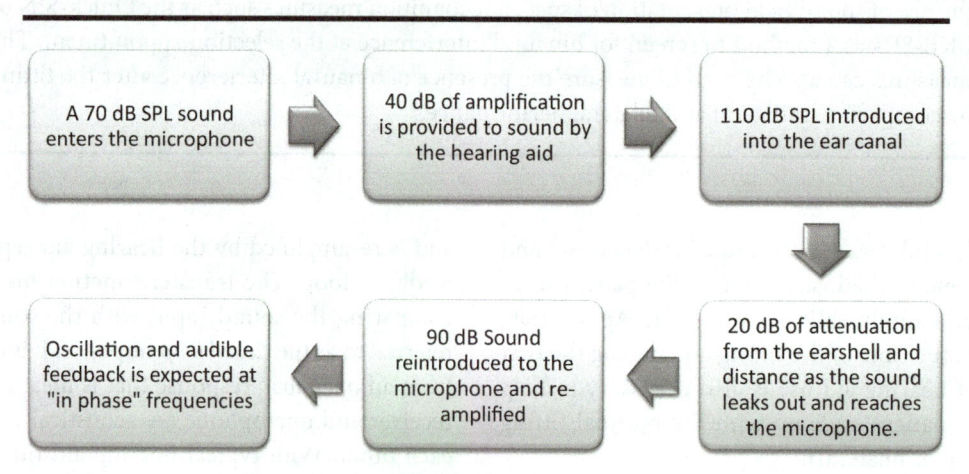

Figure 8–3. Simplified schematic of a possible feedback path with arbitrary numbers. The exact amount of gain in each case will depend on the hearing aid, and the exact amount of attenuation of the feedback loop will depend on the specific earshell and venting used.

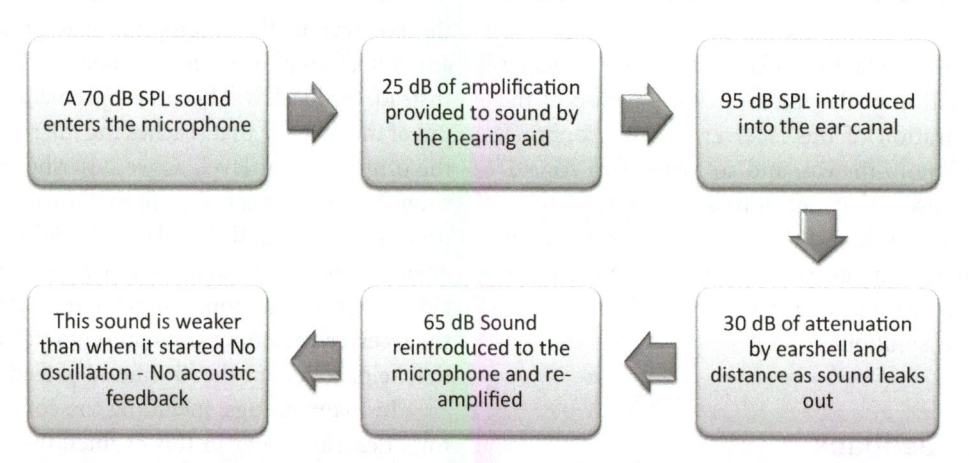

Figure 8–4. Schematic example of a hearing aid for which attenuation of sound traveling the feedback loop is attenuated through distance and limited venting, so that audible feedback does not occur.

is called *open loop* because the hearing aid signal processing path is split between microphone and receiver during this measurement, instead of sending the signals picked up at the microphone to the receiver as during typical operation. This measure provides a good estimate if feedback is probable, and changes to hearing aid gain can be made if the audiologist believes that the risk of feedback is too great (or the fitting software will make these changes automatically if that choice is selected). Basically, this measurement is the attenuation between the ear canal SPL and the microphone, and is an estimate of maximum stable gain. For example, if a tone was generated by the hearing aid with a known output of 80 dB SPL, and the microphone picks up the tone via the feedback path and it is measured to be 20 dB SPL, then we would predict that the stable gain would be 60 dB at this frequency. This value, however, should not be interpreted as the maximum gain provided by the hearing aid that was used to conduct the measurement—that is a different measure.

Examples of real-ear open loop gain measurements are shown in Figure 8–5, Panel A and Panel B. These measures are from the same hearing aid with the same hearing aid settings but using two different types of coupling systems for a patient's real ear. Note in Panel A, when an open custom tip was used, the output of the hearing aid exceeds the stable gain reference by 10 dB in the 3500 Hz region. As expected, stable gain was the lowest for the frequency region where the output of the hearing aid was the highest. This is a clear indication that feedback will be present. Hearing aid fitting software can be set so that it will automatically reduce the output for this region and minimize the potential for feedback. This usually is not a wise choice, however, as the patient needs a certain amount of gain in this region for audibility of speech (usually these automatic approaches are overly aggressive). An alternative choice would be to use an earmold with a tighter fit, which will serve to increase the stable gain values. This is shown in Panel B. All parameters of the hearing aid were set the same, except in this case, a tighter fitting custom dome was used. Note that we now have the same output peak for the 3500 Hz region, but we are 5 dB below the stable gain values—a good probability we will *not* have feedback.

Feedback Problems and Solutions

Acoustic feedback is undesirable for a number of reasons as it has the potential to lead to loudness discomfort, annoyance, embarrassment, reduced sound quality, and it will limit available gain. Individuals who wear hearing aids that are prone to feedback often will use feedback as the determining factor in adjusting the volume—they will increase the gain until they hear feedback, then turn it down a little from this point. Unfortunately, in

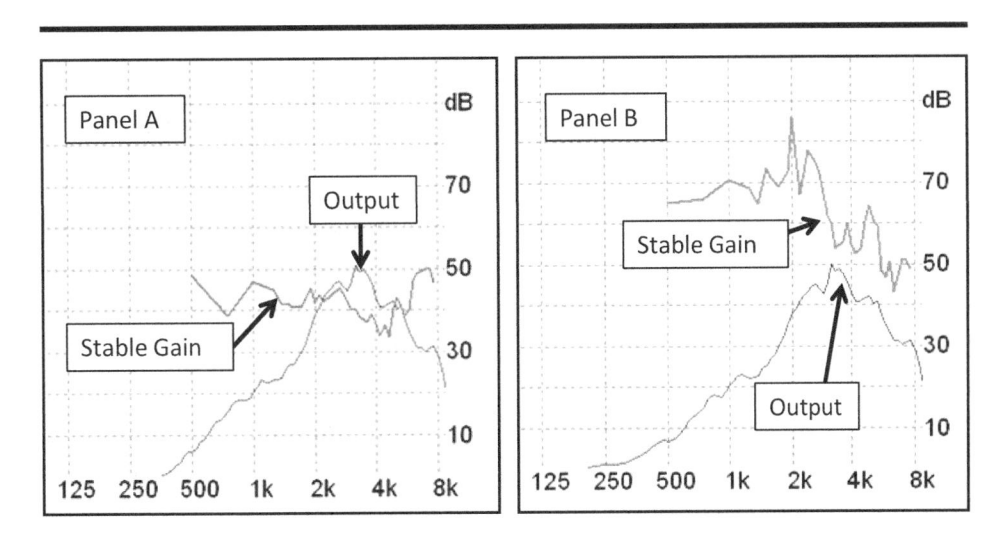

Figure 8–5. Example of open loop gain measured for the same hearing aid for an open fitting (*Panel A*) and a more closed fitting (*Panel B*). Note that the output remains similar, whereas the stable gain values change considerably.

a poorly fitted hearing aid, this setting may be less than what is needed for appropriate audibility for the patient.

In addition to the annoyance caused by audible feedback, acoustic feedback that is present at gain levels just below those resulting in oscillation (approximately 1 to 3 dB) can result in a *peaky* response (e.g., Cox, 1982). This is sometimes referred to as suboscillatory feedback. The peaky response occurs because suboscillatory feedback can cause both increases and decreases in the hearing aid output, depending on frequency. Addition will occur for in-phase frequencies (period = integer multiple of the travel time), and reduction will occur for frequencies that are exactly out of phase (period = one-half integer multiple of the travel time).

In addition to an acoustic feedback pathway, a mechanical feedback pathway is also present. That is, sound vibration from a receiver can travel through any number of mechanically linked pathways (through an earshell, up a wire and through plastic case, up tubing and through a plastic case, etc.) back to the hearing aid microphone. Although the mechanisms responsible for mechanical feedback are similar to those of acoustic feedback, other than the travel path, the solutions are different. Mechanical feedback must be accounted for in the manufacturing process by mechanically isolating the microphone from the receiver, using rubber and other vibration dampening materials to limit mechanical linkage.

To differentiate between acoustic and mechanical feedback, simply plug the microphone and/or receiver ports. If the feedback is still present, it is likely to be mechanical in nature. If not mechanical, this feedback is likely an *internal acoustic feedback* due to acoustic leakage within the case. In either situation, the solution requires a mechanical repair. Mechanical and internal acoustic feedback are not commonly observed in routine hearing aid fittings. When observed, it often is with very high gain instruments or with a hearing aid that has been damaged (e.g., dropped on a hard surface).

In contrast with solutions for mechanical and internal feedback, acoustic feedback can often be reduced by using simple clinical manipulations such as reducing leakage of the signal from the ear canal (caused by venting). All hearing aids or earmolds allow for at least a small amount of sound to leak out of the residual ear canal space (the sound that escapes around the borders of the hearing aid/earmold in the concha is referred to as *slit leak*). Venting simply refers to the *intentional* process of increasing the amount of this leakage, usually by creating an additional sound channel—see Chapter 9 for details.

Given the cause of feedback, it should not be surprising that the simplest ways to eliminate oscillation caused by acoustic feedback include reducing the hearing aid gain at the feedback frequencies or by further isolating the sound output from the receiver from sound input to the microphone (e.g., reduce venting or increasing the distance between the microphone and receiver). Both of these techniques are used in Figure 8–4. More attenuation by using a tighter earshell and greater micro-

---

THINGS TO REMEMBER: FEEDBACK AND STIGMA

We would like to expand a little on the embarrassment issue we mentioned related to feedback. Most hearing aid users do not want to draw attention to the fact that they wear hearing aids. A whistling hearing aid, especially in a quiet room, clearly works against this concept. Some patients simply then do not wear their hearing aids in these situations. This relates to the stigma issue that we discussed in Chapter 3. A driving factor related to the stigma is the common belief among average consumers that hearing aids do not work very well. A whistling hearing aid disturbing a church service confirms this belief, which then only adds to the stigma. Who among us would want to be that person known for spending thousands of dollars for something that does not work? As we explain in detail in Chapter 12, the advancement of sophisticated feedback reduction algorithms in recent years has helped us make significant strides in showing people that hearing aids really do work and can provide the desired amount of amplification without feedback.

> **TECHNICAL TIP: WHERE TO CHECK FOR FEEDBACK PROBLEMS**
>
> In our examples in Figures 8–3 and 8–4, for simplicity we used a hearing aid with linear gain. In clinical practice, however, we will nearly always be fitting hearing aids with wide dynamic range compression (WDRC). Consider that with a common WDRC fitting (e.g., 40 dB SPL kneepoint; 2:1 compression ratio), gain is reduced as input increases, to the point that at high inputs (e.g., 80 dB SPL or so) gain may only be 5 or 10 dB, and the output will be relatively similar to the input. The point where gain is the highest and feedback is the most probable is at the compression kneepoint (commonly an input of approximately 40 dB SPL). In other words, in relatively quiet environments. Why is this important for identifying potential feedback problems? Quite often, the hearing aid fitting is conducted in a room with a relatively high ambient noise level (caused by several computers running, heating and air conditioning, reverberant conditions, etc.). When the patient then goes home and uses the hearing aids in a quiet setting (e.g., his or her living room), feedback occurs. We suggest, therefore, that before you send the patient home with the hearing aids, you take them to a quiet place in your clinic or office (a test booth if necessary), sit quietly for a moment without talking, to ensure that feedback does not occur for this type of environment.

phone to receiver distance (30 dB instead of 20 dB) is a big reason. Also, gain was reduced from 40 dB to 25 dB. Reducing gain, however, could present a major problem if this patient actually requires more gain than 25 dB for this input level at this frequency and is being under fit.

Acoustic feedback can influence style selection; this most frequently happens when high levels of gain are needed. A person who desires a small hearing aid that fits totally in the ear canal (very short distance between microphone and receiver) might be served best by using a hearing aid where the microphone is above the ear (increasing the distance between the microphone and the receiver) so that the necessary feedback-free gain can be obtained. Selecting a hearing aid with a good feedback reduction system, of course, is also a big factor—yes, they do vary considerably among manufacturers.

The Occlusion Effect

Although we have described how decreasing venting can be a solution for reducing feedback, it can create a problem of its own related to the occlusion effect. Notice that we are using the term *occlusion effect*, not simply occlusion. You can have occlusion without the occlusion effect—more on that later. The occlusion effect may increase the level of sounds in the lower frequencies (e.g., 200 to 500 Hz) by up to 20 to 30 dB in the occluded ear canal when compared with the level in the open ear canal. The occlusion effect causes the hearing aid user to report, "My head sounds like it is in a barrel when I talk" or that their own voice sounds hollow or booming (see for review Mueller, 2003). In addition, this problem can make chewing food sound noisy or unpleasant. To experience this sensation yourself, simply tightly plug your ears and then speak, or better yet, chew a raw carrot or eat a few kettle-cooked potato chips.

Why the Occlusion Effect Happens

So what causes the occlusion effect? The process goes like this:

- When we talk, certain sounds, especially vowels, reach 120 to 130 dB SPL or more in the back of the throat.
- The high intensity sounds travel via the mandible (bone conduction) to the condyle, which is positioned adjacent to the ear canal.
- This bone-conducted signal then becomes an air-conducted signal by setting up vibrations (primarily low frequency) of the cartilaginous portion of the ear canal.

- In normal situations, this low-frequency energy escapes out the open ear canal and does not contribute significantly to our perception of our own voice.
- If the lateral portion of the ear canal is plugged with a hearing aid or earmold, this signal cannot escape, and the resulting trapped energy in the residual ear canal volume is reflected back to the eardrum and transmitted to the cochlea in the typical air-conducted manner.
- These sounds will then change the perception of our own voice and can also enhance sounds of chewing and even breathing.

Note that the occlusion effect process is not related to the signal going through the hearing aid. In fact, the occlusion effect will be the same whether the hearing aid is turned on or off. This is important to remember if you are ever tempted to treat the occlusion effect by turning down low-frequency gain (yes, people actually do this!). If turning down low-frequency gain solves the problem of the patient's voice sounding funny, then the problem was not the occlusion effect. The problem was too much low-frequency gain.

Magnitude of the Occlusion Effect

Prior to the common use of probe microphone measures, it was necessary to rely on the patient to describe the magnitude of the occlusion effect and inform us if our treatment strategies were working. Since the 1980s, however, we have used probe microphone measures to provide an objective measure (see Mueller, Ricketts and Bentler [2017] and Chapter 17 for a complete review). Because the effect is directly related to the energy contained in the residual ear canal cavity, it can be measured precisely by placing a probe microphone at this location.

There seems to be a general belief among clinicians that males have more occlusion effect problems than females; perhaps this simply is because their voices tend to be more booming to begin with. To examine this and to obtain general objective data regarding the average occlusion effect, Mueller, Bright, and Northern (1996) compared the occlusion effect for males and females. The subjects were fitted with custom, full-concha ITE instruments that were not vented but were somewhat loose fitting. The mean occlusion effect measured for this group is shown in Figure 8–6 (the bars represent the *range*). As shown, the greatest average effect was at 500 Hz (approximately 17 dB), although a substantial amount of occlusion also was present at the other key frequencies. Observe that, except for 125 Hz, the average occlusion effects were essentially the same for males and females. Most notable is the large range for all frequencies for both genders (see bars in Figure 8–6). The authors comment that although some individuals had 0 dB of occlusion effect at some frequencies, all subjects had at least 8 dB of occlusion effect for one key frequency. It could be that the perception that men have more problems with the occlusion effect is related to the fact that male hearing aid users are more apt to have normal hearing in the lows (e.g., a high-frequency, noise-induced loss). Although the true magnitude of the male occlusion effect may be the same as for females, it is therefore more bothersome for this population.

In the Mueller et al. (1996) research, the occlusion effect was measured by having the patient vocalize the /ee/ sound. This is a common approach in both research and clinical practice. This is because the effect is greatest for the vowel sounds /ee/ and /eye/, and not very significant at all for /ah/. This contributes to why the effect can be annoying, as not only is there the increased

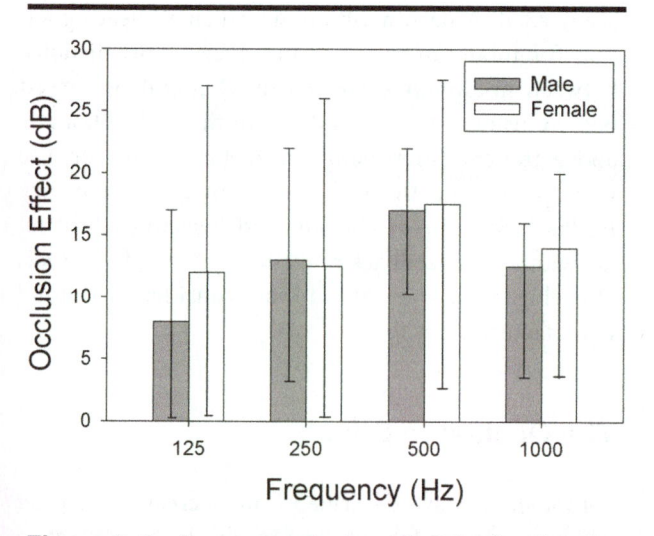

Figure 8–6. Average occlusion effect for four key frequencies comparing gender differences. Individuals were fitted with closed custom instruments. Vertical lines within each bar represent the range for that frequency. (Adapted from Mueller et al., 1996).

> **POINTS TO PONDER: AMPCLUSION—WHAT IS IT?**
>
> You might have seen the term *ampclusion* used in articles about the hearing aid occlusion effect. And unfortunately, the term has led to some misunderstanding regarding the treatment of the occlusion effect. The term was coined by Steve Painton in a 1993 article. According to Painton (1993, p. 152), ampclusion is "the combination of occlusion and low-frequency amplification that results in the 'hollowness' or 'head in the barrel' complaints." So, if we are understanding this correctly, if you know that the patient's problem is caused by the occlusion effect, then the patient *would not* have ampclusion, as there is no combined effect.
>
> We do not use the term ampclusion because usually the combined effects are not the major clinical issue. First, consider that, if the occlusion effect and the hearing aid output were at the same frequency range and the same intensity, the combined effect would be no more than 3 dB (and that is only if the two signals were equal). True, it is possible that there could be an occlusion effect problem at 200 Hz and too much gain at 500 Hz, but usually the problem is one or the other. For effective treatment and management, you really need to determine which of the two factors is the prime contributor to the problem.

emphasis of the low frequencies, but it only occurs for certain vowels. In Chapter 17, we show examples of the occlusion effect measured in the ear canal.

Identifying and Treating the Occlusion Effect

As we mentioned, it is important to differentiate between the true occlusion effect and too much low-frequency gain from the hearing aid. The easiest way to make this differentiation is to conduct probe microphone measures of the patient's vocalizations with the hearing aid turned off. Most probe microphone systems allow you to listen in, and you also will be able to hear the patient's occlusion effect yourself. If you do not have probe microphone capabilities or are pressed for time, a quick check to allow you to differentiate is to have the patient read a passage with the hearing aid turned on versus off. If the problem is amplifier gain, the "hollow voice" perception will go away when you turn the hearing aid off. If it is the occlusion effect, the voice will still sound hollow. You can use most any passage, but it helps if there are a lot of /ee/ sounds. If you want to make it a bit fun, have your patient read this passage:

"Through three cheese trees three free fleas flew."

The easiest way to alleviate the occlusion effect is to vent the space between the hearing aid/earmold/tubing tip and the eardrum. Of course, larger vents increase susceptibility to feedback. It is often a compromise. In addition, venting has little or no effect on occlusion occurring in the 500 to 750 Hz frequency region and above, unless very large vents (3 to 4 mm or greater) are used—see the effects of venting described in Chapter 9. Fortunately, a large occlusion effect in this higher frequency range is somewhat rare. The frequency-specific probe microphone evaluation of the occlusion effect will give you a quick indication of how easy it will be to reduce the output by venting—a 250 Hz or below effect can be treated fairly easily.

Open canal (OC) fittings have become popular in recent years and, although this is not venting as we traditionally know it, it is equivalent acoustically to a very large vent. And indeed, this fitting approach is very successful in reducing and, in many cases, eliminating the occlusion effect. The occlusion data from MacKenzie (2006) are shown in Figure 8–7. He compared an occluding earmold with four different sizes of vents and a totally open fitting (the open fitting data is from the mean of the open domes of three different manufacturers). Note that the occlusion effect for the closed earmolds was similar to the data shown in Figure 8–6 from Mueller et al. (1996). Also, observe that, as the vent was made bigger, the degree of occlusion decreased, especially for 250 Hz (low frequencies are most affected by venting—see Chapter 9). The effects for the open fittings,

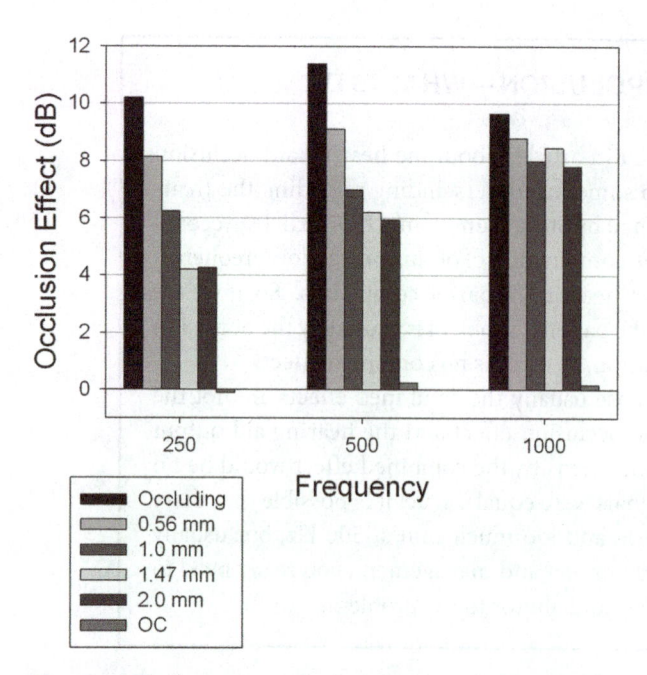

Figure 8–7. Average occlusion effect at key frequencies as a function of the tightness of the earmold plumbing. Most notable is the absence of the occlusion effect when open-fit stock eartips are used. (Adapted from MacKenzie, 2006).

however, are quite dramatic. There was essentially no occlusion effect present.

A second method for alleviating the occlusion effect is to fit the hearing aid or earmold tightly and deeply in the ear canal (down to the bony portion), very close to the eardrum (Killion, Wilber, & Gudmundsen, 1988; Mueller & Ebinger, 1996). This method decreases the magnitude of the occlusion effect by increasing impedance at the tympanic membrane, increasing the resonant frequency of the residual ear canal space and reducing how well the ear canal wall can vibrate. Although laboratory studies have shown that this method is effective, unfortunately it is uncomfortable for a large percentage of patients. Moreover, with some products, a deep earmold impression is required, which some audiologists shy away from. There continue to be new solutions for deep fittings proposed using different types of shell material, earmolds, or extended tips. None of the methods proposed prior to the time of this writing really have a proven track record of success.

We have already told you that reducing low-frequency gain is not a solution for the occlusion effect, but we mention it again, as it seems to be the most common treatment used. Part of the problem is that this notion is promulgated by the fitting software of several manufacturers—some even have a portion of the fitting software labeled "Occlusion Manger," which does nothing more than reduce low-frequency gain. As we said before, if turning down gain solves the problem, the problem probably was not the occlusion effect.

An interesting twist, however, in the treatment of the occlusion effect is to *add* low-frequency gain, rather than reduce it. This does not reduce the occlusion effect per se (it will still be the same if you measured it with your probe microphone system), but, with some patients, it reduces the complaint of the occlusion effect. Why is this? It seems that the added gain tends to mask out the annoyance—the person's voice arriving via amplification sounds more natural, perhaps because the consonant/vowel intensity ratios are better maintained with the amplified signal. The down side of course is that this extra low-frequency gain may have a negative effect on sound quality and speech understanding in background noise.

It is important to note that the occlusion effect can be a problem for any hearing aid style for which a tight fit (minimal venting) is required and a very deep fit is not desirable or possible. Therefore, the occlusion effect can be highly problematic when high amounts of gain are needed for audibility, especially when the patient desires the smallest hearing aid style possible. Sometimes patients will have complaints that are similar to those from occlusion when there is a significant amount of low-frequency amplification. This is particularly common when the patient has low-frequency hearing thresholds in the mild-to-moderate range; the close proximity of the hearing aid user's mouth to the microphone allows for their voice (particularly the low-frequency components) to be picked up and amplified more than is desirable. In this case, reducing low-frequency gain may indeed be the solution.

Hearing Aid Styles

Hearing aid styles have been grouped in various ways throughout history. The most common grouping scheme is based on where the case housing the majority of the electronic components is worn (e.g., Dillon, 2001). Specifically, instruments are categorized as behind-the-ear (BTE) or over-the-ear (OTE), eyeglass BTE, in-the-ear

(ITE), in-the-canal (ITC), and completely-in-the-canal (CIC). Using this scheme the majority of mini-BTE instruments including those referred to as receiver-in-the-canal (RIC) or receiver-in-the-ear (RITE), and receiver-in-the-aid (RITA) instruments (described in detail later in this chapter) also fall into the BTE category.

This classification scheme is commonly used by organizations such as the Hearing Industries Association (HIA) when they report the percentage of hearing aids sold for each style. More recently, the HIA has begun to differentiate RIC instruments from other BTEs; however, this still lumps mini-BTE RITA instruments with more traditional full-sized BTEs. The reason for tracking the RIC separately appears to be related to popularity, as this style has been growing by 6 to 8% over the past few years. Currently in the U.S., BTEs in general account for 81% of all hearing aid sales—the majority of this total are RIC instruments, which alone account for 66% (81% of the BTE total). The other 19% are custom instruments with the following breakdown: ITEs = 8%, ITCs = 6%, and CICs = 5%. It is difficult to determine whether the popular mini-BTE RIC earned their popularity because they are preferred by audiologists and patients or because some manufacturers initially made some of their most advanced technology available only in this form factor.

A less common, but perhaps more useful, naming scheme differentiates hearing aids by aspects of their *design* and/or *function*. It is most important to note that this scheme differentiates hearing aid styles by how they affect hearing aid *acoustics* caused by interactions between the hearing aid and user. In the following, we use this second scheme in combination with the more traditional amplifier position–based naming scheme (i.e., BTE, ITE, ITC, CIC) to provide guidance in hearing aid style selection.

If we consider the functional differences of today's hearing aids, then they tend to break down into larger classifications such as body hearing aids, traditional BTE, mini-BTE, traditional custom, and smaller custom products such as CIC instruments, but there also are several subcategories.

Body Hearing Aids

This style is mostly included here for historical reasons, although there are still one or two manufacturers that produce it. Body aids, as you might guess from the name, are worn on the body. They are relatively large and include a box-like case (approximately 2 inches high by 2 inches wide by 0.5 inches thick) that contains the microphone and amplification stages; a receiver is worn in the ear and is attached to the case by a cord. Access to the hearing aid battery and user controls, including the volume control wheel and the on and off switch, are provided on the case surface, usually on the top and/or bottom. The case can be worn in a variety of positions including on a cord around the neck, in a shirt pocket, or attached to another part of the user's clothing.

At one time, as recently as the 1950s, essentially all electric hearing aids were body aids. They were even larger than today's body aids and considerable effort was expended to make them invisible or, at the least, more comfortable to wear. Early body aids also required a rather large battery pack, which further complicated the issue.

Functionally, body aids are different than all others in that the microphone is worn on the body. The fact that the microphone is not near the position of the ear is not optimal because picking up sound or very near the normal position of the two tympanic membranes is necessary for the brain to process signals binaurally. Binaural processing of sound is necessary for optimal sound localization and also can assist with speech understanding in background noise as described earlier in this chapter. Early body aids utilized what was called a *Y-Cord* that allowed the signal to be transmitted to two receivers—a bilateral (diotic) presentation, not true binaural hearing. In later years, body aids were designed with two different microphones; however, the separation was minimal, and the effect was not what we would achieve with microphones at the two ears.

The position of the microphone on the body also leads to a so-called body-baffle effect that increases gain in the frequency region below 800 Hz and decreases amplification for the frequencies from 1000 to 2500 Hz. The body style is also problematic because of obvious cosmetic concerns. The cords are subject to breakage; there may be unwanted noise due to clothes rustling against the case; and certain wearing positions, such as around the neck, may result in food and other debris clogging the microphone port—this can be especially problematic in children and those elderly adults with limited remaining self-care abilities. Partially because of these concerns, the body aid style is rarely recommended by current practitioners.

Although the body style hearing aid represents less than 0.1% of total hearing aid sales, there are some aspects of this style that make it of some interest to some hearing aid users. One historical advantage of the body aid style relates to acoustic feedback. Specifically, the design of the body aid results in a large separation between the microphone and receiver providing the potential for the highest amplified levels without feedback of any of the available styles. The introduction of modern feedback reduction systems, however, have virtually eliminated effective advantages in usable gain and output in comparison with other large hearing aid styles. In addition to the advantage of less susceptibility to feedback, the placement and size of the user controls on the top of the case make them the easiest to see and manipulate of all the hearing aid styles.

Traditional Behind-The-Ear (BTE) Hearing Aids

By the mid-1970s, most people were wearing the BTE style because it offers several advantages over its body-worn counterpart. In traditional BTE hearing aids, all the electronics are inside a plastic case that is fitted behind the ear. Access to the hearing aid battery and user controls are provided on the case surface, usually on the back and/or bottom. Sound is routed from the receiver through an earhook that also is used to help retention. The sound is then directed to the ear through tubing and a custom-made earmold, as shown in Figure 8–8.

THINGS TO REMEMBER: AUDITORY LOCALIZATION

In our discussion of body hearing aids, and earlier on the topic of bilateral hearing aid benefit, we mention localization. Later in this chapter, we talk about localization again as it relates to CIC fittings. Here is a brief review of some localization basics:

- We are able to localize sound well primarily because we have two ears that sample sound in two different places and a sophisticated binaural processing system. The level and timing differences of a sound as it arrives at the two ears are used as the primary cues for sound location in the horizontal plane.
- Intreraural Level Difference (ILD) cues, also known as the interaural intensity difference (IID), are primarily useful for localization of high frequencies because of the contribution of head shadow—high-frequency sounds act more like a beam and do not bend around corners as well as low-frequency sounds. This is illustrated in Figure 8–1. Note that for 90 degrees, low frequencies are only attenuated a few dB, whereas high frequencies are reduced by 10 to 15 dB.
- Interaurual Time Difference (ITD), sometimes referred to as Interaural Phase Difference cues, are primarily useful for localization of low frequencies. The shorter wavelength of high-frequency sounds leads to an ambiguous phase cue essentially rendering this cue useless in the high frequencies.
- Our ability to localize in the vertical plane is primarily due to monaural filtering effects. That is, the head, shoulders, torso, and most important, the outer ear/pinna act to filter and scatter sound in different ways depending on its angle and elevation of arrival. This cue can also provide some information when localizing sounds in the horizontal plane.
- In addition to leading to accurate localization, the binaural difference cues (ILD, ITD), and monaural filtering effects are also used by our brains to aid in speech recognition in the common cases in which speech and noise arrive from different angles. That is, the accurate presence of these cues can improve speech recognition compared to having only one ear.

As discussed in detail in Chapter 9, an added advantage to the BTE design is that the earmold, tubing, and earhook can all be used to modify the frequency response of the amplified signal. Unlike the body aid, the microphone port in the BTE is nearer to the position of the tympanic membrane, as it is usually positioned between the case and the earhook placing it on top of the pinna when worn. This provides the potential for preservation of relatively natural binaural cues (i.e. similar to those provided by unaided ears with normal hearing). This design also provides the greatest separation between the sound output (at the end of the tube in the ear) and the microphone of any of the designs other than the body aid. Therefore, when used with an appropriate earmold and modern, effective, feedback suppression, this style is able to provide adequate amplification without the presence of feedback for any magnitude of hearing loss for which a listener is expected to benefit from amplification. The larger size of the traditional BTE case also makes it possible to apply various other technologies that we discuss in Chapter 12. These include directional microphones, wireless signal routing, strong telecoils, and direct auditory input (DAI). Improved miniaturization has also allowed for frequency modulated (FM) receivers to be attached directly to a BTE via a boot, shown in Figure 8-9, or be directly integrated into the BTE case. Most of these features also are available in the larger custom instruments but are often implemented more effectively in the BTE style. Because traditional BTEs can provide considerable amplification, are relatively large and easy to manipulate, and have a high degree of flexibility, they are appropriate for a wide range of hearing losses and populations. Clinically however, their most common use is for adults with severe or greater hearing loss and in children.

The fact that only the earmold is custom fitted to the ear and it contains no electronics also provides other advantages for the BTE style. Specifically, for children who are still experiencing growth of their ear canals, the earmold can be remade relatively inexpensively without requiring any change to the hearing aid itself—at some ages this is necessary every three months or so. In addition, the separation of the electronic components from the warm, moist, cerumen-producing environment of the ear canal can lead to improved durability. This is important because cerumen clogging the receiver continues to be the number one cause of hearing aid repairs for ITE, ITC, CIC, and RIC styles. The BTE tubing can still become clogged with moisture and debris, but it can be cleaned out or changed without approaching any of the electronic components. Finally, an advantage of all non-custom styles including the BTE is that they can be stocked in the clinic. This means that if necessary (or desired), a stock ear piece can be used, and the patient

Figure 8–8. External features of a BTE hearing aid with tubing and earmold attached. (Photos courtesy of Phonak and Westone).

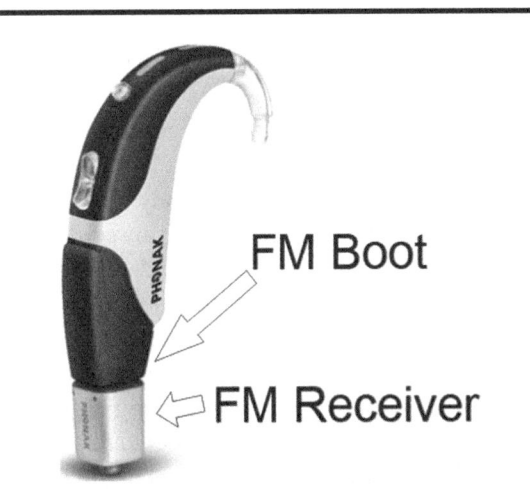

Figure 8–9. Example of a FM receiver and boot that is designed to snap onto the bottom of a BTE hearing aid. (Photo courtesy of Phonak).

can be fitted with a pair of hearing aids on the same day he or she walks in the door for a diagnostic exam.

Although traditional BTEs are among the largest of the hearing aid styles, it should be pointed out that they are not necessarily the least cosmetically appealing. The right hair style, especially those styles that cover the top of the pinna, in conjunction with the use of a clear earmold and tubing can result in an instrument that is actually much less visible than some of the custom styles such as the ITE, which completely fill the concha with colored plastic. Moreover, as we discuss later, it is now common to use barely noticeable thin tubing with mini-BTEs, and there are adaptors that allow the use of this thin tubing with the larger BTEs, making the overall fitting even less noticeable.

Eyeglass BTEs

Functionally, most *eyeglass* hearing aids also fall into the category of traditional BTEs. What are often termed eyeglass hearing aids are simply a BTE that is integrated into the temple (or bow) of eyeglasses. This style reached the height of its popularity in the 1960s, particularly in the VA/Military health care system. In some respects, the notion was logical—most people who used hearing aids also used eyeglasses, so why not have an all-in-one product? Some even saw this as a cosmetic advantage, as it was more accepted to wear glasses than hearing aids. There were problems with this style from the beginning, however. These products were heavy and uncomfortable, and did not stay adjusted. Many people needed to keep their glasses on to see well enough to change the battery. Maintenance also was a big problem, as patients would be missing their eyeglasses while their hearing aids were repaired—people did not own several pairs of glasses in the 1960s as they do now.

The BTE/eyeglass style is rarely recommended today. Reduced use of eyeglasses because of increases in contact lenses and vision surgery, changes in popular eyeglass styles leading to very thin temples, and the general miniaturization of other styles of hearing aids have further contributed to the decline of the eyeglass style. A few models of eyeglass hearing aids are still available, however. This style continues to be sometimes suggested for provision of contralateral routing of signal (CROS) amplification (described later in this chapter) and as a way to provide a directional microphone array (along the temple of the eyeglasses) that can improve speech recognition in noise performance (as described in Chapter 10). Allowing for such microphone arrays provides one potential advantage for eyeglass style hearing aids over any of the other styles. Furthermore, miniaturization has led to modern eyeglass hearing aids that are much more compact than their counterparts of the 1960s.

Mini-BTEs

A more recent incarnation of the traditional BTE instrument is the mini-BTE hearing aid. As the name suggests, these hearing aids are significantly smaller than traditional BTEs but do fit behind the ear. Mini-BTEs can be fitted in several different ways but fall into two general categories:

- RITA: These products are configured like a traditional BTE, except that the case is smaller, meaning that a smaller battery also is necessary (shorter battery life, typically less power). These products use a very thin tubing to transmit the signal to the ear, unlike the standard #13 tubing used by most traditional BTEs. There is no earhook; the tubing is attached directly to the BTE case. The ear canal coupling often is a stock eartip (many different sizes available), although a custom earmold or eartip also can be used. An example of a mini-BTE RITA product is shown in the bottom portion of Figure 8–10. These products are probably no more than 10% of total sales, or about 13% of all BTE sales.

- RIC: As the name indicates, this is a small BTE case, which is coupled to a thin wire that attaches to a small external receiver that is placed in the ear canal. This receiver is then coupled to the ear using a custom or non-custom eartip. The advantage of the RIC over the RITA is that because the receiver is removed from the case, the case can be made somewhat smaller, and more unique designs can be implemented. Also, larger receivers can be coupled to the hearing aid to provide more power than usually available with a mini-RITA. Examples of a RIC product are shown in the top portion of Figure 8–10. The mini-

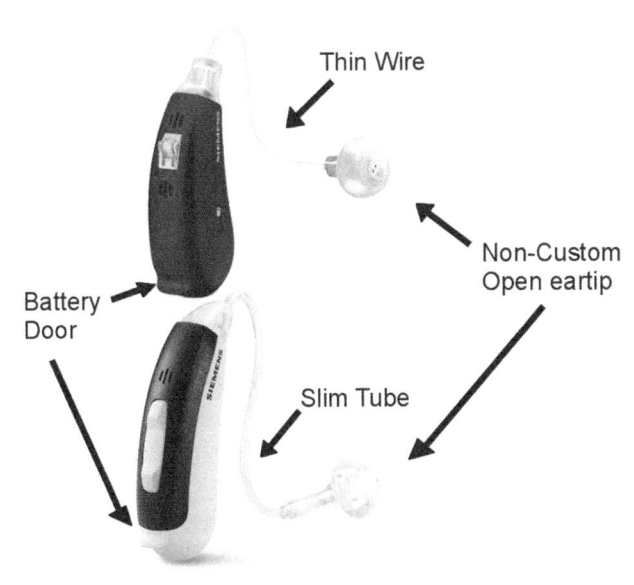

Figure 8–10. Two examples of mini-BTE hearing aids. The upper instrument is a RIC and the lower instrument is a RITA configuration. Photo courtesy of Sivantos.

sents some problems regarding what controls can be included. Many products do not have a volume control on the case. Also, there is not room for a strong telecoil, or some do not have a telecoil available at all, and it is often not possible to include a boot to accommodate FM or direct audio input. If the RIC style is used, there are additional problems related to placing a large receiver in patients with small ear canals (particularly when high levels of amplification are required).

Another limitation reported for both mini-BTE styles from at least some manufactures relates to durability of the connection between the case and the very thin wire or tube. In the case of the RITA, a breakdown of this connection can allow leakage of the acoustic signal, thus greatly increasing susceptibility of feedback. In the case of the RIC this can cause a loss of electronic connection to the receiver resulting in the hearing aid cutting out intermittently. In both cases, the problem can often be resolved by a simple and quick replacement of the tube or wire and receiver. In some cases however, a more significant repair is required. Regardless, this issue can certainly contribute to higher repair rates for mini BTE than some other styles.

Finally, with the RIC product, there is a tendency for the receivers to become plugged with cerumen. Although patients possibly could repair this themselves at home (if they were given replacement receivers), this event usually prompts a clinic visit—patients simply notice that the aid is dead. It is not uncommon for this to happen every six months or so for some patients. This of course is not unique to the mini-BTE; the same problem would occur if we used a RIC coupling with a larger BTE, except that usually is not done. The plugged receiver problem is not a minor issue. Audiologists who fit a large percentage of RIC products report a big increase in their walk-in patients needing repairs—so much so that a few have gone back to mostly RITA products. Because most audiologists use a bundled model for selling hearing aids, the time required for repairing plugged receivers normally is not billable. Depending on your status with a given manufacturer, the replacement receivers may or may not be provided free of charge to the audiologist.

It is important to note that the thin tube of the RITA also can become very easily clogged with cerumen, and this style may show more problems related to debris and occluded tubing than any other style. Fortunately, however, there is a very simple fix for this problem; the

> BTE RIC style accounts for 66% of all hearing aid sold, and about 81% of the BTE market.

The mini-BTE styles share all the potential feedback versus occlusion compromises with all other traditional BTE hearing aids. When the RIC was first introduced, some marketing material suggested that this product would be less prone to feedback, as the receiver was separated from the microphone by a much greater distance. Although this might impact mechanical feedback, this has no effect on acoustic feedback, which is what we are nearly always concerned with. The feedback path is the same whether the sound is delivered in the ear canal via the receiver or if the sound travels through a tube and is then delivered into the ear canal. Mueller and Ricketts (2006) compared two different mini-BTE products from the same manufacturer; one was a RIC and the other a RITA. The hearing aids had the same core processing, were programmed the same, and were fitted with the same level of *tightness* in the real ear. There was no difference in the maximum-gain-before-feedback for the two instruments.

Although we usually think that with hearing aids small is good, some patients have trouble handling these mini-BTEs. The small size of the case also pre-

> **POINTS TO PONDER: RIC VERSUS RITA?**
>
> There is a general perception among audiologists that when fitting a mini-BTE, RIC is better than RITA. Why is this? Maybe it is because they typically are more expensive (from the manufacturer), but are there real acoustic benefits? We have listed some potential advantages of RIC, which have been mentioned in marketing literature.
>
> - Smaller case: This is certainly true. This has allowed for smaller and more interesting case designs not possible with RITA.
> - More output flexibility: This is true. The same product can be fitted with different receivers (if they fit in the patient's ear canal), which can provide significant differences in gain (e.g., the same product could be fitted with receivers of 45, 55, or 65 dB peak gain).
> - Extended high frequencies: In theory this is true, although some manufacturers have more high frequencies in the 3000 to 4000 Hz range with their RITA than their RIC. For extended high frequencies (above 5000 Hz), RIC would appear to be the best choice because the thin tube will provide attenuation to the high frequencies—although these extended highs are unlikely to matter for most patients, as gain will not be great enough for audibility.
> - Smoother frequency response: There are some resonances of the RITA thin tube that are not present when the tube is eliminated with the RIC. These are mostly smoothed by the processing, however, and some of them are at higher frequencies that are not important for most fittings. Probably not a significant factor.
>
> While we find all these points interesting, and they are good to know, they are becoming less important each year, as the RITA style is being phased out by the majority of manufacturers—nearly all premier products introduced each year are RICs. But . . . with the current move toward over-the-counter products, we may be seeing more RITAs in the near future.

patient can insert a small plastic wire down the tube to clean it. Both the tube and wire are quite small, however, and the patient must have sufficient vision and dexterity to accomplish this task. For this reason, patients who demonstrate significant issues with cerumen may prefer the RITA style if they have good vision and dexterity, but may prefer the RIC if they do not.

Despite these limitations, the mini-BTE RIC and RITA styles continue to be very popular because of four main advantages when compared with traditional BTEs. First and foremost, as we've already stated, when a manufacturer introduces new technology, it is usually only is in this from factor. Second, there is a clear cosmetic advantage. Third, the smaller lighter case, coupled with placement of the receiver within a custom eartip within the ear canal, can lead to greater comfort and better retention. The smaller lighter case is less likely to flop off the pinna than the larger, heavier, traditional BTE case. The final advantage is a convenience issue. The mini-BTEs come with fitting kits that include stock non-custom earmold tips, which allows for a same day fitting.

Marketing experts believed these mini-BTE products would attract a younger hearing aid user, and this appears to be somewhat true, but as we discuss below, not overwhelming so. As we discuss in Chapter 3, given the same degree of hearing loss, market penetration for younger individuals is only about one-quarter of what it is for older individuals. There is a general movement to make these smaller hearing aids more fun and less old looking. To assist in attracting the younger generation, these hearing aids come in a wide range of designs and colors. Some manufacturers have replaced the traditional BTE color names of tan, beige, and brown with names like crème brûlée, snow blade, flower power, and pinot noir

Kochkin (2011b) examined the impact that mini-BTEs have had on the market:

- Mini-BTE hearing aids are expansionary (e.g., new users), influencing more affluent and more active elderly consumer segments to come forward for a solution for their hearing loss; they also tapped into segments of people with milder hearing losses.
- Most important, when the degree of hearing loss was controlled, mini-BTE hearing aids provided significant improvements in overall satisfaction, cosmetics, sound quality, and multiple environmental listening utility.
- But contrary to what was predicted, mini BTE hearing aids did not tap into younger segments of people with hearing loss. They also did not improve consumer perceptions of fit and comfort, benefit, value, or impact reductions of hearing aids not being worn; nor did they generate more positive word-of-mouth advertising or develop greater hearing aid brand loyalty.

Traditional Custom Instruments

As advances in electronic circuitry continued, manufacturers were able to reduce further the size of the hearing aid, relative to traditional BTEs and body aids, and began developing custom hearing aids such as the ITE and a more recessed version called the ITC. For simplicity, we are going to call them traditional customs (TC). The TC actually includes several sizes between and including ITE and ITC, as shown in Figure 8–11. Functionally, most ITE and ITC styles are similar enough for our purposes to fit into the TC category, although there are clear size and cosmetic differences. Although ITEs were developed in the 1960s, these early instruments

---

TECHNICAL TIP: YES, THE TERMINOLOGY IS CONFUSING

We have been talking about RIC and RITA hearing aids, as these are the terms we prefer, but it is important to point out that several other terms also are used to describe these products or similar products. RICs, for example, are sometimes referred to as RITEs. But when you think of it, neither RIC nor RITE is very descriptive. A custom hearing aid that is a CIC also is a RIC, as the receiver is indeed in the canal (except we do not call it a RIC). And all custom products would be RITEs, as the receiver is somewhere in the ear (but we do not call them RITEs). RITA does not really mean much either, as traditional BTEs and almost all custom products are all RITAs (unless they are a BTE-RIC). Some audiologists and manufacturers call mini-BTE products *thin/slim tube* hearing aids. They indeed do have a thin tube. But wait, the wire of the RIC is encased in a thin tube, but a RIC usually is not called a thin tube. And, you can take the thin tube of the mini-BTE and connect it to a traditional BTE. Is that then a thin tube product? It gets even more confusing when you start determining whether the fitting is closed or open. Here is a quick review, hopefully to clarify and not confuse:

- A mini-BTE RITA has a thin tube but so does a RIC (with a wire inside), and you can put a mini-BTE RITA thin tube on a standard size BTE (which also is a RITA).
- Both a RITA and a RIC are commonly fitted open, but they also are commonly fitted closed (or partially closed).
- An open fitting commonly is conducted with a mini-BTE RITA or RIC, but larger BTEs and even custom instruments also can be used for an open fitting.

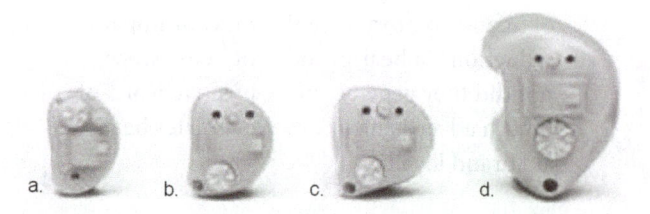

Figure 8–11. Four examples of traditional custom hearing aids ranging in size from ITC to full-sized ITE.

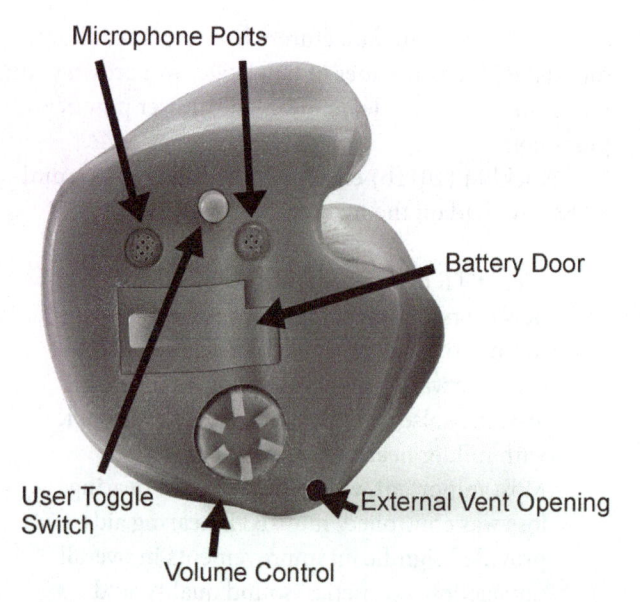

Figure 8–12. External features of a full-concha ITE hearing aid. (Photo courtesy of Siemens Hearing Instruments, Inc. All rights reserved). Photo courtesy of Sivantos.

were generally of poor quality. As a result of improved miniaturization, however, the quality of these instruments is now essentially identical to their larger siblings and currently many of the physical components and processing used in BTEs and TCs are the same.

During the 1980s, the percentage of people purchasing all styles of custom hearing aids, including TC and those described in the following sections, quickly grew from 34% in 1980 to approximately 80% of total hearing aid sales by 1990. Improved cosmetics in comparison with the BTE style is the most often cited reason for this rapid increase in popularity. It was not just cosmetics, however; but rather, the custom product was considered to be the modern hearing aid, and anything behind the ear was old-fashioned. In recent times, however, the dominance of custom hearing aids has eroded with the introduction and increasing popularity of mini-BTE products, which we just discussed in the preceding section—strangely enough, the standard custom product is now considered old-fashioned, and the BTE form factor has 80% of the market.

Like the BTE style, all the TC hearing aid electronics are contained within a plastic case. With TC instruments, the plastic case is small enough that it can be placed in the ear, however, usually within an earshell that is fabricated from an impression made of the individual patient's ear and covered with a faceplate that provides access to the battery and any user controls, as shown in Figure 8–12. With traditional custom hearing aids, the microphone port opening is on the instruments faceplate near the position of the natural ear canal opening. This placement gives the user the additional benefits over the BTE styles related to the normal acoustics provided by the pinna, including increased high frequency gain. Pinna acoustics are also important in providing sound localization cues and some natural directional effect as discussed in detail in the next section. Most full-concha instruments employ, or at least allow for, the option of using directional technology by using two omnidirectional microphones; as a result, there are two microphone ports (see Figure 8–12).

The receiver output terminates in a short tube in the end of the case within the listener's ear canal. This termination is similar to the position provided by the earmold of BTE instruments. As is the case for BTE earmolds, TC instruments can be manufactured with varying canal lengths; however, the canal portion generally extends no more than 10 to 15 mm into the cartilaginous portion of the ear canal. Longer canal portions usually are avoided because this can lead to discomfort when wearing the hearing aid as well as increase the difficulty a patient has with insertion and removal.

ITCs in this TC category differentiate from ITEs in that they are smaller and generally fill little of the concha bowl. The larger ITE fits entirely in the outer ear, filling the concha. The smaller ITC model fits mostly in the ear canal and generally does not extend beyond the tragus. The technology for manufacturing ITE shells continues to improve as does miniaturization and sound processing technology. For these reasons, current TC hearing aids are appropriate for patients with hearing loss ranging from mild through severe. When combined with modern feedback suppression technologies, in some cases ITEs may even be appropriate for some listeners with severe-to-profound hearing loss. The maximum fitting range that is appropriate, however, depends somewhat on ear geometry. In addition, the maximum severity of loss that can be appropriately fit decreases with progressively smaller instruments (i.e., ITE to ITC) because higher power instruments require larger batteries and larger receivers.

Given that these styles do not extend deeply into the canal portion, one potential problem with the TC style is that a tighter fit may lead to more problems with the occlusion effect. Although the occlusion effect can be reduced or eliminated by increased venting, this will also increase the hearing aid's susceptibility to feedback. Because of the close proximity of the microphone and receiver, the traditional ITC is usually not appropriate for patients with severe hearing loss unless the products' digital feedback suppression (DFS) is particularly effective. Even then, power is limited in half-shell ITEs and ITCs because of the use of smaller receivers and smaller batteries.

Although smaller than the BTE, the ITE and ITC styles are still large enough to accommodate directional microphones, wireless streaming technologies, and telecoils; however, DAI usually is not possible. Furthermore, because of size constraints, the telecoils in these smaller instruments are often weaker than those in BTEs or not positioned to maximize effectiveness. Finally, because of the devices' smaller size, patients with dexterity problems may have more difficulty changing batteries and operating the controls on ITEs—especially ITCs—when compared with traditional BTEs.

Traditional Custom Instruments With Recessed Faceplate

Although usually grouped together with traditional custom instruments, some hearing aids functionally and physically differ from the TC style by recessing the hearing aid faceplate and microphone deeper in the concha, traditional custom instruments with recessed faceplate (TCR). The amount of recess distance can be small, as is the case of the *low profile ITE*, or slightly more pronounced, as is the case with some deep fitting ITC instruments. Clearly, the largest effects are seen with CIC instruments. In the case of the CIC, the microphone opening, as well as the entire hearing aid

case, will be recessed into the ear canal (CIC example shown in Figure 8–13). In fact, by definition, to be a CIC, the faceplate must be recessed in the ear canal or, at the least, equal to the opening of the ear canal. Depending on the specific manufacturer, the recessed ITC or the CIC are the physically smallest instruments made. In some cases the CICs are actually slightly larger (when viewed in your hand, not in the patient's ear) because they may be made to extend deeper into the ear canal as described in the next section.

The popularity of the CIC product grew rapidly in the early 1990s as more and more manufacturers offered this model. As you might imagine, trade journals were filled with articles and advertisements extolling the many benefits of this hearing aid style. In a special issue of *The Hearing Journal*, Mueller (1994a, 1994b) reviewed 16 difference potential benefits of the CIC instrument, which he had gleaned from articles or marketing materials. Many of the potential benefits were directly linked to the deepness and tightness of the fit; something that seemed ideal from a theoretical aspect, but was not well received by most patients. In the early days, it generally was assumed that a CIC would be deeply fitted, but manufacturers soon became proficient at producing smaller hearing aids that indeed were recessed in the ear canal but were not fitted much deeper than the standard ITE. Mueller et al. (2014) review the current status of those 16 marketing claims, showing that only about one-half held true over the years.

Regardless of whether the tip of the CIC is made to extend deep into the canal or not, the fact that the

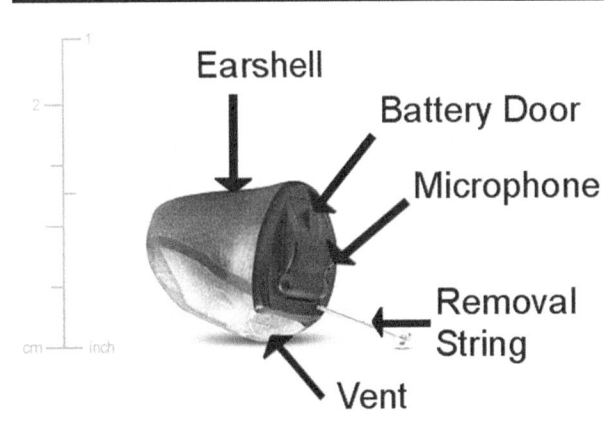

Figure 8–13. Latest generation of smaller CIC hearing aid.

faceplate is intended to be recessed inside the ear canal or at the opening of the ear canal can make the CIC the most cosmetically appealing of all the styles. In fact, in some fittings, these instruments are difficult to see without looking into the ear canal. Because of this, there is some debate as to whether the faceplate of the CIC should be skin-colored to blend in with the concha, or colored to blend with the shadow of the ear canal. On the downside, the close proximity of the microphone to receiver has negative consequences with regards to feedback. Therefore, the smallest of the recessed faceplate instruments (CIC/ITC) are usually not appropriate for patients with hearing loss falling above the moderately severe range unless highly effective digital feedback suppression is used.

Other than cosmetic appeal, the primary functional advantage provided by the ITC/CIC style relates to the more natural listening position of the microphone. Why might this provide an advantage? Actually there are a couple of reasons, namely advantages related to localization and natural directional sensitivity. Browse through the "Things To Remember: Auditory Localization" presented earlier in this chapter if you are unfamiliar with human localization.

The filtering properties related to microphone position, commonly referred to as microphone location effects (MLE), can act to change the frequency shape of sounds entering the hearing aid (See Chapter 20 for details). Simplistically, we can think of the MLE of instruments with recessed faceplates as providing *free gain*. That is, the greater the boost provided by the pinna, the less that is needed by the hearing aid amplifier. For the open ear, the average concha effect is around 5 dB at 3000 Hz with a peak at 4250 of around 10 dB (Shaw, 1966)—similar effects are therefore present for a CIC fitting. The differences in the MLE among hearing aid styles, therefore, also are predominately in the high frequencies, as the concha is the main player influencing these differences. Because the placement of the BTE microphone does not allow for pinna effects, manufacturers have attempted to build in this effect electronically (see Chapter 11).

By moving the place where sound is sampled normally (the tympanic membrane) outward to a less natural position, the change in filtering can limit or even destroy localization in the vertical plane and remove a cue that is also used in horizontal localization. For example, consider the disadvantages of placing a microphone on top of the pinna. Conversely, a microphone placed inside the ear canal can provide nearly normal filtering cues that are especially important for localization in the vertical plane. As reviewed by Mueller and Ebinger (1997), when mean minimum audible angles for vertical localization were compared for the same subjects (with mild-moderate high frequency hearing loss) fitted with ITEs and CICs, there was a significant advantage for CICs over ITEs, and aided CIC localization was not significantly worse than the unaided open ear findings. There was not a CIC advantage, however, for horizontal localization, when compared with traditional ITEs.

In addition to being important for localization, the natural filtering for this style has the (usually) desirable property of providing less sensitivity to sounds arriving from behind the user in comparison with sounds arriving in front (especially in the high frequencies). This natural directional sensitivity can help us in noisy situations like restaurants by essentially turning down the level of noise and other sounds behind us a little bit relative to the level of sounds arriving from in front. By moving the microphone outward, or in the case of a traditional BTE above the ear, we change this natural directional sensitivity. This can result in sounds being the most sensitive from the sides and even those arriving from behind.

In addition to these directional sensitivity and localization advantages, the deep faceplate placement can lead to a reduction in wind noise. The wind noise advantage varies considerably depending on the origin of the wind. This was studied extensively by Fortune and Preves (1994), who compared the wind noise from a CIC to that generated by an ITC and an ITE. When averaged across several wind source azimuths, the CIC provided a 7-dB advantage compared with the ITE and was 4 dB superior (less noise) than the ITC. Most impressive, however, was when the wind originated from directly in front of the listener. For this condition, the CIC microphone location reduced wind noise by 23 dB compared with the ITE. As we discuss in Chapter 12, modern hearing aids have wind noise cancellation algorithms, but wind noise is commonly such a high level that a combination of these algorithms and a deep placement of the microphone can be needed to optimize performance and\or comfort in wind.

Finally, if CIC instruments are fitted tightly enough and with low enough gain settings (and/or a strong digital feedback suppression algorithm is activated), effective acoustic telephone use without feedback may be possible. Telephone use typically exacerbates feedback because bringing any surface close to the hearing aid microphone can cause sound leaking out of the ear canal to reflect back toward the microphone. This increased sound reflection, also common in many situations such as hugging, scratching your ear, and so forth, greatly increases the likelihood of feedback.

Despite the positives, there are also a few potential disadvantages of the TCR style for some patients. Most notable are problems for patients without good dexterity as the instruments become smaller and insertion depth increases. Changing the smaller batteries, especially in the case of the recessed ITC and CIC styles, can be quite challenging, both for those with limited dexterity or poor vision. In addition, the instruments can be more difficult to insert and remove, although this difficulty is somewhat alleviated in the CIC style through the use of a plastic filament removal string shown in Figure 8–13. These handles also can be ordered for ITC products or custom earmolds if necessary.

The very small size of this style and their rounded shape can also be confusing to many patients. It is not unusual for patients to try to force them into their ears sideways or upside-down or even to confuse the right and left instruments before they have enough training and practice. We even know of a situation when a CIC that had been laid on a table during an intense card game was mistaken for a peanut, which then required both hearing aid and dental repair.

Differentiating between instruments made for the right and left ears can be made easier through the use of colored ink or other markers that are often added during the manufacturing process. Some manufacturers make the entire ear shells different colors (commonly red and blue) while matching the faceplate to the users' skin color and tone.

In addition to the previously stated limitations, ITCs and CICs are generally not large enough and/or are in the wrong position to implement directional microphones. This technology requires that sounds arriving from the front and the back can be differentiated. This is very difficult if the microphone ports are recessed inside the ear, as sound will hit the ports after bouncing around on the surface of the pinna and ear canal. Space limitations also prevent the effective use of telecoils, FM coupling, or DAI. However, some TCR instruments are able to accommodate modern wireless streaming technologies.

Deep Canal CIC Hearing Aids

As we described earlier in this chapter, fitting hearing aids deeply into the external ear canal has the advantage of reducing or eliminating the occlusion effect. In addition, deep canal fittings lead to an overall increase in sound pressure level (especially in the high frequencies) for the same amplifier setting (the Boyle's law principle discussed earlier). More specifically, the residual ear canal volume associated with a traditional custom instrument is about 0.7 cc. A deep canal CIC (CIC-DC) instrument, however, will have a residual ear canal volume of only about 0.25 cc. This can result in increased output of 4 dB in the low frequencies and 8 to 10 dB at 4000 Hz (Kuk, 1994). This is an advantage in that a less powerful amplifier is needed; because the amplifier gain is less, there is the potential for a reduction in feedback. Although a deep fitting can be employed with most hearing aid styles by extending the earshell, earmold, or eartip deeply into the canal, the most common application is the CIC-DC. The receivers of RIC instruments have also been fitted deeply in the canal for specific patients as described below. This deep fitting is usually accomplished with custom eartips and is particularly beneficial for listeners with more severe hearing loss.

The CIC-DC has all the advantages and limitations of the recessed CIC; however, the deep, tight fit has the additional advantages of alleviation of occlusion and reduction of susceptibility to feedback. Although many clinicians had high hopes for the deep-fit CIC style in the 1990s, the deep, tight fit is uncomfortable for many patients, particularly for CICs with hard exterior shells (which encompasses the majority of CICs). This discomfort results both from heightened sensitivity to touch exhibited by some patients and, more important, the fact that the majority of patients demonstrate significant changes in ear canal shape and volume with jaw movement resulting in increased pressure on the ear canal from the hearing aid (e.g., Darkner, Larsen, & Paulsen, 2007). Deep canal CIC fittings are therefore not that common because many patients will not tolerate them because of discomfort. Some clinicians try to counteract these complaints by ordering them slightly shorter, but this can eliminate the advantage of the deep fittings. These shortcomings clearly remain a problem because surveys suggest that many clinicians fitting the CIC-DCs have reported problems with feedback, occlusion, and the hearing aid working itself out of the ear. Otoscopy can be a useful tool when considering whether patients may be a candidate for a deep canal style.

Because they can use a softer custom or noncustom eartip, some clinicians choose to fit mini-BTE instruments deeply in the canal. These instruments share some of the cosmetic and most of the acoustic benefits of the deep fit CIC other than the fact that the microphone position (above the ear) is slightly less optimal from the standpoint of normal localization and directivity. The use of a BTE case, however, allows for the implementation of directional microphones and telecoils, as well as high levels of gain and a softer eartip, providing potential advantages over CICs.

For the rare patient with large, straight ear canals, little ear canal movement associated with jaw movement, and ear canals that are relatively insensitive to pain, the CIC-DC fitting can be used to fit up through severe hearing losses. Although certainly not for everyone, more success fitting severe hearing loss is expected for the deep canal placement when using flexible, soft tips with RICs in comparison with more traditional hard shell CICs.

Several attempts have been made to try to make deep fitted CICs more comfortable by using a softer earshell. The softer earshell has sometimes been problematic, however, because the internal components can be damaged during insertion and removal as there is not a hard shell to protect them. At least one manufacturer has attempted to circumvent this problem by making a deep fitting CIC that is intended to be professionally placed in listeners with less than severe hearing loss and left in the ear for an extended wear period (reportedly up to 120 days). According to the manufacturer, this extended wear time is made possible through the use of soft antibacterial seals and a proprietary mechanical and coating technology developed to protect the device from moisture and ear wax. Although not waterproof (swimming is not recommended), the manufacturers claim the instruments are water-resistant enough to allow the patient to shower.

In addition to the possibility of discomfort, placing the receiver increasingly closer to the ear canal and close to the medial tip of the earshell or eartip can create another difficulty. This proximity to the outer ear environment, which can be moist and cerumen-filled, increases the chances that the receiver will become clogged with debris. A number of *wax-guard* designs are currently in use, many of which are expected to help with this problem, but it certainly is not solved (the guards themselves become clogged).

Open Canal (OC) Fittings

Recall that we mentioned earlier that we would be categorizing the different hearing aid styles relative to their

---

TECHNICAL TIP:
HEARING AID SELECTION CONSIDERATIONS DURING OTOSCOPY

It is important and useful to consider hearing aid styles when performing routine otoscopy:

- Look for cerumen; even small hard pockets of cerumen can be uncomfortable when pressed on by an earmold/earshell. Depending on the position, walls or shelves of cerumen can increase feedback problems. Ask the patient if they have cerumen problems. How often do they have to have their ears cleaned?
- Ask the patient to open his or her mouth, talk, and simulate chewing. Does their ear canal move a lot, does it completely change shape? If so, a deeper and or tighter fitting may not be possible without discomfort.
- How does the patient react to the otoscope tip? If the otoscope tip is uncomfortable, or if he or she seems jumpy, a tight shell probably will be bothersome too.

function. This clearly applies for OC (for open canal) fittings, as the style could be traditional BTE, mini-BTE, or a variety of types of custom instruments. As the name implies, OC hearing aids are functionally differentiated from other styles because they leave the ear canal mostly open, which then results in the absence of the objective or subjective occlusion effect when they are fitted. In general, the occlusion effect is eliminated when the hearing aid has a vent of 4 mm or larger (e.g., Kiessling, Brenner, Thunber-Jespersen, Groth, & Jensen, 2005). Because such a large vent is needed, most OC fittings use a BTE case (usually the mini-BTE, as the gain from the larger model is not needed); however, there are some methods that use custom instruments and also keep the ear canal mostly open.

The OC style typically includes a mini-BTE case (i.e., RIC or RITA design). The success of modern OC instruments has been made possible through the advent and refinement of modern hearing aid sound processing algorithms that act to suppress or filter out feedback. These digital feedback suppression algorithms are discussed in more detail in Chapter 12.

Because nearly all OC fitting are implemented using mini-BTE hearing aids, we include some of these features in our discussion (see earlier section on mini-BTEs for more details). The physical design of this fitting provides many potential advantages including relief from occlusion and a light and expectedly comfortable fit over the ear, although also potentially providing greater physical comfort through the use of a comfortable non-occluding eartip. The non-occluding tips usually fit comfortably into the ear canal; as a consequence, when on the ear, all that is noticeable is the thin tube or wire, shown in Figure 8–14. The non-occluding eartips

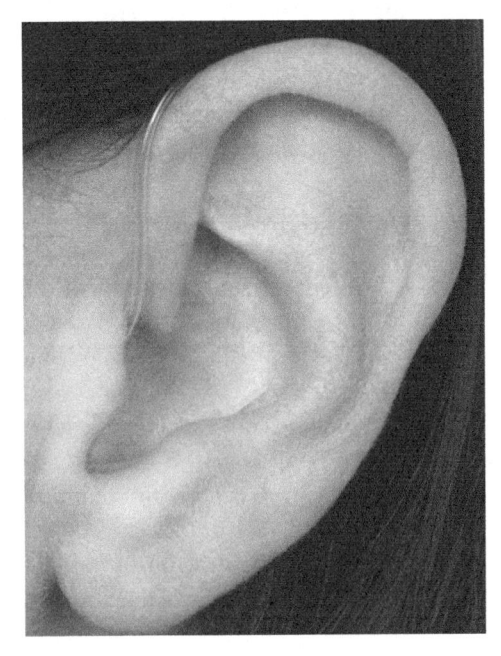

Figure 8–14. Example of a mini-BTE RITA fitted to the ear. From this view all that is visible is the thin tubing. (Photo ©2012, Unitron. All rights reserved).

TECHNICAL TIP: WAX GUARDS

- Most manufacturers have a variety of wax guards and, because there is no magical wax guard, designs continually change. The goal of these devices is to protect the receiver from being impacted with wax. Instead the wax guard will become clogged and it can be changed rather than requiring a receiver repair or replacement. You can think of it as a trap as well as a guard. In some cases, the patient is instructed to replace wax guards at home, which works fine for those patients with good vision, dexterity, and diligence.
- Wax guards differ in how effective they are. If we consider wax guards from a single manufacturer, those that protect the receiver very well tend to clog more easily and, therefore, require more frequent changing. Those that provide less protection also tend to clog less often. This of course also interacts with the consistency of the individual patient's cerumen. Therefore, the choice of wax guard is an individualized decision that requires weighing convenience and protection while considering individual patient differences.

> **POINTS TO PONDER: A LITTLE OC HISTORY**
>
> There is little documentation of the first OC fittings, but we know they received considerable attention immediately after the CROS-type hearing aids described in the next section were introduced. It was quickly discovered that the non-occluding earpieces (or in some cases, tubing only) used for the CROS hearing aid also could be used for ipsilateral high-frequency amplification (hence, the term IROS [ipsilateral routing of signals], referring to a large vent).
>
> In the late 1960s, researchers showed that OC fittings could provide useful high-frequency amplification (Green, 1969). In the early 1980s, OC fittings were attempted with *horn tubing* with some success. Over the years, clinicians more or less lost interest in OC fittings because feedback problems precluded their use for all but the mildest high frequency hearing losses. This lack of interest persisted until key technological and cosmetic factors came together to greatly increase the popularity of OC fittings:
>
> - Feedback suppression algorithms became more common and more effective.
> - Miniaturization allowed for production of cosmetically appealing mini-BTEs.
> - The mini-BTEs were coupled to the ear using a thin, cosmetically appealing tube or wire.
> - Non-custom eartips were developed that were comfortable and non-occluding.
>
> It is fair to say that this culmination of factors had a huge impact on the entire hearing aid market in the mid to late 2000s and a large portion of custom hearing aid sales moved rather quickly to the category of BTE. Specifically, BTE sales comprised only about 20% in 2004, were up to approximately 50% by 2007, and reached 80% in 2016. We do not really know what percentage of these BTE sales were indeed for open fittings, but it probably was the majority. Mueller (2009) reported on a dispenser survey that revealed that approximately 25% of dispensers stated that at least 70% of their sales were mini-BTE open fittings. We wonder if some of these actually ended up being somewhat closed when feedback problems emerged.

can be either non-custom or custom-made for an individual's ear to improve retention. Several styles of non-custom, non-occluding eartips are shown, and provided by different manufacturers. As reviewed in Chapter 16, the real ear occluded response quickly reveals whether a given tip is indeed open when placed in the ear canal. In addition to the elimination of occlusion and all of its negative consequences as reviewed earlier, the open eartip also allows natural, low-frequency sounds to leak in, which is expected to improve sound quality for patients with low-frequency hearing thresholds at or near the normal range (Cox & Alexander, 1983).

The advantages of OC hearing aids and mini-BTE instruments in both open and more closed configurations are clearly supported in current sales numbers as mentioned previously. Patients also appear to show a strong preference for this style. A recent study within the VA health system demonstrated that, after trials with mini-BTE OC instruments and traditional custom instruments, approximately 85% of the nearly 300 patients evaluated reported a preference for the OC style.

As discussed previously, one limitation that can affect a large number of potential patients relates to one of the mini-BTE instruments' primary advantages, its diminutive size and the challenges that it presents to those with limited dexterity or poor vision. In some cases, simply using a larger BTE with the thin tubing will make enough difference, and then the OC fitting is still possible.

Another limitation to an OC fitting is that the large vent allows a great deal of the amplified low frequencies to leak out. Consequently, a very high amount of low-frequency amplifier gain is needed to provide any amplification at the patient's tympanic membrane. Due

> ### TECHNICAL TIP: OC FITTINGS—IT'S THE RESULT NOT THE INTENT
>
> The style category of OC fittings is somewhat different from the other styles we have discussed, as what is important is the result of the fitting, not the intent. We explain. If you were fitting a patient with a pair of CICs, and when you put the hearing aids in the ear you saw that the faceplates were recessed into the ear canal, you indeed would know that you fitted the CIC style. But an OC fitting is only an OC fitting if the ear canal is left open (which easily can be determined by conducting probe microphone REOR measures, but often difficult to determine doing a visual inspection). The point being, simply using mini-BTEs, thin tubes, and stock eartips that are labeled "open" does not mean that the result will be an open fitting. Conversely, some eartips that are labeled closed result in so much slit leak venting in some ear canals that the resultant fitting is essentially open. The final result, of course, affects the benefit of OC fittings that we have discussed here.

> ### TECHNICAL TIP: EARTIPS FOR OC FITTINGS
>
> We review the different eartips that are available in Chapter 9. But, because we are talking about OC fittings at this time, here are some bonus points to remember:
>
> - Because no earmold impression is needed, non-custom eartips have a clear advantage in time, cost savings, and time efficiency. They typically also are comfortable, as they fit quite loosely.
> - There are several limitations to non-custom eartips though, including:
>   - Limited retention, especially in ear canals with unusual shapes. Not only does this affect the output, but the mini-BTEs are very light, and easily will fall off the ear if the eartip is not secured.
>   - Many non-custom eartips have extremely limited durability and may require changing as often as every three to six months.
>   - It may be more difficult to direct the sound outlet away from an ear canal wall, thus leading to greater susceptibility to feedback in some patients.
>   - Many patients may have difficulty consistently placing the non-custom tip in the same place. This can affect the frequency response, gain, and susceptibility to feedback. That is, the hearing aid may work better on some days than others simply depending on how well the patient is able to insert it.
>
> Although many clinicians fit the majority of mini-BTEs on patients with non-custom eartips, some clinicians have switched back to using custom eartips, even when fitting with an open venting configuration because of these limitations. These custom eartips will allow for better retention, better ability to direct the sound outlet away from the ear canal wall and reduce susceptibility to feedback, and better durability of the eartip.

in part to the negative affect high amplifier gain has on battery life and amplification of circuit noise, as well as the need for a larger receiver, some manufacturers may choose to forgo this low-frequency amplifier gain altogether and target patients with hearing loss limited to the higher frequencies (above 1000 Hz or even 2000

Hz). This can, of course, be a problem when a closed mold is added to provide additional gain at 500 Hz. As an alternative, as we mentioned earlier, manufacturers of RIC instruments will sometimes have multiple receivers available for the same model, so clinicians may select the receiver with adequate power for the patient, while still considering that the receiver and eartip must be small enough to fit in the patient's ear canal. Clearly clinicians must be careful to select instruments with adequate low-frequency gain available when fitting patients with low-frequency hearing loss. Furthermore, because of artifacts including an echo type effect and hearing a talker's voice emanating from the listeners ear, the magnitude of low-frequency amplification provided by the OC style is generally limited. One simple fix for patients with more low-frequency loss, however, is to fit a mini-BTE instrument but simply select a tighter fitting eartip.

The lack of low frequency gain also has other implications. Although presented as a limitation, the ability to provide only high-frequency gain can also be seen as an advantage for many patients. Specifically, the OC style is ideal for patients with normal or near-normal hearing in the low frequencies, but requiring substantial high-frequency amplification because of the presence of mild to moderately severe high-frequency hearing loss. This steeply sloping hearing loss configuration was quite difficult to fit prior to the introduction of OC instruments and now may be fitted quite easily.

It is important to point out that, even in patients without low-frequency hearing loss for which no gain is required, the lack of low-frequency gain will have an effect on the function of specific features. That is, certain features such as digital noise reduction and directional microphone technology only will be effective in OC instruments in the high-frequency range for which significant gain is provided. Consequently, activation of these features likely will be less noticeable by the patient in an OC fitting (see Chapter 17). Although the amount

---

POINTS TO PONDER: OPEN OR CLOSED FOR HIGH FREQUENCY GAIN?

Regarding high-frequency gain, consider that, with an OC fitting that is truly open, the patient retains all or most of the natural ear canal resonance (with a closed fitting this is not the case). This of course primarily is in the 2000 to 3000 Hz range—the very frequency range where we usually are struggling to obtain desired gain. Figure 8–15 shows an example of the average residual ear canal resonance when an open tip is placed in the ear (Mueller & Ricketts, 2006). The remaining average ear canal resonance is around 15 dB, so is this a *free* 15 dB of gain for our patients? Sound too good to be true? It is. Remember the advantages of a deep fitting that we discussed earlier—the increased SPL when we make the residual ear canal smaller? With an OC fitting, we do not obtain this advantage, which can amount to 10 dB or more, depending on how deeply the earmold goes into the ear canal.

So what is the true gain advantage of leaving the ear canal open? This was studied by Mueller and Ricketts (2006) and is displayed in Figure 8–16. By conducting probe microphone measures on real ears and changing only the earmold (open versus closed), they were able to identify the true advantage of leaving the ear canal open. This figure represents a difference curve; above the 0 dB line indicates an advantage for the OC fitting. Observe that, on average, this advantage is about 5 dB in the region of the ear canal resonance. There are individual variations depending on the patient's open ear resonance (how much do they have to lose?) and the size of the ear canal (smaller ear canals will be impacted more by a closed earmold). As expected, the closed earmold made a large difference in the average gain in the lower frequencies, especially for hearing aid A; hearing aid B did not have amplifier gain for the very low frequencies. This shows just how much gain really is leaking out with the OC fitting. Normally, this leakage is not a concern, as we would not be conducting an OC fitting if the patient needed low-frequency gain.

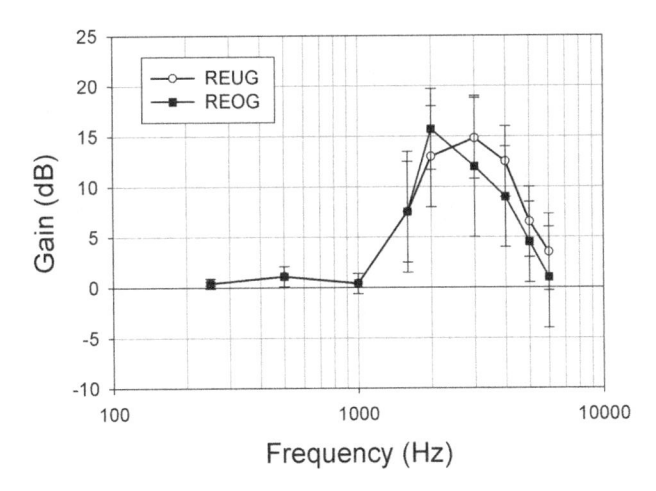

Figure 8–15. Average REUG and REOG for 14 individuals fitted with non-custom stock open eartips for the REOG measures. (Adapted from Mueller and Ricketts, 2006).

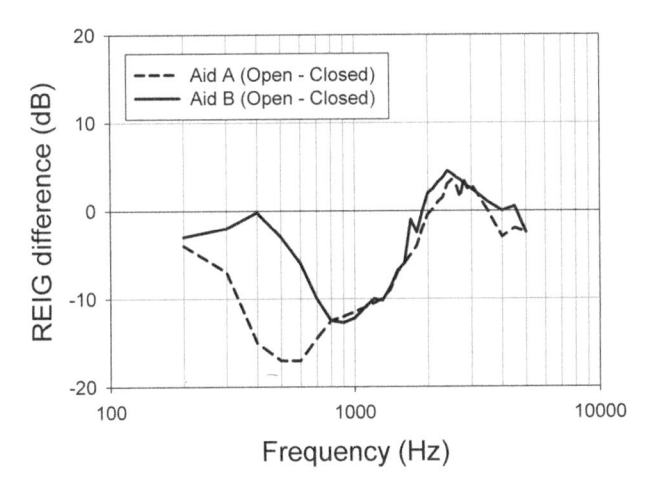

Figure 8–16. Difference in average insertion gain for two mini-BTE hearing aids measured using an open and closed fitting tip. Earmold tubing and hearing aid settings were unchanged. (Adapted from Mueller and Ricketts, 2006).

of low-frequency gain may be affected by manufacturers' design decisions, the amount of high-frequency peak gain (i.e., in the 2000 to 3500 Hz range) before the introduction of audible feedback is commonly limited by the effectiveness of the feedback suppression algorithm. Although such systems are constantly improving, current OC hearing aids are generally limited to patients with less than severe high frequency thresholds, assuming that audibility in these high frequencies is desired. In addition, large and clear differences in the effectiveness of feedback suppression continue to be exhibited across manufacturers and models. Consider that if there is a more than 10 dB difference for the gain-before-feedback between hearing aid models (and there is), this could affect the fitting range by 20 dB or more. These differences again highlight the importance of clinicians' knowledge related to the operation and limitations of the specific models they choose to fit. The effectiveness of the different feedback systems is very easy to assess on real patients using your probe microphone equipment.

Although the vast majority of OC hearing aids use a thin tube or thin wire and are designed for BTE placement of the case, at least two companies have introduced unique case placements such as those designed to fit in the fossa of the helix, and those that place the microphone in the fossa of the helix or in the ear canal. Some of these designs are quite unique and are aimed at improving the naturalness of the microphone placement and/or targeted to individuals who wish to integrate their hearing aid into their personal sense of fashion (unique case designs are available). Although there are some potential benefits, these designs all typically result in closer spacing between the receiver and microphone that can greatly limit available gain before feedback, and are therefore primarily aimed at individuals with mild-moderate high-frequency hearing loss.

Hearing Aid Style: Mini-Summary

- Selection of hearing aid style is a complex process. Although some styles can be ruled out based on the degree of hearing loss alone, many styles may be appropriate for a single hearing loss configuration.
- Style decisions can be highly impacted by cosmetics; however, the cosmetics in the hand do not always relate to the cosmetics on the head. Hair style, choice of color and material, and the exact instrument chosen can all affect the final cosmetics on the head.
- In addition to cosmetics and degree of hearing loss, the desired features should always be an important consideration because not all

features are available in all styles. Size and movement of the ear canal should also be considered, especially when considering a tight and/or deep fit.
- Finally, regardless of what *you believe* is the best style, it is important to involve the patient in this selection process. Fitting a pair of full-concha ITEs to a patient who really wants CICs, so that an extra 3 dB directional advantage can be added, is only a good move if the patient wears the hearing aids.

Special Designs and Styles

The styles we have talked about so far are all quite common in clinical use. Although the distinction is somewhat artificial, we will now talk about some styles and designs that are either less common or aimed at specific populations. This distinction is especially artificial because one could argue that few hearing aid styles we have discussed so far are really appropriate for all populations and hearing loss configurations, and certainly no hearing aid style discussed so far is optimal for all populations and hearing loss configurations. Despite this artificial distinction, it is common for new clinicians to have significantly less experience with the following hearing aid styles and configurations that include CROS/BiCROS, those that deliver sound through bone conduction (both traditional and implantable) and middle ear implants. Rather than an in-depth treatment of these options, they are only briefly introduced here for completeness and to highlight the importance of considering all possible styles as well as hearing assistive technologies when making fitting decisions. To aid in selection decisions, we have summarized all the hearing aid styles presented in a single table at the end of this chapter (Table 8–1).

Contralateral Routing of Signal (CROS) and BiCROS Hearing Aids

The contralateral routing of signal (CROS) hearing aid is designed for patients with no usable hearing in one ear, and normal hearing or a minimal hearing loss in the other ear (Harford & Barry, 1965; Harford & Dodds, 1966; Matkin & Thomas, 1972). This configuration of hearing loss is commonly referred to as *single-sided deafness*. The goal is to give the patient two-sided hearing when true bilateral hearing is not possible. Recall that one of the requirements for bilateral amplification is aidable hearing in both ears; the CROS is an alternative to a traditional unilateral fitting for these patients.

Consider this scenario. Your Monday morning patient is a 40-year-old woman who just lost essentially all her hearing in her right ear three months ago as a result of surgery to remove an acoustic neuroma. She is bothered by not hearing in this ear, is having some problems at work, and is eager to try whatever is available that might help. Her hearing in her left ear is normal. You really have five different CROS choices:

- A pair of hearing aids connected by wire (routed through an eyeglass frame)—rare in the United States
- A pair of hearing aids with the sound conducted wirelessly from the bad side to the good side
- A single hearing aid—a transcranial CROS with a microphone and air conduction receiver on the bad ear
- A single hearing aid—a transcranial CROS with a microphone on the bad side and a bone conduction receiver placed on the head in contact with bone
- An implantable bone conduction hearing aid on the bad side

Traditional Air Conduction

In the traditional CROS system, the microphone is contained within either a BTE or TC case that is located on the impaired side. The receiver is located on the side with better (normal) hearing within a BTE or TC case along with the other components necessary for signal processing and amplification. Early versions of the CROS (circa 1980 and before) often used a wire, sometimes routed through eyeglasses or a headband. Current CROS fittings, however, are commonly achieved through the use of wireless transmission that is usually in BTE, mini-BTE, or TC cases—the appearance is generally identical to those we discussed earlier for these styles. Currently, it is common for wireless streaming from one hearing aid to the other to be completed by near field induction or one of a number of radio wave protocols that are discussed in Chapter 10. The newest wireless protocols allow for wireless streaming as a built-in option across a wide range of styles; these protocols sometimes have much less interference than near field induction. Further, with the proliferation of modern wireless transmission, it is possible to configure the many standard bilateral, premiere hearing aid products to function as a wireless CROS. Some of them are limited by reduced battery life, however, although this issue continues to improve. Current typical battery life in the CROS/BiCROS streaming mode is at least three to four days and nearly two weeks in some products.

The clearest advantage for the CROS fitting is that the user can use the good ear to hear signals from the impaired side that are otherwise attenuated by head shadow. For all of these types of fittings when there is normal hearing in the better ear, sound from the receiver is usually directed into the ear using as much venting as possible so that the normal sound pathway for the better ear is not blocked. As a result of the large amount of venting, it is typical for only higher frequency signals to reach the ear with normal hearing. In general this is not a problem since it is the high frequencies that are reduced from head shadow; however, there are sometimes complaints of a tinny sound quality if too much gain is programmed. By convention, it is usual to refer to the device as a left CROS when the aided signal is routed to the left ear and a right CROS when the aided signal is routed to the right ear.

Clearly, CROS hearing aids are more successful in some instances than others (e.g., Gelfand, 1979; Upfold, 1980). It is our experience, however, that successful use of a CROS in patients with single-sided deafness (normal hearing in the better ear) requires a recognized communication need. Acceptance rates for CROS hearing aids reported in the literature generally are between 20 and 50%. While the poor sound quality, cosmetics and audible circuit noise complaints of the past have diminished with the newest CROS implementations (e.g., Hill, Marcus, Digges, Gillman, & Silverstein, 2006), the inconvenience of using two devices remains an often cited reason for rejection of CROS amplification. Successful users often report a critical communication need in an environment in which they are surrounded by important speakers and are highly motivated to hear

---

THINGS TO REMEMBER: HEARING AIDS AND HEAD SHADOW

Listening conditions change throughout the day, and input from the side without hearing can be useful for people who cannot always control the direction of the sound reaching their ears. People in the business world, for example, seem to notice the greatest handicap from single-sided deafness, as they are frequently in meetings, luncheons, and so forth, in which the talker of interest may be located on their "bad side."

- The benefit from placing a microphone on the side without usable hearing mainly relates to offsetting audibility and SNR difficulties related to head shadow. Specifically, for unaided listening, when a talker is on the impaired side, the signal will reach the good ear after the level has been reduced by head shadow.
- The amount of attenuation from head shadow is essentially zero in the low frequencies but can reach more than 15 dB in the higher frequencies (see Figure 8–1).
- If noise happens to be present on the good side, the attenuation provided by head shadow can be especially detrimental because of the decreased SNR.
- Conversely, if noise is on the bad side and speech is on the good side, head shadow can work to the patient's advantage. That is, the CROS configuration in this case can *decrease* speech recognition in noise in comparison with unaided listening. A good reason why the patient might want to have remote control for this off-side microphone.

sounds arriving from both sides equally. Due in part to the lack of acceptance of CROS hearing aids, a variety of device types that stimulate the cochlea through bone conduction have been advocated for treatment of single-sided deafness. These devices are discussed in the next section of this chapter.

BiCROS Applications. Patients with SSD who also have some hearing impairment in the better ear are more successful users of the CROS application than those with normal hearing in the fitted ear, partly because they entered the fitting with more communication problems. In cases in which amplification is provided to the better ear in addition to the contralateral routing of signals, the instruments are referred to as BiCROS (e.g., there also is a microphone for the instrument on the side of the "better" ear, thus two microphones sending signals to one amplifier/receiver). The higher success rates in patients with hearing loss in their better ear has been partially attributed to the reduced annoyance because of audibility of circuit noise, and the decreased venting typically used (to provide low-frequency amplification) improves the sound quality of signals arriving from both sides (Del Dot, Hickson, & O'Connell, 1992; Hill, Marcus, Digges, Gillman, & Silverstein, 2006). Additionally, these people are going to be wearing a hearing aid anyway (probably a mini-BTE), so adding a second aid (microphone) is not viewed as much of a difference. The general rule of thumb is that if you look at the good ear in isolation, and you consider that ear in need of amplification, then the BiCROS rather than the CROS would be selected. These products are also switchable, so the patient can turn on or off either microphone for specific listening situations—if noise is present from the side of the bad ear, this microphone could be turned off. As we discussed in the previous section, many higher level modern instruments can be configured as either CROS or BiCROS via the included wireless transmission. Thus, these instruments can include all of the modern features present in even the most advanced hearing aids as discussed in Chapters 11 and 12.

Verification. Finally, we want to mention that traditional CROS and BiCROS hearing aids need to be fitted just like all other hearing aids. That is, probe microphone testing is required to assure that the frequency response and output is appropriate. This is sometimes overlooked as the setup is somewhat different from a standard fitting. We discuss the protocol for CROS verification in detail in Chapter 17. Pumford (2005) also has written a useful review on this procedure.

Transcranial CROS

As the name indicates, in this type of fitting we are referring to sending the signal through the skull (via bone conduction). *Transcranial CROS* fittings have been proposed as a way to alleviate some of the complaints related to traditional CROS amplification (e.g., Valente, Potts, Valente, & Goebel, 1995). The goal of this type of CROS fitting is to place an air-conducted signal in the bad ear that is loud enough that it crosses over via bone conduction to the good ear. This intervention usually implements a single deep canal instrument (usually a CIC or BTE style with deep-fitted earmold), which is fitted to the ear without hearing. In true transcranial CROS implementation, the deep fit allows for mechanical coupling between the hearing aid shell and the bony portion of the ear canal. The mechanical coupling, when combined with high levels of hearing aid output, allows for transmission of sound to the contralateral cochlea through both bone conduction and air conduction (traveling around the head). In the usually less successful *quasi transcranial CROS*, the instrument is not placed tightly and/or deeply enough to achieve mechanical coupling. The transcranial CROS has the advantages of using only a single instrument on the impaired side and the fact that little, if any, circuit noise will be transmitted to the better ear. We talk about clinical methods to assess the potential success of a transcranial fitting in Chapter 17. Valente et al. (1995) also has published a useful review on this topic.

Fitting Considerations. The patient's hearing for bone conduction in the good ear and their interaural attenuation will determine what output levels are needed for this type of a transcranial CROS to be successful. We believe that it is important to first develop *fitting targets*. By using probe microphone equipment to measure ear canal SPL in the bad ear, it is possible to determine what output in this ear will cross over to the good ear. Frequency-specific, pure-tone signals are delivered from the audiometer, and the transducer used *does* matter. It is best to use an insert receiver, placed at approximately the depth of the hearing aid, using a tip that has a hardness that is similar to the hearing aid. Hard rubber immittance tips coupled to an insert earphone is one option. When the patient says they hear the tones in the good ear, the real-ear SPL in the bad ear is measured for each frequency. In general, we would like to place speech to at least 15 to 20 dB SL in the good ear, so adding 20 dB or so to the measured values will provide the ear canal SPL targets for the hearing aid fitting. For example, if the 2000 Hz signal is heard in the good ear at 80 dB RESPL (real-ear SPL), then the ear canal SPL target at 2000 Hz for an average-level speech-shaped signal would be 100 dB RESPL for this frequency. The mechanical vibrations of an actual hearing aid (which, as we mentioned will greatly influence the transmission) are different than those of the insert used for testing, so these targets still are not as precise as we would like.

Other than probe microphone testing, it is difficult to verify the effectiveness of the transcranial CROS fitting in the office or clinic. Moreover, it is probable that benefit only will occur when:

- The bone-conducted signal originating from the bad ear exceeds the air-conducted signal arriving at the good ear.
- The bone-conducted signal originating from the bad ear exceeds the background noise level at the good ear.

Because we know that the transcranial bone-conducted signal at the cochlea of the good ear probably will not be more than 30 to 40 dB SPL, for the above two conditions to occur, the patient would need to be listening to soft speech in quiet, with the speech delivered from the side of the bad ear. Because of head shadow, the amplified bone-conducted high frequencies of speech now will be louder in the good ear than the air-conducted signals traveling around the head. If this listening situation occurs frequently in the patient's everyday life and the patient considers this listening situation important, then the patient just might become a regular transcranial CROS user.

Despite the potential advantages, most patients are not appropriate candidates for this type of transcranial CROS because they find the required deep fitting uncomfortable or even painful. As a consequence, appropriate screening to determine whether the patient will tolerate a deep tight fit is critical prior to trying this fitting. This screening can be done by having the patient try a deep-fitting earplug made of a harder plastic material.

Alternative Transcranial Choices. As we have discussed, one problem with the traditional transcranial attempts is generating a strong enough bone-conducted signal. For this reason, a number of bone conduction devices also have been introduced over the years, which include those that stimulate in a number of different ways. In general, these devices have been aimed at patients with single-sided deafness who are looking for an alternative CROS application but are not interested in surgical options (which we describe in the next section). One method that has been used for many years that was originally designed for individuals with conductive hearing losses is a bone conduction eyeglass hearing aid. Historically, these have not been successful, for all the reasons we mentioned earlier in this chapter regarding why eyeglass hearing aids in general are usually not successful. Additionally, we now have a hearing aid that is even heavier and more cumbersome to use—the vibrator in the temple needs to be positioned firmly on the mastoid. There is a unique bone conduction device, however, that could be considered, the TransEar®.

TransEar®. The TransEar® was introduced in 2004 by United Hearing Systems and is now manufactured by Ear Technology Corporation. It is specifically marketed as a solution for single-sided deafness. With this device, the microphone and processing are contained within a BTE case that connects to a piece in the ear using a small wire. The configuration of this part of the device is essentially identical to that used in receiver in the ear mini-BTE devices, so we could call this a RIC hearing aid. The difference, however, is that with the TransEar® the wire terminates in a small bone conduction vibrator encased in an earmold placed in the ear canal of the poorer ear, rather than in a typical receiver. As with other transcranial approaches, the patient must be willing to accept a hard shell that is fitted fairly deeply into the ear canal. The device has modern features such as digital noise reduction and directional technology. And as with other devices, acoustic feedback can be an issue.

> **POINTS TO PONDER: HOW ABOUT A SOUNDBITE?**
>
> We know that the teeth are a good means of conducting a bone conducted signal, so how about a hearing aid that fits on the teeth? Yes indeed, that hearing aid existed for several years, was branded the "SoundBite," and was manufactured by Sonitus Medical. The company filed for bankruptcy in January of 2015, and the SoundBite has not been available since this time. This product was marketed as a solution for single-sided deafness and conductive hearing losses. In this device, the microphone and processing are housed in a mini-BTE case, then the signal is wirelessly routed to a vibrating transducer that is worn on the upper back teeth. There was little research with this product, although one early study with single-sided deafness (SSD) participants reported significant improvement in laboratory speech and noise testing, and also for real-world ratings of speech-in-noise understanding (Murray, Popelka, & Miller, 2011). They also reported no audiologic, medical, or dental complications (based on 30-day and 6-month clinical trials). Perhaps we'll see a return of the SoundBite or a similar product.

Implantable Bone Conduction Stimulation

Our final solution for single-sided deafness is a bone anchored implant (BAI). These instruments were initially designed for individuals with conductive hearing losses, so we review their clinician applications in general, including those for the patient with single-sided deafness.

Many hearing impaired patients have hearing loss that is primarily conductive in nature. Although conductive and mixed hearing loss often can be habilitated with traditional air conduction hearing aids, these aids are sometimes not appropriate because of problems with retention or other issues. For example, a patient may have physical malformation of the pinna and/or an external ear canal that makes retention a problem. In some cases, the external ear malformation (e.g., stenosis) may preclude placement of a hearing aid because of space limitations, the lack of an external ear canal, or other factors. Still other patients may find that a hearing aid or earmold placed in the ear may exacerbate an existing ear problem or result in the recurrence of a pathologic condition. It is important to reiterate that for many patients with conductive and mixed hearing loss, air conduction hearing aids may be a reasonable or even the optimal solution. The potential advantage for air conduction instruments for conductive hearing losses relates to the fact that they generally are able to provide a broader frequency response, particularly related to gain in the high frequencies. When air conduction hearing aids are problematic, however, stimulation of the inner ear through bone conduction may be a preferable alternative.

With traditional bone conduction hearing aids, a bone conduction receiver is placed on the mastoid and held in position by a headband or using eyeglasses. With these traditional bone conduction hearing aids, the cochlea is stimulated in the same way as it is during bone conduction threshold assessments. Some patients may need stronger vibrations because of unusually thick or dense skin and/or fat deposits under the skin at the stimulation site (Laitakari, Löppönen, Salmivalli, & Sorri, 1995). Therefore, although bone conduction hearing aids can be used for any degree of conductive component, only a mild-to-moderate sensorineural component may be present before providing appropriate audibility becomes difficult or impossible.

Despite the fact that some patients enjoy success with traditional bone conduction hearing aids, they have been criticized by others because of the often large, sometimes cumbersome, sometimes physically uncomfortable, and not particularly cosmetically appealing nature of their retention systems. In response to these complaints, many methods have been investigated for coupling a bone conduction vibrator to the head. To date, the most successful alternative method for patients who experience unilateral or bilateral conductive or mixed losses has been to surgically implant a titanium screw and abutment assembly into the skull that allows for the snapping on of a bone vibrator. The first BAI that received U.S. Department of Food and Drug Administration (FDA) approval in the United States is known as the Baha™ (e.g., Hol, Bosman, Snik, Mylanus, & Cremers, 2004; Wazen, Caruso, & Tjellstrom, 1998; Westerkull, 2002). The Baha™ was approved for use in the United States by the FDA for patients with bilateral conductive hearing loss in January, 1999 (FDA, 1999). Its original manufacturer, Entific Medical Systems, was purchased by Cochlear Corporation in 2005. In more recent times, Oticon Medical received FDA approval to market its devices known as the Ponto™ in 2011 and the MedTronic Sophono Alpha2™ device received FDA approval in 2013. Other devices such as the Med-EL Bonebridge are not yet available in the United States but are sold in many other countries. Each model has a *family*; the primary differences within each family relate to the amount of power available, although there are also differences in coupling.

In 2010 all approved BAIs were percutaneous (through the skin) devices, and all the hearing aid components, including a bone conduction vibrator, were inside a plastic case. The case was coupled to a titanium screw that was implanted in the upper mastoid region of the temporal bone via a titanium abutment screw that protrudes through the skin, as shown in Figure 8–17. Although the majority of BAIs dispensed continue to be percutaneous devices, BAIs that do not directly couple

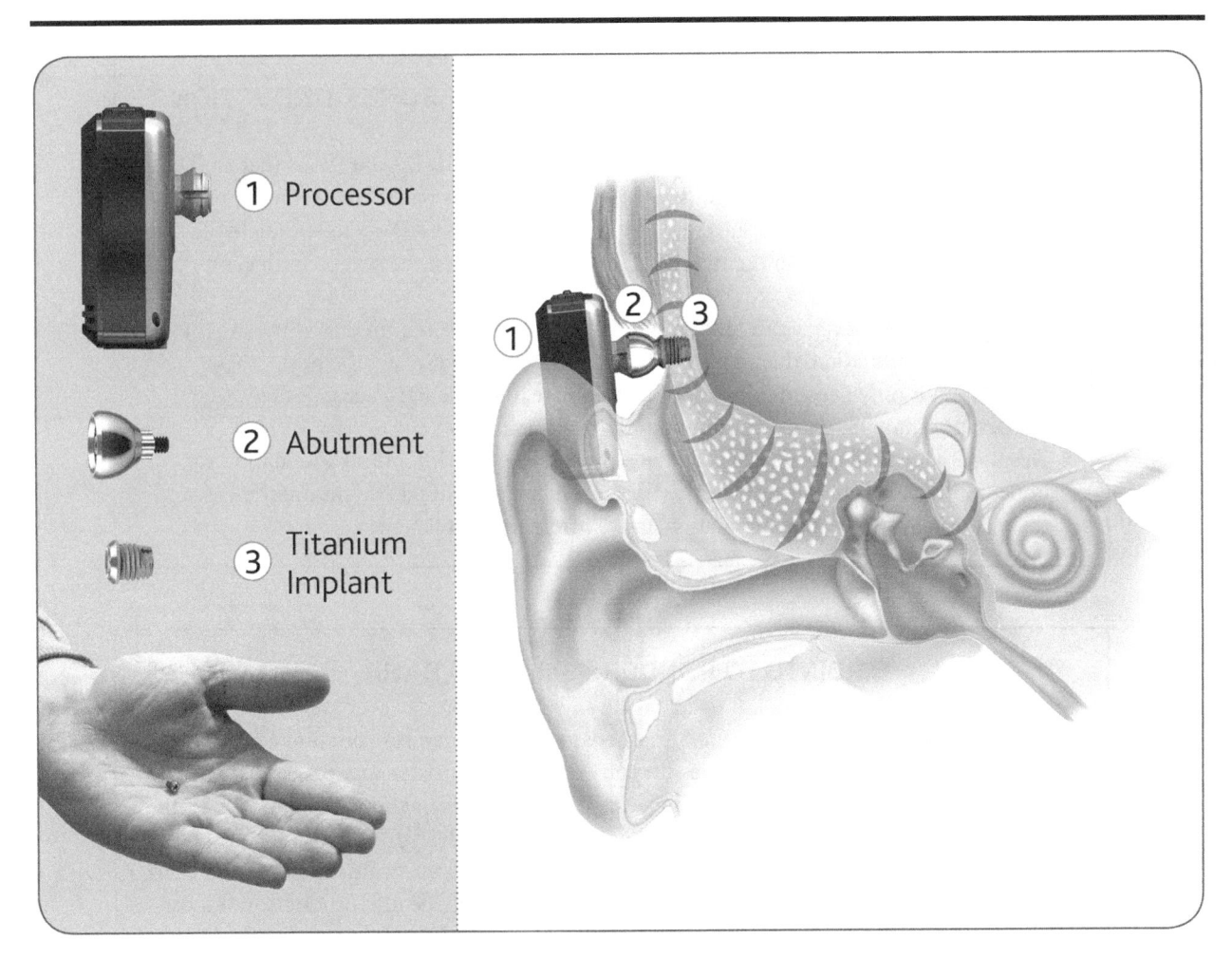

Figure 8–17. Schematic of the Baha® osseointegrated hearing device that stimulates the cochlea via bone conduction. (Photo courtesy of Cochlear® Americas).

to the implant have more recently been introduced, including the Baha® Attract, Sophono Alpha™, and the BoneBridge. These devices use strong magnets to hold the processor on the head in close proximity (through the skin) to the implant. Whereas these devices have a potential advantage for the somewhat rare patients who have issues with excessive skin growth or failure to heal when using percutaneous devices, the lack of direct coupling can limit the device output. Therefore, these magnetically coupled devices are not as appropriate when there is a sensorineural component of the hearing loss in the better ear.

Depending on the version of BAI, additional features including directional microphones and DAI are commonly available. A number of advanced processing features common in air conduction hearing aids—including multichannel directivity, multichannel gain processing, and digital feedback suppression—have also been introduced in some implantable bone stimulating devices. Although we introduced BAIs as a possible treatment for single-sided deafness, the original and continuing application for these products were for patients with permanent bilateral conductive loss and for mixed losses with limited sensorineural involvement. Data have shown that implantable bone stimulating devices can lead to a significant decrease in handicap, as well as an enhanced perception of general well-being and disease specific quality of life when compared with pretreatment across a range of conductive hearing loss etiologies (e.g., Laitakari et al., 1995; Lustig et al., 2001). BAI continues to be an effective and in many cases optimal treatment for listeners with bilateral conductive hearing loss and mixed hearing loss with at least somewhat limited sensorineural involvement. In the last few

---

KEY CONCEPT: HEARING THROUGH BONE CONDUCTION

- The bones of the skull can be stimulated directly by vibrations that are then carried through the skull to both cochleas with little attenuation.

It is interesting to note that bone conduction has been used as a way to stimulate the cochlea in patients with conductive hearing loss since at least the seventeenth century (Berger, 1976a).

- Unfortunately, however, a fair amount of vibration energy is required to stimulate the ear by bone conduction, due in part to the attenuation provided by the skin.
- Stimulation is only needed in one spot to stimulate both cochleas because the transcranial attenuation for bone conduction is usually low.
- Despite what you may have learned at one time or another, interaural attenuation for bone-conducted signals is not always 0 dB. There are individual patient differences, and there is usually significant attenuation above 5 kHz in most listeners.

POINTS TO PONDER: Baha AND BAHA

In this section we talk about the "Baha." A rather strange name, unless you think it's a botched spelling of Baja, California. Here's the story: In a former life, Baha was BAHA, which was an acronym for Bone-Anchored Hearing Aid. When Cochlear acquired the device in the mid-2000s, it was officially renamed an "osseointegrated cochlear stimulator"—a term more acceptable to insurance companies that do not reimburse for hearing aids. So today, we don't have a BAHA, but still do have a Baha, which is the name of specific products, not a class of products, amplification approach, or acronym. The original BAHA name for the class of products has generally been replaced with BAI.

decades, implantable bone stimulating devices have also been advocated for bilateral use in patients with bilateral mixed or conductive hearing loss.

Because bone conduction is able to provide stimulation to both cochleas at the same time, as we mentioned at the beginning of the section, these devices can also be used to treat single-sided deafness (Wazen et al., 2003). The Baha was FDA-approved to treat single-sided deafness in 2002, and data support these devices over traditional CROS in this population with regard to patient preference (Hol, Bosman, Snik, Mylanus, & Cremers, 2004; Niparko, Cox, & Lustig, 2003). The relative benefits for implantable bone stimulating devices and traditional CROS interventions for single-sided deafness are expected to be similar and mainly related to alleviation of some of the negative effects of head shadow.

As with other CROS applications, clinical verification is essential (see Dickinson, 2010, for review). Implantable bone stimulating devices may reduce or eliminate a number of complaints associated with traditional CROS. Specifically addressed are complaints of having to use two devices, the lack of low-frequency amplification reducing sound quality, and retention problems/discomfort from the retention mechanism associated, which are all associated with the traditional CROS. An obvious disadvantage to this surgical solution is that with a traditional CROS or the transcranial CROS options we discussed earlier, if the expected benefit is not present after 30 days, the patient can return the instrument. This is somewhat more difficult when there is an implanted titanium abutment.

As with all hearing aid styles, there are a few limitations to implantable bone stimulating devices. First, the lower power versions are primarily effective for patients with conductive hearing loss (no sensorineural component). According to the manufacturers, however, the power versions can be used with mixed hearing losses having sensorineural components of up to 50 dB HL (bone conduction average of 500, 1000, and 2000 Hz). In addition to hearing loss considerations, surgical care must be taken to ensure optimal placement on the side of the head, especially if a directional microphone is used. Finally, a limited percentage of patients will experience a few medical complications that are mainly related to percutaneous devices (Wade, 2002). The most common complications are unresolvable irritation around the abutment because of rejection of the percutaneous device or uncontrollable skin growth. We even know of a few patients for whom the abutment was completely covered by new skin growth during the healing period before initial fitting was possible. Most interestingly, some clinicians choose to implement the stimulating processor portion of implantable bone stimulating devices using a soft band or headband to avoid surgery. This appears to be particularly common for children and is required in children younger than five years. Although the soft band implementation removes the need for surgery, because the device is not directly coupled to the bone, less power will be transferred and the amount of power transfer will vary more across patients.

Middle Ear Implants

Middle ear implants (MEI) were developed for patients who have sensorineural hearing loss and are usually thought of as candidates for traditional air conduction hearing aids (Chasin, 2002). The use of MEIs for listeners with sensorineural hearing loss in lieu of conventional amplification stems from manufacturers' claims of improved fidelity, and the elimination of feedback and the occlusion effect in listeners fit with these devices (Arthur, 2002; Bankaitis & Fredrickson, 2002; Kroll, Grant, & Javel, 2002; Luetje et al., 2002; Uziel, Mondain, Hagen, Dejean, & Doucet., 2003). Results of studies investigating these claims have been mixed. It should be noted that some of the most popular MEI devices use essentially the exact same sound processing algorithms as are used in commercial air conduction hearing aids. The continued advancement of feedback suppression technologies and the OC style appears to further limit the potential advantages of this style over conventional air conduction hearing aids in listeners with mild to moderate hearing loss. The fact that these devices require surgical implantation must also be weighed against the strength of any advantages over air conduction hearing aids. The requirement of surgical implantation also precludes any usual trial period as removal also requires surgery.

In contrast, consistent patient preference has been shown for MEI devices in patients who have more severe hearing loss, particularly those who have rejected traditional air conduction hearing aids (Luetje et al., 2002; Uziel et al., 2003). The cosmetic appeal of this style would at first seem assured because of their implantable nature. Some of these devices are not fully implanted, however, and usually retain a small plastic case on the side of the head that houses the microphone and processing, shown in Figure 8–18. Regardless, these devices appear to be a reasonable alternative for some patients who are not satisfied with traditional air conduction hearing aids. This is particularly the case for those that who too much hearing loss to be fitted with open fitted air conduction instruments but desire a cosmetically appealing instrument with no occlusion effect and requiring limited care.

Other potential benefits of a MEI over conventional amplification relate to improved physical comfort (at least after surgery) because nothing is placed in the ear canal, and 24-hour hearing. That is, listeners may leave some of these devices on all of the time without ever having to worry about "forgetting their ears;" not being able to monitor for sounds during the night; or removing them during running, swimming or other physical activities during which perspiration or moisture could destroy a typical hearing aid. Current MEIs are based on piezoelectric, electromagnetic, or electrodynamics principles. Piezoelectric crystals bend in response to electrical charge, and the low power consumption and other factors in this design have led to devices that are fully implantable with a battery lasting an average of approximately five years. The other methods include mounting a very small vibrator (about the size of a grain of rice) on the ossicular chain or placing a very small magnet on the ossicular chain and *driving* it (forcing it to vibrate) with an oscillating magnetic field. Currently, three middle ear implant devices have received full FDA approval for implantation in adults, two partially implanted (Med-El Vibrant® Soundbridge™, Ototronix Maxum) and one fully implanted (Envoy Esteem®). A fourth fully implantable device is still waiting FDA approval (Cochlear™ Carina®). In some cases, it is possible to obtain third-party payment of implantation of MEIs.

Hearing Aid User Controls

Another decision that must be considered in concert with hearing aids style is the selection of user controls. In the past, small hearing aid styles were physically limited in size to such a degree that few user controls were possible. Some hearing aids in fact have no user control. More recently, possibilities related to user control have changed dramatically due to the introduction of smartphone apps, which we describe in more detail below and in Chapter 11. The need for user control of the hearing aid primarily depends on five factors:

- How well the audiologist programmed the hearing aids. If both the gain and output are set appropriately for a large variety of input signals at the time of the fitting, the patient will not need to make as many changes during use.
- How well the patient *trained* the hearing aids. If the hearing aids are trainable, and the patient actively adjusts gain for different settings during the first few weeks of use, there should be less need for a volume control once training is completed (see the section on trainable hearing aids in Chapter 12).
- The quality of the signal classification system and automatic functions of the hearing

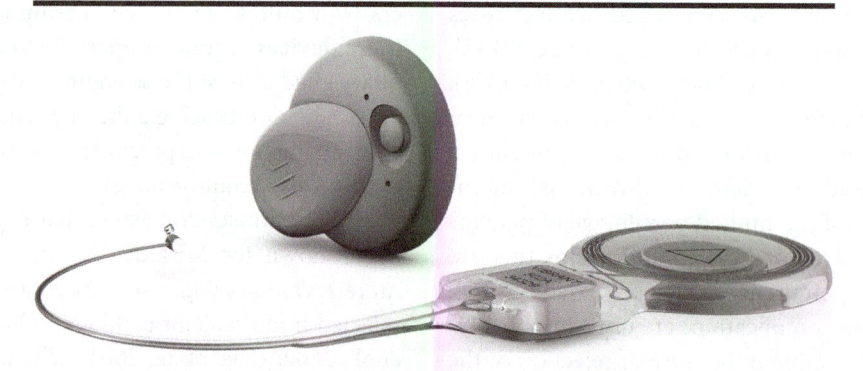

Figure 8–18. Schematic of a middle ear implant (Photo courtesy of Med-El).

aids. For example, if the classifier correctly identifies speech in noise and switches to appropriate directional and noise reduction characteristics, there is less need for the patient to change gain or programs.
- Lifestyle of the patient. If the patient has a very active lifestyle and different telephone and wireless streaming applications are included in the fitting, this will require more active program changes by the patient.
- The patient's interest in controlling the acoustic environment. Some patients like to fiddle and make discrete changes to the volume and other features as the listening environment changes.

Common physical controls on the hearing aid case include volume controls (VCs), *slider switches* (often used in BTE instruments to change user programs, activate telecoils, activate directional microphones, and turn the instrument on and off), and button/toggle switches (used in many styles to switch between programs or features or change the volume by repeatedly pushing either the same button or two different buttons). For bilateral fittings, hearing aids often are paired using wireless communication. This allows for simultaneous volume control changes on both hearing aids by only pushing the button on one of them. As an alternative, hearing aids may be fitted so the button on one side changes the gain and the button on the other side changes programs (memories).

User controls, including volume control, also can be placed on a separate remote control. Remote controls range from the extremely simple (a small magnet that can be used to activate a feature, change programs, or change volume using a magnetic sensor in the hearing aid) to the quite sophisticated (individual controls for on and off, volume and hearing aid user memories, frequency response, and special features). Today, the most common remote is an app for the patient's smart phone, which links wirelessly to the hearing aid. Because of the lack of size and processing limitations, these apps are often quite a bit more sophisticated than a simple volume and program control. For example, some of these apps include geo-tagging, which allows the patient to refine his or her settings for a number of specific locations (e.g. home, favorite restaurant) after which the app will automatically return to those preferred settings when the smartphones GPS and wireless locator systems indicate the listener has returned to the same location.

Since they were introduced in the 1980s, patient demand for remote controls has been fairly low. The low demand likely relates to complaints or concerns about keeping track of another device and cost, and/or the patient does not see any potential benefit. Today, given that most patients already own a cell phone and carry it with them, these reasons are less relevant. In general, audiologists do not seem to actively encourage the use of remote controls—they are not commonly included with the hearing aid purchase as they would be if you bought a TV or CD player. We'll see how all the new smart phone apps impact this.

In a study we conducted in the early 1990s, we found the most commonly cited patient benefit of a remote was being able to discreetly turn the hearing aid on and off (Ricketts & Bentler, 1992). For some patients, especially those who use multiple programs and are technology savvy, a hearing aid remote control or remote app can be desirable. Currently, companies are making hearing aid remote controls as part of wristwatches, pens, and key chains—although these are becoming rarer because of the increased use of smartphone apps. The increased use of smartphones for remote control stems in part from their use for streaming of audio wirelessly to the hearing aid (e.g., phone conversations, music, other apps). Other more modern uses include using the smartphone as an external microphone that allows wireless streaming from a remote location.

Over the last few decades, the routine use of amplitude compression processing has decreased the need for a patient control of hearing aid volume (level). The logic is that if the gain is programmed so that soft sounds are audible, average input levels are comfortable, and loud sounds are loud but not too loud, why does the gain need to be changed? Many patients, therefore, are perfectly happy to never have to adjust their hearing aid level using a VC. More recently, automatic systems have become increasingly sophisticated in their attempts to make accurate switching decisions for activation of hearing aid features. Previously, some features such as telecoils, different amplification characteristics for different environments (multi-user memories), and directional microphones required user input for activation. Although automatic switching systems are certainly not perfect, most patients are happy with them. Other patients who may or may not be happy with automatic systems are either unwilling or unable to switch features off and on manually because of physical limitations, inconvenience, or a host of other factors.

In contrast, some patients are willing, able, and interested in manipulating their acoustic environment. The sophistication of modern hearing aid apps is only expected to increase this interest. Such patients may be unhappy with automatic features and a lack of volume control or may appreciate sophisticated features like geo-tagging. Even before smart phone apps about half of patients if given a choice, preferred to have a VC (Dillion & Storey, 1998; Harnack, Knebel, & Bentler, 1998; Lunner, Hellgren, Arlinger, & Elberling, 1997; Surr, Cord, & Walden, 2001; Valente, Fabry, Potts, & Sandlin, 1998), and approximately one-third of hearing aid users without a VC desire one.

Whether or not a hearing aid has a VC may be key to the ultimate success of the end user. According to MarkeTrak surveys carried out over a 10-year period by Kochkin (2002), the difference in overall satisfaction ratings between consumers who need a VC and those who do not need a VC is almost 40%, and over three-fourths (75%) of hearing aid users rate the VC as highly desirable. In addition, 72% of U.S. consumers report wanting hearing aids that are easier to regulate. These data have been supported by more recent data suggesting that 77% of experienced hearing aid users wanted to have a VC no matter how infrequently they used it. For fitting success, most manufacturers have provided VCs that can be engaged or disengaged, depending upon the ultimate wishes of the consumer. The dB range of the VC also is programmable. It is important to assess each individual patient's needs relative to user controls by probing a few specific areas. Some questions that you might consider:

- Does the patient need features that need to be controlled?
- Does the patient use a smart phone and is he or she interested in smartphone control or would the patient prefer to have control by a switch? If the patient does not use a smartphone is the patient physically able to manipulate small controls?
- Has the patient used a VC in the past?
- Does the patient report frequently adjusting the volume of music and/or the television based on his or her mood or other factors?
- If the patient doesn't use a smartphone is the style under consideration too small for user switches and/or a VC? How many switches/controls are possible?

Obviously, the basic purpose of a VC is to provide patient control of amplification level. Although this seems like a good idea, it can also create problems. If the patient has dexterity problems, doesn't use a smartphone, and the VC is very small/sensitive, it may be

---

TECHNICAL TIP: MODERN HEARING AIDS AND VCS

The surveys we have reviewed were mostly conducted before hearing aids had the sophisticated switching capacitates that they have today, before smartphone apps were available, and also before the use of trainable hearing aids. As we review in Chapter 12, trainable hearing aids allow users to train the hearing aid to their desired use gain for a variety of inputs and environments. This is accomplished by storing the user's adjustments when he or she is in a given listening situation. For example, it is possible to train gain independently for soft, average, and loud inputs for speech in quiet, speech in noise, and music. Once this training has been accomplished, we would expect the need for a VC to decrease. This is especially useful for the very small products that do not have room for a VC and for which the training can be conducted using a remote. It is important to note that it has been shown that fitting to validated prescriptive targets prior to training is just as important with these modern hearing aids. That is, simply starting with minimal gain and allowing the patient to adjust the volume up to their preferred level does not lead to optimal outcomes, so appropriate verification is still critical.

> **TECHNICAL TIP: USING MEMORIES AS VC**
>
> One other method that can be very useful for patients who have poor dexterity but who desire some control over the hearing aid level is to use a program switch. Most hearing aids have three or four (or more) user memories that can be programmed to different VC settings. The level can then be adjusted by pressing a memory button on the hearing aid (most often a single button that toggles between available user memories) or on a remote control/app. We find this technique most useful if there are three to four user memories available. Two levels may not give the patient enough control (although this is fine for a few patients), and more than four levels can become confusing and/or difficult to manipulate. The audiologist will need to work with the patient to determine exactly what gain alterations are programmed, but often one memory might have gain 3 to 5 dB louder, another 3 to 5 dB softer, and if the patient has considerable low-frequency gain for the primary fitting, maybe a program that cuts some of the gain in this region. This technique, however, may not be possible if the user memories are already being used to activate other common features (e.g., wireless connectivity, bilateral beamformer, car programs, music programs).

accidentally adjusted during insertion, removal, or even through inadvertent movements. Some patients will have trouble getting the level adjusted just right or achieving a level balance between two hearing aids when using a VC on the hearing aid case. Fortunately, modern hearing aids have greatly enhanced the old-fashioned hearing aid VC. These enhancements that are available both for apps and VC on the hearing aid case include the ability to link the VC of two hearing aids together (changing the volume on one hearing aid changes both); clinician control of volume range and/or step size (e.g., volume range could be as small as 4 to 6 dB or as large as 16 dB or more); and in the case of some smartphone apps, frequency specific control of volume. Finally, for small children or others who may not be able to appropriately adjust level but for whom a VC is still desired, a screw-set VC may be used. This is simply a VC that must be set with a small screwdriver, although more commonly volume is adjusted through a smartphone app and the VC is removed from the hearing aid case.

Hearing Assistive Technology

One very important, but unfortunately often overlooked portion of hearing assessment for the purpose of (re)habilitation, is consideration of hearing assistive technology (HAT). This category includes any and all devices that are specifically used to assist patients with hearing difficulties other than the primary interventions of hearing aids and cochlear implants. A common, older term used to describe HAT that is still used by many people today is assistive listening device (ALD). We prefer the term HAT, as it is more descriptive and representative of the entire category of devices. For example, it seems odd to us to refer to a vibrating alarm clock as a listening device because this device has nothing to do with listening.

We think it is important to generally address HATs whenever considering hearing aid selection. HATs differ from hearing aids and cochlear implants in that they usually are aimed at addressing a small range of needs rather than general hearing problems. Therefore, HATs often fill a useful supplementary roll to hearing aids and, in some cases, more than one different type of HAT may be appropriate for the same patient. That is, some patients may benefit from two, three, or even several HAT devices. For some patients, however, the benefit provided by a HAT may not be large enough to warrant the cost and/or inconvenience. Trial periods may be used, but it is clear that not all patients are candidates for HAT. For still other patients, one or more HATs may be appropriate even when a hearing aid is not.

We had one such patient many years ago whose case still stands to remind us of this fact. This patient had few remaining family members, and a terminal

> **TECHNICAL TIP: COMMON USES FOR HAT**
>
> - Near-sound personal listening devices aimed at increasing the level of sounds near the listener (e.g., personal amplifiers (PSAPs), amplified stethoscopes)
> - Far-sound personal listening devices aimed at bringing sounds far from the listener effectively *nearer* (e.g., notetakers, speech-to-text systems, room loops, infrared systems, wireless routing from microphones including spouse microphone, FM microphone, sound field FM systems, and other devices that route signals of interest to the hearing aid or listener)
> - Alerting and warning devices (e.g., flashing and vibrating alarm clocks, smoke alarms, door bells, telephone ringers, and amplified telephone ringers and smoke alarms)
> - Telephone assistance (e.g., amplified telephones, teletypewriters, instant messaging translation services)
> - Smart Phone Assistance (wireless routing of cellphone conversation, music, sound from other cellphone apps to the hearing aid)
> - Television and radio assistance (e.g., closed captioning, television amplifiers—many personal listening devices can assist with television and radio listening)

illness was expected to provide him little remaining life. He desperately wanted, however, to see the Summer Olympics on television one more time before he died (something he and his deceased wife had enjoyed doing together). We set him up with a television amplifier that could also be used to amplify other voices in the room through a microphone when people came to visit. Although we are sure we did not achieve a perfect fit, the patient was able to understand the television announcer. The time and inconvenience to obtain the device was minimal on his part, and the device was quite inexpensive compared with a hearing aid. We had the satisfaction of knowing that we had enhanced his quality of life for the short time he had left.

This has just been a brief introduction to HAT, as it is something to think about while hearing aid style is selected. We devote a section in Chapter 12 to this topic, where you find a complete description of all the HAT options available.

Mini-Summary

- Many patients (as many as half) will be happier if they are given a VC, even if they have properly fitted compression. Most past VC users will want to have one in their new hearing aids. Modern hearing aids have several adjustments that can make a VC easier to use.
- Automatic systems will make more mistakes than a person manually switching (assuming the person actually switches when they should; many don't). A patient's desire to control his or her listening environment must be weighed against the patient's willingness to use controls when assessing manual versus automatic controls.
- HAT devices should always be in the back of your mind when assessing a hearing loss for the purposes of selecting hearing aids. Depending on the patient, HATs may not be needed, may be a useful addition to the hearing aid, or may be selected even if a hearing aid is not.

In Closing

Many of our patients may view differences in hearing aids style through the prism of cosmetics. Some may even go so far as to consider dexterity. In this chapter we have reviewed how style and coupling can have implications for everything from the MLE, which will affect SNR in the real world, to occlusion effect, to feedback issues and beyond. Furthermore, how important these effects are for individual patients will depend on everything from the type of signal processing used in the hearing aid, to the magnitude of hearing loss, to individual patient differences in preference and sensitivity. As we describe in Chapters 11 and 12, advanced signal processing will also interact with style and coupling. Altogether, this presents a complex clinical problem of determining the optimal feature setting/style/coupling tradeoff that maximizes benefits (speech recognition in quiet and in noise, overhearing, sound quality, localization, etc.), while minimizing annoyances and deficits (feedback, occlusion effect, background noise, unsatisfactory physical comfort, cosmetic concerns, usability and dexterity concerns, etc.) for each individual patient, based on his or her communication abilities and listening needs. Not an easy problem to solve in some cases, but our goal nonetheless.

Table 8–1. Summary of the benefits and limitations of different hearing aid styles.

Style	Main Advantages	Main Limitations
Body	Least susceptible to feedback, fit any degree of hearing loss through profound, user controls are the easiest to see and manipulate.	Unnatural microphone placement, bilateral fittings difficult, does not have sophisticated circuitry of other models, poor cosmetics.
Traditional BTE	Little susceptibility to feedback, fit any degree of hearing loss through profound, excellent venting flexibility, separation of receiver from the ear canal increases durability, good control of acoustics through plumbing, allows for directional microphone, telecoil, FM, DAI, most appropriate for children as the earmold can be remade to account for growth.	Cosmetics somewhat of a problem, considered the "old fashioned" hearing aid, tubing changes are required for maintenance.
Mini-BTE	Improved cosmetics because of size of instrument and slim tubing/wire. Use of RIC technology has potential for improved acoustics, and allows for unique sizes and shapes. Easily used for open fittings with stock eartips.	May not be large enough to accommodate all desired features, has less gain and output than traditional BTEs. Manipulation of these instruments can be quite challenging for patients with dexterity/vision problems.
Traditional Custom (ITE, ITC)	The largest sizes will be appropriate for most degrees of hearing loss, particularly when used with Digital Feedback Suppression though more susceptible to feedback than BTEs. Many allow for directional microphone and telecoil. Reducing size (ITE to ITC) may lead to improved cosmetics.	Smaller size may increase problems with manipulation for patients with dexterity problems as well as increasing problems with feedback and/or occlusion. The traditional ITC is mainly appropriate for patients with mild to moderate hearing loss.
Recessed Custom	Expected improvement of localization in the vertical plane and improved directivity in comparison to traditional custom instruments. Smallest sizes lead to improved cosmetics. May also lead to reduced wind noise and may allow more normal telephone use without feedback.	Increasingly smaller size may increase problems with manipulation for patients with dexterity/vision problems as well as increasing problems with feedback and/or occlusion. The recessed ITC is mainly appropriate for patients with mild to moderate hearing loss. Directional microphones and telecoils are not likely to be possible or available in the CIC or smaller ITC models.

continues

Table 8–1. *continued*

Style	Main Advantages	Main Limitations
Deep Canal CIC	The smaller residual ear canal volume allows for a less powerful amplifier. The DC CIC has all the advantages of the recessed CIC, but also can lead to a reduction or elimination of occlusion.	Many patients will not tolerate the deep tight fit because of discomfort. Discomfort can be minimized by using a softer tip but the subsequent "slit-leak" venting may result in feedback. Manipulation of these instruments can be quite challenging for patients with dexterity/vision problems. The DC CIC has most of the limitations of the recessed CIC, but may be fitted to patients with up-to moderately severe hearing loss if very tight.
Open-Canal Fitting	Lack of occlusion leads to a more natural sound of own voice and elimination of other problems related to occlusion, high cosmetic appeal, light and comfortable over the ear, natural sound quality for low frequency external sounds for patients with near normal low frequency hearing, often can be fit without using a custom earmold.	More prone to feedback. When mini-BTE RITA and RIC models are used, the thin tube in the RITA style can result in problems with cerumen clogging the tip. The RIC style can lead to increased problems with debris clogging the receiver as in the CIC style. The directional and noise reduction benefits will be more limited than in a closed earmold style. Limited gain makes them inappropriate for patients with severe hearing losses. Many models are only appropriate for patients with near normal low frequency thresholds.
CROS (Traditional CROS, BiCROS, Transcranial CROS)	Only for patients with profound hearing loss in one ear and either normal (CROS, TransCranial CROS) or mild/moderate hearing thresholds in the other ear. Can overcome hearing and SNR difficulties due to head shadow effects.	Benefit limited to very specific situations. Inconvenience of using two devices when there is mainly only hearing loss in one ear (CROS), poor sound quality (CROS, Transcranial CROS), physical discomfort (transcranial CROS), audible circuit noise (CROS) and poor cosmetics (CROS, BiCROS).
Bone Conduction	Directly stimulate both cochlea through bone conduction bypassing the middle and outer ears. This sound transmission path can be useful both for patients with primarily conductive hearing loss as well as patients with single sided deafness. For patients with single sided deafness fewer negatives are associated with the Baha device than with CROS or transcranial CROS (mainly related to sound quality, use of two devices and cosmetics).	As with CROS, benefit for patients with single-sided deafness limited to very specific situations. For patients with conductive hearing loss fewer negatives are associated with the Baha device than with traditional bone-conduction hearing aids (mainly related to comfort and the retention system). Surgery and appropriate placement are required for the Baha.
Middle Ear Implants	Potentially improved comfort and cosmetics compared to air conduction hearing aids for listeners with moderately severe (or better) sensorineural hearing loss. Advantages are particularly apparent in comparison to traditional, occluding custom hearing aids.	Requires surgical implantation. Benefits may be much more limited compared to some modern styles such as OC (studies still need to be done however). Much higher cost than traditional air conduction hearing aids (though patients out of pocket cost may be less due to third-party payment issues).

9
Ear Impressions, Earmolds, and Associated Plumbing

In the previous chapter, we discuss how the choice of hearing aid style not only affects cosmetics and available features but also can have important acoustic implications. More specifically, we know that hearing aid style can have considerable implications for amount of gain, potential feedback problems, and issues related to the occlusion effect. Although the general choice of hearing aid style will impact these factors, how tightly and deeply an instrument is fitted in the ear canal can also have a significant effect. That is, two different products that are both full-concha ITEs can have very different fit properties. The physical fit matters because it can affect the amount of venting (as detailed later in this chapter), as well as the overall wearing comfort for the patient. If the hearing aids are not comfortable, it is unlikely the patient will wear them.

For the majority of hearing aid styles other than the mini-BTEs, which are often fitted with non-custom coupling systems, the quality of the ear impression greatly affects how well a hearing aid shell or earmold physically fits an individual patient's ear. Therefore, we begin this chapter by discussing the process of taking ear impressions, followed by a discussion of physical hearing aid design factors affecting the acoustics of the sounds reaching the patient's tympanic membrane.

Although the physical fit can affect comfort and acoustics, the earmold or earshell is just one component of the overall sound delivery system, which also includes earhooks and/or tubing in BTE instruments, as well as damping, venting, receiver tubing, and a variety of other factors.

The sound delivered to the patient's ear(s) from the hearing aid can be significantly altered by the sound delivery system in a number of ways. We generally refer to this delivery system and the resulting physical changes as hearing aid *plumbing*, a term we think fits well, and that has been made popular in the 1970s by the publications of Samuel Lybarger and Mead Killion to refer to physical changes affecting earmold acoustics.

Ear Impressions

An ear impression is a physical or virtual cast of the outer ear and ear canal space. These impressions are used to make a negative cast of the outer ear (essentially trying to mimic the surface of the outer ear and ear canal in three dimensions), which is in turn used to make earmolds and earshells for custom instruments.

A well-fitted earmold or earshell is highly dependent on the quality of the ear impression. A poor impression-making technique can lead to custom hearing aids or earmolds that are consistently too loose or too tight, or that have uncomfortable pressure points.

The tools and techniques used to make ear impressions have changed over the years, and the technology for making these impressions, like all technology related to hearing aids, has experienced incremental improvements. Because of the different materials and techniques available, it is important to follow each individual manufacturer's instructions to ensure the best impressions possible. There are, however, some general techniques that we discuss here, that apply to all ear impression making. All methods are similar in that they require the same general steps:

- Thorough otoscopic examination of the ear and ear canal to assure that there are no conditions that would adversely affect the procedure (e.g., a large collection of cerumen, or sometimes even impacted cerumen is the most common)
- Placement of the ear dam/block (oto-dam/block)
- Preparation or mixing of the impression materials
- Insertion of the materials into the ear using an impression syringe or impression gun
- Allowance for curing time
- Careful removal and re-inspection of the ear

Syringe or Gun?

Impression material is commonly premixed and inserted in the ear using an impression syringe or automatically mixed using premeasured cartridges and mixing tips as shown in Figure 9–1. These are used with a manual or electric impression gun, sometimes called an impression pistol. Common impression syringes and impression guns are shown in Figure 9–2. Whether a syringe or gun is chosen depends on several factors, including the clinician's preference and the type of impression material. For example, extremely stiff impression material may require premixing and the use of an impression syringe. This is because the gun injectors may not be strong enough to extrude a very stiff material through the mixing tip. Cartridge guns are sometimes regarded as superior to syringes because there is an assumption

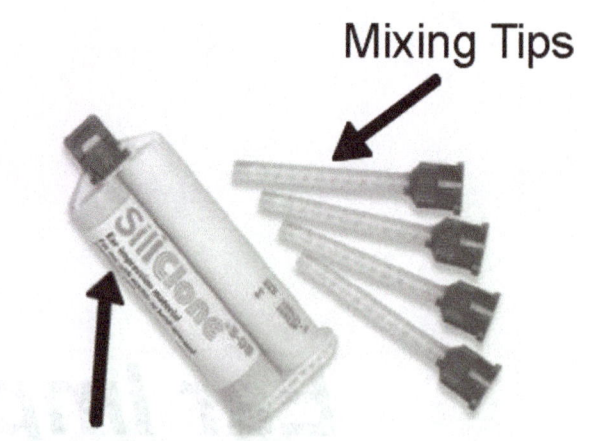

Figure 9–1. Example of one brand of premeasured cartridges and mixing tips used with impression guns. The mixing tip is attached to the end of the premeasured cartridge and then the entire assembly is attached to the impression gun as shown in the right-hand portion of Figure 9–2. (Reprinted with permission from Westone.)

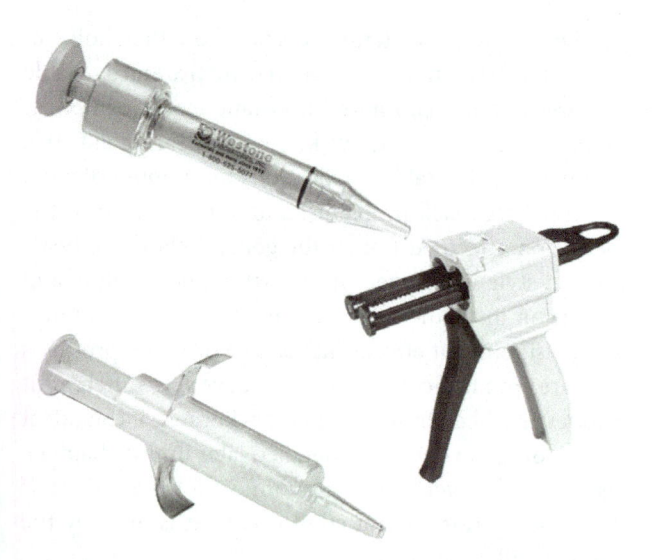

Figure 9–2. Examples of two different impression syringes (*left-hand side*) and a manual impression gun (*right-hand side*). Please note these are not to scale and the impression gun is much larger than the impression syringes. (Reprinted with permission from Westone.)

that the material flows more freely into the ear canal with this tool. However, currently available cartridge materials are designed specifically so that they do not flow freely. Regardless, we believe it is the injection technique, rather than the simple choice of material, that is most important for obtaining an optimal impression. That said, some materials will have a significantly longer time window to work with and therefore will be less exacting in the skill required to take a good impression.

> **THINGS TO REMEMBER: IMPORTANT IMPRESSION MATERIAL TERMS**
>
> **Viscosity:** A material's viscosity refers to its consistency. With regard to impression materials, this term applies to the consistency before the material hardens. In general, impression materials are often categorized as having low, medium, or high viscosity. A low viscosity material is soft and/or *runny* and flows easily; a higher viscosity material is often denser, firmer, thicker, and/or stickier. Of course the range of viscosity used in impression materials must fall within predefined limits; not so high as to distort the shape of the ear canal on insertion and not so low that it sags in the ear canal prior to hardening.
>
> - Lower viscosity materials are sometimes recommended as the default because they will lead to an impression that most accurately mimics the shape of the ear canal. Some low viscosity materials require particular care, however, because of concerns during the shipping process as described below.
> - A higher viscosity material is sometimes better to use on patients having a large amount of hair in their ears. This denser material will press down the hair, whereas low viscosity materials may flow through the hair, which can make the impression painful to remove and leave holes and flaws on the impression surface. A slightly higher viscosity is also expected to lead to a tighter fit, particularly, when taken with the jaw open using a bite block (as discussed later). Consequently, a medium or slightly higher viscosity material is often recommended as the default when used in combination with a bite block.
>
> **Shore Value:** After-cure hardness is commonly quantified using the hardness scale referred to as *Shore Value*. This is of little importance other than its relationship to damage during the shipping process. The after-cure hardness does not relate to viscosity.
>
> - There is also less of a relationship between the cured impression hardness and the ease of extraction from the patient's ear than might be expected. That is, in addition to the general hardness, the *slipperiness* of the cured impression material, which is often caused by an added material release agent, also has a large effect on the ease of impression extraction.
>
> **Contraction Ratio:** The contraction ratio describes how much an impression shrinks over time. Shrinkage of less than 3% is often considered acceptable; however, changing the recommended mixing ratio can result in shrinkage exceeding 20% (e.g., Pirzanski, 2003). Therefore, changing the mixing ratio from the recommended range in an attempt to soften the material and minimize the stretching of the ear tissue should clearly be avoided.
>
> **Stress Relaxation:** This is related to after-cure hardness and describes how well the impression returns to its original shape after being bent or stretched. It is clearly important that the impression does not change shape as a result of its removal from the patient's ear or during shipping or in-lab processing.

Impression Materials

There are three primary families of impression materials including ethyl methacrylate (powder and liquid), addition-cure silicone, and two-part vinylpolysiloxane, and each require slightly different preparation techniques. These general material types, as well as the specific products within them, also differ with regard to the specific properties of viscosity, stress relaxation, contraction ratio, after-cure hardness, and effectiveness of the release agent.

Powder and Liquid Material

The powder and liquid impression material has been available for several decades and produces a highly accurate impression if you follow a few basic rules (adapted from http://www.westone.com):

- A slight change in the ratio of liquid to powder can produce an impression that either sags because it is not stiff enough or expands in the ear canal because it is too dry. These problems can be minimized by using premeasured materials.
- Put the powder in after the liquid for easier mixing, and use a glass mixing bowl and metal spatula rather than wooden mixing spoons or other tools that may absorb liquid.
- Quickly mix the material and load the impression syringe; the curing process starts as soon as the powder and liquid come into contact.

Impressions taken with powder and liquid can prove superior to impressions taken with some of the lighter silicones described below that are applied using a gun-cartridge. This is related to the fact that mixed powder and liquid is more viscous compared with a light silicone but will expand the ear canal, enhancing acoustic seal and ensuring a secure fit for the earmold. Although generally more viscous than light silicones, the powder and liquid materials do not have a fixed viscosity; rather, they begin to increase in viscosity immediately after mixing. In addition, the powder and liquid materials have a very long shelf life compared to the silicone materials.

Although potentially yielding accurate impressions, there is a major limitation to powder and liquid materials that is significant enough that some manufacturers refuse to accept them. Namely, they produce impressions that have a low after-cure hardness and poor stress relaxation. Therefore, they are susceptible to damage during shipping or even removal from the ear canal if proper care is not taken. Shipping damage may be caused by physical trauma or heat. Furthermore, the magnitude of volume shrinkage is approximately 3% in seven days, so timely shipping is critical.

Earmold and hearing aid manufacturers suggest securing powder and liquid-based impressions to the bottom of the shipping box with an adhesive, such as household cement (e.g., Elmer's glue). In addition, nothing should be placed in the same box space with the impression to minimize distortion. Even taking these steps does not ensure there will be no distortion during shipping, however, particularly in the hot summer months.

Concern with damage during shipping is likely the reason for a decreased use of the powder and liquid impression materials. We believe, however, that given the high accuracy and low cost, these materials may see a comeback given that newer technologies allow for three-dimensional scanning of the finished impression. An electronic copy of the digital impression, which will not distort during shipping, can then be sent in lieu of a physical impression (see our section on scanning ear impressions). That is, if the impression is simply scanned immediately after it has been taken, many of the downsides of this material have been eliminated. That said, liquid and powder materials require working quickly due to their immediate and steady increase in viscosity, so if they do make a comeback, clinicians will likely need appropriate training to consistently produce accurate impressions.

Condensation-Cure Silicone

This impression material is commonly distributed in two parts: a large container containing silicon that requires use of a manufacturer-supplied measuring scoop and a tube of catalyst. This material may also be found in cartridge form for use with an impression gun. Condensation-cure, hand-mixed silicones are either medium or higher viscosity when compared with all available materials. In contrast, the lighter cartridge system materials typically exhibit low to medium viscosity. Condensation-cure silicone maintains a fixed viscosity for a brief period of time, typically less than one or two minutes, depending on the specific material.

For the hand-mixed versions, it is particularly important that the clinician always follow the specific manufacturer's instructions for preparation. In general, these instructions are similar to the following:

- Prepare the material by first flattening out a recommended measurement of impression material on a mixing surface.
- Then *draw* a line of catalyst (using the manufacturer-recommended amount) on top and mix.
- Mixing can be done in your hand, but a metal mixing blade and hard mixing surface is recommended for hygienic reasons—so your skin does not need to contact the material.
- The material needs to be mixed quickly until it reaches a consistent color and is loaded into the impression syringe. Mixing needs to be done in 20 to 30 seconds or the material will become too hard before completing insertion of the impression material.
- Using a little extra catalyst to speed things up, or a little less to slow things down, is usually not recommended because the material may harden too quickly or reach an inappropriate final consistency. It should be noted, however, that adjustment in the amount of catalyst used is sometimes necessary, as the effectiveness of some catalysts decreases with age (although, it is probably best to just throw the old catalyst away and buy new).

The relatively limited hardening time, limited shelf life, and imprecise method for obtaining the proper mixture ratio (especially obtaining the correct amount of the catalyst) have likely all led to the limited popularity of the hand-mixed condensation-cure silicone materials.

Addition-Cure Vinylpolysiloxane

This material, which is also commonly referred to as silicone, is the most popular impression material in use. It is commonly available in bulk containers, individual portion packs, or in cartridges for use in an impression gun. Addition-cure, hand-mixed silicones are either medium or higher viscosity when compared with all available materials. In contrast, the less dense (light) cartridge system materials typically exhibit low to medium viscosity. Addition-cure silicone maintains a fixed viscosity for a brief period of time. For cartridge silicones, this time ranges from one to two minutes; for hand mixed silicones, it is typically two to four minutes. After this brief period of approximately stable viscosity ends, the viscosity increases rapidly to its final cured level (sometimes referred to as the *snap* effect).

The components for all hand-mixed silicones are supplied in contrasting colors to provide means of indicating when a uniform (streak-free) mix is achieved. Addition-cure silicone has several desirable attributes that have led to its popularity. For example, these materials typically exhibit an excellent contraction ratio, shrinking from 0.1 to 0.7% in seven days, and exhibit good stress relaxation properties, with a 99.4% (±0.5%) return to original shape after application of stress (Pirzanski, 2003). As a consequence, silicone impressions do not generally need to be glued to the shipping box. These materials do have a limited shelf life of approximately one year, however. Consequently, long-term storage of an accurate ear impression requires a 3D digital image scan of the impression, regardless of the type of impression material used—a common practice by earmold manufacturers.

Making a Good Ear Impression

Now that we have discussed the different impression materials and their preparation, let's get down to the *technique* of making a good ear impression. You know the old saying, "You only have one chance to make a first impression"—so let us see if we can help you get your first one right by using this step-by-step procedure.

Step One: Before beginning the impression-making process, it is important that appropriate hand washing and other infection control procedures are followed.

Step Two: The patient's ear must first be thoroughly examined. We assume that an otoscopic examination was completed at the beginning of the assessment and that you are already familiar with these techniques from your hearing evaluation coursework. Regardless, it is important to re-inspect the ear just prior to making an impression to become familiar with the shape, angle, and depth of the individual patient's ear canal, and to determine if there are any impression contraindications. Contraindications include, but are not limited to, impacted earwax, foreign objects (should be removed prior to taking the impression), active fluid discharge, perforated eardrum, and inflammatory conditions such as swimmer's ear—which should be medically resolved prior to taking the impression. In addition, there are a host of other things you might see that may require increased care or surgical intervention prior to taking the impression (e.g., bony growths/exostosis, collapsed canal, enlarged canal, thick hair growth, cauliflower ear, mastoidectomy, or other surgical deformation). Some of these conditions can be overlooked as they will be irresolvable, but they may lead to a poor impression and may need to be discussed with the manufacturer constructing the earmold or custom hearing instrument.

Step Three: Once all contraindications are accounted for, an appropriate ear dam needs to be selected based on the otoscopic examination. An ear dam is a manufactured block that is intended to stop impression material from traveling too far into the ear canal or making contact with the tympanic membrane. Yes, we have had personal experience viewing an audiologist who forgot to use an ear dam and painfully (for both the patient and the audiologist) extracted the patient's tympanic membrane and ossicles along with the ear impression. This is a mistake you do not want to make; avoiding it is worth the trouble of carrying around this disturbing mental image. This also can happen when the ear dam is too small, as the material will go around the dam and reach the eardrum. This is referred to as *blow-by*—again, something to avoid. We have found the combination of low viscosity material combined with a round (cotton) ear dam which is too small can be particularly susceptible to blow-by. This susceptibility is because the low viscosity material can start to slide by the ear dam causing it to roll allowing more material travel further in. Fortunately, most modern impression materials have a much better release agent which prevents the impression material from bonding with the skin (including the tympanic membrane). Therefore, while extraction will likely still be painful, careful extraction even after a blow-by, typically does not result in any lasting damage.

Ear dams should be selected to be slightly larger than the ear canal. Such an ear dam is compressed slightly by the canal walls, which act to create a better barrier and hold it in place against the force of the impression material. Care must be taken, however, to make sure that an ear dam that is too large is not selected because it can lead to discomfort or stretching of the ear canal, and it can prevent you from obtaining a deep enough impression. Ear dams commonly consist of a rounded block of foam or cotton that is connected to a string or tube that aids in removal of the ear dam if it does not come out with the impression material. When a very tight impression is needed, or a material is chosen that does not have an effective release agent, there may be discomfort when removing the impression because of suction. In addition to using a proper impression removal technique (described below), this discomfort also can be alleviated by using vented ear dams. In a vented ear dam, the removal string is replaced with a thin pressure release tube that allows for pressure equalization during removal (see Figure 9–3).

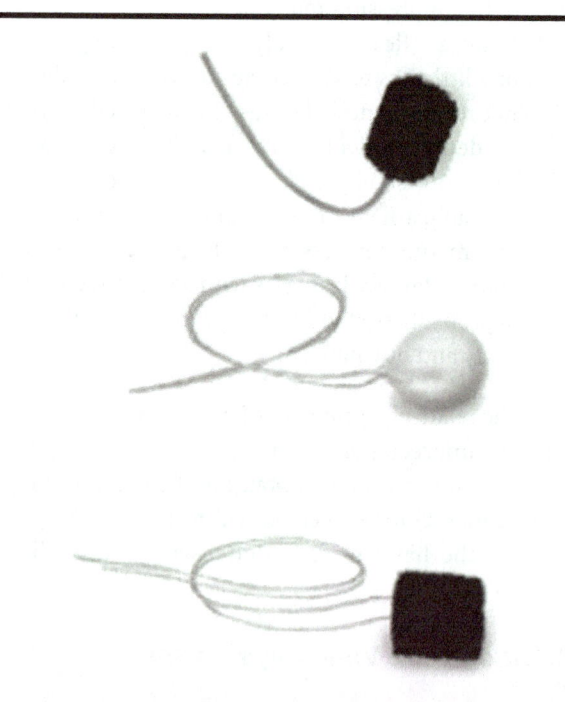

Figure 9–3. Three examples of common ear dams including (1) vented foam block with pressure release tube (*top*), (2) cotton material with string (*middle*), (3) foam block with string (*bottom*). (Reprinted with permission from Westone.)

Step Four: Once the proper size ear dam has been selected, it is placed in the ear with an ear light, as shown in Figure 9–4. Then, an otoscope is used to verify that the dam is placed properly. The ear dam should be placed beyond the second bend in the ear canal. This is the case even if a shorter canal portion is being ordered, so that the receiver can be properly angled. A receiver wrongly pointed at an ear canal wall can greatly increase the susceptibility to feedback. As with an otoscope, it is important to properly brace the ear light by making contact with the patient's head with at least one finger of the hand holding the ear light. This is critical because children can wiggle, and even adults can experience a cough or gag reflex when you touch their ear canal. To get the ear dam in place appropriately, it is often best to gently work it into place by pushing around the edges of the ear dam with the ear light. This ensures that it does not tumble sideways, as can often happen when it is simply pushed straight in.

Step Five: After placing the ear dam as described previously, mix the materials and put them in the impression syringe or gun (or prepare the mixing syringe tip). If the materials are mixed before placing the ear block, they should be thrown away and the process started over. The cost of the impression material is simply not worth a potentially bad fit because the material was too firm on insertion. The patient should be seated, with his or her head tilted slightly away from you.

- Brace the syringe using your little finger and place the end of the syringe approximately 0.25 inches inside the ear canal opening. Gently squeeze the material into the ear canal, allowing it to flow back over the syringe tip. Once the material starts to flow past the tip, start backing the tip out of the ear canal. The tip should always remain embedded in the impression material, however.
- As the tip leaves the ear canal, fill all the spaces, cracks, and crevices of the ear. We suggest you start with the concha bowl, move up into the antihelix crevice, then follow the contour of the ear, finishing at the center of the concha. This of course is not as critical for a CIC as for a full concha earmold or custom instrument, but it is best to have a full impression (a potential CIC fitting may turn into a full-concha fitting).
- Once completed, it is recommended that you leave the impression material untouched while hardening. After the impression material hardens for the manufacturer-specified hardening time, check to see if the impression has cured by pressing a plastic card or fingernail gently into the material to see if an indentation remains.

Step Six: To remove the impression, gently pull the patient's pinna up and back to break the seal. It may require a little wiggling and a couple tries. Remove the impression from the antihelix area and gently rotate forward and out. The removal string or vent tube can be used to remove the ear dam if it remains in the ear canal—typically it becomes attached to the impression.

Step Seven: Finally, after removing the impression, check the ear canal with your otoscope to assure that it is free from any material remaining from the impression process. Some slight redness may be evident and is normal.

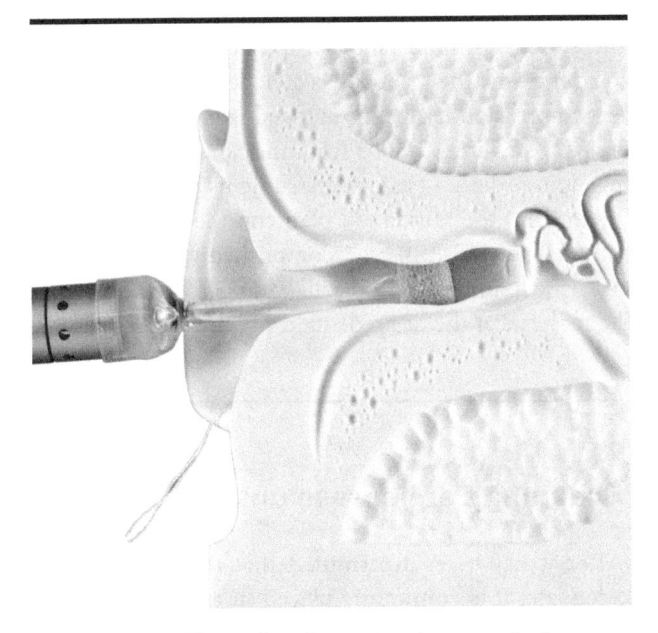

Figure 9–4. Example of proper placement of an ear dam using an ear light. The tip of the ear light is used to press around the edges of the ear dam so that it goes in straight without rolling into the ear canal. (Reprinted with permission from Westone).

> ### TECHNICAL TIP: OPEN OR CLOSED JAW?
>
> There has been a lot of debate regarding what patients should do with their jaw while the impression is being taken. This debate results from data that clearly show that patients' ear canal size and shape can be dramatically altered by jaw position (e.g., Darkner, Larsen, & Paulsen, 2007; Oliveira, 1997). Our experience leads us to believe that, for most impressions, it is best to have the patient open and close the mouth and move the jaw around during the impression. For a tighter fit, however, the patient should be required to keep his or her mouth open using a bite block. In fact, many experts recommend the bite block procedure as a default because it will lead to the best possible seal in the resultant earmold or earshell. Like others (e.g., Pirzanski, 1998), we have had the least amount of success with closed-mouth impressions.

> ### TECHNICAL TIP: MARKING EAR IMPRESSIONS FOR MICROPHONE PORT OPENINGS
>
> As we discussed in Chapter 8, the case or shell of custom hearing aids have one or two microphone port openings. When microphones are used to obtain a *directional effect*, which is the design of the majority of custom hearing aids today, there will be two port openings. The angle formed by drawing a line between these ports when the hearing aids are placed on the ear, relative to the horizontal plane, is important for obtaining the desired directional effect. When custom instruments are ordered, therefore, it is important that the manufacturer knows the horizontal plane, as this will determine how the faceplate is attached. This cannot be determined very accurately once the ear impression has been removed from the ear. The directional effect can be reduced for relatively small deviations from the horizontal plane—anything >15 degrees. For this reason, when ordering custom instruments with directional technology, we recommend *scoring* (marking) the horizontal plane on the ear impression while the impression is still in the patient's ear. This can be accomplished with a marking card, furnished by most manufacturers (most any rigid card will work). Some audiologists simply affix a plastic paper clip in the material at the desired angle. Do not use a pen marker, as this may rub off.

After making an impression, it should be inspected to make sure that the necessary canal length and all anatomical landmarks are present. If not, another impression should be taken. A bad impression results in a bad earmold or custom hearing aid shell, and this is not something our patients are content to just live with, nor should they have to. If you make a bad impression, which will happen, simply let the patient know it is important to get the impression perfect for a good fit, and it sometimes requires more than one try.

Scanning Ear Impressions

After it has been determined that the impression is adequate, it is commonly placed in a box and mailed to an earmold or hearing aid manufacturer so that an earmold or custom product can be ordered. As we have discussed, there is some concern that the important fine details of the impression can be altered through this mailing process (e.g., shrinkage, damage from excessive heat, squashing). For this reason, technologies that can perform three-dimensional scans of earmolds in the clinician's office and store the earmold as a digital image have been introduced. The first such device designed to do so was the iScan, which was introduced by Siemens in 2005. This technique of creating a *virtual earmold*, as seen in Figure 9–5, has the benefits of avoiding any shipping related deformation of the ear impression and providing a non-shrinking, permanent impression that can be easily stored and used for making future additional earshells or earmolds.

The first scanning devices that were commonly used are about the size of a computer printer and use three-dimensional technology with color-coded triangulation. The newer devices are increasingly small and very low cost, very portable 3D scanners are increasingly available. Typically the ear impression is affixed to a rotating platform where a projector illuminates it with colored light stripes from different angles. The light stripes conform to the object's surface in line with its geometry. This is simultaneously captured with a camera. The process takes about two minutes or less.

Changes, markings, or comments to assist in the fabrication can be made by the audiologist directly on the digital scan. The resulting scan can then be e-mailed to the earmold lab or the manufacturer. The reported benefits of using the scanner include:

- Elimination of the shrinkage and damage that occurs during shipping;
- A digital record of impression is available, which can be used for remakes (e.g., lost or damaged earmolds/hearing aids);
- Electronic method for indicating where changes need to be made on remakes (the audiologist can draw and write on the scan);
- Reduced turnaround time;
- Reduced cost through elimination of shipping expenses;
- Convenience (impressions do not have to be boxed-up, and orders can be placed at any time, night or day).

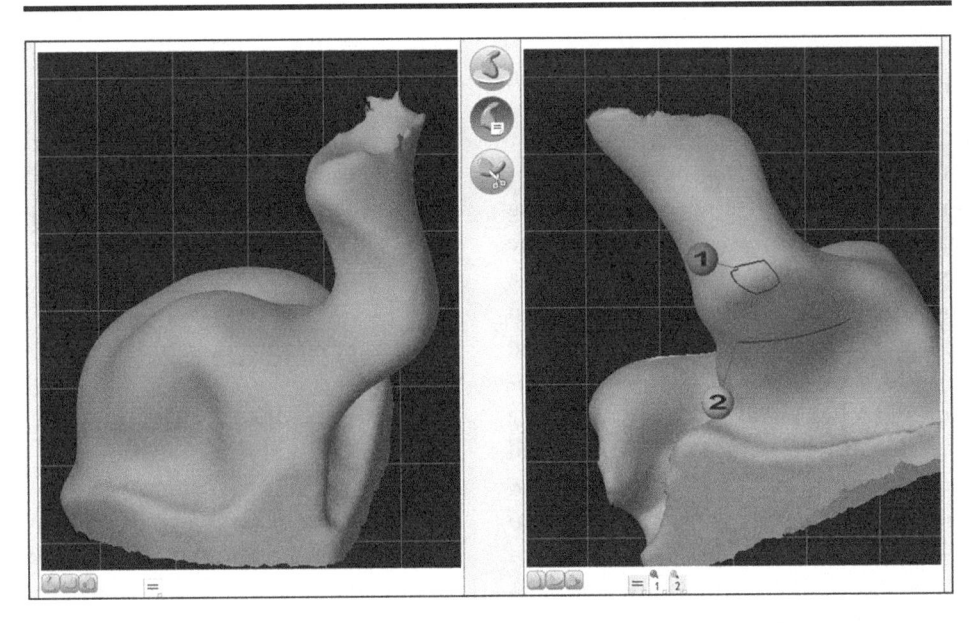

Figure 9–5. Example of a left and right scanned ear impression. These scans are three-dimensional and can be rotated so that the entire impression can be viewed. See numbering and marks on the right scan. An advantage of this procedure is that the audiologist can digitally mark the impression at specific points and make notes to the manufacturer regarding what needs to be done for these areas. Where to cut the canal is a common instruction. In this case, the previous earmold was causing irritation in the area of #1, and extra smoothing was therefore requested. Photo courtesy of Sivantos.

One manufacturer, who has had the option of electronic earmold scanning available for several years, reports that about 60% of its customers have the earmold scanning equipment, and those that have the equipment use scans for about 70 to 80% of their orders. In the past, unfortunately, the scanners have been linked to specific hearing aid and earmold manufacturers, thus limiting utility and the choice of product when ordering. This is increasingly changing. The iScan, introduced a few years ago was the first scanner to use an open data format so audiologists can transfer electronic impressions independent of the manufacturer. This technology continues to become more available and is expected to be commonplace soon.

It should be acknowledged that the effectiveness of such technology is still limited by the fact that if the ear impression is poor to begin with, the scan will simply reflect this. The true gold standard will be three-dimensional imaging of the outer ear and ear canal. We have little doubt that this technology will someday be available for hearing aids as it already exists in other fields. Currently, however, it is not cost-effective for routine clinical use.

Selecting Earmold Material and Styles

We discussed the selection of hearing aid style in Chapter 8; however, if the BTE style is selected (including both traditional and mini-BTE instruments), and if the manufacturer's modular eartips are not used, there is a secondary process of selecting the earmold or custom eartip. The choice of earmold will depend on several factors, some of which are similar to the factors considered when choosing a hearing aid style. They include the degree of hearing loss, how much venting is needed (based in large part on hearing loss configuration, low frequency gain needs and quality of the feedback suppression algorithm you are ordering), shape and size of the external ear, texture and sensitivity of the patient's skin, stiffness of the patient's external ear, and potentially other factors. Because all of these factors are important, how the choice of earmold material and earmold style might interact with the patient and the fit must be considered at every step in this process. Let us start by considering earmold materials.

Earmold Materials

There are three primary families of earmold materials including acrylic/lucite, polyvinyl chloride (vinyl/PVC), and silicone, each of which has potential benefits and limitations. A fourth material type, polyethylene, is used less often. It is similar in advantages and disadvantages to acrylic; however, it is slightly more prone to feedback, and it is also sometimes criticized for its plastic-like appearance. It is, however, the most hypoallergenic of all the materials.

Acrylic/Lucite

This material may be regular or body temperature reactive, that is it gets slightly softer when warm.

- Positives: Because it is very hard, it is possible to make thin ridges; it keeps its shape without shrinking, is very durable, and is easy to modify. The hard slick surface also makes earmolds made of this material easier to insert and remove. It is fairly hypoallergenic and the best material for many older patients.
- Negatives: Because of the hardness, it will not bend or compress to get past narrow openings on insertion, and it may be more prone to feedback. Studies suggest, however, that a tight seal can be obtained with this material as well as with softer materials. Not usually recommended for children for fear of ear injury if struck on the ear while wearing the earmold.

Polyvinyl Chloride

This material is often available in softer (recommended for children) and harder varieties.

- Positives: Softer and more comfortable than acrylic. Softness makes it appropriate for children and for hearing losses in the moderate to severe range. Although not as slick as acrylic, it is also not as tacky (sticky) as silicone, making it reasonably easy to remove and insert.
- Negatives: Not very durable, lasting from four months to two years depending on body

chemistry. Soft nature makes them much more difficult to modify than acrylic. More prone to discoloration after time. Problematic for patients with vinyl allergies.

Silicone

This material is often available in tacky/low pressure cured (recommended for greater hearing loss) and high pressure cured varieties.

- Positives: Soft and tacky nature makes this material appropriate for children and ideal for severe to profound hearing loss; it is fairly hypoallergenic.
- Negatives: Soft nature makes it much more difficult to modify than acrylic. Soft and tacky nature makes it the most difficult to insert and remove (especially difficult for floppy ears) and can cause skin abrasions in patients with fragile skin. Tubing adhesive does not bond well with some versions, leading to the need for a mechanical tubing lock. A variety of versions are now available, however, which at least partially counteract these negatives.

THINGS TO REMEMBER: MINI-SUMMARY

- There is no one best viscosity. Rather than using a single type of impression-making material for all patients, it is sometimes useful to choose a type that better addresses a patient's specific situation. For example, a higher-than-usual viscosity may be chosen for a patient with particularly hairy ear canals, whereas a medium to slightly higher viscosity in combination with a bite block may be chosen when a particularly tight fit is desired.
- In all earmold impression materials, it is desirable to have an effective release agent. A contraction ratio of less than 3% over the time period between making the impression and its use by manufacturers. Low stress relaxation is important, particularly if the impression is being mailed.
- Acrylic earmolds have the advantages of being long lasting and easy to modify but generally are not recommended for children. In contrast, polyvinyl chloride earmolds are softer, still reasonably easy to remove and insert, but are generally not very durable. Finally, silicone earmolds are soft and fairly hypoallergenic, but they may require a tubing lock and their tacky (sticky) nature can make them more difficult to insert and remove; they are generally not recommended for individuals with fragile skin.

POINTS TO PONDER: DECISIONS, DECISIONS

We have provided a relatively simplified listing of the earmold materials available—limiting it to the three general categories. On the day of the order, however, consider that it might be a bit more complicated. The following is the list of the *8 material options* for just one earmold style from just one of the major manufacturers: Acrylic Standard, Acrylic with e-Compound, Acrylic Flex Canal, OtoBlast™ silicone, AquaNot Silicon, W-1™ silicone, Formula II™ vinyl, RX™ vinyl and Polyethylene. Many of these are available in dozens of colors and finishes. Once comfortable with a manufacturer, the clinician can learn the subtleties of a particular manufacturer's material potions to select the best materials for every patient.

Earmold Styles

Now that we have considered earmold materials, let us discuss earmold styles. One of the things that makes selection challenging is that there are so many different styles, and many manufacturers use different naming schemes. Even within the same manufacturer, naming schemes are often either non-descriptive (e.g., based on numbers or letters) or inconsistent (e.g., depending on the earmold, descriptive names, inventor names, application names, and function names are used).

It is very important, therefore, that you really get to know the earmold manufacturer(s) whom you decide to use most often. Given the large number of names and the fact that we recommend you get to know individual manufacturers, we only provide a few general categories. First, let's talk about a few earmold landmarks. The earmold landmarks generally either correspond to a particular shape or landmark on the pinna or the external ear canal. Although you have probably heard all these terms before, we will revisit the pinna landmarks that are commonly used with earmolds in Figure 9–6 as a reminder. With attention to this figure, it should then be possible to match where specific portions of the earmold shown in Figure 9–7 fit in the ear. One other common earmold term not shown on this figure is *canal lock*. A canal lock is a small section encompassing only the *heel* and *antitragus* portions. There is not a complete concha portion when using an earmold with a canal lock.

With this terminology in mind, let us examine a few general categories of earmold style, as shown in Figure 9–8. Depending on your patient population, the earmold manufacturer(s) you choose, and the types of hearing aids you fit, you will likely learn many clinical tricks and shortcuts that improve your clinical skills with earmolds. We offer a few tips here that we have found to be useful over the years:

- Although seemingly logical, it is not the case that bulkier earmolds guarantee more gain before feedback. The accuracy of the earmold impression is often more important than the style of the earmold when concerned about maximum amplification.
- A variety of canal lengths are possible in nearly all custom earmold styles; longer canals are generally associated with less feedback if they fit tightly, but more feedback is possible if they terminate facing a canal wall.

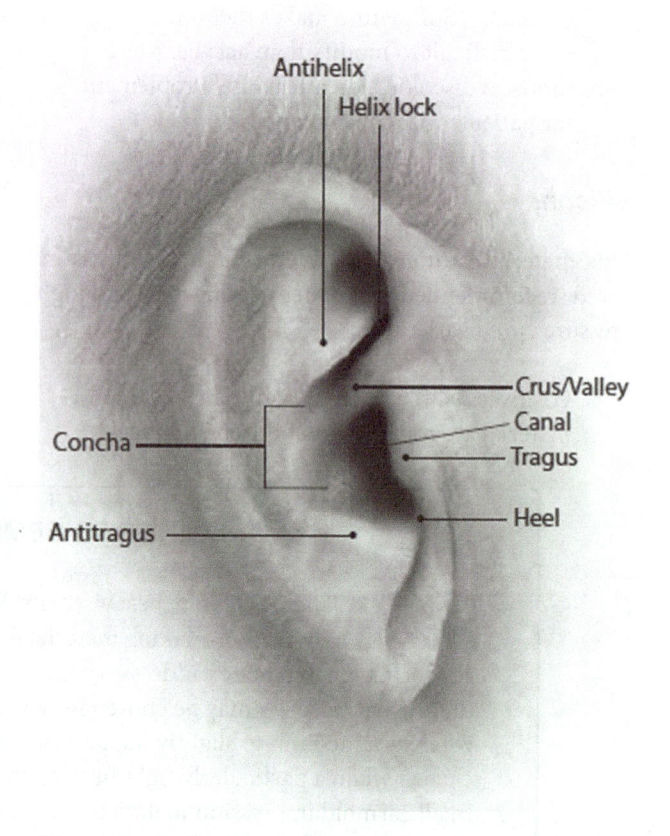

Figure 9–6. Common pinna landmarks corresponding to earmold landmarks. One can see how the earmold fits into the ear by comparing to the labeled landmarks in Figure 9–7. (Reprinted with permission from Westone.)

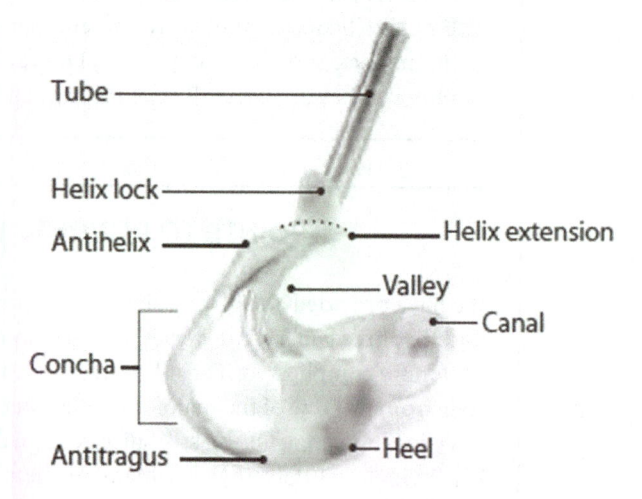

Figure 9–7. Common landmarks used when ordering and naming earmolds. These are useful when describing where problem areas are or where modifications need to be made. (Reprinted with permission from Westone.)

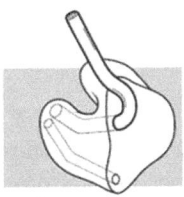

Full Shell
- Often used for more severe to profound hearing losses and younger children
- Canal portion can be made thicker (better seal), thinner (for better cosmetics), fitted with a snap ring instead of tubing (for body aid, powered stethoscopes, etc.), or the top portion of the canal can be removed (half shell).
- Can be difficult to insert if tight fitting.

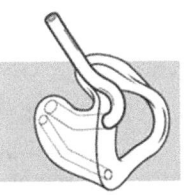

Skeleton
- One of the more common styles used with traditional BTE hearing aids.
- Can be used with a wide range of hearing loss.
- Sometimes modified to remove the middle portion of the "ring" that fills the concha bowl (semi-skeleton).

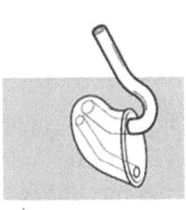

Canal
- Not usually fit as tight, so it is more suitable for mild-moderate loss. Appropriate for some patients with severe hearing loss using soft materials. Retention can be a problem, though easier insertion than many styles.
- Can be modified with a "concha lock" or by hollowing out the canal (sometimes combined with soft material for a comfort fit for patients with large changes in earcanal size with jaw movement).

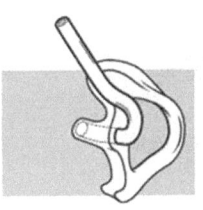

Custom Open
- Many styles with various combinations and configurations of the heel, concha and helix lock portions.
- Can be used for CROS style, open fits with BTE style or with the OC style for better retention than non-custom open.

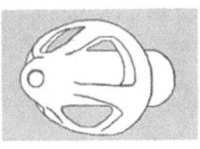

Non-Custom Mini-BTE
- Usually manufacturer specific and using tubing with a very narrow inner diameter.
- Both RITA (tube) and RIC styles available.
- Can have some problems with retention for which a custom solution is suggested.

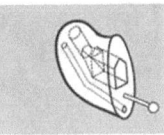

Custom Mini-BTE
- Similar to the standard canal, but intended to be used with specific models of deep canal (occluding) RIC fittings. Manufacturers often supply non-custom versions, but custom versions are often available from earmold companies when better retention is desired.
- Usually made using soft materials.

Figure 9–8. Advantages and limitations to a few common earmolds. This information is particularly useful when deciding on an earmold style within the constraints of individual patient differences, cosmetics, and gain requirements.

- Tapering the end of the canal can make insertion easier and may add comfort, but it may increase chances of feedback.
- Canal locks do not always help as much as one might think with retention. A small *wire retention adapter* (a thin stiff plastic line or plastic coated wire) can sometimes help with retention.
- Avoid tacky earmold materials for older patients with thin skin to prevent insertion abrasions.
- Buffing and grinding works well for major and minor modifications of acrylic, but use of a scalpel or razor blade (and a steady hand) is needed for softer materials, and major modifications usually are not possible in these softer earmolds.

Modular Earmold Plumbing

As we have mentioned, today's mini-BTE products come with an assortment of modular/semi-disposable earmold fittings. Originally, the mini-BTE products were designed to be fitted in an open manner, so a small supply of non-custom open tips was provided. As the fitting ranges have expanded, so has the selection of plumbing options. There is a large array of products from all manufacturers. An example of the variety of fitting tips for just one product is shown in Figure 9–9. Moreover, the mini-BTE hearing aids can be RITA or RIC, which means that different fitting kits are needed depending on the location of the receiver. The RITA also has the thin tubing, which replaces the standard tone hook/tubing that comes in different lengths. There also is a screw-on version of the thin tubing, which can be used with traditional BTEs. The RIC also has different wire lengths, as well as different size receivers (e.g., required for different maximum gain levels, such as 45, 55, and 65 dB).

Manufacturers provide kits that include all the tips and tubing that are used for these modular fittings. The fitting kits also often include tube shapers, measuring gauges, wax guards, and cleaning wires. It can be con-

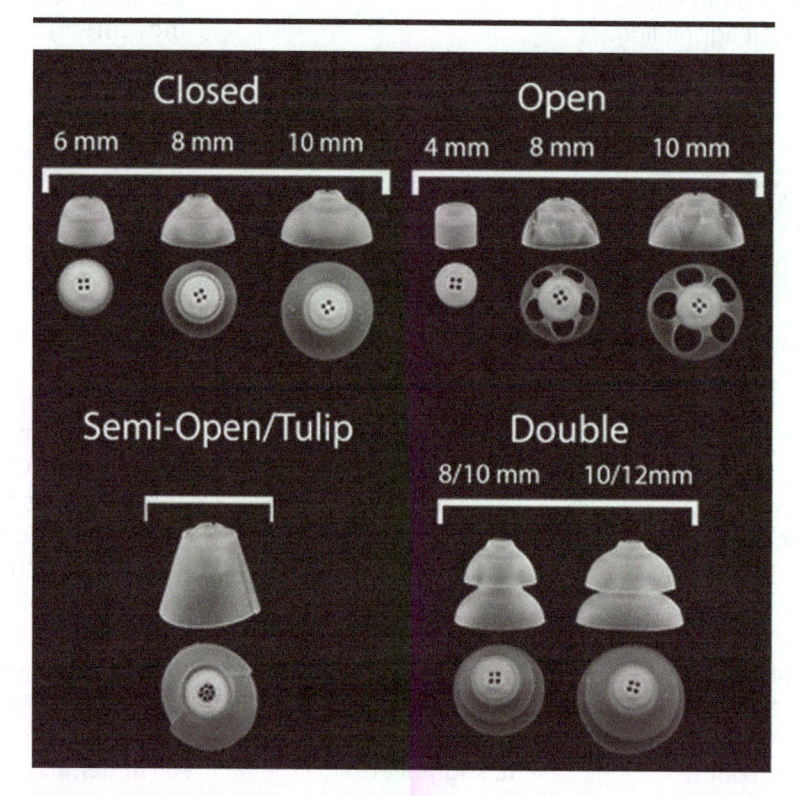

Figure 9–9. Example of eartip choices available when using modular earmolds for fitting mini-BTE products. (Reprinted with permission from Siemens Hearing Instruments, Inc.) Photo courtesy of Sivantos.

fusing, however, as a #2 tip from one manufacturer can be quite different from a #2 tip from another. Some tips are even negative numbers. Some manufacturers call the tips, tips; some call them domes; and some call them tips for some products and domes for others. Some tubing/tip combinations are named after a specific hearing aid, but they also work with other hearing aids. Consider that from just one manufacturer, for a RIC product, there are three different receiver power choices, four different wire length choices, and eight different dome choices—96 different combinations for your Monday morning patient!

Audiologists seem to be somewhat divided regarding the use of these modular fittings. The thin tube can be fitted into a custom mold, and the RIC wire/receiver also can be fitted to a custom mold, so the issue surrounds the use of the non-custom modular tips and domes versus taking an impression and ordering a custom earmold or custom eartips. Indeed, with the proliferation of RIC and RITA devices, there are an increasing number of custom eartip choices with a wide range of available venting. A recent quick scan of one earmold manufacturer revealed six to nine different custom eartips available for dozens of specific receiver types (hundreds of possibilities). Here are some of the commonly cited pros and cons for using non-custom versus custom earmolds and eartips.

Reasons Why Modular Fittings Are a Good Choice

- Openness: The non-custom open fitting tips are indeed open. It is not uncommon that the REOR (for real ear occluded response) is essentially identical to the REUR (for real ear unaided response). Not only does this eliminate the occlusion effect, but it provides some *free gain*, as the ear canal resonance is still in play. The most open custom eartips are also fairly open, although some "open" products still result in a low level of occlusion effect.
- Efficiency: The modular tips allow for same-day service. The patient can walk in the door with an appointment for a diagnostic and leave a couple hours later owning a pair of hearing aids. Assuming that these hearing aids will provide benefit for the patient, which is almost always true, this is a good thing. It also saved a patient visit, which is important for people who need to travel large distances or are required to fight traffic and parking issues coming to the clinic.
- Reduced procrastination: Related to efficiency, there is the old adage, "Strike while the iron is hot." Although not blacksmiths, audiologists dispensing hearing aids know well that when a patient says, "You know, I think I'll go home, talk to my wife about this, and get back to you," you very well might not see that patient again for five years, if ever. Or, the patient goes home, starts price shopping, and returns a week later with a bulging folder of competitive offers and Internet printouts.
- Comfort: Most of the modular tips and domes, especially the open ones, fit rather loosely and are more comfortable than a custom earmold. Some custom eartips, however, rival their non-custom counterparts.
- Cosmetics: The modular tip is typically less noticeable than a custom earmold.
- Cost: The patient does not have the $75 to $100 extra cost of the custom earmold. Many manufacturers provide the tips and domes free-of-charge to the audiologists.
- Maintenance: If the patient has good dexterity and is attentive, they can replace the tips when they become plugged or discolored. With RITAs, the tubing usually becomes stretched (because the patient uses it to take off the hearing aids), and this easily can be replaced by the patient also.

Reasons Why Modular Fittings May *Not* Be a Good Choice

- Feedback: If a patient needs considerable gain, it is sometimes difficult to find a non-custom tip or dome that will fit tight enough.
- Ear geography: If the patient has a sharp turn in their ear canal, there may be problems with the tip bumping against the canal wall. There is not the flexibility of going deeper or shallower as one would have with custom earmolds.
- Insertion: Because the non-custom tip is so small and light, some people with poor dexterity have trouble knowing when it is in

the ear canal. One of the biggest advantages of a custom eartip is they can provide a much more consistent insertion position than a non-custom eartip.

- Retention: It is fairly common for modular tips to work out of the ear canal, or partly out of the canal, when the person talks or chews. Because they are light and fit loosely, the patient sometimes does not even know that the tip is not in the ear canal.
- Anchoring: Related to retention—mini-BTEs are very light and easily can fall off the ear when a person bends over. A custom earmold will serve as an anchor, keeping the hearing aid suspended at the ear. While not as effective as an earmold, custom eartips also can increase retention compared to their non-custom counterparts. A loose fitting tip will not.
- Maintenance: In general, the non-custom tips need more maintenance (changing) than a standard custom earmold/eartip. A common problem is the plugging of the RIC receiver. This occurs more frequently when a modular tip is used than when the receiver is cased in a custom earmold.
- Overall product impression: A pair of hearing aids is the most expensive electronic devices most people purchase. Fitting them to the ear with a 50-cent disposable eartip may not seem consistent with the purported high level of technology.

The Acoustics of Hearing Aid Plumbing

We start this section by acknowledging the pioneering work conducted by Samuel Lybarger in the area of earmold acoustics. As early as the mid-1950s, Lybarger wrote the germinal Pamphlet for Radioear Corporation titled: "The Earmold as Part of the Receiver Acoustic System." At the time, he was writing about earmolds for body aid receivers, but many of the same principles apply today. Many audiologists cut their earmold acoustics teeth reading the chapters that Lybarger wrote for the different editions of the Katz Clinical Audiology Handbooks. We also want to acknowledge the impact of the 1979 monograph on earmold acoustics by Robyn Cox—for decades, it was a well-thumbed reference for audiologists fitting hearing aids.

To understand how hearing aid plumbing can affect the frequency response in hearing aids, we need to first review the acoustic behavior of air volumes and acoustic resonance:

SOAPBOX: UNDERSTANDING EARMOLD ACOUSTICS

In the modern digital age of hearing aids, it is sometimes tempting to think that earmold and earshell acoustics do not matter anymore. After all, why should we go to all the effort of learning a topic as complex as earmold acoustics when we can just fine-tune the hearing aid digitally? Although it is certainly the case that modern hearing aids are much more adjustable than their counterparts of the past, we think the argument against spending time on earmold and earshell acoustics is flawed for at least two reasons. First, it is still the case that not all hearing aids are as acoustically flexible as we might wish they would be. A dip or peak in amplitude in the wrong place can sometimes be easily remedied with simple physical changes affecting the acoustics of the plumbing. Second, and more important, we sometimes need to make adjustments to the earmold or earshell such as changing tubing size or changing vent size for a number of reasons other than acoustics (e.g., cosmetics, comfort). In such instances, it is important to know what effect these changes will have on sound delivered to the patient's ears. For these and other reasons, we will spend some time here discussing earmold and earshell acoustics, but we will focus on areas we think are of the most utility in the clinic on a routine basis.

- As you likely remember from your study of acoustics, sound is propagated through air as a series of condensations and rarefactions. Propagation of sound in response to a vibratory force occurs as a longitudinal wave of energy that oscillates molecules of air in an expanding sphere. In a closed space, the mass of the air molecules is dependent on the volume assuming the air is uncompressed.
- We can think of the sound pathway in a hearing aid as a series of tubes and cavities extending from the diaphragm of the receiver to the tympanic membrane.
- The volume of air in a tube is not compressed by low-frequency vibration, and the waveform is propagated through the volume of air in response to vibratory force. In such a volume (commonly referred to as an acoustic mass), the total impedance to sound energy increases with increases in frequency because there is compression of the air molecules at higher frequencies. Total impedance in an acoustic mass increases with increasing length and decreasing cross-sectional area of the tube.
- Unlike an acoustic mass, the volume of air in small, hard-walled cavities oscillates as a unit, undergoing compression and expansion at the frequency of the vibratory force. In such a volume (commonly referred to as an acoustic compliance), the total impedance to sound energy decreases with increases in volume of the cavity and frequency because it is increasingly difficult to compress air molecules as volume increases.
- Importantly, many cavities and tubes do not function purely as an acoustic mass or an acoustic compliance, instead they demonstrate both elements. However, they are typically dominated by one of the two physical properties.
- In addition to the reactant (energy storage) properties of acoustic mass and acoustic compliance, acoustic resistance (conversion of acoustic energy to heat) is present in the system. Additional acoustic resistance can be intentionally introduced by narrowing the tubing or introducing an object that impedes flow (e.g., a mesh screen). This is somewhat complicated by the fact that unlike mesh screens (pure resistors), narrowing the tubing (constriction) will also increase compliant reactance.

In addition to reactance and resistance, it is also important to consider resonance. The following is a review of how acoustic resonance interrelates with hearing aid plumbing:

- At some frequency or frequencies, reactance in an acoustic system will be minimized leaving only resistance to impede the flow of sound energy. These are called resonance frequencies and are seen as peaks in the hearing aid frequency response. Resonance can occur because reactance is minimized in one component (e.g., the tubing) or it is minimized by the combination of adjacent components (e.g., the residual ear canal volume and the vent volume).
- When one component (e.g., volume of air), acting as an acoustic mass, and a second component, acting as an acoustic compliance, are adjacent to each other, a Helmholtz resonance will occur. This occurs at the frequency in which reactance of the acoustic mass and the acoustic compliance are equal to each other and cancel because they are out of phase. (Recall the magnitude of reactance is proportional to frequency in an acoustic mass and inversely proportional to frequency in an acoustic compliance).
- When a component in an acoustic system has either a very high or very low impedance at the beginning and/or end (compared with the middle) such as a tube open at both ends, a wavelength, resonance will occur. The fundamental frequency of the wavelength resonance will depend on the effective length of the tube.
- Tubes (or sections of tubes) that have either high impedance or low impedance at both ends are referred to as half wave resonators and generate fundamental resonant frequencies that have a wavelength that is twice the effective length of the tube, as well as additional resonances at integer multiples of this fundamental.

- Tubes (or sections of tubes) that have high impedance at one end and low impedance at the other end are referred to as quarter wave resonators and generate fundamental resonant frequencies that have a wavelength that is four times the effective length of the tube, as well as additional resonances at odd integer multiples of this fundamental.

The previous summary was intended only to provide very brief reviews; those of you unfamiliar with these topics are encouraged to study them in more depth. With a general understanding of acoustics as they relate to volumes of air, we can then consider differences in the various portions of the acoustic system—such as the residual ear canal volume, tubes, vents, screens, and cavities in the custom hearing aid or earmold/earhook—and how they affect the frequency response of hearing aids.

In hearing aid systems, simple resonances as well as combinations of these resonances occur; the effects of length and impedance of various components, and combinations of components, are not always intuitive. For example, hearing aid receivers generally present high input impedance in the tubing to which they are attached, but this is not always the case. These issues present a challenge to engineers designing hearing aid systems, given the common goal of a broad, smooth frequency response that is relatively free of resonant peaks and unwanted dips. From a clinical standpoint, the job of the audiologist, fortunately, is to solve somewhat simpler acoustic problems. More specifically, we need only to focus on physical changes to the plumbing that have acoustic implications. These physical changes may be applied for non-acoustic reasons such as cosmetics or comfort (e.g., venting, tubing diameter) or to purposely affect the hearing aid frequency response, especially when the desired acoustic changes may be difficult to apply electronically (e.g., additional high-frequency gain).

Although very intricate effects are possible with hearing aid plumbing, these effects generally are the largest in particular frequency regions. It is useful to keep these regions in mind when making specific changes.

In the following, we consider a few specific hearing aid plumbing factors that are expected to affect acoustics of the sound reaching the patient's eardrums that we think are the most important for everyday clinical practice. These include the following:

- Differences in the BTE earhooks (these most often include specific sound bore configurations and damping materials).
- Differences in the sound bore (sound pathway from the diaphragm of the receiver to the tympanic membrane)—most importantly, the BTE earmold tubing—including internal diameter, tube thickness, and internal diameter change effects.

KEY CONCEPT: HELMHOLTZ RESONATOR

The common method for explaining the effect of a Helmholtz resonator is to use the example of air flowing over the neck of a bottle. Most of us have tried this at one time or another. The resonance will be a result of the velocity of the air, the diameter and length of the neck, and the volume of the cavity. You may recall that when applying this *scientific experiment* with a bottle containing one of your favorite beverages, if you consume some of the liquid, the volume of the cavity will become larger and the resonance then will be altered (a decrease in the resonant frequency will result). Regarding earmold plumbing, this is very similar to what happens when a closed earmold has a vent (similar to the neck of the bottle) that extends and opens to the residual volume of the ear canal (the cavity). When applied to the real ear, the Helmholtz resonator can be activated in one of three ways: external sounds going through the vent, amplified sounds from the hearing aid, or vibrations from the canal walls when the person speaks (refer to the section on the occlusion effect in Chapter 8). In the section on venting later in this chapter, we show you how alterations of the vent size and the residual cavity change the hearing aid's frequency response, all related to the Helmholtz resonance.

■ Differences in venting across all hearing aid styles—these include both intentional venting and venting differences resulting from how tightly the earmold or earshell fits in the ear.

We should point out that we do not intend to cover every possible commercially available plumbing system. Instead it is our goal to provide a basic foundation of knowledge that can be applied to any current or future plumbing system. Our thought is that commercial products come and go, but basic acoustic principles are always important, so consider each one of these three general areas.

Earhooks and Damping Effects

A BTE earhook (sometimes called an elbow or tone hook) has two primary functions: it directs sound from the hearing aid to the earmold tubing and it helps with hearing aid retention. Although retention does not directly impact acoustics, it is often the primary concern when selecting an earhook. Although retention is usually a greater issue with children than adults, it is always important to select the size of earhook that provides the best retention and the best overall fit of the instrument. In addition to the size of the tone hook, some pediatric earhooks are made of a malleable material so they can be bent for better retention on smaller and unusually shaped ears. If we were writing this text ten years ago, we may have spent several pages discussing acoustics related to earhooks. Current technology has limited the need for some of these considerations, because the smaller mini-BTEs, both RICs and RITAs (see Chapter 8) do not use earhooks. Despite these changes, one factor that should still be considered is damping.

Damping must be considered because resonant peaks are commonly present in the hearing aid frequency response. These resonant peaks are due, at least in part, to wavelength resonances. For example, the typical

---

THINGS TO REMEMBER: EARMOLD PLUMBING AND FREQUENCY RESPONSE RANGE

Residual Ear Canal Volume: How much an earshell or earmold fills up the ear canal directly affects the magnitude of the residual ear canal volume. The smaller the residual volume (the deeper the fit), the more gain that will be produced in the ear canal for the same amplifier setting (e.g., related to Boyle's law of gasses, published in 1662). This affects all frequencies but has the greatest effect for the higher frequencies.

Venting: Vents primarily affect low-frequency gain, especially frequencies below 1500 Hz—the lower the frequency, the greater the effect. Increasing vent size decreases low-frequency gain. One specific deviation of common venting rules relates to truly open fittings. The natural ear canal resonance of an open ear gives listeners not wearing hearing aids a boost in high frequencies (particularly around 2500 to 3000 Hz). This resonance typically is eliminated for this frequency region when an earmold or earshell is placed in the ear canal. If a highly vented (non-occluding earmold) is used, however, the hearing aid user may retain some or all of this natural ear canal resonance. Indirectly then, venting *increases* high-frequency gain (see the discussion of open versus closed fittings in Chapter 8).

Damping: Dampers primarily affect frequencies between 750 and 3000 Hz, although some smaller effects may also be seen in the higher frequencies. Damping acts to reduce resonant peaks, so the exact frequency of the effect depends in part on the frequency of the resonant peaks. These peaks are usually lower frequency in BTEs than in custom instruments.

Sound bore shape and size: The overall size of the sound bore can affect all frequencies, especially those above 500 Hz. Horn-shaped tubing/sound bore and reverse-horn changes to the sound bore primarily affect gain above 2000 Hz.

> **TECHNICAL TIP: DAMPED EARHOOKS**
>
> Hearing aid manufacturers commonly ship hearing aids with earhooks attached that have been acoustically modified (most commonly dampers have been added). There may be other earhooks available, however, that fit the instrument. It is important to replace earhooks with an identical match unless a change in frequency response is desired. Replacement with the wrong earhook or removal of clogged damping elements without replacement is an easy way to create an unhappy patient who is disturbed by the change in the hearing aid after it was fixed. Although the first choice would be to obtain a match, it is possible to *retune* the fitting through programming, especially if a real-ear output of the previous fitting is available.

75-mm sound bore associated with traditional BTE instruments will result in one-half-wave resonances at approximately 2300, 4600, and 6900 Hz; and one-quarter-wave resonances at approximately 1100, 3300 and 5500 Hz (Cox, 1979; Walker, 1979). Examples of peaky and smoothed hearing aid frequency responses are shown in Figure 9–10.

Frequency responses of modern hearing aids are generally smoother (less peaky) than those of old because precise digital filtering can be used to smooth the response. Nonetheless, use of dampers can still be important to limit remaining peaks. Some general points to remember include the following:

- Many modern digital hearing aids use a precise digital filter to smooth out the wavelength resonances introduced by the earhook or tubing.
- In some cases, the clinician may want to change the length of tubing for retention or other purposes. In such cases, it may be necessary to reprogram the hearing aid because the exact frequency and magnitude of resonant peaks will be affected by tubing length.
- If a nonstandard length is used, some undesirable resonances may remain that may be reduced through damping.

It is important to note that some research suggests that the frequency response associated with damping is preferred by hearing aid users (Davis & Davidson, 1996). Furthermore, limiting the *peakiness* of the response can also lead to higher overall output levels without narrow bandwidth, high-level peaks of sound exceeding the patient's threshold of discomfort (Bryne, Christen, & Dillon, 1981). That is, the hearing aid may have a peak around 1500 Hz, which exceeds the patient's LDL (for loudness discomfort level). If this peak were damped and reduced by 10 dB, as an example, it may be possible to raise the overall MPO of the hearing aid across all the other frequencies considerably, improving headroom for the peaks of speech, yet not exceeding the patient's LDL.

Dampers are commonly screens or other materials that act to provide resistance to acoustic energy. For example, before today's machined dampers were available, it was common for audiologists to use lambswool

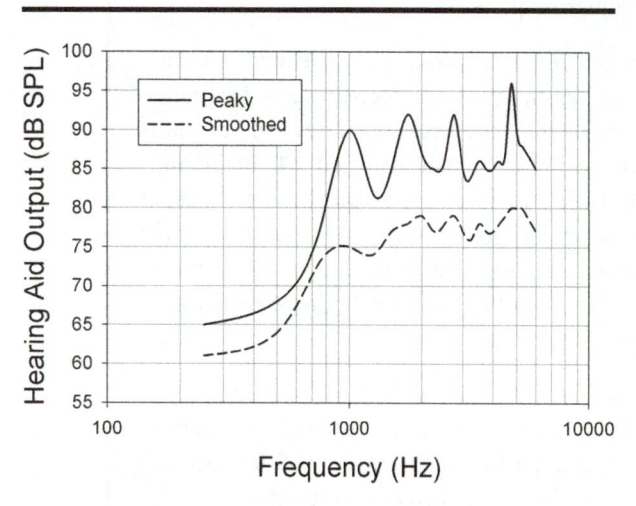

Figure 9–10. Examples of peaky and smoothed frequency responses. The smoothed frequency response was obtained by introducing a highly resistive damper near the sound outlet.

as a damper. Prepackaged dampers are available in a range of sizes, with the largest sizes usually surrounded by a metal can. Several investigations have reported the specific effects of different types of damping (e.g., Cox & Gilmore, 1986; Davis & Davidson, 1996; Studebaker, 1974). It is important to note that, because dampers provide acoustic resistance, dampers act to reduce the level (provide attenuation) of peaks in the hearing aid's frequency response. This point is important because the maximum effect provided by any specific damper will not always occur at the same frequency but will rather be determined, in part, by the frequencies of the resonant peaks in the specific hearing aid prior to damping.

In addition to the frequency at which the resonant peaks naturally occur in a hearing aid, the effect damping has on the existing resonant peaks primarily depends on two factors: (1) the impedance of the damper (measured in ohms) and (2) the placement of the damper. Generally the higher the impedance, the more attenuation. As for placement, the greatest attenuation will occur for most frequencies when the damper is placed nearest the sound outlet. For example, there will be greater damping for a placement near the tip of an earhook than near the receiver.

With today's products, the clinician's work with dampers likely will be limited—recall that traditional BTEs, the product for which dampers might be employed, are only about 10% of the market. For those who have

> **THINGS TO REMEMBER: WHAT COLOR IS *YOUR* DAMPER?**
>
> - 330 Ohms   Gray
> - 680 Ohms   White
> - 1000 Ohms   Brown
> - 1500 Ohms   Green
> - 2200 Ohms   Red
> - 3300 Ohms   Orange
> - 4700 Ohms   Yellow

> **KEY CONCEPT: COMMON CLINICAL SLANG**
>
> Some of you may be unfamiliar with some of the clinical slang we have used when referring to different hearing loss configurations. For the uninitiated, here are some explanations:
>
> - Ski-Slope: A downward sloping hearing loss, usually one that is particularly precipitous—often associated with the need for an open fitting.
> - Reverse slope: This is used to refer to patients with significant hearing loss in the low frequencies, sloping upward to normal or near-normal high-frequency thresholds.
> - Cookie bite: This is used to refer to patients with significant hearing loss in the middle frequencies (750 to 2000 Hz) and near-normal hearing in the high and low frequencies.
> - Reverse cookie bite: This is used to refer to patients with significant hearing loss in the lower and higher frequencies and near-normal thresholds in the middle frequencies. Unfortunately, some clinicians and even manufacturers have reversed our definitions related to cookie bite, so make sure to note the exact configuration when ordering special purpose earhooks and other acoustic accessories.
> - Corner audiogram: Refers to a patient who only has measureable hearing in the lower frequencies.

the interest, dampers can still be obtained from hearing aid supply stores such as Hal-Hen, who carry the Knowles fused-mesh damper. These dampers consist of a metal ferrule that contains a finely woven plastic acoustic resistance screen. They are designed to fit snugly into #13 gauge tubing. These dampers are color-coded and come in five impedances.

In addition to damping, we should also mention the availability of special purpose earhooks, which can be very useful for certain patients. Special purpose earhooks, such as those available from some hearing aid manufacturers and companies like Etymotic Research, work well for unusual hearing loss configurations such as patient's with cookie bite, reverse cookie bite, and reverse slope audiograms.

Sound Bore and Tubing Effects

In a BTE instrument, tubing serves the purpose of directing sound from the receiver to the ear canal and helps with retention by anchoring the hearing aid to the earmold or eartip. In traditional BTE instruments, the tubing is usually pushed into a hole in the earmold drilled just for the tube (typically referred to as the earmold tubing bore). The excess tubing beyond the earmold canal is trimmed off, and then the tubing is glued or held in place with a physical tubing lock (a small plastic or metal ring around the tubing). It is common to trim the tubing so that it is recessed inside the tip of the earmold. Acoustic changes resulting from tubing changes primarily relate to the internal diameter of the tubing (including changes in internal diameter over the length of the tubing).

In 1979, the National Association of Earmold Laboratories (NAEL) reached an agreement on a naming convention for tubing based on internal diameter that is still intact today—see Table 9–1. Today, the most common tubing internal diameters include the fixed bore #13 tubing, typically referred to as *standard* tubing for traditional BTE instruments and the thin tube (typically 0.9 to 0.95 mm internal diameter) commonly used with mini-BTE RITA instruments. We talk about 2-cc coupler measures in Chapter 13; however, an interesting clinical aside is that the standard 2-cc couplers aimed at BTE verification do not mimic standard #13 tubing but, rather, a 4-mm horn tubing that we describe later in this chapter.

Table 9–1. NAEL Standard Sizes for Earmold Tubing

NAEL Size	Internal Diameter (mm)	External Diameter (mm)
No. 9	3.00	4.01
No. 12	2.16	3.18
No. 13	1.93	2.95
No. 14	1.68	2.95
No. 15	1.5	2.95
No. 16	1.35	2.95
Add for "thick wall" (No. 13)		0.35
Add for "double wall" (No. 13)		0.66
Add for "medium" (No. 13)		0.15
Subtract for "thin" (No. 16)		0.79
Non-NAEL Size		
Thin Tube	0.75 to 0.95	1.0 to 1.2

Source: Blue, 1979

Bore Diameter

Reducing tubing diameter increases the effective acoustic mass and overall impedance. Although this can affect the overall frequency response, the most notable effect of decreasing tubing diameter is that the frequency of the resonant peaks resulting from wavelength resonances are slightly lowered; the exact frequencies that are affected will depend on where the resonant peaks are to begin with. It is interesting to note that these relatively small effects can actually be accentuated in modern hearing aids. Let us assume a manufacturer implements a group of *notch* filters that act to reduce gain over the narrow frequency ranges for which wavelength resonance peaks are expected. This filter will be designed for a specific internal diameter. If, however, a significantly different internal diameter of tubing is used, the frequency response could have both *dips* from the notch filter set as at the old resonant frequencies as well as *bumps* at the adjacent new resonant frequencies (see associated "Points to Ponder"). As noted previously, this can be an even greater problem if the length of the tubing is changed.

In addition to lowering the frequency of the resonant peaks, reducing the tubing internal diameter can

TECHNICAL TIP: GETTING THE TUBING LENGTH RIGHT

- Tubing length directly affects how the hearing aid case is positioned on the ear. Long tubing will result in an instrument that hangs behind the pinna. Shorter tubing may cause the hearing aid to sit too high on the top the pinna. This choice directly affects patient comfort as well as cosmetics (and maybe acoustics).
- We suggest inserting the earmold, placing the hearing aid on the ear, and adjusting for optimal position, then cutting the tubing to the appropriate length. As in carpentry, it is good to remember the motto "measure twice, cut once." Cutting the tubing too short means you will need to re-tube the earmold.
- As we discussed earlier, several predetermined lengths of tubing are typically available in the fitting kit for mini-BTE hearing aids. Because these instruments often do not use a custom earmold, correct selection of length is particularly important for fit and retention purposes (this is also true for selection of the length of wire in RIC instruments). The fitting kits usually provide a device that will assist with sizing. Better retention and reduced feedback may also require bending the thin tube to best fit an individual ear. Application of heat can sometimes aid in this process.

also lower the magnitude of the resonant peaks (dampening). The magnitude of the dampening of the resonant peaks, however, is clearly most effective with the smallest tubing diameters. Figure 9–11 shows the deviation in frequency response from a typical BTE using standard #13 tubing. The largest deviation is clearly evident for a very thin tube, such as is commonly used with the mini-BTE RITA OC style of hearing aid described in Chapter 8. For the thin tube, there is a slight 6 to 7 dB boost in the low frequencies and up to 20 dB of attenuation in the middle and high frequencies when compared with standard #13 tubing. Note that the effects will be slightly different from those shown depending on the original magnitude and frequency of the resonant peaks of the instrument in the presence of #13 tubing as well as acoustic properties of the earhook used. Also, it should be pointed out that these differences assume that you have the same coupling to the ear. Clinical fitting of the same instrument using thin tubes (RITA) versus traditional tubing and an earhook will often result in even larger differences than shown in Figure 9–11, particularly in the low frequencies, because different earmolds/eartips with different amounts of venting are usually paired with each type.

Unlike internal diameter, a tube's external diameter is not expected to affect the hearing aid frequency response. Unintentional changes, however, related to constriction of the tubing can occur, as described in the next section. The choice of external tubing diameter is usually based on how much amplification is needed (based on the degree of hearing loss) and cosmetic factors. The more amplification, the more likely it is to create

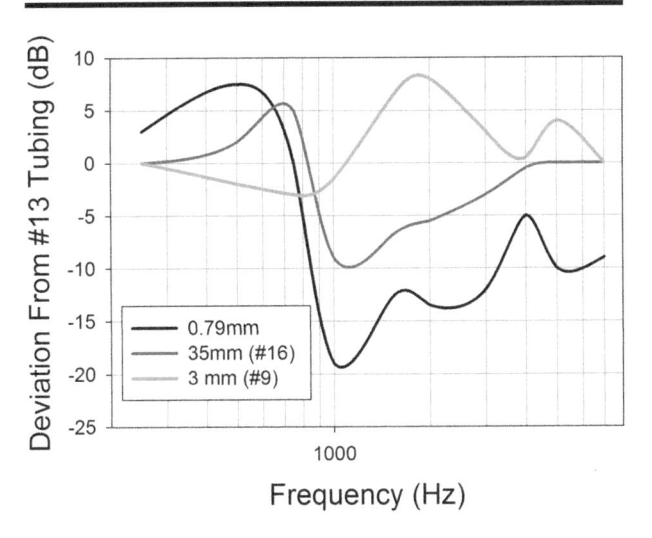

Figure 9–11. Deviation in frequency response for the same BTE hearing aid when changed from #13 (standard) tubing. It is important to note that, although this provides a view of the general effect of changing tubing length, the specific changes shown here result from the specific instrument evaluated. Instruments with different resonant peaks will show different specific effects.

> **POINTS TO PONDER: PLUMBING AND MODERN HEARING AIDS**
>
> As we described, some hearing aids will employ notch filtering to reduce the expected and unwanted effects of resonances of the earmold plumbing. If you change the plumbing and introduce a different set of resonances, an undesirable fitting may result. Here is a typical example of when this might happen: You fit a patient with a larger BTE instrument that has the standard earhook and the #13 tubing. After a few weeks of use, the patient is concerned that this plumbing is bulky and much more noticeable than the plumbing used with the mini-BTEs that the patient's friend wears. You realize that an option is for you to remove the standard earhook and use a thin-tube screw-on adapter (which will also require a new earmold for the thin-tube fitting). This indeed will be a noticeable cosmetic improvement for the patient. But what if the hearing aids fitted employ filtering to reduce the large resonant peak at around 1500 Hz that would be expected for the standard hook/tubing? What you will likely see with the new fitting is a large dip in this frequency range in the real-ear output, which will need to be accounted for with a substantial amount of added gain. But what if someone simply changed the plumbing and did not repeat probe microphone verification? How would they know that outcome? To correct this mistake it will be necessary to change the tubing configuration in the manufacturer's fitting software (so that the appropriate filtering and notch filtering/smoothing can be applied) and then refit the hearing aid using your prescriptive gain targets of choice and probe microphone verification.

vibration in the earmold tubing. This vibration can in turn set the hearing aid case and surrounding air into vibration, providing pathways that increase the likelihood of acoustic and mechanical feedback. Therefore, thicker walled tubing is sometimes recommended for patients with severe-to-profound hearing loss. Although sometimes necessary to prevent feedback, this thicker tubing is a little harder to shape and work with, so it is only used when necessary.

Horn Effects

The majority of patients that we fit with hearing aids have downward sloping losses and obtaining the desired amount of gain in the higher frequencies often is challenging. In some cases, you find that you need a little more amplification at 3000 Hz, although you already increased gain as much as the programming software will allow. This can occur despite the fact that the patient appeared to be within the manufacturer's fitting range for the hearing aid you ordered. We do not want to under-fit the patient, but yet we do not want to send the patient home to sit and wait while we reorder a different hearing aid or receiver. What can we do?

One method that has been used for many years—and is effective in changing the magnitude of amplification only in the high frequencies and only in BTE instruments using larger tubing—is a change in the bore diameter of the transmission system from the receiver to the sound outlet at the medial tip of the canal portion of the earmold or hearing aid shell. Such increases in the bore diameter can result in a boost in high-frequency gain and are generally referred to as *acoustic horns* (e.g., Killion, 1979, 1993, 2003; Libby, 1982a, 1982b; Lybarger, 1985). In contrast, decreases in the bore diameter lead to decreases in gain and are generally referred to as reverse horns or constrictions (Cox, 1979). A change in bore diameter can be achieved in a large number of ways. Two examples are shown in Figure 9–12, and lead to a variety of changes in the hearing aid frequency response, as shown in Figure 9–13. Fortunately however, acoustic horns do follow a few general rules that allow for prediction of how they will work:

- All horns have a cutoff frequency that can be mathematically derived. Little or no change in amplification level (horn effect) occurs below this cutoff frequency.

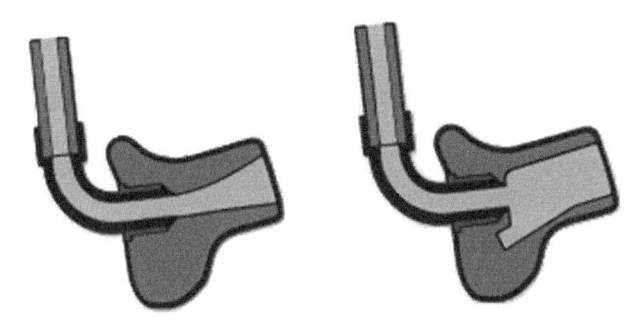

Figure 9–12. Change in sound bore diameter can be achieved in a large number of ways. This figure displays two types of CFA horns including a smoothed bore (*left-hand portion*) and stepped horn (*right-hand portion*).

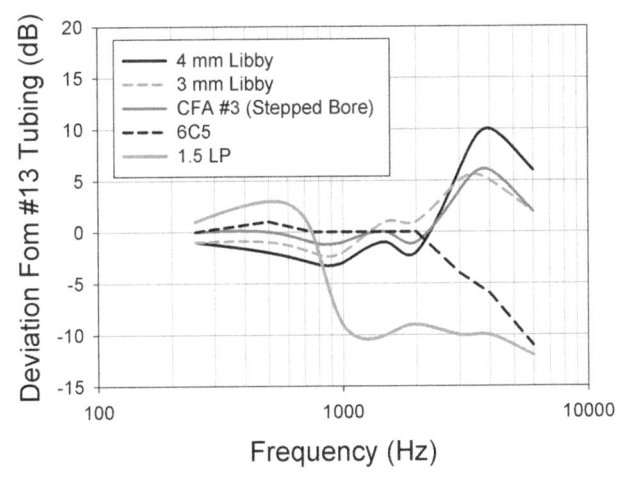

Figure 9–13. Deviation in frequency response for the same BTE hearing aid when changing from #13 (standard) tubing to one of the several available horns or constrictions. (Adapted from data presented by Dillon, 1985, 1991; and Killion, 1981.)

- The cutoff frequency in a smooth horn is calculated by (Beranek, 1954):

$$\text{Horn Cutoff Frequency} = \frac{\text{Speed of Sound} \times \text{natural log}\left(\frac{\text{outlet diameter}}{\text{inlet diameter}}\right)}{2\pi \times \text{length of Horn}}$$

- In other words, the shorter the effective horn length, the higher the cutoff frequency. For example, one of the most effective horns is a 4-mm Libby horn (22-mm long) that has a cutoff frequency of about 1700 Hz and reaches its maximum horn effect (around 5 to 10 dB) at around 3400 Hz (see Figure 9–13).
- In contrast, the same inlet and outlet diameters in a 10-mm long horn, as might be available in a belled canal of a custom instrument, move the cutoff frequency to near 4000 Hz (with a maximum not reached until almost 8000 Hz), rendering them of little use in most common hearing aids.
- Stepped horns will have a shorter effective length than smooth bores because the change in diameter occurs closer to the medial tip.

These rules clearly show that, although the change in bore diameter is important regarding the magnitude of the horn effect, having a horn with a long, effective length is critical to provide an increase in amplification that is low enough in frequency to be useful in most modern hearing aids, other than those providing extended high-frequency amplification (greater than 4 to 6 kHz). We should note, however, that sometimes introducing a belled canal or pulling the tubing back from the medial tip of the earmold, can provide a larger than expected level increase in the high frequencies. This unexpectedly large level increase usually occurs because a constriction was removed, rather than being due to the horn effect. Based on his work with Knowles Electronics, Killion (1979) introduced the idea of abutting tubes of differing internal diameter together in a *stepped horn* for hearing aids. The procedure provided the desired boost in the high frequencies very effectively, but when this new horn earmold style was rolled out for routine patient use some practical problems emerged. The dampers that had been strategically placed in the tubing for fine tuning became plugged and, after continuous use, the glued

- The magnitude of the horn effect exponentially increases from the cutoff frequency to reach a maximum dB level increase (approximately 20 log [outlet diameter/inlet diameter]) at a frequency one octave above the cutoff frequency. This peak occurs at approximately the frequency where a quarter wavelength equals the distance between the change in the tubing diameter and the medial tip of the earmold.

pieces of tubing would come apart (many patients use the tubing to pull the earmold out of the ear, which most probably contributed to this problem). Entrepreneur E. Robert "Cy" Libby (1982a) modified the acoustic horn concept of Killion by molding and manufacturing a plastic tube into a one-piece smooth horn with a stepped-internal diameter. This earmold style quickly became known as the *Libby Horn*. These horns are still in use today, which commonly are available in 3-mm and 4-mm configurations (denoting the internal diameter at the medial end of the horn). Although the best boost will be found with the 4-mm horn, this diameter is too big for the ear canal of most patients. Many clinicians and scientists have noted a small horn effect can be introduced by inserting standard earmold tubing only partially into the earmold. Although still a minimal effect compared with the other methods discussed here, this horn effect can be slightly increased by increasing the diameter of the sound bore at the medial end of the earmold or custom earshell, commonly referred to as a belled canal. It is unlikely that the belled canal approach will provide a significant high-frequency boost, simply because of the short distance of the horn length. More recently, approaches that attach a hard plastic elbow directly to the earmold or that use a snap ring have been introduced. These approaches, such as the Continuous Flow Adaptor (CFA), allow for easy attachment of tubing between the hearing aid and the ear-mold which can have a variety of horn or reverse-horn configurations built in.

In contrast with the acoustic horns designed to increase high frequencies, constrictions and reverse horns act to decrease the magnitude of high-frequency energy. Although horns are least effective when they are placed nearest the sound outlet (medial tip of the earmold or earshell), constrictions are most effective in this position. Clinically, reverse horns are rarely intentionally used because it is fairly uncommon to desire a reduction in high-frequency output because the majority of hearing loss configurations are sloping (greatest loss in the high frequencies). In addition, the majority of modern hearing aids are flexible enough to reduce gain electronically or digitally. Despite these facts, we still feel it is necessary to discuss constrictions for two reasons: (1) the rare case of an inflexible (usually relatively inexpensive) hearing aid that does not allow for enough high-frequency gain reduction in the presence of needed gain in the lower frequencies and, perhaps more importantly, (2) the inadvertent constriction of standard, constant diameter tubing.

Inadvertent and typically unwanted constrictions can happen across a variety of instrument styles with patients who have very narrow ear canals. For example, Killion (1988) reported a loss of 5 to 10 dB in the high frequencies from constriction in typical children's earmolds. Another common cause of an inadvertent constriction occurs when a tube with a larger external diameter is mistakenly forced into an earmold tubing bore smaller than that for which it was intended. This could happen when tubing is replaced, if a thick-walled tubing were mistakenly grabbed instead of standard tubing. Alternatively, larger external diameter tubing may be forced into an earmold tubing bore drilled for a smaller external diameter to try to keep the tubing from being pulled out. This is not recommended because tubing that is too large for the sound bore can cause the internal diameter of the tubing to be squeezed by the earmold sound bore. These inadvertent constrictions can significantly reduce the amplified sound level in the high frequencies in a similar manner to the intentional constriction effects of the reverse horn tubing products shown in Figure 9–13. The 6C5 and 1.5 LP tubing configurations shown in this figure are available from Etymotic Research. The 6C5 consists of #13 tubing (1.93-mm internal diameter) that is partially inserted in the earmold, followed by a small 3-mm cavity with 14 mm of #16 tubing (1.35-mm internal diameter) in the medial tip of the earmold. The 1.5 LP tubing configuration is #15 tubing (1.5-mm internal diameter) that is stepped down to a 0.9-mm internal diameter for the last 12 mm of the medial tip of the earmold.

Venting Effects

Venting is a term that simply refers to opening up an air/sound transmission pathway from the tympanic membrane to the environment outside the head. Venting is the most common alteration made to earmold plumbing by audiologists. The effects of venting can make a substantial change to low-frequency gain and output. Venting is used with hearing aid fittings for several reasons, including the following (from Mueller & Hall, 1998):

- To allow amplified low-frequency signals to escape: In some cases, the gain of the instrument in the lower frequencies is greater than necessary or what is desired by the patient. Although this usually can be adjusted with the fitting software, venting can provide an additional release of amplified low-frequency output.

- To allow low-frequency signals generated in the ear canal to escape: As discussed in Chapter 8, when a person talks, his or her voice is transmitted from the throat via bone conduction along the mandible to the condyle, which is adjacent to the ear canal. This vibrates the cartilaginous portion of the ear canal, which creates low-frequency, air-conducted energy within the cavity referred to as the occlusion effect. If this energy cannot escape (e.g., entrance is plugged with an earmold or hearing aid), it can distort the person's own voice (e.g., sounds hollow, echoes), and cause annoyance and sometimes hearing aid rejection. The most effective treatment of the occlusion effect is venting—allowing the low-frequency energy to escape (see Chapter 8 for complete review).
- To allow unamplified signals to pass unobstructed to the eardrum: When a person has normal hearing for a given frequency range (usually the lows), it often is desirable to allow speech and environmental sounds to pass naturally to the eardrum and not be attenuated by an earmold/hearing aid shell. This may improve localization, give sounds a more natural spatial perception, and improve the overall sound quality. The openness of the fitting is easy to verify using the REOR (for real ear occluded response) measure with your probe microphone equipment.
- To allow pressure relief: When earmolds or hearing aid shells are fitted tightly, there can be a buildup of pressure in the residual ear canal, and the patient will report a sensation of *fullness*. Some patients can sense this pressure increasing as the daily hearing aid use continues. A small vent can relieve this pressure, and in fact, these small vents often are called *pressure vents*.
- To allow aerations of the ear canal and/or middle ear: In some cases, when external or middle ear pathology exists, the pathology is aggravated when the normal ventilation of the ear is altered. For these patients, venting is used for medical rather than acoustic reasons, and there may need to be some compromise in the applied low-frequency gain (e.g., less than desired) to allow for the necessary aeration.

Venting can be contrasted with a *fully occluded* situation in which a sealed cavity is formed between the tympanic membrane and the medial portion of the hearing aid or earmold upon insertion. This distinction between vented and occluded is generally theoretical, however, because almost no earmold or hearing aid will entirely seal the ear canal regardless of the earmold material used. Such a fit would prove to be uncomfortably tight for most people, not to mention the problems

---

KEY CONCEPT: FIVE IMPORTANT FACTORS FOR VENTING

Not all vents are created equal, and vents that are equal can have a different effect for different fittings or for different people. When thinking about the effects that a given vent may have on the amplified signal, there are five general areas to consider:

- Length of the vent (longer results in less vent effects)
- Diameter of the vent (smaller results in less vent effects)
- Leakage of the fitting not directly associated with the vent (addition of slit leak venting to the total vent effect)
- Residual ear canal volume
- Middle ear impedance

caused relative to insertion and removal. Instead, almost all hearing aids include some magnitude of slit leak venting, which allows sound and air to pass between the residual ear canal cavity and the outside world. It is no surprise to note that the magnitude of slit leak venting is affected by the tightness of fit, the earmold or hearing aid material, the depth of the earmold/shell in the ear canal, and the degree that the earmold shell fills up the concha—ITCs will generally have more slit leak venting than ITEs and BTE earmolds. The magnitude of slit leak venting will affect the maximum available gain before feedback and will limit the use of some smaller styles with greater magnitudes of hearing loss. Fortunately, the advent of modern feedback suppression technology has extended the fitting range (available gain before feedback) of all hearing aid styles.

Although slit leak venting is certainly a consideration, particularly when selecting the hearing aid style, the term venting is most commonly used to refer to intentional air pathways that are opened between the residual outer ear canal cavity and the outside environment. Intentional venting also acts to limit the maximum gain available before feedback. This limitation is primarily found in the 2000 to 4000 Hz range—the frequencies most prone to feedback because this is where there is the largest difference between the environmental SPL (hearing aid input) and the amplified real-ear signal. Gain in the lower frequencies is more typically limited by the physical output limits of the hearing aid amplifier and receiver. The maximum available gain measured in patient's ears at 2000 and 3000 Hz across a range of hearing aid styles and venting configurations and in the *absence* of feedback suppression technology is shown in Figure 9–14. Keep in mind, however, that although these are average values, individual patients may exhibit feedback at acoustic gain values that are 5 to 10 dB less than shown here (others may receive up to 5 to 10 dB more gain before feedback). As might be expected, the magnitude of available gain decreases with increasing vent size and across styles as the microphone and receiver outlet are more closely spaced (from BTE to ITE to ITC). If you are unfamiliar with the term, *real ear insertion gain*, you can simply assume it to refer to the amount of amplification provided by the hearing aid that is greater than the patient's natural real ear unaided response.

Hearing aid vents are available in a variety of different shapes and sizes. In one common configuration, a cylindrical hole is drilled from the lateral to the medial surfaces of the custom hearing aid or earmold

> **KEY CONCEPT: INTERPRETING VENTING CHARTS**
>
> There are many charts available that illustrate the effects that a vent might have on the frequency response. For example, you might see that a vent of average length of 2 mm diameter will reduce gain at 250 Hz by 10 dB. These charts are a good starting point, but it is important to remember that this is compared with a *tightly* sealed earmold. As we discussed in this section, nearly all earmolds have slit-leak venting. Hence, there already is a vent. If there is considerable slit leak venting, the effects of adding the 2-mm vent might be significantly less than expected.

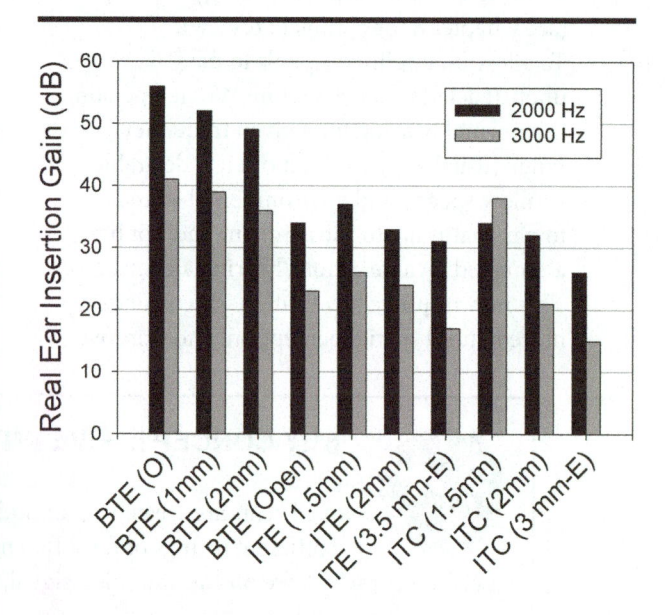

Figure 9–14. Maximum real ear insertion gain available for 2000 and 3000 Hz for various venting configurations and hearing aid styles when not using digital feedback suppression technology. In this (O) refers to a fully occluded fitting, whereas (-E) makes reference to the effective vent size resulting from the combination of slit leak and intentional venting. (Derived from Dillon, 1991; Egolf, Howell, Weaver, and Barker, 1985; and Kuk, 1994.)

in parallel to the sound bore. This is referred to as a *parallel vent*, shown in Figure 9–15. The smallest vents are the approximately 0.5 to 0.8 mm diameter *pressure relief vents*. Parallel vents as large as 3.5 to 4 mm may be possible in some earmolds if the patient has a large enough diameter ear canal. A completely non-occluding fit is also possible through several methods including (1) an open earmold, historically referred to as IROS, (2) inserting tubing with a simple *concha lock* consisting of a flexible wire or thin plastic arm that presses slightly against the concha to hold the tube in place, or (3) one of the many custom and modular eartip styles available with OC hearing aids as described in Chapter 8 and earlier in this chapter.

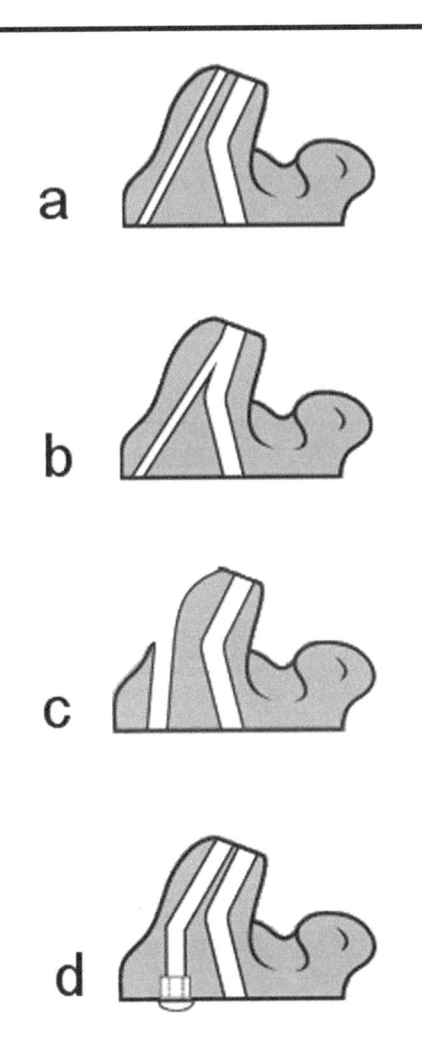

Figure 9–15. Examples of vent configurations: (A) parallel, (B) side branch, (C) trough, and (D) SAV. (Reprinted with permission from Westone.)

Because of space limitations, parallel vents are usually limited to a diameter of 2.5 mm or less in ITEs and 2 mm in ITCs. When space is particularly limited, or active drainage or other problems routinely clog the vent, a *trough vent*, sometimes referred to as an *external vent*, is used. This consists of a channel ground into the canal and concha bowl portion of the hearing aid or earmold (see Figure 9–15).

Sometimes a vent is started as a trough vent on the canal portion and then is transitioned into a parallel vent. Trough vents effectively increase the magnitude of slit-leak venting and typically behave acoustically in the exact same way as parallel vents of the same size. Trough vents are less desirable for some patients, however, as the consistency of the patient's skin and tissue can lead to the trough being filled up to various degrees, leading to a less controlled vent size. In some cases of extreme space constraints, it may be tempting to use a side-branch vent (also referred to as a Y-vent, angle vent, or diagonal vent). In this configuration, the tubing is only minimally inserted into the earmold, and then a vent is drilled from the lateral surface of the earmold to the earmold sound bore (see Figure 9–15). That is, the medial sound bore opening also serves as the medial opening for the vent. Although certainly tempting from a space conservation standpoint, we agree with many other authors (e.g., Cox, 1979) in stating that side-branch vents should not be used unless there is no other alternative or the patient has minimum need for high-frequency amplification. This recommendation is based on two negative acoustic consequences of side-branch vents: (1) decrease in the magnitude of high-frequency amplification and (2) increased likelihood of feedback. In recent years, for these small custom instruments, computer modeling using the patient's ear impression has led to better use of available real estate within the shell, and more novel, and possibly effective venting procedures.

To review, venting serves several purposes, and increasing the magnitude of venting will have several potential consequences:

- Increased susceptibility to feedback
- Decreased occlusion effect
- Reduced low-frequency gain by allowing low-frequency amplified sound to leak out, as shown in Figure 9–16
- Reduced benefit of some special noise-reduction features (because of the openness)

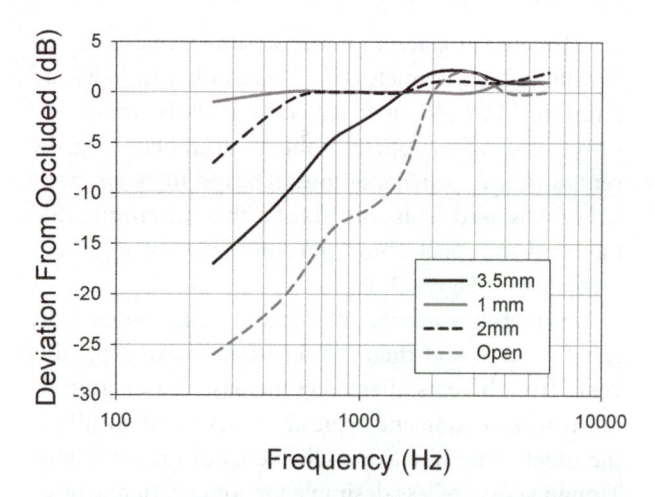

Figure 9–16. Effect of venting on the hearing aid frequency response in comparison with a tight fitting BTE earmold without intentional venting. Note both an increase in magnitude of gain reduction and an increase in the frequency at which the gain reduction begins with increasing vent size. (Adapted from Dillon, 1985.)

- Allowed unamplified low-frequency sound from the environment to leak in

Because of the acoustic consequences of increased vent size, for decades clinicians have needed to balance comfort and occlusion reduction with a loss of low-frequency gain and susceptibility for feedback. Because of slit leak venting and differences in ear geometry, it is commonly quite difficult to know *a priori* how large of a vent can be used for any individual patient. As a consequence, it is common to drill out a larger vent bore and then provide a means for blocking part of the vent (either with a small tube or valve). Commercially available versions known by names like Select-a-Vent (SAV) and Positive Venting Valve (PVV) come in a variety of sizes and allow for easy in-office modifications to the vent size without drilling. As explained below, however, it is not uncommon for the effect of changing an SAV plug on the venting effect to be more limited than might be expected. In addition to the more limited range of venting effects, another downside of the SAV is that it is a bit more noticeable than a single drilled vent.

Although the balancing problem of feedback versus occlusion exists today, the introduction of digital feedback suppression technology has moved the fulcrum of this clinical teeter-totter. Specifically, feedback suppression processing allows for more gain and more venting before feedback and has increased the available maximum gain before feedback by as much as 10 to 18 dB (e.g., Ricketts, Johnson, & Federman, 2008). If the patient has a significant hearing loss, this balancing problem remains, however, and peak high-frequency gain in an open configuration is still limited to approximately 35 dB SPL of insertion gain for a truly open fitting.

With all of these different vent configurations you might wonder how it is possible to quantify vent size and the meaning of equivalent vent size. Does the smallest constriction in the vent bore determine the acoustic properties of the vent? An important question, given the common use of SAV style plug interchange products. It turns out that short constrictions, relative to the total length of the vent, have little impact on venting. Instead, the acoustic properties of venting and their measured effect on occlusion and feedback are based on the acoustic mass of the vent.

More specifically, the greater the acoustic mass, the smaller the vent effect. From the formula for calculating acoustic mass, we can see that the smaller the cross-sectional area of the vent and the longer the vent bore, the greater the acoustic mass. That is, short wide vents will provide more venting than long narrow ones.

The concept of acoustic mass as related to vents has at least three important applications. First, it is important for understanding the effect of vent diameter. Moving from a 1- to 2-mm constant diameter vent of the

---

THINGS TO REMEMBER: CALCULATING ACOUSTIC MASS

For understanding acoustic mass, we can go back to the work of Beranek in 1954:

- Acoustic Mass = 1.18 (Air Density) × (Effective Length [m]/Cross-Sectional Area [m^2]). Where cross-sectional area = π × radius^2
- Effective Length = Length of the Vent × (0.4 × Vent Diameter at the Medial Tip)

same length will quadruple the cross-sectional area leading to an acoustic mass that is nearly one-quarter as large. (Note: It is *nearly*, rather than *exactly* one-quarter because the change in diameter also changes the effective length of the vent as shown in the second formula related to calculating acoustic mass) In contrast, moving from a 2- to 3-mm constant diameter vent reduces acoustic mass by only about one-half.

A second important consideration is how acoustic mass and venting affects our understanding of SAV plugs. When a vent channel is made up of different cross-sectional areas (e.g., a small diameter short plug in the end of a large diameter long vent bore), the total acoustic mass is the sum of the mass in each section. Therefore, if the rest of the vent has high acoustic mass (i.e., is long and thin) or the combination of the rest of the vent and slit leak venting has very low acoustic mass (i.e., loosely fit or wide and short vent), the effect of placing a short plug in one end of the vent on the overall acoustic mass will be minimal. Furthermore, similar vent plug sizes may yield nearly identical venting effects because the change in overall acoustic mass of the entire vent will be small.

Finally, acoustic mass is also important related to vent shape. For example, you might wonder if it is possible to put an effective vent in a CIC or ITC that is recessed in the ear. In this case, the faceplate area is limited by the diameter of the ear canal, and the diameter of the vent will be limited by the battery door. This may only allow a 1-mm (or smaller) vent opening on the lateral portion of the hearing aid. If the ear canal is wide enough, however, there may be room for a wider opening on the medial tip; in many cases, this wider opening is accomplished with a trough vent. This configuration is commonly referred to as a reverse-horn vent. In the example we present here, if we can halve the overall acoustic mass by using a reverse-horn vent, the effective vent size will grow to about 1.5 mm assuming a 1-mm vent opening in the faceplate.

In Closing

In this chapter, we have provided an overview of hearing aid acoustic plumbing. We hope you have gained some insight regarding how this can impact the success of the fitting. A hearing aid with the best technology on the market may be rejected if the plumbing is not right.

It all starts with a good ear impression. Although we reviewed many acoustic concerns, comfort also is very important. This ear impression is even more critical for custom instruments, as fixing the problem could mean a complete remake of the hearing aid. Indeed, the modular earmolds that have become common with mini-BTEs have several advantages, but custom earmolds are still necessary in many cases. We reviewed three different general categories when considering changes in earmold acoustics. A brief review is as follows:

- Damping with commercial dampers or other products acts to smooth the peaks in the hearing aid frequency response. The closer the damper is to the sound outlet, the more effective it will be. Damping primarily reduces resonant peaks in the middle frequencies.
- Widening the sound bore/tubing over the course of its length creates an acoustic horn. The horn effect increases the sound level in the high frequencies (generally above 2500 Hz or higher). The frequency at which the level increase begins will be increasingly lower with longer horns.
- Increasing the vent size increases the susceptibility to feedback, decreases the occlusion effect, reduces low-frequency gain, allows unamplified low-frequency sound from the environment to leak in, and allows an air exchange pathway that will decrease the buildup of moisture and increase comfort.

A Final Case Study

We close this chapter with a case study that illustrates how the understanding of venting can play an important role in the everyday fitting of hearing aids. This patient was a 72-year-old male with a mild-to-moderate downward sloping hearing loss (approximately 30 dB in the lows, dropping to 60 to 65 dB in the 3000 to 4000 Hz region) who was fitted with a mini-BTE RIC, using a modular fitting tip. Because of the degree of hearing loss in the low frequencies, the audiologist selected a dome labeled *closed* from the manufacturer's fitting kit.

As part of the pre-fitting process, therefore, she also selected "closed" from the pull-down menu in the fitting software. For this manufacturer and this particular product, there were seven choices regarding "tightness" if the modular dome was used.

In general, manufacturers do their best to make their automated fittings close to what is desired by the audiologist, particularly when the audiologist is using a standard fitting formula. In this case, the audiologist was programming the hearing aid to the NAL-NL2 prescriptive targets (see Chapter 14). The fitting software then takes into account the effects of the earmold (a dome modular tip in this case) and alters the hearing aid gain accordingly using earmold correction factors similar to those contained in the figures, charts, and tables that we have shown throughout this chapter.

Shown in Figure 9–17 (Panel A, Output A) is the output that resulted for this fitting (the real ear aided response for a 55 dB real-speech shaped input signal). The goal of the fitting was to match these average speech values to the target values. Notice that we are below our desired NAL prescriptive target output by as much as 15 to 20 dB in the 500 to 1000 Hz range and do not approach desired target until above 1500 Hz. It is unlikely this would be a successful fitting. So what happened? Because this patient's ear canal was larger than average and the fact that modular ear domes rarely fit truly closed (the kind of closed that is used in correction tables), this patient actually had a fairly open fit, although the software did not know it. To further illustrate, we went back into the software, selected the earmold setting of "open" and reprogrammed the hearing aid. The output that resulted from this adjustment is labeled Output B in Figure 9–17, Panel A. Although still not a perfect fit in the lower frequencies, note that the software has added considerable gain for the 500 to 1000 Hz region because of this earmold selection change.

To further illustrate this relationship between software adjustment, earmold fit, and resulting real-ear output, we refit this patient with a modular dome that actually *did* fit tightly (labeled *double dome*) and repeated our probe microphone speechmapping measure. These results are shown in Panel B of Figure 9–17. Note that we now have a fairly good fit to the NAL targets for all frequencies. It appears, therefore, that the manufacturer's software works, but only when the audiologist enters the correct information!

Now, you might say that because we are verifying the fit by conducting probe microphone measures, the knowledge of the earmold tightness and venting effects does not matter as much and the software does not really have to know what is going on in the ear canal, as our

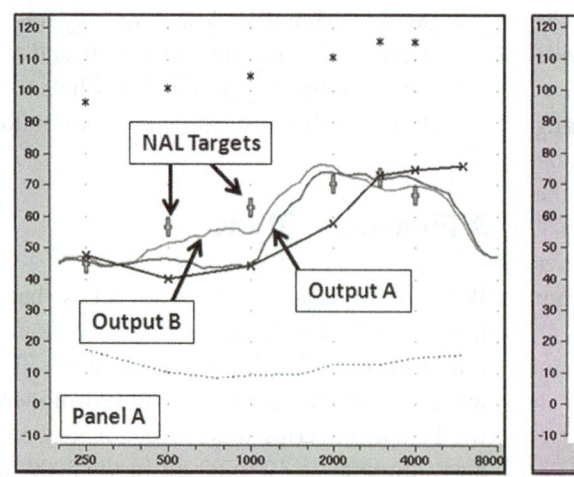

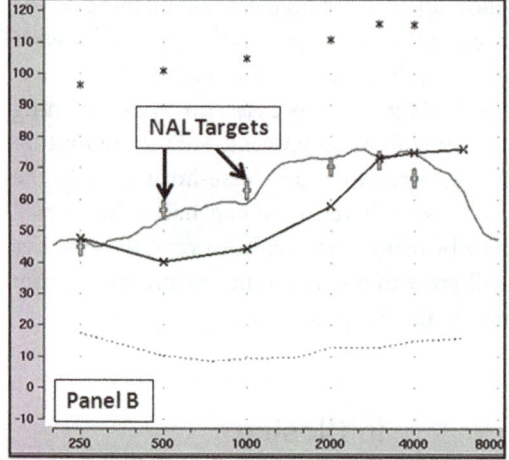

Figure 9–17. Examples of the relationship between modular eartip selection in the fitting software and the resulting changes in real-ear output (55 dB SPL real-speech input). *Panel A, Output A:* Closed tip selected in software, tip fitted loosely in ear canal. *Panel A, Output B:* Open tip selected in fitting software, tip fitted loosely in ear canal. *Panel B:* Closed tip selected in software, tip fitted moderately tightly in ear canal.

mistakes will be obvious in the real-ear output. Eventually, we will make the needed corrections to overall gain to bring us back to the desired output (e.g., match to target values). This is true, although we would have saved considerable time if we had selected the correct earmold fitting to begin with. But more importantly, what if there are audiologists who do not conduct probe microphone verification? How would they know?

10
Hearing Aid Hardware and Software: The Basics

In the preceding chapters, we focused on the incredible range and depth of important individual differences that patients bring to the fitting process, and how you can assess these aspects of communication difficulty, listening needs, personality, motivation, and so forth, prior to the selection and fitting of hearing aids. We also reviewed specific fitting considerations and applications. The time has now come to talk about the hearing aid itself.

In this chapter we will discuss the hardware and basic software that comprise modern hearing aids. It is difficult, however, to discuss hearing aid hardware and software without first understanding a little background related to electronics and signal processing. Rather than assuming all readers have been introduced to (and remember) this information, we will start with a little review. For some readers, this might seem like a hodge-podge of information already learned in classes

> **KEY CONCEPT: THEORETICAL VERSUS ACTUAL VALUES**
>
> Before we begin, it is also important to distinguish between theoretical and actual values when considering circuitry and signal processing. Specifically, almost all components and signal processing schemes will have theoretical limits based on their underlying physical and mathematic principles. For example, as we discuss later in this chapter, the theoretical limit of the dynamic range in a digital system can be calculated based on the length of the digital word. In real systems, however, the actual dynamic range, in this case referring to the range from the noise floor to the maximum input level possible of being processed, will almost always be less than the theoretical limit. Similarly, amplifiers will have a theoretical efficiency limit and directional microphones will have a theoretical limit of directivity; in real systems, however, these limits will rarely be reached due to real design and implementation limitations. We will try to differentiate between theoretical operation and actual operation of various components.

ranging from physics to computer processing. In no way is the intention of this chapter to detail the breadth and depth of these topics; rather, our goal is simply to present a few basics so that we are all speaking the same language of technology before discussing more advanced hearing aid features in the next two chapters.

If we were writing this chapter in the "old days," that is, prior to about 2000, we would likely have provided a long discussion of analog filtering, compression amplifiers, and other analog circuitry. Digital hearing aids now dominate the hearing aid market, however, and the vast majority of all hearing aids sold in the United States have been digital since 2003 or so (see Points to Ponder: A Brief History of Digital Hearing Aids). Therefore, we will limit our discussion of analog circuitry and focus more on digital sound processing.

POINTS TO PONDER: A BRIEF HISTORY OF DIGITAL HEARING AIDS

- In the mid-1980s, technology and miniaturization had progressed to a point where application of digital technology to hearing aids became viable.
- A wearable digital hearing aid was discussed in the literature as early as 1983 (Nunley, Staab, Steadman, Wechsler, & Spenser, 1983). In 1984, the Nicolet project was established with the goal of developing a commercial digital hearing aid.
- Around the same time the Nicolet project was launched (mid-1980s), a number of hearing aid manufactures developed and then marketed the first analog hearing aids with digital control. Amplification, filtering, and all signal modification in these "digitally-programmable analog" hearing aids remained analog. The use of digital switches allowed for programmability and an increased number of clinician controls without being limited by the need for case space for physical analog controls. The use of digital memory allowed for the introduction of multiple, user selectable programs in some models. The use of different programs was advocated for use in different listening environments.
- In 1988, the Nicolet project introduced the Phoenix as the first commercially available digital hearing aid (a body-style processor with ear level transducers). This group then introduced a BTE style digital hearing aid in 1989, although the size was a bit unwieldy as it was powered by three 675 batteries. Both of these instruments left the market after a relatively brief commercial run (Figure 10–1).
- Modern digital hearing aids were introduced to stay in 1996. Two ear level units, the Widex Senso and the Oticon Digifocus were the first to be introduced (at approximately the same time) in the United States; digital hearing aids represented about 6% of total hearing aid sales in 1996.
- Most modern hearing aids are digitally-programmable digital: They use digital signal processing as described below and various gain, output, and other processing parameters are programmable by the fitting clinician, typically using computer software and a programming interface. A relatively small number of digital instruments, however, are manufactured that are non-programmable. Instead they are controlled using small screw-set controls on the hearing aid case. Although digital, these controls are similar in look and operation to the potentiometers (pots) used for adjustments in analog instruments. Non-programmable digital hearing aids are mainly manufactured for use in countries where there may be limited access to computers.
- The fact that the manufacturing cost for simple digital hearing aids is at least as inexpensive as similar analog instruments, while at the same time being more power-efficient, has led to the near elimination of analog hearing aids.

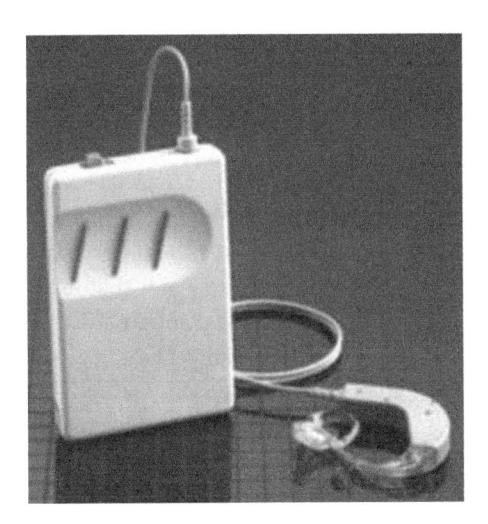

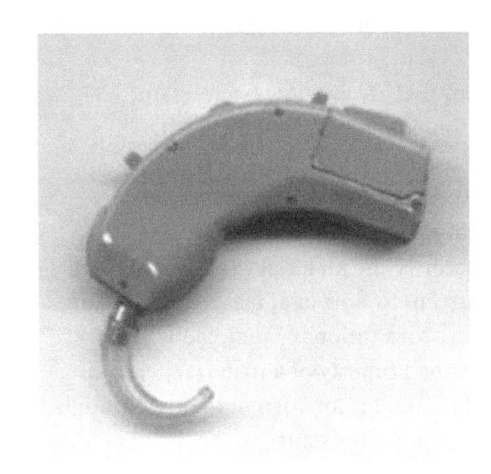

Figure 10–1. The first commercially available digital hearing aids developed by Nicolet.

Electronic Principles and Hearing Aid Hardware

Although it is certainly not our goal to turn the reader into an electrical engineer (nor could we even get close if we dedicated the entire textbook to the topic), some understanding of the fundamentals of electricity and some of the terminology commonly used is helpful for a better understand how hearing aid components operate. Most of you likely have some sense of the basics of electricity, but let's review a few definitions:

- Voltage, conventionally denoted as E, is an electromotive force, typically supplied by a battery or power supply, that causes a unit of electrical charge to move toward a unit of opposite charge. Voltage is something that pushes electrical charges around.
  - The unit of electromotive force is the VOLT (V).
- Current, conventionally denoted as I, is the flow of electrical charges through materials that allow charges to pass (called conductors). For convenience the direction of the flow of conventional current is usually defined as the flow of positive charge. With this convention, current has a direction of flow that is always from positive to negative. At the same time there is a flow of negative charges (electrons)

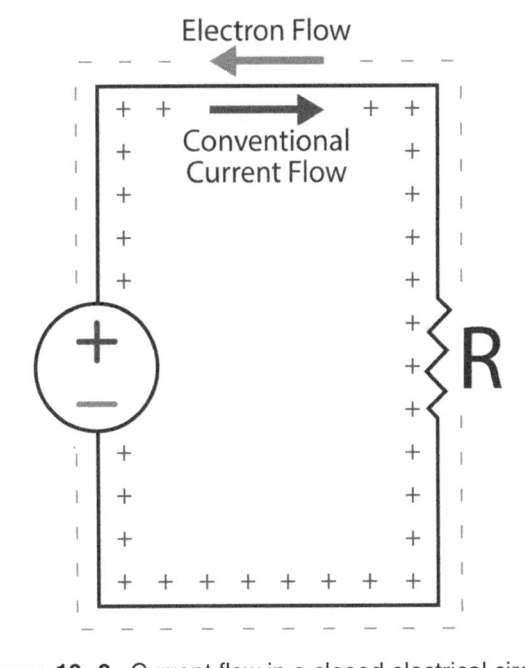

Figure 10–2. Current flow in a closed electrical circuit.

in the opposite direction (Figure 10–2). The unit of electrical current is the ampere (A). A current of 1.0 amps is a flow rate of 1.0 Coulomb/sec. (A Coulomb is the standard unit of electrical charge and is a very large number, specifically, 6.2425×10^{18}, or 6.24 quintillion; named after Charles-Augustin de Coulomb, a French physicist,

one of the 72 names inscribed on the Eiffel Tower).
- Current that always flows in the same direction is called direct current (DC), whereas current that flows first in one direction and then the other is called alternating current (AC).
■ A conductor is any material (e.g., a wire) that allows current to flow in at least one direction.
■ Resistance, conventionally denoted with an R, describes the property of a material pertaining to how difficult it is for current to flow through it. The higher the resistance of the material, the lower will be the current for any given voltage difference that exists "across" the material. Electric components with a defined amount of resistance are commonly used in electrical circuits and referred to as resistors. The unit of resistance is the Ohm (Ω). The Ohm is defined in terms of the other two variables: One ohm of resistance is that resistance that has one amp flow through it when one volt of electrical potential is placed across it (named after German physicist Georg Simon Ohm, who researched the new electrochemical cell, invented by Italian scientist Alessandro Volta).

> **KEY CONCEPT: A LITTLE BASIC ELECTRONICS TERMINOLOGY**
>
> ■ A *transducer* is any device that changes or transduces one form of energy (e.g., physical movement) to another (e.g., electrical current). Microphones and loudspeakers are two types of transducers. The small loudspeaker used in hearing aids is commonly referred to as the *receiver*. This is a throwback to the old term used for the small loudspeaker used in telephones.
> ■ A *power supply* is a device that supplies electric energy. This can be contrasted with devices that store electric energy for delivery, including *batteries* and *fuel cells*.
> ■ The *frequency response shape* refers to the relative signal level as a function of frequency (see Chapter 13). If there is equal energy at all frequencies over a defined range, the frequency response is commonly referred to as *flat*.
> - Components or processes that affect the frequency response, especially in an undesirable or intended manner are said to "color" the frequency response.
> - The shape of the frequency response in hearing aids is intentionally modified during the hearing aid fitting through filtering and other processes.
> - Components or processes may also affect the frequency range, typically referred to as the *bandwidth*. The term "broad bandwidth" is commonly used, but not very precise, in that is typically is used to mean that the frequency bandwidth of interest is generally preserved. Depending on the sound amplification, however, the term broad bandwidth has been used to describe bandwidths from as small as 4000 Hz to more than 20,000 Hz. For hearing aid applications it is also important to contrast physical bandwidth (the physical frequency range) with audible bandwidth (the range of frequencies delivered to the patient's ear that are audible), which will depend in part on the patient's hearing thresholds.
> ■ A *filter* is any device or processing that is used to change the frequency response shape.
> ■ An *amplifier* is a device that is used to increase the level of an electronic signal. The amount the signal is increased in dB is referred to as *gain*.
> ■ *Distortion* is the introduction of any part of a signal that was not there originally. We discuss distortion in much greater detail in Chapter 13.

- A *fundamental law* of electricity is that current has to flow in a loop. Whatever current leaves one side of a voltage source has to be matched by current returning to the other side of the voltage source.
- For many types of materials (commonly referred to as Ohmic resistors), the value of the resistance, defined as the ratio between voltage and current, is a constant (commonly referred to as Ohm's Law). Algebraically, this is expressed as Resistance = Voltage / Current or R = E/I.

The fundamentals of electricity are also helpful to keep in mind as we describe a few other electrical principles including capacitance and electromagnetic induction. At this point you might be wondering why we would discuss these principles at all in a hearing aid textbook, but there is a good reason. The principle of capacitance is used in the electret and microelectromechanical systems (MEMS) microphones commonly used in hearing aids. In addition, the principle of electromagnetic induction is important for everything from t-coils, to receivers, to room loops. Before we go any further though, let's consider a few more common terms that will be helpful as we discuss hearing aid components and circuitry (see associated Key Concept: A Little Basic Electronics Terminology).

Capacitance and Microphones

So what are capacitors? The simplest description is that these are devices that can store charge as a voltage difference across two plates. Physically, capacitors are made of two "plates" made from conductive material that are physically separated by a gap of non-conductive material (Figure 10–3). Capacitors were originally called condensers and their basic operation was first described by a German scientist named Ewald Georg von Kleist in November 1745, although our modern understanding of the devices took about another 100 years.

So how does capacitance relate to microphones? Just stay with us a little bit longer and we will explain. If one plate of a capacitor is set into motion towards the other, the spacing between the plates will necessarily

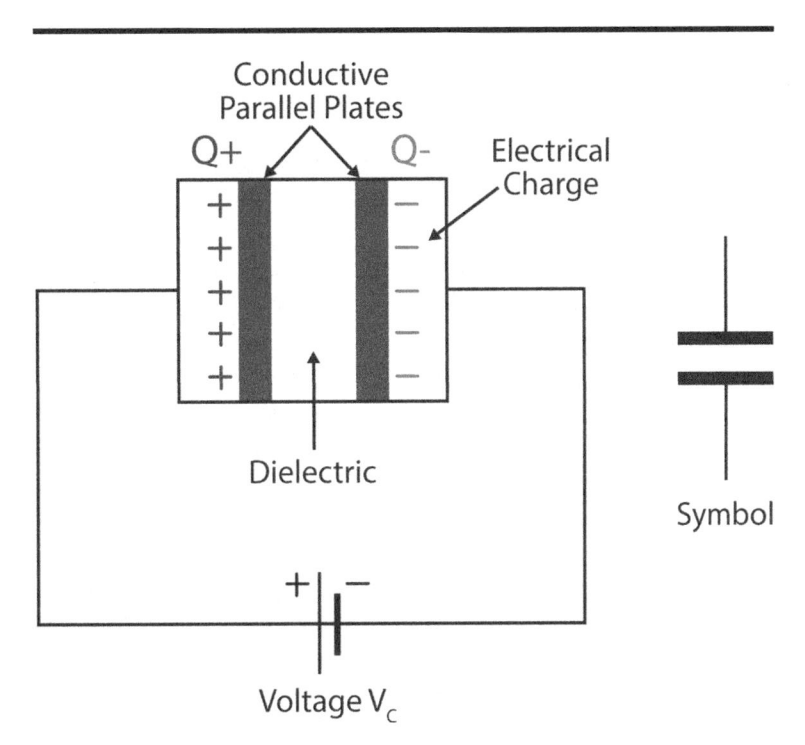

Figure 10–3. Schematic of a capacitor (*left*) and its circuitry symbol (*right*).

> **KEY CONCEPT: CAPACITANCE BASICS**
>
> - The non-conductive material that fills the gap between the plates is called the *dielectric*. In some cases the dielectric is simply air. Positive and negative electrical charges have a strong attraction for each other (positive charges will try to get to the negative pole and negative charges will try to get to the positive pole). When voltage is applied, therefore, one plate will fill with negative charges (electrons) and the other plate will fill with positive charges, creating a voltage difference across the plates. The number of charges that can be stored across the plates of a capacitor depends linearly and exactly upon the voltage difference between the plates.
> - The unit of capacitance is the Farad. A one Farad capacitor can store one Coulomb of charges at a voltage difference between the plates of one volt. For our applications, it turns out the Farad is an extremely large value and capacitance that is generally quantified in micro-Farads.
> - Capacitance depends upon three physical features of the capacitor: (1) surface area of the plates, in which increasing area increases capacitance; (2) size of the gap, in which increasing gap size decreases the capacitance; and, (3) nature of the dielectric, in which nonconductive materials that can polarize their molecules lead to increased capacitance, compared to nonconductive materials that are nonpolarizable.

be reduced, resulting in reduced voltage across the plates (assuming the total charge remains the same). This principle can be exploited by fixing a back plate and suspending a very light and movable diaphragm near the back plate in the same electrical configuration as a capacitor. Sound vibrates the diaphragm, causing changes in distance between it and the back plate, and generating voltage fluctuations, which in turn follow the sound pressure variations. Referred to as a condenser microphone in tribute to the original name for the capacitor, this type of microphone was developed at Bell Labs in 1916 and is still used in expensive sound level meters, some sound test equipment, and some other applications.

Using a very similar principle, the electret microphone was developed in 1961 and has been the primary microphone used in hearing aids for the last several decades. In a condenser microphone, the voltage difference across the two plates is created by voltage supplied from a battery or power supply. Conversely, in an electret microphone, one of the plates is a very thin light piece of synthetic polymer (plastic) with metal flecks in one surface and the other plate is a rigid piece of metal coated with a thin material that holds a permanent electric charge called an electret. One can think of an electret as the electrostatic equivalent of a permanent magnet, that is, a voltage difference is permanently "stuck" across the plates. Consequently, the microphone does not require a power supply aiding in miniaturization, thus decreasing complexity and increasing durability when compared to true condenser microphones.

More recently, we have seen the *MEMs* microphones, commonly used in cell phones, introduced into hearing aids. These silicon-based microphones are manufactured by depositing and removing semiconductor materials from a silicon wafer to form a capacitor. The rest of the parts are then etched out and include a flexible diaphragm, a stiff backplate, and damping holes with an electrical charge on the backplate, just as we see with a conventional electret microphone.

The interest in MEMS microphones relates to the potential of optimizing the interaction between sensitivity and size. The sensitivity of an electret microphone is based in part on the size of the diaphragm: the smaller the diaphragm, the lower the sensitivity and the higher the noise. In contrast, silicon microphones can be made that are highly sensitive with extremely small diaphragms. This design offers the potential for lower noise floors and better resistance to vibration (Figure 10–4). Apart from being made of silicon and the MEMS'

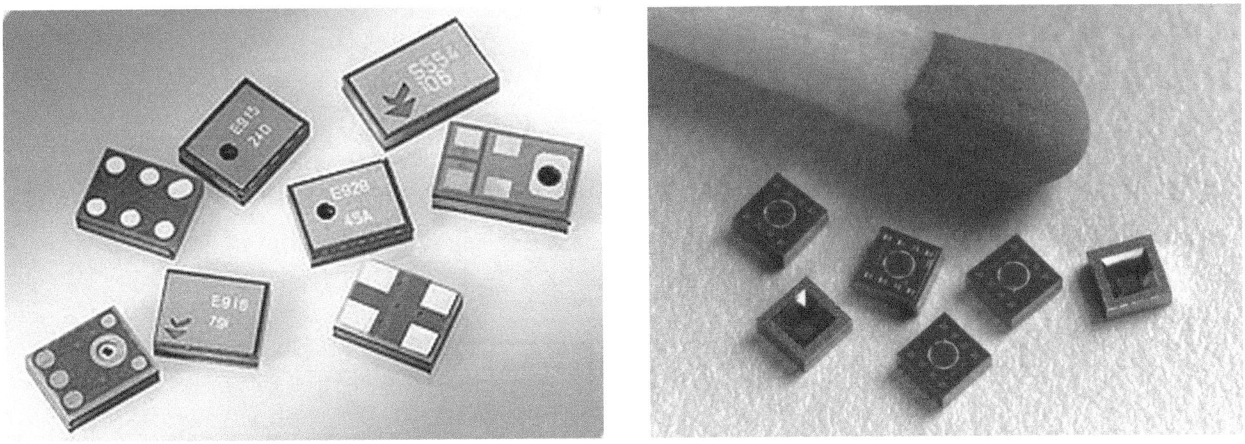

Figure 10–4 Examples of microelectromechanical system (MEMS) microphones.

potential for a much smaller size, the largest difference between the operation of electret and MEMS microphones involves how the charge is maintained on the backplate. A MEMS microphone does not have a charge when first manufactured; instead the charge is "pumped" onto the backplate via a complementary metal oxide semiconductor (CMOS) circuit. The chip restores this charge whenever the microphone is activated.

Inductance, T-Coils, and Receivers

When you wrap a coil of wire around an iron bar and provide voltage so that current flows through the wire, an electromagnet is created which generates a magnetic field. In 1831, Michael Faraday discovered that you could, in fact, induce current in a conductor by exposing it to a moving magnetic field. This property is referred to as electromagnetic induction and the amount of voltage generated is predicted by Faraday's law, which is described mathematically by the Maxwell–Faraday equation. The unit of inductance is the Henry, named after Joseph Henry (1797–1878), the American scientist who discovered electromagnetic induction independently of, and at about the same time as, Michael Faraday (1791–1867) in England. Understanding completely how electromagnetic induction works requires a number of formulas and a fair bit of math. Rather than going down that path in a clinical audiology textbook, we will just summarize the process in very general terms (without the math):

- Pushing electric current through a coil generates a time-varying magnetic field (Figure 10–5). The lines of magnetic force rotate in concentric circles around the wire. This results in a flow of magnetic energy referred to as magnetic flux.
- The direction of magnetic flux relative to current is often described by the right-hand rule. Close your right hand and point your thumb straight out like you are giving a thumbs up. If the direction of the current flow is the same as your thumb, the rotation of magnetic flux is the direction the fingers of your closed hand are pointing.
- As you move to concentric circles that are further from the wire, the strength of the magnetic flux reduces.
- The time-varying magnetic field generates current in opposition to the primary current in the coil (see Figure 10–5).
- Similarly, physically moving an external magnetic field through a coil that is part of a closed electric circuit will generate an electromagnetic force (e.g., a time-varying magnetic field) that, in turn, will result in the induction of current in the coil. An example is shown in Figure 10–6. If we move a fixed magnet into a coil of wire we can generate current in the wire.
- Magnetic flux generated by any source can induce current in a coil of wire when the coil

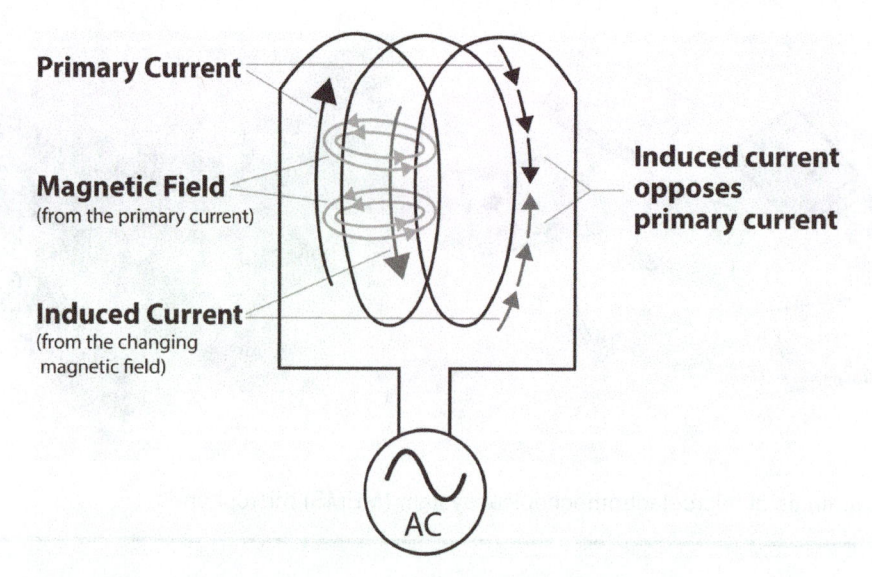

Figure 10–5. Schematic of the relationship between primary current, the time-varying magnetic field generated from the primary current, and the induced current following in the opposite direction generated from the time-varying magnetic field.

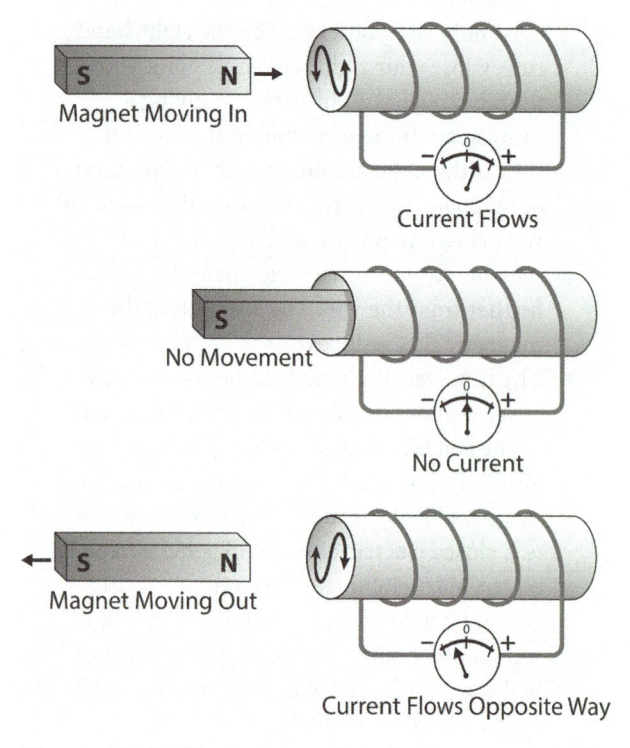

Figure 10–6. Electromagnetic induction generated by moving a fixed magnet relative to a coil.

is positioned to intersect the magnetic lines of force.

So how is electromagnetic induction used in hearing aids? One way relates to how the receiver operates. One common loudspeaker design is to coil wire around a tube that is attached to loudspeaker diaphragm. This coil and diaphragm are then suspended by a magnetic field generated by strong fixed magnets that surround, but do not touch the coil (Figure 10–7). When current is forced in one direction through the coil, a magnetic force is generated, and the coil and the attached diaphragm are forced in the other direction. You can see in Figure 10–7 that the current is forcing the diaphragm to move in—as would happen with a sine wave as amplitude goes down. The current direction is reversed to push the diaphragm out—as would happen with a sine wave as amplitude goes up. In short, an alternating current acts to push and pull the diaphragm back and forth, generating condensation and rarefaction of air molecules producing sound.

A significant challenge in loudspeaker design relates to the interaction between the mass of the dia-

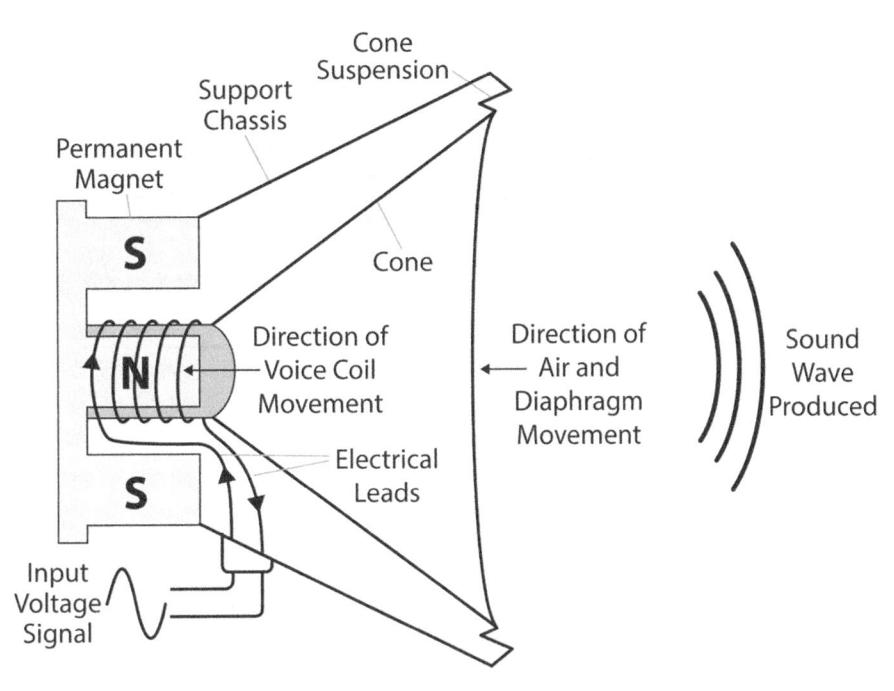

Figure 10–7. A schematic of how pushing current in one direction through a wire can cause the wire to move if the electrons are held in place by strong magnets that are fixed in space and the coil of wire is very light, not fixed to any unmovable surface, and can move easily.

phragm and frequency. Given the long wavelengths of low-frequency sounds, a lot of air needs to be pushed to produce high sound levels, so a large diaphragm is desirable for low frequencies. Conversely, the wavelength of high-frequency sounds is much shorter, so the coil and diaphragm have to be able to move very quickly, so a very small and light diaphragm is desirable. With too much mass the diaphragm cannot be moved quickly enough to produce the higher frequencies because the movement is "sluggish" compared to the changes in current applied to the coil. This frequency dependent effect is the reason many loudspeakers designed for music listening include more than one speaker in the same box (e.g., tweeter, midrange, and woofer drivers) to reproduce a wide range of frequencies accurately. Another popular technique is to use multiple drivers of the same (typically middle) size. With this design, the sound power adds up across the drivers, and then a filter is applied to turn down the middle frequencies so the frequency response is flat. As we describe later in this chapter, the small speaker used in hearing aids uses the principles of electromagnetic induction with elegant design elements that help to overcome some of the limitations resulting from its diminutive size.

Other applications for electromagnetic induction in hearing aids take advantage of the fact that current is generated in a coil that is proportional to the electromagnetic force generated by a time-varying magnetic field, as described earlier. A simplified example of this process is shown in Figure 10–8. Specifically, a time-varying magnetic field is generated by spinning a fixed magnet. The magnetic field lines (flux) rotate through the coil creating an electromagnetic force in the coil, which through induction produces electric current. As we described, current can be induced in a coil by exposing it to any time-varying magnetic field. In this specific case, the relative orientation of the magnet results in a circular rotation of the magnetic flux through the coil as the magnet spins. Consequently, the voltage produced exhibits a sinusoidal pattern from positive to negative with each rotation.

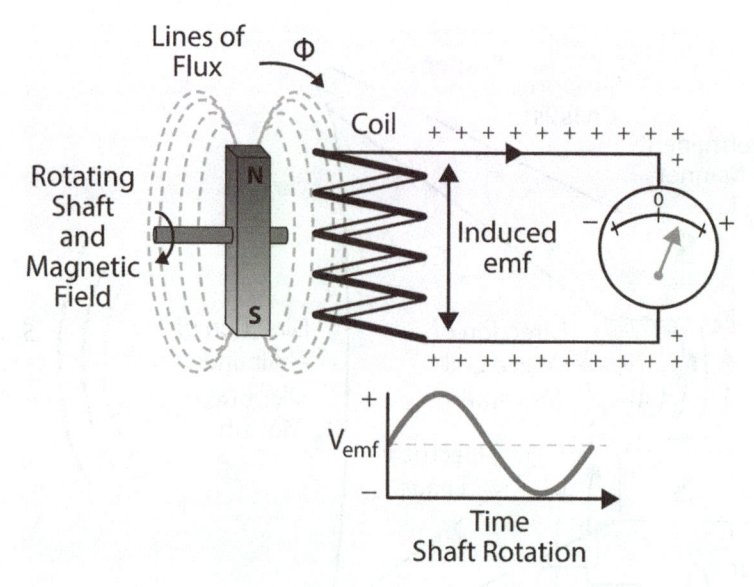

Figure 10–8. An example of how a time-varying magnetic field can induce a current in a coil of wire.

In practice, time-varying magnetic fields are generated in several useful situations including (1) as a by-product of the operation of dynamic loudspeakers, including the old receivers used in the telephones of the past and a few current telephones (such as specially designated payphones for individuals with impaired hearing); (2) intentionally using analog signals as is the case with Hearing Assistive Technology (HAT) devices (e.g., neckloop, room loop, silhouette, as shown in Figure 10–9); or (3) intentionally using sound that is coded as a digital signal and then transmitting this signal through a series of electromagnetic pulses. The latter method is used by some bilateral hearing aid configurations (i.e., for communication between hearing aids) and with some wireless linking devices (Figure 10–10). In this final case, signals are first delivered to the bridge transmitting device via direct wiring, Bluetooth, or other wireless techniques, and then the signal is retransmitted to the hearing aid using near-field magnetic induction. Although there is a considerable distance limitation to

---

TECHNICAL TIP: BLUETOOTH TECHNOLOGY?

You perhaps noticed that when we just talked about wireless techniques we mention *Bluetooth* technology—a term commonly used by people of all ages, but maybe not always so well understood. The technology was invented by Ericsson Telecommunications in 1994 as a method to transmit data over short distances, initially as a replacement for RS-232 cables. We discuss how it works in a little more detail later in this chapter. The name Bluetooth, coined in 1997, is taken from 10th century Scandinavian king Harald Bluetooth (*Blåtand* or *Blåtann*). One of the original goals of Bluetooth technology was to unite systems together, somewhat like King Bluetooth helping unite the Danish tribes into a single kingdom. These technologies are managed by the Bluetooth Special Interest Group, which has more than 25,000 member companies. Bluetooth is among the IEEE family of technologies, 802.15.1.

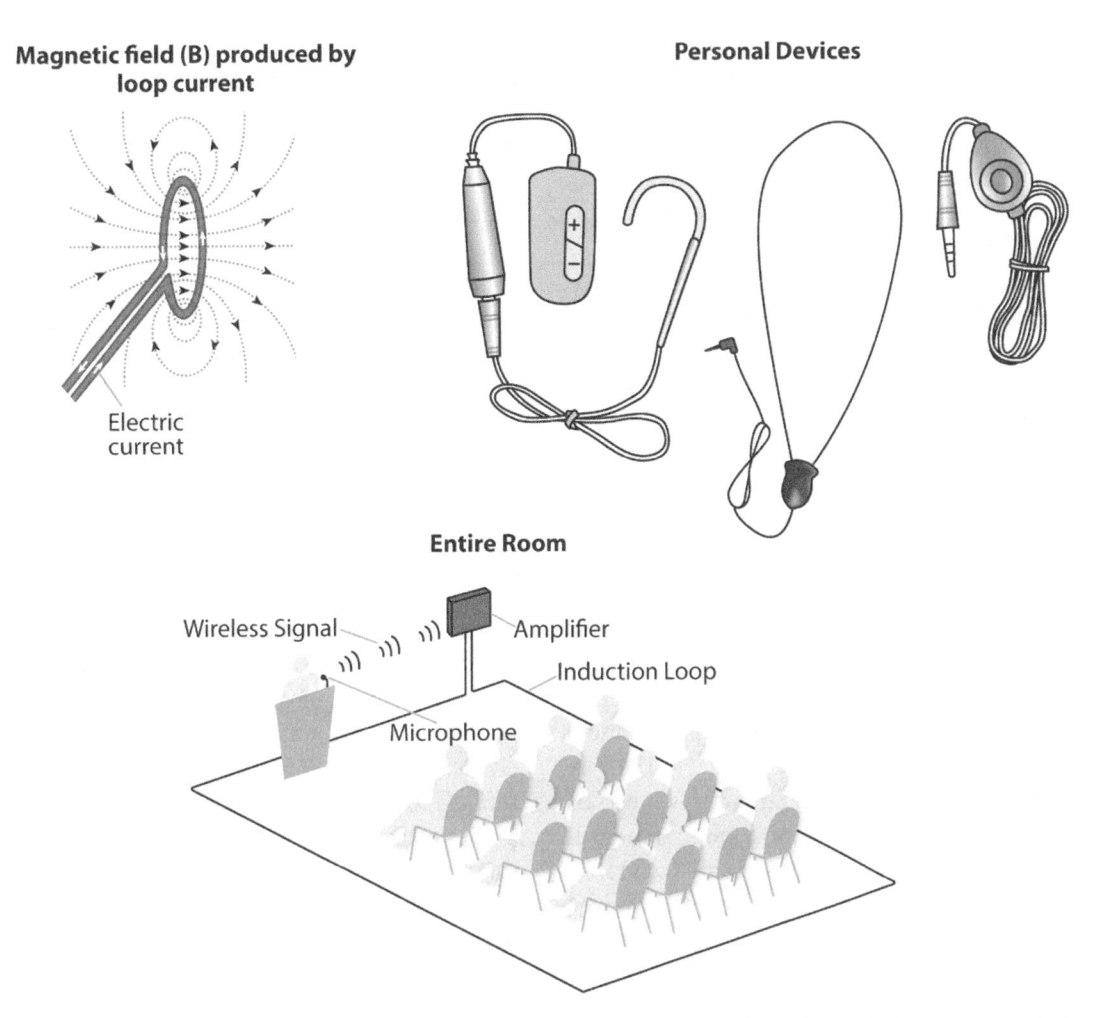

Figure 10–9. Examples of analogue induction field generators. The schematic in the upper left demonstrates how electric current applied to a single loop can generate a time-varying magnetic field. Note the strongest EMF is generated inside the loop.

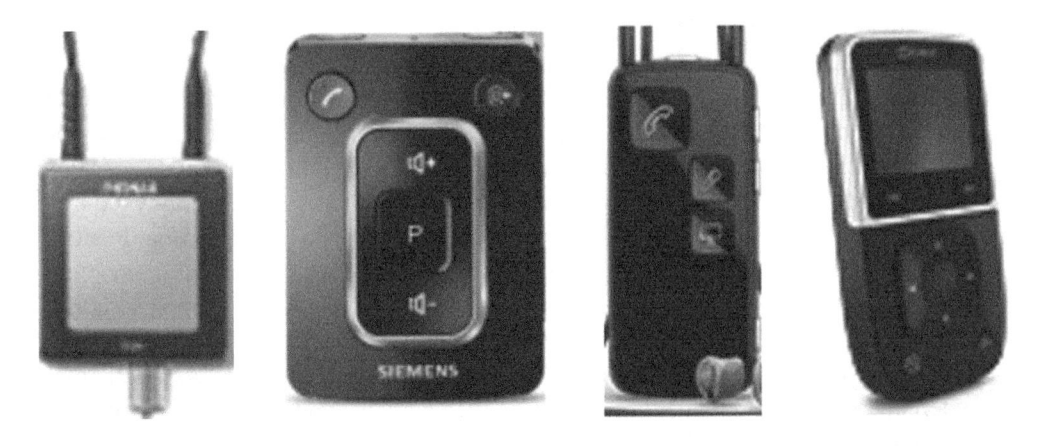

Figure 10–10. Examples of induction based wireless hearing aid linking devices used with hearing aids.

near-field magnetic induction, this method is much more energy efficient (less hearing aid battery drain) than many other wireless communication techniques.

The current produced by electromagnetic induction is always proportional to the electromagnetic force; however, more current will be generated if more electromagnetic field lines (flux) move through more coils (loops) of wire. That is, the more "turns" in the coil of wire, the more current that will be generated. As a consequence, higher output from a coil (greater sensitivity to the time-varying magnetic field) will occur with a coil having a larger number of turns. In addition, the orientation of the coil is critical to maximize sensitivity. Not only is the angle of orientation important, the magnetic field lines must pass through the coil, so the coil needs to be relatively close to the generator source of the time-varying magnetic field. For many hearing aid applications this translates into a length of about 12 to 24 inches from the generator source. In the case of a wire loop the magnetic field strength is inversely proportional to the diameter of the loop. Standards specify that the long-term root mean square (rms) field strength of room loops is at least 100 mA/m; however, not all room loops achieve this level at all positions.

Transistors and Amplifiers

One of the most important breakthroughs in making electricity more useful for the consumer was the transistor. Electronic devices ranging from amplifiers to computer processors rely on transistors to function. There are many different transistor designs; however, we will focus on their function here, rather than the details of their design. Those of you who are interested in transistor design can find many detailed descriptions on the web.

Both digital and analog output amplifiers are comprised of transistors and a number of other electronic components. Historically, the analog amplifiers used in hearing aids came from three main classes, A, B, and D. The class A output amplifiers used in hearing aids were simple, small, and relatively cheap to manufacturer. Class A amplifiers have relatively low power efficiency, in that only a maximum of about 50% of the input power from the battery is evident in the signal power of the amplified output. They are designed so that there is a steady amount of current flow regardless of input signal level. When current is applied to the coil of a dynamic loudspeaker it acts to push the position of

---

KEY CONCEPT: A LITTLE BACKGROUND ON TRANSISTORS

- Bipolar transistors can provide amplification by using the small current or voltage present at their input (for example the output of the hearing aid microphones buffer amplifier) to control the flow of a much larger current (the hearing aid battery voltage applied to the receiver coil).
- A second transistor technology is commonly used in digital circuitry where they essentially function as a switch. Most commonly, many transistors are packaged together along with other electronic components including resistors and capacitors in a complete electronic circuit. In modern hearing aids, transistors and other components are etched onto a block of silicon referred to as a complementary metal oxide semiconductor (CMOS) or simply a *chip*. Often these are packaged together with other components on a miniature circuit board referred to as an *integrated circuit*.* The central processing unit (CPU) in your computer or tablet is one such chip, although it is a complex one, sometimes containing more than one or two billion transistors spaced less than 50 nanometers from each other (less than 25% of the wavelength of light). As a point of reference, the diameter of a human hair is in the neighborhood of 18,000 to 180,000 nanometers (according to the *Physics Factbook*).

*In 1964, Texas Instruments provided the first integrated circuits used in a consumer product, a hearing aid. The semiconductor industry surpasses $1 billion in sales for the first time.

the diaphragm out a bit. As we saw in Figure 10–7, the loudspeaker diaphragm will move inward or outward depending on the direction of current flow. In general, Class A amplifiers can provide high levels of distortion free amplification if they are provided with sufficient current. For this reason, high-quality Class A amplifiers are prized by some audiophiles and still are used in some music systems when considerable heat dissipation and high current draw are not considered problematic. Unfortunately, hearing aid batteries provide very limited current, which led some authors to describe the Class A amplifier as implemented in hearing aids of the 1990s and before as "starved" (Palmer, Killion, Wilbur, & Ballad, 1995). The effect of current starving a Class A amplifier is that they are unable to provide very much amplification without physically limiting or "peak clipping" the negative amplitude peaks of the signal (see related Points-to-Ponder). It was possible to provide the Class A amplifiers used in hearing aids of the past with a higher constant current level (referred to as a higher biasing current); however, this would result in greatly reduced battery life. In order to alleviate some of the

POINTS TO PONDER: ANALOG CLIPPING

- All analog electronic components have physical limitations. That is, they will generally continue to transduce, filter and amplify signals as current, voltage, or pressure is increased as a function of input level. Once the input level to the component becomes high enough, however, the component will no longer be able to perform its intended function in the same way.
- In many components, the signal will simply be limited at the highest level the component can handle. This is referred to as physical clipping. Peak clipping refers to limiting the maximum current (positive, negative or both) to a specific level and includes the unintentional physical clipping and intentional clipping introduced as a method of limiting output. The use of intentional peak clipping as a way to limit a hearing aid's peak output so that it does not exceed a listener's threshold of discomfort creates considerable distortion and is generally avoided.
- Clipping has two main consequences: It limits the output signal level and introduces distortion. You may remember from acoustics that a square wave is made up of a fundamental frequency and its odd numbered harmonics (3rd, 5th, 7th, etc.). By clipping or "squaring off" the sine wave harmonics are introduced as shown in Figure 10–11. By definition, these newly introduced harmonics are a distortion since they were not in the original signal.
- Clipping can be symmetric (maximum current excursions are clipped in both the positive and negative directions) or asymmetric (current excursions in only one direction are clipped). Asymmetric clipping occurs with starved Class A amplifiers and has been shown to introduce high levels of intermodulation distortion, which is more bothersome than the typical harmonic distortion which is the dominate distortion introduced by symmetric clipping (Palmer et al., 1995).
- In a hearing aid and other systems, clipping may be introduced intentionally as a way to limit the maximum signal output.
- Although we usually think of clipping as an analog problem, similar phenomena can happen when we use digital signal processing (DSP). Every digital system has a finite word length. Word length is synonymous with the largest number that can be represented. If the underlying math tries to produce a result greater than the maximum allowed by the word length, then distortion results from the inherent limits.

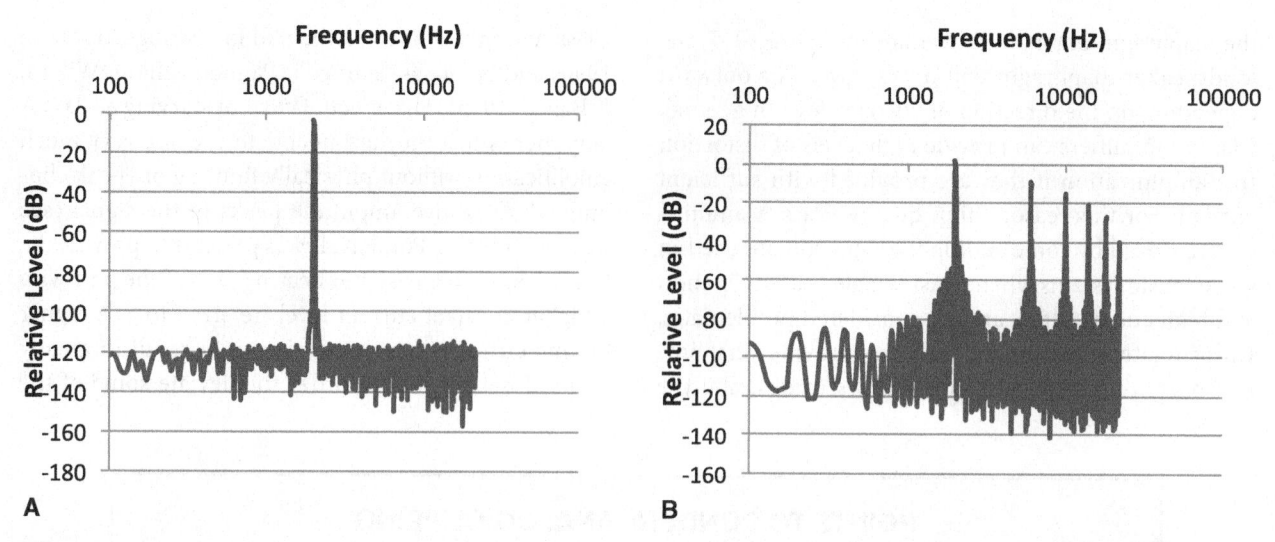

Figure 10–11. Frequency analysis of a 2000 Hz pure-tone before (**A**) and after (**B**) clipping or "squaring off."

problems with Class A amplifiers as used in hearing aids, a number of other techniques were used in the analog hearing aid realm including Sliding Class A/Class H, Class B (sometimes referred to as a "push-pull" amplifier) and Class D.

Analog Class D amplifiers work on an entirely different principle from Class A and B amplifiers. We will spend a bit more time discussing Class D because the principles used in analog Class D amplifiers are very similar to those used today in common digital amplifiers. The Class D amplifier was first designed in the 1960s, and was miniaturized and brought to hearing aids in the 1980s. Class D amplifiers had two major advantages compared to previous amplifiers used in analogue hearing aids. They could be made very small (could even be placed inside the metal can that also housed the hearing aid receiver) and they had high theoretical efficiency (almost all of the battery power could be used for amplification and there was little or no current drain when there was no input). The specific design implemented inside the hearing aids receiver case also presented a clinical advantage in that peak gain and output shifted to the higher frequencies (around 3000 Hz) making it more suitable for patients with sloping hearing losses. Unlike Class A and B amplifiers, Class D amplifiers do not directly provide amplification to the analog signal. Instead, current from the battery is applied to the receiver using an ongoing stream of high-frequency pulses.

TECHNICAL TIP: USING A CLASS D AMPLIFIER TO DRIVE THE RECEIVER

- The amplifier constantly sends current pulses at a high rate (typically around 80–100 kHz or higher) to the receiver. Each pulse is sent with the maximum possible voltage.
- When there is no input to the amplifier, the width of each pulse is extremely narrow and the total current provided to the receiver is very low (Figure 10–12).
- In the typical analog configuration referred to as Pulse-Width Modulation, the pulse is left on for a longer duration (wider pulse width) when a signal is present. The higher the target output level, the wider the pulse.
- A second common configuration is referred to as *pulse-density modulation*. Some argue this is not a true Class D amplifier and refer to it as a *digital amplifier* or *direct digital*

drive (DDD). In this configuration more pulses are sent per unit time (higher pulse density) when a signal is present. The higher the target output level, the more pulses that are generated per unit time (see Figure 10–12).

- Importantly, the pulses are switched on and off so quickly that the receiver diaphragm is simply unable to move fast enough to respond to each pulse individually. So instead of jerking back and forth with each pulse, the electrical force from adjacent pulses adds up to push the diaphragm of the receiver. Therefore, we can think of the total electrical force being applied to the receiver, and the total amount of movement generated by the diaphragm of the receiver in response to this summed force as proportional to the area under the pulses over a fixed unit of time (×).
- The relationship between the signal amplitude in sound pressure at the diaphragm, the electronic signal amplitude at the output of the microphone pre-amplifier, the desired signal amplitude at the output of the amplifier (displayed as the average voltage applied to the coil as a function of time), and the corresponding voltage pulses out of the amplifier applied to the receiver coil for two snapshots in time are shown in Figure 10–13.

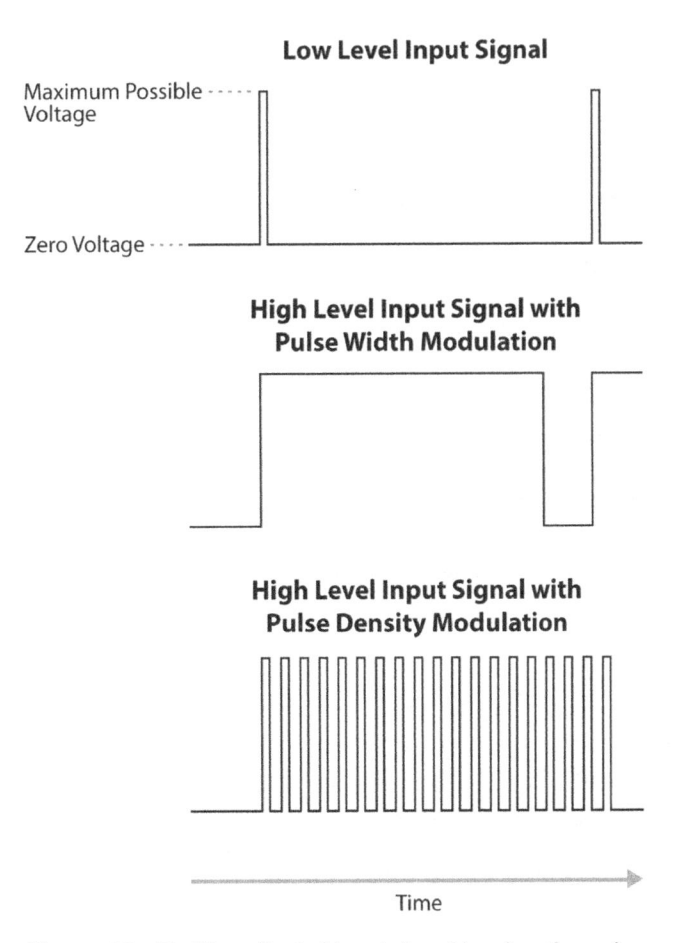

Figure 10–12. The effect of input signal level on the pulse configuration in PWM and PDM Class D amplifier outputs.

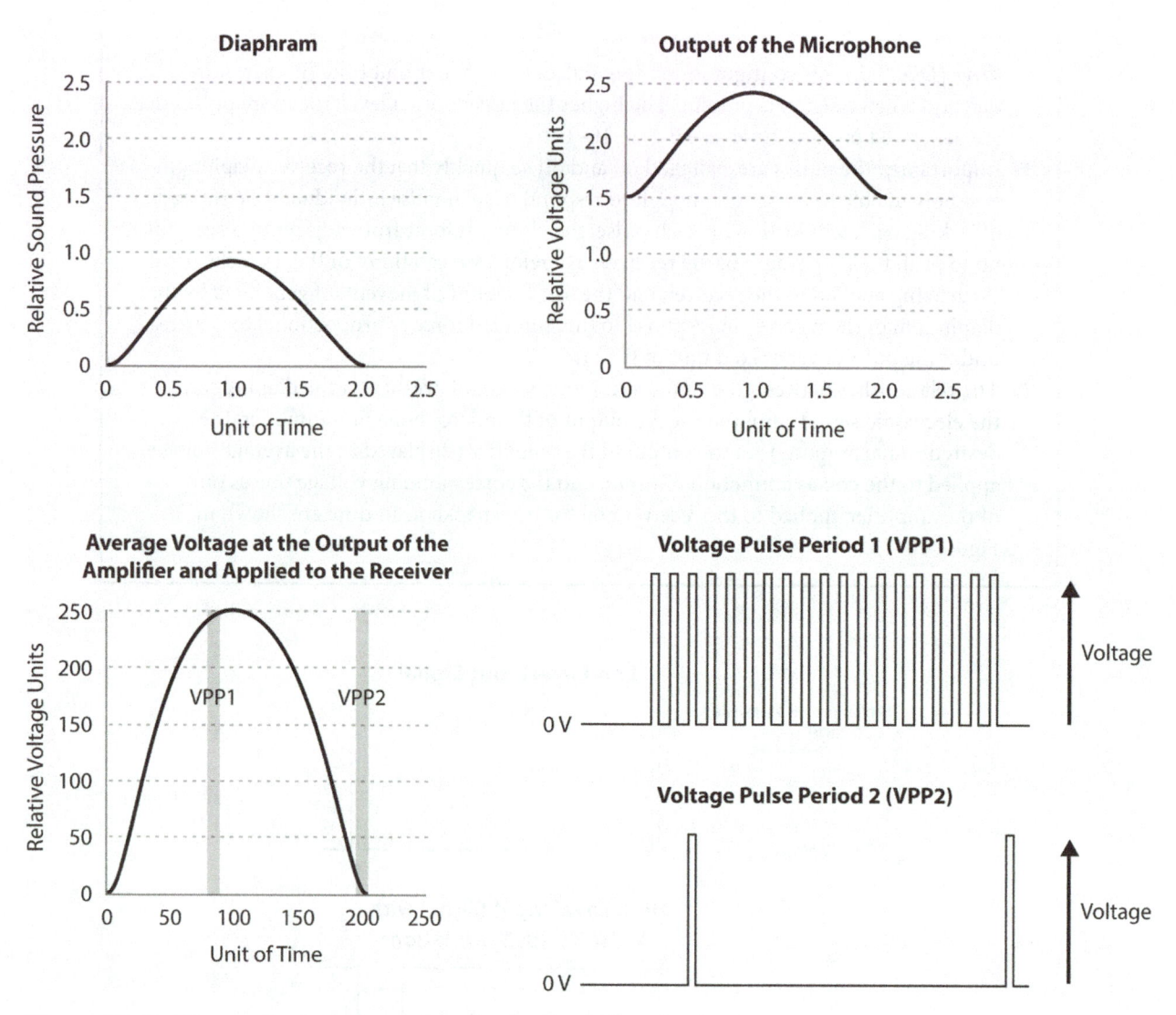

Figure 10–13. The amplitude time waveform for the first half cycle of a sine wave as measured at the microphone input and the microphone output are displayed in the top two panels. The average voltage applied to coil of the receiver is shown in the bottom left panel. A schematic of the voltage pulses from a PDM amplifier for two very brief units of time is shown in the bottom right panel.

The pulses in a Class D amplifier are typically generated by using four output transistors to switch rapidly between maximum voltage and off (no voltage). By using four transistors, Class D amplifiers are designed to drive the receiver coil first with one polarity of voltage from the battery, then the other. This makes them extremely efficient. At the theoretical maximum, 100% of the input power from the battery is evident in the signal power of the amplified output in a Class D amplifier (Benson, 1988), although they are a little less efficient than this in practice. The switching in Class D amplifiers also allows for nearly twice as much voltage to be applied to the receiver as in the case of a Class A. That is, like a Class B, a Class D amplifier is capable of higher outputs before reaching its physical limits compared to a Class A, given equivalent power consumption.

Radio Frequency Transmission and Wireless Applications

We have already discussed one method for wireless transmission in which the audio signal is converted into electric current flowing in one coil in order to generate current in a second coil through electromagnetic induction. Another group of wireless techniques uses radio frequency (RF) transmission. Until recently, most hearing aid manufacturers used near-field induction both for communication between hearing aids and for communication between the hearing aids and an intermediary bridge device that was used to connect to external devices, such as personal music players. Today, however, all major manufacturers have switched to RF transmission methods when streaming sound from the smartphone and other devices using a standard 2.4 GHz technology (outlined later in this chapter), at least in their premium products. It would seem to be of considerable interest for manufacturers to use a standard method for the end user, in that it would then make it much easier for manufacturers of other devices (e.g., cell phones, wireless microphones), to build in a single method for wireless streaming directly to hearing aids without the need for additional modification. Proprietary, manufacturer-specific methods have often been applied, however, because of limitations of standardized methods including everything from power consumption and delay concerns to increased costs due to technology licensing fees. Moreover, marketing thrives on having a feature that is not available from all other manufacturers. We have repeatedly seen important technologies like hearing aid programming move from proprietary methods to standardized methods, so we expect an increasing unified wireless approach moving forward.

While FM systems using the technology described below have been in use for several decades, it wasn't until very recently that digital RF technology had matured to the point that it could be used viably by the majority of manufacturers. The use of RF methods are of considerable interest because they have the benefit of not requiring the intermediary bridge device required for near field induction. RF transmission methods use the electronic signal of interest to modify (modulate) a high frequency electromagnetic sinusoidal carrier wave. Radio frequencies include the electromagnetic wave frequencies from about 3000 Hz to 300 GHz, which are generated by RF oscillators (transmitters) and can be picked up by an antenna and decoded using an RF receiver using wireless transmission algorithms (software). We will denote this type of receiver as RF (although engineers typically do not), in order to differentiate it from the miniature hearing aid speaker that is also referred to as a receiver. Confused yet? Stick with us and we will explain further. It will be worth our efforts because this type of wireless transmission system is used in everything from radios, to Wi-Fi, to wireless speakers, to hearing aids. By the way, given that we use the term "Hi-Fi" for high fidelity, you might think that Wi-Fi stands for "wireless fidelity." It does not. It's simply a made-up word developed by a marketing team for the Wireless Ethernet Compatibility Alliance.

There is a very large range of RF modulation techniques that fit into three general categories (see related Key Concepts). In all techniques, the receiver is set up to reconstruct the original signal from the modulated signal in a process called demodulation. These radio transmitter and receiver combinations are designed to work in relatively narrow and precisely defined frequency bands called transmission channels, which are specifically regulated within each country. Transmission channels are defined for everything from AM and FM radio, to FM systems used in hearing aids, to various types of Wi-Fi, with the goal of keeping these channels from interfering with each other or getting too crowded. Too many devices attempting to use the same transmission channel can get in the way of each other or interfere with adjacent channels, and there is the potential for picking up the wrong transmission or introducing noise and interference. It is common to label these techniques by the specific methods or standards implemented (e.g., frequency modulation, Bluetooth™, ANT, UWB); however, sometimes they are labeled by their transmission channel base frequency (e.g., 900 MHz, 2.4 GHz).

Now that we have some general structure, let's drill down a little deeper into the operation of two general methods used commonly for the type of short-range transmission used in hearing aids, frequency modulation (FM) and frequency-hopping spread-spectrum (FHSS). With FM, the carrier frequency can be modulated by the analog signal of interest, as shown in Figure 10–14. As you can see in this figure, the frequency of the carrier is increased and decreased as the amplitude of the signal of interest (modulator) changes over time.

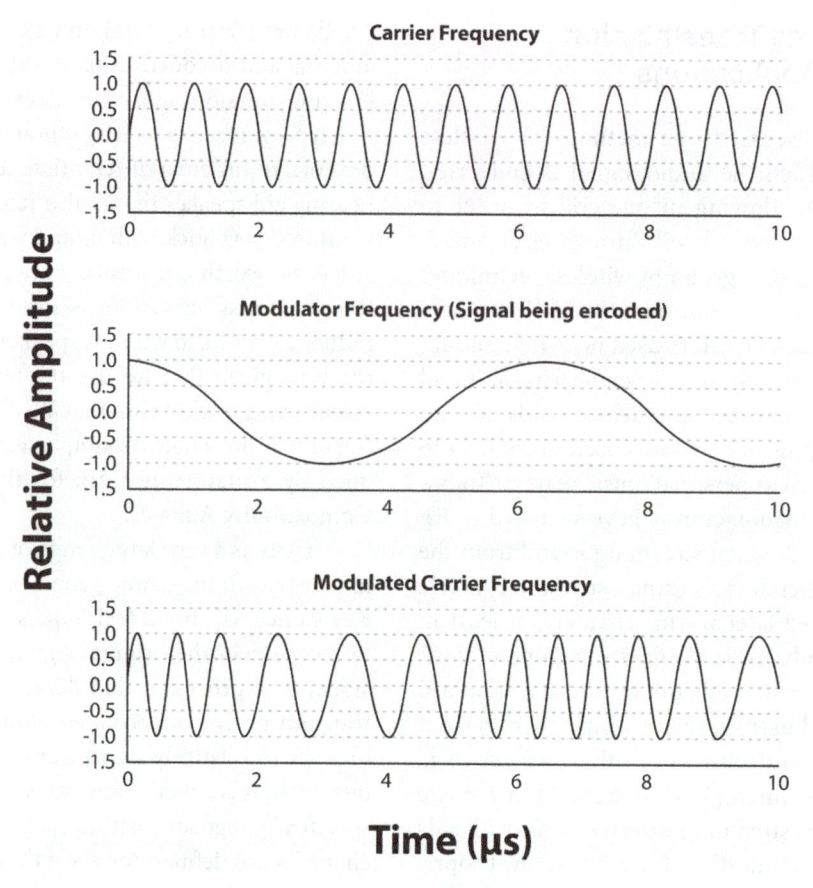

Figure 10–14. Example of how a carrier frequency is modulated by a signal of interest (in this case, a sine wave).

Once modulated and transmitted, the receiver applies demodulation resulting in a signal virtually identical to the original. One strong advantage to FM compared to some other analog signal transmission methods is that, even when there is a weak carrier signal, the embedded signal of interest is still preserved (although it can become so weak that it ceases to be picked up at all). The presence of interference from other electromagnetic fields in the same channel will add noise, however, particularly if the strength of the carrier is relatively weak. Depending on the country, the frequency bands used by FM systems and hearing aids using wireless FM include those ranging from about 30 to 900 MHz and 2.4 GHz. For example, 216 to 217 MHz is commonly used for narrow-band analog FM systems in North America. They are called "narrow band", because they operate using a relatively narrow band of carrier frequencies (e.g., 25 kHz in North America). Some modern FM systems are designed so that multiple transmitters can be picked up by the same receiver, allowing one hearing aid wearer to receive signals from multiple talkers. To further decrease interfering noise and improve performance, digital spread-spectrum techniques in the 900 MHz and 2.4 GHz transmission bands (wideband FM; wFM) have also been introduced.

There are a large range of FHSS in use and new techniques are constantly being adopted. Some of the biggest differences in the techniques used are the algorithms used for hoping between frequencies in the transmission band and modulating the carrier. Rather than go into all of the details, we will just leave it at there are lots of different standardized, as well as a variety of proprietary, techniques. Much goes on with these techniques before the signal of interest can be encoded and sent, including ensuring that the RF transmitter and receiver find each other, they lock onto each other's sig-

> ## KEY CONCEPT: RF MODULATION TECHNIQUES
>
> - A number of signals of interest can be used to modulate the carrier. Related to hearing aids, the signals of interest include (1) analog representation of sound; (2) digital representation of sound; and (3) digital packets of information that range from information about sound, to the state of the hearing aid (e.g., as is used for bilateral control discussed in Chapter 12) and beyond. Digital representation of sound is described later in this chapter.
> - The earliest RF modulation techniques were analog and include frequency modulation, amplitude modulation, and a host of other techniques. In *analog RF modulation* techniques the carrier is modulated using the continuous analog signal.
> - *Digital RF modulation* techniques are similar in many ways to the analogue techniques, but the modulation is accomplished by discrete digital signals. This type of modulation and demodulation can be thought of as a form of analog-to-digital and digital-to-analog conversion discussed later in this chapter. Digital RF modulation techniques are used in digital modems and other digital signal transmission systems.
> - In traditional narrow-band wireless techniques, like the original FM systems, the transmitter and receiver are locked into one carrier frequency and will interfere with any other devices at that same frequency. As you might be able to tell by the name, *spread-spectrum RF modulation* techniques take the bandwidth of the original signal of interest and purposefully increase its frequency range. By spreading out the frequency spectrum there is less likelihood there will be interference with a large number of devices. There are a large range of spread spectrum technologies used for RF transmission; however, many function using one of two basic ideas. One is to spread the spectrum but stay within a fixed sub-band (e.g., *direct sequence spread spectrum*; *DSSS*), which includes Wideband FM. The other is to hop around to constantly changing frequencies within the transmission channel using specific algorithms (e.g., *frequency hopping spread-spectrum*, or *FHSS*), which encompasses many commonly used wireless transmission techniques including Bluetooth™. Spread-spectrum techniques include those which send both analog and digital signals, although most common current techniques are digital. The general ideas around frequency hopping have been around since the early 1900s and there is an interesting and unique history surrounding the people who initially invented and patented the technologies. If you have a little time, we encourage you to search terms that include actress and mathematician Hedy Lamarr (not a combined career that you hear of occurring very often; not to be confused with *Hedley Lamarr* for you Blazing Saddles fans), the company Telefunken, and Polish inventor Leonard Danilewicz, for the storied history!
> - One subgroup of wireless transmission techniques has been specifically designed to send digital information, including digital representation of sound, back and forth over short distances. This subgroup includes Bluetooth™ and other techniques used in hearing aids which establish wireless personal area networks (WPAN).

nal, they synchronize their hopping frequencies, and so on. In general, new and improved techniques are generally aimed at continually reducing interference with other devices within the transmission channel, performing functions automatically, improving power consumption, improving signal fidelity, and reducing delay. The techniques used also differ in a number of other important ways, including the strength of the carrier allowed.

Some of these techniques like Bluetooth™ have a variety of additional features including (1) the use of transceivers (transmitter and receiver on the same chip) so data can be sent in both directions (WPAN); (2) after initial "pairing," the ability for the transceivers to quickly and automatically find each other and synchronize; (3) interconnectivity of up to eight different devices in a single group referred to as a *piconet* (which gets its name from "pico," which means very small, and "net" which is short for network). One fairly unique feature of this design is that it allows for the combined function of different devices rather than just simple one-way, or even two-way, data transmission. The groups of algorithms performing specific Bluetooth functions are arranged in *layers* which are grouped together into upper and lower *stacks*. How the stacks interact with each other to accomplish the desired task is defined by the *Bluetooth Protocol*. The original Bluetooth standard applied a large range of protocols that are used to accomplish everything from delivery of sound to wireless headphones and loudspeakers to computer peripheral usage like a mouse and keyboard. The original sound delivery protocols and the associated hardware were not really suitable for sharing signals directly with hearing aids for two reasons. The delay was long enough to be disruptive to communication (e.g., the mouth and sound don't line up precisely enough) and, although designed for portable devices, the power consumption was still too high. More recently, a low energy (LE) Bluetooth standard was approved and was initially used for transferring data (not sound), primarily in medical devices. Even more recently, some very clever engineers have determined some ways of transmitting sound with minimal delay while maintaining low power consumption based on this standard. As of 2016, a small number of proprietary methods using similar techniques were being applied for wireless transmission from external devices directly to hearing aids. As of this writing standardized, nonproprietary LE 900 MHz or 2.4 GHz wireless transmission methods were not yet in use in all hearing aids, but some of the important first steps towards this expected outcome have already occurred.

Digital Signal Processing (DSP)

We have been throwing around the terms digital and analog in this chapter but have not yet clearly differentiated between them; we will do so now. As we demonstrated in the top portion of Figure 10–13, the electronic signal at the output of the microphone is intended to mimic the pressure changes of the sounds in the environment that impinge on the microphone diaphragm. In analog hearing aids this continuously varying voltage at the microphone output is filtered, amplified, and delivered to the receiver coil. This process is very quick; however, any desired changes to the signal such as filtering, providing input level dependent amplification (compression and amplification), and so forth are achieved through the introduction of physical circuitry. The introduction of new physical circuitry limits how many things we can do in an analog hearing aid before size, internal noise, and battery drain become significant problems. Modern digital hearing aids differ in that the electrical output of the microphone is converted to a string of representative numbers. The advantage of representing the analog signal by a string of numbers is that changes to the signal can be introduced by applying math functions. Furthermore, the changes made can be based on ongoing analyses of properties of the incoming signal. Groups of math functions intended to perform specifically defined actions are commonly referred to as *digital algorithms* or just *algorithms*. Together these algorithms when applied to digital representations of sound are referred to as *digital signal processing (DSP)* or just *processing*. After the representation of the signal is in the form we want, it is converted back into an analog signal for delivery to the listener. Before going into more detail regarding these processes, let's review how analog signals can be represented digitally. Unlike us older folks writing this, we know that some of you probably learned the foundation for these basics in grade school, but let's review for those of you that have not thought about this in a long time.

Basics of Digital Representation of Sound

The digital representation of a sound includes the numeric representation of the amplitude level at each discrete time interval (sample) and a way to define the length of the discrete time interval. Digital systems however, don't use the standard 10-base number system that we commonly use in everyday life (e.g., 24 + 79 = 103). Instead, **bi**nary dig**its** (*bits*) are used, which instead of having 10 possible states (0,1,2,3,4,5,6,7,8,9), only have two possible states (0,1). So if we can only represent two states with one bit, how many can we represent with two bits?

Bit #	2	1
0 =	0	0
1 =	0	1
2 =	1	0
3 =	1	1

So we can represent four different values with two bits. What if we had four bits?

Bit #	4	3	2	1
0 =	0	0	0	0
1 =	0	0	0	1
2 =	0	0	1	0
3 =	0	0	1	1
4 =	0	1	0	0
5 =	0	1	0	1
6 =	0	1	1	0
7 =	0	1	1	1
8 =	1	0	0	0
9 =	1	0	0	1
10 =	1	0	1	0
11 =	1	0	1	1
12 =	1	1	0	0
13 =	1	1	0	1
14 =	1	1	1	0
15 =	1	1	1	1

We can represent sixteen values with four bits. From this pattern we can see that the quantity of values that you can represent with any quantity of bits is the value two raised to the number of bits. So, if we have eight bits, $2^8 = 256$ values; with 16 bits, $2^{16} = 65,536$ values. So increasing the number of bits provides many more numbers to quantify accurately the amplitude of the signal at each sample. The group of bits used to represent a single quantity like signal amplitude is commonly referred to as a digital word. That is, an 8-bit system has digital words that have eight binary digits. For comparison, in 2017 the operating systems of laptop computers typically used a 64-bit word.

One of the limits of this process, however, is that the digital representation of sound is in discrete steps rather than a smooth and continuous (perfectly accurate) representation of the original signal over time. This misrepresentation of the continuous amplitude change in the original signal introduces roundoff error and quantization error. In simple terms, the original smooth continuous signal is squared off in stair steps and the amplitude of the signal is not perfectly represented at many instants of time (Figure 10–15). These errors introduce quantization distortion, which is functionally a noise floor that limits the dynamic range of the DSP. Importantly, the more bits available (the larger the digital word), the smaller the error and the larger the maximum dynamic range. The dynamic range of DSP is defined as the difference between the largest signal that can be digitized and the noise floor resulting from quantization distortion.

Theoretically, each additional bit will double the number of possible values and, in doing so, provides a

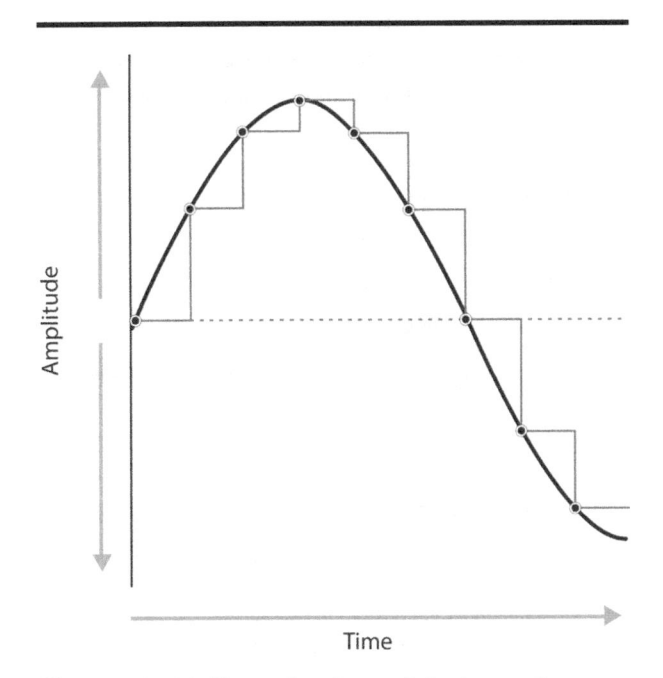

Figure 10–15. Example of an original smooth waveform and the "squaring-off" of the signal that results from digitization.

6 dB increase in dynamic range. Therefore, a 16-bit system will have a theoretical dynamic range of 16 × 6 dB = 96 dB, whereas a 12-bit system will have a theoretical dynamic range of 12 × 6 dB = 72 dB. In practice, however, the dynamic range of digital hearing aids, as well as other digital sound delivery systems are typically 3 to 10% less than the theoretical limit. For reference, commercial compact discs (CDs) are typically 16 bit, while commercial DVDs and Blu-Ray DVDs can use up to a 24-bit process for audio. Typical modern hearing aids use processes that have equivalent bit values of 12 to 24 bits. Some early hearing aids introduced a problem by using too few bits in that the dynamic range of sounds of interest in the environment was larger than the dynamic range of the hearing aid. Because it is important to provide amplification to very low input levels, the limited dynamic range also resulted in a limited input ceiling. In order to prevent digital clipping with high level inputs, sounds in the environment above levels as low as 83 to 88 dB were not allowed into the hearing aid. This was accomplished with a "front end" input compression limiting system. This aggressive front-end compressor used in early digital instruments may have prevented digital clipping, but it did have some interesting side effects related to the hearing aid fitting. Mueller and Hawkins (2006) report on an interesting case regarding a patient who was professional golfer and was fitted with CIC hearing aids. Interestingly, because of this front-end compressor, he could hear the "ping" of his golf drive unaided, but could not hear it when he was wearing his hearing aids!

Fortunately, modern hearing aids typically use a number of techniques including higher numbers of bits and/or input level dependent microphone pre-amplifier gain to avoid this limitation. We therefore believe that clinicians should not worry about the specific bit rate used in hearing aids, and generally assume the dynamic range is large enough to accomplish the speech recognition goals of each manufacturer's specific instruments. This issue can still provide an important and noticeable limitation, however, when listening to music that has a large dynamic range and a high input level. We are not just referring to rock concerts either. Live classical and jazz music can have instantaneous peaks as high as 115 dB SPL.

It is important to note that it is not the simple case that the more bits used (the longer the digital word) the better. Processing longer digital words requires more processing power and will result in greater battery drain. Therefore, engineers must balance having enough bits for an accurate representation without more bits than necessary. How accurate the representation needs to be not only depends on the desired dynamic range, but also on the specific requirements of the signal processing algorithms of interest.

Our description of DSP thus far has focused on integer-based (whole numbers) sound representations. The class of DSP that works this way is referred to as fixed point, which refers to the fact that numbers are represented using a fixed number of digits to the right and the left of the decimal point. This can be contrasted with DSP that is based on floating-point representation and manipulation of rational numbers using at least 32-bits. As is evident from the name, floating-point representations allow for the number of digits before and after the decimal point to vary. As a consequence of

---

THINGS TO REMEMBER: INPUT CEILINGS OF TODAY'S HEARING AIDS

Input ceilings in modern hearing aids are both variable in level and flexibility. The default input ceiling in some current instruments is as low as 92 dB SPL, although several other models/brands are much higher (from approximately 106 all the way up to 113–115 dB SPL). We say default level because another technique used is to change preamplifier gain for specific programs/input levels. That is, the analog to digital converter's dynamic range is not increased, but the input ceiling (and floor) are increased. This increased input ceiling is most commonly applied for the user-selected music program or when input levels consistently remain above some predefined level.

these two designs, the gap between numbers in fixed-point processing is always one, meanwhile the gap between numbers in floating-point processing varies, which can provide a more accurate representation of amplitude, reduce round off error, and lower quantization noise. Although these benefits for floating-point processing can be realized in a hearing aid, the decision is not so simple because the chips that support this sort of processing will always be larger and consume more power than fixed-point DSP designs. Furthermore, the entire set of DSP algorithms selected must be written for one type or the other. That is, one cannot simply port an algorithm from floating point to fixed point without a considerable rewrite. This type of processing also has higher complexity. How difficult is the choice? Articles in engineering magazines with titles like "Fixed vs. floating point: a surprisingly hard choice" point to the answer. Manipulations in these designs can become extremely complicated, so let's just leave it with the knowledge that engineers must first select the optimal type of processing for their needs and then be very careful and precise when manipulating the math to minimize quantization noise.

The sampling rate, also referred to as the sampling frequency, is the number of samples per second (measured in Hz) and is used to define the discrete time intervals of the digital representation of the sound. The time between each sample is referred to as the sampling period and is the inverse of the sampling rate. For example, if the sampling frequency is 1000 Hz, the sampling period is 1/1000 samples per second or 1 ms. Sampling rate limitations are described by a theory first described by Harold Nyquist in 1927 referred to as, you guessed it, the Nyquist Theorem. This work was later expanded and enhanced by Claude Shannon and is now referred to as the Nyquist-Shannon Theorem.

In Figure 10–16, we sampled a signal every millisecond, or at a sampling rate of 1000 Hz. Therefore, the sine wave represented has a period of about 16.6 ms, so its frequency must be around 60 Hz (1000 divided by 16.6). This is a pretty low frequency and thus has a long wavelength. We therefore had a little more than 16 samples for every period, giving us a nice representation of the waveform. What would happen if we sampled a higher sound frequency using this same sampling rate? If the sine wave were 250 Hz, we would only be sampling four times for each period using a 1000 Hz sampling rate. Could we still represent the waveform appropriately with only four samples? If the sine wave of interest were 2000 Hz, we would only be sampling once every other period. We hope it's obvious that this wouldn't be often enough, but what would a high enough sampling rate be? According to the Nyquist-Shannon Theorem, any sound that has been sampled can theoretically be perfectly reconstructed from the samples if the sampling rate is at least twice the highest frequency of interest and the sound does not include any frequencies that are higher than or exactly equal to one-half the sampling frequency. Importantly, this theorem expresses a theoretical limit; real signals and sampling techniques are generally slightly more limited. It is therefore typical practice to sample at slightly more than twice the frequency of interest. For example, the frequency range of human hearing is commonly thought of as 20 to 20,000 Hz. In other words, frequencies as high as 20,000 Hz may be of interest. This assumption led to the use of a sampling rate of 44,100 Hz for commercial CDs. DVD audio uses a sampling rate of 96,000 Hz, although rates as high as 192,000 Hz are sometimes used in Blu-Ray DVDs. The term Nyquist frequency refers to the upper frequency of interest (also the bandwidth of interest). In the example of CDs just given, the Nyquist frequency would be 22,050 Hz. This should be differentiated from the Nyquist rate, which is defined as double the Nyquist frequency (and very near the sampling rate in traditional sampling algorithms).

So what happens if a sound is sampled that has a higher frequency than half the sampling rate? For instance, let's say our sampling rate is 12,000 Hz, and

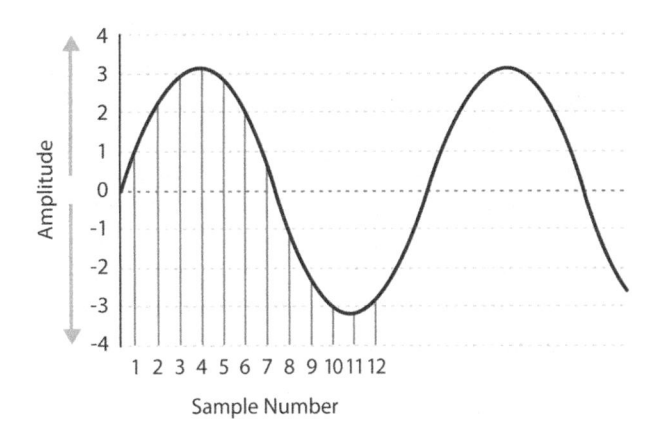

Figure 10–16. Schematic of the process of A-to-D conversion in which a signal is sampled every millisecond.

we are interested in a pure tone that is 9000 Hz. In this case, the DSP system doesn't know that it was originally a 9000 Hz signal at the input, and it may fit the sampled points with a lower frequency signal. The inability to tell the correct higher frequency signal from a lower frequency that fits the same sample points is referred to as aliasing. An example of two different pure tones that fit the same two sample points is shown in Figure 10–17. In this case the higher frequency cannot accurately be represented because there are not at least two samples for every period. Consequently, one typical way to avoid aliasing in digital equipment is to use a low-pass anti-aliasing filter that does not permit frequencies equal to or above half the sampling rate to be sampled. This is not quite as simple as it sounds, however, because the most desirable anti-aliasing filter would let in all frequencies up to the Nyquist frequency and no higher frequencies. To do so perfectly, the slope of the filter skirt would need to be infinite.

Analog to Digital (A/D) and Digital to Analog (D/A) Conversion

The process of obtaining a digital representation of sound through sampling and quantization is called analog-to-digital conversion (A/D), sometimes called digitization or A-to-D for short. Sampling is the process of measuring the signal amplitude at discrete points in time. Measurement of amplitude and assignment of numeric values at each sample is a process referred to as quantization. Here is an example of a simplified analog-to-digital conversion:

- Assume we have a simple sine wave as an input as shown in Figure 10–16.
- Also assume we have an A/D convertor that can sample the signal amplitude every millisecond.
- Further assume that we can represent the amplitude of the signal using a total of nine numbers as shown, −4 through +4 (including 0).
- Our digital representation of this signal would then be pairs of numbers consisting of the representation of time in milliseconds and amplitude using discrete steps. In this specific case the result would be time 1, amplitude 0; time 2, amplitude 2; time 3, amplitude 3; time 4, amplitude 3. In a real digital system, however, we would represent these standard numbers with a binary number system as described above.

From our simple example above, we can immediately see some problems. First, we clearly don't have enough numbers to represent the amplitude of the signal at any point in time very accurately. For example, at 3 ms, we really need an amplitude number between two and three and a roundoff error is created. To decrease this error to reasonable levels, we need more numbers for our amplitude representation than the nine in our example. In other words, we need more bits as we described above. As we noted above the low sampling rate used would also create a possible problem in our example. Clearly, we need to have a digital representation of sound that is accurate, but how accurate is accurate enough?

We could use a simple A/D convertor with a high number of bits, a high sampling rate, and the requisite anti-aliasing and anti-imaging filters. Then we could use a powerful processor like the CPU in your computer to complete the complex math that is required for the signal analysis, filtering, multi-channel gain processing, and application of the desired features that we discuss in the next chapter (e.g., various types of digital noise reduction, microphone array processing, digital feedback suppression). We could then use a digital-to-

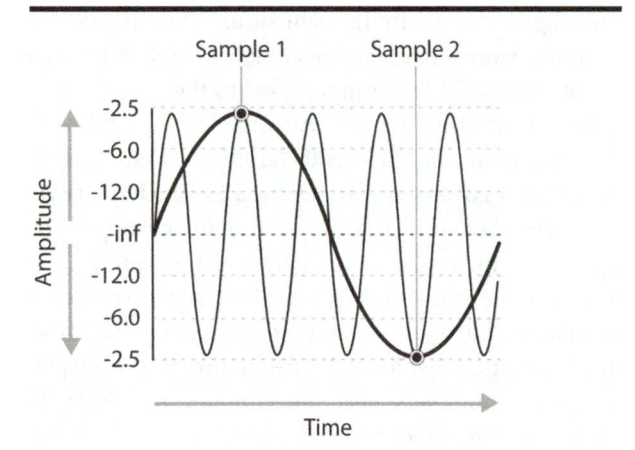

Figure 10–17. An example of two different pure tones that fit the same two sample points. The two sample points are represented by the two large dots.

analog (D/A) convertor (D-to-A for short) to convert the digital representation of our processed sound back into an analog (continuous) current that we could then send to "steer" the current from the battery to provide a higher voltage representation of our processed signal to the coil of the receiver so that it could be transduced to acoustic sound pressure and delivered to the ear.

The D/A convertor performs an action just the opposite of the A/D convertor. That is, it uses strings of numbers that precisely represent the amplitude of the processed signal to update the assigned voltage sent to the output transistors at discrete points in time corresponding to the sampling rate. One limitation of traditional D/A conversion is that the output voltage is only updated at precise intervals determined by the sampling rate, and is held at a constant value between sample points (over the sampling period) as shown in Figure 10–15. This "staircase" reconstruction has two negative effects. First, it introduces a constant delay equal to one-half the sampling period. Given the sampling rates used in hearing aids, this delay is rather minor compared to the processing delay. Secondly, this reconstruction introduces new harmonics above the Nyquist frequency referred to as images. These are sort of the D/A counterparts to aliases described as part of the A/D conversion. A low pass anti-imaging filter is typically used to remove this distortion. Once the signal is back in the form of an analog voltage, it is routed to the hearing aid amplifier (output transistors) for amplification.

This simplified conversion and signal processing structure can be a real problem in hearing aid design for several reasons. The first problem is that the signal processing will require more and more electrical power from the battery as we increase the bits used and the sampling rate. Furthermore, both A/D and D/A consume electricity from the battery. General purpose CPUs like those used in computers are also relatively inefficient when it comes to electrical consumption compared to a processing unit specifically designed for the desired hearing aid signal processing, or even one designed specifically for optimizing sound processing. Even if we did not have the limitations of the hearing aid battery, there would be another major problem with this design, and that is *delay*. We discuss the delay problem in more detail below, but clearly we need the hearing aid to operate in real time and not have noticeable delays between the time a sound is picked up at the hearing aid microphone and when it is delivered to the ear.

Given the need for accurate digital representation of sound, real-time signal processing with limited delay, and making sure we can do all of this using a hearing aid battery that we would like to last more than five minutes (hopefully a week or more), a variety of complex and, in some cases, proprietary methods are used. We discuss a few general methods below.

Some types of A/D and D/A methods used in modern hearing aids implement processes referred to as oversampling and upsampling. The oversampling ratio, a bit of information you sometimes see advertised on commercial audio gear as well as associated with hearing aids, is calculated by dividing the actual sampling rate by the desired Nyquist rate (double the maximum bandwidth of interest).

One group of A/D and D/A conversion processes used in hearing aids implements oversampling and upsampling via so-called Delta conversion (e.g., a form

---

POINTS TO PONDER: EXAMPLE OF OVERSAMPLING

So how is oversampling ratio calculated?

- If it is desirable to amplify frequencies through a hearing aid up to and including 8000 Hz (Nyquist frequency), the Nyquist rate would be 16,000 Hz.
- If the actual sampling rate is 384,000 Hz, the oversampling ratio would be 384,000/16,000 = 24.
- This is typically expressed and advertised as 24× oversampling (read as 24 times oversampling).
- Its not uncommon for today's hearing aids to have oversampling rates of 128× or 256×.

of oversampling referred to as Sigma-Delta A/D conversion and a form of upsampling referred to as Delta-Sigma D/A conversion are common). These methods sample at such a high rate that as little as a single bit can be used to assign amplitude values as either lower or higher than the previous sample. After oversampling in the A/D stage, the sampling rate can be lowered to the desired Nyquist rate without losing information using a process called decimation. Because such a high sampling rate is used and there are so many samples within a single wavelength, these oversampling processes have the advantage of limiting problems with aliasing and imaging. In addition, Delta convertors implement a digital filter, which allows specific and known noise sources that are introduced during the conversion process to be effectively targeted and controlled using processes typically referred to as noise shaping.

Another method of converting a signal from a digital to analog representation that is aimed at overcoming the limits of the hearing aid battery avoids using a D/A convertor altogether. Instead, one of several possible processes is used to prepare the digital signal to drive the receiver directly. This process exploits the fact that digital signals are binary (numerically either a 1 or 0). Electronically, they can be represented as single brief pulses of voltage that are either all on (1) or all off (0). What would happen if we sent the digital signal as a train of voltage pulses to a Class D amplifier as we described earlier? Similarly to the analog Class D, we could send a lot of pulses (high-pulse density) or a few pulses (low-pulse density) to produce high and low intensities respectively. In this way we could directly drive the output transistors with a digital signal, bypassing D/A. Of course, a few steps will need to occur to change our digital representation of the processed sound to create a pulse train that can be used to drive the digital amplifier directly. Just prior to sending the digital signal to the output transistors, the digital signal needs to be upsampled and converted to a useful form using digital-to-digital (D/D) conversion. The digital signal must be converted to reflect the pulse density corresponding to the appropriate summed voltage we want to deliver to the speaker coil (Figure 10–18). Upsampling allows us to have much greater control on the range of possible pulse densities. Specifically, the more pulses we are able to generate over the duration of one period of a waveform, the finer control we will have over the summed voltage applied to the speaker coil and therefore the exact position of the loudspeaker diaphragm at each instant in time. Another benefit of upsampling techniques like Delta-Sigma conversion is they generally limit the need for complex anti-imaging filters. These filters may be necessary for simple non-oversampled D/A convertors; in some cases the natural high-frequency receiver roll-off can provide sufficient low pass filtering so that traditional anti-imaging filters can be avoided altogether.

There are a very large number of ways that A/D and D/A conversion can be accomplished. All of the available methods generally operate within the constraints related to the number of bits and the Nyquist-Shannon Theorem discussed earlier. The specific choice

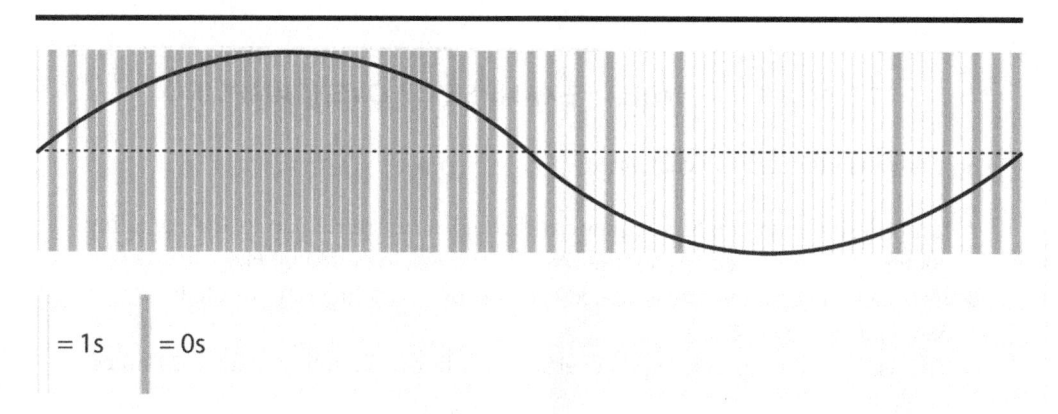

Figure 10–18. Example of using a digital signal to provide the pulse density required to produce a sine wave using a digital amplifier. Filled bars represent 1s and unfilled bars represent 0s.

of methods when a hearing aid is designed is based on several factors including battery drain, aliasing and imaging issues, limiting noise, cost, and so forth. Fortunately, these choices are generally an engineering rather than clinical concern. Consequently, rather than going into more complex details regarding A/D and D/A, we will continue by discussing general DSP terminology and processes.

Processing of Digital Signals

To understand the operation of DSP in much depth, considerable knowledge of mathematics is required. Fortunately, we do not believe that clinicians need a deep understanding of DSP to understand the general operation of digital hearing aids, so we will keep things relatively simple. It is our intention to give enough explanation of common terminology to provide you with a working vocabulary of DSP fundamentals and a general understanding of the benefits and limitations of DSP. For a more detailed treatment of signal processing for hearing aids the interested reader is referred to a variety of other sources including Kates (2008), Lyons (2010), or any more recent DSP textbook.

Changes to the signal in a digital hearing aid that are made by the processor are achieved in the software, rather than through physical changes in components (hardware) as is the case with analog instruments. For each patient, we can modify how the signal processing algorithms within the hearing aid are applied based on patient information. The step-by-step procedure for determining the appropriate settings is referred to as the fitting algorithm. Fitting algorithms are described in detail in Chapter 14. Briefly, in order to achieve the desired signal processing, a programming algorithm that resides on a computer is used to define the desired parameters for the signal processing algorithms and hearing aid controls. The programming algorithm is part of a software package that is typically referred to as the manufacturer's programming software. The patient-specific desired parameters for the signal processing algorithms are downloaded from the computer to the hearing aid memory through a specific mechanism for connecting the hearing aid to the computer, generally referred to as a programming interface. The software, hardware, and methods used to program hearing aids also are discussed in more detail in Chapter 14. In addition, we will describe several types of signal processing algorithms in more detail in Chapters 11 and 12 when we talk about hearing aid features, so for now let's just stick to the basics.

The complexity and speed of the algorithms that can be performed, as well as the current drain associated with these processes, are related to the design of the processing chip. The processing chip in modern hearing aids is a very small circuit board that typically includes a processing unit and the memory we describe above. In order to improve efficiency, it is typical for the processor to include some sections within the processor dedicated to specific functions like filtering (commonly referred to as hard-wired digital processing) and some parts of the processor dedicated to manipulating math (commonly referred to as software processing or general arithmetic processing). There are benefits and limitations to each type, so both are commonly applied. The earliest digital hearing aids used hardwired digital processing for essentially all functions. We have also seen products for which nearly all functions are completed in the software (commonly referred to as open platform). The primary advantage of hardwired processing is the significantly lower current consumed, but it comes at the expense of limited algorithm flexibility.

Manufacturers commonly refer to the collection of digital processing circuitry as a platform and the major hearing aid manufacturers typically use one platform for an entire line of products from their most basic model to their premium technologies wherein all advanced features are activated. Twenty years ago, the major hearing aid manufacturers released a new platform every three years or so. We have seen this pace increase since 2010 or so, and some manufacturers have released a new platform in as little as 12 to 18 months after the previous generation.

The speed and power consumption of the chip are dependent on the manufacturing process and the chip's clock speed. All chips have an embedded clock that provides the timing for the overall digital logic as well as all individual processing algorithms. As with the CPU in your computer, generally the higher the clock speed the faster the processing and the greater the battery drain. Shrinking the size of the components on the chip (referred to as feature size) generally reduces the power drain at the same clock speed. As we noted earlier in this chapter, the current feature size in digital hearing aids is quite small (Figure 10–19). Increased processing speed

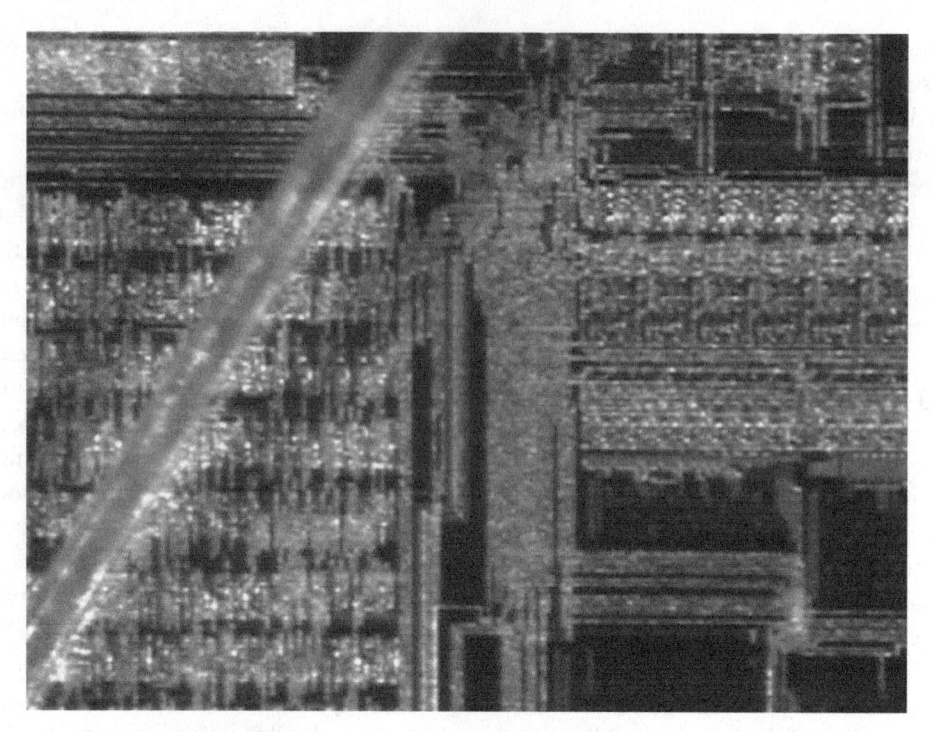

Figure 10–19. A zoomed in view of a processing chip. Notice the close feature spacing. The very thin silver lines are connected transistors and other features etched in the silicon. The large pipe-like structure crossing the chip on the left side is a human hair (about 100 μm thick)! (Used with permission from Steve Armstrong.)

allows the chip to perform more complex processes because more calculations can be done within the same time frame. The calculations that are completed are usually relatively simple and based on a defined instruction set. A chip's processing power is typically expressed in terms of instructions per second. These values are often difficult to compare across chips, however, because not all systems use instruction sets of the same complexity. Let's take a simple example to illustrate that point: A chip that could only add or subtract but could do so at 3 billion instructions per second may actually use less processing power for performing mathematical operations than a chip that is only capable of 2 billion instructions per second but also includes multiplication and division in its instruction set, or even perform multiplication and addition in a single instruction. Make sense?

Digital Delay

While additional processes do not require additional hardware, as is the case in analog systems, more accurate digital representation of the sound, greater numbers of algorithms, and more complex algorithms will all increase processing time. It is important to clarify, however, that the amount of time sound is delayed by the hearing aid, referred to as total delay, is dependent on a number of factors in addition to processing speed. For example, both A/D and D/A conversion require some processing time (approximately 0.5 ms each). The number of frequency ranges (channels) used for processing and how those frequency ranges are broken up can also have large effects on processing time. For example, the delay may be frequency independent (essentially the same delay at all frequencies) or frequency dependent (typically more delay in the low frequencies falling to less delay in the higher frequencies), depending on the type of digital filtering used.

Frequency-specific delay related to DSP is referred to as group delay. We discuss the effect filtering can have on delay in more detail later in this chapter. In addition, some signal processing algorithms require more time than others, depending on whether analysis and processing are completed sequentially or in blocks. As recently as 2005 to 2008, the total delay measured in our laboratories for some digital hearing aids was as large as 11 to 12 ms. Today, the total delay we measure is typically between 2 and 8 ms. According to data reported by Alexander (2016b), delays have remained in this range over the last several years. Delay times were also relatively constant across products from the same manufacturer and over time. Based on past research, values of less than 9 to 10 ms are generally considered too small to be problematic. Delays in the range of 10 to 15 ms have been shown to be objectionable to listeners with normal hearing (e.g., Agnew and Thornton, 2000). Listeners with hearing loss, however, have been shown to tolerate longer delays of 14 to 30 ms (Stone and Moore, 1999; 2005). Other work has suggested, however, that delays as short as 5 to 6 ms may be noticed by listeners when fitted with hearing aids using open eartips (Stone, Moore, Meisenbacher, & Derleth, 2008)—patients might report this as an echo. Additionally, localization may be negatively impacted by delays of 10 ms, even when listeners are provided a period of acclimatization (Simon et al., 2008). Understandably, therefore, keeping group delay to a minimum is also a design concern when manufacturers introduce new algorithms.

Frequency Specific Analysis and Processing Techniques

To state the obvious, patients do not typically have the same magnitude of hearing loss at all frequencies. Consequently, it is often necessary to apply different processing at different frequency regions. In order to apply the frequency-specific processing algorithms for control of gain, output and many of the features described in Chapters 11 and 12, the digital input must be analyzed and processed as a function of frequency. Once the digital signal at the output of the A/D convertor is decomposed into its frequency components, they can be analyzed in a variety of ways (e.g., amplitude, phase, changes compared to previous samples) to make processing decisions. For example, in a compression system the amount of gain depends on the input level, so analysis of the input level in each frequency range is used to determine the appropriate compressor gain values. Once the input signal has been analyzed and calculations made to determine the desired changes, each of these components can be processed using math functions (for example, gain may be applied using simple multiplication).

The digital representation of sound at the output of the A/D convertor is in the *time domain*. That is, the digital information represents how the signal changes over time (consider the time-amplitude waveform way of graphing sound). One general type of hearing aid processing keeps the representation in the time domain throughout, and all desired changes to the sound at the hearing aid output that are due to signal processing result from math applied in the time domain. A second general type of processing is to transform the time domain representation into a *frequency domain* representation (think of the spectral representation of sound on an amplitude-frequency graph). One common method for doing this transform is the Fast Fourier Transform (FFT) described in more detail below. Math can then be applied in the frequency domain to accomplish the desired processing. Once this is completed, the individual frequency components can then be transformed back into the time domain by using the Inverse Fast Fourier Transform (IFFT) prior to D/A conversion.

When working in the time domain, it is possible to bring in a sample and apply all mathematical steps for processing in a step-by-step fashion on each sample. This method is very fast and referred to as *sequential processing*. In hearing aids using sequential processing, the specific processes applied to each sample (e.g., magnitude of gain applied) are typically determined based on the values of preceding samples, but no information about the specific sample in question is used. Alternatively, it is sometimes of interest to bring in a block (group) of samples first, and apply processing to the entire block. This second method is referred to as *block processing*, *frame processing*, or *windowing*. Block processing may be applied to time domain processing; however, it is always used in frequency domain processing because the transform into the frequency domain requires a group of samples prior to calculation.

There are a couple of potential advantages to working in the frequency domain, as well as at least two potential limitations. On the plus side, it is more computationally efficient. That is, rather than calculating what you want to do relative to processing for every sample, the calculations are made on a group of samples all at once and applied to a group of samples all at once. This allows the hearing aid processor, which is typically pushed to its limit in terms of processing complexity, to

> ## POINTS TO PONDER: WORKING WITH FREQUENCY DOMAIN PROCESSING
>
> As we mentioned, there are some potential negative consequences of working in the traditional frequency domain. Here are some general techniques used in hearing aids aimed at offsetting problems with traditional frequency domain real-time sound processing systems:
>
> - Design the processing chip and/or instruction set to perform FFTs using fewer mathematical operations. That is, use an instruction set for which some of the processes are essentially "built in."
> - Place a dedicated FFT processor on the hearing aid processing chip.
> - Carefully design the processing so that one fewer FFT is needed, though this can increase quantization noise.
> - Use a group of techniques that are generally referred to as side-branch or parallel processing. A large number of specific techniques of this type have been proposed that differ in a variety of ways that are beyond the scope of this text.
>   - In general, many of these approaches can be thought of as hybrid approaches that combine frequency and time domain approaches in order to decrease processing complexity, meanwhile decreasing total delay when compared to traditional frequency domain approaches.

calculate more complex algorithms with the same total processing power. In addition, frequency domain processing provides blocks of frequency-specific data that can be sequentially compared. Analyzing blocks of data is useful for application of many hearing aid features such as wind noise detection, feedback suppression, as well as some sound classification techniques (discussed in Chapters 11 and 12).

On the negative side, working in the frequency domain requires a transform and reverse transform that take time and, consequently, total delay is increased. In addition, these transforms also require considerable processing power. As Kates explained in 2008, the calculation of a total of four FFTs (including inverse FFTs) are necessary in an optimal FFT based multi-channel compression hearing aid. This requires more processing power than desirable, however, considering the total processing power available. Several techniques are used in modern hearing aids to combat this problem.

Working in the Time Domain: Filter Banks

Even when processing in the time domain, it is still of interest to analyze the input and apply DSP in a frequency-specific manner. In such systems it is common to use a *digital filter bank* to separate the digital representation of sound into adjacent frequency bands, commonly referred to as *channels*. Often the digital filter bank applied is similar in function and design to the analog counterpart that was used in analog hearing aids. That is, it functions as a series of overlapping band pass filters (Figure 10–20).

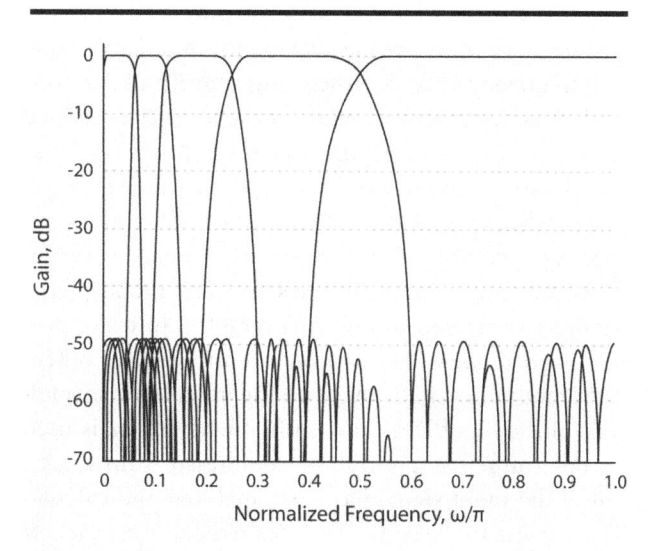

Figure 10–20. An example of the frequency response of a digital filter bank.

> **KEY CONCEPT: A LITTLE MORE ON DIGITAL FILTERS**
>
> As we've discussed, in signal processing in general, a digital filter is a system that performs mathematical operations on a sampled, discrete-time signal to reduce or enhance certain aspects of that signal. Here are some specific aspects of digital filtering in hearing aids:
>
> - Filtering is any processing or circuit used to change or limit the frequency response. Specifically, filters are intended to reduce the level of unwanted frequency components or enhance the level of desired frequency components (by attenuating other frequencies).
> - In hearing aids, filters may be used to reduce gain or output over a particular frequency range, or more commonly, to divide the frequency range into *frequency bands* for control of gain and/or *frequency channels* for frequency-specific processing, including control of gain or output as a function of input level (*compression and expansion*).
> - Filters are typically classified as high-pass (providing attenuation to the lower frequencies), low-pass (providing attenuation to the higher frequencies), band-pass (attenuating both lower and higher frequencies while passing a band in the middle), or band-stop (the opposite of band-pass).
> - Filters are defined by their 3 dB or 10 dB down *cut-off frequencies* and the *filter slope* (also referred to as the filter rejection rate). In the case of band-pass and band-stop filters, the filter is also defined by the center frequency and bandwidth.
> - Analog filters, sometimes referred to as an RC circuit, are composed of a resistor and capacitor placed in series (in a row). In an analog filter, every RC pair, is referred to as a "pole" or an "order" and provides 6 dB of attenuation per octave beyond the cut-off frequency. That is, the filter skirt has a slope of 6 dB per octave. Increasing the number of pairs acts as a multiplier, so a third order filter has a filter skirt slope of $6 \times 3 = 18$ dB per octave. It is convention to continue to describe filter slopes in terms of order, even in digital filters when the attenuation is provided through math.
> - In analog hearing aids, filters were generally limited to third or fourth order (no more than 24 dB/octave filter slope) in part because of the increase in circuit noise and phase distortions associated with increasing the number of physical components. In contrast, digital filters can be constructed with filter slopes of 80, 100 or even 1000 dB/octave. Phase distortions near the cut-off frequencies, however, also limit the desired rejection rate in digital filters.
> - In both digital and analog filters, the steeper the filter slope (filter order), the greater is the group delay associated with a given filter.

In modern digital hearing aids, filter banks are sometimes designed using steep filter skirts, so that it is possible to have processing within the channels operate relatively independently. More commonly, however, the filter bank is designed with considerable overlap (shallow filter skirts), and the processing algorithms consider not only the input signal in each sub-band of frequency within each filter, but also aspects of the broadband sound. Digital filters are very powerful, in part, because they can achieve any filtering effect that can be expressed as a mathematical algorithm.

> ### THINGS TO REMEMBER: QUANTIFYING A DIGITAL FILTER
>
> - The shape of a digital filter is typically expressed by the filter output when presented with a very brief input signal. Engineers call this the systems *impulse response*.
> - Since digital filters are applied using math, and the math functions are based on a processor clock, digital filters can be quantified in terms of duration. That is, it is useful to characterize a digital filter by its impulse response, and then describe the *digital filter* duration or *filter length* (how long that impulse response lasts, typically a certain number of samples).
> - In order to design a specific digital filter, several values that serve as constant multipliers in the filter math function must be derived. Engineers call these number constants *digital filter coefficients*. There are several techniques for deriving coefficients, and these methods are generally intended to minimize the maximum deviation from the ideal output. Changes in filter coefficients affect the operation of the filter and a number of filter parameters (e.g., cutoff frequencies, filter skirt slope).

There are a large number of different types of digital filter designs implemented in modern hearing aids. These designs are intended to balance several potential trade-offs which include, but are not limited to (1) speed (e.g., the delay they introduce), which is ultimately limited by the speed of the processor clock; (2) interaction between frequency and phase; (3) cost; (4) computational complexity, which will be limited by the processing power and the effect on battery life; and (5) desired frequency resolution, which limits the size of the frequency block that signal processing can be applied and can limit the amount of control the fitting clinician has in adjusting the frequency response.

Rather than discuss the wide range of designs in detail, let's only consider the basic design categories. There are two general categories of digital filters that are commonly used in sound processing, *infinite impulse response (IIR)* and *finite impulse response (FIR)*. An IIR filter, also called a *recursive filter*, is so named because its impulse response can last an infinite amount of time. IIR filters are relatively fast and are capable of extremely complex filter shapes. An example of two different filter transitions for filters with the same filter skirt slopes is shown in Figure 10–21. The group delay of an IIR filter is also generally shorter than other filter designs. If a bank of IIR filters is used, however, the fact that group delay is frequency dependent creates interactions. In such filter banks the group delay usually peaks in the lower to mid frequencies and then rolls off to smaller values in the higher frequencies (Figure 10–22). Consequently, construction of an IIR filter bank requires very careful consideration because the differing delays combine to affect the *filter phase response*. Consider a frequency range that is processed by two overlapping filters. If the group delay characteristics aren't matched, then a phase mismatch is also likely. The implication here is that there is a risk of peaks or dips in the overall frequency response due to constructive and destructive interference effects. Careful design choices can eliminate this phenomenon.

IIR Filters are contrasted with FIR filters, also called *nonrecursive filters*, which have an impulse response that is limited in duration to a defined number of samples. FIR filter duration is described by the filter order. This use of the term "order" should not be confused with its typical use in describing the slope of the filter skirt. The number of samples that an FIR filter lasts corresponds to its order plus 1. For example, a fifth order FIR filter will have a duration of six (5+1) samples, meanwhile a second order FIR filter will have a duration of three (2+1) samples. One of the largest advantages for using FIR instead of IIR filters when designing a filter bank is that FIR filters can be designed so that the change in filter phase is proportional to frequency, referred to

Typical Skirt Transition Region (Bessel Filter)

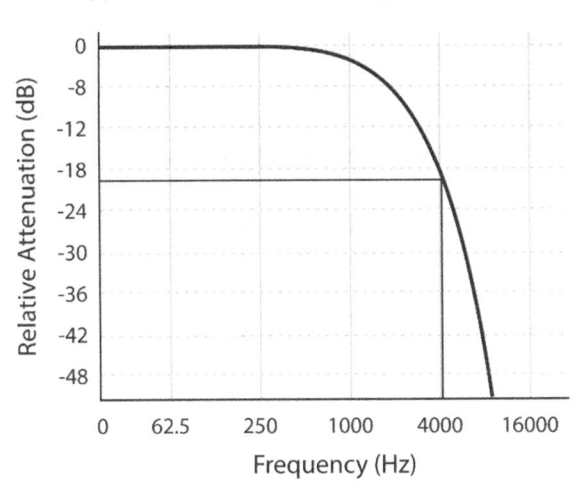

Sharp Skirt Transition Region (Chebychev Filter)

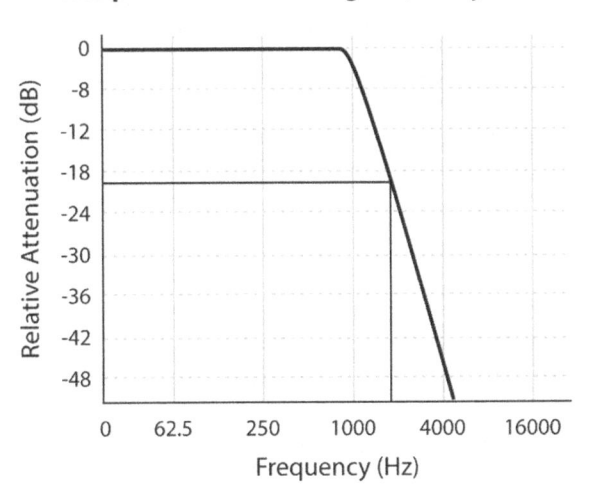

Figure 10–21. Different filter slope transitions for two low-pass filters matched for cutoff frequency (1000 Hz) and slope of filter skirt (6th order). Remember the cutoff frequency is defined as the 3 dB down point.

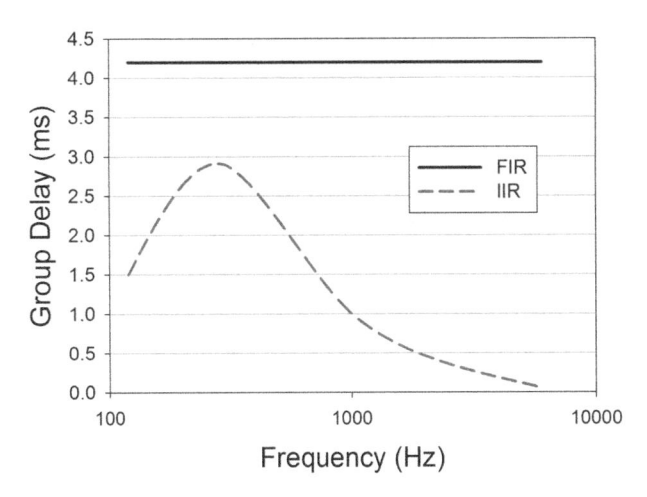

Figure 10–22. An example of group delay for two similar FIR and IIR filter banks, each consisting of five overlapping band-pass filters.

as *linear phase*. FIR filter banks of this design result in minimal phase distortion and, therefore, minimal dips in the frequency response in the regions where the filters overlap. Although this is a clear benefit of linear phase FIR filters, these filters of course have a few downsides when compared to IIR filters having similar function (e.g., similar slope of the filter skirts). First, FIR filters are typically more than an order of magnitude more computationally demanding than IIR filters. In addition, although the group delay is typically fixed as a function of frequency, the fixed magnitude of group delay in an FIR filter bank is somewhat higher than the group delay at *any* frequency for an IIR filter bank. A theoretical example of group delay for two similar FIR and IIR filter banks consisting of five band-pass filters each is shown in Figure 10–22.

The desired frequency resolution is also of interest across all filter bank designs. A high-frequency resolution means we are interested in analyzing and processing the frequency content within very small sub-bands of frequency. In other words, a hearing aid with a large number of channels is desired. Increasing frequency resolution with a filter bank requires increasingly more and more narrow filters, each with steeper roll-off rates. This will increase the total delay and the battery drain in the hearing aid, however.

A number of sophisticated filtering techniques are applied in current hearing aids aimed at minimizing the relative limitations of traditional FIR and IIR filter banks. The complexity of the design of these filter banks and the associated processing for applying compressor gain result in rather unique platforms for each manufacturer. These unique implementations comprise what might give different platforms a uniquely different sound impression, even when they are matched as closely as possible to the same prescriptive gain targets.

Working in the Spectral Domain: Fast Fourier Transform (FFT)

Processing and/or analysis in the spectral domain requires transforming the digital representation of the signal from a time waveform to a representation of the frequency content. The decomposition of the digital math function representing the discrete frequency components is typically completed in hearing aids using a process called Fast Fourier Transform (FFT). It is not necessary—or typical—to decompose complex signals into every possible frequency component using FFT. The calculation of an FFT will be based on a number of samples. Remember, however, sound in the environment will typically be changing over time, so essentially the output of FFT is spectral "snapshots" that are provided for time periods defined by the number of samples. The actual number of samples collected for each FFT are referred to as FFT points. That is, if 128 samples are collected, it is referred to as a 128-point FFT. The number of samples collected for each FFT directly affects frequency resolution. In simple terms, if the FFT is calculated based on 128 samples, there will be 128 frequency components and the frequency resolution will be the analysis bandwidth, as determined by the sampling frequency divided by 128. Some common techniques such as overlap-add can improve the efficiency of this process, but the general relationship between the number of samples, the delay introduced, and the frequency resolution will typically maintain the same ratio relationship. An example of 32-point versus 128-point FFT calculations performed on the same signal is shown in Figure 10–23. From this figure you can clearly see the fine scale level information present in the 128-point FFT sample that is not present in the 32-point FFT. As with the filter bank approaches, however, increasing the FFT frequency resolution will not only increase the total delay, it will also require increased processing power and therefore increase battery drain in the hearing aid.

Digital Signal Processing (DSP): Memory

The processing portion of the chip in a hearing aid is the workhorse, but it needs access to a number of pieces of information including (1) the user settings, (2) the processing algorithms, (3) the instruction sets, and, (4) the timing and sequencing information related to the processing algorithms. Consequently, all chips include blocks of memory that store data. There are at least three general types of memory that are commonly used in hearing aids and are coupled to the hearing aid processor. For our purposes these three types will be categorized based on the type of data they are intended to store and how they need to be used. The physical type

---

KEY CONCEPT: QUICK REVIEW OF FOURIER ANALYSIS

- The decomposition of the varying time domain series of audio samples into a series of functions representing sinusoids (pure tones) is called Fourier analysis.
- A Fourier transform is the process that is used to transform the complex function into its simple components (individual frequencies).
- The simple components may be recombined into a complex waveform using a process called Fourier synthesis.
- The Fourier transform is an analog function. In digital hearing aids, we have a discrete digital signal rather than a continuous one. An equivalent Fourier transform in the digital realm is referred to as a discrete Fourier transform (DFT).
- Calculating a DFT requires complex math and is time-consuming. Therefore, a number of different types of DFT calculations have been proposed. A specific DFT calculation that is more computationally efficient and is commonly used is the fast Fourier transform (FFT). The computationally efficient, digital counterpart to Fourier synthesis is referred to as an inverse FFT (or reverse FFT).

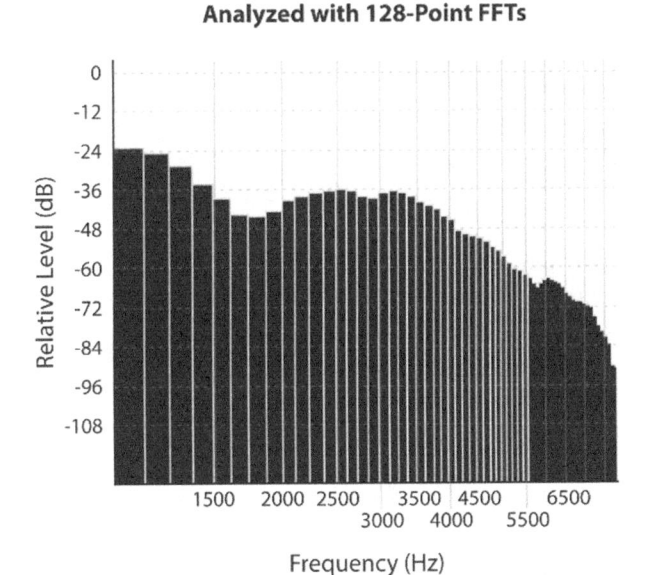

Figure 10–23. An example of the same sound, originally sampled using a 16 kHz sampling rate and subsequently analyzed (level by frequency) with 32-point (*upper panel*) and 128-point (*lower panel*) FFTs. Note the differences in smoothing of the shape of the frequency response due to averaging.

of the processing algorithms, commonly referred to as firmware. This information is typically permanently stored in a memory chip that is not typically intended to be written to by the clinician. In many modern hearing aids and hearing assistive technologies, however, these instruction sets can be overwritten if necessary to improve or modify hearing aid or device function after initial fitting. Although not tremendously common, occasionally an error in the software will be discovered after a product is released. In such cases the manufacturer can sometimes correct this error by a firmware update that can be applied (in some cases automatically) when the hearing aid is connected to the computer and programming interface. In other cases, a manufacturer will either add a processing feature or improve processing of a current feature using a firmware update. For example, we know of one case for which support for an additional type of streaming devices was added to the intermediary streamer using this method. In at least one case, a manufacturer has designed a hearing aid system so that the overall range and operation of hearing aid features can be purposefully affected. That is, a single hardware version of the hearing aid is provided and the clinician can activate specific feature sets depending on the level of technology selected. In this way the level of features can be selected at the fitting appointment or during the trial period based on a patient's listening needs without changing the physical hearing aid. This design exploits the fact that feature differences in modern hearing aids really are much more based on software than hardware.

The second general type of memory stores the user-specific settings for the hearing aid algorithms as well as the individual user programs. This is what we use to store data when we program a hearing aid during fittings. Multiple memory hearing aids are made possible by storing more than one set of user settings (typically between two and five) in this second type of memory. Individuals wearing hearing aids can then switch between these preprogrammed settings, typically using a toggle switch on the case of the hearing aid or an external remote control, such as an app on a cell phone.

The third general type of memory is used during active processing of the sound signal. Specifically, it may be used to hold the changing digital representation of the sound as successive processing algorithms are applied. This is similar to the RAM used in a computer that temporarily holds data and programs during processing.

of memory used, however, can be from one of several available options.

The first general type of memory used in hearing aids stores the instructions related to general operation

> ### THINGS TO REMEMBER: A LITTLE ABOUT MEMORY
>
> - One general category of memory is designed to contain data that can only be read. This general memory type includes read-only memory (ROM).
> - A second category of memory is designed both to be read from and written to, in contrast to the previous read-only memory. This second general category includes random access memory (RAM), static random access memory (SRAM), dynamic random access memory (DRAM), and synchronous dynamic random-access memory (SDRAM). In 2017 the RAM used in most computers and tablets was one of many forms of SDRAM.
> - A third category, a hybrid type of memory, can easily be read from, but can only be written to slowly. This type includes programmable read-only memory (PROM), erasable programmable read-only memory (EPROM), electrically erasable programmable read-only memory (EEPROM), and others.
>   - For reference, flash memory—commonly also referred to as "memory sticks," "flash drives," or "thumb drives," which are in common use in personal computers and tablets—are similar to EEPROM memory but consume more power.
> - The various types of RAM generally differ in how long they are able to store data even when power is applied, and how fast they are at accessing and moving data. The various types of ROM generally differ in how difficult it is to erase existing data and how quickly and easily new data can be written.
> - Memory also differs as a function of what happens when you remove the power supply. One general category is only able to store data when power is applied. This category of memory which includes all types of RAM is called *volatile* because all data is lost when not provided with power.
>   - Despite the inability of use for data storage due to volatility, RAM is particularly useful because the high speed at which data can be read and written to this type of memory allows it to essentially be used as short term memory" that holds data the processor can work with very quickly.
> - Volatile memory is contrasted with nonvolatile memory, which is designed to continue to store data even when no power is applied; this includes all types of ROM.

Hearing Aid Hardware

Whew, that was a lot of background to work through! Now that we have a few fundamentals under our belts, let's discuss hearing aid hardware in a little more detail. As we already mentioned, a hearing aid's job is to pick up, amplify and process, and then deliver sound to the listener. In the following sections of this chapter we will go through the physical components used to accomplish this process. The first step is getting the sound into the hearing aid. In order to determine the best way to pick up signals, we must first identify which signals are of interest. By far, the most common are acoustic signals present in the air. But other useful signal types include the electromagnetic leakage from a telephone or induction loop and wireless RF transmitted sounds. Picking up these wireless signals directly can be particularly useful for a hearing aid wearer because the signal can be accessed directly without also picking up acoustic background noise present in the environment. In addition, since a microphone is not used, some common problems (most importantly feedback) can be eliminated. Microphones (used to pick up sound from the air) and coils (used to pick up electromagnetic fields) fall in the general category of transducers. A transducer can be defined as "a device actuated by power from one system and supplying power to a second system." So in the case of a hearing aid microphone, it is actuated by acoustic power from the environment and supplies a voltage to the A/D convertor. Wireless RF sound transmission works a bit differently so we will discuss it in more detail later in this Chapter and also in Chapter 12.

Getting a Signal Into the Hearing Aid: Microphones

In a hearing aid it is of interest to have a microphone that is modular to simplify the manufacturing process. The microphone also needs to be as durable as possible. Consequently, the electret microphones themselves, along with a miniature microphone pre-amplifier, are typically manufactured inside a metal case (Figure 10–24). It is the job of this amplifier, commonly referred to as a *pre-amplifier* or *buffer amplifier*, to provide amplification to the very small voltage produced by the microphone, producing a signal that is better suited for amplification by the main hearing aid amplifier while keeping the main amplifier from loading down the microphone. Engineers often refer to the microphone buffer amplifier as the FET because it is sometimes comprised of a single field effect transistor. Microphones also typically include, spacers, shielding materials, and other components not shown in Figure 10–24. Together, the entire microphone and its housing are sometimes referred to as the *microphone can*. The ability to miniaturize hearing aid microphones continues to be impressive. Microphones with dimensions smaller than 2.6 × 2.6 mm have been introduced, as have thin and wide microphones that are less than 1.5 mm thick across their narrowest dimension (Figure 10–25). Building a microphone inside a can certainly achieves the design goal of modular miniaturization.

One advantage of placing the microphone in a metal can is that some shielding from electromagnetic interference is provided. Another advantage is that the most fragile piece of the microphone, the diaphragm, can be oriented so that it is somewhat protected from objects directly entering the microphone port. Of course this doesn't stop a motivated patient from occasionally destroying the microphone diaphragm by jamming a paperclip into a microphone port while trying to clean it. It also doesn't prevent the microphone port from being clogged by the dirt and debris that occur in the patient's environment. Another advantage of the design is that the metal case can be suspended inside the hearing aid case using soft rubber materials. A short section of rubber tubing connects the sound tube of the metal case to the sound outlet port, typically referred to as the microphone port, on the case of the hearing aid. The rubber tubing and suspension system acts to minimize

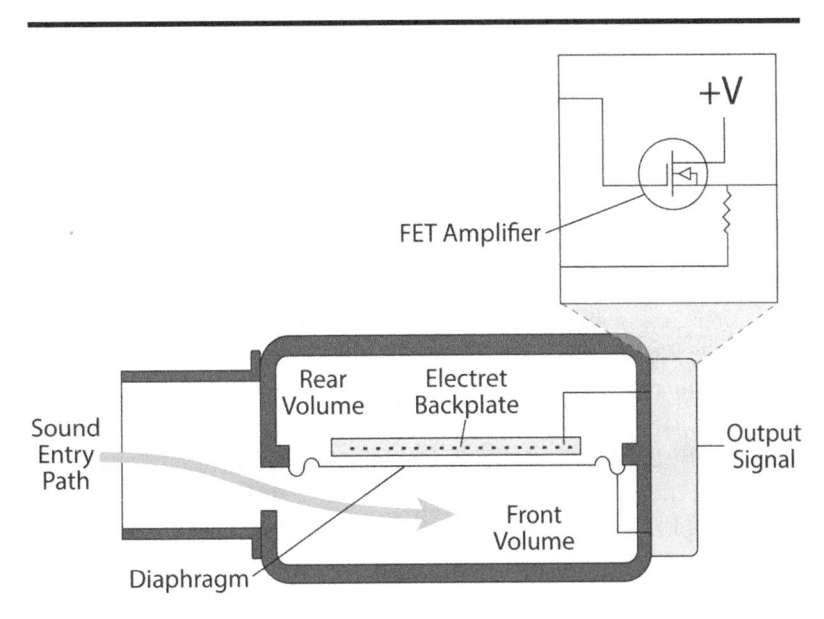

Figure 10–24. Schematic of an electret hearing aid microphone.

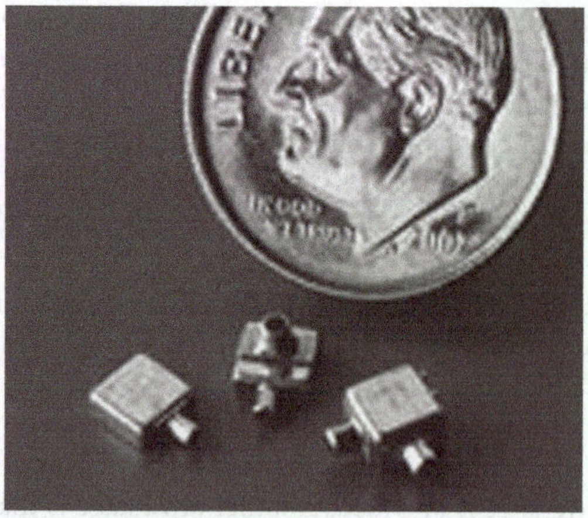

Figure 10–25. Examples of electret hearing aid microphones.

the transfer of vibration into the microphone, which in turn minimizes problems with mechanical feedback. If too much vibration energy from the receiver is allowed to travel back to the microphone through mechanical coupling, feedback will occur regardless of how well the microphone and receiver are acoustically isolated from each other. The most popular hearing aid style currently fitted are mini-BTEs with the receiver in the canal (usually called RICs). Since the receiver is typically coupled to the case with a plastic covered wire, this style is particularly susceptible to mechanical feedback when high output is applied. Furthermore, the plastic covering on the wire can stiffen with age, thus increasing the likelihood of feedback, so routine follow-up may be prudent when programming gain that approaches the limit allowed by feedback.

Limitations of Common Electret Hearing Aid Microphones

Hearing aid design is often a series of well-considered tradeoffs. A large number of hearing aid microphone designs with different goals and limitations are therefore used in hearing aids. One continued limitation is microphone size. Although modern hearing aid microphones are quite small, there is continued demand to make them even smaller. In addition to size, design considerations also affect the hearing aid microphone frequency response. Modern hearing aid microphones are usually assumed to have relatively flat and broad frequency responses. For a variety of reasons, however, it may be of interest not to have a completely flat response or an extremely broad response. Typical modern microphones vary in output by less than +/− 5 dB over a range from 100 to 7,000 Hz (Figure 10–26). More specialized microphones have been introduced that exhibit frequency responses that extend down to approximately 50 Hz, as well as those that extend up to more than 12,000 Hz. Microphone sensitivity indicates how well the microphone converts acoustic pressure to output voltage. In a microphone with high sensitivity, less amplification is needed by the main amplifier. This is a practical concern but not directly an indication of microphone quality; in fact, "sensitivity" is a bit misleading since true sensitivity (the lowest intensity sound the microphone can pick up) is generally dependent on the microphone noise floor.

THINGS TO REMEMBER: THE MICROPHONE NOISE FLOOR

- The microphone noise floor is due to random motion. Thermal energy creates a small amount of random motion of the electrons within the electrical circuitry (generally referred to as electrical noise) and a small amount of random motion of air particles in the air volume adjacent to the diaphragm (generally referred to as acoustic noise).
- Noise generated by the electrical circuit, including the FET, combines with acoustic noise generated within the microphone and lead to the measured microphone noise floor.
- In current microphones the level of the noise floor, which is generally dominated by acoustic noise, peaks in the lowest frequencies and rolls off at about 3 to 6 dB per octave.
- The microphone noise floor in modern hearing aids is around 25 to 30 dB SPL.

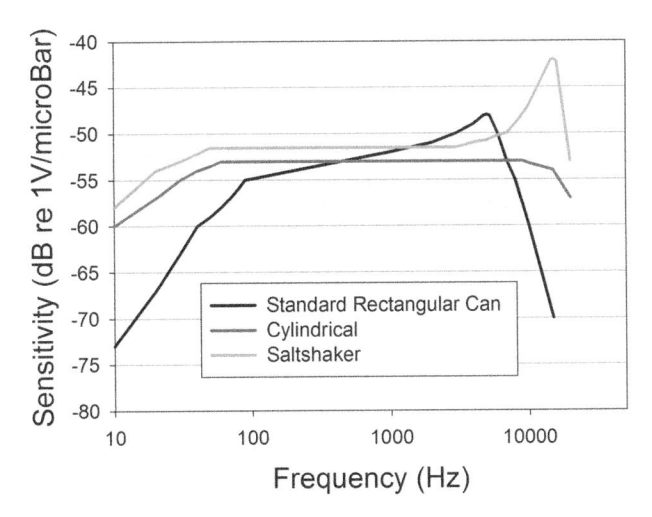

Figure 10–26. Examples of sensitivity plots for three different hearing aid microphones.

A low microphone noise floor is particularly important when we wish to provide amplification to low-intensity sounds. Importantly, when amplification is applied to the microphone output, both the noise floor and sounds in the environment are amplified. The noise floor in hearing aid microphones is typically quite low, around 25 to 30 dB SPL. Since the peak energy of the microphone noise floor is typically found in the lowest frequencies, the combination of relatively good low-frequency hearing, some low-frequency amplification, and high microphone noise floor can lead to patient complaints about hissing or circuit noise. As we describe later in this chapter, this problem is only exacerbated when using directional microphones and microphone arrays.

The advantages of placing a hearing aid microphone in a metal case were discussed, but this design also has a consequence that is sometimes undesirable. Specifically, the air inside the can will have a have a characteristic resonance frequency, which is based in part on the volume of air in the container and the size of the opening (Helmholtz resonance). Modern hearing aid microphones commonly produce resonant frequencies (observed as a bump in the frequency response as shown in Figure 10–26) at around 4 to 5 kHz or higher.

One of the biggest limitations to traditional microphone technologies used in hearing aids is that they can't read the patient's mind when the hearing aids are being worn. Although this statement is made partially in jest, picking up signals of interest is often complicated because listeners may desire to hear only one or a few of the many available signals (e.g., their spouse across the table at a busy restaurant). The fact that the hearing aid wearer can often hear sound, but not the specific sounds he or she wants, continues to be one of the most common complaints of hearing aid wearers.

Efforts to Improve and Enhance Hearing Aid Microphones

Traditional hearing aid microphones have their limitations, so is there any progress in combating some of these problems? Over the past decade, there have been a number of clever enhancements to traditional electret microphones that have helped broaden frequency response and lower noise. In fact, the hearing aid microphone is one of the most refined parts of the hearing aid. The resonance peaks present in hearing aid microphones have even been essentially eliminated in some microphone systems by using very small cylindrical designs that move the resonant peak above the frequency range that is usually amplified by the majority of hearing aids. In terms of further miniaturization and further reduction of noise floor, the MEMS microphones used in some models demonstrate considerable improvements in these areas.

What about that mind-reading issue? Have we come up with hearing aids that can do that yet? Unfortunately no, however, microphones have been developed that don't pick up all sounds, but rather are differentially sensitive based on the angle and elevation of the arrival of sound. Traditional microphone designs are approximately equally sensitive regardless of the angle or elevation of sound arrival. Microphone designs without directional sensitivity, such as this, are referred to as *omnidirectional*. It should be noted, however, that when an omnidirectional microphone is placed in a hearing aid case and placed in or on the ear, it ceases to be truly omnidirectional. That is, the microphone is more sensitive to some angles than others because of the effect of sound shadow and sound reflection from the head and pinna. An example of the directional sensitivity of an omnidirectional microphone BTE hearing aid placed on the head is shown in Figure 10–27. This type of figure is called a polar plot, and it shows relative hearing aid output as a function of the angle of the source loudspeaker

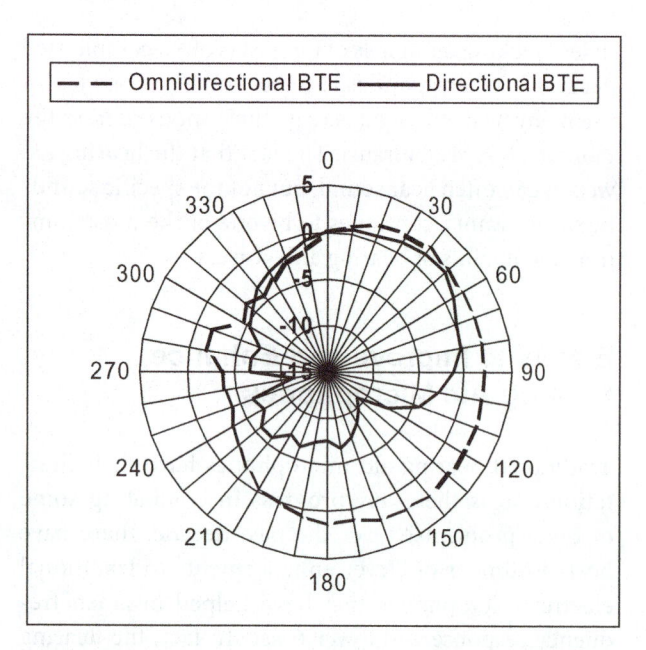

Figure 10–27. Two examples of directional sensitivity patterns measured in a single horizontal plane. These plots were measured at the output of a hearing aid in an acoustic simulator mounted in an acoustic manikin.

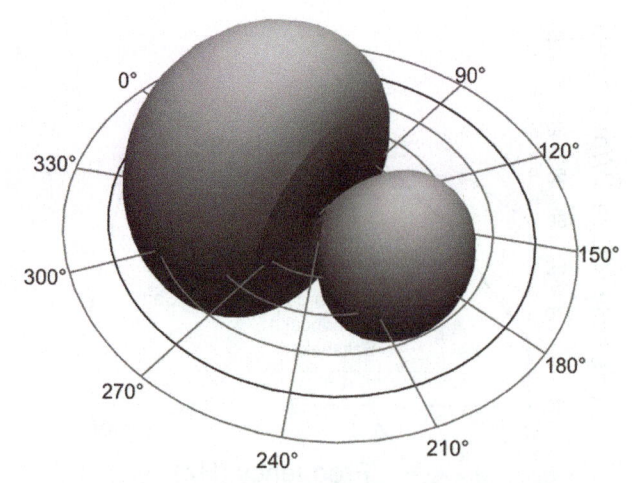

Figure 10–28. An example of a spatial directivity pattern measured from a directional microphone hearing aid in the free field (not on a KEMAR). (Reproduced with permission from Daniel Warren, GN Advanced Science).

in the horizontal plane. Points closer to the center of the circle denote a lower relative level. Polar plots are typically measured in a room that is free from any reflections (anechoic chamber). In the simplest measurement configuration, a single loudspeaker is placed a fixed distance from an acoustic manikin, which is fitted with the hearing aid. The manikin is then rotated by fixed increments and a measure of hearing aid output is taken at every increment. This type of plot is often sometimes called a directional sensitivity pattern, though that term is sometimes reserved for three-dimensional sensitivity measures, which cover the full range of elevations in the vertical plane as well as the full range of angles in the horizontal plane (Figure 10–28).

The directional sensitivity of the omnidirectional BTE shown in Figure 10–27 may not be desirable, especially when the listener is surrounded by noise and facing the signal of interest. That is, this hearing aid is nearly equally sensitive to sounds arriving from 150 degrees (behind the listener) as to sounds arriving from 30 degrees (in front of the listener). For the environment described, a more desirable behavior would be a microphone that picked up sounds in front and attenuated sounds from behind (when placed on the ear), as shown in the directional BTE plot also shown in Figure 10–27. This intentional directional focus is in fact the design goal of directional microphone hearing aids.

Directional hearing aids were introduced in 1971, and have been available from nearly all manufacturers since that time. Basic directional hearing aids work by comparing incoming sounds sampled at two different locations. Sound at the two locations can be either directed to a single microphone through the use of two inlet ports (once the common approach but rarely used today) or can be directed to two separate omnidirectional microphones (approach used by most larger manufacturers today). In either case, the directional characteristics of the microphone are related to two factors that we will describe as internal delay and external delay. In modern directional hearing aids, the microphone ports are typically separated by 4 to 12 mm, and are located on the case of the instrument. Let's take a look at how this works in the single microphone, two-port approach through the use of a schematic of such a microphone (Figure 10–29).

This schematic shows a microphone that has been modified so that sound energy can be directed to both sides of the diaphragm. Sound traveling through the rear microphone port travels down and impacts the bottom of the diaphragm, meanwhile sound traveling through the front" microphone port impacts the top of the diaphragm. If we imagine this microphone placed in

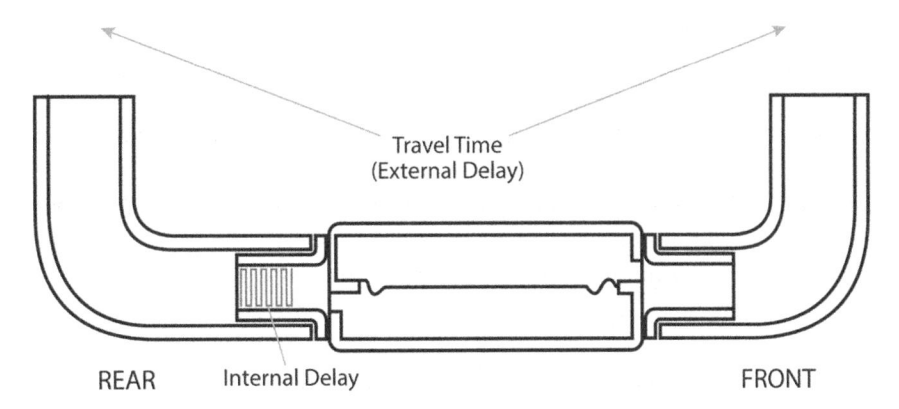

Figure 10–29. A schematic of a simple directional microphone with two port openings, which are directed to either side of a single diaphragm. This design will provide the greatest relative attenuation at specific angles depending on the exact relationship between internal and external delay values.

a hearing aid case on the side of the head, sounds arriving directly from the listener's side (90° azimuth noted by the position of the sound source) would enter both microphone ports at the same time. Let's ignore the section labeled "internal delay" for now. Since the sound would have the exact same distance to travel down both ports, it would affect both sides of the microphone diaphragm at the same time. Since sound in the air is really just condensation and rarefaction of air molecules, the effect is that the diaphragm gets pushed from both sides and then pulled from both sides at the same time, with a net effect of cancellation. This design is typically referred to as a pressure gradient directional microphone because cancellation is based on phase difference between the sound pressure impinging on either side of the diaphragm.

In the example just provided, we described a microphone that cancelled sounds arriving from the side. When sounds arrive from other angles, the phase of the condensations and rarefactions don't line up at the diaphragm (the sound traveling down one port is slight delayed relative to the sound traveling down the other port because it has further to travel) and the cancellation effect is reduced. The more perfect the phase match at the diaphragm the more attenuation. If the timing between the sound when it arrives at both sides of the diaphragm is desparate enough, there will be no attenuation. However, the attenuation

---

THINGS TO REMEMBER: DIRECTIONAL CANCELLATION

- In real directional hearing aids cancellation is never perfect, so the sound doesn't ever get completely wiped out at any angle, though we may see attenuation of sound by up to 25 to 30 dB over a very narrow range of angles, typically referred to as a null. Slightly further away from the nulls the magnitude of attenuation will typically only be in the range of 5 to 15 dB.
- The fact that nulls are very narrow is important because in many typical environments, particularly indoor environments, the angle of arrival from a sound source is often not from only a single direction because of reflection (reverberation).
- Since the interaction between phase and timing is frequency dependent, the pattern and magnitude of attenuation (across angles) will be different depending on the frequency we examine.

pattern is affected by other factors (see associated Things to Remember).

Although cancellation of sounds from the side of the head may sometimes be useful, it is often more useful to concentrate on cancellation at other angles. Let's first assume we are interested in attenuating sounds arriving from directly behind the listener. If a sound arrives at the hearing aid from 180° azimuth, it will enter the rear opening first, then require extra time (based on the speed of sound) to travel to the front. We will call this travel time *external delay*; the further the openings are spaced apart, the longer the external delay (see Figure 10–29).

In order to offset the travel time in this example, we introduce *a time delay acoustical network* to mechanically slow down the speed of the sound traveling through the rear microphone port. This network (in this case a wire mesh referred to as acoustic damper) increases travel time for sound resulting in an internal delay. What happens when the internal and external delays are set so that sounds arriving from the rear travel through both microphone openings and hit both sides of the diaphragm at the same time? The condensations and rarefactions of acoustic pressure will push and pull on opposite sides of the diaphragm at the same time, and the sound will again be cancelled. The relationship between these internal and external delays gives rise to specific patterns of spatial attenuation. In a free field (a sound field with no reflections), the angles for which a directional hearing aid attenuates sound, as well as the theoretical limits of the magnitude of this attenuation, can be mathematically predicted based on the relationship between external and internal delays. Terms like cardioid, bidirectional, supercardioid and hypercardioid are used to describe these patterns (Figure 10–30). The use of these terms is a bit misleading for hearing aids, however, since directional microphones designed with these theoretical patterns placed in a hearing aid case and placed on the listener's ear have very different patterns of attenuation (see Figure 10–29).

Importantly, the pressure gradient directional microphone design is not the only one that is possible; in fact, currently it is seldom used. Rather than using a single directional microphone, the same effect can be achieved by using two omnidirectional microphones for phase inverting the signal from the rear microphone and summing the output. In this dual microphone or twin microphone directional design (actually more accurately described as a microphone array) the internal delay becomes a delay placed on the signal from the rear

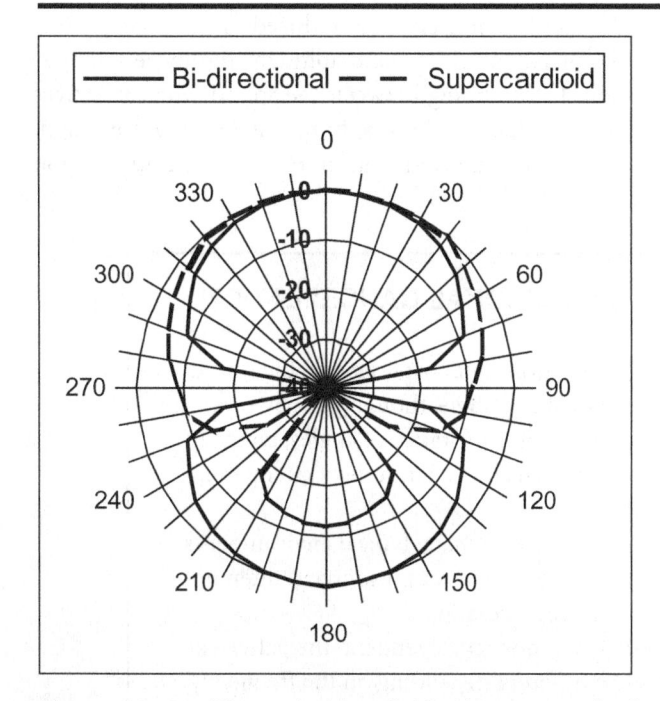

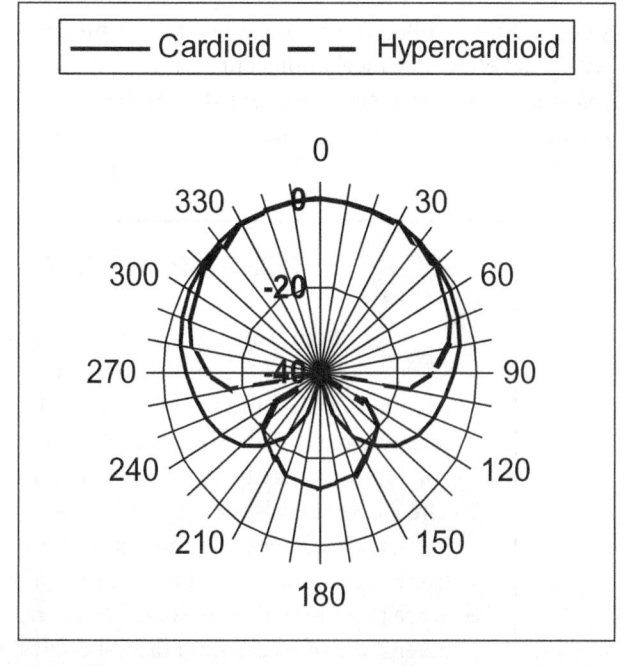

Figure 10–30. Theoretical free field polar patterns for first-order directional microphones.

microphone. This delay can again be achieved mechanically (as with a traditional directional microphone), it can be applied electronically (prior to summing the electronic output of the two microphones), or it can be applied digitally provided that the output of both microphones undergoes analog-to-digital conversion prior to summation. In the two-microphone approach, effective cancellation requires that the two microphones are acoustically matched to provide identical outputs when provided with the same input. In the case of either single or dual microphones, the response of the directional microphone hearing aid is tuned to provide maximum directivity across frequencies within the theoretical limits of the particular design implemented.

Regardless of design (single or twin microphones, mechanical, electronic or digital delay), the spatial attenuation provided by directional hearing aids is dependent on the relationship between internal and external delay. Consequently, all these designs have the same theoretical limits related to the maximum overall attenuation they can provide. Specifically, they are able to provide a maximum of approximately 6 dB of attenuation for a sound arriving at all angles and elevations in comparison to the same sound if it arrived only from directly in front of the listener, a value referred to as *directivity index* (DI). We will summarize a few aspects of the DI. Readers interested in greater detail are encouraged to see Ricketts and Dittberner (2001) and ANSI S3.35 (2004) for further details.

The DI can be defined as the ratio of sound intensity (measured at the output of the hearing aid) for an "on-axis" sound source (arrives from directly in front) to that produced in response to a diffuse sound source of the same total acoustic power. The term "diffuse" is often overused, so it is important to note that in this case we are assuming the specific acoustic definition: statistically uniform energy density and for which the directions of propagation of the noise waves are randomly distributed. The DI is a ratio of outputs for on-axis versus diffuse sound source locations. Therefore, equal sensitivity at all angles, as we see from omnidirectional microphones in the free-field, leads to a DI of 0 dB. Increasingly positive and negative DIs are indicative of increasingly more and less directivity, respectively. Negative DI values are possible in hearing aids if the average sensitivity to sounds at angles other than 0° is greater than the sensitivity of sounds at 0°. As we demonstrated above, omnidirectional microphones are not truly omnidirectional when placed on the head. Indeed, the measured DI will be affected by where the omnidirectional microphone is positioned (e.g., Ricketts, 2000). Data have shown that the average directivity provided by an omnidirectional completely-in-canal (CIC) instrument is approximately equal to that of an

---

POINTS TO PONDER: DI VERSUS AI-DI

It has been suggested that the preciseness of the DI can be enhanced by using a weighting system based on the frequency-specific importance function of speech (Killion et al., 1998). One method that has been suggested, and used in some research, is based on the audibility index (AI) of the Mueller and Killion Count-The-Dots audiogram that we discussed in Chapter 5. As you might recall, the density of the dots (frequency importance for understanding speech) is much greater in the 2000 Hz range than at lower frequencies such as 500 Hz. It is possible then, to use a weighting system so that the DI for 2000 Hz counts more heavily toward the average DI than the DI for 500 Hz. This is referred to as the AI-DI. Specific weighting for key frequencies is as follows: 500 Hz = 20%, 1000 Hz = 23%, 2000 Hz = 33%, and 4000 Hz = 24%.

Using this weighted method, it is clear that a hearing aid with a DI of 5.0 dB at 2000 Hz and 2.0 dB at 500 Hz would have a larger average DI than a hearing aid with 2.0 dB at 2000 Hz and 5.0 dB at 500 Hz. For most hearing aids, however, the difference between the average AI-DI and the average DI is small because most products have a similar DI at all frequencies. Manufacturers and researchers today are split between use of the AI-DI and the equally weighted average DI.

unaided open ear, with DI values that are negative in the low frequencies, positive in the high frequencies, and an average of about 0 dB. An omnidirectional ITE will also provide similar average DI values to the open ear, albeit DI values will be lower in the highest frequencies because there is less sound shadow from the pinna. A very different directivity pattern is present for omnidirectional BTE instruments. In this case DI values are negative across the frequency range and the average DI is approximately −1.5 dB. Consequently, omnidirectional BTE hearing aids are expected to provide a SNR *disadvantage* compared to the open ear. Consequently, many manufacturers default to a slightly directional setting (positive directivity in the high frequencies), in lieu of a truly omnidirectional setting in their BTE and mini-BTE instruments.

The DI of the theoretical directional patterns presented in Figure 10–30 can also be calculated. This calculation reveals that the cardioid and bidirectional patterns will yield a maximum DI of 4.8 dB, whereas the supercardioid and hypercardioid designs will yield maximum DI values of 5.7 and 6.0 dB, respectively. Greater off-axis attenuation than 6 dB in the free field can and has been achieved in hearing aids; however, it requires the use of an array of more than two microphones. It is common to describe microphone arrays by order, which is defined as the number of microphones minus one. That is, a first-order microphone array has two microphones and a third-order array implements four microphones. Second-order arrays using three microphones oriented in a BTE case were introduced in the mid-2000s, but only achieved limited commercial success. This may have been, in part, due to its somewhat larger size, and the fact the case had to be modified with small plugs differently depending on whether the instrument was used on the left or right ear. More recently, third-order arrays using all four microphones from bilateral hearing aids (bilateral beamformers) and first-order

---

TECHNICAL TIP: APPLYING GENERAL MVDR IDEAS TO A FIRST-ORDER MICROPHONE ARRAY

- Assume a first-order microphone array (e.g., two-microphone directional BTE hearing aid) is pointed at a speaker of interest and surrounded by noise speakers in an anechoic chamber.
- If the output of the two microphones is arranged so that the configuration is a reverse cardioid, the speaker of interest will fall squarely in the null so the output will be almost completely made up of the noise (i.e., a good estimate of the noise signal).
- In contrast, the output of the single omnidirectional microphone nearest the front of the case will include both the talker of interest and the noise.
- We then subtract the reverse cardioid output from the omnidirectional output. What is left is mostly the talker of interest. The effect is to greatly reduce the strong noise signals (effectively placing nulls at the angle of arrival for noise signals).
- The omnidirectional (speech + noise estimate) and reverse cardioid (noise estimate) are rapidly and continuously updated so the system can adapt to changes in position of the strong noise signals (e.g., effectively move the cancelation nulls to the position of the strong noise sources).
- When the hearing aid is placed on the listener, the front facing null in a unilateral beamformer, such as the one described in this section, will likely not be pointed directly at the talker of interest because of head shadow. In addition, reverberation will cause some of the talker energy to arrive from other angles and become part of the noise estimate, so effectiveness in the real world will be somewhat limited.
- Similar techniques can be applied in a bilateral beamformer allowing it to function adaptively. The use of four microphones, however, allows for more accurate speech and noise estimates and a greater number of nulls, thus leading to improved directivity when compared to unilateral adaptive beamformer techniques.

arrays using both of the single microphones in bilaterally fitted CIC instruments have been made possible through full band wireless signal sharing between hearing aids. Second and higher order arrays have also been introduced in remote and FM microphone systems, which are routed wirelessly to the listeners' hearing aids.

In addition to these higher order arrays, some two microphone arrays currently utilize more sophisticated techniques than those used in the directional hearing aids of the 1990s, as well as many of the current models. For example, some advanced methods are based on minimum-variance distortion-less response (MVDR) beamformer techniques (e.g., Vorobyov, 2014). The details of these techniques are well beyond the scope of this book, but they have been used in a wide range of beamformers, including radar, as a way to improve SNRs and signal detection. As applied in hearing aids, they differ from the simple delay, invert, and cancelation method we described above by using multiple versions of the microphone array output to provide essentially directionally focused "acoustic snapshots" of the total signal input. Although these methods are generally somewhat proprietary as they are applied in specific products, we can give you a general idea of how they can be effective.

The directional patterns of higher order microphone arrays are significantly different in terms of the magnitude and pattern of attenuation. The number of polar nulls in higher order designs is generally one less than the number of microphones. So the directional pattern of a four-microphone beamformer will usually have three polar nulls. DI values as high as from 10 to 12 dB have been reported for fourth- and fifth-order beamformers, although average reported DI values for current bilateral beamformers are approximately 7 dB. DI values depend on specific manufacturer design decisions, quality control, and other factors.

DI values also vary considerably as a function of frequency. Figure 10–31 provides an example of frequency specific directivity averaged across five different ITE and five different BTE models for directional and omnidirectional microphones settings and the open ear. Importantly, the DI is often assumed to provide a reasonable estimate of the *effective SNR* if the signal of interest is in front and near the listener, and the competing noise field surrounds the listener and is reasonable uniform.

It is of interest to provide both directional and omnidirectional microphone modes in the same hearing aid. Twenty to thirty years ago or so, when the

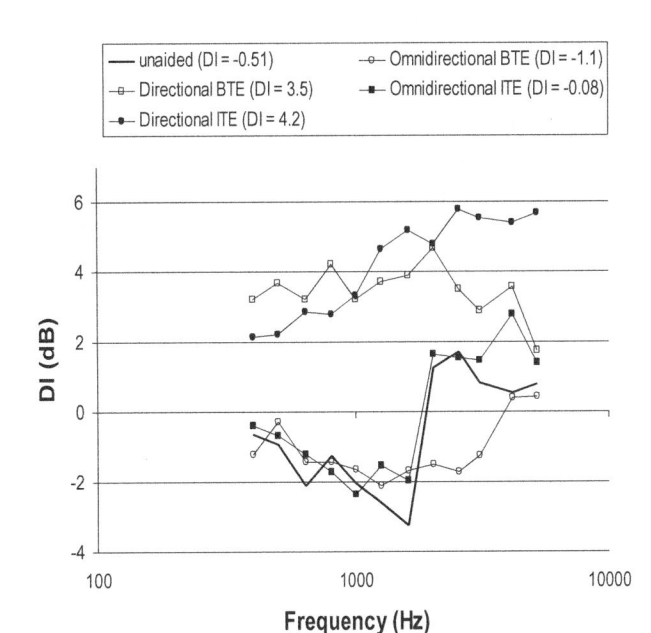

Figure 10–31. The frequency-specific and average DI as a function of microphone setting and hearing aid style.

POINTS TO PONDER: DOES DI EQUAL SNR ADVANTAGE FOR SPEECH?

It is tempting to think of the DI as being equivalent to an SNR advantage for understanding speech in background noise—that is, if a hearing aid has a DI of +5.0 dB, then we might expect a 5 dB SNR advantage for speech recognition (e.g., on a test such as the HINT). Although there certainly is a relative relationship (bigger is better), research that has examined this has shown that the SNR advantage is not as great as the DI. For example, Ricketts and Dittberner (2002) combined data from different studies and showed a relationship of SNR benefit to be around 60% of the change in AI-DI. That is, if the AI-DI increases 5 dB, we would predict that the SNR benefit would be about 3.0 dB (3.0 = 60% of 5.0). As we discuss in Chapter 11, however, the specific relationship is affected by the magnitude of hearing loss consistent with hearing loss desensitization.

single microphone directional system was commonly used, this was commonly achieved by adding an omnidirectional microphone to the hearing aid. In this system there were two microphones (one directional and one omnidirectional) for a total of three microphone ports in the hearing aid, although only one microphone was active at a given time. Another approach was to use a slider on the top of the BTE hearing aid, which closed off the back port of the directional microphone, eliminating the cancellation effect (Mueller & Johnson, 1979). Today, switching between microphone modes is accomplished by enabling either one (omnidirectional) or both (directional) omnidirectional microphones of a two microphone array.

Although using two microphones instead of a single directional microphone does not provide an advantage in terms of maximum spatial attenuation, the microphone array design does allow for additional useful processing. Specifically, using an array of two or more microphones allows the manufacturer to develop algorithms that effectively vary the specific spatial attenuation pattern, depending on the environment. Traditional fixed microphone arrays, also known as delay-and-sum beamforming, achieve a fixed directional pattern by keeping constant the transfer functions of the microphone signals. In other words, the signal of each microphone is processed according to a desired algorithm involving filtering, amplitude weighting, and time delay, and then is summed together prior to the output. In adaptive array techniques, the array weights are determined by actual noise field conditions instead of a theoretical, ideal noise field. Hence, the processing of microphone signals is continuously adjusted and will depend, in part, on the properties of the signal being received. For example, if the noise source moves from one region in space to another, adaptive processing can manipulate the summed output of the separate microphone signals by suppressing the sensitivity from the particular direction the noise source is being received. Theoretically these traditional adaptive directional hearing aids and more recently introduced adaptive bilateral beamformers will "find" a specific noise source (within the rear hemisphere), then will switch to the spatial pattern that provides the most attenuation to the angle of the competing sound source. Whereas this processing has substantial additional benefits when a single noise source is present in the environment, less utility has been shown in environments with multiple noise sources. Fortunately, however, it is expected that adaptive arrays will always function at least as well as their fixed counterparts, regardless of environment.

A second useful processing algorithm that can be applied to microphone array hearing aid systems is automatic switching—something that is available in nearly all directional products. Based on a sophisticated signal classification system, automatic directional hearing aids are programmed to automatically switch between directional and omnidirectional microphone modes depending on the listening environment. Most recently, microphone-based noise reduction has become increasingly sophisticated and may include (1) algorithms that smoothly switch from slightly directional to directional as possible based on the acoustic input, or even, (2) adjust the direction of attenuation or "look" depending on either user adjustment or automatically based on directionally sensitive features in the acoustic environments (e.g., reverse directional, microphone steering). These much more sophisticated methods will be discussed in detail in Chapter 11.

While microphone arrays represent an enhancement to traditional omnidirectional designs in terms of reducing background noise in some situations, their design also introduces a couple of additional limitations. One interesting dichotomy is that even though directional microphones reduce background noise, they themselves are noisier than omnidirectional microphones. This limitation occurs because microphone arrays are less sensitive in the low frequencies than their omnidirectional counterparts for sounds that arrive on-axis. This reduction in sensitivity results in directional microphones having 5 to 15 dB greater levels of equivalent input noise than their omnidirectional counterparts. Unfortunately, low-frequency sensitivity is further decreased in microphone arrays with increasing order. The reduced sensitivity is commonly referred to as directional rolloff and it occurs because of frequency dependent differences in phase alignment. Consider a simple first-order design. Since the low-frequency signals have longer wavelengths, when they are sampled at the two microphone ports they are more similar (resulting in greater cancellation when the two signals are added together after phase inversion of the signal from the rear) than shorter wavelength, high-frequency signals. The frequency at which the low-frequency rolloff begins is predictable based on the spacing between the microphone ports, with increasingly smaller separation resulting in the reduction in sensitivity occurring at increasingly higher frequencies. That is, the closer the microphone ports the greater the potential for reduced audibility of low-frequency sounds unless gain compensation is provided. Consequently, it is expected that if directional rolloff is a problem, the effect will generally be greater for ITE and miniature BTE styles, where space on the faceplate is limited, than for traditional full size BTE instruments. Regardless of port spacing, the theoretical magnitude of low frequency roll-off is a relatively constant 6 dB per octave. In practice, the directional roll-off of a hearing aid may be less; however, due to venting effects or low-frequency gain increases that are programmed to compensate for the directional roll-off (typically referred to as gain equalization or directional equalization).

Since a reduction in low-frequency gain is associated with switching to directional mode, it may seem logical to fully compensate for this change. The gain that is applied to compensate for this loss of low frequencies, however, is also applied to the noise floor. This increase in gain has the potential to increase microphone noise to a level that is audible or perhaps even bothersome to a listener in quiet environments (although we would assume that the hearing aid will automatically switch to omnidirectional for a quiet situation).

Another important consideration is related to microphone matching. In the case of dual omnidirectional microphone design for directivity it is important that the two microphones are matched in terms of the output they provide—they are purchased in pairs from the microphone vender by the manufacturer. The microphones must be matched as closely as possible since a sensitivity difference between the two microphones as small as 1 dB can eliminate nearly all the directional advantage (e.g., Ricketts & Dittberner, 2001). While microphone matching is a design consideration, problems in this area are one of the reasons we advocate for measuring directional microphone performance clinically, as discussed in Chapter 13, in order to maintain quality control.

In addition to concerns related to microphone mismatch in the manufacturing process, there is some concern that microphone sensitivity may drift over time, potentially causing a mismatch that was not present at the time the hearing aid was manufactured (Thompson, 1999). Although the potential for microphone drift exists, the magnitude of this drift, and whether it actually occurs in hearing aids in real-world settings, has not been demonstrated. Further, some authors (e.g., Thompson, 2001) contend that microphone drift rarely, if ever, occurs. One of the desirable characteristics of MEMS microphones is related to drift. Both temperature and humidity drift are significantly reduced when this technology is used. We believe a greater concern relates to the fact that microphone diaphragms, microphone ports, or the screens covering them, may become partially or completely covered or clogged by debris (dust, hairspray, and the like) resulting in a mismatch insensitivity. Unfortunately, concerns related to dirt and debris apply to both dual microphone and single microphone design. Because of the potential problems with debris, audiologists are encouraged to check and, if necessary, clean the microphone ports during routine, periodic hearing aid evaluations.

With dual microphone designs, technology exists to counteract a limited amount of microphone mismatch. That is, several manufacturers incorporate circuitry in their digital hearing aids that measures and offsets small differences in microphone sensitivity. Some modern DSP circuits can be used to calibrate the relative outputs from the two microphones. It should be noted however that this circuitry is generally quite limited and a large enough mismatch will still result is a reduction in directivity. Therefore, regular clinical evaluation of directivity is still important.

Wind noise presents another significant problem for directional hearing aids because the annoying noise sounds louder through a directional microphone than through its omnidirectional counterpart (Dillon, Birtles, & Lovegrove, 1999). This may seem surprising given we just discussed that directional microphones reduce sensitivity, particularly in the low frequencies. However, this reduction is for signals in the far field. In contrast, when a spherical wave front hits both microphone openings at the same time (as is the case with wind), there is instead a low-frequency boost in comparison to the omnidirectional setting. As a result of this boost, most listeners prefer the omnidirectional setting in windy environments. While wind noise has a fairly broad frequency spectrum, it is most prominent in the low frequencies. Therefore, one technique of wind noise management is to switch the low-frequency range to omnidirectional mode and reduce amplification in the low frequencies when wind is detected. As we discuss in Chapter 12, more recent wind noise reduction algorithms have been designed to provide some cancellation of the wind noise.

A related issue occurs for a talker's own voice. The close proximity of the talker source to the microphone also results in a spherical wave front. Commonly referred to as the Proximity Effect, an increase in low-frequency energy of as much as 16 dB can be realized. As a consequence, some hearing aid wearers, particularly men with deep voices, may complain about a "boomy" quality to their own voice when the directional microphone is active. Appropriate counselling may therefore be necessary to reassure patients this is a sound quality artifact and not an actual change in the patient's voice. A recent feature available from at least one manufacturer is a hearing aid algorithm that detects when the hearing aid wearer is talking (after some training), and then automatically adjusts the gain to the degree determined by a pre-fitting adaptive procedure conducted by the audiologist at the time of the fitting. This processing can help reduce complaints related to own voice level and quality when using microphone arrays with low-frequency gain equalization.

One final issue specific to bilateral beamformers and higher order arrays relates to binaural cues. Binaural advantages and the potential benefits associated with bilateral amplification are discussed throughout this text. Since most listeners experience considerable benefits from wearing two hearing aids, a trial with bilateral amplification is typically recommended for the majority of patients clinically. Without additional processing, bilateral beamformer processing, which combines the input from all four microphones, would result in presentation of the exact same, highly-directional signal to both hearing aids. If unaided audibility through the hearing aid vent does not occur, this diotic presentation will eliminate all interaural difference cues with clear negative consequences. As a result, all commercial implementations of bilateral beamformers preserve or restore some of the interaural information. In one technique, the frequency region over which the bilateral beamformer provides a diotic signal is band-limited to the higher frequencies and a dichotic signal is presented in the lower frequencies via traditional directional processing. In a second and more common technique, the ITD or ILD cues are estimated at the input to the two hearing aids and partially reintroduced after beamformer processing by convolution with an average head-related transform. In one commercial example the ILD is reintroduced across all frequencies (rather than just in the high frequencies as would occur in listeners with normal hearing) in an attempt to provide a more consistent interaural difference cue.

Getting a Signal Into the Hearing Aid: T-Coils

A second major way to introduce signals into a hearing aid is through a telecoil, commonly referred to as a *t-coil*. T-coils have existed in hearing aids since the late 1940s. Hearing aids that have t-coils often have a user control that can be switched from microphone (M) to t-coil (T) modes and, in some cases, activate both the t-coil and microphone at the same time (MT). Some modern t-coils are automatic. That is, they are automatically activated and deactivated based on the presence or absence of a magnetic field. Hearing aid t-coils work on the principle of inductance and their most basic form is simply a ferrite (iron) rod surrounded by a coil of very thin copper wire (Figure 10–32). Specifically, current generated in the coil as magnetic waves—which were generated by dynamic loudspeakers, room loops, or other sources—pass through the coil.

In comparison to a microphone, there are a few specific advantages related to the use of a t-coil. First, whereas the microphone on a hearing aid picks up all sounds, the t-coil will only pick up electromagnetic signals. Noise in the wearer's environment will not be picked up and amplified if the hearing aid microphone is deactivated. T-coils are also useful for telephones because placing any surface, including a telephone, near an active hearing aid microphone increases the

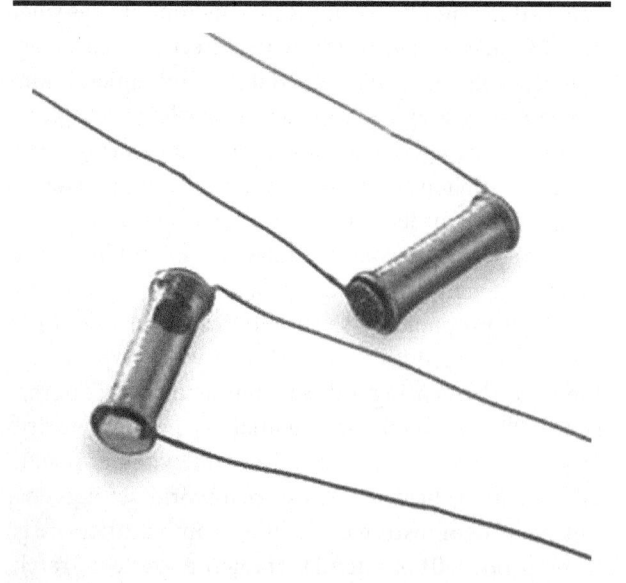

Figure 10–32. Examples of hearing aid t-coils.

likelihood of acoustic feedback. This feedback can be eliminated when using a t-coil by disabling the hearing aid microphone. Many individuals with hearing impairment and associated groups, including the Hearing Loss Association of America (HLAA), are strong advocates for inclusion of t-coils in hearing aids. Although the utility of t-coils for telephone use has long been recognized, these advocates point out their additional utility for easily bringing signals directly and economically from an external microphone to the hearing aid through the use of an induction loop in the room, meanwhile avoiding picking up acoustic noise near the listener. Since hearing aids are generally equipped with t-coils (at least upon request and assuming sufficient case size), the listener has little additional expense.

Limitations of Common Hearing Aid T-Coils

As we discussed earlier in this chapter, the smaller the t-coil, the weaker it will be. All other things being equal (wire diameter, shape), halving the size of the t-coil results in a reduction of sensitivity of approximately a factor of four. For this reason, t-coils are primarily present in the larger BTE and ITE style hearing aids. We also discussed how important orientation is to the strength of induced current. A telephone is typically placed facing the ear and the magnetic field is often oriented directly outward from the receiver; however, a good deal of variation is evident in modern telephones. With the typical orientation, the strongest field moves from the side of the head to the center. However, the biggest limitation for t-coils is that most modern telephones, including most cellular phones, do not produce an electromagnetic field at all. Consequently, careful consideration of the telephones available and even the purchase of a new telephone may be necessary for individuals interested in using the t-coil. Although they are becoming increasingly rare, many public telephones work with t-coils. Public phones that work with t-coils are mandated in some public spaces (like airports), and public telephones that can be used with t-coils are marked by a blue grommet around the cord at the place that it attaches to the hand piece.

In contrast, induction generators (neck loops, room loops, silhouettes, wireless receivers and transmitters) generate and propagate electromagnetic fields in a number of different directions, including from the floor upward. The bottom line? The optimal t-coil orientation for one application may not be the same as for another, necessitating that the clinician determine the primary use for the t-coil for each individual and be prepared to provide coping strategies for use in other environments. The influence of environment is further complicated by the fact that the strength of the electromagnetic field often varies considerably with small changes in position. Therefore users must be trained to orient the telephone or themselves (in looped situations) in order to obtain the most satisfactory response. Often the hearing aid user must use trial-and-error to obtain the best position.

A final limitation is the presence of stray electromagnetic fields that create interference. These unwanted fields from fluorescent lights, power lines, electrical transformers, and other sources, including those generated intentionally, can be picked up by the t-coil and amplified. These stray fields are generally in the 50 to 400 Hz range and are perceived as buzzing or humming sounds, although in some cases it can extend to 10 kHz or beyond and is heard as a hissing. These signals are commonly not only annoying but can lead to reduced speech recognition and, in many cases, they can also completely obscure the signal of interest, thereby rendering the t-coil useless. It is sometimes possible for hearing aid wearers to lessen this interference by tilting their head or moving.

Efforts to Improve and Enhance T-Coils

The facts that smaller t-coils are weaker and that hearing aid wearers often wish to have the smallest instrument possible for cosmetic reasons have presented obvious problems for quite some time. The popularity of the mini-BTE style (see Chapter 8) only has served to exacerbate the problem. In the smaller sizes, the signal out of the t-coil can be quite a bit weaker than the signal out of a microphone, necessitating increasing the amount of amplification provided (either by adjusting the volume or programming the amplifier for more amplification). One increasingly common technique that improves this problem is the use of t-coil pre-amplifiers. Some modern digital hearing aids allow this preamplifier to be programmed for differing amounts of amplification so that it can be more easily matched to the microphone output.

Another technique that has been developed to improve t-coil performance is to wrap the copper wire around a curved or rounded surface rather than a straight bar. By doing this, coils have been developed that offer similar sensitivity in both horizontal and vertical orientations.

Attempts have also been made to counteract the electromagnetic interference created by sources such as power lines, fluorescent lights, industrial equipment, appliances, and other household electrical and electronic equipment. Generally these techniques attempt to identify and reduce interference through cancellation of magnetic fields that are not deemed to be near the person. Whereas such processing is expected to improve t-coil use with telephones, it is also expected to interfere with t-coil performance in looped room situations. Consequently, processing aimed at cancellation of far-field EMF must be disabled in room loop situations.

Finally, technology continues to be refined that automatically switches the t-coil on and off in the presence and absence of electromagnetic fields. These automatic t-coils can provide a convenience for many users. Determining the most appropriate sensitivity for switching is, however, still problematic for manufacturers. If the sensitivity is set low, they will only activate in the presence of a strong magnetic field and may not switch on for some magnetic fields of interest. If the sensitivity is set high, they may activate in the presence of extraneous and unwanted fields. The ultimate utility of these devices may therefore depend in part on the individual hearing aid wearer's environment. The most common compromise is to set the sensitivity low and provide a strong fixed magnet with an adhesive surface that can be placed on the phone to ensure activation.

Getting a Signal Into the Hearing Aid: Other Methods

A third major way to introduce signals into a hearing aid is through a direct electronic connection referred to as *direct audio input (DAI)*. DAI requires a physical connection via a proprietary snap-on connector commonly referred to as a "boot" or "shoe" (Figure 10–33). This method is commonly used to connect the hearing aid to a frequency modulated (FM) system, some wireless microphone systems, and other HATs. DAI is usually only available in BTE and mini-BTE hearing aid styles Wires connecting the hearing aid to a device need to be well-shielded as they can unintentionally act as antennas for nearby radio transmitters.

A final way of getting the signal into the hearing aid is the use of wireless receivers built into the hearing aid case. These include both FM receivers, which have been available for quite some time, and the more recently introduced wireless receivers, including the coils used with near field induction systems and some of the wireless protocols discussed previously. We will discuss wireless technologies in considerable detail in Chapter 12.

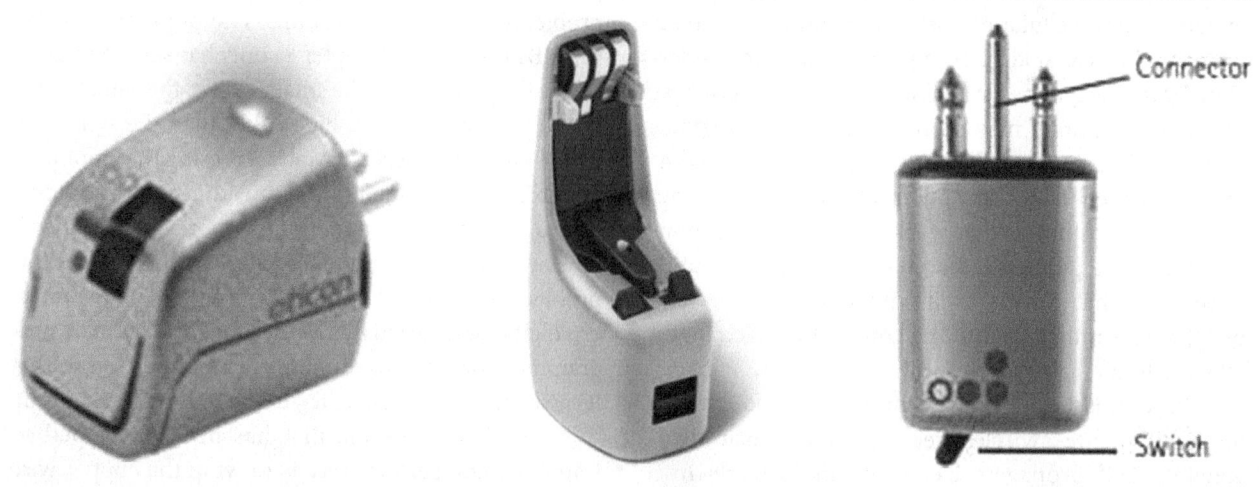

Figure 10–33. Examples of hearing aid "boots" or "shoes."

Batteries

All the sophisticated circuitry in the world won't work at all without electrical energy. In hearing aids, current is provided by the energy storage device commonly referred to as the hearing aid battery. The hearing aid battery is critical because it provides electrical power for all the hearing aid circuitry. On a side note, a hearing aid battery is not really a battery at all, and is more accurately described as a power cell.

Hearing aid batteries typically produce about 1.25 to 1.5 V of electric force. In the not so distant past, hearing aid batteries using mercury and silver-oxide technologies were not uncommon. Due to cost, safety, and other concerns, these technologies are no longer used. Instead, most hearing aids in 2017 used *zinc-air* technology. Zinc-air batteries are favored over other hearing aid battery technologies for two other reasons. First, they are able to provide more energy per unit of volume (typically referred to as a higher energy density) than many other technologies. Secondly, rather than providing high voltage early in their life which then decays over time, zinc-air batteries provide a nearly constant 1.25 V over nearly their entire life, then completely fail rapidly. This relatively constant voltage supply is desirable when designing circuitry, in part because it results in more stable operation of the DSP, amplifier, and other components. Some circuitry will require a minimum voltage for proper operation. When the voltage drops, rather than simply ceasing to work, distortions, noise, or other errors may be introduced.

As the name suggests, zinc-air batteries mainly contain zinc and are activated by removing a paper tab covering a hole in the back, which allows air from the atmosphere in to complete the necessary electrochemical reaction. Once the battery has been activated in this way, it will typically last for no more than six weeks, even if it is never used. Extremes in relative humidity deviating from around 40 to 50% can further shorten the battery life both when not used and when used in a hearing aid. Even if the tab is never peeled off shelf life is typically between one and two years.

Hearing aid current drain will depend on the type of circuitry, type of processing, activation of special features, required gain and maximum output, bandwidth,

---

POINTS TO PONDER: A BATTERY OR A CELL?

- By strict definition, a battery is a collection of two or more electrochemical cells.
- Each of these cells generates voltage and current through chemical reactions.
- In the case of a hearing aid only a single cell, rather than a collection of electrical cells, is present.
- Currently, however, it is common across hearing aids and other industries that use single electrical cells to refer to them as batteries.

THINGS TO REMEMBER: BATTERY LIFE

The life of a hearing aid battery when in use will depend on the hearing aids *current drain* in milliamps (mA) and the *battery capacity* in milliamp hours (mAH).

- Suppose we have a hearing aid with an average current drain of 1.3 mA.
- Furthemore, suppose we use a battery in this hearing aid with a capacity of 190 mAH.
- This battery should last 190/1.3 = 146 hours.
- If a patient uses the hearing aid 16 hours a day, this translates into a little more than nine days.

and other factors. Furthermore, the hearing aid current drain may or may not be stable over time. That is, with the majority of modern circuitry, battery drain will depend on factors such as the gain and output level, the signal input level, and the activation and operation of various processing features. As we describe earlier, digital amplifiers, like their analog Class D counterparts, use much less electrical power in quiet than when a signal is present. Therefore, it may only be possible to estimate the average current drain for a hearing aid, or measure it for a specific configuration using techniques described in Chapter 13.

Battery capacity is specified on each battery and is generally related to battery size. That is, the smallest hearing aid batteries will only have a capacity of 35 mAH or so, meanwhile the largest may have a capacity of approximately 575 mAH.

Hearing aid batteries are typically described by a number which refers to their type and indirectly to their size and approximate capacity (Table 10–1). To ease in identification, the removable tabs covering the air holes are typically color coded. An example of sizes of typical hearing aid batteries is shown in Figure 10–34. Figure 10–35 provides a rough indication of the range of expected battery life as a function of hearing aid battery size and average hearing aid current drain.

Rechargeable batteries in ear level hearing aids have been available for about 10 years, but recently we have seen an influx of rechargeable technologies in the hearing aid sector. Rechargeable battery technologies including nickel metal hydride (NiMH), nickel cadmium (NiCad), silver zinc, lithium ion (Li), and others have been introduced, as shown in Figure 10–36. Even refillable fuel cell technologies are being investigated for use in hearing aids. Differences across these technologies relate to recharge time, operating temperature, ability to provide a consistent voltage, and most impor-

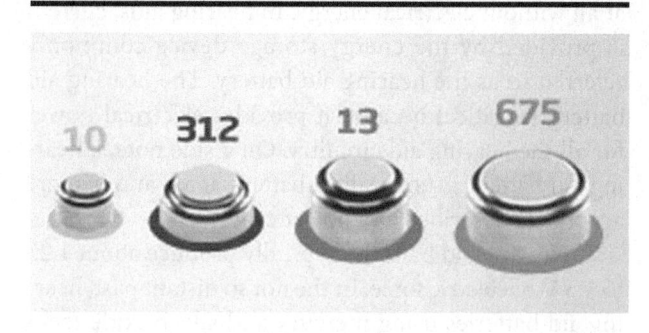

Figure 10–34. Examples of common hearing aid batteries.

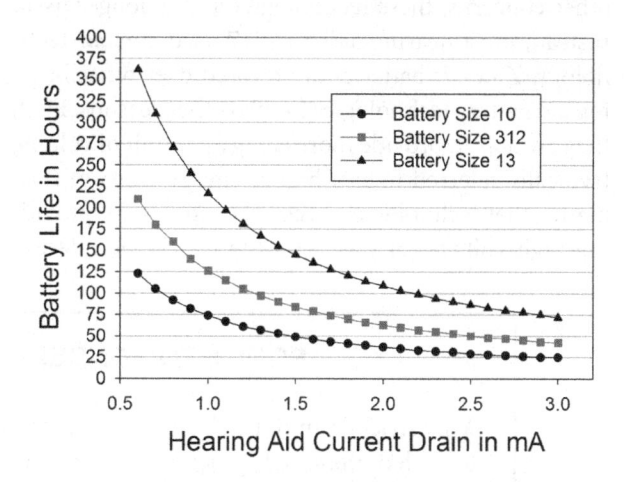

Figure 10–35. The range of expected battery life as a function of hearing aid battery size and average hearing aid current drain. Adapted from W. Stab (2016). http://hearinghealthmatters.org/waynesworld/2016/hearing-aid-battery-life-can-vary-widely/

Table 10–1. Capacities, Color Coding, and Uses for Typical Hearing Aid Battery Types

Battery Type (Size)	Typical Capacity (mAH)	Color Code	Typical Hearing Aid Styles
675	530	Blue	BTE
13	230	Orange	Mini-BTE, BTE, ITE
312	120	Brown	Mini-BTE, ITE, ITC
10 (A10, 10A, 230)	65	Yellow	Mini-BTE, ITC, CIC
5 (A5, 5A)	35	Red	CIC

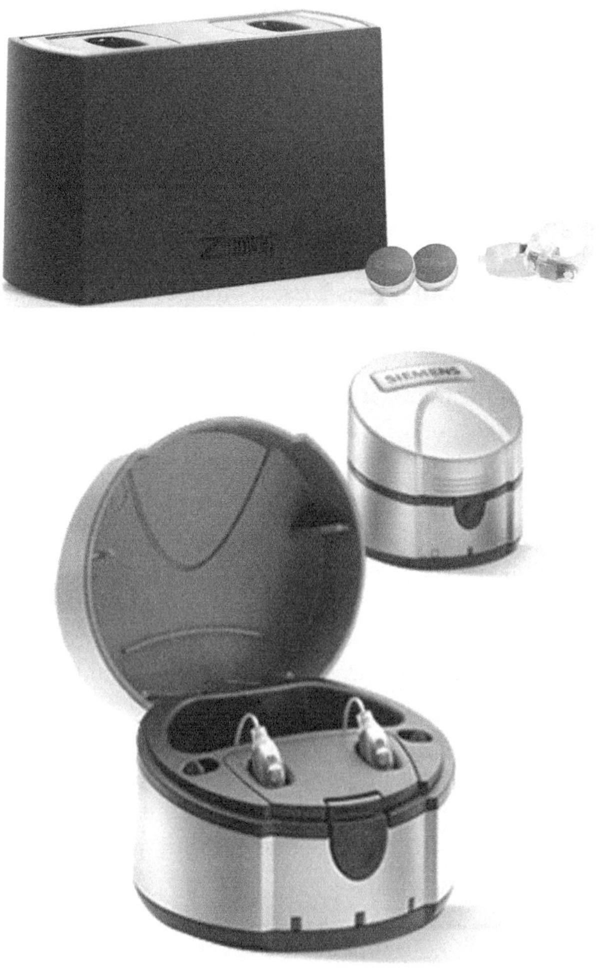

Figure 10–36. A few examples of rechargeable hearing aid battery systems.

Rechargeable battery life is typically defined by both the capacity when new (which determines the number of hours the hearing aid can operate without needing to recharge the battery) and the number of charge cycles before there is a significant decrease in capacity (typically 30%). All rechargeable batteries have battery capacities that are a fraction of their non-rechargeable counterparts. To be viable for hearing aid use, it is important that a rechargeable battery last all day (16–18 hours). Optimally, this capacity would be available for at least 6 to 12 months. Early versions of rechargeable hearing aid batteries suffered from insufficient life, particularly after several charge cycles. Battery life after six months in some early examples we evaluated was as little as six to eight hours. Fortunately, by 2015 we saw examples of rechargeable products that routinely lasted longer than 18 hours even when activating wireless features during routine use. Not surprisingly given these findings, many manufacturers have introduced products that are rechargeable. A number of third-party battery manufacturers have also entered this market. One challenge for some of these companies is providing consistent voltage and current for the hearing aid. Some manufactures have introduced clever methods for ensuring optimal operation including application of control circuitry built into a replacement battery door. In our opinion we have finally reached the stage where some rechargeable battery technologies are truly viable for use in hearing aids and, consequently, we expect the use of these technologies will continue to grow rapidly.

Presenting the Signal to the Listener: Receivers

After we have the signal located within the hearing aid, our most basic goal is to provide gain (amplification) to all or some of the frequency range. We discussed basic amplification, filtering, and DSP in the first part of this chapter. We will discuss compression and expansion at the end of this chapter and a host of other signal processing features in more detail in Chapters 11 and 12. Whether we have accomplished amplification and signal shaping in the analog or digital realm, we have picked up sounds and processed them and now have a voltage out of the output transistors that reflects all desired amplification, signal shaping, and processing that were

tantly, battery life. These technologies are all of interest because rechargeable technologies produce much less waste and can be considerably more convenient to use than disposable batteries (it's estimated that 1.4 billion disposable batteries go into landfills each year). Greater interest in rechargeable batteries is also related to concerns over the increased current drain resulting from activation of some modern wireless features. Some current hearing aids exhibit current drain as low as 0.8 mA when all features are disabled. Hearing aids commonly exhibit current drain in the 1.0 to 2.0 mA range, however, with standard features activated. When activating wireless technologies that stream sound between hearing aids we have measured current drain in the 4.5 to 5.5 mA range or even higher.

applied. Now we need to transduce this electronic signal back into a form that the hearing aid wearer can receive. The most common output transduction is from an electric signal to an acoustic signal using a tiny loudspeaker commonly referred to as a receiver. Less commonly, the signal may be transduced into mechanical vibration as is the case with bone conduction hearing aids, bone anchored implants, middle ear implant, and a host of other techniques described in Chapter 8. In this chapter, however, we will focus on the much more common method of sound delivery, the receiver.

The hearing aid receiver operates on some of the same principles of electromagnetic induction we described earlier in this chapter as applied to dynamic loudspeakers (e.g., Figure 10–7). The most common receiver design is the *balanced armature transducer* shown in Figure 10–37. There are several variations in the exact construction and operation of receivers of this type, especially as a function of size.

In the general design, the current from the amplifier is applied to the coil making the armature an electromagnet. The *armature,* sometimes referred to as the "reed," is made of an iron alloy and shaped like a U. The bottom of the armature is fixed to the metal case of the receiver. Application of positive and negative current to the coil results in a time-varying magnetic field that varies from north to south magnetic pole. In magnetic fields, like poles repel each other and opposite poles attract each other. The arrangement of the strong fixed magnets around the armature causes the time-varying magnetic field to drive the free arm or the armature up and down. Since there is room between the coil and the armature, the armature is able to freely vibrate up and down as current changes are applied to the coil. Together, the armature, coil, and fixed magnets are sometimes referred to as the *motor*. Vibration generated in the motor is carried up a thin stiff wire called the *drive rod*, to a flexible membrane referred to as the *diaphragm*. The diaphragm typically is held in place by a *support ring*. Together the diaphragm and its support ring act to seal acoustically the space above the diaphragm, referred to as the *front volume*, from the air space around the motor, referred to as the *back volume*. Pressure changes in the front volume resulting from the vibration of the diaphragm travel out the sound outlet, through tubing, to the ear canal.

The schematic shown in Figure 10–37 is somewhat simplified compared to actual receiver construction. One typical design that is not shown in this figure places the output transistors (amplifier) within the metal case

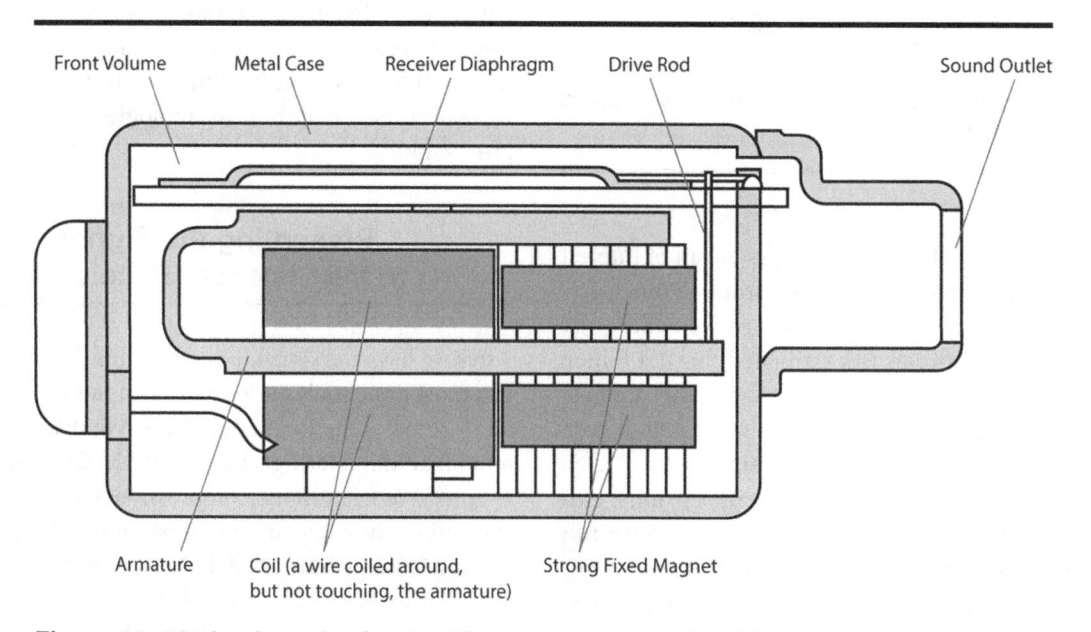

Figure 10–37. A schematic of a simplified hearing aid receiver. The volume of air above the diaphragm is referred to as the front volume, whereas the volume of air under the diaphragm is referred to as the back volume. Note how the position of the diaphragm acts to protect it from objects entering the sound outlet.

of the receiver. A second group of typical structures that is not represented includes various mounting brackets, spacers, and vibration dampers. These structures serve multiple purposes, which are intended to optimize the function of the receiver. One of the most important functions is to limit vibration in an attempt to limit mechanical feedback. In addition to the traditional rubber damping material, other more sophisticated methods for reducing vibration are sometimes used. One method injects a viscous liquid, which is a mixture of rust particles and mineral oil (ferrofluid), into the receiver's motor, typically in the space between the fixed magnets and the armature. This liquid acts to dampen vibration of the armature near the receiver's resonance frequency. Even though this method doesn't directly target vibration, it limits the peaks in the receiver output, thus reducing the output level at resonant frequencies. The use of a ferrofluid to dampen output peaks both reduces vibration at higher levels and helps reduce problems with the hearing aid output peaks exceeding the listener's threshold of discomfort at specific frequencies. At least one receiver manufacturer has designed receivers for which the metal case is further mechanically isolated by placing it inside a second, larger, metal case. Rubber damping material is then used to isolate the outside metal case mechanically from the vibrations generated by the inside metal case. The higher the desired output from the receiver, the more likely that vibration will be present, and the greater the need for clever solutions for dampening vibration.

Both mechanical feedback and acoustic feedback were described in some detail in Chapter 8. The receiver also introduces the possibility of a third type of feedback that we have not discussed previously: magnetic feedback. Magnetic feedback, like acoustic and mechanical feedback, occurs because energy at the output finds its way back into the input and is re-amplified repeatedly in a loop to a point of oscillation. A magnetic feedback loop can occur because the tiny magnetic field generated by the receiver coil and armature can be picked up by the hearing aid t-coil. Since magnetically shielding the t-coil would prevent it from picking up desired signals, it is therefore necessary for the engineers who design receivers to provide magnetic shielding around the receiver (or at least the receiver motor). In addition, it is of interest to shield the coil from magnetic fields occurring in the environment. Magnetic shielding is typically achieved by using a metal receiver case made of materials that act to partially block magnetic fields (typically a nickel iron blend), a metal foil wrapped around the magnetic components (typically copper or gold), and/or shielding plates.

Hearing aid receivers are available in a number of different sizes and configurations (Figure 10–38). Different receivers may be selected based on the desired gain and output, frequency response, frequency range, and size. Because high output intensities require the movement of a lot of air, larger receivers with larger magnets, coils, and diaphragms are generally able to provide a higher output level than smaller receivers before saturation (i.e., the point just before mechanical failure or when no more output is possible regardless of input). Typically however, the phrase "hearing aid saturation" is used to describe a level well below that leading to mechanical failure. Specifically, saturation describes the output level prior to the point for which unsatisfactory levels of distortion are reached, commonly when total harmonic distortion reaches 10% or more.

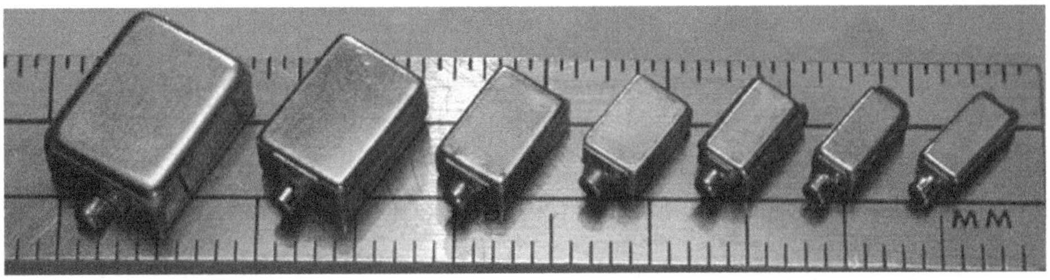

Figure 10–38. Examples of several hearing aid receivers. The maximum output before saturation ranges from 145 dB SPL for the largest receiver on the far left to 110 dB SPL for the smallest receiver on the far right. (Reproduced from Knowles Electronics.)

Depending on their size, receivers often saturate at outputs between approximately 100 dB SPL to more than 140 dB SPL. Since the receiver coils are driven with the battery, it should not be surprising that between 50 and 90% of the total battery power can be consumed by the receiver. Unfortunately, the efficiency of smaller receivers is lessened compared to larger receivers because of the use of a smaller diaphragm (air is moved less efficiently) and a back volume of air which is stiffer due to its small size. Consequently, a smaller receiver will consume more battery power than larger receivers given the same desired output.

In cases of very high power requirements, especially when a broad bandwidth is desired, two *drivers* (essentially sets of receiver components) may be used (Figure 10–39). This is similar to home loudspeakers, which may include one low frequency speaker (bass driver) and one high frequency speaker (tweeter) within the same case. The use of a larger receiver will increase the overall size of the hearing aid case, which may be of particular concern in smaller custom instruments, however. Another size consideration is specific to receiver-in-the canal (RIC) mini-BTE instruments in that larger receivers may be too large to fit in smaller ear canals. This may be especially problematic if an open fitting is desired in that there must be enough room between the receiver and the ear canal wall to place an eartip to help with retention without occluding the ear canal or causing discomfort.

The receiver usually is the limiting factor relative to hearing aid bandwidth. It is especially challenging to obtain a receiver that has both a high output and a broad bandwidth. The frequency response of a range of common, single-driver hearing aid receivers is shown in Figure 10–40. This figure demonstrates that even receivers that are considered "wideband" typically have limited output available above 7 or 8 kHz. For example, the receiver in the bottom panel in Figure 10–40 has a maximum output of approximately 77 dB SPL at 9 kHz. For comparison purposes, normal hearing thresholds at 9 kHz are approximately 16 dB SPL, meanwhile listeners between 61 and 70 years of age with pure-tone average thresholds in the normal range (<25 dB HL) have been shown to exhibit average hearing thresholds of approximately 60 dB SPL at this same frequency (Dreschler & van der Hulst, 1987; Matthews, Lee, Mills, & Dubno, 1997). Therefore, providing an audible output at 9 kHz to an older listener with even a mild hearing loss would be challenging at best. The situation can be improved through the use of a dual driver (see Figure 10–39). Current drain and size are necessarily increased compared to a single driver. It should also be noted that it is possible to provide more high frequency output through plumbing changes as we describe in Chapter 9.

In addition to limiting bandwidth, receiver failure is also the most commonly reported cause for hearing aid repair, especially in custom and RIC instruments that place the receiver in the ear canal. The receiver is the weak link relative to hearing aid durability, mainly because of two factors: sensitivity to being dropped and impaction by dirt, cerumen, and other debris.

Since a receiver must have parts that are both small and can easily and freely be sent into motion, they can

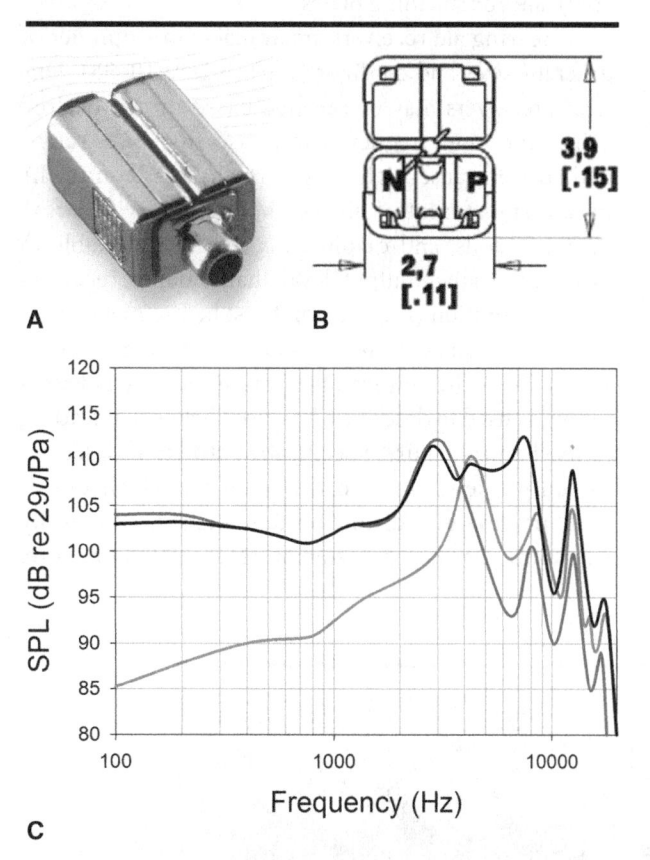

Figure 10–39. A dual driver balanced armature transducer (**A**), cross-sectional schematic (**B**), and associated frequency response of each individual driver and when combined (**C**) (Knowles TWFK-30017. Reproduced from Knowles Electronics).

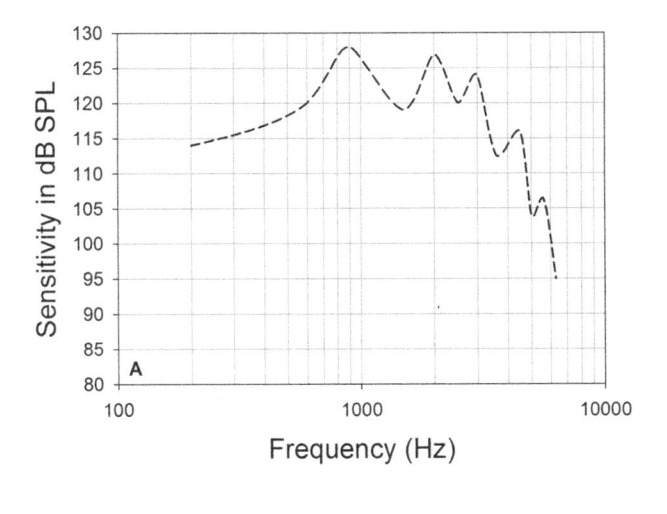

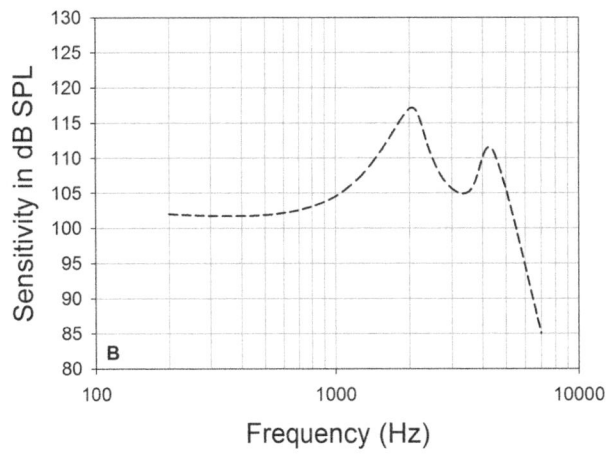

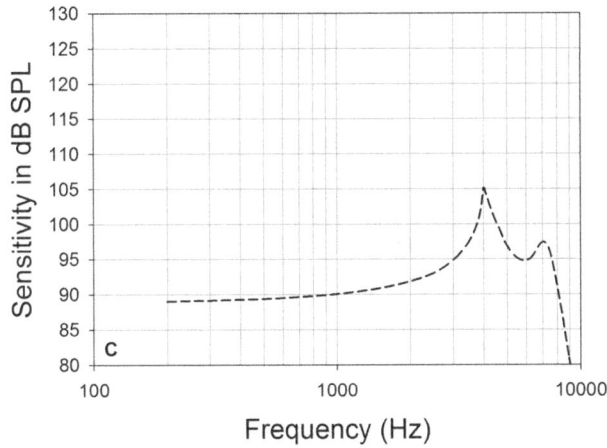

Figure 10–40. Examples of the frequency response limitations of several hearing aid receivers; ranging from a large powerful receiver with somewhat narrower bandwidth (**A** – Knowles CI), to a typical receiver (**B** – Knowles ED), to a wider band receiver (**C** – Knowles WBFK). (Reproduced from Knowles Electronics).

be damaged by physical shock, such as dropping them on a hard surface. A measure of increased distortion in a hearing aid is commonly caused by mechanical shock damage to the receiver. Fortunately, receiver manufacturers have introduced several techniques that reduce the risk of mechanical shock damage to hearing aid receivers, although some susceptibility remains.

Cerumen, debris, and moisture are all problematic for receivers, but this issue is exacerbated in receivers that implement dampers. Damping screens can become easily clogged in patients who generate large quantities of cerumen. Even if no damper is present, cerumen can migrate into the receiver, clogging the sound outlet or impeding vibration of the diaphragm. Although it is possible in some cases to train hearing aid wearers to clean cerumen from the sound outlet, such cleaning can result in pushing cerumen further into the receiver and even cause damage to the receiver components or damper if the cleaning tool (typically a wire loop) is forced too deeply into the receiver. In addition, cleaning the receiver sound outlet is limited to patients that have good manual dexterity. Once the cerumen gets deeply impacted into the sound outlet, it is typically preferable to have the patient bring the hearing aid in for cleaning by a trained clinician or return the instrument to the manufacturer for receiver cleaning and/or replacement. Sometimes the wax can be removed through the use of one of many available vacuum or suction devices. In the popular min-BTE RIC devices, the approach simply is to replace the receiver. For a full-time hearing aid user, it is not uncommon to replace the receiver every six months or so. Some patients do this themselves, but usually it is a quick office visit. Most dispensing audiologists maintain a large supply of replacement receivers for the hearing aids from their favorite hearing aid manufacturers. And yes, the receivers from some manufacturers tend to go bad much more frequently than the receivers from other companies.

Another technique to limit damage from cerumen is the use of a wax guard. Wax guards are typically plastic inserts placed in the hearing aid sound outlet (Figure 10–41). There have been many different designs of wax guards, and new designs are continually introduced. This fact should tell us that no optimal solution has yet been found. The difficulty is that the wax guards themselves are usually susceptible to clogging. This is not to say that wax guards aren't useful, however, as they can provide some protection from wax for the receiver components. Therefore, it is typical to use wax guards and change them regularly when they become plugged. Even though not the maintenance-free operation we would like to see in hearing aids, changing a plugged wax guard is certainly easier and less costly than repairing or replacing a receiver—and can significantly reduce receiver-related repairs. As with cleaning, patients with poor dexterity will commonly need you, a technician, or a more dexterous spouse or caregiver to change the wax guard for them.

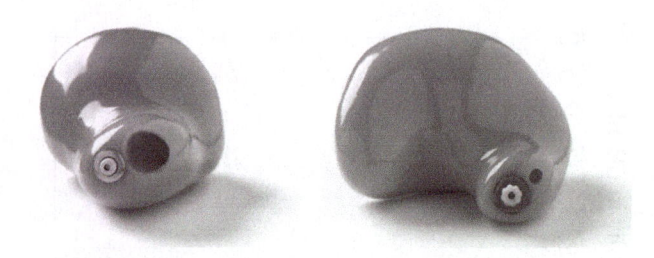

Figure 10–41. Two examples of commercial wax guards placed in the sound outlet of custom hearing aids. These styles are intended to be changed by the hearing aid wearer.

Gain Processing and Compression Basics

In Chapter 4 we discuss the importance of audibility and quantifying the speech signal at length. In this chapter we have discussed how hearing aids work and the physical components and processing used to perform a hearing aids most fundamental job, to increase the intensity of sounds in a frequency-specific manner to offset the loss of audibility resulting from hearing loss. In Chapters 11 and 12, we discuss hearing aid process-

---

POINTS TO PONDER: DO HEARING AID COMPANIES MANUFACTURE THEIR OWN PARTS?

Whereas some manufacturers do make their own transducers, amplifiers, and processors, a great number are manufactured by other specialty companies. Increasingly with digital technology, hearing aid manufacturers are in the business of software rather than hardware. As of this writing some of the largest hearing aid transducer companies include Knowles Electronics (estimated at about 80% of the world market), Tibbets Industries, and Global Coils SAGL. Manufacturers of amplifiers and processors include Etymotic Research, ONsemi, Taiwan Semiconductor Manufacturing Corporation (TSCM), and Zarlink Semiconductor. Company acquisition continues to change this landscape rapidly. For example, DSPfactory was bought by AMI, which in turn was acquired by ONsemi. SoundDesign Technologies (formally part of Gennum) was also purchased by ONsemi. Onsemi supplies DSP chips to Intricon, which has developed a number of algorithms and sells preconfigured DSP chips to the market, as does ONsemi, which also sells blank chips. ONsemi doesn't actually fabricate the DSP chips in-house. As does almost everyone else, ONsemi uses chips from TSMC in what is called a fabless semiconductor model (Personal Communication from Steve Armstrong).

ing and features aimed at doing more than simply making sounds louder. Since we have already have reviewed the acoustic quantification of the speech signal, it might seem logical to discuss how we might optimally assign the amount of amplification for each individual listener, typically referred to as a prescriptive gain method, but actually we won't get to that in detail until Chapter 14.

First, we need to discuss how level-specific amplification is assigned as a function of frequency and how this affects speech and other sounds. In modern digital hearing aids, the sound level in each channel or over a range of frequencies when working in the spectral domain is analyzed prior to applying DSP. These levels are then used to assign the level-specific magnitude of amplification (gain) within each target frequency group, commonly referred to as defining the compressor gains (see our following discussion of input compression). In some systems, compressor gains may also be defined as a function of predicted output level by first applying linear gain to the input signal and analyzing the predicted output level (input plus gain) and then applying the desired compression (see our discussion of output compression).

So what is compression? It is simply the act of reducing the degree of amplification of a signal as its level is increased. This acts to reduce the dynamic range from the lowest to highest levels at the output of the hearing aid relative to this same range at the input to the hearing aid. When we combine gain and compression processing in a hearing aid, we describe the resulting amplification as *nonlinear gain*. Nonlinear gain (compression) is applied to offset the reduction in the residual dynamic range of hearing in listeners with sensorineural hearing loss and make sure that high-level sounds are not too loud. We will explain these ideas in much more detail in the second half of this book.

Nearly every hearing aid today uses at least one type of compression, and most use at least two different types. Understanding how the various types of compression works is essential for fitting and fine tuning all hearing aids. Compression is often referred to as automatic gain control (AGC) because the gain of the hearing aid changes automatically as the input intensity changes. Because there is no one simple way to describe compression in a modern hearing aid, it helps to contrast different types of compression to each other, and discuss how each type of compression is designed to contribute to a successful fitting. Before we do that though, let's first start with the basics of how we describe compression. Then we will discuss the effect different types of compression can have on the speech signal.

Input/Output (I/O) and Input/Gain (I/G) Functions

Input/Output (I/O) and Input/Gain (I/G) functions can be a good way to introduce many compression concepts. Once you understand these functions, your knowledge of compression will fall into place (we think). As you already know, input + gain = output. For the input/output function, we use a chart that has input on the x-axis and output for the y-axis. The input/output function of a given hearing aid is then displayed by the diagonal line. At any point on this line, gain can be determined by subtracting the input values from the output. The place on this line where it bends or changes angle (deviates from 45 degrees) is called the compression kneepoint (with a little imagination the entire function can be viewed as a very thin leg with a bent knee but missing a foot.). The kneepoint is where compression begins, and is also referred to as the compression threshold. You might see abbreviations such as CT for compression threshold, CK for compression kneepoint, or TK for threshold of kneepoint; all mean the same thing. We can also plot gain as a function of input. These I/G functions do not provide any information that is not already in the I/O plot, they are just a different way to visualize the same information.

The I/O and I/G functions shown in Figure 10–42 show the difference between linear amplification and a few different compression hearing aid settings. For the hearing aid providing linear amplification, notice how the output grows in a linear manner as the input increases up to 90 dB SPL. In other words, the gain stays the same as the input increases Observe that a 70 dB input equals 90 dB output (20 dB of gain) and, likewise, an 80 dB input equals 100 dB output (again, 20 dB of gain). When an input signal of 90 dB SPL is reached, notice that this hearing aid reaches its MPO (think of this as a ceiling, determined by the setting of the AGCo kneepoint). This means that the output will not significantly increase for higher inputs, which then indirectly reduces gain. As we mentioned earlier, it is important

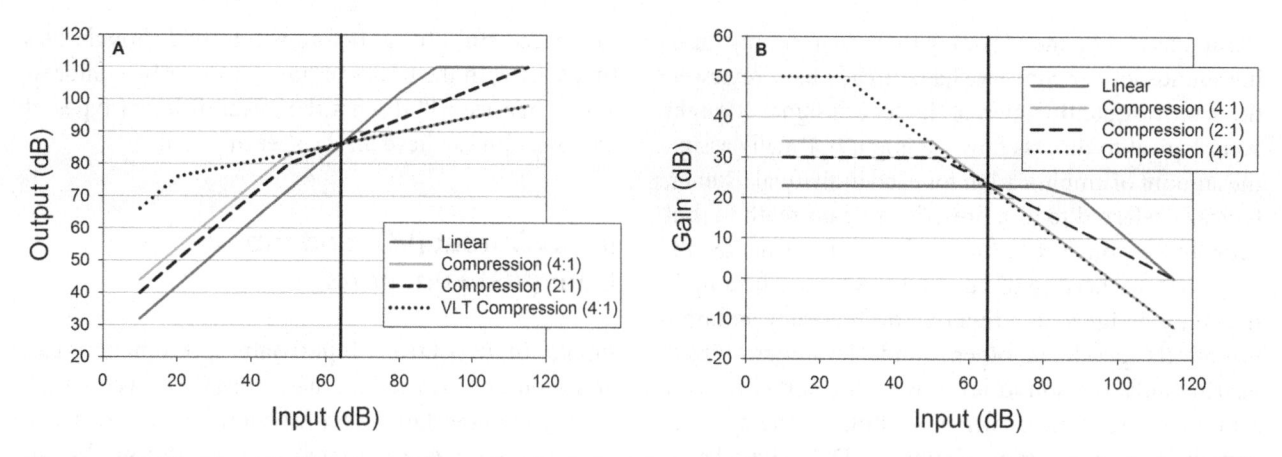

Figure 10–42. The I/O functions (at one frequency) of four well-fit hearing aids that apply linear, WDRC with a 2:1 CR, WDRC with a 4:1 CR, and very low threshold (VLT) compression with a 4:1 CR gain processing (**A**). The corresponding I/G functions are also shown (**B**).

to remember that the MPO (OSPL 90) varies with each hearing aid and must be set by the hearing aid fitter, based on the patient's measured frequency-specific LDLs.

In contrast, hearing aids with input compression vary the gain as the input changes, once the input is above the compression kneepoint. The graphs in Figure 10–42 show this. Notice how now the output change is not a straight line. This is because as the input increases, the amount of gain applied also varies, starting at inputs of either 20 or 50 dB SPL. When the input level goes above these input levels, there is no longer a one-to-one relationship between input and output, and the input/output function no longer progresses along at a 45-degree angle. That is, the hearing aid becomes nonlinear for a high input level. This is even clearer in the I/G graph on the right-hand side of Figure 10–42, where we can see gain going as input increases above the kneepoint. The input compression kneepoints vary considerably across manufacturers and among channels in the same hearing aid. AGCi kneepoints could be as low as 20 dB SPL or as high as 70 to 80 dB SPL depending on the manufacturer and the channel(s) involved. In contrast, output compression kneepoints are typically assigned through clinician adjustment of maximum output in the hearing aid fitting software during the fitting—the procedure we outlined in Chapter 5.

When input compression kneepoints are relatively low, this is referred to as wide dynamic range compression (WDRC). What this means is that a wide portion of the average speech signal is being compressed. There are no hard-and-fast rules regarding what kneepoint levels constitute WDRC, but typically we would consider any input compression kneepoint of 50 to 55 dB SPL or lower as falling into this category. Obviously, once a kneepoint reaches 65 to 70 dB SPL or so, there would no longer be a "wide" portion of the average speech signal in compression.

Compression Ratio

The compression ratio describes the amount of compression, or in simple terms, the squash effect. Compression ratio can be calculated by dividing the change in input by the change in output. For example, if an input signal change of 10 dB results in an output change of 10 dB, the ratio is 1:1, or linear. If the change in input of 10 dB results in an output change of 5 dB, the ratio would be 2:1. Input/output functions for various compression ratios are illustrated in Figure 10–43.

When thinking about the amount of compression that is appropriate, we must also think about overall gain. In some instruments, it is possible to adjust kneepoints, ratios, and overall gain to obtain the desired loudness perceptions for the patient. To accomplish this effectively, it is important to think of these perceptions for three areas: soft, average, and loud inputs. If a patient only has problems with loud inputs, your adjustment

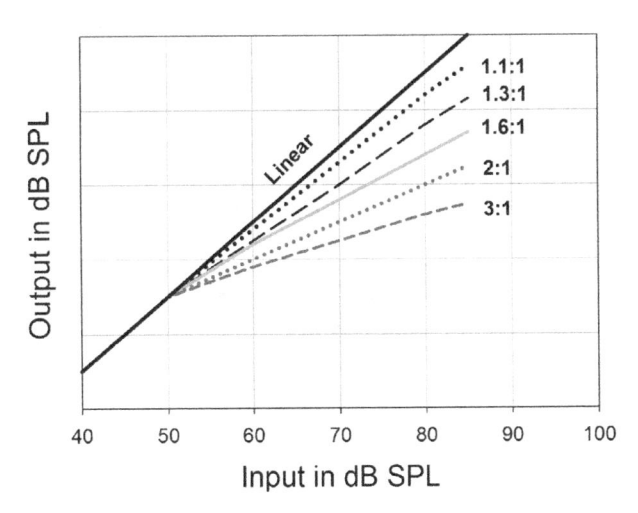

Figure 10–43. Input/output functions for various compression ratios. (Used with permission from Taylor and Mueller, 2017. © Plural Publishing, Inc.)

will be much different than if he or she has problems with soft, average, and loud inputs. In Chapter 17, we provide you with a "cheat sheet" for adjusting soft, average, and loud sounds based on the patient's complaints. However, most modern hearing aid software provides indirect compression control, using loudness tabs for different levels.

Attack and Release Times

As we briefly described earlier, the compression attack and release times tell us how long it takes the hearing aid to respond to changes in input. With many hearing aid fittings, a very low CK is used, so the hearing aid is nearly always in compression. Consequently, it is important that we do not mistakenly think that compression

---

POINTS TO PONDER: CONTROLLING GAIN AND COMPRESSION—BEHIND THE SCENES

You might think that controlling compression would be a matter of clicking on different kneepoints or ratios. Although this might be possible with some digging through the software, manufacturers often confuse things, as they handle compression adjustment differently in their software:

- You usually will have the option of clicking on a term that describes what you want to do, rather than specifically changing a kneepoint from 45 to 55 dB, or making a ratio 2.3:1 when it was formerly 2.7:1.
- You might see labels like "gain for soft", "gain for loud", "gain for average," and sometimes even "gain for very soft" and "gain for very loud." Adjusting these controls typically affects both gain and compression at the same time.
- Exactly how they control compression and gain parameters differs substantially across manufacturers, so you still (sort of) need to know what is happening behind the scenes.
  - Let's say you have a patient who needs more gain for loud inputs. In some software, you would increase gain for loud inputs by increasing gain for loud, in other software you would raise the WDRC kneepoint, in other software, you'd make the WDRC ratio smaller, and in yet other software you'd raise the MPO. Which one of these actions does your favorite manufacturer use? What happens if you use the wrong control?
- With all of these differences we always encourage you to play with these controls while looking at the hearing aid output so you have the best understanding of how the brand(s) of hearing aids you use control gain and compression.

time constants refer to how long it takes for the hearing aid to go in and out of compression. Instead, they refer to how long it takes to readjust gain in response to a specific change in input level.

As the names suggest, *attack time* is the time it takes to turn gain down in response to an increase in signal level, whereas *release time* is the time it takes to turn gain up in response to a decrease in signal level. Compression attack and release times are measured electroacoustically using a standardized format (ANSI S3.22), which involves stepping up then stepping down frequency-specific input signal levels from 55 dB SPL to 90 dB SPL and back looking, for the time it takes to reach stable output values (within +/−3 dB). Figure 10–44 demonstrates the effect of compression attack and release times on an input signal. The upper part of this figure shows the signal prior to entering the hearing aid, and the bottom part shows the signal being amplified by a compression hearing aid. Time A to Time B shows the signal amplified before compression. The intensity increase that occurs at Time B triggers the onset of compression. This takes a few milliseconds for the signal to become compressed. The distance between Time B and Time C is the attack time of the instrument. Modern hearing aids have attack times varying from

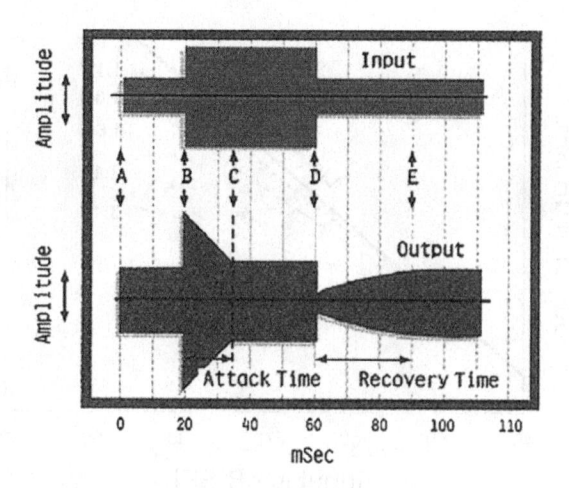

Figure 10–44. Schematic of the effect of compression attack and release time on an input signal that steps up and down in amplitude. (Used with permission from Taylor and Mueller, 2017. © Plural Publishing, Inc.)

less than one millisecond to a few seconds, although the majority of manufacturers apply relatively short attack times (approximately 1 to 20 ms), at least for sudden high intensity sounds, to help ensure that these brief bursts are not uncomfortable for the patient. We can

---

POINTS TO PONDER: ATTACK, RELEASE, AND A "WOOF"

To help you think a little bit about hearing aid attack and release times in the real world, here is a short case study (modified from Taylor and Mueller, 2017):

- A patient has hearing loss of around 50 dB HL, and has LDLs around 100 dB HL.
- The hearing aid has a compression kneepoint of 40 dB SPL, and you have programmed it to deliver 25 dB of gain for a 50 dB SPL input (soft sounds) and 10 dB of gain for an 80 dB SPL input (loud sounds).
- The patient is sitting listening to his wife talk softly at around 50 dB SPL, and his dog barks—an 80 dB SPL "woof." Would the hearing aid deliver 25 or 10 dB of gain for the woof? This depends on the attack time. If the attack time is fast, the hearing aid will quickly readjust compression, and only deliver 10 dB of gain.
- The patient's wife continues talking in her soft voice following the woof. Will her voice now receive 25 or 10 dB of gain? This depends on the compression release time. If the release time is long, five seconds or so, her voice would not receive the full amount of programmed gain until this time has passed and the patient may complain the hearing aid has dead spots. If the release time is very short (<100 ms), the full amount of gain would be restored very quickly.

see that the intensity of the input signal in Figure 10–44 decreases to its initial intensity level at Time D. The loud signal is no longer present, so the hearing aid needs to return gain back to the level appropriate for this lower input level. The time it takes to do this, the compression release time, is shown as the distance from Time D to Time E. Modern hearing aids vary tremendously with regard to release times. Ranging from as short as 20 to 30 milliseconds or less to as long as five seconds or more. If the release time is too short, the hearing aid may have slight distortions. Although rare in current hearing aids, these short release times can sometimes result in an audible pumping of ambient noise in a quiet room—the increased gain in gaps in speech makes ambient noise audible to the user. If the release time is too slow, the hearing aid gain may not be restored quickly enough, resulting in dead spots. If speech rapidly drops from 85 to 50 dB SPL, the patient will need considerably more gain for the 50 dB SPL input, and may need this quickly or he or she may miss things. In addition to carefully selecting compression time constants to minimize distortions, some companies have introduced a variety of techniques—including using different time constants for different types/levels of signals—as we describe later in this chapter.

Input Versus Output Compression

So why would it matter if we assign compression based on the level before or after amplification? The most important factor relates to how AGCi and AGCo interact with a volume control. Even in hearing aids without manual volume controls, input versus output compression is still an important theoretical consideration as we discuss soon.

Figure 10–45 schematically shows the difference between AGCi and AGCo I/O functions for three different volume control settings. For AGCo (left side of the figure), we can see that because compression behavior is based on the sound level after linear amplification, compression is activated above the same 85 dB SPL output across all three volume control settings. As a consequence, as the user increases the volume, gain increases for input levels below the MPO, but there are no changes to maximum output.

The effects of changes in the volume control with AGCi are considerably different (see Figure 10–45, right side). We can see that because compression behavior is based on the sound level at that the hearing aid input (before linear amplification), compression is activated above the same 40 dB SPL input across all three volume

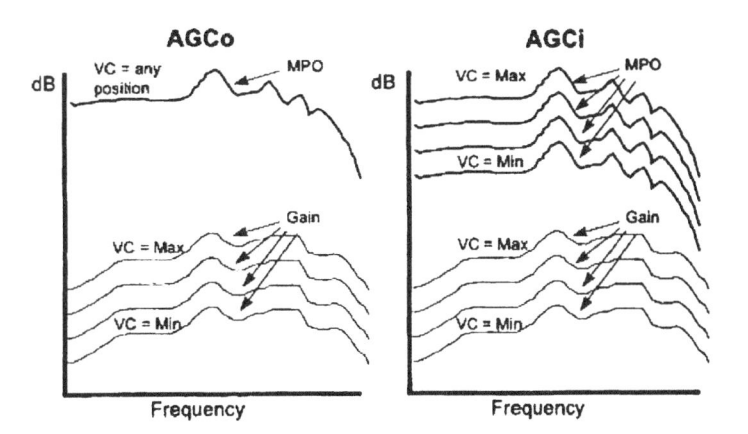

Figure 10–45. The I/O functions for AGCi and AGCo systems at three different volume control settings. (From *Compression for Clinicians* by Ted Venema. Copyright © 1998, Singular Publishing, Inc. All rights reserved. Used with permission, p. 64.)

control settings. Consequently, when the VC is changed using AGCi processing, both the gain and MPO are affected.

As we detail in Chapter 14, we often want to control the amount of gain assigned across soft, average, and loud sounds based on their level in the environment (input level). From a conceptual standpoint, it is straightforward to do this using AGCi with a low CK. That is, ACGi is used to ensure the desired loudness relationship for soft, average, and loud inputs. Conversely, we are also interested in ensuring that loud sounds are not too loud at the hearing aid wearers' ear, so conceptually AGCo with a high CK makes sense for limiting the MPO. Think of it as setting the ceiling for loud sounds—ensuring that those loud sounds fall below the patient's LDL. Consequently, it is quite common for hearing aids to implement both AGCi and AGCo. Depending on the aggressiveness of the AGCi, it's possible that in some cases, the sound leaving the amplifier will never reach the kneepoint of the AGCo. In these cases, the AGCo circuit becomes sort of an idle bystander for the entire amplification operation. If the AGCo kneepoints are set correctly, however, then this probably would not be an efficient fitting, as the patient's headroom would be unnecessarily restricted. Of course if a hearing aid does not have a user VC, both low threshold level control and high level limiting could be accomplished with either only AGCo or only AGCi through the use of two knee points and two different CRs. Since a VC is still at least an option for many models, however, it makes sense to continue to implement AGCo for limiting and AGCi for gain control across a wide range of input levels.

Compression Applications

Now that we have described some basics, let's introduce some terms and general compression applications. We describe the application of compression in much more detail when we cover prescriptive methods in Chapter 14, so our purpose here is only to provide a general framework. We'll start with explanations of a few terms:

- **Headroom:** For a given input signal and gain setting, the dB range available between the upper level of the amplified signal and the hearing aid's MPO. In general, we try to optimize headroom, so that the peaks of speech (and other signals) can fluctuate but yet stay below the patient's LDL.
- **Compression limiting (CL):** A fitting application which utilizes compression to limit the output; requires relatively high kneepoint and high ratio. Commonly AGCo but can be AGCi.
- **Low threshold compression (LTC):** Compression that utilizes frequency-specific kneepoints that are low enough so that a sizeable portion of the dynamic range of speech is in compression. Typically, CKs are 50 dB SPL or lower but could be as high as 70 dB SPL or slightly higher. Most commonly, LTC is referred to as wide dynamic range compression (WDRC); however, depending on the manufacturer and the generation of the dynamic range compression, full dynamic range compression, whole range syllabic compression and full range compression have been used in some cases to emphasize the level of the CKs or the range of time constants implemented.
- **Slow acting automatic volume control (SAAVC); sometimes just called automatic volume control (AVC):** A fitting application of LTC that utilizes a long release time. The term "long" can mean as short as 500 ms or as long as several seconds.
- **Syllabic compression:** A fitting application of LTC that utilizes a short release time in order to control the level of sounds the approximate length of a syllable, typically, 50 to 150 ms.
- **Phonemic compression:** A fitting application of LTC that utilizes a short release time in order to control the level of sounds the approximate length of a phoneme, typically, 5 to 40 ms.
- **Adaptive compression and dual compression:** Two similar fitting applications of LTC that combine long and short release times. The release time is related to the duration of the input signal and sometimes the level. For most inputs, a long release is in effect, but if a short duration signal occurs, particularly one that is high intensity (e.g., door slam), shorter release times will be activated and temporarily replace the long release. These are

two different patented technologies that differ in a few ways, including the fact that only two release times (one short and one long) are used with dual compression, whereas release times are varied adaptively over a range with adaptive compression.[1]

- **Sliding linear window:** A fitting application of LTC that utilizes a moving linear window, typically with a range between approximately 7 and 15 dB. When input levels fall inside this window, linear amplification is applied (gain remains constant). When inputs consistently fall outside the window, the amount of amplification changes rapidly to "slide" the window to a new range and gain is again held constant. This can be thought of as a combination of linear processing and very fast compression. The first processing of this type used commercially was Automatic Dynamic Range Optimization (ADRO™), first used in cochlear implants. This processing determines when to slide the window based on probabilities of the signal being inside the window (e.g., constant gain is applied as long as 90% of signal inputs fall in the target range). More recently, sliding linear window processing referred to as SpeechGuard™ was introduced, which changes gain based on signal level averaged over short windows in time rather than probabilities.
- **ChannelFree™ gain processing:** Gain is applied in conjunction with a wideband filter for frequency specific control of nonlinear amplification. The filter shape is based on frequency domain analysis of the input signal.
- **High-level compression (HLC):** Typically refers to the type of compression used to accomplish compression limiting. It has also been used to describe LTC with a higher than usual CK (above 70 dB SPL).

Clinically, WDRC typically implements AGCi with a relative low compression threshold (~55 dB SPL or below) and CRs below 4:1 (typically 3:1 or less). As previously mentioned, it is called this because a wide range of the input dynamic range of speech (see review in Chapter 4) falls above the CK. This characteristic of WDRC is shown in the curve labeled VLT (very low threshold) compression in Figure 10–42. The simple rule to remember is that as input goes up, gain goes down. Recall that most people with mild-moderate cochlear pathology have LDLs similar to people with normal hearing. In most WDRC applications, little or no gain will be applied for loud inputs, but significant gain can be applied to soft inputs, making them audible. As we detail in Chapter 14, the fitting result of WDRC compared to well-fit linear amplification is that soft sounds are more audible, meanwhile loud sounds are less likely to be too loud. All of this is accomplished while providing enough amplification for sounds with average loudness levels to remain near a patient's MCL—that is, average-level sounds typically receive the same amount of gain for a WDRC fitting as for linear.

To some, it is counterintuitive that "compression" makes soft speech *louder*. After all, shouldn't compression, compress? To explain, it isn't compression per se that makes soft sounds louder, it is the adjustments related to the compression activation. See if this makes sense:

- A patient is using linear amplification and has the gain of the hearing adjusted so that average speech falls at his MCL.
- We implement WDRC, with a kneepoint of 45 dB SPL and a ratio of 2:1. This will reduce the output for average speech by 10 dB.
- Because the output has been reduced by 10 dB, we increase the hearing aid gain during the fitting by 10 dB, to get the output back to his MCL.
- While this 10 dB increase in gain will result in the same output level for average speech, it will also have the effect of increasing the level of soft speech by 10 dB. So indirectly, yes, compression makes soft sounds louder.
- Once compression is activated, gain will continue to decrease with increasing input level. So by the time we reach loud speech inputs, compression we result in a lower level than we had for the linear fitting.

Compression limiting typically consists of AGCo with high compression ratios (typically 10:1 or higher)

---

[1]Adaptive compression was developed by David Hotvet who worked with Harry Teder at Telex.

and high compression kneepoints (typically 95–100 dB SPL output or greater when converted to 2-cc coupler values). These high levels correspond to the LDL of the average hearing impaired patient (mild to moderate loss). The high 10:1 CR means that there is only a 1 dB corresponding increase in output for a 10 dB change in input, once the signal is above the kneepoint. Although that might sound like a lot of compression, it occurs at a high kneepoint, and at that point you need to turn things down a lot with increasing input to stop things from getting too loud.

Most current hearing aids include output-limiting compression used as a partner with WDRC. WDRC takes care of the soft to loud speech sounds; output limiting takes care of the very loud sounds. As we discuss in detail in Chapter 17, it is important to know which is which when you start making "mouse clicks" during post fitting visits. Start changing the WDRC when the problem really is with the AGCo, and the patient who walked in with one problem, might just leave with two! WDRC does most of its work for soft and average level sounds, particularly conversational speech, by providing appropriate gain to maximize listener comfort with loudness and provide audibility for soft sounds. It's generally not the purpose of WDRC to control maximum output (although it will do this if you program it that way). For higher level inputs, the high compression kneepoints and aggressive ratios of output compression limiting are well-suited for protecting the user from uncomfortably loud sound.

Multiple Channels

As we mentioned earlier, today's products have multiple channels. Recall that, within a channel, it is not only possible to have independent control of gain but also compression (both kneepoint and ratios). Imagine a patient who has a downward sloping hearing loss (most do) going from 30 dB HL at 500 Hz to 70 dB HL at 4000 Hz. His LDLs range from 100 dB HL to 110 dB HL, and therefore his dynamic range varies from 70 dB (lows) to 40 dB (highs). Since part of our fitting goal is to "repackage the world" into the listener's dynamic range, we will need more aggressive compression in the high frequencies than in the lows. This clearly is the advantage of multiple channels. In a case like this, your prescriptive fitting approach will provide you with suggested compression ratios, and the manufacturer's fitting software will program the hearing aid accordingly; in a 20-channel instrument, you might have 20 different settings of compression. This is a huge gain control advantage over the single channels devices used as recent as the 1990s.

If you keep the kneepoint relatively low for all frequencies (to maintain the benefits of WDRC), you probably will end up with compression ratios of ~1.4 to 1.7 in the low-frequency channels, 1.8 to 2.4 for the mid-frequency channels, and 2.5 to 3.0 for the high-frequency channels. The goal, of course, is to maximize the audibility of soft sounds without making loud sounds too loud, and to accomplish this across the entire amplified spectrum of sound.

Multichannel for AGCo

Multichannel compression is not just for WDRC instruments. We've always known that multichannel processing would be helpful in limiting programming compression for some listeners, but for many years we were forced to work with single-channel AGCo, even in hearing aids that may have had 20 channels of AGCi. In recent years, multichannel AGCo has become available in most instruments. Just as we don't want the same gain for all frequencies, we also want to individualize the maximum output. Multichannel compression limiting allows us to set the kneepoints in different channels to correspond to the patient's LDL for that frequency range. For example, if you see that the MPO exceeds the patient's LDL at 2000 Hz by 5 dB, in the "old days" of single channel AGCo (only ten years ago), you would have to turn down the kneepoint by 5 dB for *all* outputs, just to tackle that 2000 Hz problem. Today, all you have to do is go to the corresponding MPO channel for 2000 Hz, turn down that kneepoint 5 dB, and all the other outputs more or less stay the same. Headroom is not unnecessarily reduced.

The key is to get the AGCo kneepoint set pretty close to correct during your pre-fitting programming. Don't expect the automated programming to do this for you; you'll have to make a few mouse clicks on your own for this one (see Chapter 5).

Effects of Compression on Speech

In Chapter 4, we discuss the speech signal in considerable detail, in part because audibility of speech is one of the most commonly cited reasons patients pursue amplification. In Chapter 14, we discuss how we assign compressor gains as a function of level in considerable detail. Exactly how compression interacts with the frequency-specific levels of the speech signal within each channel, however, can differ depending on whether we are considering the effects over the long term or the effects from moment to moment. In Chapter 14, we will discuss the fact that most prescriptive methods have attempted to amplify average speech input levels to a comfortable range. Consequently, it is the case that a well-fit compression hearing aid will provide similar gain for average speech input levels to a well-fit linear hearing aid. With WDRC instead of linear processing, however, it is also possible to make soft speech more audible meanwhile improving comfort for loud sounds (making sure loud is not too loud). What does this mean in terms of the impact of low-threshold compression on the output level of speech, if we assume similar fitting rationales for linear and compression hearing aids?

- Compression and linear hearing aids will have similar output levels for average speech intensity input levels (i.e., an input level of approximately 62–70 dB SPL, depending on the procedure).
- The output level in response to soft speech input intensities will be greater for compression versus linear hearing aids.
- The output level in response to loud speech input intensities will be less for compression versus linear hearing aids.

For example, consider the I/O functions of three well-fit hearing aids that differ as a function of the type of gain processing displayed in Figure 10–42. We can see that all input/output curves intersect at 63 dB SPL (average speech input intensity). Importantly, we applied different amounts of gain before compression in all three fittings to make sure we achieved this fitting goal. Remember here that compression turns the output signal level down above the CK, so we need to apply more linear gain in the WDRC hearing aid with a low kneepoint to make the amplified signal level for a 63 dB SPL input level to equal that achieved with linear processing. In this example, if we examine the 20 dB SPL input we can see the linear instrument provides about 23 dB of gain (output = 43 dB SPL). In contrast, the hearing aid with 2:1 compression provides about 30 dB of gain (output = 50 dB SPL). With the 4:1 CR, the amount of gain before compression reaches 34 dB (output = 54 dB SPL). This effect is exacerbated even more when we reduce the CK as we see in the dotted line on the VLT compression 4:1 curve. When we lower the CK to 20 dB SPL, the gain for a 20 dB input rises to more than 55 dB (output approximately 75 dB SPL). In other words, the maximum amount of amplification (gain) required for a well-fit hearing aid increases as we use increasingly more compression. From a design standpoint, if we want a hearing aid capable of very low CKs and higher CR, we will need an amplifier that can produce a lot of gain. Fortunately, however, this will not change the maximum output we need, so a larger receiver may not be required. The other trend that we can see in this figure is that, for a fixed CK and after adjusting gain so that there is the same gain for average speech levels, the output dynamic range shrinks with increasing CR. Consider 50 and 80 dB inputs in this figure. With the linear hearing aid the range of outputs for these inputs remains 30 dB. It is reduced to 15 dB for 2:1 compression, however, and only about 7.5 dB for the 4:1 CR. Of course this change is expected given the compression ratios. That is, 30 divided by 2 for 2:1 and 30 divided by 4 for 4:1.

Compression and Speech: Dynamic Properties

The dynamic (changes over time) interaction between speech and LTC depends on the length of the speech signal of interest and the compression time constants (attack and release times). In Chapter 4, we discussed how the amplitude changes in speech could be described in terms of modulation rate and depth. For example, we can think of phonemes as having a modulation rate of about 30 Hz (short phonemes have a duration of around 33 ms) and a modulation depth of about 30 dB (reflecting the difference between the lower and higher levels of phonemes produced with the same vocal effort—that is, the frequency-specific dynamic range). In addition, recall that speech produced with soft, average, and shouted vocal efforts have an average overall level of about 52, 62, and 82 dB SPL, respectively.

Rather than using real speech, let's use a narrow band of noise modulated on the order of phonemes as a stand-in for real speech (Figure 10–46, top panel). In this example, the three average amplitudes at the input

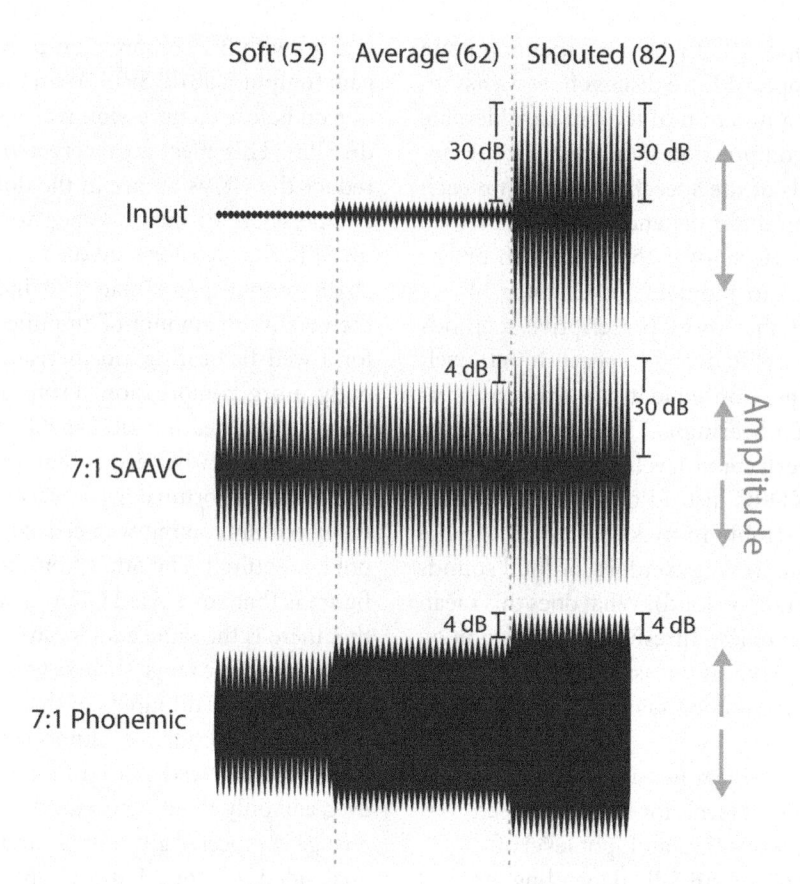

Figure 10–46. A demonstration of the effect time constants have on relative amplitudes over shorter and longer durations. *Note.* Because of scaling, the distance on the y-axis is proportionally larger as the amplitude approaches zero. Therefore, even though it does not look like it, there is a 10 dB amplitude difference between the soft and average input in the top panel.

were 52 (soft), 62 (average), and 82 dB SPL (shouted). At each of these three average amplitude levels the noise is modulated at 30 Hz, with a modulation depth of 30 dB, reflecting the maxima and minima of running speech. In the middle panel, we see the output after applying SAAVC compression (attack time = 5 ms, release time = 500 ms, CK = 50 dB SPL) to the input. In this case we applied a very high CR (7:1) in order to visualize changes in amplitude easily. After compressing the signal we applied gain, so we can see large increases in amplitude for the soft and average input levels compared to the original signal. Another change that is easy to see is that the difference between soft and shouted speech is now much smaller. That is, the SAAVC processing affected the relationship between the overall levels of speech that

was expected, given the CR applied. We can also see, however, that the modulation depth (speech minima to speech maxima) was unaffected (still 30 dB). Why? The release time was long enough that every time the signal level went down, the gain change was too slow to actually occur before the signal level was back up to the higher level. We like to think of this as a 110-year-old man running the gain change lever that is controlling the release time. He just can't move quickly enough, and by the time he starts moving, the input is already back up. SAAVC is effective at controlling the level for sounds over long durations but not for amplitude changes that occur very quickly.

In the bottom panel, we see the output after applying phonemic compression (attack time = 1 ms, release time = 20 ms, CK = 50 dB SPL) to the input, using the same CR and gain settings. Similar to the middle panel, we again can see that the intensity level difference between soft and shouted speech has been reduced by the compression by exactly the same amount. A large difference can be seen, however, when examining the distance from the speech minima to maxima (rapid amplitude fluctuations). Specifically, the 7:1 CR effect is now also evident in these segments in that the amplitude difference is now much smaller, 4.3 dB (30/7) instead of 30 dB. We can see the short-term amplitude changes for the soft speech segments are considerably larger than for the average and shouted speech. This reflects the fact that the CK = 50 dB. Given the minima are 15 dB below the average level of 52 (33 dB) not all of the speech fell above the CK.

One way other authors have discussed the interaction between the length of sound segments and the effect of time constants is the concept of effective compression ratio (ECR). We are going to describe ECR a little differently from the way it was defined initially by Neal Viemeister in 1979 and Michael Stone and Brian Moore in 1992, but the basic principles are the same. Conceptually the ECR refers to the fact that the effect the compression ratio has on the change in gain with changes in level depends on signal length and time constants. For example, the nominal CR in the example we just gave was 7:1. When considering the SAAVC processing in this example, the changes in level for the long-term signals were as expected and the effective CR was 7:1 (30 dB input dynamic range / 7:1 ECR = 4.3 output dynamic range). Conversely, when looking at the amplitude changes over the length of phonemes, there was no change in the relative level and the effective CR was essentially 1:1 or linear (30 dB input dynamic range / 1:1 ECR = 30 dB output dynamic range).

To further make this point, we have plotted the effective CRs for the same frequency channel after applying SAAVC, syllabic compression, and phonemic compression (Figure 10–47). All three compression processes have the same 4:1 nominal CR, the same 10 ms attack time, the same 50 dB SPL CK, and only differ with regard to release times. We can see from this figure that many longer release times will not lead to effective compression for the shortest phonemes, and gain processing for these shortest segments is essentially linear for all but the shortest release times. Specifically, the phonemic compression hearing aid that was evaluated maintained

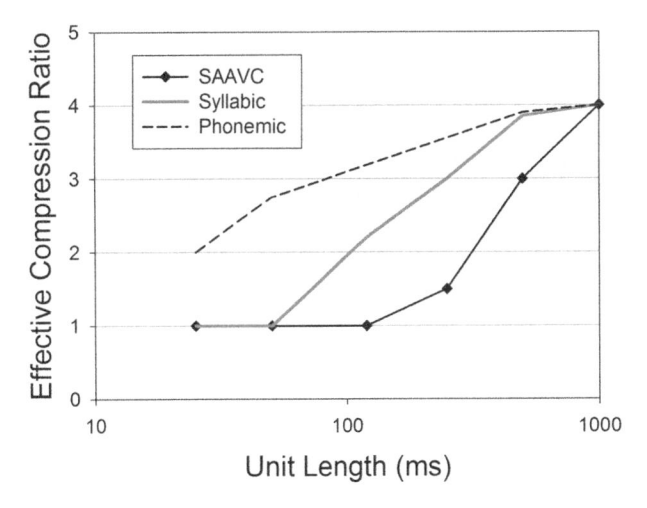

Figure 10–47. The compression ratio effectiveness for three different time constants as a function of signal length.

some compression (CR <2:1) for all segments of speech. In contrast, the SAAVC system had no compressive effect (ECR = 1:1) for all signals with a duration of less than 200 ms or so.

Dynamic Compression Properties and Audibility

Given our discussion of ECR, it seems obvious that faster time constants have the capability of compressing things more, and should result in increased audibility in a listener with a small residual dynamic range of hearing. In Figure 10–48 we have plotted an individual's thresholds in dB SPL against the entire (conservative) dynamic range for soft through shouted speech (see Chapter 4). As you can see, audibility is pretty limited. Even if we apply linear amplification, the listener would miss either much of the soft speech or the shouted speech would fall above saturation and be limited. At the maximum, a total of 62% of speech information would fit into this listener's residual dynamic range with linear amplification. How much could we improve audibility with compression? To simplify things we will only use two-channel compression because, for our purposes, the results would not change very much by going to a higher number of channels. To make things somewhat clinically realistic, we limited the maximum CR to 3:1 (we will explain more in Chapter 14). The amount of the

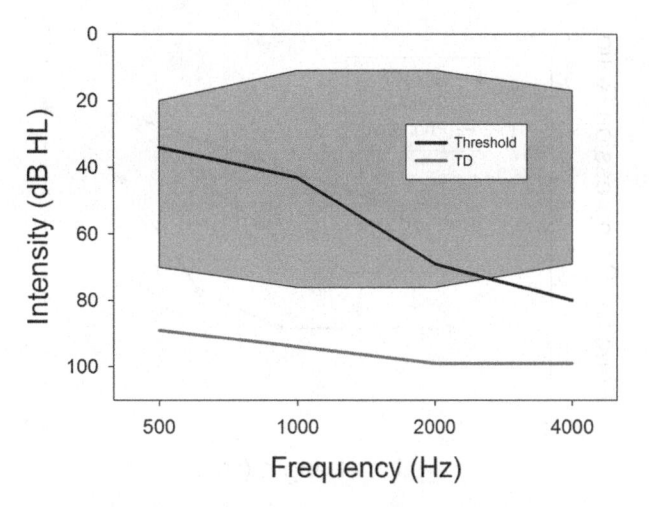

Figure 10–48. An example of an individual's thresholds in dB SPL plotted against a conservative estimate of the entire dynamic range for soft through shouted speech.

entire dynamic range of speech we can fit into the listener's residual dynamic range for SAAVC (release time 500 ms), syllabic compression (release time = 80 ms), and phonemic compression (release time = 10 ms) are shown in Figure 10–49. As we move from left to right and speed up the release time, we can see that audibility improves from 62% of total energy for the linear system to 82, 88, and 94% for the three compression release times.

So should we be fitting more phonemic compression to maximize audibility? There is some suggestion that the gains in audibility that result from fast-acting compression may be offset by the fact that these systems distort the amplitude relationship of speech segments and this may have a negative impact on speech intelligibility. In fact, some studies have shown that fast-acting compression actually reduces speech intelligibility (as compared to linear) for listeners with extremely reduced (less than 25 dB) dynamic ranges (i.e., those with severe/profound hearing losses). Of course this is the very population for which audibility will be most compromised. So what is the best way to apply compression? More importantly, does it matter? At this point the jury is still out. Importantly, most hearing aids do not have a provision for clinician adjustment of time constants and dynamic effects. In other words, the way the dynamic behavior of compression is chosen for our patients is by selecting specific products or, in some cases, manufacturers that have the gain processing we want.

Fortunately, the data to date suggest that, with regard to speech intelligibility in large groups of listeners, compression specifics seem not to have large effects for many listeners; however, as we will soon describe, they can have effects for some. In addition, we do know that the specific structure of compression processing can certainly affect sound quality and is expected to be an important player in a patient's preference for the sound of one hearing aid over another. The proprietary (default) fittings of nearly all manufacturers are to use minimal compression, much less than is called for by validated prescriptive methods. We suspect that this is so that the first-time listener has a good first impression of hearing aid processed speech, a fitting goal which may be counter to the audiologist's desire to make soft speech audible, or to fit soft, average and loud inputs to prescriptive targets.

Compression Benefits and Limitations: Differences Across Designs

When compared to linear amplification, one benefit present in all types of compression from SAAVC to phonemic is that compression will reduce the overall intensity differences between sounds of different levels. That is, the level of Little Suzy's voice will be increased to improve audibility, meanwhile the level of Uncle Steve's booming baritone will be reduced to a more comfortable level. So do time constants matter given that data have shown little if any average difference across compression types in quiet? A study by Stuart Gatehouse and colleagues in 2006 drummed up considerable interest when it showed faster time constants appeared to help some postlingually impaired listeners in noise. Specifically, those listeners with better gap detection performed better with faster time constants and many speculated that a listeners' cognitive skills may be useful in selecting compression parameters (Gatehouse, Naylor, & Elberling, 2006; Yund & Buckles, 1995). In addition, slower time constants (less compression) are sometimes preferred with regard to sound quality (Moore, 2012). In an excellent clinically applied study, Souza and Sirow (2014) examined speech recognition in performance on the Quick-SIN across different time constants ranging from very slow to very fast using three commercially available hearing aids. Their results demonstrated that older patients with more hearing loss demonstrated better performance with slow time constants (cogni-

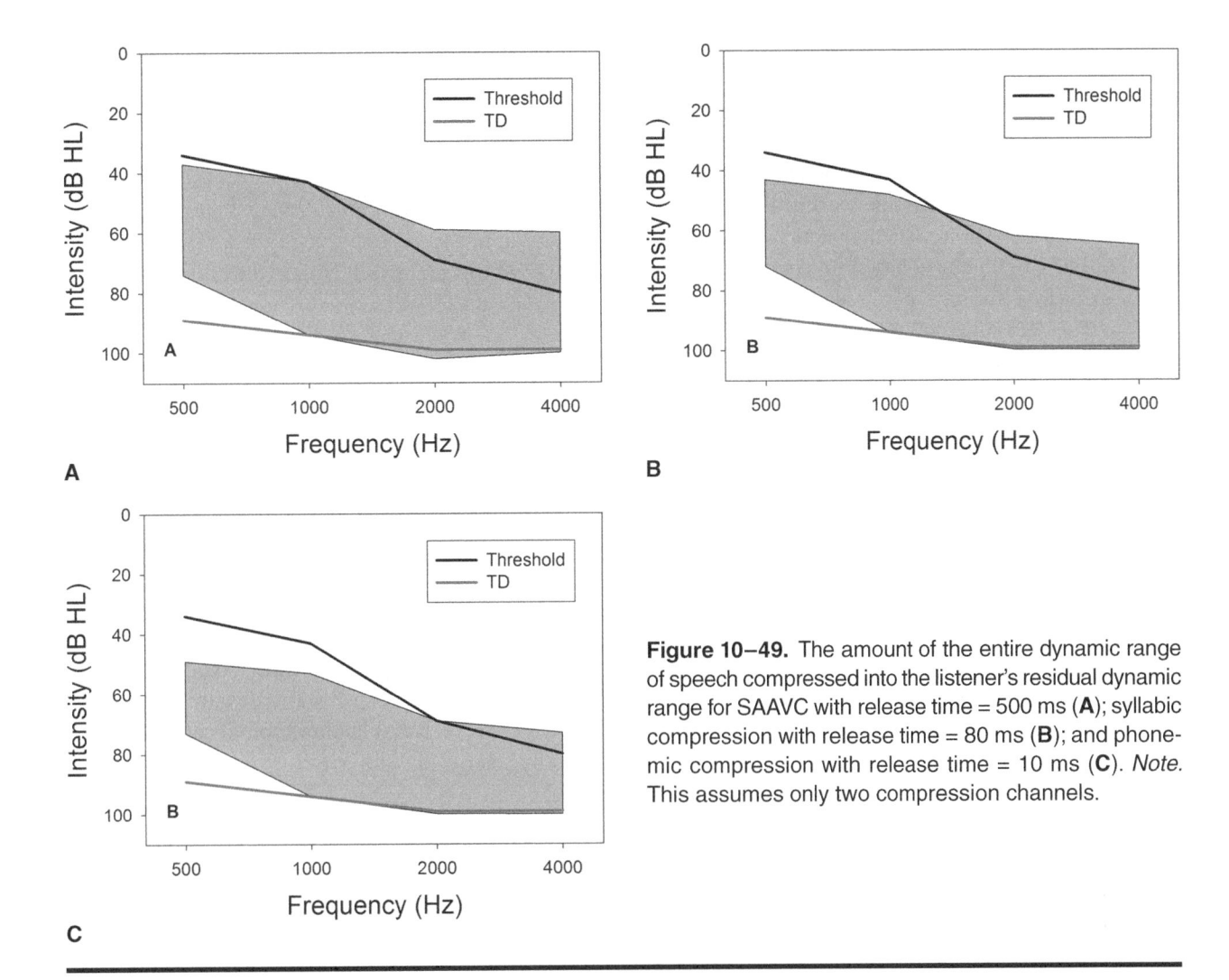

Figure 10–49. The amount of the entire dynamic range of speech compressed into the listener's residual dynamic range for SAAVC with release time = 500 ms (**A**); syllabic compression with release time = 80 ms (**B**); and phonemic compression with release time = 10 ms (**C**). *Note.* This assumes only two compression channels.

tive ability was not a significant predictor). Conversely, younger listeners with less hearing loss and higher working memory were more likely to perform best with faster time constants. In other words, our older patients with the most hearing loss may be better served with slower time constants. Emerging work also has suggested that children with more hearing loss may also perform better with either slower time constants or sliding linear window technologies.

We cannot just apply simple SAAVC in these individuals, however. Remember the "Attack, Release, and a 'Woof'" case study from earlier? Fast attack times used with long release times can temporarily cause the hearing aids to seem as if they have "gone dead" after high-intensity transient sounds. Fortunately, there are a few fixes for this problem. Some of the first methods were to use the adaptive release time or dual time constant methods mentioned above. Both of these methods essentially operate like SAAVC systems for most speech level inputs, meanwhile operating more like a compression limiter for short duration signals (particularly with higher intensities). There is considerable variability in exactly how these systems function with regard to time constants for low level and higher level inputs (some even use slow attack and release times for lower level inputs); all have loosely similar effects. Another group of techniques use a sliding linear window. We know of no studies that have compared sliding linear window technologies to dual time constant technologies, but limited work has shown these technologies can lead to improved speech recognition compared to syllabic compression in some listeners. As we have already mentioned, the bottom line is that differences across different types of compression processing in large groups of listeners are often small or nonexistent (Plyler, Reber, Kovach, Galloway, & Humphrey, 2013). There do, however, seem to be fairly large performance differences in some individuals. Considerable work still needs to be completed to determine whether compression selection can be individualized based on cognitive factors, age, hearing loss, and/or other predictive variables. The work to date does suggest this type of optimization may be worth the effort in at least some listeners.

Ending With Something Simple

We recognize that understanding compression can sometimes be difficult or, at the least, a bit confusing. We'll therefore end this section with a simplified analogy to help summarize the different ways compression is applied—making the point that compression really is as simple as driving a car (modified from Mueller & Hall, 1998b):

- You are driving down a city street going 35 miles per hour, no doubt listening to some good music.
- You see a stop sign one block away. Think of that stop sign as your patient's LDL (i.e., UCL, TD), and the speed of your car as the gain of the hearing aid. The LDL (stop sign) = 100 dB.
- The stop sign is for a very busy highway; cars traveling 65 mph. You need to stop at the sign to avoid an accident. So, you're going to use your brakes.
- Think of the point that you hit your brakes as the compression kneepoint (one city block = 60 dB), and the pressure that you apply on the brakes as the compression ratio.

Choice #1: You continue driving 35 miles an hour until you are only 100 feet from the stop sign. At this point you slam on the brakes as hard as you can. There is a squealing of tires, your car slides sideways, you bump your head on the windshield, you chip your tooth on the steering wheel, but you do not slide out into traffic. This happened to a teenager in Ryder, ND, about 50 years ago.

Type of circuitry? This is linear processing with output limiting using peak clipping. (It's nasty, but it does get you stopped at the stop sign without serious injury.)

Choice #2: You continue driving 35 miles an hour until you are only 100 feet from the stop sign. At this point you slam on the brakes as hard as you can. This time you do not slide sideways, your ABS works fantastically, no bumped head, no chipped tooth. You stop cleanly at the stop sign.

Type of circuitry? This is linear processing with output limiting using AGCo, kneepoint = 110 dB SPL, ratio = 10:1 (equivalent to slamming on the brakes). (It's an unusual way to drive, but sometimes it's necessary to go that fast until the very end. Other times, it simply happens due to a lack of attention or driving instruction.)

Choice #3: Starting a block away, you put your foot on the brake at a constant pressure. The pressure is such that it allows you to come to a rolling stop at the stop sign.

Type of circuitry? This is WDRC, linear compression, kneepoint = 40 dB SPL, ratio = 2:1. (It works pretty well but remember that the pressure on the brake is directly related to the point when you first start braking and the location of the stop sign. Had you stepped on the brake midway through the block—e.g., a kneepoint more like 60 dB SPL or so—you would have had to apply more pressure—e.g., a ratio around 3:1.)

Choice #4: Starting a block away, you put your foot on the brake. This time, however, you start with a very light pressure, and then, the closer you get to the stop sign, the more pressure you apply. Again, you come to a rolling stop at the stop sign.

Type of circuitry? This is WDRC, curvilinear compression, kneepoint = 40 dB SPL, ratio = variable from 1.5:1 (soft inputs) to 6:1 (loud inputs), effective ratio = 2:1. The same could be accomplished using two kneepoints between 40 and 80 dB SPL inputs. (This is an alternative method to linear compression for stopping at the same place—utility depends on the driver or dispenser, the vehicle or hearing aid, and road conditions or patient's loudness growth function.)

Expansion

Another feature that is usually combined with WDRC compression is audio expansion. Expansion reduces the level of signals below the kneepoint and is used to minimize annoyance from amplified microphone and processing noise and low-level environmental sounds. Expansion often allows the patient to use the gain necessary to make soft speech audible without the negative side effects of excessive amplification of ambient noise.

You can think of expansion as compression in reverse: When sound is *below* the kneepoint, it is squashed. It has no effect whenever the signal is above the kneepoint. If you want to make soft sounds softer, you raise the kneepoint (more sounds in expansion). It will squash any sound below the kneepoint including speech (so don't put the kneepoint too high). The kneepoint usually is placed around the SPL level of soft speech, which also tends to be around the WDRC kneepoint for most fittings.

It is probably easiest to understand expansion if you think of an input/gain function, rather than an input/output function (Figure 10–50). Notice, that as the input increases below the expansion kneepoint, gain is expanding. One of the main patient benefits is to reduce microphone noise; in fact, some manufacturers label the feature "microphone noise reduction," some manufacturers call it "soft squelch," and others call it "low level noise reduction." Many manufacturers call it nothing, as it usually does not show up in the software, and you

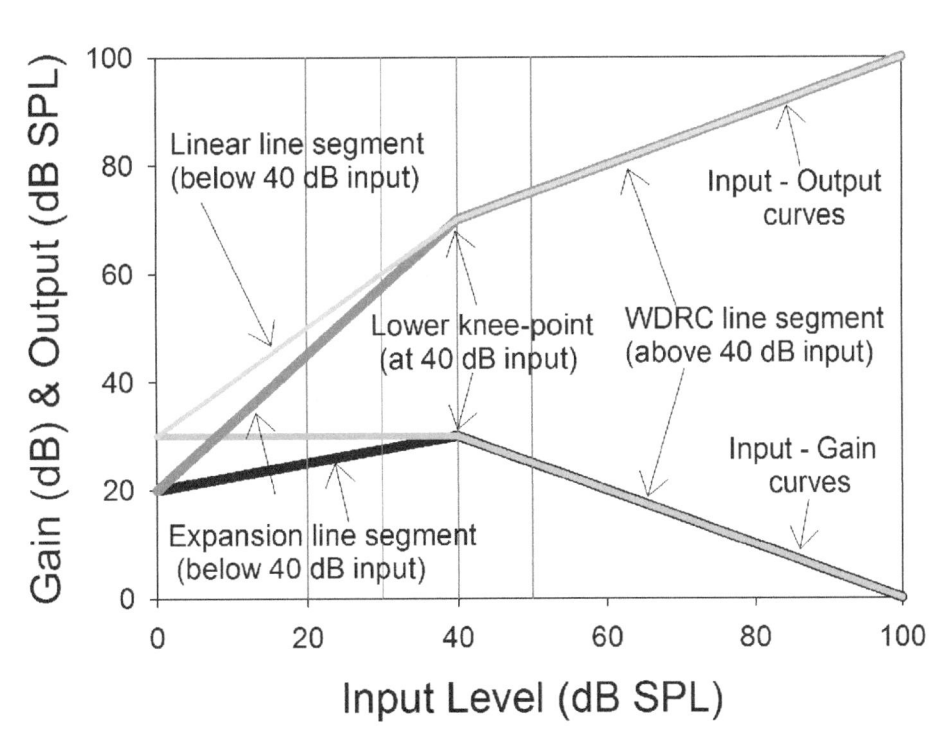

Figure 10–50. Input/output and input/gain curves for compression and expansion. The top two curves are input/output curves, and the bottom set are input/gain curves. Note the compression kneepoint (CK) is 40 dB. The lower line on the chart illustrates the effects of expansion for inputs below the 40 dB SPL kneepoint. (Used with permission from Taylor and Mueller, 2017. © Plural Publishing, Inc.)

cannot turn it off. It is controllable in some manufacturers' software, however, typically by a gain control handle labeled "gain for very soft" or through an on-off toggle of "microphone noise reduction."

Summary

In this chapter we discuss some of the basic principles of electronics and digitization, as well as the physical components used to take signals in the environment, apply desired changes to these signals, and then deliver these modified signals to the hearing aid wearer. The journey that a signal takes through a digital hearing aid is briefly summarized in Figure 10–51. By understanding DSP basics and how the individual physical components work, we hope to have provided the reader with a better understanding of the potential benefits and limitations. With this foundation we can move forward to describe a number of advanced hearing aid features. We discuss how we derive desired compressor gains in some detail when we discuss prescriptive methods in Chapter 14.

Microphone
- Acoustic pressure changes from sound in the environment are picked up by the microphone and transduced into an alternating voltage that mimics the original pressure changes. This tiny electrical signal is then typically provided a very small amount of amplification using a preamplifier.

A/D
- The current changes are then sent to an A/D convertor which represents the current level measured at discrete time intervals using strings of binary numbers referred to as digital words given a defined sampling rate. The digital signal consists of tiny transient pulses of voltage. For example a "1" may be represented by a higher (but still tiny) voltage and a "0" may be represented by no voltage.

DSP
- Changes to the digital representation of the signal are made to reflect filtering, amplification, compression and other processing using DSP via the processor and different types of memory which act to hold the digital signal at various stages as well as hold the instruction and timing information.

D/A or D/D
- The digital signal is then either converted to an analog electrical signal using D/A conversion or digitally converted to a very high rate digital signal which represents the electrical amplitude of interest within very small adjacent blocks of time with amplitude represented by the digital pulse density. The D/A conversion leads to a low voltage analog signal, while D/D leads to a low voltage digital signal.

Amplifier
- After either D/A or D/D conversion, the low voltage analog or digital signal is sent to the output transistors (amplifier) which use the low voltage to control the flow of the much higher voltage from the battery. This provides a higher voltage amplified output.

Receiver
- This much higher voltage is then routed to the receiver coil. The receiver then acts to transduce the electrical signal into an analog change in sound pressure for delivery to the patient's ear.

Figure 10–51. Summary of a signal's simplified path through a digital hearing aid.

11
Signal Classification and Sound Cleaning Technologies

Hearing aids have been designed to be amplifiers since their inception. More specifically, the most fundamental goal of hearing aids is to amplify sounds at each frequency to improve audibility for each individual's hearing loss configuration, however, listening comfort must also be maintained. As we describe in Chapter 10, modern hearing aids are complex and sophisticated devices and their basic application as a frequency-specific amplifier has been accomplished very successfully in the past 20+ years. Bandwidth has been improved and distortion reduced. The use of compression amplification, applied using the current fitting prescriptions we describe in Chapter 14, results in audibility for the majority of speech signals without allowing loud sounds to become too loud.

But there has to be more to a hearing aid than just making sounds louder, right? Modern hearing aids include a number of different, but integrated, processing features with goals ranging from enhancing speech to reducing feedback to eliminating specific types of distortions to logging environmental acoustics and beyond. Even "basic" hearing aids of today are expected to include multi-channel compression, at least a basic version of digital noise reduction, and directional microphone technology. These features are even available in a few of the more advanced Personal Sound Amplification Products (PSAPs), which like the most basic hearing aids, are available for around $500 or less.

One of the most often cited difficulties expressed by hearing aid wearers relates to listening in noise. We have, therefore, dedicated the majority of this chapter to hearing aid processing aimed at reducing unwanted noise. We differentiate "reducing unwanted noise" from "improving SNR" because many types of noise reduction will generally not improve speech recognition in noise, but instead provide other benefits including improved listening comfort, reduced annoyance of noise, preferred sound quality, improved listening effort, and so forth.

Before discussing sound processing aimed at reducing unwanted noise, however, we will first describe sound analysis and classification schemes. For many features in modern hearing aids, it is not desirable to have them operate the same way at all times. For example, we do not want a directional microphone to be active in quiet environments. Consequently, nearly all modern hearing aids use an input classification scheme that, in turn, is used by one or many decision rules controlling feature activation and/or adjustment with the goal of environment specific optimization. Regardless of how effective they are in isolation, the benefit provided by noise reduction technologies in the real world will always be limited by the accuracy of sound classification and how optimally decision rules are implemented. We will therefore begin by describing how signal classification schemes work and how they differ across manufacturers.

Input Analysis and Classification

Modern digital hearing aids typically include several processes aimed at analyzing incoming signals so that various automatic functions can occur. These analyses range from simple (e.g., intensity level in a channel) to

---

TECHNICAL TIP: ACOUSTIC FEATURES USED TO CLASSIFY SOUND INPUTS

As we mentioned, several factors can be used to classify an acoustic environment. The list below includes many of them:

- Overall level
- Band-specific level
- Spectral peaks
- Spectral location of base envelope modulation rates.
- Channel specific amplitude modulation depth and amplitude modulation rate of the base envelope or short term changes in signal energy (useful for speech identification—speech typically falls in the 3–6 Hz range).
- Co-modulation, that is, amplitude modulations that occur with the same timing in different channels/frequency ranges.
- Short term spectral changes over time and frequency relationships between the spectral peaks (e.g., spectral flux and Mel-Frequency-Cepstral Coefficients [MFCCs]). These are essentially nonlinear spectral representations of the spectrum. Yes, it is complicated but also very useful for sound and speech identification.
- Spectral and temporal signature of both lower and higher level portions of the input, that is, separate estimates of the higher level signal of interest (talker) and the lower level background (noise).
- Relative amplitude of the portion of the input signal estimated to be speech versus that estimated to be noise (typically based on level and modulation information). This is used as an estimate of signal-noise ratio (SNR).
- Identification of tonal signals in the high frequencies (e.g., feedback detection).
- Unilateral and Bilateral input signal comparison: Examples include (1) comparing the signal measured at each of the two microphones in the same hearing aid as is done when identifying wind noise, (2) comparing the signal measured at both hearing aids in a bilateral pair including tonal stimuli (differentiate external tonal stimuli from feedback), (3) comparing the same signal after applying different types of microphone processing (e.g., omnidirectional, directional, reverse directional to help identify the direction of the loudest talker and contribute to decisions regarding directionally sensitive noise reduction), (4) comparing the input from the two hearing aids to help define unique polar patterns for CROS and BiCROS processing, and (5) comparing the input from the two hearing aids to help determine when speech is originating from the hearing aid user and not external talkers.

quite complex (spectral modulation rate and depth). Typically, information from various analyses are combined into a complex processing stage aimed at classifying the input signal type. This stage is commonly referred to as a classifier or signal classification scheme. These analyses are then used to affect signal processing in an ongoing fashion. For example, simple level information might be used for the purpose of setting the gain in each compression channel. In parallel, classifier information may be used to determine when to activate omnidirectional, directional, or bilateral beamformer microphone settings as well as the magnitude of gain reduction of the digital noise reduction processing.

Classifiers now offer the opportunity to obtain direct measures of input characteristics based on acoustic information. The usefulness of that capability in the establishment of management strategies for the hearing aid user seems obvious. That is, once classification is completed, it would seem relatively straightforward to simply amplify and possibly enhance sounds of interest (speech) and ignore or attenuate sounds that are not of interest (noise). Unfortunately, identifying and separating various sound sources that comprise the total sound input at the ear turns out to be a fairly difficult task. In his seminal text on the topic, Albert Bregman (1990) detailed the difficulty in identifying and separating the mishmash of acoustic information that impinges on the ear into "auditory streams," using a process he referred to as *auditory scene analysis*. Bregman points out that it is really rather remarkable that humans are able to pick out one talker or other sound of interest from a mix of several talkers, background noise, and other sounds.

Also amazing is the human ability to recognize specific speech sounds even when they are spoken by different talkers who are likely to produce them at different pitches and levels. Bergman described a large number of acoustic cues that contribute to the perception of auditory streams but also pointed out these cues are sometimes in competition with each other when identifying an auditory stream.

No matter how advanced computer algorithms that attempt to mimic human's amazing auditory scene analysis ability become, there is a human factor that precludes perfect accuracy when completing *computational auditory scene analysis*. One reason for this is that the specific stream of interest within an auditory scene depends on the listener's interest or listening intent. That is, perfect operation would require the algorithm to also read a listener's mind! Believe it or not, investigators are working on ways to do just that. Perhaps future hearing aids will be able to "steer" or adjust based on listener attention as measured via an electroencephalpgram (EEG) or on the direction the eyes are pointed. While progress is being made, it will likely be some time before such methods are in commercial products and appropriately optimized. Consequently, listener intent in environments that are acoustically identical continues to present a significant challenge in the automation of hearing aid algorithm operation. Acoustic scene analysis has advanced significantly, however, in modern hearing aids.

There is considerable variability in the signal classification schemes used across manufacturers, but in general these algorithms take the simplified approach of attempting to classify the entire sound input within and

---

KEY CONCEPT: SOME ACOUSTIC FACTORS THOUGHT TO BE USED IN HUMAN STREAM SEGREGATION

- **Frequency Factors:** Frequency regions of complex sounds tend to have a harmonic relationships and/or have a specific formant ratio relationship.
- **Timbre Factors:** A complex sound has a particular and identifiable sound quality (e.g., it is easy to differentiate a clarinet from an oboe even though the spectral content of their sounds are quite similar).
- **Change Factors:** All frequency regions of a complex sound tend to undergo changes in frequency and level as a group.
- **Timing Factors:** All portions of a complex sound tend to start and stop at the same time.
- **Spatial Factors:** A complex sound tends to originate from a single location.

across specified frequency ranges (e.g., speech, noise, speech in noise, music), rather than attempting the much more difficult task of identification and separation of auditory streams within the same environment. One advancement toward this more advanced goal, however, is the ability of some modern classification schemes to use information from both hearing aids at the same time to identify the general direction of the talker with the highest input level at the hearing aid microphones. That is, is the person with the highest level in front, to one side, or behind the listener? Modern classification schemes may also be used to identify the acoustic "signature" associated with very specific signals or signal characteristics of interest such as feedback, wind turbulence realized as wind noise, reverberation, identification of the talker's own voice, high-intensity transients/impulse sounds, and so forth. In most of these cases, these specific signals are problematic and/or annoying for the hearing aid wearer, so the goal of identification is application of processing to cancel or reduce the negative impact.

The primary goal of most classification schemes is to estimate the types of signals in the input and acoustically describe these signals in terms of SNR, level, frequency, and other acoustic factors. For example, is the signal speech, speech in noise, quiet, music, only noise, or some other signal? Is speech present in the signal? If noise is present, what type of noise is it: nonamplitude modulated (steady state), very rapidly modulated, brief burst (transient) such as that which is generated by clanking dishes, an echo, some other noise type? If speech and noise are both present, what is the SNR? What is the frequency-specific level of the input? What is the acoustic relationship of the input across frequency channels, and in some cases, what is the signal's spectral signature? To complete these signal classification estimates, manufacturers use a combination of many possible acoustically based analyses.

Since it can be quite difficult to identify the individual (or even the predominate) signals from many different sounds all occurring at the same time (which may then be further modified by reverberation and other environmental effects), sound classification is typically accomplished using a probability-based system. That is, based on the acoustic analyses, the classifier algorithm calculates the probability that the input signal is each of several predetermined types. Since a probability system is used, it is important to realize that sound classification is not absolute. For example, the classifier output might identify a signal as speech in noise. This final classification might result from the following probabilities: (1) 55% probability that the signal is speech in noise, (2) 30% probability that the signal is music, and (3) 15% probability that the signal is noise without speech.

Examples of two manufacturers' classification categories are shown in Figure 11–1. Note that hearing aid A only considers speech and noise signals, whereas hearing aid B also includes music. Although there are clearly more and less complicated systems, the level of complexity does not necessarily translate to advantages for patients or clinicians. Manufacturers differ not only in the exact classification scheme they use—including the number and type of environments which they attempt to identify—but also in how they use this information to affect operation of features (commonly referred to as decision rules). Decision rules are manufacturer-specific algorithms that activate or change the operation of various features based on input analyses and the output of the sound classifier. We propose that, in order for sound classification and the subsequent changes to signal processing to be beneficial to an individual listener, at least four things must go right:

- The sound input is accurately classified.
- The appropriate sound processing algorithms are activated via an accurate set of decision rules.
- The processing algorithms produce a more positive outcome by enhancing wanted signals and/or reducing or eliminating unwanted signals. This is something that may be much more difficult than it sounds because the signal of interest and unwanted signal may be acoustically similar and only differ in terms of the listener's interest.
- The processing algorithm does not produce artifact, interact negatively with other algorithms, and does not negatively impact other parts of the input (e.g., enhance unwanted signals, suppress wanted signals) to a degree which offsets any potential benefits achieved. Current data suggest that the tradeoffs between potential positive and negative effects likely vary as a function of an individual listener's listening needs and hearing abilities.

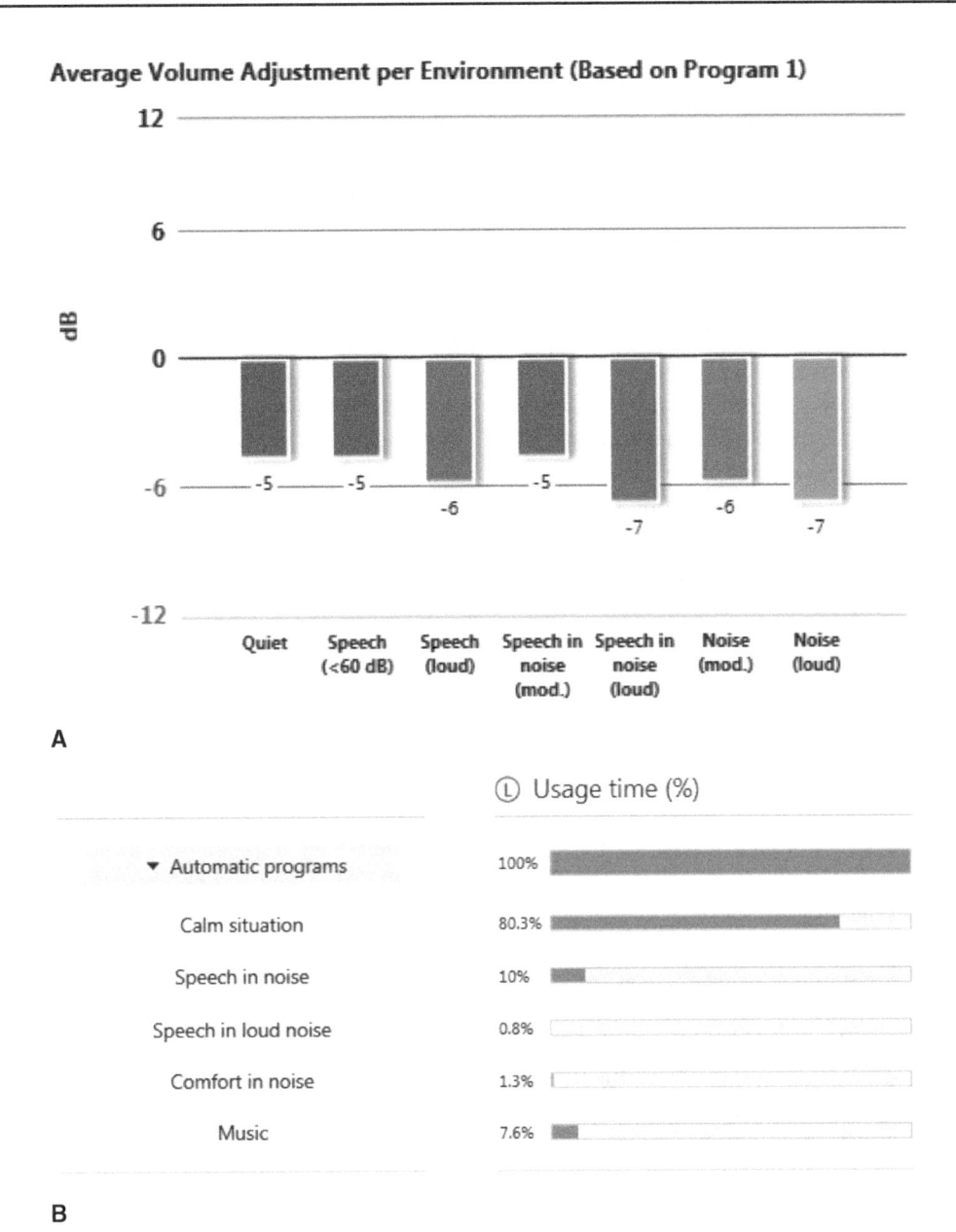

Figure 11–1. Examples of two manufacturers' environmental classification categories. Panel A also shows the average user gain adjustment for each estimated environment, while Panel B also shows the use time for each estimated environment.

Clearly, it is not enough to have a good, or even perfect, classifier. Instead, much of the burden for providing additional benefit is related to the operation of hearing aid features and the decision rules used for their control. That said, it is equally true that even the most beneficial signal modification features can be rendered useless, or even result in decrements, if the signal isn't appropriately classified to begin with. For example, let us assume the hearing aid input is a speech signal of interest in a background of noise. If this input is mistakenly classified as only noise, features may be mistakenly evoked that suppress the entire input, potentially rendering the desirable speech less audible. The validity and reliability of classification systems across manufacturers has been shown as quite variable (e.g., Büchler, 2002; Taylor & Hayes, 2015). We have seen cases in which the same speech presented at a poor signal-to-noise ratio in the presence of a very complex background noise was classified as (1) noise, (2) speech in noise, or (3) music, depending on the specific hearing aid model. Fortunately, however, modern classifiers perform quite well in relatively simple environments, such as those containing only speech in quiet, speech in low level noise, or noise alone, which is amplitude modulated at rates either higher or lower than is typical of speech (e.g., less than 0.5 Hz or greater than 15 Hz).

Finding differences in accuracy across signal classification schemes in more difficult environments is not that surprising given the large number of acoustic cues that could be used to classify an incoming stream and the probability-based algorithms used for sound classification as described above. For example, consider music. How classical music or a single singer are classified as music instead of noise based on acoustic differences is reasonably straightforward, but what about rock music or percussion? Given the importance of speech audibility to communication, classifying signals that have speech in them appropriately so that the speech level is not inadvertently reduced in level is clearly quite important. We listed many of the analyses used to identify speech/voice in a previous technical tip, with modulation rate, co-modulation, and temporal fine structure being among the most common methods used. Detecting voice activity is an analysis that has really improved in modern hearing aids, and many advanced hearing aids can identify the presence or absence of speech quite well, as long as the SNR is not too adverse.

TECHNICAL TIP: SIGNAL CLASSIFICATION AT ITS BEST!

Because we focused on how difficult signal classification can be—and what can go wrong—we may have given you the impression it doesn't work very well. Although environmental identification is rarely 100% accurate, many products are accurate in all but the most complex listening environments. Furthermore, modern classifiers have implemented an incredible range of techniques to counter some of the limitations of earlier generations. From identification of the direction of voice to differentiating feedback from tonal music, current classifiers really can figure out some very complex acoustic environments. Some examples of a classifier getting it right in the day of a patient are offered here:

- Wind was appropriately identified and wind noise reduction was activated, decreasing annoyance during the patient's early morning walk and allowing the patient to hear traffic better and feel safer.
- A talker in the back seat was properly identified and directional steering was activated, allowing the patient better communication with her child on her way to daycare.
- The noise from the air conditioner in the office was properly identified and digital noise reduction was applied, decreasing annoyance and total sound level throughout the day, meanwhile still allowing for communication with co-workers with less listening effort.
- Speech and noise were accurately identified and adaptive directional processing was maximally activated, allowing the patient to understand the floor manager's update while walking through the factory floor.
- The symphony orchestra was accurately identified as music. Gain processing was made more linear to preserve dynamics and tonal sounds were not cancelled by feedback suppression processing, allowing the patient with an open fitting to enjoy an evening concert while still having the benefit of no feedback and appropriate gain control for speech throughout the day.

Digital Noise Reduction (DNR)

Since we now know a little bit about signal classification, let's go on to discuss hearing aid features that have the goal of reducing noise levels. Understanding how these features work, including potential benefits and limitations, is important for appropriate expectations counseling and adjustments based on individual listeners' needs and abilities. For example, if a patient expects a technology to "move that background noise off into the distance" based on a hearing aid advertisement, we need to make sure the patient doesn't also expect improved speech recognition if this technology is not capable of such a feat. In some cases, we may even disable specific features because interactions with the patient or the environments they are in may result in negative consequences that outweigh the intended positive ones.

> **THINGS TO (MAYBE) REMEMBER:**
> **A LITTLE "NOISE REDUCTION" HISTORY**
>
> On September 7, 1983, it was announced that President Ronald Reagan was wearing a hearing aid in his right ear. A barrage of public press coverage concerning hearing aids ensued, ranging from TV coverage and interviews to full-page articles in *Time* and *Newsweek*. A few years later, on February 16, 1988, Reagan again made audiologic news when the story broke in *The Washington Post* that the President had just been fitted with a pair of new hearing aids—this story was picked up by the AP and published nationally, with a subsequent photo on the front cover of *Parade Magazine*. The statement in the 1988 news article that caught the eye of many current and potential hearing aid users was this: "The device, which fits within the ear canal and is virtually invisible, contains an electronic circuit to help filter out the crowd noises that often prevent individuals with hearing loss from discerning conversations in a crowded room."
>
> The special hearing aid mentioned that "filtered out crowd noises" was the Siemens ASP (ASP stands for automatic signal processing). The article went on to say that these were innovations not available from other commercial hearing aid manufacturers. Although you might think that this endorsement was a terrific boon for Siemens business, in the long term just the opposite was true. The company received an overwhelming number of orders for the new ASP hearing aid (a custom product), mostly from audiologists who previously were not Siemens customers, creating an unmanageable backlog, which of course disrupted service for long-time loyal Siemens customers. For the record, this special noise reduction circuit was simply input compression that was only activated for the lower frequencies. This compression strategy later became known as bass increase for low levels or BILL processing (although more accurately described as bass decrease for high levels but with the less desirable and more difficult to pronounce acronym of BDHL).
>
> Speaking of BILL processing, around the same time as the emergence of the Siemens ASP, we had the Argosy Manhattan circuit (which later became Manhattan II), a BILL processor that also was considered noise reduction by many. It became a very popular product among audiologists in the early 1990s until research showed that, although BILL processing could improve listening annoyance in noise, there was no effect on speech recognition. In case you're curious, the name for this circuit came from a "Name-The-Circuit" contest at a 1980s ASHA national convention at which a 3′ × 3′ blow-up of the circuit was displayed. The winning entry related to the fact that the circuit diagram looked like an aerial view of downtown Manhattan.

One general class of hearing aid features, which really includes several technologies, is often referred to as *digital noise* reduction or *processing-based noise reduction*. In the past, there were a number of analog signal processing schemes applied to hearing aids in an attempt to improve speech recognition in noise. Several of the earliest attempts were based on the notion that reducing the level of high-intensity, low-frequency sounds would reduce the negative effect of upward spread of masking, resulting in increased speech recognition in noise (Lybarger, 1947). This processing was shown, however, to be ineffective, whether achieved through low-frequency tone controls (e.g., Fabry and Van Tasell, 1990) or through compression (e.g., Tyler and Kuk, 1989). Likewise little benefit was found for other more complex analog techniques such as the Zeta Noise Blocker™ (Bentler et al., 1993a; 1993b). As we detail later in this chapter, current processing based DNR techniques also generally do not directly improve speech recognition in noise because they do not improve the SNR at any instant in time. Instead, they generally reduce noise during instances in time and in frequency ranges for which speech is not the dominant signal. All current DNR technologies share the general goal of reducing the level of sound identified as noise and/or unwanted signal distortions through frequency-specific gain reduction, cancelation, or filtering, while not changing gain in the frequency regions where speech is the dominant signal. DNR algorithms are differentiated both by the type of noise they are designed to counteract and, specifically, how they operate. Importantly, the noise identified will be based on the classifier determination, so one way to describe different DNR algorithms is based on classification of the target noise.

Gain-Reduction Digital Noise Reduction (G-DNR)

The most common and oldest method of DNR used in hearing aids reduces steady-state noise; more specifically, it reduces the gain when the signal in a channel is dominated by noise. There may also be speech or music present, but the level either is so low or the acoustic signature is so similar to noise that it won't be identified by the signal classification system. We will refer to this general method as gain-reduction DNR (G-DNR), although it has also been referred to as steady-state noise reduction, modulation-based noise reduction, or simply noise reduction. We discuss speech modulation rate and depth in detail in Chapter 4, and it is easy to visualize the difference between these envelope modulations and those of a more steady-state noise (Figure 11–2). Whereas most of the original hearing aid based G-DNR algorithms were confined to noise classification based on envelope modulation rate and depth, current versions may also include overall level, center frequency, spectral tilt, and other acoustic parameters during sound

---

TECHNICAL TIP: COMMON NOISE CLASSIFICATIONS

- Steady-state (non-fluctuating) noise in isolation within a processing channel: The level does not fluctuate by more than 5 dB over a defined time period; no signals identified as speech or music within the same channel as the noise over the same time period.
- Noise occurring in the time gaps between speech segments: Typically, the noise must have a different spectral signature than speech and must not include components that are harmonically related. Also, it is more easily identifiable if it is steady state.
- An impulse or brief, typically higher-level, transient: For example, clinking dishes, sharp tapping sounds.
- Sounds which exhibit the spectrotemporal characteristics of reverberation.
- Noise associated with wind turbulence: Typically identified by the spectral signature; enhanced identification through establishment of a lack of signal correlation at the two microphones in the same hearing aid.

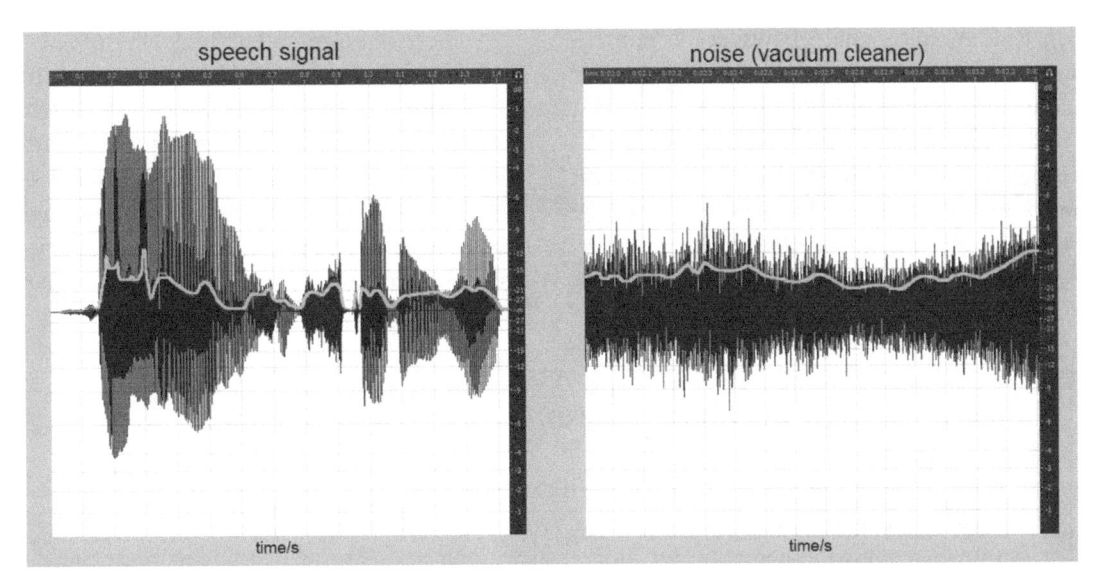

Figure 11–2. Example of the amplitude envelope modulation rate and depth for speech and noise signals.

classification. In addition, some systems use additional information from input analyses aimed at speech and music identification, with the goal of ensuring gain is not inadvertently reduced in channels dominated by signals of interest. For example, unlike typical noise, the spectral peaks of speech and many types of music are often harmonically related. The classifier algorithm uses this information to determine the likelihood that the signal of interest is dominated by unwanted noise.

A decision rule is then applied to invoke a reduction in channel specific gain. This decision rule not only defines when DNR is activated, it also may adjust the magnitude of the gain reduction depending on acoustic properties of the noise (e.g., overall level, classifier probability, estimated SNR). Generally, the decision rule used to activate DNR is based on a criterion total sound level (e.g., input to the hearing aid must exceed 70 dB SPL) and a criterion SNR (e.g., estimated SNR must be poorer than 0 dB). Once activated, gain is typically decreased more as sound level increases and as SNR decreases, reaching a maximum level at a high sound input when the sound input is judged to contain only steady-state noise (Figure 11-3). The timing of G-DNR is based on multiple time constants. Three time periods combine to form what we refer to as the total DNR attack time:

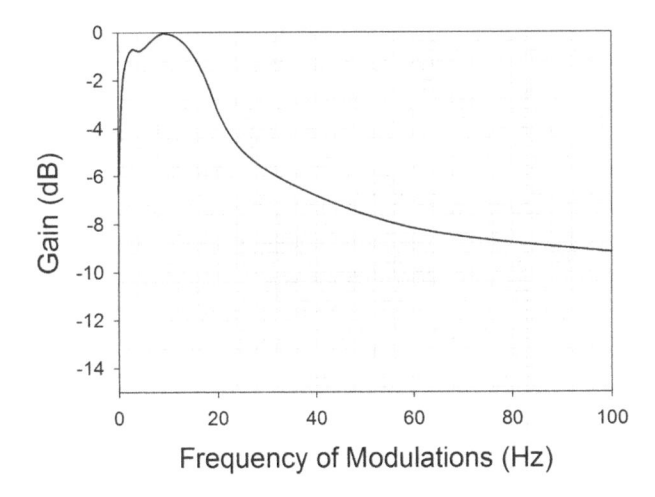

Figure 11–3. An example of increased gain reduction as a function of decreased amplitude modulation frequency.

1. The time it takes to identify that noise is the dominant signal in a channel
2. The time allotted after noise is detected before gain reduction begins (i.e., manufacturer determined wait time)
3. The time period from the beginning of gain reduction to the instant of maximum gain reduction

When a dominant signal of interest is reintroduced, two time periods combine to form what we refer to as the total DNR release time:

1. The time it takes to identify that a signal of interest is the dominant signal in a channel
2. The time period from the beginning of gain recovery to full gain recovery (0-dB gain reduction)

There is no manufacturer-determined wait time introduced during the DNR release time, since it is of interest for it to be as short as possible to avoid loss of audibility for signals of interest. Since the introduction of G-DNR, several studies have repeatedly shown the specific decision rule, the concomitant magnitude of gain reduction, and the DNR attack time vary considerably across manufacturers and products, in part because

> **KEY CONCEPT: CLINICAL QUANTIFICATION OF G-DNR**
>
> We recommend clinical quantification of the operation of G-DNR to obtain a sense of how it interacts with different inputs. The resulting information can be useful when adjusting operation for individual patients and counseling patients regarding the effects.
>
> - If you consider a single manufacturer, DNR typically operates similarly across styles and models, and it does not interact with ear geometry. When there are differences across models this is usually well publicized. Therefore, you really only need to quantify operation in one or two devices, and you really do not need the patient there. You can complete this in the test box as we describe in Chapter 13.
> - Since steady-state noise is quantified as noise by virtually all DNR systems we are aware of, simply playing a white or pink noise and comparing the output for the various DNR settings including "off" (disabled) will provide a quick picture of how much gain reduction can occur in a frequency-specific manner. The magnitude of gain reduction depending on signal level, signal type, frequency, manufacturer, and setting can range from as little as 2 to 3 dB to as much as 20 to 25 dB in current instruments (Figure 11–4). Furthermore, for most products a minimum total sound level must be exceeded before the G-DNR reduces gain. Consequently, we recommend testing at a few different levels (e.g., 55, 65, and 75 dB SPL). In addition, some test systems will allow for presentation of speech in steady-state noise at different SNRs. This can be used to assess if audibility might be affected at some SNRs.
> - Since classification is never 100% accurate, it is also sometimes useful to look at hearing aid output for music and other sounds that are important to your patients. It is important clinically to know if the DNR inadvertently decreases audibility for these important sounds (see Figure 11–4).
> - In addition to paying attention to how much the signals are turned down, it is also useful to obtain a sense of the time course of the DNR gain change. How long does it take to turn things down? Does it happen in stages or continuously over time? If speech is introduced, does the gain get turned back up rapidly?
> - Finally, given the popularity of open fittings, keep in mind that many of the DNR effects that you see in the coupler in the low frequencies will not be present in the real ear when the ear canal is left all or partially open (as is discussed further in Chapter 17).

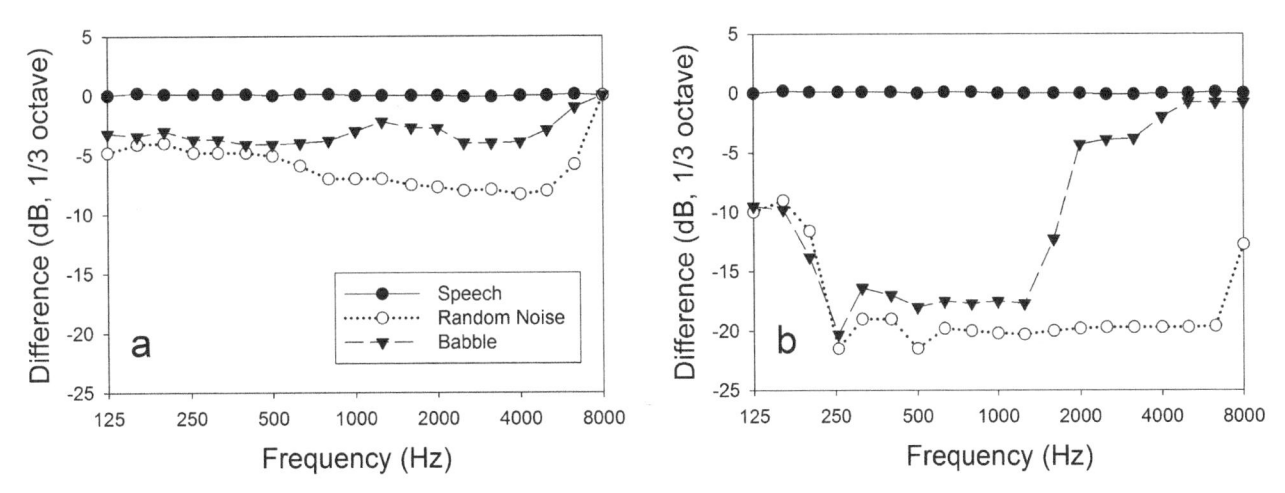

Figure 11–4. The frequency specific gain reduction provided by two different commercial products for three different signals presented at 70 dB SPL.

there is no clear evidence supporting an optimal setting. Indeed, recent work has shown that the speed and maximum magnitude of gain changes for current DNR systems continue to vary dramatically across manufacturers (Scollie et al., 2016). Specifically, maximum gain reductions can be as little as 6 dB to up to more than 20 dB. Furthermore, the DNR attack time varies from a few seconds to more than 20 seconds. Some manufacturers also implement gain reduction in multiple stages. For example a small amount of gain reduction may be applied very quickly, and then more gain reduction applied after an additional period of time.

The magnitude of gain reduction can be modified in many products by the audiologist. In some products, the clinician controls are as simple as weak, moderate, and strong. Other products use as many as five to seven levels of strength. Others offer separate adjustments for simple and complex environments, and provide control for the maximum amount of gain reduction (e.g., −3, −6, or −12 dB). Other manufacturers make adjustments to the G-DNR operation based on patient-specific input such as lifestyle or activity level rather than providing direct control of DNR strength.

Given all of the potential differences in how G-DNR is applied, it is useful to quantify the behavior of G-DNR across all possible settings in order to more effectively counsel and make adjustments for individual patients. Fortunately, it is relatively simple to assess the behavior of G-DNR systems of this type using a hearing aid test system or probe microphone system as we discuss in more detail in Chapters 13 and 17 respectively.

Traditional DNR (T-DNR)

In addition to G-DNR, many modern hearing aids also include an algorithm that reduces noise through one of a number of different traditional DNR techniques. We refer to these methods as "traditional" because, despite being introduced in hearing aids after G-DNR techniques, they were some of the first noise reduction methods introduced in signal processing outside of the hearing aid industry. In addition, the goal of G-DNR is to simply reduce gain when speech is not the dominant signal, whereas the goal of T-DNR techniques is to remove noise from the combined speech and noise signal. Unlike G-DNR, T-DNR techniques reduce noise between segments of speech, even in gaps that are very short (e.g., between words). Clinically, when T-DNR is available, it is nearly always used along with G-DNR. Sometimes both are activated through the same clinician controls. In other cases, a toggle button allows the clinician to turn T-DNR on and off independently from G-DNR. In still other cases the DNR control may only affect operation of the G-DNR, and the T-DNR may always be active.

Wiener Filtering

The majority of T-DNR techniques used in hearing aids are based on calculation and application of a filter (typically a Wiener filter; pronounced "Weener"), spectral subtraction, or techniques that combine the properties of these two methods. The Wiener filter, named after Missouri-born mathematician Norbert Wiener, considered the originator of cybernetics, was developed in the early 1940s and first publicized in 1949. The original application was removal of steady-state noise from the speech signal in telecommunication devices.

To implement the Wiener filter, the power spectra of the original image and the additive noise must be estimated. The input to the Wiener filter is assumed to be the signal $s(t)$, corrupted by the additive noise $n(t)$. The output $x(t)$ is calculated by means of the filter $g(t)$, using the following convolution:

$$x(t) = g(t)*(s(t) + n(t))$$

In Chapter 10 we describe how some hearing aids convert the input from a time representation (time domain processing) to a spectral representation (frequency domain processing). Wiener filtering techniques have been applied both in the time domain and in the frequency domain. Application in the time domain was of great interest originally in digital hearing aids because of the decreased time required compared to conversion into the spectral domain and back. These concepts are already complicated, and adding more math is not going to make this better for many readers. If we ignore the math and consider the theoretical basis, however, gain is reduced with decreasing SNR and the result is a filter shape that results in an output waveform as similar as possible to the signal of interest at the input. In other words, noise is reduced as much as possible across the frequency spectrum without removing speech information. If you have a perfect representation of the speech, application of this type of filter as described mathematically earlier can be extremely effective. Of course, this type of filter does not work perfectly in hearing aids in the real world because the speech signal has to be continually estimated from the total incoming sound (that is, the exact representation of the speech of interest is not known a priori), and the subsequent filter must be adaptively adjusted in an attempt to filter out as much noise as possible.

In one adaptive Wiener filtering scheme used in hearing aids, the input is continually analyzed within relatively short blocks of time (e.g., three seconds). These analyses are used to estimate the speech and noise signals under the assumption that speech and noise are relatively stable within short blocks of time. Alterna-

---

KEY CONCEPT: WHO WAS NORBERT WIENER?

Wiener filtering, which was named after Norbert Wiener (Figure 11–5). Wiener was a child prodigy who graduated from high school at the age of 11 and obtained his first degree in mathematics from Tufts University at the age of 14. Despite his personal shortcomings (vision problems, poor social skills), he went on to teach philosophy at Harvard (his Jewish roots denied him a permanent position) and mathematics at MIT until his death at age 69. He is well known for his groundbreaking work in cybernetics, robotics, and computer science, which he readily shared with other scientists around the world. These included Soviet researchers, a connection that placed him under suspicion during the Cold War. He was adamant in his refusal to accept government funding or work on military projects. One biographer, Freudenthal (1992), describes him as follows:

> In appearance and behavior, Norbert Wiener was a baroque figure, short, rotund, and myopic, combining these and many qualities in extreme degree. His conversation was a curious mixture of pomposity and wantonness. He was a poor listener. His self-praise was playful, convincing and never offensive. He spoke many languages but was not easy to understand in any of them. He was a famously bad lecturer.

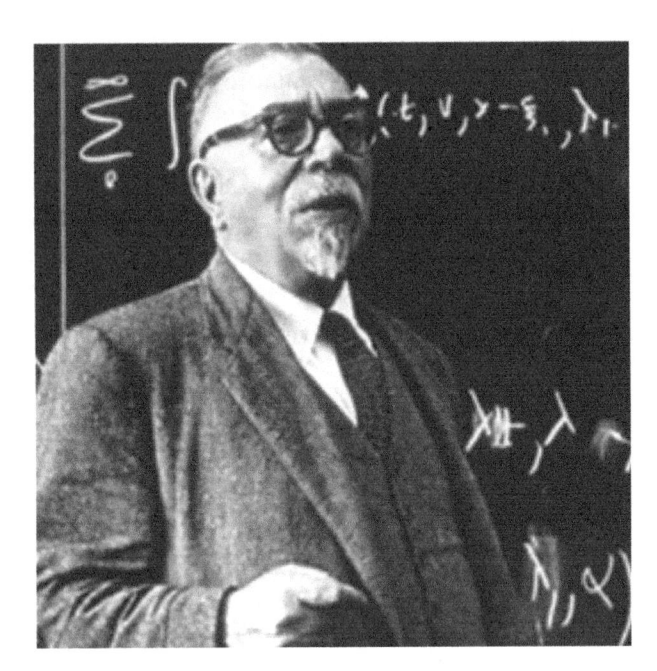

Figure 11–5. Norbert Wiener circa 1962.

tively, analyses are constantly ongoing and spectral estimates are updated if significant changes are measured over blocks of time, looking backward over a fixed window of time from the sample for which the estimated change was discovered. In the time domain, estimation of the speech can be accomplished by comparing the long-term SNR estimated from the average amplitude modulation depth in each channel/frequency range to the short-term SNR based on the ongoing (near instantaneous) amplitude modulation depth. This modulation-based method for estimating SNR is quite similar to the techniques used to estimate SNR for G-DNR. Given this approach it is not surprising that estimates are pretty good for steady-state noise and a single talker, but increasingly poor when the speech and background noise are more temporally similar (e.g., fluctuating background noise, multiple talkers). Given this potential for error, most manufacturers use their own decision rule, which limits the amount of filtering instead of applying the most aggressive Wiener filter.

Spectral Subtraction

Although not as old as Wiener filtering, spectral subtraction techniques have been around for quite some time as well. They were first introduced as a noise reduction method in digital signal processing in 1979. Spectral subtraction was introduced as a frequency domain based process that subtracted the magnitude of the estimated noise spectra from the magnitude of the total spectra. If we assume noise $d(n)$ adds to the speech signal $x(n)$, the speech in noise $y(n)$ can be represented by the formula: $y(n) = x(n) + d(n)$, for time indexes falling between 0 and the number of samples minus 1. The objective is to solve for the cleanest speech signal from $y(n)$, assuming the speech and noise spectra are uncorrelated. Once the speech spectra is estimated it is used to estimate the noise spectra from the total spectra. Then the estimated noise spectra is subtracted from the total spectra. Unlike traditional Wiener filtering, the analysis window for spectral subtraction is quite short, typically 3 to 8 ms. Of course similar to Wiener filtering, a key to making this work is accurate estimation of the speech spectrum. One technique to improve this estimation is to use a voice detector to determine when speech is present. Once speech is identified, the noise spectrum is estimated during segments for which no speech is present. Although this method can be used to then estimate the speech spectrum accurately, the phase will be distorted by the noise. Perceptually, this is often heard as "musical noise" and can significantly decrease sound quality.

Whereas the details of spectral subtraction require some math and are beyond the scope of this chapter, we think it is enough to understand that the outcome of the process is to reduce the noise that is present within short time blocks for which speech energy is not present (or at least at a very low level) on a frequency by frequency basis. As is the case with Wiener filtering, the general spectral subtraction techniques also work best with steady-state noise. In this case this is because, if the noise is changing over time, the spectral representation that is based on segments during which no speech is present may be completely wrong.

Modern T-DNR techniques have been modified and enhanced using a wide range of techniques, often based in perceptual psychoacoustics, to reduce noise as much as possible without introducing undesirable artifacts, such as generation of musical noise. In addition, combination techniques including subtraction of a noise spectrum that is estimated based on the Wiener filter have been applied. Consequently, it is often not very useful clinically when a manufacturer advocates for its chosen T-DNR technique over another unless the details of the various implementations are known. More important are the potential benefits and limitations from the techniques applied, which we describe in more detail in a later section.

As we have described, a perfect spectral subtraction could be achieved if there is a perfect spectral representations of the speech signal of interest and the competing noise. In fact, if spectral subtraction is aggressively applied when the speech and noise spectrum are known a priori speech recognition can actually be improved (although sometimes at the cost of a significant decrease in sound quality). Since we have to rely on spectral estimates in the real world, however, it is generally desirable to err on the side of caution. That is, if the noise spectrum estimate actually contains some speech energy, spectral subtraction can negatively affect audibility of the speech of interest. This fact, combined with the potential for reduced sound quality, has generally led hearing aid manufacturers to limit the aggressiveness of spectral subtraction techniques.

Spatially-Based DNR

As we describe in Chapter 10, it is now possible for hearing aids utilizing microphone arrays to identify the general direction of the loudest talker of interest. With directional technology (unilateral beamformer comprised of two omnidirectional microphones) the loudest speech signal can be categorized as falling in the front or back hemifield. With bilateral wireless communication between the hearing aids, the possibility of identifying the loudest talker on the left or right side is also added. Both unilateral and bilateral MDVR beamformers (see Chapter 10) can also be designed to generate two or more "acoustic snapshots" based on the direction of sound arrival (e.g., omnidirectional, front pointing directional, rear pointing directional). Speech identification analysis is completed on each of these snapshots. When there is not a strong speech representation in the rear facing snapshot, it can be used to derive the noise estimate, providing a more accurate estimate than traditional classifier estimates based on the total hearing aid input (e.g., Jensen and Pedersen, 2015). Furthermore, since the noise estimate is spatially based, manufacturers can use more aggressive noise reduction techniques without fear of reducing the speech information arriving from the front. Some manufacturers also use this method to gain a better representation of speech arriving from the front in an attempt to preserve or even enhance the speech signal while reducing the noise as much as possible. Techniques include those which estimate the noise and speech spectra and apply spatially based spectral subtraction and those that rapidly estimate the noise and speech in multiple channels and apply subtraction in the time domain. Both techniques operate very quickly. Therefore, this processing is able to reduce noise levels at frequencies where speech is not the dominate signal and also selectively attenuate noise between speech segments in time (e.g., between words).

Evidence-Based Benefits

There have been many studies of G-DNR technology, often in combination with T-DNR. For this section, we will refer to this combination simply as digital noise reduction (DNR). Generally (as expected) these DNR studies did not demonstrate improved speech recognition in noise for adult listeners with impaired hearing (e.g., Boymans & Dreschler, 2000; Ricketts & Hornsby, 2005; Sarampalis, Kalluri, Edwards, & Hafter, 2009;). Similarly, no significant effects (either positive or negative) have been demonstrated for children's speech recognition in noise (e.g., Stelmachowicz, et al., 2010; Pittman, 2011). The fact that G-DNR does not enhance speech recognition is expected because the instantaneous signal to noise ratio at any frequency is never affected. With G-DNR, gain for all signals (potentially both speech and noise) within each channel is either decreased or not in unison. Unfortunately, changing the level of noise in channels where speech is not present has been shown repeatedly to have little or no effect on speech recognition using G-DNR techniques, except in fairly contrived cases of extremely high-level narrow band noise. In contrast, a few studies have shown a speech recognition in noise advantage for some T-DNR techniques, but these benefits have generally been limited to listeners with normal hearing.

Why are these benefits generally not demonstrated in listeners with hearing impairment? It is hypothesized that benefits in listeners with normal hearing relate to reduction of temporal masking and masking at adjacent frequencies. This type of masking has the largest effects, however, when the masking noise has a higher level than speech (i.e., negative SNR). Unfortunately, most listeners with hearing loss are unable to understand speech until the SNR reaches fairly positive values (e.g., Wilson, McArdle, & Smith, 2007). Consequently, the SNRs at which T-DNR can provide significant speech recognition benefits are generally not accessible for many listeners with hearing loss.

There are several studies that have examined benefits for DNR processing (G-DNR + T-DNR) that are unrelated to speech recognition. For example, laboratory studies have demonstrated that patients exhibit a preference for DNR when listening to speech presented in noise, including higher subjective comfort ratings in comparison to conditions for which DNR is not activated (e.g., Bentler, Wu, Kettel, & Hurtig, 2008; Boymans & Dreschler, 2000; Ricketts & Hornsby, 2005;). Indeed, data collected across a range of noisy conditions revealed that, as the SNR delivered to the patient decreased, preference for DNR increased (Figure 11–6). In the highest noise condition, patients indicated a preference for DNR in 85% of the presentations. Although there has not yet been a systematic evaluation, it has been speculated previously that improved comfort is likely related to both G-DNR and T-DNR processing. In contrast, improved sound quality, particularly in cases for which the noise and speech are spectrally matched, likely results from T-DNR processing and is not affected by G-DNR.

The sound quality and comfort benefits for DNR technology measured in the laboratory have also been demonstrated in real world listening. Specifically, in a double-blinded study patients' subjective ratings on the Averseness subscale of the APHAB improved significantly when DNR was activated (Bentler et al., 2008). Not surprisingly, the DNR benefits for sound quality and comfort stem in part from making noise in the environment more acceptable. This was directly quantified by Mueller, Weber, & Hornsby (2006), and confirmed more recently using a second manufacturer's product (Lowery & Plyler, 2013). Activation of DNR resulted in improved acceptable noise levels (ANLs) of approximately 4 dB. In addition, those listeners with the lowest noise tolerance unaided (poorest ANL scores) demonstrated the largest improvements.

More recently, research has suggested there may be DNR benefits related to a reduction in use of cognitive resources. As we describe in Chapter 15, one of the definitions for listening effort that we like is "the cognitive resources necessary to understand speech". The researchers that have adopted this working definition have concluded that in some cases DNR can reduce listening effort. For example, Desjardins and Doherty (2014) used a dual task paradigm to evaluate the effect of activating DNR processing (a form of spectral subtraction) in 12 adults who were experienced hearing aid users. Both low- and high-probability R-SPIN sentences were presented to participants in a female, two-talker babble. The SNR was individualized to achieve percent correct scores corresponding to "moderate" (76%) and "difficult" (50%) listening conditions. The secondary task was visual motor tracking of a circle-shaped target that rotated along an elliptical track. Consistent with past research, the DNR algorithm used did not improve or degrade speech recognition scores, but performance on the secondary task improved significantly for the difficult listening conditions (Figure 11–7). The assumption is that fewer cognitive resources were required for the primary speech recognition task, allowing for better performance on the secondary task. This decrease in cognitive load is expected to have a range of potential benefits associated with use of DNR ranging from more time on task, to longer hearing aid use per day, to possibly lower fatigue.

Evidence that some types of DNR processing reduce cognitive load is also provided by the research of Ng and colleagues (Ng, Rudner, Lunner, Pedersen, & Rönnenberg, 2013; Ng, Rudner, Lunner, & Rönnenberg, 2015). Specifically, these authors demonstrated

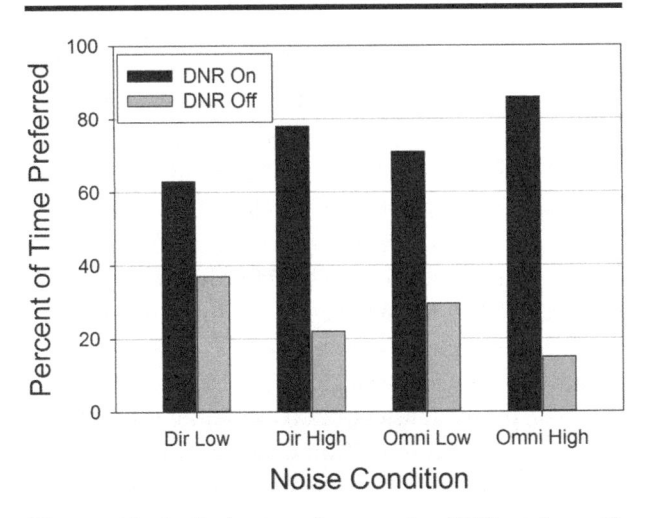

Figure 11–6. Patient preference for DNR at two different SNRs with and without directional microphone. (Adapted from Ricketts and Hornsby, 2005.)

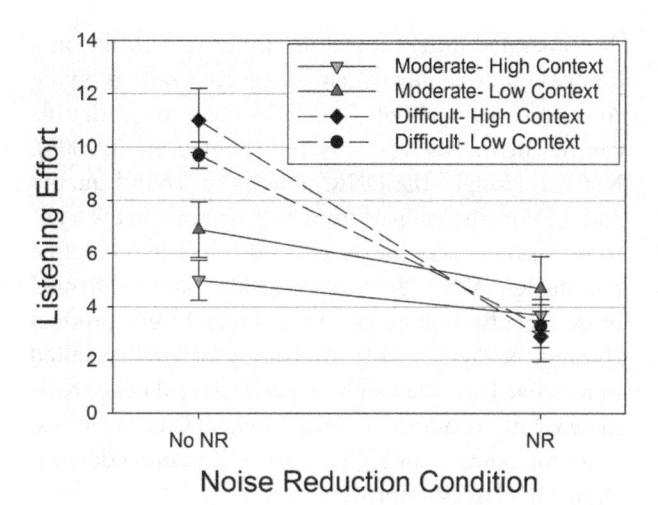

Figure 11–7. The effect of one type of DNR on secondary task performance in a dual task listening effort paradigm. (Adapted from Desjardins and Doherty, 2014.)

word learning speed in noise increased when DNR was activated. Likewise, Pittman (2011) demonstrated that the rate at which children learned novel words increased when DNR was activated. It was speculated that this improvement may have been related to a decrease in listening effort.

DNR: Limitations and Clinical Adjustment

Unfortunately, some patient complaints, including reduced speech recognition, are associated with specific DNR implementations. For example, a patient who worked in an office with a noisy window air conditioning unit indicated that when people walked into her office and started talking it "sometimes takes a while before I can catch onto what they are talking about." Another patient contacted us because she felt as though her hearing aids were intermittent at home. She was very concerned because she had a newborn baby and was afraid she might not hear her—hearing the baby was the very reason she obtained hearing aids. In both cases, the hearing aids had been fitted in another office to the strongest DNR setting, resulting in more than a 20 dB gain reduction. In addition, for this manufacturer, the DNR release time was a couple of seconds or more. We know in both cases that the DNR was the culprit, in part because turning the DNR off alleviated the problem. In the case of the office worker, after some counseling we adjusted the DNR setting to "medium" and the patient was satisfied with the balance of understanding speech and lowering the level of the annoying air conditioner noise when no talkers were present. If these patients had been initially fitted based on a listening needs assessment and the fitting clinician had full knowledge of how the DNR systems operated in the fitted instruments, there is a good possibility that these problems might have been avoided altogether. Although it is unusual to find DNR processing that is as aggressive and slow in modern instruments, knowledge of how DNR reacts to different sounds can still be highly useful.

Transient Noise Reduction (TNR)

The DNR algorithms described above have a number of advantages; however, they typically do not provide relief from transient sounds such as a door slamming, the clinking of dishes, or even computer keystrokes. One-third of environmental noise experienced by hearing aid users have transient duration and are considered to be annoying (Keidser, O'Brien, Latzel, & Convery, 2007; Chalupper & Powers 2007). Many of these sounds are soft in level. Several manufacturers have developed transient noise reduction algorithms (also referred to as impulse dampening) to target non-speech inputs and reduce the annoyance of such sounds—you may see marketing terms for this technology like "Sound Smoothing" or "Sound Relax." TNR algorithms first calculate the temporal properties with a very short processing delay (<1 ms) in order to minimize reaction time to the transient sounds. Next, envelope features are extracted and factors such as steepness of the envelope slope (relative to that of a speech signal) are used to activate a gain reduction. Such algorithms can be implemented in any or all frequency channels of the hearing aid. Transient identification and gain reduction necessarily occur extremely quickly in order to dampen the transient signal (Figure 11–8). Anything that disrupts the rapid rise time (e.g., reverberation for repeated transients at a distance, background noise that approaches the level of the transient peaks) will limit the effectiveness of this processing. Consequently, it is most effective in specific listening situations—for example, dishes clinking together or banging/tapping near the listener when other background noise levels are low. We have not heard any patient complaints relative to TNR arti-

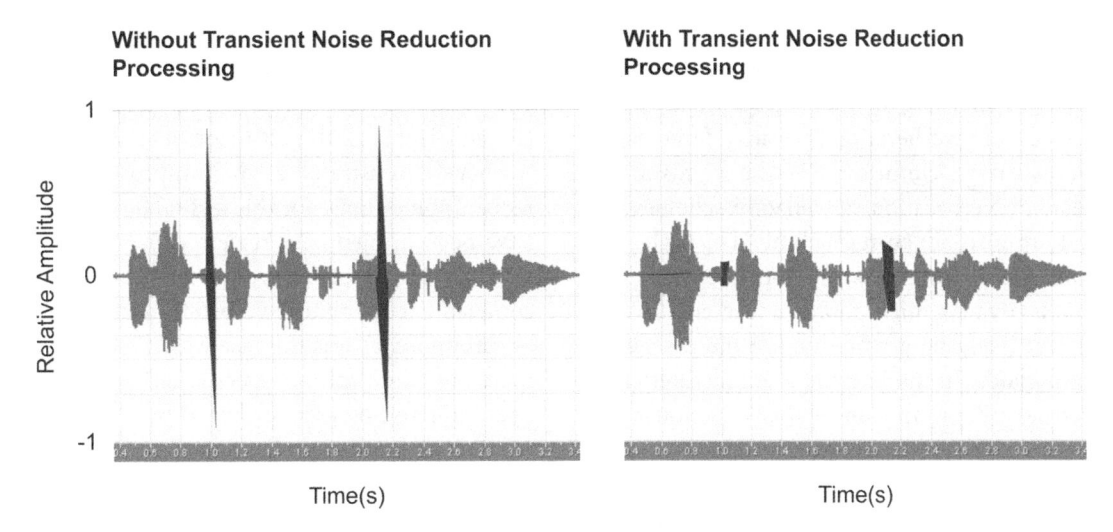

Figure 11–8. An example speech and impulse signal with and without application of transient noise reduction (TNR) processing.

facts, although when set to maximum, there have been patient comments that some environmental sounds are a little too dull.

It is clear from behavioral data that different manufacturers do not use the same TNR processing. For example, Liu, Zhang, Bentler, Han, and Zhang (2012) demonstrated significantly lower ratings of transient noise loudness when TNR was active with no changes in sound quality for speech. An evaluation of another manufacturer's product revealed no changes in speech recognition but significantly better sound quality for transient sounds when TNR was activated (Korhonen et al., 2013). Conversely, a study comparing two additional manufacturer's products revealed significant speech recognition benefits for both types of TNR processing but no differences in subjective ratings (DiGiovanni, Davlin, & Nagaraj, 2011). Specifically, this latter study demonstrated improved speech recognition in the presence of multi-talker babble, chair clang transient noises, and when combining these noises for one manufacturer and only when the transient noises were present for the other manufacturer. Although these data suggest that some types of TNR can improve speech recognition in transient noise, the largest average improvement reported was approximately 13% for the multi-talker babble condition. Given the basics of TNR operation, one might not expect benefits in multi-talker babble, and benefits for TNR processing in this noise background have not been shown for any other manufacturer. This finding demonstrates a common issue when evaluating a manufacturer's proprietary processing algorithms: It is sometimes difficult to assess what specifically is leading to the measured benefits. Despite this uncertainty, TNR appears to have a variety of potential benefits ranging from improved sound quality, to reduced loudness, to improved speech recognition, and this processing is quite effective in some environments and less effective in others. Our advice is to consider using TNR for any patient that is bothered by transient noise but recognize that the type and magnitude of benefits are manufacturer specific.

Reverberation Suppression

As we detail in Chapter 4, high reverberation has a number of negative consequences including significantly decreased speech recognition, particularly beyond the critical distance. In addition, long reverberation times can reduce sound quality and listening comfort. Perhaps surprisingly, recent research suggests moderate levels of reverberation may not increase listening effort, however, even when speech recognition is negatively affected (Picou, Gordon, & Ricketts, 2016). Long reverberation times generate self-masking noise. Specifically, the temporal delay results in an unwanted echo that can mask the original signal of interest. In addition, reverberation can act to temporally fill the gaps between fluctuating noises, thereby increasing masking effects. Reducing the negative effects of reverberation is clearly of interest for hearing aid wearers. Unfortunately, the sophisticated, experimental, reverberation cancellation schemes that show great promise, are currently limited by high computational power requirements and increased computational complexity with microphone movement. In other words, it will likely be a while before these schemes reach hearing aids. In the interim, manufacturers have introduced reverberation suppression techniques that operate in a way that is somewhat analogous to classic DNR. That is, when the signal in a specified time window and frequency channel is identified as primarily consisting of an echo, gain is reduced. The goal is to apply these gain reductions without reducing gain when the signal in the channel is not an echo. Consequently, this processing is expected to be most effective for long reverberation times.

Even though this type of processing has existed for some time, peer reviewed reports of benefits have been limited. Anecdotal reports suggest improved sound quality but little effect on speech recognition. In addition, some recent data suggest reduced listening effort may be associated with this technology. Specifically, subjective and physiologic listening effort were both shown to decrease by approximately 20 to 25% (objective EEG) and 10% (subjective) in a multi-center study (Froehlich et al., 2017; Littmann et al., 2017). These data further demonstrated a small improvement in speech recognition in noise for this technology. Although there have been limited peer-reviewed publications demonstrating clear benefits, we have not heard any patient complaints relating to reverberation suppression either. Furthermore, as was the case with TNR, it is likely that there are manufacturer-specific differences in the core operation and benefits provided by reverberation suppression technologies. Based on the data to date, we see no reason to not recommend trying reverberation suppression, however, patients should be counseled regarding realistic benefits.

Wind Noise Reduction (WNR)

Wind crossing the hearing aid microphone port openings creates turbulence. These fluctuations of air vibrate the diaphragm of the hearing aid microphone, generating relatively high noise levels that are highest in the lowest frequencies (Figure 11–9). Because wind noise is high level, it is not only very annoying to the listener but is also effective at masking speech. Furthermore, dou-

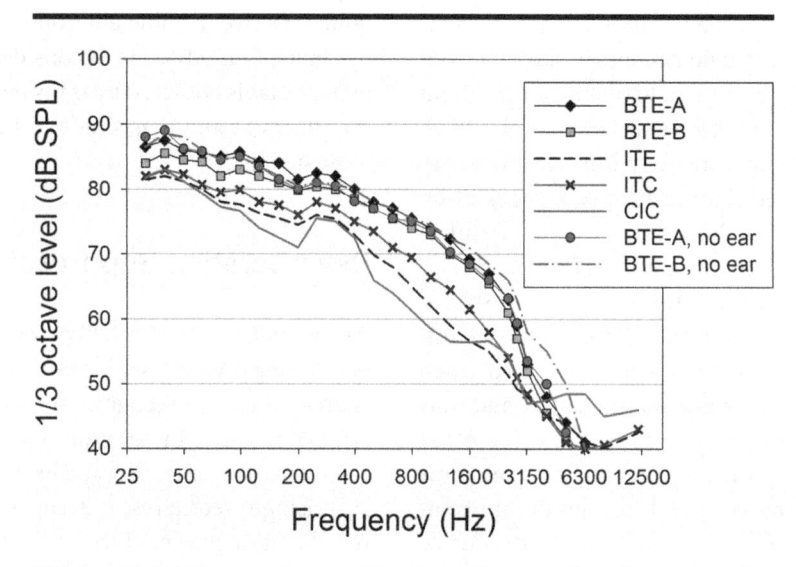

Figure 11–9. Frequency-specific wind noise as a function of hearing aid style for wind generated directly from the side (Adapted from Dillon, Roe, and Katch, 1999.)

bling wind speed increases the wind noise realized by more than 12 dB (Kates, 2008; Morgan & Raspet, 1992). Wind noise is also affected by direction; with most styles of hearing aids presenting the highest wind noise readings when the wind arrives from the front.

We have certainly heard many patients complain about difficulties with communication while wearing their hearing aids in windy situations. In fact, MarkeTrak VIII data (Kochkin, 2010) revealed that a smaller percentage of hearing aid wearers were satisfied with their hearing aids' performance in wind noise than in any other type of noise listed! Wind noise can be identified by a combination of factors including its general spectral shape (more energy in the low frequencies) and uncorrelated energy present at the two microphones within the same hearing aid (due to the fact that it is generated from turbulence rather than being an actual noise present in the environment). Data from Zakis and Hawkins (2015) have also shown that wind noise levels can vary significantly across mini-BTE device designs, revealing that small differences in microphone location, shell design, and/ or wind shielding can result in large differences in wind noise levels. In addition, these researchers demonstrated that wind noise had the potential to reduce speech intelligibility at 3 meters per second (m/s), and totally mask speech at 6 m/s, across BTE and mini-BTE devices. Clearly processing that can reduce the negative effects of wind noise in hearing aids is highly desirable.

Several techniques have been applied to reduce wind noise in hearing aids. Some of the most effective are physical wind screens and wind deflectors. Although these methods can reduce the apparent level of wind noise by up to 18 dB, they are still limited and complaints about wind noise persist even though these physical techniques have been applied for decades. As for processing-based techniques, several have been introduced and evidence of effectiveness in patients is still limited. Wind noise can be identified via level and spectral information; however, it is difficult to do so accurately. One much more accurate method is to use both microphones in a single hearing aid or, more recently, through examining the input for all four hearing microphones (two on each side) in a bilateral array. Identifying wind noise is more accurate using multiple microphones because wind has the unique property of being uncorrelated at the two microphones within the same instrument despite their close proximity to each other. Most other signals will be highly correlated at the two microphones because they originate from sound rather than turbulence.

Unfortunately, even though the lack of correlation helps dual-microphone hearing aids better detect wind noise, detection is there is only half the battle. One additional problem is that activation of directional processing will actually boost low-frequency wind noise compared to omnidirectional settings. The boost is similar in magnitude and frequency range to the boost described for talkers' own voices in Chapter 10 (e.g., 5–10 dB in the lowest frequencies). Therefore, some hearing aids offset this additional problem with wind noise by switching to an omnidirectional setting when wind is detected. If multichannel directivity is available for a given product, the switch to omnidirectional processing in wind is typically only made for the low-frequency channels so that directional processing can continue to provide benefits for higher frequency speech sounds.

Many of the processing-based methods for reducing wind noise identify wind noise in a channel and then, similarly to G-DNR, reduce gain in that channel (sometimes through filtering). Although these methods greatly reduce the annoyance from wind noise, the benefits are limited because wind noise is reduced at the cost of low-frequency audibility. That is, amplification for both the low-frequency wind and any desired signal at the same frequency are both reduced. Consequently, speech recognition will not be improved, and the loss of low frequencies can reduce sound quality, particularly for music. Therefore, it is important that patients are counseled, as to realistic expectations.

One WNR strategy that has been shown to be more effective is wireless sound sharing between bilateral hearing aids. Essentially this method identifies the hearing aid with less wind noise and routes the signal from this better SNR ear to the other hearing aid to replace the signal with more wind noise. Indeed, research has shown that wind noise can be up to 25 dB higher in one ear than the other at some frequencies (Figure 11–10). This WNR strategy has been shown to significantly improve speech recognition up to 27% when a fan was placed on one side of the head (270°) and speech was presented from the other side at 60° (Latzel & Appleton, 2013). Smaller benefits were reported for other angles, although overall, lower ratings of loudness and

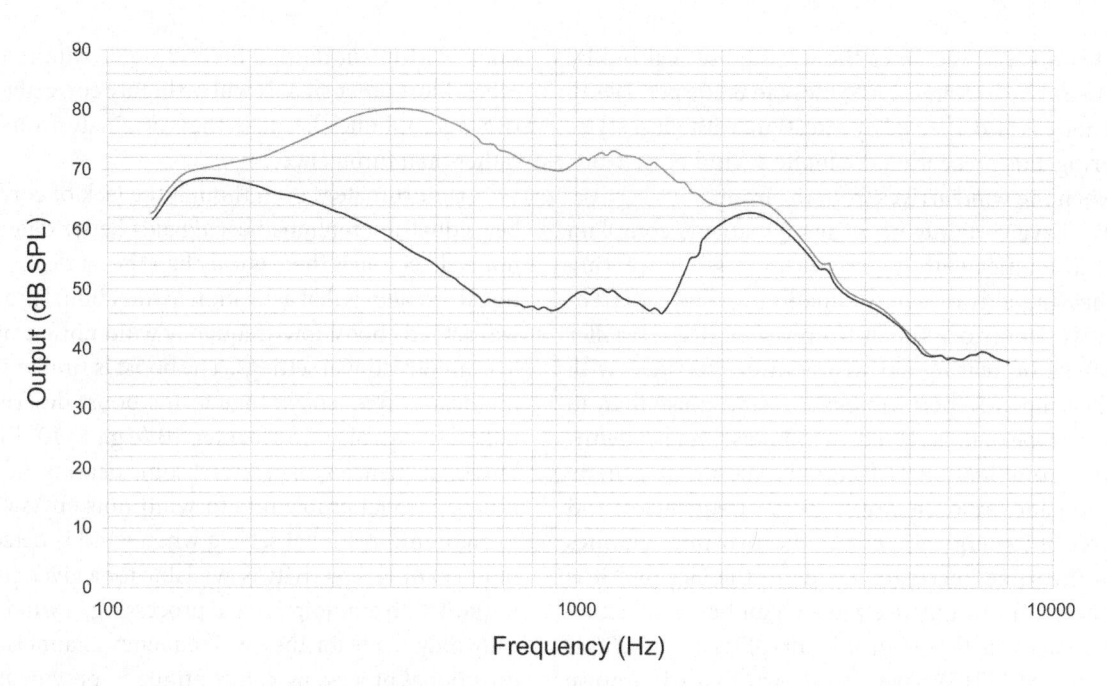

Figure 11–10. Differences in wind noise level for bilateral hearing aids for an angle for which wind noise is maximal on only one side (Adapted from Freels, Pischel, Wilson and Ramirez, 2015).

annoyance were reported. Unfortunately, data demonstrating benefits from this type of processing in the real world are still somewhat limited, so the overall magnitude effects on the listening experience are still unclear.

Because wind noise results from turbulence, it is highly uncorrelated over time and at different sample places, so estimating the noise spectrum for cancellation is problematic. Consequently, many traditional noise reduction strategies, including spectral subtraction, are largely ineffective against wind. A number of other methods for separating fluctuating broadband signals like wind and speech have been proposed. The idea is to model both signals independently and then model the combined signal. Modeling of this type has been based on the hidden Markov model with a Gaussian mixture, vector quantization, non-negative sparse coding, and other techniques. Once modeled, filtering is applied to reduce the unwanted signal. If you model the speech and the wind noise before filtering accurately, these approaches can work rather well. Unfortunately, models are limited in accuracy in the real world where modeling must be done on estimations completed while the wind and speech is ongoing.

A relatively recent method using a similar approach exploits a property of Least Mean Square (LMS) filters. These filters are designed to identify the filter coefficients that minimize the squared error between the desired and the actual signal. Since this occurs when the desired and actual signal correlate, and filter coefficients cannot be identified when these signals are uncorrelated, LMS filters have been shown to reduce uncorrelated noise. Investigators realized this technique had promise for reducing wind noise because it is uncorrelated at the two microphones, meanwhile the desired speech signal is typically highly correlated.

Data examining benefits for LMS wind noise reduction revealed this type of processing reduced wind noise by up to 15 dB (Korhonen, Kuk, Seper, Mørkebjerg, & Roikjer, 2017). Importantly, this technology was most effective at reducing wind level when wind arrived from directly in front of the listener, an environment for which the bilateral sound sharing method is largely ineffective because wind noise is similar at the two ears. Indeed, the LMS strategy reduced subjective annoyance for wind from this angle was by approximately 14% for wind speeds of 4 to 7 m/s. This study also reported a large and significant

> **TECHNICAL TIP: IMPORTANT PRACTICAL ISSUES REGARDING WIND NOISE**
>
> In your day-to-day fitting of hearing aids, here are three issues to consider regarding wind noise:
>
> - Wind noise annoyance easily can be caused by rapid movement of the patient, even when there is no wind per se. This is a big issue for bicycle riders, joggers, and even people who walk briskly.
> - Our discussion here has mostly been based on the use of BTE instruments. One of the best ways, however, to reduce wind noise is simply to place the microphone port deeper in the ear (at the entrance of the ear canal) rather than above the ear. CIC hearing aids, therefore, are an effective method of reducing wind noise (see Chapter 8); research has shown a reduction of wind noise by over 20 dB with a CIC microphone location.
> - Our discussion here has mostly been based on closed-ear fittings. With open fittings, there is less wind noise in the lows because of the absence of amplifier gain (and leakage), but for the same reasons, the wind noise reduction algorithms will be less effective (e.g., transferring the audio signal from the non-wind side to the wind-side only will be effective if the signal does not leak out of the ear on the wind side).

phoneme recognition in wind noise benefit. It should be noted, however, that whereas the measurement conditions included several different speech presentation levels, only wind presented from 0° and speech presented from 270° was evaluated. The magnitude or even presence of speech recognition benefits at other angles and in other realistic environments are as yet unknown.

A number of proprietary strategies for reducing wind noise, including modifications of the above techniques, have been introduced. Data in support of WNR techniques are still limited, but improvements in sound quality and, in fewer products, speech recognition are expected in specific yet realistic listening environments. As we describe, the orientation of wind and speech for which benefits are maximized depends on the specific type of processing applied. Therefore, it is important to counsel patients to orient themselves appropriately for the specific WNR technology being used to maximize benefits. That is, patients should be told to "point your nose into the wind" for the LMS-based WNR strategies and "face your ear toward the wind" for the sound-sharing WNR strategies.

Microphone-Based Noise Reduction

In Chapter 4 we described in detail how background noise can greatly reduce speech recognition, especially in listeners with hearing impairment. One group of technologies that have repeatedly been shown to improve the effective SNR and associated speech recognition in a wide range of noisy environments are microphone-based. In hearing aids, these technologies include remote microphones (e.g., spouse microphones, personal FM systems, and other remote microphones), directional microphones (also referred to as first-order microphone arrays and unilateral beamformers), advanced directional microphones (including lobe steering and reverse directional), and higher order microphone arrays (most commonly bilateral beamformers). We described the basic operation of remote microphones, directional microphones and microphone arrays in Chapter 10, so we won't repeat those details here. Instead we will focus on how these features are activated and used in current hearing aids as well as potential benefits and limitations.

TECHNICAL TIP: ARRAYS, BEAMFORMERS, AND DIRECTIONAL MICROPHONE TERMINOLOGY: NO WE ARE *NOT* USING ALL OF THE STANDARD TERMS

For our purposes we will treat the terms "microphone array" and "beamformer" synonymously. By definition a beamformer is a general term describing an arrangement of two or more sensors such that the phase of the signal at each sensor can be used to enhance signal level from some directions and suppress it from others. A microphone array is a more specific term denoting an arrangement with the same goal; the beamformer "sensors" are microphones. As we describe in Chapter 10, a directional microphone picks up sound at two locations using either two microphone ports, which open up to either side of a single diaphragm (pressure gradient approach), or two omnidirectional microphones. If this is all clear, the following should make sense:

- A directional microphone (using two omnidirectional microphones with fixed internal delay) and a pressure gradient directional microphone (using two microphone ports with the same spacing and fixed internal delay as the twin mic design) will operate identically.
- In the above example, the pressure gradient design is a directional microphone, but it is not a beamformer or microphone array because there is technically only one microphone.
- Twin microphone systems are also referred to as a directional microphone, but in the modern designs it is also technically correct to refer to them as a first order microphone array or unilateral beamformer (denoting beamforming is being completed within one hearing aid).
- A bilateral beamformer uses all four microphones from both hearing aids to create a higher order microphone array.
- The majority of engineers and manufacturers working in hearing aids have typically referred to the higher order microphone arrays we have labeled bilateral beamformers as binaural beamformers. We assume this is because the commercially available examples either reintroduce or preserve some binaural cues. In addition, the technology we have labeled unilateral beamformers have been instead labeled bilateral beamformers when a patient is fitted with a pair of these devices. We believe that even though these terms have been in common use, both are a little misleading. We take a psychoacoustic and physiologic view of binaural processing; it is the cognition applied by humans that provides binaural benefits based on differences in the signal arriving at the two ears. We also have the viewpoint that the words before beamformer refer to the information used when beamforming. When two microphones are used within the case of one instrument, the beamforming processing is based on the signals in that single hearing aid (i.e., unilateral beamforming). That is true whether a person uses one or two of these instruments. Indeed, many listeners exhibit good to excellent binaural hearing abilities when fitted bilaterally with unilateral beamformers. In comparison, the beamforming processing in a bilateral beamformer is based on the input to all four microphones. Human binaural processing is not used to enhance this beamforming. In addition, the natural binaural cues are distorted

> by this processing leading to typically poorer binaural performance when fitted with these devices than when fitted bilaterally with unilateral beamformers. As a consequence, we prefer and use the term bilateral beamformer to describe binaural cue preserving higher order microphone arrays, despite the fact that many publications to date have labelled them binaural beamformers.

Remote microphones place the microphone input much closer to the target source. This can greatly improve SNR because this close proximity can raise the input level of the target talker relative to the noise in the room. Microphone arrays are designed to maintain the input levels for sounds arriving from specific directions (most commonly the front), while reducing the levels for sounds arriving from other directions (most commonly to the sides and behind). SNR and speech recognition are therefore improved for many hearing aid wearers using microphone arrays in environments for which the talker of interest is in front—and competing signals (noise) are either concentrated in the opposite direction or surround the listener. In contrast, hearing aids using standard omnidirectional microphones, although effective at increasing audibility for speech and other sounds, are largely ineffective in improving the SNR.

Remote Microphones

The more basic approach of placing the microphone and sound source in close proximity is by far the most effective if the goal is enhancement of SNR for a single talker. We will generally refer to these technologies as remote microphones because the microphone is placed a distance away from the hearing aid wearer. A hardwire remote microphone was used by listeners with hearing impairment more than a century ago, but less cumbersome wireless techniques have been used for many decades (Figure 11–11). Both digital and analog wireless microphones, including FM systems, have been shown to significantly improve SNR by as much as 16 to 20 dB in noisy environments; however, several studies over the last few decades have demonstrated that the magnitude of SNR advantage greatly depends on the specific configuration (e.g., mix ratio, use of fixed versus dynamic microphone gain, directivity of the microphone) and may be as little as 4 to 5 dB for some situations.

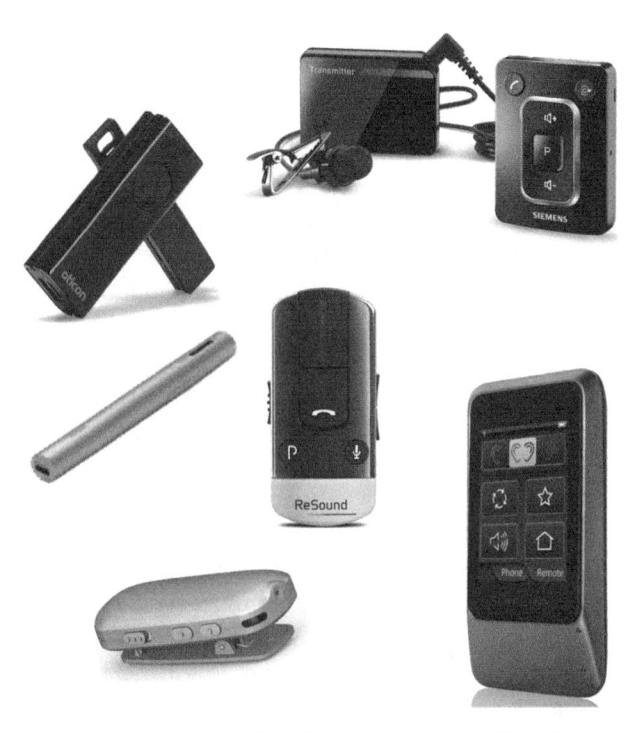

Figure 11–11. Examples of wireless remote microphones used with hearing aids.

When wireless microphones are used without activation of the hearing aid microphones, the SNR at the ear is determined primarily by the SNR at the location of the remote microphone. In other words, SNR is optimized by placing the remote microphone in close proximity to the talker's mouth and/or using microphone array technologies to improve directivity. In contrast, when both the wireless microphone and the hearing aid microphones are activated at the same time, as is typical, SNR is determined by the highest level of the speech (e.g., location of the remote microphone) and the highest level of noise, which can be either at the location of the remote microphone or the hearing aid microphone (e.g., Norrix, Camarota, Harris, & Dean, 2016). As a

TECHNICAL TIP: REMOTE MICROPHONE TERMINOLOGY AND CLINICAL TIPS

There are a few terms that have been used when describing adjustment of FM systems over the years, but they really can apply to any remote microphone technology. Details of these effects are beyond the scope of this chapter, and the interested reader is pointed to any current hearing assistive technology textbook. Importantly, not all remote microphone systems include these technologies or include the same level of adjustment.

- Remote Microphone Type: As we discuss in the next section, the benefits from remote microphone technologies are limited in part by the SNR at the remote microphone. Consequently, performance is sometimes improved through the use of directional microphones or microphone arrays in lieu of omnidirectional microphones. Highly directional beamformers are sometimes used to allow a user to hold the microphone so it can be pointed to talkers of interest in multi-talker environments. Use of an omnidirectional microphone placed in the middle of several talkers (e.g., on a conference table) can actually reduce performance compared to using a directional hearing aid without a remote microphone if the SNR at the remote microphone location is poor.
- Remote Microphone Frequency Bandwidth: The bandwidth that can be carried by a wireless system is limited, in part, by the transmission method. For example, in traditional narrow band FM systems the design must consider that there is a trade-off between frequency bandwidth and dynamic range. Therefore, the amplitude dynamic range is typically limited to ensure a frequency bandwidth of 6 to 7 kHz. The original LE Bluetooth audio transmission bandwidth was even more limited (i.e., less than 5 kHz), although efforts are ongoing to increase this bandwidth.
- Mix Ratio: It is common to leave the hearing aid microphones active for monitoring, and mix in the remote microphone signal at a higher level. FM system best practice guidelines typically aimed at children, recommend a mix ratio of 10 dB. That is, after already assuming a higher talker level at the remote microphone, the talker voice from the remote microphone is delivered to the listener at a level that is 10 dB higher than the signal from the hearing aid microphone. One technique used in some modern systems is to dynamically adjust the level of the signal from the remote microphone based on the estimated SNR. Speech recognition benefits for this technique have been demonstrated for several noise environments over traditional fixed level techniques. As we discuss in the next section, the optimal mix ratio for adult listeners using remote microphones will depend on listening needs.
- Venting: Increasing vent size will limit the low frequency amplification that can be provided by the remote microphone signal. Little or no audible low-frequency energy will typically be transmitted with an open fitting. This may be acceptable, however, in patients with near normal low-frequency thresholds and relatively good speech recognition in noise.

result, benefit from a wireless microphone when the listener is surrounded by noise will be greatly reduced by activating the hearing aid microphones, even if the SNR at the remote microphone is very good. Because of these tradeoffs, the optimal configuration for a remote microphone is a balance for each individual patient between the following factors:

- The amount of difficulty communicating in noise—how much help does the patient need?
- The need, desire, and ability to monitor sounds other than the primary talker (which might differ from time to time, location to location).

Clearly, these issues need careful consideration when the hearing aids are programmed and the patient is counseled. Some of these issues might be difficult to predict. Multiple options could be provided, and some real-world field trials might be needed.

When considering a typical FM system configuration, electroacoustic evaluation and behavioral data demonstrate a clear SNR advantage for remote microphone technologies over hearing aid based microphone arrays (e.g., Lewis, Crandell, Valente, & Horn, 2004). What then, are the potential disadvantages? One of the most obvious disadvantages for remote microphones is they require an external device that must be worn by a talker. Even though this is not a problem in and of itself for some hearing aid wearers, most express concerns about cosmetics and drawing unwanted attention to their hearing loss. Another disadvantage related to the use of the remote microphone is that benefits are typically limited to conversing with a single talker of interest. Remote microphones may not be optimal when listening to multiple talkers or when overhearing other conversations is the listening goal. As we described, combining the input from the remote microphone placed near the speaker of interest with the input from an "environmental microphone" placed near the listener (e.g., activating the hearing aid microphones) has long been advocated to overcome this problem. Data have shown that this combination provides an improvement in SNR that is far smaller, however, resulting in limited benefit in noise from this configuration (Lewis et al., 2004). Indeed, we have recently found that using a omnidirectional remote microphone in a center table location in a noisy environment can decrease speech recognition compared to simply using the hearing aids without remote microphones. Multi-channel remote microphones allowing for automatic switching between two or more microphones have been in development for some time and likely will be routinely available to hearing aid wearers very soon. Even these devices limit the number of sources of interest to less than perhaps four to five talkers. Furthermore, the listener cannot enhance the SNR for secondary sources of interest with a simple head turn as is possible with microphone arrays.

Traditional Directional Technologies and Higher Order Microphone Arrays

Microphone arrays are advocated as a potential method for improving SNR in noisy environments while providing greater portability (since hardware external to the hearing aid is not needed) and alleviating some of the monitoring difficulties associated with wireless microphone systems. Although they differ significantly in the benefit provided in noise (much less for many listening conditions), the reality is that there is no "one size fits all" when considering microphone based technologies for improving SNR; all have both potential benefits and limitations. Modern hearing aids use a range of array processing and a variety of different decision rules when activating directional microphones and microphone arrays. The most basic devices activate these technologies when the overall input level is above some criterion (e.g., 55–65 dB SPL; adjustable on some models), and the estimated SNR falls within a range that ensures both background noise and speech are present and identifiable. When these criteria are *not met*, the hearing aid uses an omnidirectional setting. These rules are applied in an attempt to minimize potential negative consequences of activation of directional technology discussed later in this chapter. In addition to continued improvements in sound classification and the associated decision rules, advances in first-order microphone array designs have continued—including adaptive null-steering in the rear hemisphere, which became popular around 2005, and an automatic reverse-cardioid pattern, which was introduced in 2010.

As we describe in Chapter 10, a number of different higher order microphone arrays have been developed for hearing aid wearers. For example, in 2002 a second-order array utilizing three microphones oriented along the side of a full-sized BTE case was introduced. More recently, improved wireless streaming between hearing aids allowed for the introduction, in 2011, of the first bilateral beamforming instruments utilizing all four microphones of a hearing aid pair. Current instruments with bilateral beamforming technology also include more traditional adaptive directional microphone technologies (e.g., unilateral beamformers), as well as omnidirectional and (in some products) the slightly directional technologies described below. The use of multiple microphone technologies within the same instrument relates to limiting potential negatives associated with increasingly enhanced SNR.

Activating a directional microphone may be done through a dedicated user program; however, surveys suggest the vast majority of clinical fittings use automatic activation and adjustment of directional processing based on classifier information. Rather than defaulting to automatic activation, bilateral beamformer function varies by manufacturer and clinical settings, in part because some manufacturers target these technologies at the individuals that have the greatest difficulty understanding speech in noise. In some cases, there is a dedicated program that requires activation by the hearing aid wearer, or the user can adjust the "narrowness" of the beam using a smart phone app. Other products allow the bilateral beamfomer to be activated automatically. In automatic switching systems, the exact activation threshold level used for directional microphone and bilateral beamformers differs across manufacturers. In most cases bilateral beamformer activation only occurs at high levels with poor SNR (very difficult listening conditions). In some products, activation of directional microphones also does not occur until there are relatively high total sound levels (e.g., 70 dB SPL or higher). Data have shown that many noisy environments have much lower speech in noise levels, however, suggesting the potential for directional benefit with lower activation thresholds (Wu, Stangle, Zhang, & Bentler, 2015; Ricketts, Picou, & Galster, 2017). Due to these factors, a variety of complex decision rules and techniques are currently applied to directional microphones and bilateral beamformers. The goal of these advanced techniques is to limit the known problems of being in the "wrong" microphone setting for a particular environment, while at the same time maximizing performance whenever possible.

The most advanced microphone-based and DNR technologies do not operate in discrete states. Instead, they fluidly move from little to no sound cleaning for environments estimated to include speech in quiet (e.g., omnidirectional/real ear sound with no DNR) to very high degrees of sound cleaning for environments estimated to be quite loud with very poor SNR (e.g., bilateral beamforming and maximal DNR). These systems typically have either a number of discrete combinations of intermediate levels of sound cleaning (e.g., 3, 5, or 7 different levels) or a capacity for smooth transition from slightly directional/omnidirectional to fully directional or bilateral beamforming (i.e., variable strength of directivity depending on the acoustic environment).

A few manufacturers also allow the clinician some freedom to adjust the behavior of the microphone processing within predetermined limits. In some models,

---

TECHNICAL TIP: METHODS AIMED AT MAXIMIZING FIRST-ORDER DIRECTIONAL BENEFIT WHILE LIMITING POTENTIAL DECREMENT ACROSS COMPLEX LISTENING ENVIRONMENTS

- Automatic switching between multiple levels of directivity, including omndirectional
- Clinician control of the aggressiveness of the decision rules
- Use of limited, high-frequency directional processing in place of omnidirectional processing in BTE and Mini-BTE styles to offset negative microphone location effects on SNR
- Asymmetric microphone settings

the clinician control affects microphone array activation and strength of directivity (in systems with multiple levels of sound cleaning). These clinician adjustments may affect the level activation threshold, the SNR activation threshold, and/or the aggressiveness with which the processing moves through multiple directivity levels in response to changes in the acoustic environment. That is, these methods provide the clinician control of how aggressively sound cleaning is applied in response to increasing noise contamination of the speech signal. Some sophisticated clinician control schemes also effect switching aggressiveness and maximum strength of advanced DNR techniques at the same time, including the spatially based T-DNR described early in this chapter. To make things even easier, this does not even have to be done in the clinician's office.

Another technique aimed at minimizing error, which is applied by one manufacturer, is an asymmetric microphone setting. An asymmetric directional setting simply refers to use of omnidirectional processing in one hearing aid and directional in the other when listening in noise. The original asymmetric systems used a fixed asymmetric setting. In the second generation, the hearing aids remained in an asymmetric configuration in noise, but the directional microphone was activated on the ear with the poorer estimated SNR. In the most advanced current generation, asymmetry is applied even more judiciously.

TECHNICAL TIP: USER ADJUSTMENT OF DIRECTIONALITY

With the explosion of advanced smartphone control of hearing aids, user controls of microphone technologies have become simple and sophisticated. One example of the types of controls for advanced microphone technologies is shown in Figure 11–12. In addition to this type of control, many manufacturers also offer smartphone apps, which the patient can use to give his or her audiologist remote control of hearing aid adjustments so that problems with gain, output, and a variety of features can be addressed through distance programming. For example, the patient who finds he or she doesn't like manual control of the bilateral beamformer after all, can contact their audiologist and, after providing control through the app via the Internet, allow the clinician to program for automatic activation in the default listening program. All this without ever leaving their living room!

TECHNICAL TIP: IS OMNI REALLY OMNI?

As we describe in Chapter 10, the omnidirectional BTE microphone location results in an SNR that is poorer than the open ear. Given this limitation and the current popularity of mini-BTE devices, these products are often designed to use a slightly directional setting instead of an omnidirectional setting to prevent decreased performance for speech recognition in noise when listening at levels below the directional activation threshold. Depending on the manufacturer, this "slightly directional" setting has been labeled in many ways including real-ear sound, pinna sound, and TruEar. Hence, omni isn't really omni. The directivity index (DI) values associated with these techniques are similar to the unaided open ear. Therefore, resulting speech recognition performance is expected to be similar to that achieved using an omnidirectional CIC.

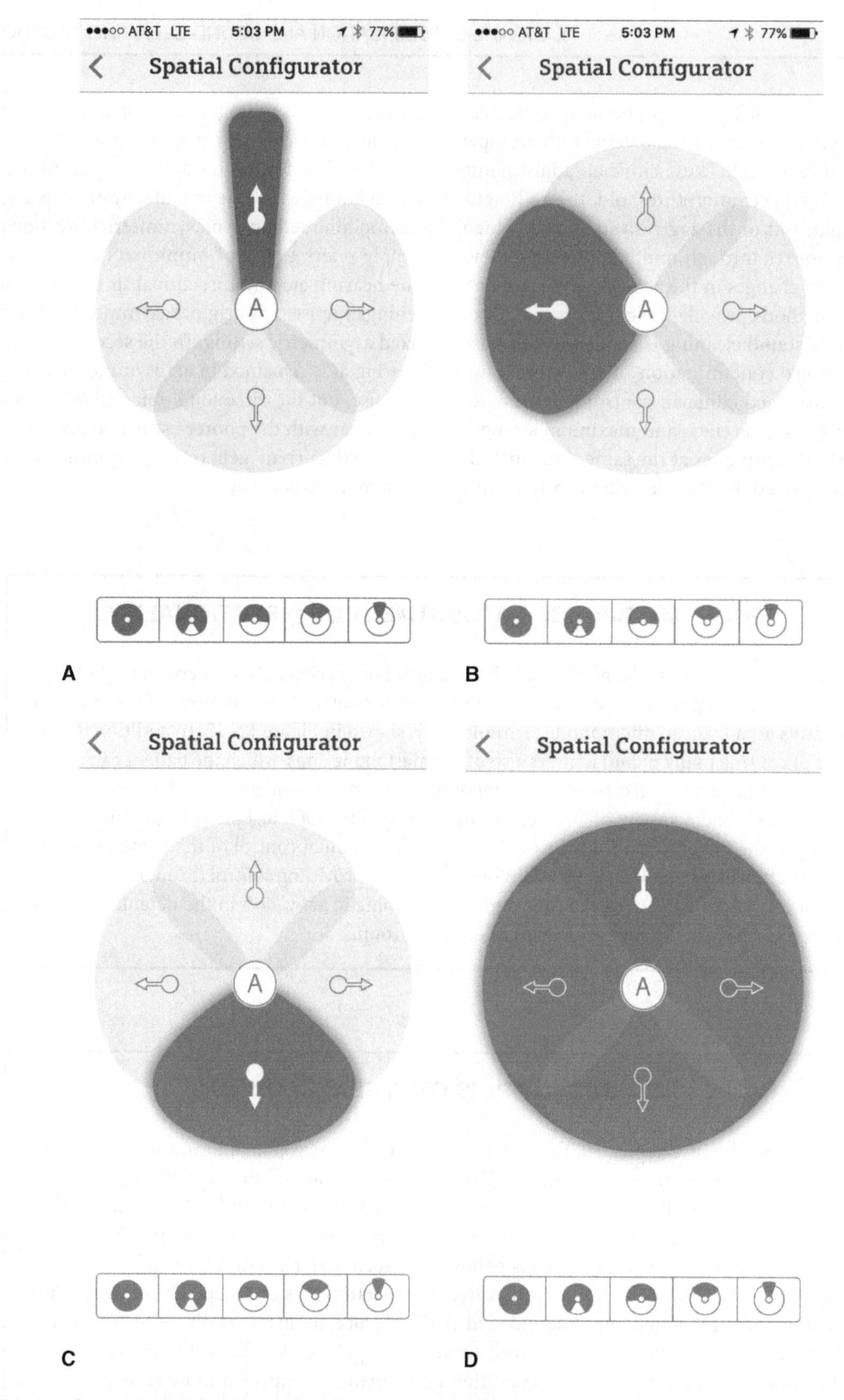

Figure 11–12. An example of patient smartphone controls for one manufacturer's advanced microphone technologies. **A.** Narrow focus bilateral beamforming. **B.** Lobe steering left. **C.** Reverse directional. **D.** Omnidirectional with pinna effect.

> **TECHNICAL TIP: ADVANCED ASYMMETRIC SWITCHING TECHNIQUE**
>
> - When the classifier suggests a high probability that the omnidirectional mode will be optimal (e.g., speech in quiet environment), the omnidirectional setting is activated for both hearing aids.
> - When the classifier suggests a high probability that the directional mode will be optimal (e.g., conditions of speech in front in the presence of high-level steady-state noise, poor SNR), the directional setting is activated for both hearing aids.
> - When the classifier suggests a complex environment that is difficult to classify accurately (e.g., speech in speech, considerable modulation), the hearing aid with the poorer estimated SNR is set to directional and the other hearing aid is set to omnidirectional.

Evidence-Based Benefits

Given that directional technology in hearing aids has been available since the late 1960s, considerable research has been conducted with these instruments. The primary focus has been related to improvements in speech recognition, but subjective ratings also have been obtained. More recently, there has been an interest in the potential for this type of processing to reduce listening effort and listening fatigue. Unfortunately, over the years the majority of this research has been based in the laboratory, where experimental design easily can influence the outcome (e.g., azimuth of target speech, azimuth of competing noise, number of noise sources, types of noise). There have been some well-designed field studies, however, which we review in the following section.

Speech Recognition in Noise

Benefits from microphone technologies are most often described by changes in speech recognition in noisy environments. The positive effects of these technologies on word recognition has been reported in terms of absolute scores, as well as difference scores (i.e., relative performance for directional and omnidirectional settings). We will refer to these two constructs respectively as speech recognition performance and directional, remote microphone or beamformer benefits. As we mentioned previously, there have been several studies over the decades demonstrating the benefits of FM systems and how these benefits are affected by environments, configurations and settings (e.g., Boothroyd, 2004; Thibodeau,

2014). There are fewer studies demonstrating the benefits of newer wireless remote "companion microphones," which commonly use an omnidirectional microphone and are sometimes packaged with the hearing aid purchase. Our own evaluation of an omnidirectional companion microphone placed near the talker's mouth in a typical noisy room suggests a remote microphone benefit of around 5 to 7 dB SNR on tests like the BKB-SIN are reasonable to expect in the absence of visual cues when the hearing aid microphones were also active (+10 or +12 dB mix ratio). These benefits are similar, or slightly larger, than we have measured for a bilateral beamformer if we assume the listener is facing, and is relative near the talker. These remote microphone benefits are also similar to those reported in the literature in a comparison of four different wireless technologies using the HINT (Rodemerk and Galster, 2015).

As we discussed in Chapter 10, some remote microphones are available with first or higher order microphone arrays. By activating the microphone array within the remote microphone, additional speech recognition benefits can be achieved (Thibodeau, 2014). Remote microphones with microphone arrays can also be held in the listener's hand and pointed at multiple talkers of interest. Rodemerk and Galster (2015) demonstrated that by disabling the hearing aid microphones, and using only the remote microphone, benefits increased to 11 to 15 dB. Those patients who really struggle with communication in noise may require this configuration if they are not successful with a less aggressive intervention. However, they should be counseled relative to the lack of monitoring ability in this setting, and also, safety concerns should be addressed. For example, you certainly would not want to disable the hearing aid microphones for a patient environment that included walking on a busy street.

One clear advantage of remote microphone over bilateral beamformers is that the listener position relative to the talker does not have a large effect on the SNR improvement. For example, the talker could be 12 feet away, and the listener could have his or her back turned, and similar benefits would still be expected. On the other hand, the beamformer has the advantage of changing the direction of focus with a simple head turn, and therefore is often the preferred intervention when there are multiple talkers of interest. However, when there are a few known talkers of interest, use of multiple remote microphones in network can be quite beneficial for those listeners with very poor speech understanding in noise (e.g., De Ceulaer, Bestel, Mülder, Goldbeck, de Varebeke, & Govaerts, 2016).

Studies have reported a wide range of directional benefit provided by hearing aids using first-order microphone arrays. When measured in traditional laboratory settings, directional benefit values ranging from negative values (decrement) up to 11 dB SNR-50, and 70 percentage points have been reported in the literature. Some of this variability is related to the DI of the instruments evaluated and a number of different patient factors. However, the majority of the variability is due to the test environment. For example, considerably more directional benefit will be measured using a single noise loudspeaker in a sound booth placed carefully at the angle corresponding to the directional null. This is very different than a more typical listening situation, where there are multiple noise sources surrounding the listener, and different levels of reverberation.

So what can we expect in a difficult but realistic listening situation? Let's assume we start with a hearing aid with a directional microphone that is functioning well (average DI in the range of 3.5–5.5 dB). If we consider listening distances of 4 to 10 feet, moderate reverberation, and noise surrounding the listener, significant directional advantages of approximately 2 to 4 dB on an SNR-50 test (e.g., HINT or BKB-SIN) have been reported for both children and adults for a wide range of hearing loss.

So how often are adults and children in these listening environments? Walden, Surr, Cord, and Dyrlund (2004) evaluated patient preference for directional and omnidirectional hearing aid modes over a six-week period. Individuals were asked to identify and describe at least one listening situation each day in which the directional and omnidirectional settings performed best. Overall, listeners reported a preference for the directional setting for about one-third of active listening time. The environmental factors associated with directional preference were consistent with those identified in laboratory-based studies: facing a talker who is near in a room with moderate or less reverberation. A variety of other studies suggest the potential for directional benefit in about 30 to 50% of active listening time in adults.

What about children, can they also benefit from these technologies? In order to receive benefit, children, like adults, must be able to point their nose in the general direction of sounds of interest. Fortunately, data support that younger and older children are capable of accurately orienting to a primary talker (Ching et al., 2009; Ricketts & Galster, 2008). Orientation is not perfect, however, in that the children directly oriented to talkers during about 30 to 50% of active listening time. Children were the most accurate when listening was the most difficult, however, suggesting that when they really need help, they will look where they are listening (thus likely to also obtain visual cues). Broadly consistent with the data in adults, observer judgments in school envi-

---

TECHNICAL TIP: WHAT IS A "DIFFICULT BUT REALISTIC" LISTENING ENVIRONMENT?

1. The listener is facing the talker of interest.
2. The talker is relatively near to the listener (the more reverberation the smaller the distance consistent with the effects of critical distance).
3. SNR is relatively poor, typically +10 or poorer.
4. Competing noise of at least a moderate level (~50–65 dB SPL) is surrounding the listener.

ronments have demonstrated that the directional microphone setting is expected to provide an SNR advantage during approximately 42% of the active communication time (Ricketts et al., 2017). Although not true for some advanced designs we describe later in this chapter, traditional directional microphones and bilateral beamformers will limit audibility from the back and the sides, even when a signal of interest arrives from those directions. Depending on the microphone design this can greatly limit speech recognition in environments where the talker of interest is behind the listener. Microphone arrays can also limit off-axis overhearing and monitoring in both children and adults, particularly in listeners with severe and greater hearing loss and/or those with very poor speech recognition in noise abilities. An example of the effects that talker location has on directional benefit is shown in Figure 11–13. These data, adapted from Ricketts, Galster, and Tharpe (2007), reflect the directional benefit measured in 26 children with hearing loss in a variety of simulated classroom environments. As you can see, SNR-50 performance on the HINT-C was approximately 2 to 3 dB using the directional setting whenever the talker of interest was in the front hemifield (teacher front, teacher front while completing desk work, simulated discussion with presentation from three different talker locations around a table). Performance using the directional setting was more than 2 dB poorer when the teacher was behind, however, and on the average the directional setting did not help or hurt in a simulated bench seating lunch room (when talkers were near and directly from the sides). Similar directional decrements for off-axis talkers have also been reported in adult listeners when using traditional directional technologies (e.g., Wu, Stangl, Bentler, & Stanziola, 2013).

Although it has been demonstrated that the degree of hearing loss does not greatly affect directional benefit as measured by changes in SNR-50, benefit measured by percent correct performance at a fixed SNR will be affected consistent with the hearing loss desensitization factor (Ricketts & Hornsby, 2006). Indeed, multiple studies using AI/SII calculations have shown that, as the degree of hearing loss increases, the benefit obtained from the same improvement in SNR decreases. Specific to directional benefit, data collected using the Connected Speech Test showed the speech recognition in noise score of those with moderate hearing loss improved approximately 7% for every one dB increase in DI, whereas scores for those with severe hearing loss only improved approximately 3.5% per dB (Ricketts, Henry, & Hornsby, 2005).

The vast majority of directional hearing aids in use now, are adaptive. As we describe in Chapter 10, adaptive directional hearing aids operate by automatically varying the physical directional properties until an attenuation pattern that results in the lowest output intensity is obtained. The original adaptive directional microphones were based on the total signal bandwidth, meanwhile many current hearing aids include frequency specific adaptive processing that operates independently in multiple frequency channels. Multichannel adaptive processing has the potential to reduce noises arriving from different angles that have different frequency content. Given how adaptive directional hearing aids function, it is not surprising that the benefits are identical to a fixed directional microphone that is optimized for that same environment. In other words, if a fixed directional microphone is optimized for noise surrounding a listener, an adaptive directional microphone will provide equivalent speech recognition performance in that same environment. Alternatively, if a fixed directional microphone is optimized for noise arriving from directly behind, the adaptive system will provide equivalent benefit in a listening environment for which there is a single noise source behind the listener (e.g., Ricketts, Lindley, & Henry, 2001; Ricketts et al., 2005).

A few studies, have demonstrated an additional directional benefit for adaptive processing over a fixed

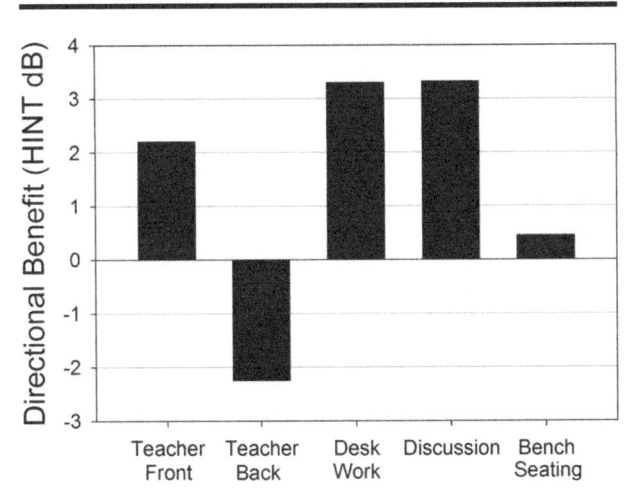

Figure 11–13. Directional benefit across five listening environments.

directional setting (referred to herein as an adaptive advantage). Not surprisingly, this advantage is seen in environments for which the "fixed" directional pattern is not optimized. Fixed directional systems are typically optimized for listening environments in which noise surrounds, or is concentrated behind, the listener. Consequently, performance using fixed and adaptive systems are often similar in these environments. The largest and most consistent adaptive advantages have been observed when the noise sources were placed at the listener's side (i.e., at 90° and 270°). The typical magnitude of the adaptive advantage in these environments is approximately 1 to 2 dB, or up to 20 percentage points of speech recognition improvement.

A specific advantage to adaptive directional processing is the ability of the adaptive null to follow a moving noise source. One situation in which this has been found to be helpful is when the wearer is having a conversation on a busy street with moving car noise in the background—it has been reported that some hearing aids can track a noise equivalent to a car traveling at 40 to 50 miles/hour, if the hearing aid is already in the adaptive directional mode. Ricketts et al. (2005) found a 2 dB SNR advantage for adaptive versus fixed for a moving noise source, and a 7 dB advantage versus omnidirectional for this listening condition.

Adaptive directional microphone technology also can be used to construct an anti-cardioid or reverse-directional polar pattern—that is, noise reduction is the greatest for signals from the front, rather than the back. The efficacy of this technology was reported by Mueller, Weber, & Bellanova (2011), who conducted clinical testing using a listening setting favorable for this type of processing—noise from the front and speech from the back. Their results revealed a significant effect, showing that when the anti-cardioid pattern was automatically activated, there was a 5 dB SNR advantage compared to omnidirectional, and a 10 dB SNR advantage when compared to conventional adaptive directional. A similar study by (Chalupper, Wu, and Webber, 2011) at the University of Iowa showed almost identical findings. This technology along with two other advanced array microphone techniques are compared later in this chapter in a real world setting.

As we noted earlier, one manufacturer has advocated an asymmetric microphone configuration. Speech recognition in noise outcomes for asymmetric fittings have been mixed. For adults with mild-to-moderate hearing loss, some investigators have found that asymmetric fittings can result in as much directional benefit as a symmetric directional fitting (Bentler et al. 2004; Kim & Bryan, 2011). Other studies have found asymmetric fittings provided 1.5 to 2 dB less directional benefit than symmetric fittings in adults and children with mild-to-moderate hearing loss (Hornsby & Ricketts, 2007; Ricketts & Picou, 2013). Listeners with severe hearing loss have shown equal speech recognition benefits from symmetric and asymmetric directional microphone configurations (Picou & Ricketts, 2017). In addition to degree of hearing loss, the test environments also differed across the studies completed to date. We speculate based on these findings that additional speech recognition benefits for symmetric directional fittings over their asymmetric counterparts may be limited to adults and children with mild-to-moderate hearing loss in particularly difficult listening situations, including those with moderate or higher reverberation.

Increasing the DI through the use of higher order microphone arrays also increases the magnitude of benefit. Both fixed and adaptive bilateral beamformers have been shown to provide an additional 1 to 2 dB SNR-50 advantage compared to traditional directional microphones for a wide range of hearing losses in environments for which the noise surrounds the listener. Research at Vanderbilt University revealed that this 2 dB advantage over adaptive directional technology also was present for individuals with severe hearing loss (Powers & Littmann, 2016). This benefit also is not limited to the BTE form factor. Further Vanderbilt research showed the same 2 dB advantage over adaptive directional when beamforming was used in the ITC hearing aid style (Froelich & Powers, 2015). In this latter study, results also revealed that when hearing impaired users were fitted with beamforming instruments, their speech recognition in background noise was significantly superior to that of a group of individuals with normal hearing. This same finding has been found in two other studies (see report of Froehlich, Freels, & Powers, 2015). As expected given these SNR-50 results, significant improvements in percent correct speech recognition have also been shown for bilateral beamformers, particularly in difficult reverberant environments (Figure 11–14; Picou, Aspell, & Ricketts, 2014).

The original bilateral beamformers implemented a fixed pattern and were generally optimized for conditions for which noise surrounded the listener. Con-

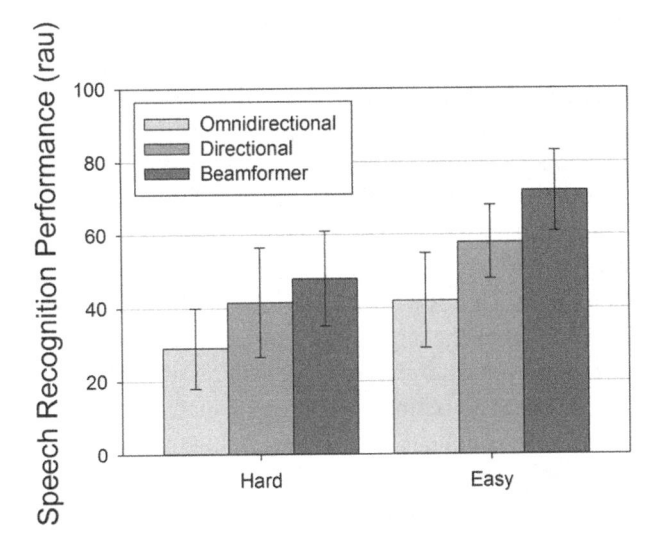

Figure 11–14. Speech recognition performance measured using the CST for three different microphone technologies measured in two environments.

loss (Picou & Ricketts, 2017). Further, there was no difference between the listening effort measured across the directional and bilateral beamformer settings. This suggests that the additional speech recognition in noise benefits associated with bilateral beamforming are not at the cost of increased listening effort measured via dual task paradigms.

Subjective Benefit

In comparison to the large number of investigations that have examined directional and bilateral beamforming technologies in the laboratory, relatively few studies have examined subjective benefit in the real world. Furthermore, automatically activated directional processing is now commonplace in the vast majority of hearing aids dispensed, whereas most studies examining subjective benefit were completed several years ago when manually activated directional processing was commonplace. Unlike the large and clear speech recognition benefits demonstrated in the lab, formalized self-assessment studies of directional benefit have demonstrated more limited support. For example, Valente, Potts, Valente, and Goebel (1995) measured hearing aid benefit using the PHAB and APHAB in 50 listeners who had been fit with directional hearing aids and compared the benefit to normative data. The authors reported better PHAB scores for the directional hearing aids on the background noise (BN) and reduced cues (RC) subscales at one site, and better APHAB scores on the BN and aversiveness (AV) subscales at the other site. Additionally, the authors reported a general preference for the directional hearing aids as compared to the participants' current omnidirectional hearing aids at one of the two experimental sites. In a more direct comparison, Walden et al. (2000) compared, omnidirectional, directional, and noise reduction in combination with directional user memories in 40 hearing aid wearers during a six- to nine-week evaluation period. Despite a large speech recognition in noise advantage, there were no significant differences on the PHAB across the user memories. One issue with many of these studies was that noisy situations, for which both directional advantages (talker front) and directional decrements (e.g., talker behind) would be expected, were included within the same subscale of the standardized measures used. Ricketts, Henry, and Gnewikow (2003) demonstrated that significant subjective directional benefit could be

sequently, little or no speech recognition benefit was measured for conditions in which there was only noise from the side (around 90° and/or 270°). Indeed, speech recognition performance in noise arriving from only the side for a fixed bilateral beamformer was significantly poorer than that achieved with an adaptive unilateral beamformer (adaptive directional microphone). More recently, adaptive bilateral beamformers have been introduced. These adaptive systems have the advantage of not only providing additional benefit for listeners surrounded by noise, but also providing similar benefits to unilateral beamformers in environments where noise only arrives from the sides.

Listening Effort

In addition to improved speech recognition performance, microphone-based technologies have the potential to decrease listening effort because performance is improved. Alternatively, introduction of distortion, such as that measured for the interaural difference cues, could offset other advantages and increase listening effort. Fortunately, recent data has shown both directional and bilateral beamformer technologies can reduce behavioral and subjective listening effort in comparison to the omnidirectional setting both in listeners with moderate (Picou, Moore, & Ricketts, 2017; Mejia, Carter, Dillon, & Littmann, 2017) and severe hearing measured through the use of a subscale that focused questions specifically on talker front in noise listening situations. Wu and Bentler (2010b) further demonstrated that microphone setting preference was affected by the specific listening situation. Moreover, even in situations that patients identified as having noise that was louder than the speech, the directional setting was only preferred approximately 20% of the time. In these same environments, approximately 60% of the preferences reported were for the omnidirectional setting with no preference in the remaining 20%. Together these data suggest the directional setting is only preferred in some portion of noisy environments. In addition, individual differences in preference for microphone setting is expected based on the emerging data we'll soon discuss.

Factors That May Affect Directional Effectiveness

Can the specific listening environment affect benefits? Are there choices made during selection and fitting that can affect benefits? Understanding the answers to these questions not only help ensure the best counseling relative to use and expectations in provided but also inform us clinically as we weigh potential benefits and limitations against other fitting decisions.

Physical Orientation

As we describe in Chapter 10, directional microphones and bilateral beamformers are most sensitive to sounds in the front and can generate nulls of greatly reduced sensitivity to the sides and back. Consequently, we counsel patients that they can optimize performance in noisy environments by "pointing their nose where they want to listen," and, if there is a concentrated noise source, "try to get it behind you." Distance and reverberation can also affect benefit in noise. We discuss reverberation time and critical distance in Chapter 4. Remember that the benefit from directional hearing aids and bilateral beamformers is based on the angle from which the sound and noise arrive (e.g., speech from the front and noise surrounding/behind). In a reverberant room this does not necessarily correspond to the same angle from which these signals originated, however, particularly if they are far away. The speech of interest as well as competing sounds will be made up of both direct energy arriving from the angle of origin and reflected energy arriving from a number of angles after bouncing off the floor, walls, and ceiling. By definition, increases in directivity index can be viewed as decreasing the level of the diffuse field (reflected energy) as well as direct energy arriving off-axis. Consider a noisy, highly reverberant room. If the talker of interest is close (inside the critical distance), direct energy from this source dominates, and the directional benefit provided is similar to that measured when there is much less reverberation. Once the talker is well outside the critical distance, however, energy from the talker is dominated by the reflected portions and the benefit provided by directional microphones and bilateral beamformers will be greatly reduced (Ricketts & Hornsby, 2003). If this seems complicated, think of it as the talker energy arriving from all around and the noise energy also arriving from all around, so turning down the energy from behind no longer helps. The greater the reverberation, the closer the patient needs to get to the talker, an important counseling point. Getting closer to the sound source will not only improve the SNR and speech recognition in noise in general, based on distance and reverberation effects, it will also improve the benefit provided by unilateral and bilateral beamformers.

Microphone Port Orientation

Another factor that can affect how much benefit a patient receives is microphone port orientation (Rick-

---

THINGS TO REMEMBER: FACTORS THAT INTERACT WITH DIRECTIONAL AND BILATERAL BEAMFORMER PROCESSING

- Physical orientation
- Microphone port orientation
- Venting
- Gain "equalization"
- Localization and monitoring

etts, 2000a). Making sure the microphone ports are in the intended orientation (typically horizontal or near horizontal) is necessary to maintain the desired external delay. Remember from Chapter 10 that the relationship between external delay (sound travel time difference to the microphone ports) and the designed internal delay generates the intended attenuation pattern. Deviation from the horizontal plane can occur with ITE hearing aid fittings if the ear impression is not appropriately marked (most manufacturers provide a preferred method for doing this) or if the manufacturer is not able to orient the microphone ports appropriately due to the constraints of an individual's ear geometry. Fortunately, most manufacturers will now contact you if ear geometry forces an orientation that is outside their predefined standards.

Port deviation from the optimal plane can occur in BTE and mini-BTE hearing aids because microphone port angle is affected by the length of the tubing (BTE, RITA) or receiver wire (RIC). Ricketts (2000a) reported that placement of the case of a BTE hearing aid so that it is in contact with the back of the pinna over the entire length of the hearing aid can result in a microphone port orientation that deviates from the horizontal plane by as much as 24 degrees. Since this finding we have seen the emergence of BTE and mini-BTE hearing aid designs that consider the actual average angle on the ear, rather than calculating external delay based on port spacing. We have also seen a number of interesting case designs in mini-BTE instruments that have the goal of raising the rear microphone opening to more closely approach horizontal (Figure 11–15). Based on the work to date a few important clinical considerations are offered:

- Small deviations from the optimal plane (approximately +/−10°) do not significantly impact DI for either BTE or ITE style instruments.
- Deviations of approximately +/− 20° from horizontal significantly reduce directivity by up to approximately 1 dB; however, the DI even in the worst conditions is still greater than for omnidirectional.
- BTE and mini-BTEs, directivity can be reduced up to approximately an additional 1 dB when the close proximity of the microphone ports to the helix of the pinna creates "sound shadow." In other words, tucking the instrument too far behind the ear to improve cosmetics can reduce benefit.
- On-ear directivity measures can be useful to get an idea how/if port orientation is affecting directivity on an individual patient (see Chapter 17).
- Particularly for BTEs and in a few mini-BTEs, the patient may find the position that provides maximal directivity is either uncomfortable or reduces retention. Consequently, on-ear directivity measures are not intended to aid in optimal placement. We are not going to send the patient out the door with an ill-fitting instrument! Rather, they are intended

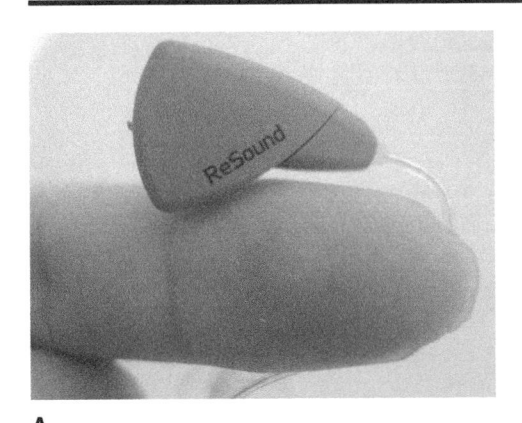

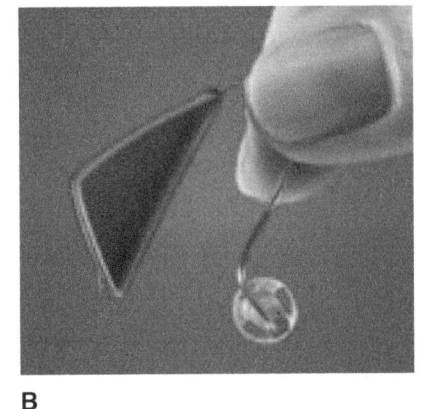

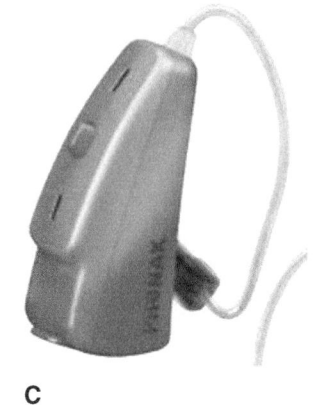

A B C

Figure 11–15. Creative mini-BTE designs aimed at improve microphone port orientation for directional processing.

to provide information about the potential reduction in speech recognition in noise benefit when the instrument is appropriately fitted to an individual's ear.

Venting

Increasing venting also can greatly reduce directivity, particularly in the low frequencies. The data shown in Figure 11–16 were collected using a full shell, acrylic earmold with no venting and #13 tubing without an earmold for the comparison (open fit) condition. As you can see from the figure, going from no venting to an open fit decreases directivity (AI-DI) by 40%. When we consider modern mini-BTE hearing aids that are often fit open and have very small, cosmetically appealing cases that are sometimes tucked behind the ear, it is not surprising that average directivity is about half of what is measured in traditional BTE and ITE instruments with less than 2 mm venting (Figure 11–17). Given these data it is not surprising that speech recognition performance in noise for open fit mini-BTE instruments has been shown to be approximately 1 to 2 dB poorer than for devices with more limited venting (Magnusson, Claesson, Persson, & Tengstrand, 2013; Valente & Mispagel, 2008). Whereas some studies have suggested very little reduction in benefit when increasing venting in specific products, it is nonetheless important to recognize that the amount of reduction will be dependent on frequency-specific DI. For example, an instrument with DI values in the low frequencies near zero (ineffective directional microphone in the low frequencies) when fitted closed may have no reduction in directional benefit with increased venting. The lack of decrease, however, is not because the directivity was somehow preserved, but because there was no directional benefit in the low frequencies to begin with—so nothing could be lost!

Importantly, a 1 to 2 dB reduction in speech in noise performance also occurs when open fittings are used

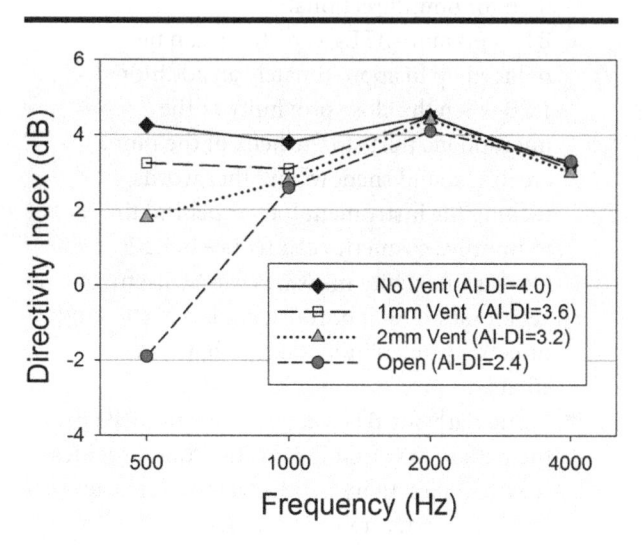

Figure 11–16. Changes in low frequency DI and AI-DI as a function of venting in BTE instruments. (Adapted from Ricketts, 2000a.)

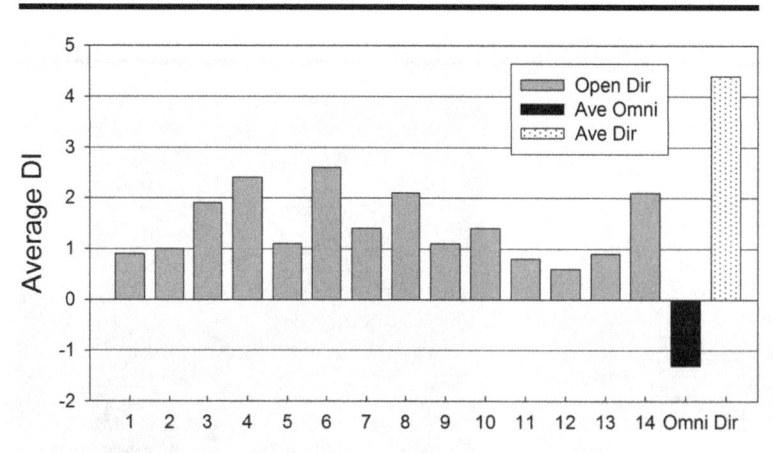

Figure 11–17. Average DI for 14 commercial open mini-BTE hearing aids in comparison to average omnidirectional and directional in three models with limited venting.

with wireless microphones, including FM systems. Are we suggesting using very small vents when they are not needed for other purposes? Not at all. There are considerable benefits to open fittings, as we detail in Chapter 8. However, with many mini-BTE instruments, it is possible to use a "closed" eartip to increase microphone array and remote microphone benefits while maintaining many of the benefits of a fully open fitting, including greatly reduced occlusion effect because of considerable residual slit-leak venting. Consideration of the tradeoffs in speech recognition in noise benefits relative to the magnitude of venting and its associated benefits is important, particularly for listeners who struggle the most communicating in noise.

Gain Equalization

As we describe in Chapter 10, one byproduct of activating directional or bilateral beamforming is decreased microphone sensitivity in the low frequencies. Gain equalization, the act of offsetting this decreased sensitivity with increased low-frequency gain, can eliminate loss of audibility. This equalization will also increase the likelihood that patients with relatively good low-frequency hearing will hear microphone noise, however, and increase the possibility that patients with deep voices and limited venting will complain about their own voice quality (e.g., boomy-ness) due to the proximity effect. Based on measured and calculated effects on audibility previously reported (Ricketts & Henry, 2002) we therefore recommend beginning to offset lost audibility through directional equalization for individuals that have low-frequency thresholds poorer than about 35 to 40 dB HL. Gain equalization is not necessary for those with less hearing loss because calculated audibility will not be significantly affected. For listeners with more severe-to-profound hearing loss, however, equalization is required to avoid decreased speech recognition in noise performance due to decreased audibility. With equalization, these listeners may also experience poor voice quality due to the proximity effect, and therefore counseling will often be warranted. Explaining that their boomy voice quality is not being heard by others, and that decreasing low-frequency gain to improve the artifact is likely to decrease audibility for other talkers, can be helpful. Usually a combination of counseling and partial directional equalization will provide an acceptable solution.

Localization and Monitoring

Another consideration when fitting remote microphones and microphone arrays are the potential effects on localization and monitoring. We previously discussed how decisions regarding activation of the hearing aid microphones in tandem with the remote microphone interact with monitoring and the magnitude of benefits. The directional setting can limit the patient's ability to monitor or understand speech and other sounds that are behind him or her, particularly in patients with the most hearing loss or only some difficulty understanding speech. Higher order beamforming can make it even more difficult to monitor off-axis sounds. In extreme cases "tunnel hearing" is reported by some listeners (Mejia et al., 2015). This complaint has generally been associated with high-order beamformers (e.g., fourth order and higher) and not the bilateral beamformers currently available in commercial hearing aids. In patients with less hearing loss, the activation of a microphone array in a quiet setting might make the hearing aid sound "noisy," see Chapter 10. In total, if speech recognition ability is acceptable to the listener because the noise level is low enough, the omnidirectional setting is often preferred since in addition to decreased microphone noise, monitoring off-axis sounds will be much easier than when using a microphone array for many listeners with limited audibility.

Another microphone array distortion is of the inter-aural difference cues that are important for localization. Research has demonstrated that ILD cues are distorted slightly by directional processing and both ILD and ITD cues may be distorted by bilateral beamforming (Figure 11–18; Picou et al., 2014). From this figure we can see that the ILD deviates from normal in that it stops increasing beyond 60 degrees for the slightly directional and adaptive directional processing that was evaluated in this study. The ILD for the bilateral beamformer deviates from normal beyond 30 degrees. In addition, while ITDs were not distorted for the slightly directional and adaptive directional processing, the bilateral beamformer processing resulted in an ITD of 0 degrees, regardless of angle. The actual interuaral distortion effects observed depends on the specific design. Therefore, the pattern of distortion in some systems is different than described here. However, all bilateral beamformers we have evaluated to date result in much greater interaural cue distortions than observed for unilateral beamformers.

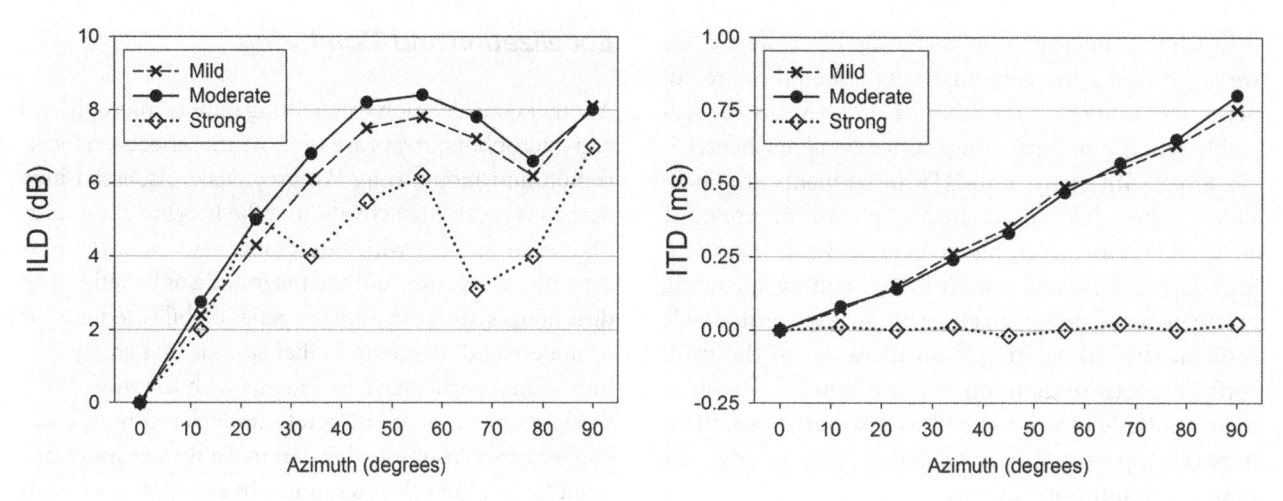

Figure 11–18. Interaural cue preservation in one hearing aid model using slightly directional, adaptive directional, and beamformer processing.

Given this interaurual cue distortion, it is not surprising that decreased horizontal localization performance has been reported for both directional microphones (Keidser et al., 2006; Van den Bogaert et al., 2006) and bilateral beamformers (Van den Bogaert, Doclo, Wouters, & Moonen, 2008). Localization difficulties when fitted with first order microphone arrays tend to be fairly limited in magnitude, however, and typically only occur at the sides (approximately 70–110 degrees). In addition, improvements in front-to-back reversals are found for this first order setting in comparison to the omnidirectional setting, so in total we expect little, if any, localization decrements for listeners out in the real world when using directional technologies. Conversely, localization distortions for bilateral beamformers are much more pronounced. For example, reduced performance in a simple frontal hemifield localization task has been reported when visual cues were not available (Picou et al., 2014). Specifically, listeners were generally able to determine the correct quadrant of the source but sometimes selected a source position closer to midline than the accurate position. Despite these limitations, it is important to point out, that the same localization decrement (compared to a traditional, adaptive directional microphone setting) was not present when visual cues were available—we assume that when having a conversation at a dinner table in a noisy restaurant, most people have their eyes open! More importantly, a very limited, 20- to 30-minute real world trial revealed that more than two-thirds of hearing aid wearers preferred the bilateral beamformer over traditional, adaptive directional microphones. Furthermore, when the bilateral beamformer was not preferred, reasons given generally related to sound quality or loudness and not issues with localization.

Factors That Do Not Have a Significant Impact

A number of other issues have been evaluated that do not appear to significantly affect speech recognition in noise performance when using directional or bilateral beamformer technologies including (1) type of gain processing, (2) hearing aid style, (3) unilateral versus bilateral fitting, and (4) presence or absence of visual cues.

Since the gain processing (e.g., WDRC) used in the majority of current hearing aids varies gain as a function of input level, we might question whether this would affect directional benefit. Consider that sounds—including speech and noise—arrive at the directional microphone or bilateral beamformer from a number of angles at the same time, and then gain processing is applied to the total signal. The SNR at any instant in time is, therefore, not affected by the gain processing. If, in the real world, the signal of interest occurred during one instant in time, at one azimuth, and noise occurred during a different instant in time, at another azimuth (as is the case with the clinical directivity measures described in Chapters 13 and 17) there would be no need for directional microphones. We can think of microphone arrays as a type of "front end" processing that results in changes to the SNR prior to all other processing. Nearly all subsequent hearing aid processing has no effect whatsoever on the instantaneous SNR, and therefore will not affect the magnitude of benefits from these technologies, assuming equal audibility.

As we describe in Chapter 10, the average directivity provided by the directional processing in BTE, ITE, and ITC styles is fairly similar if the same venting is used. Therefore, speech recognition in noise is similar across styles, both when considering directional processing as well as the additional benefit provided by bilateral beamformers. Because the average DI measured for omnidirectional BTEs is significantly less than for omnidirectional ITEs/ITCs (because of pinna effects for the latter), studies report less directional benefit for custom instruments compared to BTEs, even though speech recognition in noise performance in the directional setting is typically similar (Pumford, Seewald, Scollie, & Jenstad, 2000; Ricketts, Lindley, & Henry, 2001). As the omnidirectional setting will typically be used in quiet and the directional setting in noise, real-world speech recognition performance is expected to be quite similar across BTE, mini-BTE, and ITE/ITC styles, assuming a well-designed directional microphone or bilateral beamformer is implemented.

A few studies have also examined potential interactions between bilateral fittings and directional benefit. Bilateral speech recognition advantages of 1.5 to 3.4 dB have been reported; however, the bilateral advantage was not significantly different for directional and omnidirectional conditions. That is, the same amount of directional benefit was present whether the patients were fit with one or two hearing aids (e.g., Henry & Ricketts, 2003). Clinically, this means we expect patients to receive similar benefits from microphone technologies regardless of whether they are fitted unilaterally or bilaterally. For patients fitted unilaterally it is important to remember that the angle of maximum sensitivity for most hearing aid styles using directional processing is approximately 30 to 45 degrees (not directly in front). Therefore, even though many patients will discover this on their own, it can sometimes be useful to counsel patients to turn their head slightly in noisy environments to improve speech recognition in noise. Data have shown this can provide about a 1 dB advantage for patients who wear a single hearing aid (Henry & Ricketts, 2003).

One limitation of many studies examining microphone array speech recognition in noise benefit is that they are typically completed without visual cues. Concerns about this limitation were highlighted by research demonstrating that, in realistic SNRs, the speech recognition performance of listeners using omnidirectional processing could approach maximum (ceiling performance) in a laboratory environment, essentially eliminating any possibility for directional benefit (Wu & Bentler, 2010). Fortunately, subsequent work has shown that when other realistic factors that limit performance (e.g., reverberation, poor speech understanding abilities) are introduced, significant directional and bilateral beamformer benefits are observed when visual cues are present, even at SNRs as favorable as +9 to +12 dB (Aspell, Picou, & Ricketts, 2014; Wu & Bentler, 2012).

Individualization of Microphone Technologies

As we detailed above, remote microphones, directional technologies and bilateral beamformers all significantly improve communication in noisy environments. Given the interactions between these technologies and an individual patient's listening needs and abilities, it seems likely that there is no "one size fits all" application and patients may benefit from some individualization when selecting and adjusting these technologies.

Despite clear benefits, the data to date suggest that at least some listeners prefer omnidirectional processing in many noisy listening environments, even though remote microphones, directional technologies, and bilateral beamformers will provide a significantly better SNR for the signal of interest. Recent work at Vanderbilt has shown a number of factors may contribute to this preference difference, including the individual patient's speech understanding in noise abilities, ability and need to monitor sounds in the environment, noise tolerance, and individual listening needs. The factor that is most important for selecting and adjusting these technologies is the relationship between the patients' listening in noise abilities and their listening needs.

We can illustrate this issue with a married couple we saw as patients several years ago. Mr. and Mrs. Carhart (Ray and June) have similar hearing losses and

POINTS TO PONDER: SUMMARY OF MICROPHONE TECHNOLOGY TRADEOFFS

	Wireless Microphones	Adaptive Directional Processing	Bilateral Beamformers
Clearest Benefits (with a few caveats)	Largest SNR improvement resulting in the best performance in noise for a single talker of interest. Not affected by source-to-listener distance and relative source position like the other technologies.	Best for spatial monitoring. Performance in noise is typically only 1 to 2 dB poorer than with bilateral beamformers.	Better speech in noise performance than traditional directional microphones, while still providing SNR improvement for multiple sources of interest based on head angle.
Important Limitations	Benefits typically limited to one source of interest or multiple known sources). While benefits decrease, monitoring is improved when hearing aid microphones are activated. Requires external device which can lead to embarrassment.	Less SNR improvement than the other two techniques. Can limit overhearing for sources from behind, although not as much as the bilateral beamformer.	Decreased localization when visual cues are not available. Can limit overhearing. Use can decrease hearing aid battery life (at least slightly).

are fitted with identical directional hearing aids. Clinical evaluation using the BKB-SIN showed that both were obtaining about 6 dB of directional benefit, so we know the instruments are working well. When they came to our office, they ended up completing the COSI together—not something we usually recommend, but this was a retired couple who indicated they do everything together. They indicated the most difficulties at the shopping mall and at weekly poker games. Results from a follow-up COSI after wearing the hearing aids were surprising at first. Ray reported good benefit at the shopping mall but no improvement at the poker game. In contrast, June says she still can't understand anything at the mall but gets a lot of help playing cards. After we look back at their *unaided* BKB-SIN scores though this makes sense. Ray's score was 0 dB SNR loss, whereas June had a 12.5 dB SNR loss. If we assume around a 10% change in performance for every 1 dB change in SNR, we can plot the performance/SNR function for both patients (Figure 11–19). (Note: Figure 11–19 is really just a rough estimate. Individual patients often do not have a smooth change in performance with changing SNR and, instead, can exhibit plateaus for which there are few or no changes in percent correct performance, even though the SNR changes by a couple of dB).

Let's also assume that the average SNR at the mall is about 0 dB and the average SNR at the card game is about +10 dB and show these on the same figure. Although 0 dB seems like a very adverse SNR for a mall, this is a very busy tourist mall in the Nashville area and, because June has a soft voice, it reaches 0 dB SNR, particularly on a Saturday. We can see that in the mall, Ray's performance improves from 50 to 85% when activating directional processing. He was near ceiling performance already at the card game and really doesn't need directional processing there. Something we missed by allowing them to fill out the COSI together! In contrast, when playing cards June's performance increases from 10 to 80%. Unfortunately, she is still can't understand at all while in the mall and a companion microphone is recommended in that setting to provide the needed improvement in SNR.

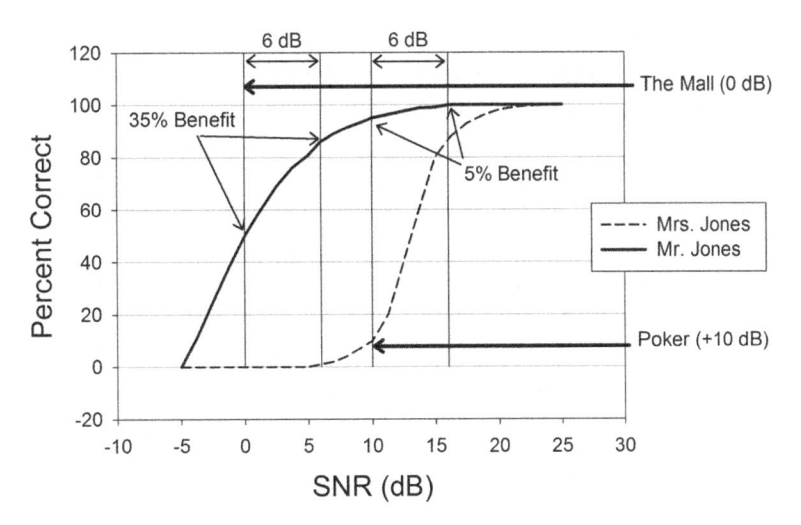

Figure 11–19. Individual patient differences effects on directional benefit as a function of SNR.

TECHNICAL TIP: CLINICAL FACTORS WHEN SELECTING AND ADJUSTING MICROPHONE TECHNOLOGIES

- Very good speech recognition in noise (e.g., SNR-50 <5 dB)? Probably prefer omnidirectional in all but the most difficult listening situations. Adjust directional switching to be the least aggressive possible.
  - Caveat: If there is very poor tolerance of noise (low ANL score), more aggressive settings are likely to be preferred.
- Very poor speech recognition in noise (e.g., SNR-50 > 12–15 dB)? Probably prefer aggressive directional switching. Likely prefer bilateral beamforming in more difficult conditions. May require remote microphone in the most difficult listening situations.
  - Caveat: If monitoring sounds outside the field of vision is important, a little less aggressive settings are likely to be preferred.
- Moderate speech recognition in noise abilities? Probably prefer moderately aggressive switching. However, preference likely to be affected by:
  - Good speech understanding for talkers outside the field of vision (less aggressive).
  - Poor tolerance for noise (more aggressive).

Situation-Specific Microphone Array Techniques

We have described a range of techniques that have been applied in an attempt to provide the most optimal microphone setting (omnidirectional to fully directional/beamforming) for a variety of complex environments. There also are advanced techniques that are aimed at further improving SNR in specific listening situations.

As we described earlier in this chapter, there are listening environments in which talkers of interest are in front of the listener. These include a wide range of group environments from cocktail parties to classrooms. In many of these environments, however, hearing off-axis is mainly important for monitoring purposes. Noisy environments—with the primary talker of interest behind or beside the listener—are less common, but certainly exist. For example, conversational partners, when watching

TV, typically do not face each other. We do not usually face each other while having a conversation walking down a street or while in a store shopping. Another common situation is driving; conversational partners are beside or behind the driver, who is surrounded by noise. Difficulties understanding speech while driving are exacerbated by the lack of visual cues. Use of visual cues for speech understanding while driving seems like a sure way to end up in an accident. Consequently, to improve speech understanding in these environments, it is of interest to either steer the direction of focus toward the primary talker and/or suppress noise from directions other than the talker of interest.

Technologies specifically designed for enhancing communication in these environments include (1) side suppression, (2) reverse directional, and (3) bilateral lobe steering. The benefits of these technologies have been demonstrated in a few laboratory studies including the reverse directional studies we mentioned earlier. In addition, the relative benefits of all three technologies were compared in an interesting study using recordings made in a vehicle in a real-world situation conducted by Wu, Stangl, Bentler and Stanziola in 2013. Specifically, sentence recognition (CST) was assessed based on signals recorded using a KEMAR, fitted with hearing aids implementing these three technologies and, seated in a van driving down Interstate 80 in Iowa. Sentences were presented from both the side and back. The background noise was the actual road noise of the vehicle. We will refer to these study results throughout this section.

Side suppression operates by reducing amplification for some frequencies of sound arriving from the opposite direction of the signal of interest when speech is identified as arriving from one side of the listener. This differs from traditional, adaptive directional hearing aids in that the two hearing aids work together by wirelessly sharing data, both to identify the talker direction and to suppress noise. Only data are shared between instruments; this is not a type of full-band signal sharing such as that used in bilateral beamformers and bilateral lobe steering. With side suppression, if the talker is in quiet, an omnidirectional pattern will typically be activated. If the talker is in the front and in noise, a typical directional pattern will be activated (Figure 11–20, top row shows an example). If the talker is on the right, the side suppression algorithm will place the null of the right hearing aid to the listeners left. At the same time, the side suppression algorithm will also place the null of the left

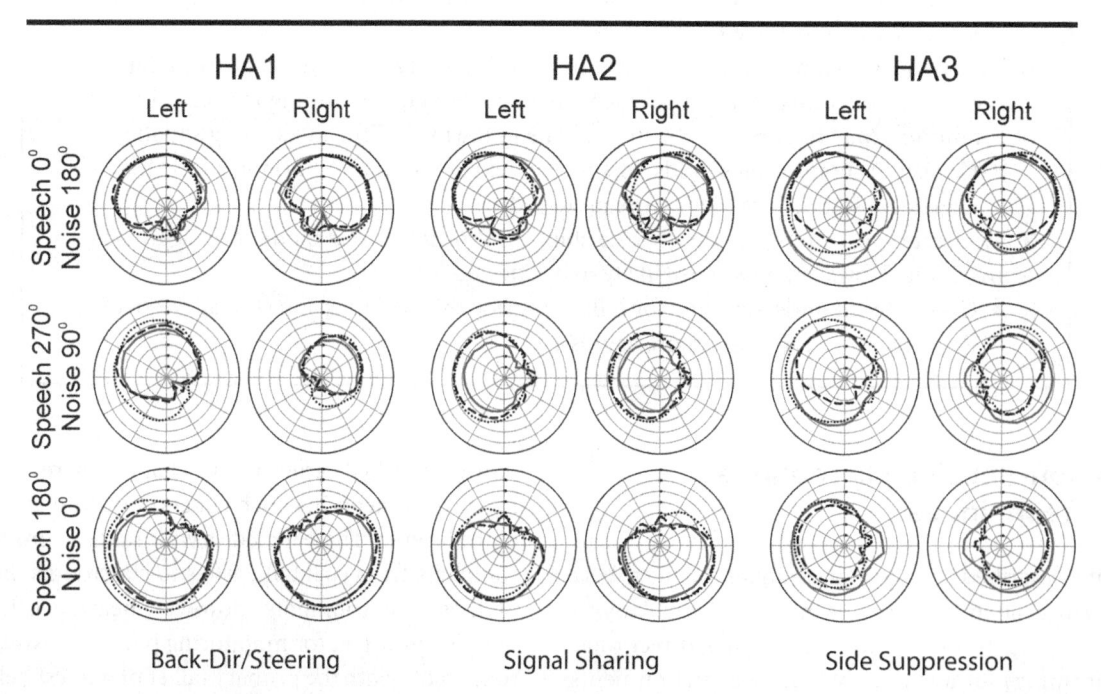

Figure 11–20. Polar patterns for three hearing aid technologies for listening while driving. (Adapted from Wu et al., 2013)

hearing aid to the left but may also reduce overall gain for the left instrument to further suppress signals arriving from the left (see Figure 11–20, middle row, for an example). As with all directional technology, side suppression works in a frequency-specific manner. Because low frequencies travel around objects easily due to their long wavelength, side suppression is most effective in the higher frequencies. In the commercial example we show in Figure 11–20, when the talker was identified as coming from the back, omnidirectional processing was activated. This is much preferred over activation of directional processing, which would occur in a traditional, automatic directional instrument because there is less suppression of the talker from behind. The data from Wu et al. (2013) support the effectiveness of this technology in the real world. Specifically, there was an approximately 10 and 20% improvement over directional and omnidirectional processing for speech presented from the side. When speech was presented from the back, side suppression did not provide an advantage over omnidirectional processing.

Two other technologies essentially steer the direction of focus and consequently are sometimes both referred to as "lobe steering." Reverse-directional technologies essentially flip the direction of focus of a traditional, unilateral beamformer. In other words, the nulls are placed in front of the listener and the direction of focus is steered behind. Essentially, the reverse-directional technologies work just like traditional, unilateral beamformers (directional microphones) except the assignment of "front" and "back" microphones are reversed. Current versions of reverse-directional technologies can be activated manually or automatically whenever the highest level talker is identified in the rear hemisphere. When the highest level talker is in the front hemisphere, the direction of focus is flipped back to the front and the hearing aids operate like traditional, adaptive directional instruments (see Figure 11–20, top row). In the commercial example we show in Figure 11–20, when the talker was identified as coming from the left, slightly less directional processing was activated in the left instrument, and gain was reduced for the right instrument. The data from Wu et al. (2013) support the effectiveness of this technology in the real world. Specifically, there was an approximately 30% and 15% improvement over directional and omnidirectional processing for speech presented from the back. Since a traditional, automatic system would typically activate directional processing in this environment, the identified benefits are quite clear. When speech was presented from the side, reverse directional suppression did not provide an advantage over omnidirectional processing.

Bilateral lobe-steering technologies typically operate like traditional and reverse directional instruments when the highest level speech signal is from the front and back, respectively (see the top and bottom rows of Figure 11–20). When the speech is from the side, however, a different strategy is used. First, data shared wirelessly between the hearing aids are used to modify the directivity pattern of the unilateral beamformer nearest the speech signal (better SNR) to focus toward the speech and minimize the noise as much as possible. Then the resulting signal is wirelessly transmitted to the other hearing aid, much as is done with a wireless BiCROS—except in this case, the same optimized signal is then delivered to both ears at the same time. This effect can be visualized in the middle row of Figure 11–20, which reveals identical directivity configurations in both bilateral lobe steering hearing aids. The data from Wu et al. (2013) support the effectiveness of this technology in the real world. Similar to the reverse directional technology, there was an approximately 30% and 15% improvement over directional and omnidirectional processing for speech presented from the back. In addition, there was an approximately 35% and 20% improvement over directional and omnidirectional processing for speech presented from the side.

Difficulty understanding speech in a vehicle is reported by many patients. Data suggests that all three of the technologies described above have the potential to improve understanding in some specific situations including listening in a car. Because some technologies only improve speech recognition for speech from the front and either only for speech from behind (reverse directional) *or* from the side (side suppression), it is important to know where talkers are relative to the individual in his or her typical vehicle environment prior to selecting the technology. In this case, you are selecting a manufacturer when you are selecting a technology, as each of these three technologies are specific to certain manufacturers. In addition, with automatic implementation of these technologies, it is particularly important to counsel patients on operation and understand their listening needs. For example, in a noisy restaurant the highest level talker might be at a table behind the hearing aid wearer. In this case, the reverse directional may focus on a talker who is "noise" and reduce sensitivity for the talkers of interest at the listener's table. If this error is a possibility for a patient, it may be worthwhile to have a dedicated "car" user program and remove this type of processing from the general use program, which is the approach taken by many audiologists.

Summary

Although there is typically no effect on speech recognition in noise, DNR can improve the total listening experience by improving sound quality, enhancing listening effort, and reducing annoyance for a number of specific noise types. Conversely, remote microphones, directional hearing aids, and bilateral beamformers represent some of the only hearing aid technologies that have been shown to improve SNR consistently for listeners across a wide range of environments. Data supporting the use of these technologies to aid the speech understanding of listeners with hearing loss in noisy situations are overwhelmingly positive. It is equally clear, however, that a number of factors can affect directivity and benefit. Due to individual differences, some patients may not achieve significant benefit. Venting and the orientation of the microphone ports are known to reduce directivity. In addition, benefit may be much more limited in some environments, especially those with high reverberation and large speaker-to-listener distances. In some situations, such as listening to talkers who are not in front of the hearing aid wearer, directional microphones and bilateral beamformers may be undesirable or even detrimental. Despite these limitations, it seems clear that the use of sound cleaning technologies, combined with appropriate adjustment, counseling and expectations, can lead to increased speech understanding in noise, decreased listening effort, increased hearing aid satisfaction, and an overall improvement in the total listening experience for many listeners with hearing impairment.

12
More Hearing Aid Features and Algorithms

Hearing aid design has always had the goal of addressing the listening needs of individuals with hearing loss. As we discuss throughout this text, the most basic need is the loss of audibility due to each individual's hearing loss, which is offset by selectively increasing sound level. We will detail the current rationales for achieving this goal in Chapter 14. The second most common complaint relates to listening in noise and we describe technologies aimed at decreasing the negative effects of noise in the previous chapter. In this chapter, we describe other important areas, the wide range of hearing aid features aimed at addressing other listening needs, at overcoming specific hearing aid limitations, or aimed at counteracting the negative side effects of other processing. Understanding these features in some detail can improve clinical practice in several ways. Although we discuss "selecting" features in this chapter, it is important to note that many of these features will be available with all, or nearly all, models. We believe it is still important to discuss these features from a selection standpoint for at least two clinical reasons. First, it is imperative that we understand the potential benefits and limitations of each hearing aid feature that we fit if we are to counsel patients appropriately with respect to use and expectations. For example, if a patient expects the DNR technology we describe in the last chapter to "move that background noise off into the distance," as some manufacturers advertised in the early days of this technology, we need to make sure the patient doesn't also expect improved speech recognition because DNR is generally not capable of such a feat. In some cases, we may even disable specific features because interactions with the patient or the environments they are in may result in negative consequences that outweigh the positive attributes that are intended. In addition, many features provide the clinician with adjustment options (e.g., different strengths or aggressiveness). We must therefore understand the technology in order to adjust each feature in the best way for the individual patient's communication needs.

Manufacturers have a myriad of proprietary names for their signal transmission and modification features. Sometimes these names are intended to differentiate an algorithm from others based on specific parameters. At other times, however, a manufacturer will change the name of a feature when it is introduced in a new model for marketing purposes, even if the underlying algorithm really hasn't changed at all. These practices and the desire to differentiate one hearing aid model from another have led to a dizzying array of names for algorithms. To cut through the confusion that this may create, we will offer a limited number of categories of patient goals and then describe the general benefits and limitations of each feature aimed at addressing each goal. We will also discuss manufacturer differences in implementation of features, particularly when data demonstrate that those differences can affect patient outcomes.

> **THINGS TO REMEMBER: GOALS AND THE SPECIFIC FEATURES THAT ADDRESS THEM**
>
> - Quantifying patient behaviors and allowing for-patient directed individualization
>   - Data logging
>   - Automatic gain increase (AGI)
>   - Output learning via volume control
> - Overcoming traditional hearing aid limitations
>   - Digital feedback suppression (DFS)
>   - Bilateral data sharing for feature and hearing aid control
>   - Wireless streaming
>   - Smartphone integration and telephone listening
> - Signal modification for specific listening needs
>   - Selective speech enhancement
>   - Extended high-frequency amplification
>   - Frequency-lowering technologies (frequency compression, frequency transposition, frequency fill)
>   - Tinnitus masking
> - Targeted hearing aid interventions
>   - Light actuated amplification
>   - Extended wear technologies

Quantifying Patient Behaviors and Allowing for Patient-Directed Individualization

Data Logging

In Chapter 11 we discuss the operation of signal classification schemes and how they can differ across manufacturers. The classifier information is not only used in conjunction with decision rules to affect hearing aid operation, it is also typically stored in the hearing aid memory along with a range of other information. This information storage feature is generally referred to as data logging. This feature allows the hearing aid to store information concerning hearing aid use, listening situations encountered by the user, and the degree and frequency of changes in user gain and user memories. This information can be downloaded into the fitting software. The first commercially available hearing aid with a data logging feature was the 3M Memory-mate™, first marketed in the late 1980s. This product had eight memories, and it used data logging to record how often each memory was accessed and for how long each memory was used. When this product disappeared from the market we didn't think too much about data logging until it was re-introduced in modern digital hearing aids. Since around 2000, many hearing aids have included data logging. The additional information stored typically includes some information about the amount of time the hearing aid is on per day, percent of time the various features (e.g., noise reduction, directional microphone) are activated, the use of any manual programs, as well as information regarding user changes to the volume control.

Data logging provides a useful review of the actions of the classification system. For example, if the hearing aid has six different classifications such as quiet, speech in quiet, speech in noise, noise, music, and car, the audiologist easily can review what percent of the time each one of these situations were classified for a given patient. Since the classifier also aims to describe the auditory input, it can also estimate the type and distribution of various auditory inputs. Consequently, data logging systems may provide the clinician with information ranging from the number of hours the user was wearing the hearing aid each day, to the estimated percent of time spent in quiet listening environments, or even the average level of the incoming signal for a given period of time. Although studies have shown that signal classification is not perfectly accurate, it has improved considerably over the years. Indeed, the most sophisticated systems can even correctly identify music at a very high rate of accuracy, at least for many of the most popular genres. One manufacturer decision that can affect the accuracy realized is the definition of quiet. For example, based on the desired processing, a manufacturer may identify soft speech in a background of low level noise as "Speech in Quiet." This is often not a limitation of the classifier, but instead a conscious decision; however, we need to be aware of such decisions when discussing environments with patients.

There are a several important uses for data logging information: counseling during the follow-up visits ("*You don't seem to be using your hearing aid as much as you thought you would." "You report your daughter wears the hearing aid all day at middle school, but the data logger shows an average use of 2 hours a day."*), troubleshooting patient complaints and adjusting features (*"The data logger shows you spend a lot of time in noisy environments and you indicate you are still bothered by how loud the noise is. Let's turn up the noise reduction effect."*). The potential utility of data logging is affected by at least four factors: (1) the specific patient issue, (2) the quality of data logging information, (3) avoiding overreliance on the accuracy of data logging information, and (4) the willingness of the dispenser to access and use this feature.

Indeed, even though data logging is available in the majority of modern hearing aids, not all audiologists use this feature. We're not certain of current data, but things probably haven't changed much since a Mueller (2007) survey when the use rate was only about 40% (interestingly, significantly more so for female audiologists than male audiologists—we'll let you draw your own conclusions on that one).

Even though we know the data log may not be terribly useful for every patient, a quick check, particularly for newer users and children can often be illuminating. If nothing stands out in the data log, checking only took a few seconds. Due to imperfect accuracy, the data log is often best used in conjunction with counseling. The data log from one patient we had a few years ago indicated he or she spent considerable amount of the day in a "speech in noise" environment. This seemed curious because the patient had not mentioned it previously. Through conversations, however, we determined that the classifier was likely wrongly classifying music as speech in noise. Had we relied on the log as being perfectly accurate, we might have mistakenly activated an aggressive DNR, something that we expect would have made this musician a very unhappy patient. One other common mistake is to assume that usage is always accurately represented. A clever child avoiding using his or her hearing aid can turn it on and stuff it in a gym bag. An elderly patient might forget to turn the aids off at night. Just because the hearing aids are on does not necessarily mean they are being worn!

The patient issue for which we have found data logging useful most often is usage, particularly in children, although usage information can also be useful in adult listeners, particularly some of our more elderly patients. Indeed, we saw a patient who seemed very happy when she left the office, but then reported limited benefit at a six-week follow-up appointment. She brought the hearing aids into our office in a box with the batteries removed. Data logging revealed very limited use time despite the fact that she reported wearing them "all the time." Further counseling and demonstration revealed that she had been inserting the batteries upside down and the hearing aids had not actually been active since the first set of batteries had died after about two weeks. This case also reveals an issue with the quality of information from some data loggers. The majority calculate use time by taking the total time since last connected for programming and dividing by the number of days. In the case of this patient, all we had was a report of a low number of hours of use per day. Data indicating full time use for two weeks, followed by no use for four weeks would have been more illuminating, but we were able to figure this information out through counseling.

As we alluded to above, use time can be a good conversation starter when discussing usage in children. For example, Gustafson et al. (2017) compared estimates by parents and teachers of use to data logs for 13 seven-to-ten-year-old children. In agreement with similar studies, parents overestimated hearing aid use by about one hour per day. Interestingly, parent's estimates of usage in the classroom were fairly accurate and in some cases overestimation of use could be directly attributed to instances outside of school. One large discrepancy in use time led to a discussion with the parent that revealed that the family had recently taken several vacations during which hearing aid use was not enforced. This led to fruitful discussion with the parents about the importance of hearing aid use during leisure time. Again, having time-stamped use time would have made this issue easier to identify, but it was discovered nonetheless through counseling in combination with available data logging information.

Automatic Gain Increase Algorithms

Most practicing audiologists who routinely fit to prescriptive targets have encountered patients who are not happy with the gain and output provided, which is, of course, expected given that they are targets for the "average" person. Often, new hearing aid patients' complaints center on the fact that there is too much gain. Probably all of us have used the counseling technique that goes something like this: "You will get used to it in no time. You are just used to living in a quiet world. You're really just hearing what all of us with normal hearing commonly hear." We talked about this earlier in the section on adaptation to loudness. Some patients, however, do not "get used to it" and simply stop using their hearing aids or return them for a refund during the trial period.

A possible solution is to automatically gradually increase gain over time. This approach is based on the notion that, if we introduce something gradually, it will be more acceptable than if we introduce it all at once. Manufacturers have marketing terms for algorithms that increase gain incrementally and automatically and, like most terms used in hearing aid marketing, some make sense and others do not. We simply refer to these algorithms as automatic gain increase (AGI) because that is essentially what happens.

AGI differs from the patient-trainable approach that we discuss in detail later. With traditional patient-trainable hearing aids, you program to a validated prescription that is close to what you believe is best but then allow the patient to fine-tune the fitting to be louder or softer depending on his or her preferred listening level. For AGI, the audiologist makes a determination as to what he or she thinks is best and then programs the hearing aid to less gain. Then the AGI is programmed to automatically increase gain gradually over weeks or months so that, at the end of this training, the gain is at the level that was initially desired (by the audiologist, not the patient).

Potential Advantages of AGI

Some new hearing aid users seem to be gain-shy, and it is pretty obvious on the day of the fitting that they are not willing to use the gain that seems to be appropriate. Although you might feel guilty sending them out the door with the gain that they desire, you also sense that if you were to send them out with the correct gain, they may never wear their hearing aids. AGI is a reasonable compromise. It allows the audiologist to initially program hearing aids at a level below what is desired but at a level that is acceptable to the patient. Then depending on where you want your final gain to be, you can set the AGI to increase the gain in small increments. For example, if you start 8 dB below the desired setting, you can program a 1 dB/week increase over the next two months.

Here is a fitting tip: Before you send the patient out the door, be sure that the final gain destination will not create a feedback problem. This is relatively easy in most products if you are completing probe microphone verification of a validated prescriptive target, because you fit to desired targets and then activate the AGI scheme that begins by decreasing gain from those final targets.

Some audiologists use this feature with hearing aids that have active volume control adjustments. In our opinion though, it makes more sense to deactivate the volume control during this initial gain-increase period. After the period is over, the volume control can be reactivated, perhaps even in conjunction with a trainable algorithm. If patients have control of the gain, they may reduce gain without giving themselves a chance to get used to the higher sound levels that were automatically introduced.

The data supporting the use of AGI is sparse. We propose that the utility of the feature depends not only on the specific patient but also on the clinician. If you typically counsel patients in such a way that they accept the prescribed gain after a period of adjustment with good success, AGI may be useful for only a small number of patients. On the other hand, if your clinical style is to start with lower gain levels and help the patient adjust up over time, you may find AGI a very useful feature for the majority of new hearing aid wearers. In either case, it is likely that this feature is not particularly useful for experienced hearing aid wearers because they are already used to amplified sound levels, unless they have been under-fit in the past.

Trainable Hearing Aids

As technology advanced, it was recognized that data logging information could be used to alter the hearing aid fitting, which leads us to what we now call *trainable hearing aids*. In fairly simple terms, the hearing aid can "remember" what user adjustments are made or are in use at a given time through the data log. Over time, gain will be altered from the original programming to the desired settings of the patient when the hearing aid is first turned on. We should mention that this does not have to happen automatically. In some products, the hearing aid can be programmed to simply store the new settings, and audiologists can then decide whether the learning settings should be implemented.

The key to the effectiveness of this process is that the user has to make an adjustment to the volume in order for the hearing aid to collect useful information regarding desired changes to the original fitting. Some products collect data that allow for the training of gain, the frequency response—particularly the high frequencies—and some products also allow for training of the strength of the noise reduction or other special features. In conjunction with the signal-classification system, these training-related data sets can be categorized as a function of the listening environment. That is, totally independent training can be implemented for speech in quiet, speech in background noise, music, and so on. This type of logging can either be time-based or event-based, depending on the company or products that you are using (see related Technical Tip).

Whether the training is time-based or event-based, the hearing aid is recording three critical pieces of information that potentially can be used to alter the original hearing aid settings:

- The *acoustic listening environment* as identified by the sound classifier. Was the patient listening to speech in quiet? In background noise? Was the signal simply noise with no speech present? Some models of hearing aids conduct independent training for five or more different listening environments.
- The *intensity of the input signal*. It is important for today's products to train independently for different input signals, sometimes referred to as *compression training,* rather than just train overall gain. We consider this approach desirable because it's very possible that many patients will want to alter gain for soft inputs differently from gain for loud inputs.

KEY CONCEPT: TRAINING HEARING AIDS—TIME- OR EVENT-BASED?

Trainable hearing aids can collect data points based on timing wherein data points are stored every X seconds or minutes or based on events wherein data points are stored whenever the patient makes a change. Here is a brief review of the two different methods:

- Time-based means that the hearing aid records the situation, the input level, and the gain setting at periodic intervals, perhaps once every minute. For example, if the patient adjusts his or her hearing aid to a comfortable setting and sits for an hour listening to music, the hearing aid will record this continuously. If the patient does not make any adjustments to the hearing aid during this time, it keeps recording the same values. Although we know of no research to directly support this notion, it seemingly might be best for a patient who spends a considerable amount of time in a limited number of situations. The downside of time-based training algorithms, depending on how often they record, is that if a person is going in and out of different situations and making several changes, the timing of the logging might miss a change. Likewise, if a person prefers to change the hearing aid a lot within a given situation, these changes may not be recorded.
- Event-based training means that every time the patient makes a change to gain or the frequency response, the hearing aid records what is happening. In other words, the user has to do something for the event to be recorded; otherwise, no data helpful for training are available. We might predict that the event-based strategy will be better for a person who is in many different situations and is good at making changes to the hearing aid.

- The *action of the hearing aid user*. Was gain turned up or down? By how much? Was the frequency response altered?

As more and more samples are gathered, the hearing aid develops a preference profile for the listener. It evaluates all of the adjustments over time and predicts what setting the listener prefers on average. The training is typically based on cumulative use over several weeks, because we expect that the same listener may not pick the exact same setting every time. Ideally, the more information that is collected for more inputs and listening situations, the better the average prediction will be. These stored data points could be for average speech, loud speech, speech in background noise, and so on, depending on the level of sophistication of the product that the patient is using. As we have mentioned, many products train specifically for different input levels and classifications. Therefore, it is important that the product has a good classification system or situation-specific training will not work very well. Some situations are fairly easy to classify, such as speech in quiet; you can expect that this listening condition will be classified correctly in 95% to 100% of the cases. For various types of speech-in-noise situations, however, correct classification will not be this accurate.

We have found that some audiologists report that they really like trainable products and use them regularly, whereas other audiologists dispense hearing aids equipped with the trainable feature rarely or never implement it. Why is this? Over the past few years, we have collected opinions on this topic from audiologists on both sides of the fence. The following is a summary of those opinions.

Trainable Hearing Aids Are a Good Thing

Here are some reasons why audiologists say they like trainable hearing aids:

- Gain and output adjustments. We know that prescriptive fittings are an average and that probably one-third or so of our patients will have preferred listening levels that are somewhat different from what is determined by these prescriptive algorithms.
- Loudness for different inputs. Compression training allows patients to shape the aided loudness-growth function to match their specific levels. Many fittings are based on a linear growth function when, in fact, some patients may have a curvilinear pattern (e.g., their MCL is closer to their LDL than to their threshold).
- Hands-free operation. Training for different listening situations means that it is less likely that patients will have to physically switch programs when they move from one setting to another. If they prefer 5 dB less gain for loud noise than for loud speech and have made

---

TECHNICAL TIP: INTERPOLATION USED IN TRAINING ALGORITHM

As we mentioned, the training algorithm will "fill in" samples that are missing for the profile for a given hearing aid user. That is, the patient does not have to listen to all possible inputs in all listening environments for the training to be complete. Here is an example of how this process might work for a couple who listen to music in their home: The patient's wife likes to listen to music in their family room at different input levels, depending on the artist, the time of day, and her mood. The husband, who uses hearing aids, on the other hand, tends to prefer a fairly equal SPL for music all the time. He adjusts his hearing aids accordingly, and the hearing aids remember what he does. Over several weeks, the husband sets his hearing aids for 25 dB of gain for the 60-dB SPL music input, 20 dB of gain for the 65-dB input, and 10 dB for the 75-dB input. Assuming that training was complete, when his wife turns on music of 70 dB SPL, the hearing aid applies about 15 dB of gain for the 70-dB signal, as predicted from the training that occurred from the other input signals (e.g., he tends to prefer an output of about 85 dB SPL).

this adjustment during training, the change in loudness will happen automatically.

- VC replacement. Many hearing aids are fitted without a VC control. For these patients, a loaner remote control device or a smart phone app during the first few weeks of use will allow them to zero in on their desired gain and loudness levels through training.
- Taking ownership. The training process allows the patient to be part of the overall fitting and to "buy into" the outcome. The fitting process is now a partnership, and the patient is partly responsible for the success.
- Reduced patient visits. Many patients return to the clinic several times, often without appointments, during the first few weeks of the fitting for minor tweaking. Audiologists using trainable hearing aids speculate that the number of patient visits may decline because some of the fine-tuning is accomplished through training.

Trainable Hearing Aids Maybe Are NOT Such a Good Thing

Although the items listed in the previous section all sound pretty good, many audiologists do not routinely use trainable hearing aids. Why is this?

- Mental and physical skills. Many patients do not have the cognitive or dexterity skills to do the training. In some cases, patients will *not* prefer their trained gain and will instead prefer the original gain. If they are lost to follow-up, such patients may be less satisfied with their hearing aids, receive less benefit, or both.
- Hassle factor. It's just one more thing to explain to a patient who often is confused already by the technology. Patients want things to be simple.
- Who is doing the work? Patients are already paying the audiologist to program the hearing aid. They might question the audiologist's abilities if they have to do much of the work.
- Turning a good fitting into a bad one. Considerable time often is spent on the day of the fitting getting everything programmed

correctly. What if the patient messes everything up with training (note: research has shown that this rarely happens)?

- Reduced patient visits. In theory, if training works, the patient will require fewer post-fitting visits. Although some consider this good, other audiologists do not. It is during these post-fitting visits that they get to know their patients and demonstrate to the patients that they are problem solvers, which then leads to follow-up purchases and word-of-mouth referrals.
- Reduce need for audiology? Some audiologists believe that trainable hearing aids are just another step in eliminating audiologists from the dispensing process.

Research With Trainable Hearing Aids

Most of the reasons provided in the preceding section are either clinical speculation or beliefs based on patient comments. Given the field's increasing focus on evidence-based practice, the implementation (or not) of trainable hearing aids should be based on data. There is not much published research on this topic, however, which may be one reason why there are so many conflicting opinions concerning the benefit of trainable hearing aids. We have summarized four studies below that help us begin to form evidence-based recommendations for this technology.

Mueller, Hornsby, and Weber (2008) used a crossover design to study the first generation trainable product, which had training only for overall gain. Each of their 22 participants was initially fitted to either 6 dB above or 6 dB below NAL-NL1 targets, which was verified with probe microphone measures. The participants trained for this fitting for two weeks, returned and were fitted to the other condition, and trained for two more weeks. The two primary research questions were as follows: (1) Will the subjects tend to train toward the NAL-NL1 prescription targets? (2) Will the starting point influence the end point for gain training? The investigators found large variability among participants—for example, one trained to 14 dB above the NAL target and another trained to 14 dB below the NAL target. Interestingly, however, when the two sets of data were combined (6 dB above and 6 dB below), the mean and the median trained gain for the group were within a dB or so of the current NAL-NL2 prescription. When the participants were initially fitted 6 dB above the NAL, they tended to train to 2 to 3 dB above the NAL. When the same participants were fitted 6 dB below the NAL, they trained to 5 dB below the NAL. These trends were not influenced by what condition the participant had first. There was also considerable variability in the magnitude of change within patients across the two trials. The positive slope of the regression line in Figure 12–1 nevertheless at least indicates that patients who decreased gain less for the +6-dB condition were more likely to increase gain for the −6-dB condition.

- Take Home Points: For the participants in this study, there appears to be a wide range of acceptable gain, and the starting point for training can have a significant impact on the final trained gain. Remember that speech recognition benefit is highly dependent on audibility, and patients in this study trained down in gain much more than they trained up. Therefore, we view these results as indicating a strong need for initially fitting patients using validated prescriptive targets *even* when they subsequently use a trainable hearing aid.

Palmer (2012) studied trainable hearing aids with new hearing aid users, all initially fitted to the NAL-NL1. She questioned whether the starting time for training had an impact on the outcome. For the control group ($n = 18$), training was turned off at the initial fitting and then activated a month later at the second visit. The experimental group ($n = 18$) had training activated from the very beginning. Accordingly, the first group had only one month of total training, whereas the second group had two months of training. Prior to training the aided Hearing in Noise Test (HINT) was administered to both groups, and there was no difference between groups on the pre-training HINT. The

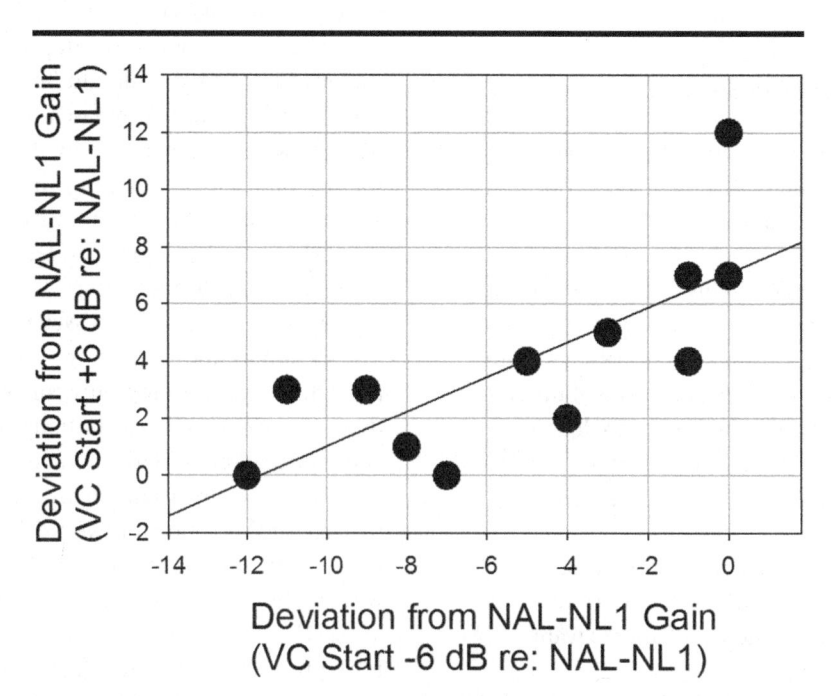

Figure 12–1. Deviation of trained gain from the starting VCW position for the +6-dB and −6-dB conditions. It is clear from the graph that when the participants were initially fitted 6 dB above the NAL (*abscissa*), they tended to train to 2 to 3 dB above the NAL. When the same participants were fitted 6 dB below the NAL (*ordinate*), they trained to 5 dB below the NAL. (Adapted from Mueller et al., 2008, with permission.)

findings revealed that gain for soft sounds was reduced slightly for both groups. The speech intelligibility index (SII) for soft-level sounds for the control group was reduced by about 2%, as calculated by the AudioScan Verifit. The SII for soft-level sounds for the experimental group that trained for two months was reduced by about 4%. Unfortunately, we do not know if this was simply because the experimental group had an extra 30 days to train or if the initial use of the NAL-NL1 fitting influenced the subsequent training for the control group. Post-training HINT performance was the same for both groups, and it was not significantly different from pre-training scores for either group. Following a real-world comparative trial of the trained setting versus the NAL-NL1, 65% of the participants favored the trained setting.

- Take Home Points: When new users are initially programmed to the NAL prescription, on average, they do not train far from this gain setting. Using the gain prescribed by NAL-NL1 for a month may influence training. Group findings show that allowing patients to alter their gain and frequency response through training does not reduce speech recognition in background noise. Interestingly, about one-third of participants did not show a significant preference for their new "trained" gain setting. Of course, if their trained gain was similar to the NAL-NL1 (and it was for many), then when forced to choose one or the other, we'd expect a 50/50 split.

Keidser and Alamudi (2013) reported on 26 hearing-impaired individuals (experienced hearing aid users) who were fitted with trainable hearing aids, initially programmed to NAL-NL2. Following three weeks of training, they examined the newly trained settings for both low and high frequencies, for six different listening situations (the training was situation-specific). The participants did tend to train down from the NAL-NL2, but only by a minimal amount. For example, for the speech in quiet condition for the high frequencies, the average value was a gain reduction of 1.5 dB (0.95 range = 0 to −4 dB), and for the speech in noise condition, there was an average gain reduction of only 2 dB (0.95 range = 0.5 to −4.5 dB). The trained gain for the low-frequency sounds for these listening conditions was even closer to the original NAL-NL2 settings (Figure 12–2).

- Take Home Points: When initially programmed to the NAL-NL2, individuals tend to train to values similar to the NAL-NL2. Training does not vary significantly for different listening situations such as speech in quiet versus speech in background noise. Importantly, the authors repeated training and found only about 60% of patients reliably trained to similar settings.

Mueller and Hornsby (2014) questioned whether experienced hearing aid users will train to the gain that they had previously used when fitted to the NAL-NL1 using new trainable instruments. They studied 20 experienced hearing aid users: 6 females and 14 males between the ages of 52 and 80 years (mean age of 68.3 years). On average, these participants had been using hearing aids that were programmed about 10 dB below NAL-NL1 targets for soft sounds and 5 dB below for average speech inputs. The hearing aids used in this research had compression training, so it was possible to train the gain for soft sounds without impacting gain for loud inputs. As shown in Figure 12–3, these authors found that, after two weeks of training, the participants did not train to their previous use gain, but rather trained to gain similar to the NAL-NL1. For soft-level inputs, 45% of the participants trained at least a 3-dB gain increase, and the overall findings showed that 55% were using 10 dB or more gain following training than they had previously been using.

- Take Home Points: Individuals who have been using gain substantially below NAL-NL1 targets and then are fitted to NAL-NL1 prescriptive targets do not train to their previous use gain.

In general, we conclude that the results of all these studies are favorable regarding patient-controlled trainable hearing aids. Of course, the people who participated in these studies all had the ability and expressed a willingness to use trainable hearing aids; this will not be the case for all clinic patients. In three different studies, we see that individuals do not train very far from

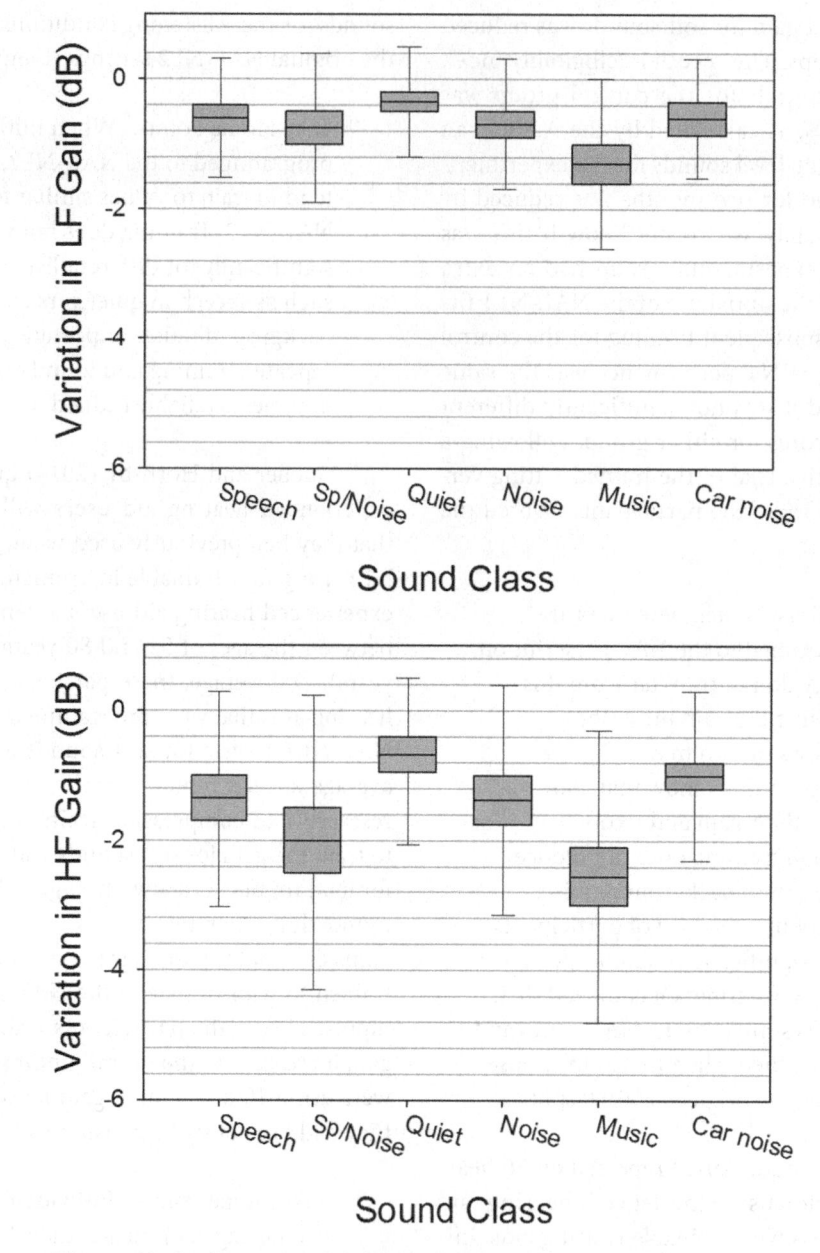

Figure 12–2. Average trained deviation from baseline for experienced, bilateral hearing aid users following a training period. Negative values indicate that the participants preferred less of the low-frequency (LF) or high-frequency (HF) gain than was prescribed. The boxes show +/−1 SE, and the bars show +/−0.95 times the standard deviation. (Adapted from Keidser and Alamudi, 2013, with permission.)

the NAL targets. We really don't know, however, if that is because these are the preferred gain settings or if it is related to the fact that the individuals were initially fitted to the NAL in each of these studies. In both the Palmer (2012) and Mueller and Hornsby (2014) studies, however, the individuals were using hearing aids that

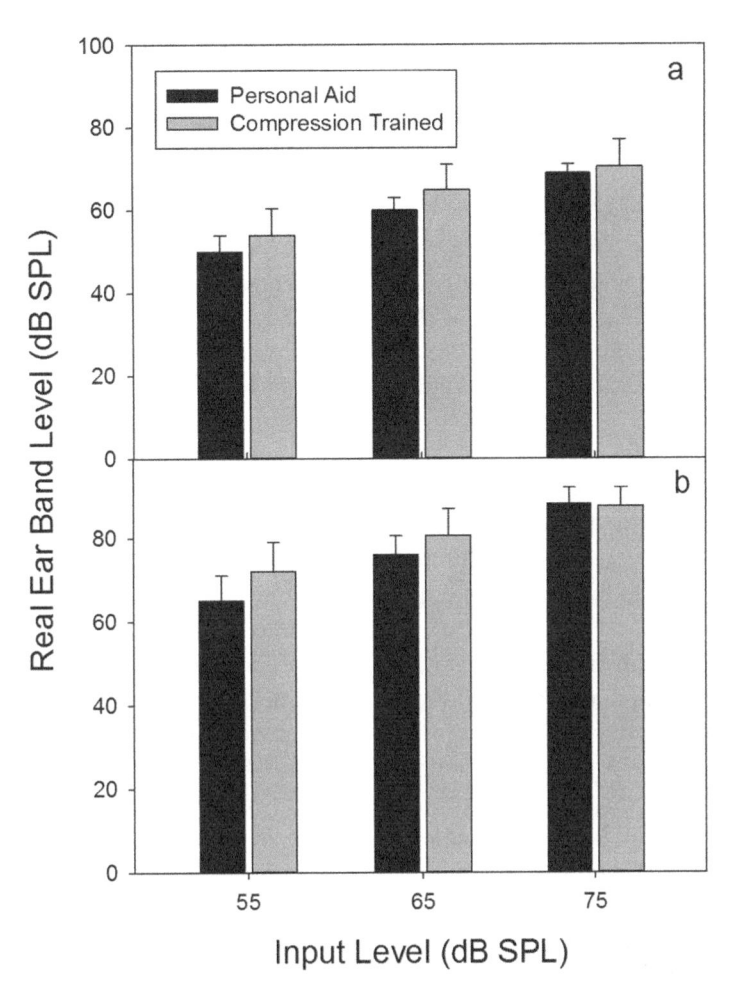

Figure 12–3. Average real-ear band level measured across 20 experienced hearing aid users after two weeks of training. The top panel (*Panel A*) is the average of the low-frequency band, and the lower panel (*Panel B*) is the average of the high-frequency band. The different shaded bars show the average output for the participants' own hearing aids and the trained gain. (Adapted from Mueller and Hornsby, 2014, with permission.)

had the capability of training +/–16 dB away from target, so deviating significantly from NAL certainly was possible. Finally, these and other studies show a sizable portion of patients either cannot train reliably and/or end up not preferring their trained gain setting. These findings suggest training is not for everyone, and we discourage the use of trainable algorithms in patients without an interest. Keidser and Alamudi (2013) offer some additional clinical recommendations related to trainable hearing aids that seem appropriate to us:

- A satisfied patient who has trained significantly large changes should continue wearing the trained devices as they are.
- A satisfied patient who has little or no trained changes is assumed to be happy with the prescription and should have training deactivated to avoid inadvertent changes.
- An unsatisfied patient who has little or no trained changes should be encouraged to continue training the devices for longer.

- An unsatisfied patient who has trained significantly large changes should be reset to the prescription, and the reason for dissatisfaction should be explored.

AGI and Trainable Together?

We have talked about AGI and trainable hearing aids and suggested one way of implementing both within the same fitting on the same patient. However, we really have three options (from Mueller, 2014b and Ricketts & Mueller, 2014):

1. We could implement both patient-training and AGI at the time of the fitting. That seems like a poor choice to us because you have two different things going on, which could be working in opposite directions.
2. We could use AGI first. This might help us push gain to a higher level than patients might initially accept, which might take a couple of months. Then after they arrive at that higher level, we could implement training to fine-tune compression and obtain preferred gain for different listening situations. This seems reasonable to us and would be good for the patient who initially is not fond of much gain; which will be true of most patients who are good candidates for both technologies.
3. Our third option is to use patient-training first for patients who initially accepted an appropriate amount of gain—recall that the gain starting point does influence the ending point. We allow the patient to settle on a preferred gain for different listening situations, which might take a couple of weeks. Once preferred gain is established, we conduct probe microphone testing to determine how the fitting looks. If audibility is not optimal, we could then implement AGI. Although this might make sense for some patients and some clinicians, it seems less efficient to us because it may require multiple office visits to recheck the fitted gain values.

AGI is something that you have in your back pocket to pull out for either Option #2 or Option #3, and the use seems to depend on the patient's first perceptions or the outcome of training. We are mostly talking about new hearing aid users for these scenarios. We assume that experienced users are fairly settled on their preferences. This might not be true, however, if they were under-fit for gain initially and have been using hearing aids that did not have gain adjustments. Recall from the Mueller and Hornsby (2014) data, experienced users were using considerably more gain after training (when they were refit to more gain). Implementing these training procedures does usually involve a few more trips back to your office, but that is not necessar-

---

KEY CONCEPT: TRAINING LESS GAIN AND OUTPUT?

In this section, we talk about the need to encourage patients to use more gain, which will increase audibility and, one hopes, speech understanding. There are some instances, however, in which we want the patient to adapt to *less* gain and/or *less* output. Some patients with longstanding severe-to-profound hearing loss and who have used high-power hearing aids for many years have a desire for a significant amount of gain, which can be made possible only by using a high MPO. For some of these patients, the additional gain is not improving speech recognition; it is simply what they have become used to, and it "sounds right" to them. The concern is that, in some cases, this gain/output is so great that it potentially could cause increased hearing loss. This is then a dilemma for the audiologist programming the hearing aids. Set the gain/MPO to what the patient wants or to what is "safe?" To address this problem, at least one manufacturer allows for audiologist-driven training that automatically reduces gain/MPO over time. As with the gradual increase of gain, the notion is that if the change happens gradually, the patient will adapt, and at the end of training both the patient and the audiologist will be happy.

ily a bad thing. Furthermore, given current advances in distance-based telehealth technologies, it is likely that completing follow-up services related to trainable hearing aids may be increasingly less cumbersome for both patients and clinicians.

Clinical Implementation of Patient Training

To successfully implement trainable hearing aids, you first have to ensure that patients agree that this strategy is good for them. You also have to ensure that the patient is able and willing to make the necessary changes in real-world settings. Research studies on this topic are somewhat misleading, as we tend to recruit only patients who we are fairly sure can conduct the training. In the clinical world, we would say that about 60 to 70% of people could effectively do the training. As you've noticed, even the elderly use smartphones and various remote controls more now than they did 10 years ago, and many people are more capable than you might think.

Our recommendation is to start with a fitting that is as close to your desired ending point as possible. Remember, the starting point does matter. There is no reason to start well below a desired level and think patients will train up. Research shows that they probably will not (Mueller et al., 2008). Here are some other considerations from a Keidser, Dillon, and Convery (2008) study:

- When they surveyed a typical clinical population about trainable hearing aids, they found that 59% of adult hearing aid users were interested in training their own hearing aids.
- They found that the people who would be most successful were younger adults who have a strong interest in technology, people who have a milder hearing loss, and people who have less symmetrical hearing loss.
- They also found that 54% of those surveyed wanted to train using a remote control, whereas 46% wanted on-board controls. The use of remotes is becoming increasingly common given the current trend of using smartphones as remotes.
- Interestingly, 82% of all those surveyed, whether they used training or not, thought that training would make the hearing aid fitting better.

When initiating training, we encourage you to give patients detailed instructions. Ask them to go to different listening situations, and suggest they make gain changes whenever necessary to optimize loudness, listening comfort, and intelligibility. Doing so should result in a better overall fitting. We suggest giving them a diary where they can make a checkmark if they listen to loud music, soft music, loud noise, soft noise, and so on, which will give them some structure for the training process. This approach has worked well in our research projects. We also suggest monitoring the progress at about two weeks post-fitting. Look at the data logging to make sure that they have been in different listening situations and see what changes are being made. At a one-month interval, assuming all is well, training likely can be discontinued if the patient is satisfied with the trained response.

At periodic intervals, you may want to implement training again for at least three reasons:

- The patient's hearing loss has changed.
- The patient's listening situations have changed. Maybe the fellow who was retired is now working part-time and is in a lot of background noise. If so, he may need new training.
- You will also need to account for overall adaptation for loudness. At some point, new users will become experienced users. It is difficult to determine exactly on what day or what year users become experienced, but when they do they probably are going to want more gain.

In summary, validated prescriptive fittings are a good starting point, but they are mostly geared toward certain attributes of amplification for the average patient, with an emphasis on intelligibility and appropriate loudness. Those may not be the attributes that your patient believes are most important, or your patient may not be average. The patient may like more gain, less gain, have a different loudness contour, or have different listening interests. Trainable hearing aids will allow your patients to train the fitting to their environments and to their fitting goals and can be an important aspect of the post-fitting process.

Overcoming Traditional Hearing Aid Limitations

Digital Feedback Suppression (DFS)

As discussed in Chapter 8, one of the greatest sources of frustration for past clinicians was the task of eliminating the "squeal" of feedback. Although acoustic feedback can be reduced by minimizing the vent size, changing the tightness of the fitting, or reducing gain, these changes all have the potential to create new problems such as limited audibility, increased occlusion effect, or an uncomfortably tight fit. Fortunately, these limitations can be greatly offset by modifications allowed by activating a digital feedback suppression (DFS) algorithm (also referred to as automatic feedback reduction) in the fitting software. Specifically, effective DFS algorithms can provide clinical benefits, either by allowing for more gain while maintaining appropriate venting (potentially leading to improved audibility if the patient is under-fit due to feedback limitations), or by allowing for increased venting without decreasing gain (potentially leading to improved sound quality and comfort).

The advent of effective DFS algorithms led to the introduction of the modern version of the open-canal hearing aid style and the increased use of non-custom eartips, which are in large part responsible for the current popularity of the mini-BTE style. As we discussed in Chapter 8, the benefits of open fittings to individuals with normal or near normal low frequencies are wide ranging and include allowing natural low-frequency sounds to leak in improving naturalness of sound quality, elimination of occlusion effect, provision of gain only in the high frequencies where hearing loss is present and improved wearing comfort. DFS allows for increased use of non-custom eartips for a wide range of hearing losses because relatively high levels of gain can be provided in the presence of considerable slit-leak venting without feedback. Even though non-custom eartips are not always optimal due to limitations related to consistent fit, limited retention, and very high-gain requirements that result in feedback even with DFS active; their use in a large segment of hearing aid wearers improves service efficiency because an ear impression and subsequent custom manufacture is not needed. Every manufacturer uses at least one DFS algorithm; however, there are variations in how they are implemented and how effective they are. General DFS techniques include (1) notch filtering, (2) phase cancellation, and, (3) frequency shifting.

Identifying and Modeling Feedback

Prior to applying DFS techniques, feedback, or the potential for feedback, must be identified. Feedback detection algorithms are used to monitor for sustained narrow-band oscillations (e.g., tonal signals). These techniques can identify the presence of feedback quite quickly once it occurs. As we describe in Chapter 11, modern versions of these techniques use data sharing to differentiate feedback present in one hearing aid from tonal signals in the environment that are present at similar levels for both hearing aids.

Regardless of the DFS technique applied, initialization is commonly applied during the hearing aid fitting. During DFS initialization, a broadband or swept pure tone signal is generated by the hearing aid receiver. The output of the hearing aid microphone is monitored to determine how much of the generated signal is leaking out of the ear and reaching the microphone input. As we describe in Chapter 8, this is referred to as open-loop gain measurement and it is used to obtain the frequency and phase response of the feedback pathway on the individual patient with the hearing aid, coupling, and any venting in place—sometimes referred to as the external feedback path (Figure 12–4).

Notch Filtering

Much like you might expect based on the name, notch filtering methods simply lower gain in a narrow frequency region, for which feedback is detected or expected, to a level below unity gain. Because it is the goal to reduce gain in the narrowest frequency region possible to ensure audibility, a very narrow *notch filter* is used. If feedback occurs at multiple frequencies, multiple notch filters may be applied. If the feedback signal changes frequency, the frequency of the notch filter is often also altered to match—commonly referred to as a *roving notch filter*. Notch filtering was the first processing-based feedback suppression technique, but reduced audibility presents a clear limitation. That is, the notch filter can reduce or eliminate feedback but will do so at the expense (slight though it may be) of audibility of the surrounding frequencies. In some early versions

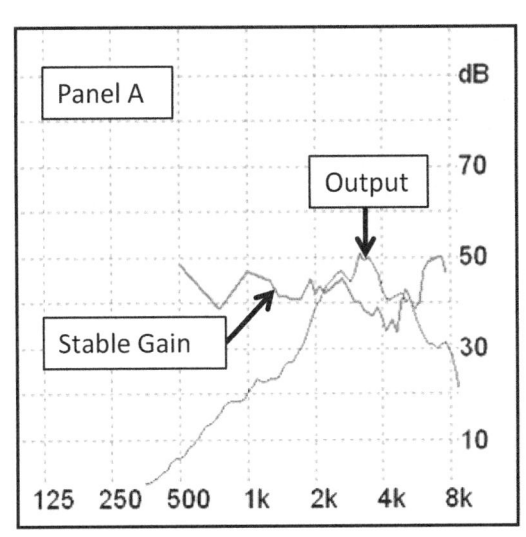

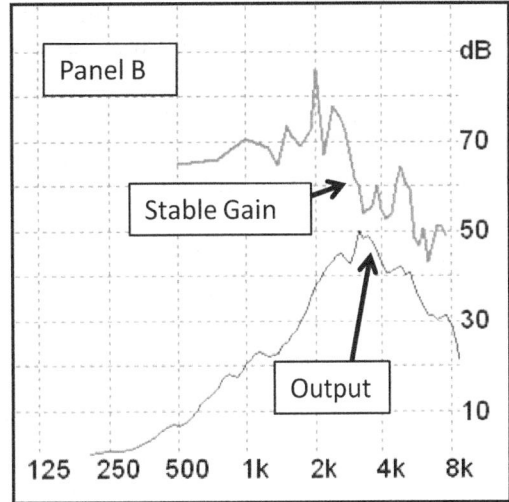

Figure 12–4. Example of open-loop gain measured for the same hearing aid for an open fitting (*Panel A*) and a more closed fitting (*Panel B*). Note that the output from the open loop gain measurement remains the same, whereas the stable gain changes considerably.

POINTS TO PONDER: WHEN IS DFS REALLY DFS?

Once DFS initialization has been completed, it is possible for the clinician to make a mouse click that will then simply limit gain below unity gain so that oscillations resulting in audible feedback do not occur. Manufacturers sometimes refer to this technique as feedback suppression or feedback limiting, but it really doesn't provide any benefits to the hearing aid user compared to having the audiologist just limit the amount of gain below feedback for this frequency range during fitting. After all, no clinician is going to send the patient out the door with active, audible, feedback! There is, however, a benefit to the clinician. The technique is quick, easy, accurate, and efficient. That is, gain in the frequency region responsible for feedback is quickly and automatically targeted without having to use a little trial and error when adjusting frequency-specific gain. It is important to remember, however, that this manner of "feedback reduction" might also be referred to as "audibility reduction," as the gain often is reduced to below optimal levels for patients with considerable hearing loss.

---

of this technique, the notch could be rather broad. In addition, sometimes the roving notch would remain in effect after the feedback frequency changed, resulting in an even more deleterious effect on audibility. Due in part to these limitations, manufacturers typically do not use notch filtering as the only processing-based method of feedback control. Notch filtering does have one strong advantage though: It can be made to operate very quickly. Consequently, some manufacturers implement notch filtering as a secondary DFS technique that is effective in limiting or reducing occasional feedback, which occurs due to a rapid change in the feedback path; for example, getting a hug or bringing a hand up to the ear.

Feedback Path Cancellation

Feedback path cancellation controls feedback by using an approach that capitalizes on the fact that shifting a signal by 180° will cause it to be precisely out of phase with itself and cancellation will occur. Conceptually, this approach uses the frequency and phase response obtained in the DFS initialization routine to model an "internal feedback path" (i.e., processing done in the hearing aid) that exactly mimics the external feedback path. The earliest techniques generated a tonal signal out of phase with the feedback as the internal feedback path, resulting in cancellation. This technique had some undesirable side effects, however, including generation of audible tones in response to tonal signals in the environment that were misidentified as feedback; it is no longer used. Modern techniques replace the tone with a filter used to cancel the feedback. Like the tone, this filter is generated based on the frequency and phase of the feedback obtained during DFS initialization. One limitation of this static approach is that changes to the feedback path, such as those resulting from additional slit leak venting due to jaw movement or bringing a hand close to the hearing aid, are not accounted for and can result in feedback. Consequently, some manufacturers instead use non-static (adaptive) filter approaches instead, or at least make them available as an option.

In the adaptive filter cancellation approach, the continuous temporal correlation between the input signal and the feedback signal is monitored. This information is used to adjust the cancellation filter coefficients (i.e., the math that describes the exact properties of the filter) so that the correlation between the microphone input signal and the amplifier output signal is minimized. In theory, this will cancel as much of the feedback as possible when there are changes to the static feedback path. In some systems, the speed of adaptation is changed depending on the environment. For example, adaptation rate may be reduced when the classifier identifies music as the primary signal or when a music program is selected. Some adaptive approaches introduce an additional disadvantage in that the level of tonal signals in the environment, including some music, may also be reduced, or canceled out.

The most advanced DFS systems use information sharing between the two hearing aids to better differentiate feedback from external tonal signals as we describe in Chapter 11. Unlike external tonal signals, feedback will be present at much different levels at the two ears and have a phase relationship consistent with the distance between the hearing aids, therefore this information sharing scheme can greatly improve accuracy of feedback identification.

Frequency/Phase Shifting

The third general technique capitalizes on the fact that if the similarity of the sound entering the hearing aid and that amplified version of this same sound leaking out of the hearing aid is disrupted, the addition of these two versions which lead to oscillatory feedback will be compromised. One way to disrupt similarity is to shift the frequency or phase of the amplified sound. In order to limit negative effects on sound quality, the amount of frequency shift is typically rather small (e.g., 10–20 Hz) and limited to the high frequencies where feedback is most likely. Alternatively, small, rapidly changing adjustments are made to the phase. In either case, the mismatch in frequency or phase between amplified and re-amplified versions of the same sound can introduce a "roughness" in the sound quality that may be noticeable for some listeners. Generally, larger frequency shifts will have increasingly detrimental effects on sound quality.

Benefits and Limitations

Although we described notch filtering, phase cancellation, and frequency shifting separately, it is common for current hearing aids to use two or even all three approaches at the same time. In some cases, the clinician has some control over activation of the approach. For example, some manufacturers will have a toggle button in the fitting software for the type of cancellation (static versus adaptive) or the speed of the filter adaptation (e.g., turbo, dynamic, fast). Other manufacturers allow for switching between "standard" and "advanced" DFS. This may activate secondary DFS processing such as frequency shifting or notch filtering. In nearly all cases, this control is made available because even though activation of non-standard settings often improves performance, it may also introduce audible artifacts for at least some patients.

The potential benefits and limitations of activating DFS algorithms are quantified in several ways including (1) the magnitude of maximum gain before feedback or the additional gain available before feedback, commonly referred to as "gain margin," "added stable gain," "added gain before feedback," or a host of other terms; (2) the duration required to eliminate feedback after introducing a physical object or sudden change to the feedback path, referred to herein as "feedback adaptation time"; (3) the misidentification of an external signal as feedback and introduction of artifact or distortion by attempting to cancel this signal, commonly referred to as "entrainment", maladaptation, or a number of other terms; and (4) the introduction of other signal artifacts or distortions.

Although it is clearly important that the DFS algorithm not introduce unwanted side effects, the most commonly discussed attribute related to performance is the magnitude of additional gain available before feedback. The magnitude of additional gain available before feedback (AGBF) has been previously defined in a variety of similar ways. For example, several years ago we defined it as the REAR values measured 2 dB below audible feedback with the feedback suppression system activated minus those measured 2 dB below audible feedback with the feedback suppression system deactivated, while maintaining the same frequency response shape (Ricketts, Dittberner, & Johnson, 2008).

Another common measurement is added stable gain (ASG) which refers to the additional gain provided by DFS processing prior to a loss of stability (start of suboscillatory feedback). When measured using different criteria, the magnitude of AGBF is generally the same as, or nearly identical to, that of ASG. The magnitude of AGBF and ASG values that have been reported to range from 0 dB to more than 20 dB and have been shown to vary widely as a function of manufacturer and specific product (e.g., Freed and Soli, 2006; Ricketts et al., 2008). Interestingly, these data also demonstrated that, even though measuring AGBF in an acoustic manikin can provide reasonable information, the relationship between outcomes measured in this way and average AGBF measured in real ears is not constant. That is, the AGBF measured in an acoustic manikin tends to be better than that measured in real ears for some manufacturers and worse in others. Consequently, we like to obtain these measures in real ears when making across-product comparisons.

No cross-manufacturer studies of DFS performance have been published recently, but Steven Marcrum collected data as part of a NIH T35 project (Marcrum & Ricketts, 2011), and we collected follow-up data on improved products in 2013 and 2014. In this series of studies, we asked manufacturers to identify their products that they believed had the best DFS. We then purchased these products. In total we measured AGBF across 14 different models (all RIC devices) from seven different manufacturers (the "Big 6" plus one smaller company) in at least 16 listeners. All participants were fitted with non-custom pediatric open eartips to obtain as open a fitting as possible. In addition, the receiver wire was shaped whenever necessary to ensure the receiver outlet did not terminate near an ear canal wall. We have found ensuring the receiver is "pointed" away from any earcanal surface (we apply a little heat from a hair dryer or other device to the receiver wire or thin tubing to make the adjustments) can help improve DFS performance in individual listeners.

Although AGBF is useful information from a scientific standpoint regarding how well a DFS system performs, from a clinical standpoint, it is more useful to know the maximum gain we can achieve with DFS active and the hearing aid in place on the ear. It is these values that really describe how much hearing loss we can fit with open eartips. We have mentioned AGBF, but perhaps a more meaningful measure for clinicians is the maximum real ear insertion gain (REIG) that can be obtained before feedback. The maximum REIG we were able to obtain across the seven manufacturers with their best performing open-fitted RIC device is shown in Figure 12–5. There are at least two striking factors associated with these data. First, while the average maximum REIG across all manufacturers is consistent with AGBF of around 8 to 10 dB, large intermanufacturer differences remain. The large range of maximum REIG before feedback greatly affects the range of open fittings possible. Specifically, if you fit to NAL-NL2 targets using the products from manufacturer A or G, you will likely find you can continue to use an open eartip with high-frequency thresholds up to 70 dB HL or more. Conversely, use of open eartips for manufacturers D and E is likely limited to high-frequency-thresholds of no more than 50 to 55 dB HL.

In addition to manufacturer differences, individual differences in hearing aid, eartip or earmold fit, ear geometry, and ear canal impedance can also affect AGBF (Ricketts et al., 2008). The maximum REIG averaged across 2000 to 4000 Hz for 16 listeners using six different products is shown in Figure 12–6 (Marcrum & Ricketts, 2011). These data demonstrate that we cannot expect average values on every patient. Instead the range of average AGBF within a product may vary from less than 10 dB to more than 15 dB. This same group of

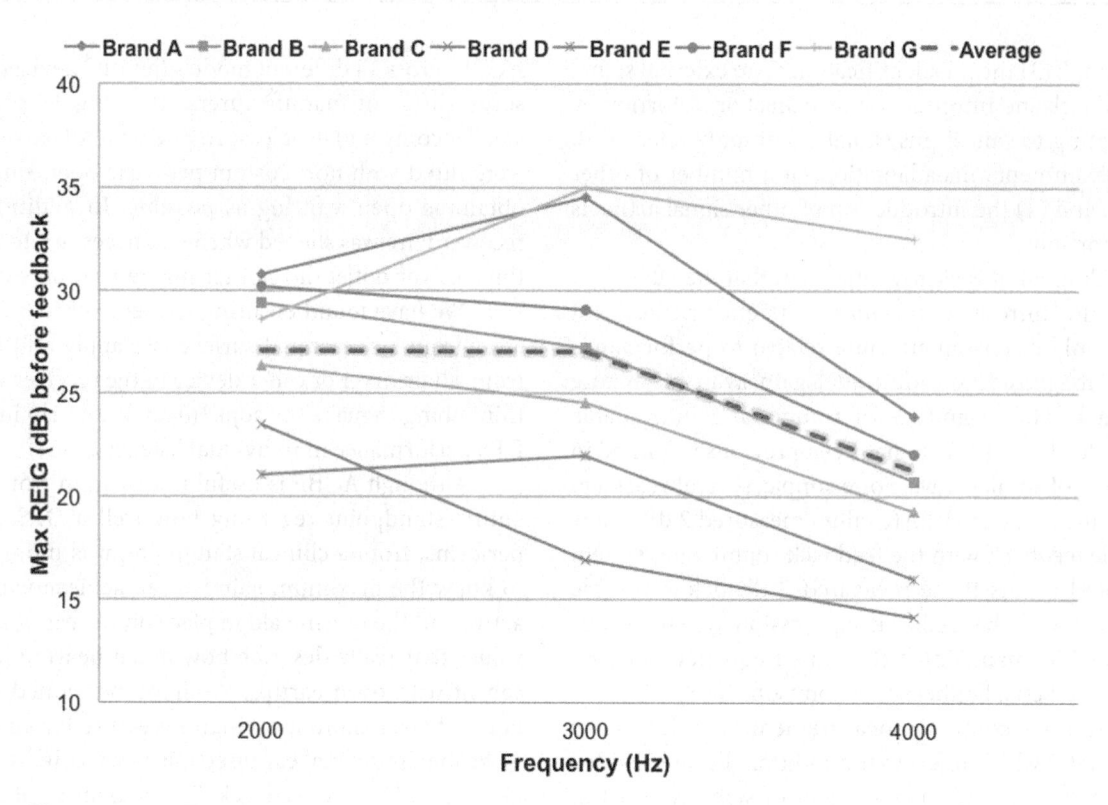

Figure 12–5. The maximum, average, high-frequency REIG obtained using an open RIC device from seven manufacturers. All measures reflect the average data from at least 16 ears.

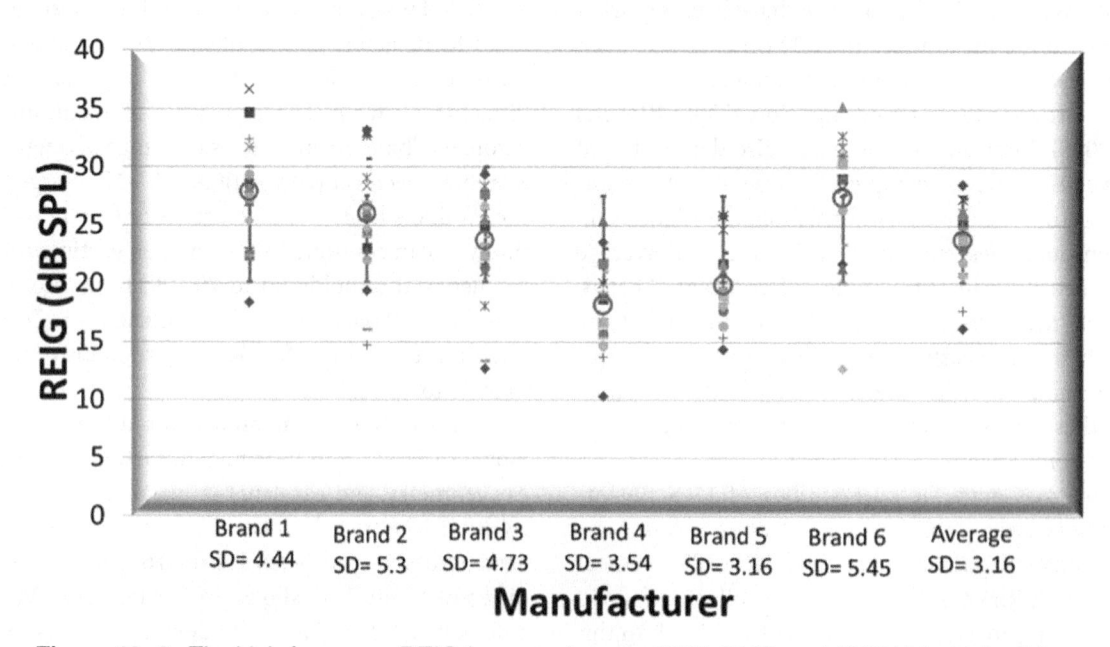

Figure 12–6. The high-frequency REIG (averaged across 2000, 3000, and 4000 Hz) obtained from 16 ears using an open RIC device from six manufacturers.

studies also examined how quickly systems could adapt to a large change in the feedback path associated with quickly bringing a phone up to the hearing aid. As we noted above, several techniques have been applied to adapt to this type of change including adaptive cancellation and notch filtering. Prior to 2010 or so, most systems adapted quite slowly and many required more than a second or two to adapt to a new path. Since that time, many systems have become much faster, often resulting in no more than a brief chirp (<500 ms) before feedback is again eliminated in response to bringing a phone up to the hearing aid. Importantly, some adaptive cancellation systems vary the adaptation speed based on total signal classification or the user program selected.

Individualization of DFS Technologies

Clearly, there are large differences across current DFS algorithms in terms of AGBF. The story is not always as simple as simply choosing the product that allows the most gain possible before feedback, however. Complicating selection and adjustment of DFS technology further is the fact that the model with the most effective DFS may not have other features that are desired for a specific patient. Consequently, when attempting to individually optimize selection and adjustment of DFS technologies, it is important to first consider the relative importance of a large AGBF value relative to other hearing aid selection considerations. Then we can weigh a variety of issues that may affect patient outcomes. Several clinical considerations follow:

1. The magnitude of AGBF will ultimately be limited in all models. Combinations of increased hearing loss and increased venting will always exceed DFS limitations. Use of models with the greatest AGBF may be necessary when large vents are desired for patients with greater than moderate hearing loss. In some cases, however, it may be preferable to reduce venting rather than select a different hearing aid model in order to retain maximal performance of other desired features.
2. Sound quality will be reduced for some adaptive cancellation systems and systems employing frequency/phase shifting. Whereas we certainly do not want to send a patient out the door with inferior sound quality, it is important to note that many studies demonstrating sound quality differences across DFS algorithms have been completed in individuals with normal hearing. Research on patients with impaired hearing and commercial products demonstrated no significant differences in the sound quality provided by DFS-on versus DFS-off conditions for speech and music stimuli (Johnson, Ricketts, & Hornsby, 2007). Clinically, however, it is sometimes useful to assess differences in sound quality as a function of DFS setting, particularly when multiple DFS settings are available within the same product and more aggressive DFS settings are necessary to obtain the desired gain.
3. The time required to eliminate feedback in response to dynamic changes to the feedback path varies considerably across products. Knowledge of adaptation time in the products dispensed is necessary to select and adjust DFS optimally and counsel patients regarding expectations in situations such as bringing a phone to the ear or hugging.

Bilateral Data Sharing for Feature and Hearing Aid Control

In previous sections of this book, we discussed how modern products share digital representations of the actual audio signals across a hearing aid pair for the purposes of bilateral beamforming, enabling other unique directional patterns, and for CROS and BiCROS applications. This full-audio sharing technology is a fairly recent development and, even today, is not available from all major manufacturers. Data transfer between hearing aids, however, is much more widespread and has been available since 2004 (see Herbig, Barthel & Branda, 2014 for review). In data sharing, digital information that can be used to adjust or control processing is transferred between the two hearing aids. Benefits from these technologies include those aimed at feature control in order to overcome limitations imposed by other processing and those that improve convenience. The primary benefits to the patient, from a convenience standpoint, include the following:

- Synchronous adjustment of gain for both instruments by only pushing a button or toggle on one instrument
- Simultaneous change of listening programs in both hearing aids (e.g., switching to programs

designed for listening to music) by only pushing a button or toggle on one instrument
- On-ear adjustment by patient while still fitted with very small custom instruments where there is only room for one button or switch (because a single button or switch can control both instruments)

How It Works?

Since the time of the first aid-to-aid communication, near-field electromagnetic transmission has been used as we describe in detail in Chapter 10. You may recall this type of transmission has a rapid rate of attenuation, which allows for accurate transmission of data between the hearing aids, but does not have a signal strength that is high enough to interfere with other near-field devices (transmission distance is limited to about 25–30 cm). It also benefits from low power consumption when compared to other wireless transmission methods such as Bluetooth technology.

Bilateral Data Sharing for Feature Control

We've already mentioned the patient convenience benefits of being able to change gain and programs for both instruments simultaneously with one control. These benefits are quite straightforward. What is not so straightforward relates to the communication between the signal classification systems of the two hearing aids. A signal classification system is like the coach of a sports team making decisions what players (e.g., directional processing, feedback reduction, DNR) should be playing in the game at any given time. When we have two hearing aids, we have two coaches. Should we allow each coach to simply handle his team (hearing aid) independently or should the two coaches put their heads together and make a joint decision? And, if the latter is the case, should this joint decision be for all features or only some?

Over the years, manufacturers have not been unanimous regarding their decisions regarding the shared signal classification system. Here are some examples:

- Directional processing. The decision for a hearing aid to switch automatically from omnidirectional to directional processing is based on some combination of the overall SPL, the content of the signal(s) present, and the estimated SNR of the environment. For some environments, these might be somewhat different from one side of the head to the other. Is it okay if one hearing aid is omnidirectional and the other is directional? If so, is it okay if the ear-specific microphone setting is allowed to change independently across environments? At least one manufacturer thinks so, but for most products, directional processing is either phased in or out simultaneously for both instruments or a fixed asymmetric microphone setting is used. The data supporting these different configurations were discussed in detail in Chapter 11.
- Digital noise reduction. Like directional processing, the strength of the DNR will be based on a shared decision using information from both hearing aids, and then that degree of DNR will be applied bilaterally. This seems reasonable to us as it will provide a more consistent listening experience.
- Amplitude compression. Because of head shadow, it is possible that the input signal could differ significantly from one side of the head to the other, especially for the high frequencies. From a loudness and audibility standpoint, it makes sense to us *not* to link compression and to have each hearing aid respond independently. There have been products, however, that have had compression adjustment linked. Why? Perhaps because data have shown, at least in some products, that bilateral compression control can lead to improved localization in the horizontal plane.

Clinical and Real-World Research

Early studies of aid-to-aid connectivity focused on the convenience factor. For example, Powers and Burton (2005) showed that 95% of experienced hearing users reported that changing programs on both instruments with one button was useful, and 70% preferred this feature for changing gain. From a user convenience standpoint, this technology is really straightforward and only requires that users are properly counseled on use and function.

We know that binaural processing is enhanced when bilateral gain is set optimally, which hopefully occurs during the initial fitting process. Indirectly then, from a binaural processing standpoint, it would seem to be an advantage for gain to be controlled simultaneously and equally for both ears. Hornsby and Mueller (2008) found that after gain had been set according to prescriptive methods and balanced, some individuals made gain adjustments between ears resulting in significant "gain mismatches." These mismatches were often inconsistent across trials, suggesting that these adjustments were unreliable, although speech recognition results from their study showed no significant decrease for the mismatched settings.

There also is limited data suggesting that directional processing should be linked and activated or deactivated simultaneously for both hearing aids. Keidser and colleagues (2006) studied the effect of nonsynchronized microphones on localization for 12 hearing-impaired listeners. Results showed that left/right localization error was largest when an omnidirectional microphone mode was used on one side and a directional processing one was on the other. If the microphones were matched, the localization error decreased by approximately 40%.

There have been few real-world studies comparing linked hearing aids to unlinked. One study, however, did show significant benefit for linking, with simultaneous changes in directional processing and DNR. In research by Smith et al. (2008), in a crossover design, 20 participants used hearing aids in the real world for both the linked and unlinked conditions (Figure 12–7). The outcome measure used was the Speech, Spatial, and Qualities (SSQ) of Hearing Scale. When individual SSQ questions were analyzed, there were higher scores for the linked condition. This was especially true for the speech domain, in which linked was rated the highest for 12 of 14 questions, and for the spatial domain, in which linked was rated the highest for 14 of 17 questions. Despite this overwhelming preference, only one item reached statistical significance: *"You are sitting around a table or at a meeting with several people. You can't see everyone. Can you tell where any person is as soon as they start speaking?"* When asked to state a preference for linked versus unlinked, 65% preferred linked with only 15% preferring unlinked.

If you notice, most of the research mentioned here was in the earlier days of aid-to-aid wireless linking. Today, it has become a common practice for all manufacturers, and we don't see this changing. Indeed, recent research has shown that modern hearing aids can affect the relationship between ITDs and ILDs, in some cases introducing large ITD–ILD conflicts, particularly for bilateral beamforming (Brown, Rodriguez, Portnuff,

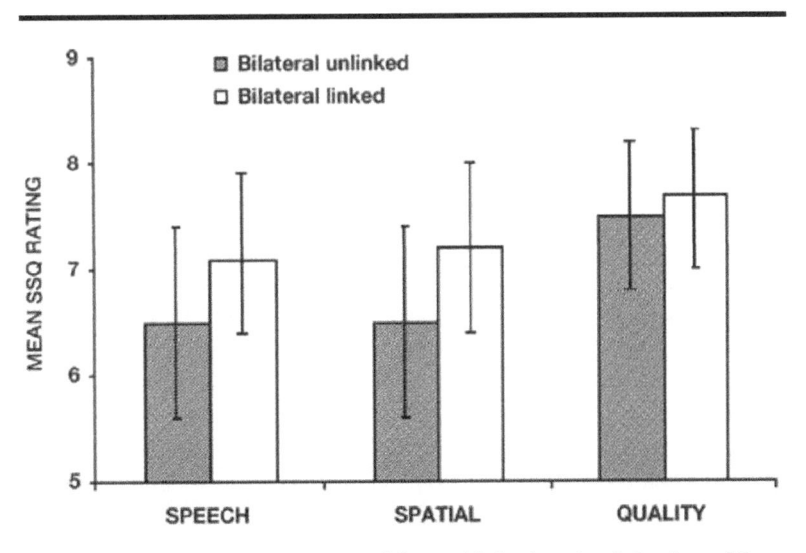

Figure 12–7. Rated score across bilateral linked and unlinked conditions on the Speech, Spatial, and Qualities (SSQ) of Hearing Scale after real world trials with each setting. (Adapted from Smith, Davis, Day, Unwin, Day & Chalupper, 2008).

Goupell, & Tollin, 2016). These data support the utility of bilateral control in that it will limit some of these distortions. There have also been efforts to enhance binaural cues with the goal of improving localization and speech recognition performance in listeners with impaired spatial abilities. These studies have generally found little or no benefits related to "binaural enhancement." It seems that, despite the complexity of some of these processing algorithms, increasing the magnitude of ILD and ITD cues to exaggerate interaural differences does not appear to help individuals with reduced sensitivity to these same cues.

Wireless Streaming

In addition to sharing data and audio between hearing aids, most hearing aid systems can wirelessly receive audio signals from other sources. We will consider streaming from remote microphones, television, home theatre, and other sound delivery systems here. Telephone communication has a few other considerations, so we will discuss it separately in the next section. While, hearing aids alone can provide sufficient audibility for talkers, television and other signals in the environment for many listeners, a portion of our patients are unable to obtain desirable sound levels or SNRs for external sources using hearing aids alone. In addition, there can be considerable convenience associated with streaming signals from an external device directly to a patient's hearing aids across a wide range of hearing loss configurations. We discuss general methods for wirelessly streaming audio signals including FM, LE Bluetooth, and near-field electromagnetic induction (NFEI) in Chapter 10. The specific method used still differs considerably, however, depending on the manufacturer and what is being streamed.

Dual Streaming

One common technique first uses common commercial techniques, typically hardwire and/or the audio Bluetooth standard, to bring signals to an intermediary router. This intermediary router then delivers the signals to the hearing aids using near-field electromagnetic induction (NFEI). As we describe in Chapter 10, NFEI techniques have low latency from the intermediary router to the hearing aids (they are fast) and are power efficient. They do require, however, that the user wear the intermediary router very close to the hearing aids (e.g., around the neck, in a shirt pocket, or under clothing) because of the limited transmission distance These relatively small (silver-dollar size) NFEI intermediary devices can function as a Bluetooth streamer, remote control, and in some cases a remote microphone.

Radio Frequency (RF) Streaming

Alternatively, other manufacturers use a variety of proprietary radio frequency (RF) techniques (e.g., those based on LE Bluetooth) to deliver sound from intermediary devices. As we detail in Chapter 10, these techniques allow for considerably longer transmission distances, allowing RF devices to be placed on or within

---

TECHNICAL TIP: HOW MANY WIRELESS SYSTEMS IN THE SAME HEARING AID?

The earliest attempts at data sharing between hearing aids used NFEI to send data between hearing aids directly or via an intermediary router. RF sound streaming from external sources to the intermediary router was then added. Now that RF streaming directly to hearing aids is being used by nearly all manufacturers, it is reasonable to wonder how data and/or sound are transferred between hearing aids. The answer, as always seems to be the case with emerging technologies, it depends on the manufacturer. Specifically, some manufacturers use the same RF strategies for all of their streaming needs, whereas others have retained NFEI streaming for communication between hearing aids. This second group cites latency advantages as the primary reason for including both IE and RF communication within the same hearing aid.

the device that is streaming (i.e., remote microphone, television, personal music device, etc.) rather than on the user. Although not employed by all manufacturers, some RF techniques are also capable of wider transmission bandwidth than typically applied with NFEI, potentially improving signal fidelity for some listeners. ReSound was the first manufacturer to introduce modern, digital RF techniques in hearing aids, but all other manufacturers have since followed suit, at least for smartphone streaming. We expect all manufacturers will continue to adopt spread-spectrum, digital, RF streaming methods for increasingly more wireless streaming applications.

Benefits and Limitations

We discussed the operation and benefits of remote microphones in Chapter 11. As a reminder, the effective reduction in distance to the talker can provide considerable benefits associated with better audibility and improved SNR. They can also improve understanding by delivering sounds directly to the ear without reverberation. Environments with long reverberation times can greatly reduce speech recognition, as we discuss in Chapter 4. These listening benefits are also present when streaming television, music, and other audio signals. In

---

POINTS TO PONDER: WIRELESS SIGNAL DELIVERY FROM EXTERNAL DEVICES

Technology is constantly changing, especially in this area. Our review below is early 2018 vintage. If you are reading this a few years later, things very well could be different. We review smartphone connection separately later in this chapter.

Dual Streaming Techniques.
- Widex. NFEI streamer accepts Bluetooth, direct connections, or input from other compatible far-field streamers that can be placed on devices such as television.

Dual Streaming and Radio Frequency Techniques.
- Sivantos (Signia). NFEI streamer accepts Bluetooth, direct connections, or input from proprietary remote microphone. An RF television streamer is also available.
- Sonova (Phonak). NFEI streamer accepts Bluetooth, direct connections, or RF input from proprietary remote microphone. Propriety boots and some hearing aid models without boots will directly accept input from a propriety RF remote microphone that includes beamforming technology. The RF remote microphone can also be used with a hub device to relay transmission from television and other sources directly to the hearing aid or boot. One model will pair directly with a Bluetooth enabled Hub which can be placed near the device being streamed.

Radio Frequency Techniques.
- ReSound. Intermediary RF streamer placed on the remote device (e.g., television) via direct connection. An inexpensive RF remote microphone (spouse mic) is also available, which can stream directly to the hearing aid. More advanced remote microphones are also available that have increased transmission range (up to 80 ft.) and can include multi-microphone technologies.
- Starkey. Intermediary RF streamer placed on the remote device (e.g., television) via direct connection. A second type of streaming device is available that adds, Bluetooth and remote functions, and can also serve as a remote microphone.
- Oticon. Intermediary RF streamer placed on the remote device (e.g., television) via direct connection. An inexpensive RF remote microphone (spouse mic) is also available, which can stream directly to the hearing aid or to an NFEI intermediary device.

addition, there can also be benefits for television and music streaming that we would describe as very real but somewhat indirect. Clinically, we have all heard complaints from spouses about the television being turned up "way too loud." The need for television and music to be loud enough for a family member with hearing impairment when the rest of the family has normal hearing can be a source of family strife and embarrassment. Sometimes, the hearing aid alone is not enough to fully remedy this problem, particularly if it is a noisy household. In addition, streaming music to the hearing aids "on the go" can be quite convenient and effective because the listener does not have to remove his or her hearing aids to use headphones, and the hearing aids provide frequency shaping that is appropriate for the individual's hearing loss.

Special consideration must be made when streaming television or other AV sources, however. Even standard Bluetooth audio (the type used in Bluetooth headsets, not the LE Bluetooth used in hearing aids) is not optimal for television streaming because its high latency can create a mismatch between the audio and video timing that is unacceptable to most listeners. Consequently, specialized television streamers aimed at minimizing audio delay are sometimes employed. Delay continues to be an issue for some devices, however, and devices currently have delays ranging from a quite acceptable 10 ms (or less) to more than 150 ms. Another alternative that can be applied with a streamer that has an unacceptably long latency is to adjust the video delay. That is, some modern televisions allow the user to delay the video signal relative to the audio by a range of fixed amounts. Although this can produce acceptable results, many elderly hearing aid wearers may not be capable of making these adjustments to their televisions without assistance, even if they own a television with this capability.

Technologically, the simplest way to limit wireless latency is to use an intermediary near-field NFEI streamer that is worn around the listener's neck for streaming from the hearing aids while also employing a low latency streaming protocol from a streamer connected to the television to the intermediary streamer. Of course, this requires the user to wear the intermediary streamer rather than simply place a single streamer on the television. The setup, number of required streamers, and delay all differ in current solutions. Consequently, it is important that we understand the delay present in the television streamers we provide clinically and recognize the potential benefits and limitations.

Coupling must also be considered when streaming from television and music players as it can affect audible bandwidth (discussed in Chapter 8), which in turn can drastically affect sound quality. The frequency response of the same selection of music delivered from a personal music player to a commercial, partially occluding earbud and streamed to a mini-BTE hearing aid fitted with an open eartip is shown in Figure 12–8. The lack of low-frequency energy through the open eartip is easily visualized. Consider a patient with normal or near normal low-frequency hearing, as is often the case when an open eartip is used. If the patient is streaming from a remote microphone being used by a talker who is relatively close or from a television or other device that is also delivering the same sounds using loudspeakers, the low frequencies delivered to the ear through the air will act to fill in the low frequencies providing an appropriate frequency response and sound quality. For signals that are only delivered through streaming (e.g., music from a personal music player, or a talker using a remote mic who is far away), however, the low frequencies will either be greatly reduced or eliminated entirely resulting in a "tinny" or harsh sound quality. Audibility of low frequencies is known to be highly important for overall sound quality. Indeed, even moving the low frequency cut-off from around 100 Hz to around 200 Hz has been shown to significantly reduce the rated naturalness of sound (Moore & Tan, 2003).

Wireless routing from external devices is limited not only by latency and coupling, but also by the quality of the stream. Often times, the audio stream is quite compressed and fairly low bit rates are used in an attempt to reduce power consumption and latency. Consequently, even though some wireless streamers deliver a bandwidth to the ear that extends from around 100 Hz to more than 8 kHz, others are much more limited. We measured one that only delivered signals from about 300 Hz to about 4.5 kHz. Also remember that the bandwidth delivered to the ear doesn't just depend on the limitations of the streamer. Ultimately, it will also be limited by whatever audible bandwidth the hearing aid is capable of delivering to the listener.

The various transmission methods also provide greatly varying noise floors and, in some cases, an audible hiss may be present, particularly in listeners with a range of normal or near normal threshold.

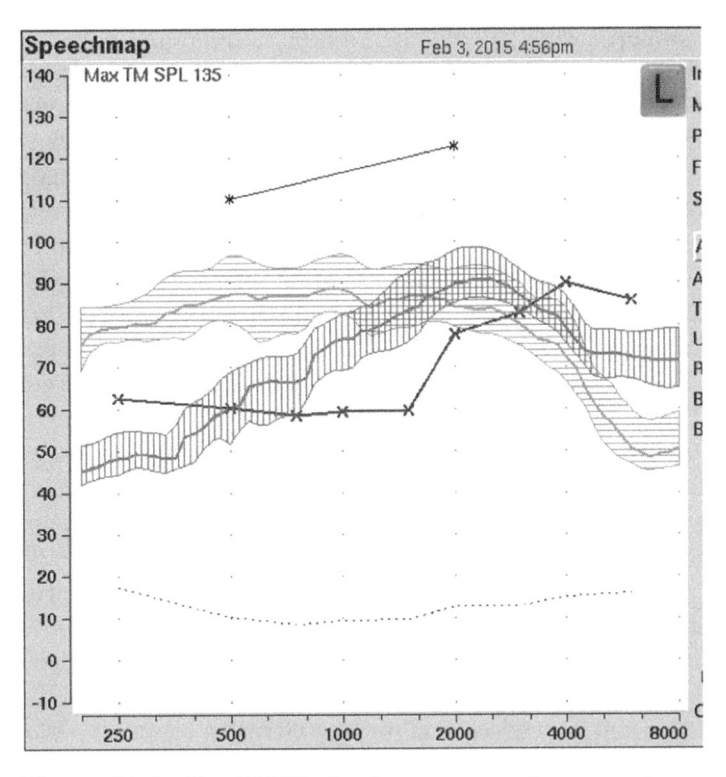

Figure 12–8. The REARs for the same music segment presented to a patient through a commercial, partially occluding earbud and streamed to a mini-BTE hearing aid fitted with an open eartip (much less low frequency energy)

Peer-reviewed literature in this area is lacking, in part because new and improved devices are constantly being introduced. There are, nonetheless, clearly large differences in the quality of streamed signals resulting from differences in the specific techniques used. We encourage audiologists who recommend these technologies to spend a few minutes with your probe microphone system (while "listening in" over headphones) to assess the bandwidth and general sound quality of the signal being delivered. We have never been big fans of using our own normal hearing ears to make clinical decisions for our patients, but in the case of wireless streaming this information, combined with the measured bandwidth can provide general guidance relative to the limitations of streaming systems.

Tips for Candidacy

Of course, the primary reason wireless streaming may be recommended to a patient is that he or she wants it. By probing for details about listening needs, however, we are able to better counsel patients related to use and benefits. Here are some questions to consider:

1. Are you pursuing streaming for your smartphone?
    a. If so, many of these other streaming options are a simple addition.
2. Do you watch television/listen to music with others in the room? If so, do they have normal hearing? Do you have trouble understanding or need to turn up the volume a lot?
    a. If yes to all three, streaming will likely help.
3. How noisy is it in the room where you watch television/listen to music?
    a. If it is noisy, streaming will likely help.
4. Are the patient's coupling needs aligned with his or her listening needs?
    a. If a patient has relatively good low-frequency hearing but also desires streaming, it may be worth experimenting with a closed dome. As we describe in Chapter 8, sometimes there is enough slit leak venting with a closed dome to limit the

occlusion effect to low levels while still limiting venting enough to be able to provide acceptable low-frequency audibility for streamed signals.

b. Also ask questions related to how sound is delivered. Particularly in the case of TV listening, sound may be delivered through streaming and speakers. In that case, open eartips in combination with streaming may provide acceptable sound quality and performance in listeners with near normal low-frequency hearing.

Smartphone Integration and Telephone Listening

For people who grew up with computers that were terribly slow and not very portable, it's hard to believe that today most all of us, over 2 billion people worldwide, carry around a very fast and powerful computer—our smartphone. In 2017, this translated into about 44% of the world's adult population and over 80% of adults in the United States, and this increases substantially each year. This is not just a young adult phenomenon. In the 65-years and over age group, nearly half own a smartphone. Importantly, over 80% of this group own a cell phone of some type (including smartphones), so we expect the smartphone percentage will continue to increase substantially with future cell phone purchases.

Even individuals who are not particularly tech-savvy use their smartphones for a variety of purposes in their daily lives. If you live in a cold climate, starting your car remotely to warm it up is helpful—this easily is accomplished with a smartphone. Around your home you can use your smartphone to control the temperature, monitor security, change the lighting, and even remotely operate your pet feeder. By pasting a sensor on your back, your smartphone will help you control your posture. So if we can use our smartphone to control all of this, why not use it to control hearing aids too? Of course control is not the only application of smartphone integration with hearing aids, there are a number of other potential benefits as well.

How It Works

How the telephone and other sound functions of the smartphone are used with hearing aids depends on two major factors. First, does the hearing aid have the capability to connect directly and wirelessly with a smartphone via RF or is an intermediary NFEI streamer needed? Currently, all of the big six manufacturers offer at least one hearing aid model with direct connection to Apple brand devices (both smartphones and tablets), and at least one manufacturer also has direct connection to any Bluetooth enabled smartphone including Android and Windows based devices. For the other manufacturers, non-Apple devices (e.g., Android or Windows), are typically connected using a small RF transmitter that is placed on the smartphone for communication with the user's hearing aids. These small devices pair with the smartphone via Bluetooth or plug into the smartphones headphone jack. Some manufacturers also have some models that do not yet have built-in Apple connectivity and instead use these small dedicated telephone streamers for all smartphone brands.

Another technique applied in some hearing aid models is to use a small, battery-powered, Bluetooth receiver that relays signals to and from the smartphone and then streams these signals directly to the hearing aid using NFEI. These neck-worn receivers are the same devices we describe in the previous section on wireless streaming. All manufacturers initially used this method of telephone streaming, but it is being phased out and replaced by direct-to-hearing aid streaming.

Streaming sound back and forth from a smartphone directly to hearing aids is a challenging feat, in large part because of the amount of data that must be transferred in real time. In contrast, application functionality—including using smartphone apps as a remote control, for distance support, for geo-tagging, and so forth—requires the transfer of considerably less data. Consequently, this functionality existed well before direct-to-smartphone streaming. Using a smartphone app to control a hearing aid was initially accomplished in one of two ways, both of which have their own advantages and disadvantages and are still used.

The first technique uses a control sound that is a recognized code. The hearing aid then decodes these sounds into the appropriate command. Typically, the phone is close enough to the hearing aids to be easily detected. The control sounds are typically audible, however, and some users report that they can draw (sometimes unwanted) attention. The greatest advantage for this method is that, because sound is used as a control, no pairing or extra equipment is needed, so they can be made to work with a wide range of smartphone brands.

The second technique is to use Bluetooth pairing to a near-field NFEI streaming device worn by the listener. Yes, this is the same intermediary streaming device we have already discussed a few times. Information is sent back and forth between the smartphone and the intermediary device, which then relays this information back and forth with the hearing aids. The biggest advantage to this method is that there can easily be two-way communication of data and, because standard Bluetooth is implemented, the majority of smartphones with Bluetooth capability can use the app. Of course, this technique has the disadvantage of having to use an intermediary streamer.

The newest methods use the direct connect LE Bluetooth protocols to send data back and forth in addition to streaming audio. This method has clear advantages over the previous techniques because it allows for two-way communication without the need for an intermediary device. It is currently available in many hearing aid models and depending on the hearing aid manufacturer, may only work with specific smartphone brands. Given the advantages, however, we expect to see continued increasing use of this control method.

Potential Benefits for Both Patients and Audiologists

We have discussed acoustic telephone programs, telecoils, and wireless streaming solutions throughout this textbook. In addition, we will discuss troubleshooting telephone issues in detail in Chapter 18. It is nevertheless important to consider telephone solutions here, as the potential benefits and limitations of wireless streaming interact with individual patient differences and listening needs. Consequently, there is not a single telephone configuration that is optimal for all patients.

The increased use of cell phones has greatly limited the utility of t-coils for telephone listening. In addition, we know from considerable data that the best speech recognition in noisy environments in children and adults occurs when the telephone signal is streamed to both ears (e.g., Picou & Ricketts, 2011; 2013; Wolfe, Mills, Schafer, John & Hudson, 2014; Wolfe, 2013). The benefits from bilateral over unilateral streaming in noise can be as much as 20 to 40% on average if the hearing aid microphones are not activated. We also know that use of an open fitting greatly reduces streaming benefits in noise, as does activation of the hearing aid microphones. Streaming to both ears without activating at least one of the hearing aid microphones, however, will make it more difficult to monitor the listening environment. Finally, we know that listeners with relatively good low-frequency hearing and an open fitting can perform well on the phone by simply holding it up to their ear. Armed with this knowledge, we can consider a few questions that may allow us to better optimize the selection of an initial telephone solution without relying so heavily on troubleshooting at follow-up appointments:

- Is it an open fitting? If so, is the patient satisfied with telephone performance when simply holding the phone up to the ear?
  - If yes, encourage the patient to continue telephone usage as they have been doing.
  - If, because of the convenience, they desire streaming anyway, consider streaming to both ears and disabling the hearing aid microphones to maximize performance; however, ensure environmental monitoring is adequate through the open earmold. Counsel that performance may be reduced in noisy environments and that sound quality will likely be poor, as we described previously. Remember, the voice bandwidth delivered through a telephone is only 300 to 3000 Hz. With an open fitting and normal low-frequency hearing it is quite possible to only deliver audible telephone signals to the ear from 1200 to 3000 Hz. Clearly this can have very negative effects on sound quality and speech recognition over the telephone.
- Alternatively, consider using a closed tip to improve sound quality and performance. Streaming to only one hearing aid or leaving the hearing aid microphones active may lead to acceptable telephone performance in this configuration, while still allowing for monitoring, if the patient has good enough speech understanding. Also, ensure that the use of a closed eartip does not result in an unacceptable increase in the occlusion effect and associated

decreases in sound quality for the patient's own voice and when chewing.
- Is the listener often on the telephone in noise? If so, how poorly does the listener perform on the telephone in noise?
  - If performance in noise is very poor, bilateral streaming may be required.
- How important is monitoring sounds in the environment for safety or awareness?
  - If very important, consider leaving the hearing aid microphones active or only stream to one ear (with the hearing aid microphone deactivated on that side), and allow for monitoring with the other hearing aid. It is sometimes a balancing act between monitoring and performance in noise issues. Many models will also allow the clinician to adjust the mix ratio between the telephone stream and the hearing aid microphones. Manipulating this mix ratio may be necessary to optimize the relative importance of monitoring and understanding the telephone streamed signal.

In the next sections, we talk about some potential benefits related to smartphone connectivity for both the patient and the audiologist in addition to the previously described improved communication over the telephone. Note that we use the word *potential*. Most of them have not been carefully researched, and the benefits we state often are simply based on speculation, limited field trials, and patient testimony. We also need to mention that not all features we discuss are available with all products. For example, some of these potential advantages are only possible if two-way communication is available — check with your favorite manufacturer to see what they have to offer. At the time of this writing, we still have patients who continue to report difficulty with pairing and making everything work. Still, these issues continue to improve and some systems walk patients through pairing using a very small number of steps.

Potential Benefits for the Patient: Signal Processing

- Ability to override automatic functions of the hearing aid. For example, most products will not switch to narrow directivity unless the overall SPL is at a certain level. For a given listening situation, however, a patient, using his or her smartphone, can change the processing from omnidirectional to narrow directionality, to everything in between, to optimize speech understanding.
- Geotagged memories. Such memories will automatically switch modes when the smartphone GPS feature detects the patient is in a tagged location (e.g., the patient has a specific program and settings that works the best in his or her favorite pub—the hearing will automatically switch to that program and settings when the pub location is detected).
- Motion detection system of the smartphone. The hearing aids will alter their signal processing when the patient is moving. For example, one might assume that, when the patient is walking, he or she will be interested in surrounding sounds in the environment to promote situational awareness. The hearing aid processing, therefore, would be more apt to stay in omnidirectional processing mode rather than to go to narrow directivity when a voice is detected.

Potential Benefits for the Patient: Convenience, Information, and Care

- Apps are easily used to change volume, programs and frequency response (e.g., turn up or down the bass or treble). In Chapter 11, we describe some apps that can even control advanced hearing aid microphone settings so that the user can "point" the hearing aid sensitivity in the direction the or she wants to listen.
- Advanced functions for streamers are also available. These range from remote control of the streamer settings (i.e., adjusting the relative level of a TV streamer versus the hearing aid microphones) to giving specific information about lost connection between hearing aids, streamers, and devices.
- Patients can review amount of daily hearing aid use and type of listening situations. These

data are stored, several months of data can be reviewed, and the patient can then monitor his or her activity. It is speculated that this might encourage hearing aid use, much as a step tracker might encourage walking.

- If the hearing aid has an "own voice" detection system, the patient can use this to track their vocal participation in various listening conditions—are they active or just a listener?
- The hearing aid calculates the patient's projected daily listening effort and, based on the use, the overall SPL and SNR experienced during the day. The patient can compare this to his or her own assessment of the day.
- Many smartphone apps can be streamed directly to the hearing aid. Providing audio access to everything from music listening, to video streaming, to hearing the sound of your favorite mobile game can offer entertainment and educational value.
- The smartphone can be used as a remote microphone. This is a handy feature for a noisy restaurant or maybe even to "listen in" to a conversation around the house.
- Instructions on use and care of the hearing aid are available as part of an app.
- Auditory training programs can be accessed.
- Battery strength can be monitored.
- Just as you might change the ring tone of your smartphone, the patient can select what alert signals he or she would like to hear for program change, low battery, and so forth.
- Distance support is one of the newer features we are starting to see show up in apps. Using these systems, a patient can send an electronic message to their audiologist about a problem, complaint, or question. The audiologist can then respond with a message and, in some cases, remotely make changes to the hearing aid settings so problems can be fixed efficiently and directly without having the patient return to the office. We expect these telehealth applications will continue to expand and allow for enhancement of patient care and improved access for patients. We describe them in a bit more detail in the next section.

Potential Benefits for the Audiologist

- The smartphone/hearing aids pairing can be used for an on-the-spot assessment of a listening condition, a watered-down version of ecological momentary assessment or EMA (Wu, Stangl, Chipara, Hasan, Welhaven & Oleson, 2017). The patient can do a

---

TECHNICAL TIP: A PASTURAL STORY

We mention that a feature available today for the patient using his or her smartphone is the ability to find a misplaced hearing aid. Now, you might think that this is simply to track it down in the patient's home, but there are other applications. A rancher in western North Dakota bought a pair of new hearing aids with this feature and, fortunately, his audiologist trained him regarding its use. A couple of days after the purchase of the hearing aids, he decided to walk the fence line of his 160-acre pasture—a common thing for ranchers to do (to check for possible breaks in the fence caused by the cattle, known to think that the grass on the *other side* of the fence is greener). He decided to wear his new hearing aids on his walk, thinking that maybe he could hear the call of the meadowlarks occupying the pasture, which he had been missing for many years. He indeed found some places needing repair and stopped a few times to do mends. When he returned to his pickup, he realized that one of his hearing aids was missing. He activated his "find hearing aid app" and repeated his walk around the pasture. He found his lost hearing aid. No report is available on whether he heard the call of the meadowlarks.

real-time rating regarding how they are doing for variety of listening situations in their daily life. This can then be reviewed by the audiologist as an outcome measure, and to facilitate counseling.

- The patient can take a "snapshot" of a given listening situation that is difficult for him or her. This can be remotely viewed by the audiologist or shown to the audiologist on the repeat visit, and provide information such as the overall SPL, the SNR, and the hearing aid settings (e.g., activation of directional features). Armed with this information, the audiologist can develop treatment and/or counseling strategies. For example, if the overall SPL is 85 dB, the SNR is +3 dB, and the audiologist knows the patient's QuickSIN score is +10 dB, the treatment is likely counseling and not reprogramming.
- Through internet access of the smartphone, the hearing aids can be programmed remotely by the audiologist if the patient has installed this app. Whereas today this might not be popular for many audiologists, who typically would like their patient to come back to their office, this certainly is a feature that might become more popular with groups like the VA, who often have hearing aid patients who live 100 miles or more from the nearest clinic. Moreover, given the passage of OTC hearing aid legislation, let's think a little bit about what the delivery system in future years could be. Perhaps the patient picks up a pair of hearing aids from the neighborhood drug store after having his or her hearing tested in a kiosk. The patient downloads a free programming app (provided by the manufacturer of the OTC product). The app does a quick search for a nearby participating audiologist who does online programming. And we're off and running.
- We know that the average patient forgets about one-half of what we say about his or her hearing aids on the day of the fitting. Smartphone apps are available that can provide the patient access to all this information at home following the fitting.

Potential Limitations

To state the obvious, the patient must have a smartphone and the hearing aid must be able to connect with the patient's smartphone. Although not specifically a limitation, a consideration for the dispensing audiologist is that fitting the patient with a product with direct smartphone streaming might mean that a different desired feature is not available. For example, a patient who wants both direct streaming and a rechargeable battery may only be able to have one or the other (at least from some manufacturers). And of course, the patient must have the cognitive ability and motivation to use the features available. Certainly, some of the advanced features will only apply to a small group of hearing aid users, but almost all patients have the skill set and general cognition to use their smartphones simply for such things as volume adjustment or checking their battery life.

TECHNICAL TIP: A LITTLE MATH ON BATTERY LIFE

Here is a little battery life example adapted from Barry Freeman (2016). Corrine is a teenager with a mild-to-moderate hearing loss. She wears hearing aids that have the capability of direct streaming from her iPhone. Corrine wears her hearing aids 12 hours per day with wireless streaming to her iPhone for an estimated three of those hours. During normal operation without streaming, the current drain of each hearing aid is 2.0mAh and while streaming it is 5.5 mAh. Therefore, total daily battery drain is 34.5 mAh (2.0 mA × 9 hours + 5.5 mA × 3 hours = 34.5 mA of daily current drain). If she uses a disposable 312 zinc-air battery with a functional capacity of 126 mAh, she will have an estimated 3.6 days of battery life (126 mAh/34.5 mA per day = 3.6 days). Without the iPhone streaming, she would expect her batteries to last nearly twice long, although she very likely would consider this a small price to pay (literally) for the streaming advantage.

Speaking of battery life, this is another factor to consider. As most of you know from your smartphone use, streaming features significantly shorten battery life. Let's take a modern high-end hearing aid with a 312 battery. Without streaming, in general use we might have battery drain of about 1.0 mAh (milliamp/hour). With streaming but idling, we would expect a drain of about 2.0 mA. But, with phone or music streaming, we now would have a drain of around 5.0 to 6.0 mAh. For people who use the streaming function for several hours a day, it's obvious that battery life will be shortened significantly. Given the relatively low cost of hearing aid batteries (18 cents/battery at big box stores), this is not a major issue for most patients. There are always, of course, the patients who return frequently to the office complaining that the batteries in their new hearing aids just don't last as long as they did in their old hearing aids. Savvy audiologists just give these people a year's supply and the problem goes away (well, at least for a year). There are patients who do not have the dexterity to change the battery, and this is a different issue. The drain from streaming has been reduced in recent years, and as we move more and more to rechargeable hearing aid batteries, battery life will be less of an issue (see section on batteries in Chapter 10).

Speech Enhancement

Over the years there have been a large number of techniques aimed at enhancing speech to try to improve speech understanding in listeners with hearing loss. One group of techniques that has enjoyed considerable popularity recently is frequency-lowering, which we discuss in a later section. We will discuss a number of other techniques here. One of the more common speech enhancement techniques is spectral sharpening (spectral contrast enhancement). The goal of this processing is to use filtering and other methods to reduce spectral valleys, thus providing greater contrast relative to the spectral peaks. The point is to try to make peak frequency energy stand out more sharply. Unfortunately, even though these techniques can enhance detection of speech peaks, they do not appear to improve intelligibility, even in listeners with normal hearing. The only time when speech recognition performance is improved is if the speech enhancement increases peak energy from a point of inaudible to audible. Of course, for this to happen, loudness would also be increased and the same benefits would be achieved by simply increasing gain. Such increases in gain for low-level speech can and are already accomplished using multichannel amplitude compression (i.e., WDRC) which is considerably simpler than some complex speech enhancement methods that require detection of speech sounds prior to enhancement. These technologies are even less compelling when we consider that sensorineural hearing loss reduces frequency resolution, making it even more unlikely that listeners with hearing loss could use or even detect spectral sharpening. A number of other types of speech enhancement have been attempted, and whereas a few have shown modest improvements in listeners with severe-to-profound hearing loss, the magnitude of these improvements is typically far less than the average benefits provided by cochlear implantation in this population.

"Extended" High-Frequency Energy— Importance and Amplification

We discuss the acoustics of speech in detail in Chapter 4, pointing out that research related to the SII has shown that the importance of speech energy above 4 kHz is limited. Indeed, this is one of the reasons that the bandwidth of telephones remains around 300 to 3000 Hz, despite the use of a number of very advanced processing techniques used in many modern smartphones. In addition, data has clearly demonstrated that individuals with both flat and sloping high-frequency hearing loss demonstrate a poorer-than-normal ability to use amplified speech information in the extended high-frequency region (e.g., Ching, Dillon, Katsch, & Byrne, 2001; Hornsby & Ricketts, 2003; 2006). Despite the small effect, this same work demonstrated speech recognition still improves significantly with increasing high-frequency audibility through 7 kHz. Work with children suggests that audibility of high-frequency speech energy may be even more important. For example, Stelmachowitz, Pittman, Hoover and Lewis (2001) demonstrated that both adults and children with impaired hearing demonstrated large and significant increases in speech recognition performance when the maximum high-frequency energy was increased from 6 kHz to 9 kHz and the target was a female talker. Performance increases in adult listeners were as much as 50 percentage points; however, increases of more than 70 percentage points were reported for children. As we discuss in Chapter 4, even patients with high-frequency dead regions can benefit from, and indicate a preference for, audible energy above 3000 Hz. The effect of restricted access to high-frequency information is not limited to decrements in speech recognition. For example, data have shown that production of some high-frequency consonants (/s/ and /z/) is 15 to 18% worse for children with significant high-frequency hearing loss who use hearing aids, than for their peers who use cochlear implants (Grant, Bow, Paatsch, & Blamey, 2002). In addition, data have shown that increasing audible bandwidth above 5 kHz can improve localization (e.g., Brungart and Simpson, 2009), improve spatial release from masking (Moore, Glasberg & Stone 2010), and decrease listening effort (e.g., Karlsen, Flynn & Eneroth, 2006).

Perceived sound quality is also highly dependent on the audible frequency bandwidth, at least in listeners with normal hearing. For example, Moore and Tan (2003) reported that perceived sound quality of music was rated highest for the widest tested bandwidth of approximately 16.5 kHz. A significant degradation in sound quality was noted for both speech and music when the upper cutoff frequency was decreased below 10.8 kHz and when the lower cutoff frequency was increased from 123 to 208 Hz. Listeners with impaired hearing demonstrate a different pattern, however. Franks (1982) demonstrated that increasing the high-frequency cutoff in a hearing aid from 4 to 10 kHz significantly improved sound quality in a group of normal hearing listeners, but not in 20 listeners with hearing loss (ranging from 10–85 dB HL for frequencies above 750 Hz). Other research however, has demonstrated individual differences in performance and sound quality preference as a function of audible gain and bandwidth in listeners with impaired hearing. Ricketts et al. (2008), demonstrated that preference for either a higher or lower high-frequency cut-off frequency (9 or 5.5 kHz cutoff frequency, respectively) was correlated with the slope of hearing loss from 4 to 12 kHz, with steep threshold slopes associated with a preference for narrower bandwidths. Specifically, listeners with thresholds no poorer than 75 dB HL and a high-frequency threshold slope of less than 12.5 dB per octave or less demonstrated preference for the higher cutoff (Figure 12–9). Furthermore, preferences were strongest and most consistent when the amplification applied ensured the high-frequency content was approximately 10 dB above threshold. Less amplification (3 dB of audibility) eliminated preference differences and more amplification (20 dB of audibility) resulted in decreased preference.

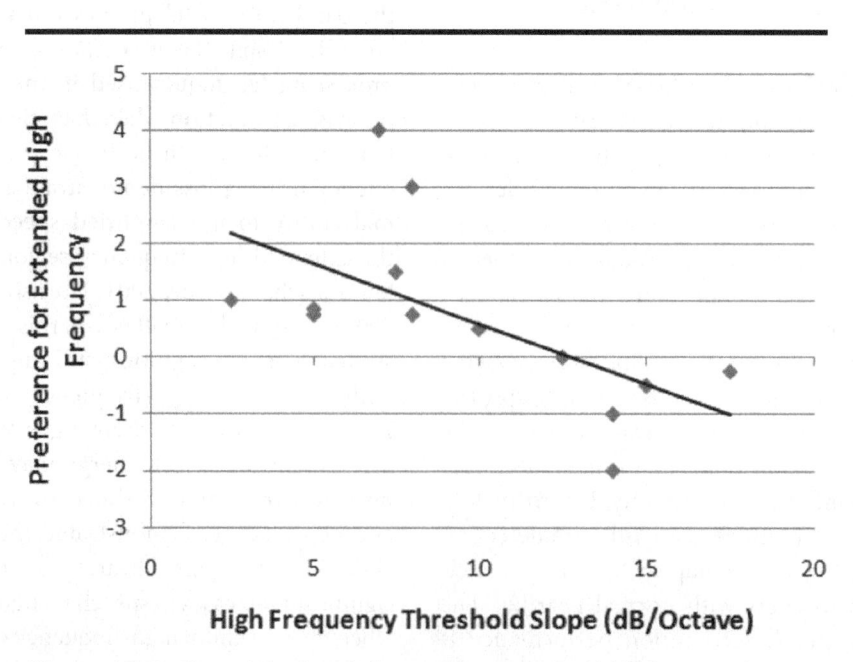

Figure 12–9. Sound quality preference for extended high frequencies as a function of hearing loss slope (2 kHz–12.5 kHz).

Individualization of "Extended" High Frequencies

While increasing access to sound above 4 to 5 kHz, sometimes referred to as extended high-frequency information, can lead to improved performance, one hallmark of previous studies is considerable individual variability. That is, some individuals appear to benefit from this extension, meanwhile others receive no benefit or even perform more poorly. In addition, these extended high frequencies can also differentially affect sound quality. Although more work in this area is needed, a few considerations are offered as a clinical starting point when considering provision of extended high-frequency amplification:

- Degree of high-frequency hearing loss matters: Those listeners with high-frequency thresholds that exceed 75 dB HL will be less likely to prefer extended high-frequency amplification. In addition, given that sound energy in this frequency range is typically fairly low level, providing audibility for this extended frequency range might not be possible using conventional air conduction technologies for those with greater hearing loss.
- Slope of hearing loss probably matters: If you measure thresholds from 2 kHz through at least 10 kHz, those with slopes less than 12.5 dB per octave are more likely to exhibit a preference for audible extended high frequencies.
- Age probably matters: Children (prelingually impaired) are more likely to benefit from extended high-frequency audibility than adults with acquired hearing loss.
- High-frequency dead regions probably don't matter, but in adults you can measure performance differences. In Chapter 6 we discuss the use of the Quick-SIN for assessing utility of high-frequency speech information. Listeners with significantly poorer performance on the high-frequency emphasis version are likely not good candidates for extended high-frequency amplification.

Frequency-Lowering (FL) Algorithms

While the importance of audibility for sound energy in the extended high-frequency range may depend on the individual, the importance of sound energy in the more traditional high-frequency range (e.g., 1.5–5.5 kHz) has been clearly demonstrated. Access to this high-frequency energy is often limited, however, particularly in listeners with steeply sloping hearing loss (e.g., Kimlinger, McCreery, & Lewis, 2015). Indeed, this research revealed the highest audible frequency for eight commercial BTE hearing aids, which were specifically chosen based on their ANSI specified high-frequency band limits, was less than 4000 Hz for a speech signal, assuming profound high-frequency hearing loss. The highest audible bandwidth increased to between 6 kHz and 8 kHz when high-frequency thresholds in the severe range were assumed. Importantly, these estimates should be considered conservative, in that tight coupling without any slit leak venting or possibility of feedback was assured.

For many listeners with significant hearing loss, high-frequency energy may not be accessible due to audibility constraints. Even if available, it may be undesirable, due to degree or slope of hearing loss, decreased performance, or decreased sound quality. Since audibility for sloping hearing loss is expected to be most limited in the highest frequencies, it is not surprising that the idea of shifting sounds from a high-frequency range, for which audibility is limited or absent, to a lower frequency range for which audibility is achievable has been around for many decades (see Simpson, 2009, for a review). Historically, a wide range of different techniques have been used. The history is actually pretty interesting, but we will refer you to other sources rather than spend the time to review it here in detail because modern devices use somewhat different techniques and are aimed at slightly different populations.

Early frequency-lowering techniques were focused on patients with very little usable hearing, at least in the high frequencies. Processing was first introduced in analog devices and then later digital control and DSP processing were applied. Several problems were noted in these early devices including greatly reduced sound quality, limited benefits, and shipping issues for repairs (one company using this technology in the 1990s was in Israel). These factors combined to greatly limit the use of frequency-lowering by the early 2000s. Furthermore, advances in cochlear implants greatly reduced interest in frequency-lowering techniques for many listeners with limited usable hearing (i.e. profound hearing loss).

How It Works

Modern frequency-lowering techniques were first introduced in the mid-2000s. Specifically, Widex introduced a technique it referred to as "Audibility Extender" in 2006. This was followed by Phonak's introducing "SoundRecover" in 2008. Currently, all of the big six manufacturers have frequency-lowering processing; Widex and Phonak have introduced updated versions of their original techniques (see Alexander, 2016a, for review). In addition to the reported benefits, the interest in these technologies across manufacturers was also likely spurred by the fact that some countries now require that some form of frequency-lowering be available in all new hearing aids fitted to children. Although there are many variations, modern frequency-lowering implements three general techniques: frequency transposition, frequency compression, and high-frequency reinforcement. All three general techniques have a low-frequency limit (LFL) and an upper-frequency limit (UFL), which define the high-frequency source region that is being lowered or analyzed. The manufacturer-specific terms used for these limits and regions vary widely. With a few exceptions described later, the UFL is typically the highest frequency processed by the hearing aid (typically limited by the microphone). In addition, all have a target frequency region that is the frequency region that will be in some way modified to introduce energy based on the content of the source region. In current hearing aids, all methods also have a range of low-frequency speech energy which is not altered because it is already audible without the need for lowering. Compared to the original frequency-lowering techniques, preservation of the lower frequencies helps maintain better sound quality and limits frequency distortion that can reduce recognition of speech segments that are dominated by low frequency energy, especially vowels (e.g., Alexander, 2016)c. As we detail later in this section, the target region may fall above the LFL, may fall below the LFL, or may overlap the LFL, depending on the specific lowering technique used.

The modern frequency-lowering techniques currently available from major manufacturers and their sister companies are summarized in Table 12–1.

TECHNICAL TIP: GENERAL FREQUENCY-LOWERING TECHNIQUES

- Frequency transposition. One band (or more) of high-frequency input energy is identified above the LFL limit and then lowered to a frequency range that overlaps with existing low frequency energy (below the LFL). The lowered high-frequency band(s) is mixed with the existing low frequency energy and delivered to the ear together as a combined output.
- Frequency compression. One (or more) high-frequency range(s) of the input signal is compressed into one (or more) smaller target range(s) of output frequencies. In most systems, the LFL is held constant and the UFL is lowered to compress the range of frequencies.
- High-frequency reinforcement (envelope replication). This technique differs significantly from the other two in that no energy is actually moved. Instead, the spectral envelope of the high-frequency content is derived when energy in the source region is present. This envelope is then applied to existing (acoustically related) energy below the LFL to provide a boost and reinforce the total amount of high-frequency energy.
- Combinations of these techniques are also applied in modern hearing aids. The exact process for lowering or compression, the relative frequency relationships, and the scaling of the relationships all vary by manufacturer. The general processes are shown conceptually in Figure 12–10.

Table 12–1. Modern Frequency-Lowering Techniques by Manufacturer and General Method

Manufacturer	Feature Name	Frequency-Lowering Method
Widex	Audibility Extender	Transposition
	Enhanced Audibility Extender	Transposition (adaptive)
Phonak	SoundRecover[a]	Compression
	SoundRecover2	Compression (adaptive)
Starkey	Spectral iQ[b]	High-Frequency Reinforcement
Signia	Frequency Compression[c]	Compression
ReSound	Sound Shaper[d]	Compression
Oticon	Speech Rescue[e]	Transposition (adaptive)

Note. Techniques labeled "adaptive" modify general operation based on the content of the input. Manufacturers are listed in chronological order.

[a]Also offered by Unitron as "Frequency Compression." [b]Also offered by Microtech as "Sound Compression." [c]Also offered by Rexton as "Bandwidth Compression." [d]Also offered by Beltone as "Sound Shifter." [e]Similar to, but not the same as, what is offered by Bernafon as "Frequency Composition" and by Sonic as "Frequency Transfer."

Source: Adapted from Alexander (2016c).

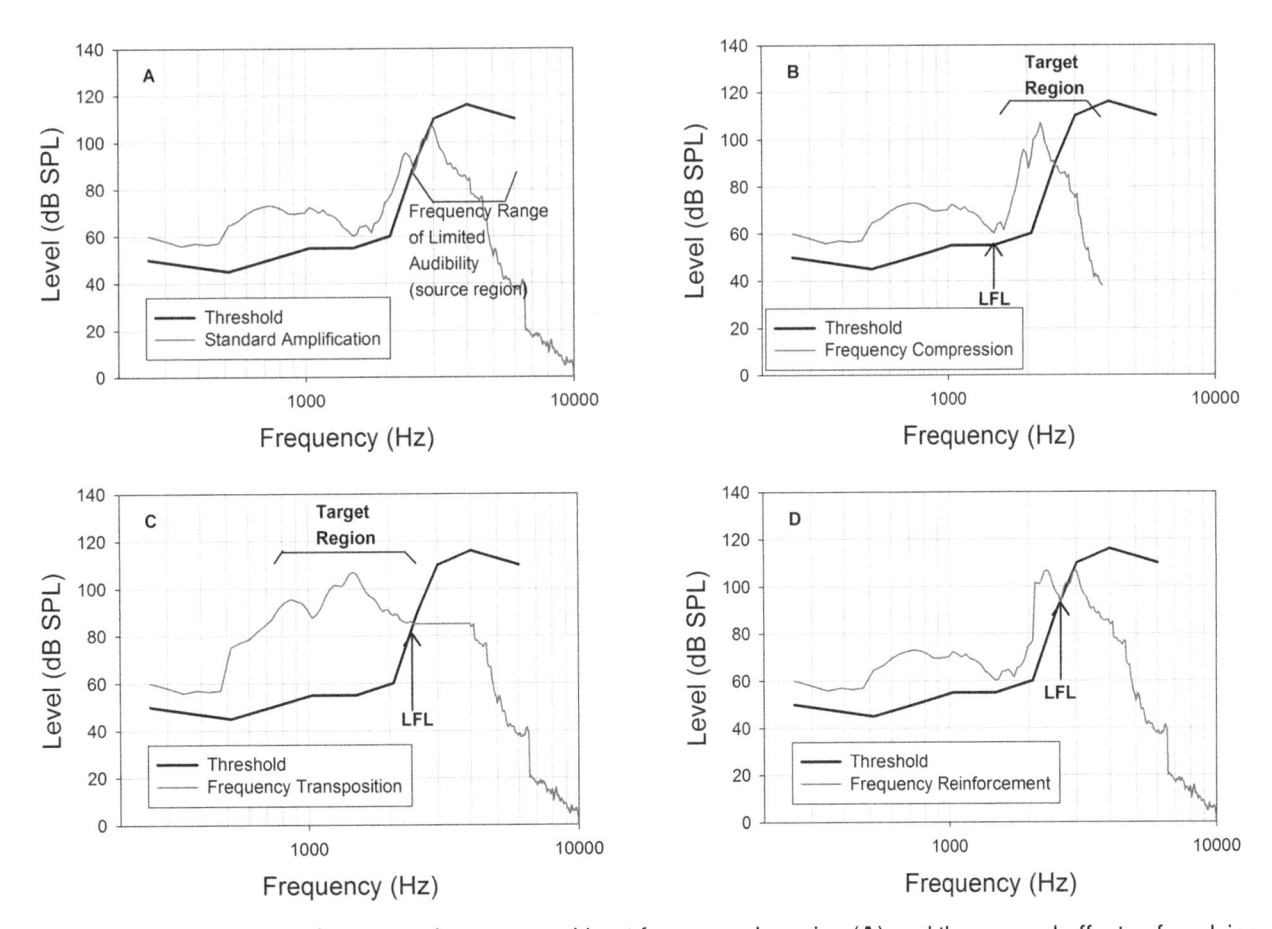

Figure 12–10. The REAR for a speech segment without frequency-lowering (**A**) and the general effects of applying frequency compression (**B**), frequency transposition (**C**), and high-frequency reinforcement (**D**).

Frequency Transposition (FT)

In general, FT techniques begin by identifying the energy peak above the activation frequency. In the original Widex version one octave around this peak energy was copied and transposed down (moved) by one octave (one-half the frequency of the energy peak). For example, if the peak energy was an octave centered around 3000 Hz, this high-frequency energy was moved down one octave relative to this peak to 1500 Hz and mixed with the existing signal. In the current Widex processing there are two overlapping high-frequency source regions targeted for lowering. One can choose to lower only the lower frequency source region by one octave, similar to the original version. Optionally, the second higher frequency source region can also be lowered, albeit by a greater amount (one-third the peak frequency). For example, a peak in the higher frequency region centered at 6000 Hz will be transposed down to 2000 Hz. In addition, the clinician has the option of setting the bandwidth of the low-frequency region that is not subject to lowering. In other words, audibility of frequencies above the LFL can be preserved even when that same speech energy is also targeted for lowering.

The current Widex processing also includes processing that adaptively changes the behavior of the frequency-lowering algorithm based on signal classification—specifically, whether incoming high-frequency speech energy is identified as harmonically related or not (e.g., noise). In other words, the classifier is designed to differentiate voiced from voiceless phonemes (Kuk, Schmidt, Jessen, & Sonne, 2015). This information is used to provide less gain to the lowered signal if it includes voiced phonemes. Processing is also applied, given the goal of keeping the harmonics of these voiced phonemes aligned with the harmonics already in the low frequencies (Kuk et al., 2015). According to the manufacturer, these techniques are applied to improve sound quality, reduce distortion of the harmonic content, and increase distinction between voiced and voiceless energy.

The current FT algorithm employed by Oticon also moves high-frequency energy (without compression) to lower frequencies while also preserving high-frequency energy above the LFL, but it does so using very different techniques from those employed by Widex (Angelo, Alexander, Christiansen, Simonsen, & Jespersgaard, 2015). First, there are either two or three subregions within the source region that are broken up differently as a function of setting. More aggressive settings have three source regions that span into slightly lower frequencies (e.g., 3 or 4 kHz), and less aggressive settings have two source regions that are generally limited to the highest frequencies. Multiple subregions are identified because, rather than just lower the entire source region by the same amount, each subregion is linearly lowered by a different amount so that the energy from each subregion overlaps in the destination region. For example, in one setting, input energy from 4000 to 7000 Hz is divided into three 1000 Hz wide subregions and then all three are linearly transposed by different amounts to result in an overlapping target region that is only 1000 Hz wide in total (i.e., 1600–2600 Hz). According to the manufacturer, use of a narrow target range has the potential to reduce distortion of the existing low-frequency information, as well as provide better frequency resolution for the lowered signals, because a wider frequency range of signal is distributed over a narrow region of the cochlea.

Frequency Compression

As we noted in Table 12–1, there are three companies that use a form of frequency compression (FC) for frequency-lowering. They are similar in that all move the frequencies downward by compressing energy below the UFL toward the target LFL. That is, there is a different input UFL for the input (source region) and the output (target region). Manufacturers refer to this output UFL using terms like "Fmax" and "upper cutoff." FC processing squeezes the source region into a smaller target region, reducing frequency bandwidth. One easy way to visualize this effect is to plot the relationship between input and output frequency, much as we plot input-out functions for amplitude compression. Another way that can be even more illustrative is to plot both the changes in level and in frequency (Figure 12–11). Unlike amplitude compression, there is unfortunately not an accepted nomenclature for FC. It is important to understand these nomenclature differences because, unlike amplitude compression, fitting an individual with the same compression kneepoint and compression ratio will not necessarily result in the same fitting across different manufacturers. This can make things complicated when adjusting settings across manufacturers. Whereas one company has only three possible FC settings, more than

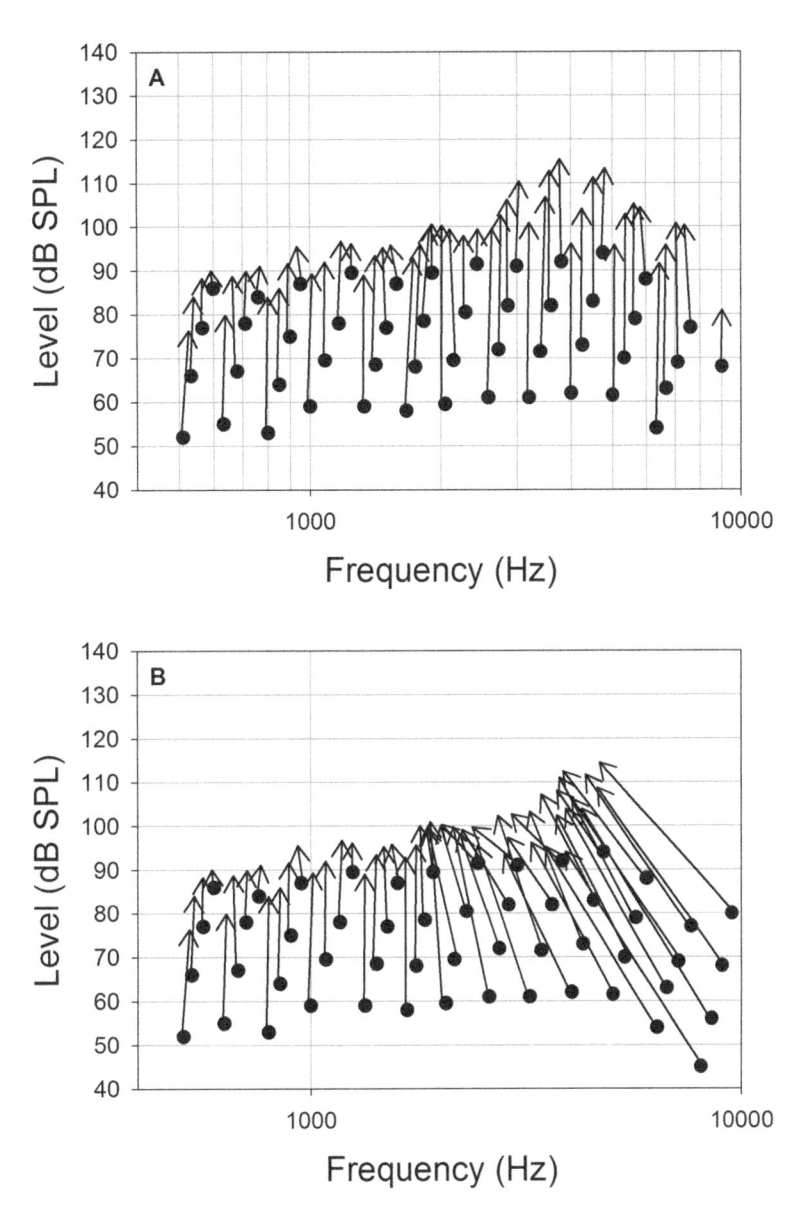

Figure 12–11. An example of the change in frequency and level for one setting of one manufacturer's frequency compression processing. (Adapted from Kokx-Ryan, et al., 2015).

80 possible combinations are possible from another company, so understanding what the company-specific terminology means matters.

One example of manufacturer specific terminology differences is the FC equivalent of the amplitude compression kneepoint, which we generically refer to as the LFL. It is referred to when using terms like "start frequency," "minimum frequency," or "cutoff frequency" depending on the manufacturer. The differences are even less straightforward when considering the relationship between the input and output frequencies. All three companies use the same term to refer to this relationship: compression ratio; however, the nature of the relationship is different depending on the manufacturer. Furthermore, the UFL of the source region differs across manufacturers (from approximately 7000 to 11,000 Hz). In Phonak's original processing the relationship between input and output frequency was logarithmic. If, for example, we assume a compression ratio of 2:1 and a source region that is two octaves wide (e.g., 2000–8000 Hz), the compressed output would be one octave wide (2000–4000 Hz). In contrast, the relationship between input and output frequency for the ReSound algorithm is proportional. If we assume a compression ratio of 2:1, frequencies move 50% closer to the LFL. For example, if we assume a LFL of 4000 Hz and a CR of 2:1, energy at 5000 Hz moves to 4500 Hz. The frequency compression ratio in Signia products is defined in another manner altogether. Rather than being a fixed logarithmic or proportional relationship, the target frequency region is adjusted directly by manipulating the LFL and output UFL. The compression ratio is then defined by the resulting relationship between the frequency bandwidth of the source region and the resulting bandwidth of the target region. Although this is quite easy to calculate, the relationship across settings is not a constant on a linear or logarithmic scale.

The second generation of Phonak's FC algorithm differs from the others currently available because it functions in an adaptive manner as a function of input signal frequency dominance (Rehmann, Siddhartha, & Baumann, 2016). Specifically, a higher LFL is applied when the incoming speech is dominated by lower frequency energy. In this case, a low-frequency limit of the source and target range is applied which is referred to as the lower cutoff. When the incoming speech is instead dominated by higher frequency energy, however, a much lower LFL is used (referred to as the higher cutoff). Even though the compression ratio depends on the setting applied by the clinician, once the ratio is set it is applied consistently regardless of whether the lower or higher LFL is used. In other words, frequencies above the higher cutoff are always compressed, whereas frequencies between the lower and upper cutoff are only compressed if the total input signal at that instant in time is dominated by high-frequency energy. In order to make things manageable, clinician controls are limited to two different types: (1) twenty steps that progressively increase the lower cutoff of the LFL and the UFL (decreasing FC aggressiveness) and, (2) four steps that progressively increase the upper cutoff of the LFL (decreasing how much FC is applied to low-frequency dominated sounds).

The implementation of two different LFLs was in response to data showing that, if the LFL is set low enough when vowels and other low-frequency dominated sounds are present, recognition of these sounds decreases (Alexander, 2016a; Parsa, Scollie, Glista, & Seelisch, 2013; Souza, Arehart, Kates, Croghan, & Gehani, 2013). This two stage scheme aims to circumvent this problem and prevent distortion of low-frequency formants by using a higher LFL when those speech sounds are present, while at the same time allowing for a much lower LFL when high-frequency energy dominates, than in the first-generation product. The objective is to allow for better audibility for patients with hearing loss in the severe to profound range, particularly when there is considerable hearing loss beginning in the middle frequencies (750 to 2000 Hz). In addition, the use of two, context-sensitive LFLs allows for increased audibility without implementing very high compression ratios. This is important: Data from Alexander (2016a) also suggests that those listeners with the smallest dynamic ranges (generally more severe hearing loss) are especially vulnerable to decreased performance from using aggressive FC settings (lower LFL and high-compression ratio).

High-Frequency Reinforcement

The frequency-lowering method implemented in Starkey hearing aids doesn't actually move the higher frequency signal to lower frequencies. Instead, when high-frequency energy is present in the source region, energy is added to a lower frequency region to reinforce the audibility of the higher frequencies. This works by first identifying whether high-frequency energy in the source region is present (if no energy is present in the source region, nothing is done). If energy is present, it continues to be amplified, but the spectral envelope of this energy is also derived. This envelope is then applied to existing energy at harmonically related lower frequencies to provide a boost and reinforce the total amount of high-frequency energy (Galster, Valentine, Dundas, & Fitz, 2011). The harmonic relationship between the source region and the target region is chosen to mimic the natural harmonic structure of voiced speech.

Benefits and Limitations

Outcomes for FL technologies relative to speech recognition have been mixed to date. It is difficult to obtain a complete picture of the benefits and limitations of

> **POINTS TO PONDER:
> FREQUENCY REINFORCEMENT FOR MUSIC PLAYBACK**
>
> Conceptually, high-frequency reinforcement is very similar to the bass reinforcement that was introduced into commercial audio systems in the 1970s. These systems added higher harmonics (mi-bass and high bass) to help reinforce the low bass to make it more audible on small speakers that were incapable of reproducing the lowest frequencies. This type of processing still exists today and is implemented using everything from standalone mixers to digital plugins for mixing software. It is particularly in making sure the low-bass energy is audible (albeit at higher frequencies) through devices that have limited bandwidth like laptop computer speakers and cheap earbuds.

frequency-lowering technologies because versions continue to be modified, new versions are introduced to address limitations, optimal fitting methods are sometimes unclear, and it may require a period of listening experience with a specific frequency-lowering technology before maximum benefits are realized.

As pointed out in a 2012 and a 2016 review of fre-quency-lowering evidence, Ryan McCreery noted that about 90% of the studies examining FL benefits by 2016 were completed on Phonak's first-generation frequency compression algorithm. Very few peer-reviewed studies have been published yet for any of the current frequency-lowering algorithms. Furthermore, the FL setting that optimizes speech recognition may decrease sound quality, and studies examining how FL can affect factors like sound quality and listening effort are only beginning to emerge. Lau, Kuk, Keenan, and Schumacher (2014) demonstrated that the sound quality of extended high frequencies was preferred over that provided by a more limited bandwidth or provided by frequency transposition in a group of listeners with mild-moderate hearing loss. Indeed, frequency transposition led I believe to the lowest sound quality ratings in this population. Similarly, Parsa et al. (2013) demonstrated that application of strong FL settings can result in much poorer ratings of sound quality than conventional amplification. In contrast, at least one study demonstrated similar sound quality for extended bandwidth and FC, both of which were rated higher than a limited bandwidth condition (McCreery et al., 2014). It is clear that there is much more to learn regarding current FL techniques, but the data to date do provide a few important insights.

Variability is clearly present across studies and within studies. For example, Alexander, (2013a) reported average benefits for FC, but decrements for FT. Miller, Bates & Brennan et al. (2016) reported no average benefits for FC and speech recognition decrements for two types of FT. A few studies demonstrate small but significant FL benefit for average listeners; however, these same studies demonstrate some listeners receive larger benefits, some demonstrate no benefit, and a small sub-set have decreased speech recognition (e.g., Souza et al., 2013; McCreery et al., 2014). Not enough data exist yet to ascertain whether current FL technologies lead to increased average benefit or decreased individual variability in outcomes when compared to the earlier modern technologies.

Outcome differences within and across studies are likely to be at least partially attributed to individual differences in audibility after lowering, given differences in hearing loss configuration. That is, some FL technologies will provide very limited increases in audibility for some hearing loss configurations. Unfortunately, many of the earlier studies of FL technologies did not quantify the effects of FL on speech audibility. This may be one reason why support for these technologies to date is mixed. In other cases, clinical methods that ensured improved audibility were not yet well developed or applied. For example, Bentler, Walker, McCreery, Arenas, and Roush (2014) evaluat-ed 66 children, who were between approximately one and eight years of age with at least six months of experience with either FC or conventional amplification, and found no differences in speech and language outcomes. Although this result may be viewed as dis-appointing, it was not surprising because the two cohorts also were shown to exhibit no differences in audibility. That is, if audibility does not change, there is no potential for benefit from frequency lowering. It is also important to recognize, however, that while improved audibility is an important initial criterion, it does not ensure benefit. Too much lowered audibility has been shown to result in poor outcomes (e.g., Souza et al., 2013). This finding is perhaps not that surprising, given that frequency lowering distorts the original speech signal by design. As a result, many authors have advocated for using the weakest FL setting that can provide increased audibility (e.g., Scollie et al., 2016; McCreery, 2016).

In addition to individual variability, it has also been suggested that a period of acclimatization may be needed in order to optimize FL speech recognition outcomes. The data to date however, do not universally support this contention; in fact, the need for an adjustment period may depend in part on the type of processing and the type of task. Data examining the first generation of FT have shown a clear need for an acclimatization period. For example, Kuk, Keenan, Korhonen, and Lau (2009) demonstrated that performance on some classes of speech sounds (e.g., affricates, approximates, nasals) initially decreased with activation of FT and then improved over time to result in equivalent or better performance compared to conventional processing. Indeed, studies of FT show marked improvements in performance after training and adjustment period in both adults and children (e.g., Auriemmo et al., 2008; 2009). In contrast, the need for an adjustment period and training is less clear when applying other frequency-lowering technologies. For example, some work has shown speech recognition benefits from frequency compression can occur immediately in both children and adults who have never previously used this technology (McCreery et al., 2014). This same work demonstrated that even listeners with less hearing loss could benefit from using FC technology if audibility is improved through its application. Indeed, a number of studies have demonstrated that well-fit FC typically does not result in performance decrements in most listeners without an acclimatization period, typically will not degrade sound quality, and may provide a benefit in reducing susceptibility to feedback (e.g., Picou, Marcrum, & Ricketts, 2015). Some work in adult listeners has demonstrated no average improvement over time for speech in quiet or noise using FC (Ellis & Munro, 2014; Hopkins, Khanom, Dickinson, & Munro, 2014). Other work suggests increasing benefits over time in children when listening in noise, but not in quiet (Wolfe et al., 2011). Still other work suggests children can show continued improvement over at least a few months' time, but whether experience provided additional benefit depended on the specific task (Glista, Scollie, & Sulkers, 2012).

Another issue that remains unclear is the relative benefit provided to adults versus children. A number of earlier studies suggested benefits for children were likely

---

POINTS TO PONDER: WHY ISN'T THERE MORE BENEFIT?

One question we often get asked is why there is not more benefit from frequency lowering. After all, aren't we moving sounds from a range of inaudible to audible? Whereas it might make sense conceptually to think we are taking a phoneme like /s/ or /sh/ and moving it down, the high-frequency speech energy is actually primarily bands of noise. So all we are really doing in most cases is adding some noise energy to a lower frequency. Indeed, the reason too much lowering leads to confusions between /s/ and /sh/ is that they are primarily distinguished by the peak frequency and frequency bandwidth of their noise spectra. That is not to say that increasing audibility of this noise energy can't be very useful. This point was nicely illustrated by Josh Alexander (2016b). As shown in Figure 12–12, he plotted the time waveform of the sentence "The dog sleeps in a basket" under three conditions: without alteration, after low-pass filtering to simulate a severe to profound high-frequency hearing loss, and after applying FL. You can see from this comparison that FL was able to reintroduce much of the temporal envelope energy, albeit at a different frequency. Despite the frequency distortion, this can provide a strong temporal cue to help reinforce speech recognition.

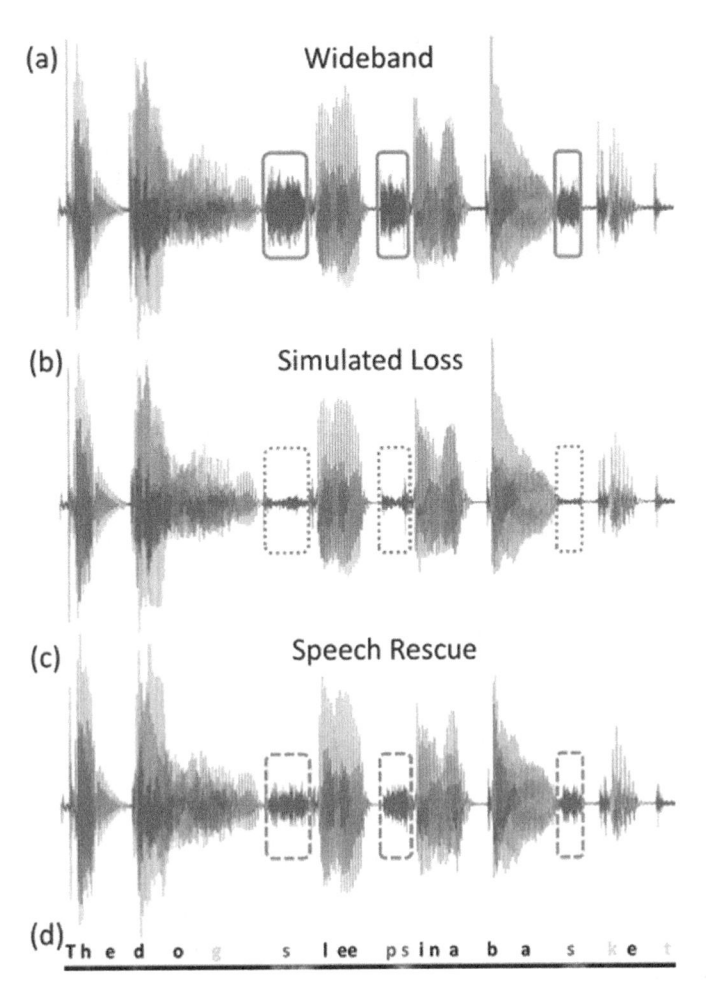

Figure 12–12. The time waveform of the sentence "The dog sleeps in a basket": **A.** Without alteration; **B.** After low-pass filtering to simulate a severe to profound high-frequency hearing loss; and **C.** After applying FL. Courtesy of Joshua M. Alexander, PhD.

larger than benefits for adults. In addition, the majority of studies which reported no average benefit from FL technologies were completed in adults (e.g., O'Brien, Keidser, Yeend, Hartley, & Dillon, 2010; Kokx-Ryan et al., 2015; Souza et al., 2013). A more recent study, however, demonstrated small but similar speech recognition benefits for adults and children when similar audibility increases were present (McCreery et al., 2014). These authors concluded that the potential for benefit from FL was similar in adults and children. It may be the case that because children are typically fitted with more gain, the change in audibility across FL studies may have been different in the two groups, thus affording children more benefit in some studies.

Frequency-Lowering Goals

As we just reviewed, speech recognition benefits from frequency lowering depend on the presence of a hearing loss configuration for which audibility can be improved through frequency lowering and having the right amount of audibility. In addition, emerging data suggests that listeners with better spectral resolution and higher working memory capacity may be more likely to benefit from FL technologies. The specific FL setting can also differentially affect speech recognition and sound quality. Consequently, clinical fitting of these technologies in adult listeners often requires evaluation of lowered audibility, measures of distinction between different speech sounds, and sound quality comparisons. Every manufacturer has its own recommended process for accomplishing these goals. We discuss fitting and verification of frequency-lowering techniques in Chapter 17, but should point out that not all manufacturers or researchers agree on the optimal goal. Scollie et al. (2016) have published a detailed fitting guide for FL technologies, albeit the focus is on FC. In addition, Josh Alexander has a number of FL "fitting assistants" that are a handy way to determine which settings can increase audibility using FL and can help prevent excessive lowering. He suggests considering the following goals when applying FL technologies:

- The audible bandwidth after frequency lowering is activated should not be less than it was before it was activated. In other words, frequency lowering should not restrict the existing audible bandwidth.
- The lowered information should be audible.
- The "weakest" frequency-lowering setting should be used to accomplish your objective.

Tinnitus Masking

The diagnosis and treatment of tinnitus is generally outside the scope of this text; however, we wanted to provide a little guidance relative to hearing aid processing here. One long-standing benefit from using hearing aids for some users is that amplified sounds can help to partially mask tinnitus, thus making it less noticeable and bothersome (e.g., Kochkin & Tyler, 2008; Searchfield, Kaur, & Martin, 2010). A subgroup of individuals with tinnitus do not receive adequate relief simply from using hearing aids, however. For these individuals some form of counseling, signal generation to partially mask the tinnitus, or a combination of these techniques are often recommended. Relatively recently, most manufacturers have introduced some form of tinnitus masking into their hearing aids. In many cases the level, frequency, bandwidth, and in some cases type of signals and/or temporal properties can be manipulated. Research supporting the use of tinnitus maskers as part of hearing aid processing is still limited; however, benefits are expected to be at least equal to stand-alone (nonamplifying) masking devices. Although a "try it and see if it will help" approach can be applied relative to tinnitus masking, it may not lead to optimal outcomes. For example,

using too much masking can overly mask the tinnitus and also reduce audibility. Furthermore, those with tinnitus often have greater aversion to sound when using hearing aids. Consequently, we encourage audiologist to apply tinnitus maskers used in hearing aids in a manner consistent with tinnitus best practices.

Targeted Hearing Aid Interventions

Light Actuated Amplification (EarLens™)

We describe MEIs, BAIs, and a few other nontraditional hearing aid technologies in Chapter 8. One device that we have not yet described, because it does not directly fit into the other previous categories, is the Earlens™ (Figure 12–13). Much of this device (the processor) is essentially an open-fit mini-BTE; however, it differs in the mechanism for sound delivery (the lens). Rather than using a receiver to generate sound, a laser in the open tip is used to drive a light receiver, which is supported by a deeply placed ring, and a small lens that rests on the tympanic membrane, much like a contact lens adheres to the surface of the eye. This approach of directly driving the eardrum with vibration is somewhat analogous to how some MEI devices deliver sound; however, no surgery is needed. Although peer-reviewed data supporting the benefits from this device are lacking, some interesting theoretical possibilities are supported by preliminary data. First, since the tympanic membrane is driven directly, the open eartip can be used without significant loss of low frequencies. Consequently, this device has the potential to deliver the benefits of an open fitting, meanwhile also providing enough gain to ensure appropriate audibility to listeners with significant low-frequency hearing loss. In addition, this device has been shown to be capable of very high levels of gain in the extended high frequencies. Preliminary data suggest more than 40 dB of gain is possible through 10 kHz, a feat that is not possible in current air conduction devices. Of course, there are some candidacy considerations relative to this device as well. For example, fitting the device requires an impression of the entire ear canal including the tympanic membrane. Furthermore, at least some wearers report being able to feel the lens (although many do not). In addition, similarly to BAI and MEI devices, probe microphone measures are not

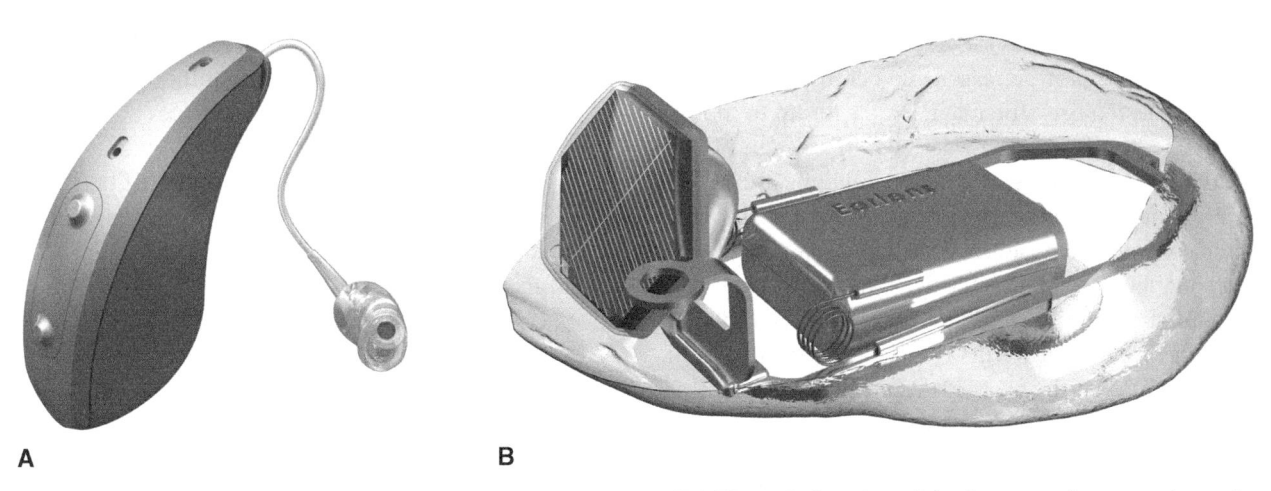

Figure 12–13. The Earlens™ sound processor (**A**) and lens (**B**). The relative size of the lens was increased greatly for easy visualization. Photos courtesy of Earlens Corporation.

possible, making precise gain verification more difficult. Although more data are needed to further quantify the potential benefits and limitations, this device offers some potential benefits not available in current air conduction hearing aids.

Extended Wear Technologies

Extended wear devices represent another interesting group of technologies that appear to provide somewhat unique benefits. Extended-wear hearing aids are placed in the ear canal by a hearing healthcare provider. The devices fit deeply into the ear canal, making them very discrete (Figure 12–14). Because they are seated so deeply in the ear canal, the space between the receiver and the eardrum is very small. This allows the devices to use less gain. Also, because they are housed within the ear canal, they use the natural acoustic cues of the outer ear, for example, the spectral pinna cues that allow for localization in the vertical plane. Also because they use less gain and take advantage of the ear's natural sound shaping, less processing of sound is needed and they therefore consume less energy. This allows the devices to be worn for months at a time without removal or replacement of batteries (Banerjee, 2016). In addition, they are covered with a water-resistant nanocoating, so that even though swimming is not recommended, they can be left in during showering and in other conditions under which they may get wet.

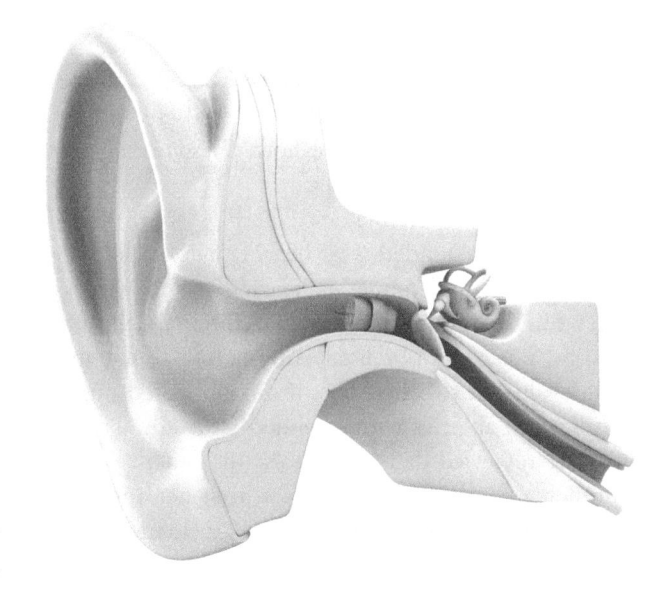

Figure 12–14. An example of an extended-wear hearing aid (Lyric™) as it would be placed in the ear canal.

Benefits and Limitations

There are few studies evaluating extended-wear hearing aids. A study on the data logging of 6,696 children (birth to 18 years.) found that few children wear their hearing aids throughout their waking hours (Jones & Feilner, 2014), which may be due to maintenance and cosmetic reasons. Thus for older children, an extended-wear option might be reasonable because they are less visible and require little maintenance for up to months at a time. Wolfe, Schafer, Martella, Morais, and Mann (2015) evaluated extended-wear and daily-wear hearing aids use in children (10 to 17 years of age) with mild to moderately severe SNHL. Children used their personal hearing aids in the daily-wear condition. The extended-wear HA were worn for four to six weeks. Speech recognition results revealed no significant difference between the participants' own daily-wear hearing aids and the study extended-wear hearing aids for CNC words at 50 and 60 dB HL; BKB-SIN threshold was significantly better with the extended-wear HA from a statistics standpoint but likely not clinically significant. The APHAB results showed that extended-wear HA was rated significantly better in the background noise subscale than the daily-wear HA, meanwhile all other subscales and global scores were not statistically significant. The SSQ-C result showed that ratings indicated a greater perceived benefit for the extended-wear HA than the daily-wear HA (no statistics cited). All participants were tested with their personal HA first and then the extended wear device, however, so testing order might have affected outcomes.

Brungart, McKenna, and Sherlock (2015) examined whether extended-wear hearing aids would allow soldiers with mild-moderate hearing loss to return to service in situations under which traditional daily-wear hearing aids cannot be used. Although this pilot study only evaluated two listeners, it demonstrated normal localization abilities with extended-wear HA. There is no peer-reviewed data to support this benefit yet, but another potential advantage is 24-hour hearing. This, for example, allows individuals the ability to monitor for sounds during the night.

As with all technologies, these devices also have some limitations:

- Extended-wear HA do not fit all ear canals. They are semisoft and flexible but can be particularly problematic for individuals with sharp bends in their ear canals, very small ear canals, or hearing aid wearers who exhibit a lot of ear canal deformation with jaw movement. Careful otoscopy can help establish patient candidacy relative to fit.
- There is limited gain compared to daily-wear instruments, which limits the fitting range to not much more than a moderate loss.
- Even though they are made to seal in the ear, the facts that they are not custom-fitted devices and the distance between receiver and microphone is smaller, mean that there is a greater chance for feedback, particularly when considerable slit leak venting is present.
- As we mentioned above, it is not recommended that patients swim with the device and, unlike traditional amplification, they are not designed for simple removal and reinsertion.
- If the battery dies, the user cannot change it. Instead he or she must see an audiologist to have the device replaced. Fortunately, the devices are made so that the user can remove them when they fail, so they are not stuck walking around wearing earplugs.

In Closing

Modern hearing aids typically include a wide array of features that are aimed at improving outcomes, easing adaptation, or off-setting limitations of other processing. In addition, some features have the potential to indirectly improve outcomes through provision of information to the clinician or through automatic feature adjustment. Feedback from many of our patients suggests that these advances provide an excellent listening experience through automatic adjustment for a wide range of listening conditions. However, not all patients need or even want all features. Individualized adjustment of some features will allow for tailoring to personal listening needs. Indeed, a small subset of patients report a dislike for automatic processing in general. These individual differences may contribute to findings of equivalent outcomes across basic and premium level hearing aids (e.g., Cox, Johnson, & Xu, 2014). In addition, counseling is important to ensure that patients have appropriate expectations relative to benefits and limitations. They must also be advised how to optimize benefit for specific technologies. A good example of the need for this type of counseling is for wind noise reduction processing. Specifically, the angle the patient needs to hold his or her head relative to the wind for optimal speech recognition benefit depends on which brand they are fitted with. Technological advances in hearing aid processing provide the ability to address a very wide range of listening needs. Because of these advances, our patients may initially believe that a hearing aid purchase is like choosing between a Mercedes, Cadillac, Ford, Chevy, or a Kia, but it is certainly not. Professional selection, adjustment, and counseling focused on addressing individual listening needs can be at least as important as the technology itself.

13
Electroacoustic and Other Quality Control Techniques

Hearing aids must meet reasonable and expected quality standards prior to scheduling the patient for the hearing aid fitting and verification. Current best practice guidelines recommend that all hearing aids (new and repaired) be assessed electroacoustically to provide a benchmark against which future quality control measures can be made (AAA, 2006; ASHA, 1998). In addition, the guidelines say that confirmation that the features are functional and the physical parameters are adequately constructed should be carried out prior to the patient's arrival. We agree.

Quality control is important to ensure that we do not waste our time or the patient's. Many patients are older and traveling to the clinic can be challenging; parking is often difficult to find and expensive. Younger patients often have the added inconvenience of taking time off work or finding child care. If our patients arrive at their fitting appointment only to find a new, but "broken" hearing aid, such an occurrence is not only an inconvenience but also has negative consequences for patient rapport and perceptions of our professionalism.

Our pre-fitting quality assessment may include confirmation that the shell color/style and processor are appropriate to the order, and that the operation of the volume control and/or user switches, basic processing, receiver, directional microphone(s), t-coil, and so on, are all adequate. Several decades ago a number of these quality assessment measures, specifically the electroacoustic evaluation, were completed by clinicians to aid in the selection and fitting of the hearing aid; that is, they were a form of verification. Although no longer necessary in this way, except for some pediatric applications, electroacoustic evaluation is still a critical component of quality control.

Early History of Quality Checks

Early history indicates that, prior to national and international standards, all hearing aids were evaluated for acceptability by the Council on Physical Therapy of the American Medical Association (Davis et al., 1946). The Council was charged with evaluating each new model, a process that took several weeks. A referee would evaluate each submitted hearing aid and submit a report to the Consultant on Audiometers and Hearing Aids. The requirements for acceptance included the following:

- identification by model number;
- written guarantee and instructions for the consumer;
- engineering data to support claims of "acoustical amplification," effectiveness of tone controls, and battery drain. Adequate acoustical amplification meant that the hearing aid was required to have 30 dB of gain between 300 and 3000 Hz, and without high inherent noise;
- appropriate marketing, that is, "the firm shall be responsible for the ethical merchandising practices, financial dealings and contracts of its agents, sales representatives, and service men with the purchasers of instruments" (Davis et al., 1946).

As history has it, this final requirement was the cause of the most denials for acceptance, although a "certain amount of self-satisfaction, optimism and general puff (was) allowable" (Davis et al., 1946, p. 219). The report from the Council was published in the *Journal of the American Medical Association*. The list was updated year-by-year, and even month-by-month, as new models became available and were deemed acceptable. A portion of that list is shown in Table 13–1.

Table 13–1. Hearing Aids Evaluated for Acceptability by the Council on Physical Therapy of the American Medical Association

Trimm Distributors, Inc. 1770 W. Berteau Ave., Chicago, Illinois	
Trimm Vacuum Tube No. 300	1947
Vacolite Company 3003 N. Henderson, Dallas, Texas	
Vacolite Model D	1942
Western Electric Co., Inc. 300 Central Ave., Kearny, New Jersey	
Western Electric Audiophone Ortho-Technic Model (Carbon)	1939
Western Electric Telephone Type Audiophone, Model J-1 (Carbon)	1944
Western Electric Model 63	1946
Western Electric Model 64	(Report not yet published)
Zenith Radio Corporation 6001 Dickens Ave., Chicago, Illinois	
Ravox (Semi-Portable)	1939
Zenith Radionic Model A-2-A	1945
Zenith Radionic Model A-3-A	1945
Zenith Radionic Model B-3-A	1945

Source: Reprinted from Davis, H. (Ed.) (1947). *Hearing and Deafness: A Guide for Laymen.* New York, NY: Murray Hill Books, Inc.

SOAPBOX: YOU WON'T KNOW ABOUT THE PROBLEM IF YOU DON'T TEST IT!

Our conversations with several current clinicians suggest a disturbing trend of *not* completing electroacoustic analysis. In other words, hearing aids received from the manufacturer are never evaluated prior to when they are fitted on the patient. There may be several reasons for this, but one commonly offered is: "these modern sophisticated digital instruments will function as expected." Unfortunately, this simply is not true. In fact, with increasing sophistication, additional features including directional microphones may not function appropriately or not work at all, even in a new instrument, and therefore require careful testing. Will a patient alert you if the directional microphone technology isn't working the day of the fitting? Unlikely. And yes, like analog instruments of old, new digital hearing aids will come out of the box and be intermittent or even "dead." Unfortunately, many clinicians believe that quality control of modern hearing aids using electroacoustic measures is too complex or takes too much time. Quality control remains critical, and we must continue to encourage manufacturers to deliver consistent and easily testable instruments.

Also, the early days of hearing aid dispensing saw involvement from the Federal Trade Commission (FTC) in the 1940s. It was investigating the franchise system of the hearing aid industry. The FTC brought action against several companies for violating federal laws such as the Clayton Act. The Clayton Act of 1914 made procedural modifications to federal antitrust law (e.g., the Sherman Act of 1890). The purpose of the Clayton Act was to capture anticompetitive practices in their incipiency by prohibiting particular types of conduct not deemed in the best interest of a competitive market. Several manufacturers fought this—and lost. Although we still have franchise hearing aid offices today, in order to get around the law, the dispensers at these offices are allowed to sell hearing aids from other manufacturers (but usually don't).

Since those early days, a number of regulations and regulating bodies have evolved and are aimed at ensuring the quality control of the manufacturing process, the marketing process, and the clinical provision of amplification systems. In this chapter we will look at those entities in greater detail.

Governmental Regulating Bodies

Oversight of the manufacturing and selling of hearing aids falls within three government regulating bodies: the FTC, the Food and Drug Administration (FDA), and the Federal Communications Commission (FCC). Each organization deals with somewhat different aspects of the overall hearing aid fitting process.

Federal Trade Commission (FTC)

The FTC is an independent agency of the United States government, established in 1914 by the Federal Trade Commission Act. Enacted by President Woodrow Wilson, its principal mission is the promotion of consumer protection and the elimination and prevention of what regulators perceive to be harmfully anticompetitive business practices, such as coercive monopoly. The FTC has the authority to take action against hearing aid companies (and dispensers) that attempt to mislead or deceive consumers. This can occur through deceptive advertising, falsifying hearing loss diagnoses, overrating hearing aid performance, false statements of warranty, and refund policies (Kaplan & Hesse, 2000). Its activities include investigations, enforcement actions, and consumer and business education.

The FTC also monitors mail order hearing aid sales. Although such sales are not prohibited by federal law, some state laws preclude the practice. The FTC does monitor the timeliness of such purchases and requires companies who do mail order sales of hearing aids to

---

KEY CONCEPT: INTERNATIONAL ORGANIZATION FOR STANDARDIZATION (ISO) CERTIFICATION

You probably have noticed that some hearing aid companies will promote the fact that they are "ISO 9001 Certified." Although this sounds like it is something controlled by the government, it is not. Do these companies have higher quality hearing aids? Maybe, maybe not.

The ISO 9000 family of standards is related to quality management systems and designed to help organizations ensure that they meet the needs of customers while meeting statutory and regulatory requirements related to the product. ISO 9000 deals with the fundamentals of quality management systems; ISO 9001 deals with the requirements that organizations wishing to meet the standard have to fulfill. Although ISO 9001 does relate to quality, it does not relate directly to the product itself (e.g., hearing aids) but rather to the quality of the process behind the development, manufacturing, sales, and service of the product.

Third-party certification bodies provide independent confirmation that organizations meet the requirements of ISO 9001. More than a million organizations worldwide are independently certified, making ISO 9001 one of the most widely used management tools in the world today.

give customers the option of canceling their orders if products are not supplied in the promised time frame. Today, when we say mail order sales, we primarily refer to hearing aids purchased on the Internet. In Chapter 1, we discuss the pros and cons of internet sales for the consumer, and how this delivery method relates to the audiologist's role in the dispensing process. Whether or not it's legal in a given state, of course, is a different matter. The laws on this vary from state to state, and often change; however, on the companion website, we have a summary of the states that do not allow this practice at the time of this writing. Realistically, given everything that falls under the FTC jurisdiction, we doubt that the internet sale of hearing aids has a high priority—no hearing-aid-sniffing-beagles have yet to be spotted at the Miami airport! Of course this landscape is rapidly changing with the passage of OTC hearing aid legislation.

Although the FTC does not enforce individual consumer complaints against companies, it does monitor business patterns and have the authority to take action against any company for repetitive illegal practices. Secondary to its industry-monitoring role, the FTC also has the charge of educating the public regarding the legislation and regulation of consumer rights. On the Consumer Protection portion of its home page (http://www.ftc.gov), information to help the consumer "determine whether a hearing aid will work for you and what to look for when shopping for one" is available.

Where to Go for FTC Complaints

The information from the FTC website reads as follows:

> The FTC works for the consumer to prevent fraudulent, deceptive, and unfair business practices in the marketplace and to provide information to help the consumer spot, stop, and avoid them. In the case of hearing aids, we assume the consumer could be the audiologist buying the hearing aids from the manufacturer, or the patient buying the hearing aids from the audiologist. To file a complaint or to obtain information on consumer issues, visit ftc.gov or call toll-free, 1-877-FTC-HELP (1-877382-4357); TTY: 1-866-653-4261. The FTC enters consumer complaints into the Consumer Sentinel Network, a secure online database and investigative tool used by hundreds of civil and criminal law enforcement agencies in the United States and abroad. Website: http://www.ftc.gov/bcp/edu/pubs/consumer/health/hea10.shtm

Food and Drug Administration (FDA)

Whereas the FTC monitors the business practices of hearing aid dispensers and vendors, the FDA enforces regulations that deal specifically with the sale of hearing aids, which are considered a medical device. The FDA has established classifications for approximately 1700 different generic types of devices and grouped them into 16 medical specialties that are referred to as panels. Each of these generic types of devices is assigned to regulatory classes based on the level of control necessary to ensure the safety and effectiveness of the device. Devices are classified into three categories: Class I, Class II, and Class III:

- Class I devices are deemed to be low risk and are therefore subject to the least regulatory controls. For example, dental floss and conventional air conduction hearing aids are classified as Class I devices.
- Class II devices are higher risk devices than Class I and require greater regulatory controls to provide reasonable assurance of the device's safety and effectiveness. For example, condoms and hearing aid tinnitus maskers are classified as Class II devices.
- Class III devices are generally the highest risk devices and are therefore subject to the highest level of regulatory control. Class III devices must typically be approved by the FDA before they are marketed. For example, replacement heart valves are classified as Class III devices.

Because the FDA recognizes traditional hearing aids as Class I medical devices, there is regulatory authority over their sale. Following a series of Senate hearings held in 1975 and 1976 by the Subcommittee on Government Regulations of the Select Committee on Small Business and the Senate Permanent Committee on Investigations, Senator Charles Percy of Illinois, recommended the promulgation of regulations specific to hearing aid sales. These so-called "FDA regs" were in effect and held the "force of the law" through 2016.

These regulations did not apply to the instruments themselves, but rather delineate the now well-known conditions that must be met by all dispensers before selling a hearing aid:

- Dispensers must obtain a written statement from the patient, signed by a licensed physician. The statement must be dated within the previous six months, state that the patient's ears have been medically evaluated, and that the patient is cleared for fitting with a hearing aid.
- A patient 18 years and older can sign a waiver for the medical examination, but dispensers must avoid encouraging the patient to waive the medical evaluation requirement. Dispensers also must advise the patient that waiving the examination is not in his or her best health interest.
- Dispensers must advise patients who appear to have a hearing problem needing treatment to consult promptly with a physician.
- An instruction brochure must be provided to the patient with the hearing aid that illustrates and describes its operation, use, and care. The brochure must list sources for repair and maintenance, and include a statement that the use of a hearing aid may be only part of a rehabilitative program.

There were repeated efforts to have these 1977 regulations overhauled, and slight revisions made in 2012. A more substantive change was made in 2017.

Related to the current FDA requirements, the National Institute on Deafness and Other Communication Disorders/National Institutes of Health (NIDCD/NIH) sponsored a working group on *Accessible and Affordable Hearing Health Care for Adults with Mild to Moderate Hearing Loss*. The working group was held in 2009 from August 25 to 27 in Bethesda, Maryland. The purpose of the working group was to develop a research agenda to increase accessibility and affordability of hearing health care for adults with mild to moderate hearing loss, including accessible and low-cost hearing aids. That group addressed two of the most contentious components of the current FDA regulations:

- Do the existing FDA requirements for medical evaluation and clearance prior to hearing aid procurement provide significant protection to patients or do they create a significant barrier to access? Is the protection necessary for all patients?
- Are the current "red flag" conditions (requiring medical consultation) appropriate for different service delivery models: face-to face versus Internet versus telephone?

As we discussed in Chapter 1, this led to two major changes: (1) the sudden and immediate elimination of the requirement for medical clearance for adults early in 2017; and, (2) the creation of the law authorizing the FDA to create a new category of OTC hearing aids for individuals with mild or moderate hearing loss in August 2017.

The 1993 Uprising

Things had been going along fairly quietly between the FDA and the hearing aid industry for several years, but that all changed abruptly in April of 1993. These events have an impact on our products and sales practices today, so we'll briefly review the history. On April 16th of that year, a letter went out to six major hearing aid manufacturers, instructing them to stop making misleading claims about products. As you might guess, this was great fodder for the press, and news releases found their way into all major newspapers. Soon, the person spearheading the process, FDA Commissioner David Kessler, was being quoted and appearing on TV news shows to talk about the issue. Discussions on the topic, particularly the July 6, 1993 airing of NBC Dateline, also addressed current sales practices, which indirectly related to the misleading advertising. As this continued, the final message that seemed to be resonating with the average consumer was that "hearing aids don't work very well and watch out for the people selling them." All companies, products, and individuals selling hearing aids were more or less lumped into the same category, and hearing aid sales took a serious nosedive. Even those who did purchase during this time frame often had an "it probably won't work" attitude.

So what prompted the letter? Feature articles and advertisements in Florida Sunday newspapers did indeed make unrealistic claims about improvements for speech understanding in background noise. And of course, there was the constant bombardment from

Miracle Ear television ads, which would make a respectable audiologist cringe, and the FDA commissioner, too, no doubt. The directive from the FDA was straightforward: If you're going to say it, it needs to be supported by research. Other advertising issues pointed out by the FDA were not as egregious. Siemens Hearing Instruments, for example, was included because of the tagline it used for some of their products that stated, "Better hearing is better living." The FDA questioned whether this was supported by research. Now as audiologists we don't really find that statement to be contentious, but in 1993, was there substantial research showing that this indeed was true?

In the FDA letter Kessler stated, "The FDA will not tolerate misleading claims on hearing aid products. These companies have overstepped the line with their advertising. They must comply with the law, or the agency will take further action."

The FDA told the companies to remove all misleading promotional literature and advertising immediately, and warned that continued distribution of the hearing aids with misleading claims could result in enforcement actions such as seizure, injunction, and civil penalties. The agency also advised the firms to correct the misconceptions they had created by their misleading promotion and advertising. The firms were given 15 days to inform the agency of corrective action they would take to bring their products into compliance. In August 1993, a general notification letter from the FDA went out to the entire hearing aid industry, stressing the importance of advertising compliance.

Hearing Industries Association (HIA) Task Force

With a dark cloud hanging over the industry, the HIA took proactive measures. In case you're not familiar with this organization, the HIA is the national trade association of manufacturers of hearing aids, assistive listening devices, component parts, and power sources. Today there are about 25 members, including all of the "Big Six" manufacturers; the members of the HIA represent about 85% of all hearing aids sold in the United States. The proactive measure we're referring to is that the HIA formed a self-regulating board to address the advertising issues raised by the FDA. Specifically, the FDA had mentioned three different problem areas:

- Advertisements with misleading performance claims, referred to as "misbranding" of a product;
- Testimonials from hearing aid users without proper substantiation (see related Key Concept);
- Speech understanding in background noise is a "new intended use" and therefore required a 510(k) (see related Key Concept).

This all changed, however, when the FDA Modernization Act became law in 1997. This was the result of congressional legislation to deregulate low-risk medical device companies. Nearly 200 Class I devices were removed from the list that required a 510(k) submission. This included hearing aids, and therefore the 510(k) requirement for preclearance of speech-in-noise claims no longer applied. With this background, the HIA formed a taskforce for substantiation of performance claims to develop a document which could be used to negotiate with the FDA. The FDA had identified two key areas: Type 1—Technical performance claims, and Type 2—Wearer benefit claims. The HIA document, however, broke the two types into three tiers summarized below:

1. Type 1 Claim
   - Definition: Claims that are generally accepted by the clinical and user communities.
   - Example: "Many hearing aid wearers find that when using hearing aids it is easier to communicate with friends and family."
   - Substantiation: Minimal.
2. Type 2 Claim
   - Definition: Performance claims, supported by information, valid for the device in the context of the claim.
   - Example: "This hearing aid circuit helps to make soft sounds audible and loud sounds comfortable."
   - Substantiation: Clinical data, benchtop data, published research on the topic, and so forth, as deemed appropriate by manufacturer.
3. Type 3 Claim
   - Definition: Direct or implied claims involving improved speech recognition in noise with a given product.

> ## KEY CONCEPT: TESTIMONIALS FOR ADVERTISING
>
> You don't have to watch many television commercials to notice that testimonial advertising is very popular. A testimonial from Joe-the-Plumber from Toledo that a product is good often works better than evidence from an article in *Brain and Science*. The hearing aid industry, of course, recognizes this, and frequently uses testimonial advertising. But because of the FDA guidelines, there's a catch: When the comments relate certain benefits, such as speech understanding in background noise, the testimonial comment from the delighted patient cannot contain reference to something that has not been proven by that manufacturer in research, even if the given patient really made the comment (without coaxing). For example, a patient could not state, "Ever since I started using my ZIPPO3 hearing aids with ShutDown noise reduction, I can understand my friends a lot better at parties," unless the manufacturer had completed research at two different sites, and these data show that the ShutDown noise reduction does (significantly) improve speech understanding in background noise. What you'll often read in newspaper advertising (or see on the Internet), therefore, are testimonials that are more general and talk about audibility, listening comfort, a better social life, and so forth—things that do not fall directly within the scope of speech in noise understanding. The same rules tend to apply to testimonials used by dispensers in newspaper ads and postings on their websites; if they have an affiliation with a given manufacturer (as most do), and use the manufacturer's name in the same advertising, the manufacturer could be pulled into the potential violation.

- Example: "For many people, speech understanding in a group situation will be much easier using this product."
- Substantiation: Clinical research data, per the FDA guidance document; product must be precleared through 510(k) process.

With these three tiers in place, the HIA task force went about developing a document that would clearly spell out what was needed for the Type 3 Claim—the one of primary concern for all parties. The main points of this document were as follows:

- Supporting research for a speech-in-noise claim must be based on research from at least two sites (one site can be the manufacturer's laboratory).
- The same protocols must be used at all sites.
- Norm-referenced, standardized testing materials must be used.
- Statistical significance must be at least at the 0.05 level.

Since the 1993 uprising, there have been three different HIA taskforces that addressed this topic. The above guidelines have been modified somewhat in recent years; however, they really haven't changed significantly, and have driven industry research for more than two decades.

Today, a manufacturer's advertising claim is probably more closely scrutinized by competing manufacturers than by the FDA, audiologists, or consumers. It would of course be counterproductive for one manufacturer to tattle to the FDA on another, as that only would bring increased scrutiny to the industry as a whole. We suspect that any minor discrepancies that might occur are handled within the HIA task force. Our casual observations of advertising materials in recent years suggest that the current method is working well.

Where to Go for FDA Complaints

Complaints to the FDA are typically not lodged by individuals, as individuals are more typically impacted by the actual dispensing process (FTC) than the manufacturing and labeling process (FDA). Yet, an audiology

> **KEY CONCEPT: WHAT IS A 510(K)?**
>
> In our discussions about what has been happening with hearing aid products and the FDA, you'll notice we mention the 510(k)—pronounced *Five-Ten-Kay*. Although 510(k) sounds like some government tax form or retirement account, it's actually a process not a form. The process is so named because in the Food, Drug, and Cosmetic Act of 1938—amended in 1976 to include regulation of medical devices—Chapter V, Section 510(k) describes the clearance of medical devices. The 510(k) process applies to most of the Class II medical devices sold in the United States and a small number of Class I and Class III devices as well. Technically, the FDA does not *approve* medical devices; it *clears* them for sale. When a product is cleared, the FDA has determined that the device is substantially equivalent to legally marketed predicate devices, which already have been cleared for sale by the FDA. For example, if a hearing aid that had been for sale, and had the primary purpose of amplifying sound, now has a tinnitus masker added as an option, the product would no longer be "substantially equivalent to legally marketed predicate devices."

coalition, made up of the Academy of Dispensing Audiologist (now the Academy of Doctors of Audiology), Academy of Rehabilitative Audiology, American Academy of Audiology, American Speech-Language-Hearing Association, and Educational Audiology) approached the Commissioner of the FDA in 1994 with concerns relative to the 1977 regulations. Key points of those concerns included the following:

- Persons interested in obtaining a hearing aid should undergo a thorough evaluation by a licensed audiologist to determine the degree and type of hearing loss, site of lesion, and the potential need for a medical evaluation.
- Neither a medical evaluation nor warning signs are necessary components of a prepurchase hearing evaluation when conducted by a licensed audiologist.
- At the minimum, the qualifications that health care professionals must possess to perform and interpret the prepurchase audiologist assessment include a postgraduate professional degree with emphasis in hearing from an accredited institution of higher education.

The FDA did not respond to the lodged complaints in a manner that altered the current regulations. As a result, the 1977 version remained law until 2017. Have the standards the FDA recognizes for evaluation of hearing aids also been updated? In short, no. Since the summer of 2009, the ANSI S3.22 (2003 version) standard for hearing aid specifications has been recognized by the FDA as the measurement standard despite updates and revisions by ANSI. More information is available from the FDA website (http://www.fda.gov/MedicalDevices/Safety/ReportaProblem/default.htm).

Federal Communications Commission (FCC)

Finally, the FCC has involvement in hearing aid provision. The FCC is an independent federal government agency responsible for the development and implementations of regulations for interstate and international communications, such as radio, television, telephone, cable, and satellite systems. For example, the Hearing Aid Compatibility Act of 1988 required that the FCC ensure that all telephones manufactured or imported for use in the United States, and all "essential" telephones, are hearing aid-compatible. (See related Technical Tip.) The FCC is also responsible for portioning radio frequency bands for manufacturers and users of frequency-modulated (FM) and the higher radio frequencies used in many modern wireless communication systems used in hearing aids. Recent controversy has again arisen relative to the use of FM bands by multiple entities, thus increasing the likelihood of interference problems. Since personal FM systems are low-powered (typically <1 milliwatt), one-way transmission systems, the broadcasting frequency bands are not licensed. The receivers are highly sensitive to interference if it occurs in the same frequency band to which the personal FM system is tuned. This controversy is quieting, however, with increasing moves to higher frequency two way transmission systems (e.g., 2.4 GHz wireless).

What Are the FCC's Requirements?

As we've stated, the FCC has requirements regarding hearing aid compatibility for both landline and wireless telephones. Here is a summary from its website:

Requirements for Hearing Aid Compatibility (HAC) for Wireline Telephones: FCC rules require that phones subject to the HAC Act: (1) produce a magnetic field of sufficient strength and quality to permit coupling with hearing aids that contain telecoils; and (2) provide an adequate range of volume. FCC rules also establish technical parameters to ensure that telephones are compatible with hearing aids.

FCC rules also require that telephones allow volume to be increased to accommodate individuals with hearing disabilities, whether or not they use hearing aids. Telephones allowing high-volume levels must automatically reset to a lower volume each time the handset is returned to an on-hook condition. Telephone equipment manufacturers may request a waiver permitting high volume telephones to remain at the high-volume setting under certain conditions. If you need a volume higher than the 18-dB volume limit specified in the FCC's rules, you must reset the volume each time you use the telephone, even when you are the primary user of the telephone.

Requirements for hearing aid compatibility for digital wireless telephones state that analog wireless telephones usually do not cause interference with hearing aids. Digital wireless telephones, on the other hand, sometimes cause interference because of electromagnetic energy emitted by the telephone's antenna, backlight, or other components. Therefore, the FCC has adopted specific hearing aid compatibility rules for digital wireless telephones.

The standard for compatibility of digital wireless phones with hearing aids is set forth in the American National Standard Institute (ANSI) standard C63.19. ANSI C63.19 contains two sets of standards: an "M" (originally a "U") rating from 1 to 4 for reduced radio frequency (RF) interference to enable acoustic coupling with hearing aids that do not operate in telecoil mode, and a "T" (originally a "UT") rating from 1 to 4 to enable inductive coupling with hearing aids operating in telecoil mode. A digital wireless handset is considered hearing aid-compatible for acoustic coupling if it meets an "M3" (or "U3") rating under the ANSI standard. A digital wireless handset is considered hearing aid-compatible (HAC) for inductive coupling if it meets a "T3" (or "U3T") rating under the ANSI standard.

In addition to rating wireless phones, the ANSI standard provides a methodology for rating hearing aids from M1 to M4, with M1 being the least immune to RF interference and M4 the most immune. To determine whether a particular digital wireless telephone is likely to interfere with a particular hearing aid, the immunity rating of the hearing aid is added to the rating of the telephone. A sum of four would indicate that the telephone is usable; a sum of five would indicate that the telephone would provide normal use; and a sum of six or greater would indicate that the telephone would provide excellent performance with that hearing aid.

How to File a Complaint With the FCC

A complaint to the FCC must be specific to accessibility (telephone, radio, etc.) using a personal hearing aid.

TECHNICAL TIP: WHAT ARE "ESSENTIAL" TELEPHONES?

"Essential" telephones are defined as coin-operated telephones, telephones provided for emergency use, and other telephones frequently needed for use by persons using hearing aids. Examples of telephones in areas where people with hearing disabilities may be isolated in the event of an emergency include elevators, tunnels, highways, and workplace common areas. Also included would be some workplace phones, phones in confined settings (e.g., hospitals and nursing homes), and phones in hotel and motel rooms.

> **TECHNICAL TIP: TELEPHONE LABELING REQUIREMENTS**
>
> Telephone manufacturers are required to clearly label their telephones and the telephone packaging containing hearing aid compatible handsets (Table 13–2). They must also make information available in the package or product manual, and require service providers to make the performance ratings of hearing aid compatible telephones available. For example, the letters "HAC" should be permanently affixed to the telephone. The HAC labeling is usually found on the base of the telephone along with other required information. Telephones are not required to have volume control or "VC" labeling, however, because whether or not the telephone has a VC will be evident upon inspection.

The agency recommends that if you have a problem using a hearing aid with a digital wireless phone that is supposed to be hearing aid-compatible, for example, you first try to resolve it with the equipment manufacturer or your wireless service provider. If that approach is not successful, a formal complaint can be filed with the FCC. There is no charge for filing a complaint. You can file your complaint using an online complaint form (https://consumercomplaints.fcc.gov/hc/en-us), emailing (fccinfo@fcc.gov), or calling the FCC Consumer Center: 1-888-CALL-FCC (1-888-225-5322) voice; 1-888-TELL-FCC (1-888-835-5322) TTY; or 1-866-418-0232) fax.

Non-Government Regulation of Hearing Aids

In the preceding section we reviewed three government agencies that in one way or another have some control over the manufacture and sale of hearing aids. In day-to-day practice, however, audiologists are more involved in the standards that directly relate to the electroacoustic measurement of hearing aids. Quality control of hearing aids has undergone significant evolution since the Council on Physical Therapy era. Three main bodies have developed and disseminated standards for quality control measures:

- Hearing Aid Industry Council (HAIC)
- American National Standards Institute (ANSI)
- International Electrotechnical Commission (IEC)

Hearing Aid Industries Council (HAIC)

HAIC began in 1955 as an industry organization whose charges included public relations, as well as market share analyses and public dissemination of total market sales data. About one-third of the original charter members were not actually hearing aid manufacturers, but manufacturers of components, batteries, and trade magazines (Berger, 1974). Perhaps the major contribution of HAIC was the development of a standard description of hearing aid acoustic measures. The first HAIC standard was approved by the membership in 1960. In 1967 this standard became the ANSI Standard S3.8-1967.

Table 13–2. Label On a Telephone

Hearing Aid Compatibility = M4

TTY compatible. This is an all-digital phone. Digital Service is not available in all areas, and when not available your phone will not operate or be able to make 911 calls. Activation and use of this phone are subject to Verizon Wireless' customer agreement, plans and additional charges.

Bluetooth capable for certain profiles. See http://www.verizonwireless.com/Bluetooth for details.

The American Engineering Standards Committee (Now ANSI)

The American Engineering Standards Committee was organized as a nonprofit group in 1918 with the intent to develop and encourage broader use of standards in the field of engineering. The group expanded to become the American Standard Association (ASA) in 1928; one product of its efforts included the first standard for audiometer calibration (ASA-1951). In 1966 they became the United States American Standards Institute, but due to the misperception that the body was a government organization, it renamed itself the American National Standards Institute (ANSI) in 1969. It continues today as the private, nonprofit organization that coordinates the work of standards development in many fields, including the measurement of hearing aid characteristics. The first hearing aid standard related to quality control measures was approved in 1976 and is known as ANSI S3.22. It has undergone revisions resulting in new versions in 1982, 1987, 1996, 2003, 2009, and 2014. The original purpose of the standard was "to provide a means of determining whether a production hearing aid as shipped was as stated by a manufacturer for a given model" (p. iv). Since 1976 this standard has been incorporated into the FDA regulations. As of 2017, the FDA recognized only the 2003 version of the standard. The body of the ANSI S3.22 standard describes measurement techniques intended for quality control purposes, and to provide tolerances for these measures. Annexes are provided for informational purposes only. More detail about the measurement steps and stages is provided later in this chapter under Electroacoustic Measures.

International Electrotechnical Commission (IEC)

The IEC was formed in 1904, and in 1947 affiliated itself with the newly formed International Organization for Standardization (ISO). The last published count noted more than 60,118 documents or standards governing areas of electronics and related technologies (Preves

---

POINTS TO PONDER: THE STANDARDIZATION OF STANDARDS

The standardization process is an ongoing effort carried out by volunteers with expertise and/or industry involvement in design and measurement of hearing aids. Once an ANSI standard has been approved, it is required that the working group revisit the standard every five years to reaffirm, modify, or make it obsolete. Procedures contained within the standard do not require mandatory compliance unless they are mandated by a federal regulatory agency as was S3.22 (Specifications of Hearing Aid Characteristics), which were adopted by the FDA as a set of required measures for hearing aid manufacturers.

All voting is conducted by letter ballot, rather than at meetings, to provide all committee or subcommittee members the opportunity to vote. The following actions require a ballot and are considered approved if a majority of the consensus body casts a vote (counting abstentions) and at least 80% of those voting approve (not counting abstentions):

- Approval of a new standard
- Approval of revision or addendum to part or all of a standard
- Approval of reaffirmation of an existing standard

In the process of standards development, the committee must respond to comments from the public review period. Anyone who has a direct and material interest has the right to appeal any procedural action or inaction. A procedural action can include the question of whether or not comments were properly handled. It cannot include the technical decision, however (ANSI Accredited Operating Procedures, 2008).

& Curran, 2000). In the 1980s, the group formulated a standardized set of hearing aid measures that differed from the ANSI 1976 standard in several ways that included coupler requirements and frequencies of test, among others. Because manufacturers of hearing aids adhere to quality control standards in their production and marketing, this has created additional effort for marketers who export their product internationally; that is, one effort in accordance with ANSI S3.22 for products marketed in the United States and Canada, and another effort for marketing in the other international countries (e.g., Europe and Asia) that require the IEC series of standards.

How does all this work in your clinical practice? For all clinicians and clinical practices, it is important to know that there are rules in place for the measurement of sound, sound spaces, hearing aids, and so forth. If each company—or each clinician—had a specific, independently defined set of rules for determining quality control, there would be no real regulation of anything we do. That could result in no confidence or value in our quality control measures. Although it is easy to complain about the standards that are in place in hearing aid evaluation and fittings, it is important to note the necessity of the regulations.

Measurement Couplers

One of the cornerstones of many quality control procedures is the development of a testing process that is highly repeatable. For example, it would be of little use to have a quality control procedure to ensure that all floor tiles were a very specific size if we could not agree on the scale used to conduct the measurement of each tile.

So how should we test a hearing aid? We could put it in an individual's ear; however, ears vary dramatically in their shape, size, and a variety of other ways. Therefore, we would first have to agree on whose ear it would be; certainly testing every hearing aid in that same ear would be a logistical nightmare for that person. Fortunately, from the standpoint of quality control, it is more important to have a procedure that is repeatable and consistent than it is to have one that perfectly reflects what happens in a real ear. Consequently, testers very early on began using a metal cavity (or coupler) for quality control measures of hearing aids. By specifying the exact properties of a coupler, many can be manufactured to this standard and distributed. In this way, all individuals agreeing to use them in the same specific way (e.g., hearing aid manufacturers and audiologists fitting hearing aids) are able to evaluate instruments in a repeatable and reliable manner regardless of where they are located (e.g., on a manufacturer's assembly floor or in an audiologist's office).

The use of a 2cc coupler for quality control measures of hearing aids was introduced by Romanow in 1940 in a paper presented at the Acoustical Society of America that was published in 1942. Although his intention was to provide a measurement technique that would "compare the sound that reaches the ear first through the air path and then through the hearing aid" (p. 294) for evaluating the function of a hearing aid, that procedure was deemed to be too "laborious and time consuming." Instead, Romanoff proposed coupling the receiver of the hearing aid—external from the cases in those days—to a small closed cavity, as shown in Figure 13–1, and measuring the ratio of the pressure in the coupler to the undisturbed input pressure at the position of the hearing aid microphone with the following formulation: C.C. = P_3/P_1

Where C.C. refers to closed coupler calibration, P_1 is the "undisturbed acoustic field pressure" at the microphone entrance in a planar field, and P_3 is the pressure developed in the closed coupler. Although an

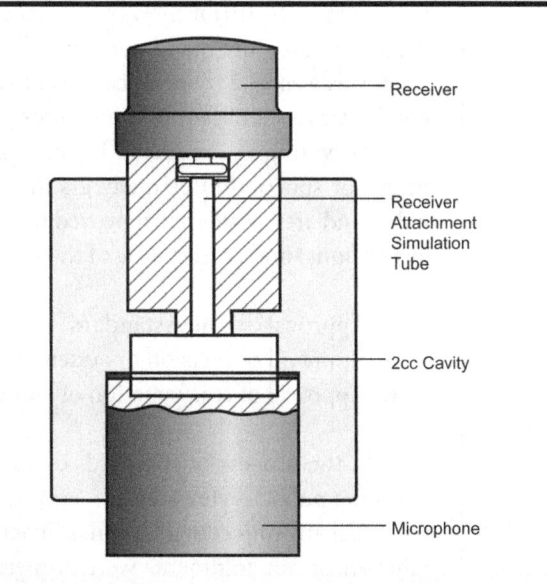

Figure 13–1. Original coupler design of Romanow (1942).

artificial ear with acoustic impedance very near that of the human ear was in development at that time (Inglis, Gray, & Jenkins, 1932), the construction and calibration of that form of coupling device was considered to be too difficult and expensive. The cavity size was chosen to simulate the average volume of the human ear "after the insertion of the earpiece" with appropriate length and diameter to prevent "extraneous longitudinal or transverse resonances." And so the 2cc coupler for measuring hearing aid performance was born.

Today, it sometimes is assumed that the 2cc coupler can mimic the human ear's response to hearing aid amplification. As we'll discuss later, that is not the case. And this is okay, as we have better ways of determining real-ear performance. Rather, the intention of the 2cc coupler measure is for quality control purposes only. That is, does the new/used/repaired hearing aid function as the manufacturer intended it to function? When used for that purpose, the coupler works as well today as it did when developed over 70 years ago.

Standard Hearing Aid Couplers

A number of different hearing aid couplers are specified in current standards. The couplers differ both in their size and their compatibility with different models of hearing aids. The HA-1 coupler is used to measure the acoustic pressure generated by an in-the-ear (ITE) hearing aid. Figure 13–2 shows the basic configuration and standardized dimensions of this coupler. Most in-the-canal (ITC) hearing aids can also be attached to and measured using this coupler. It is important to note that the opening of the hearing aid receiver inlet is to be placed flush with the opening in the cavity wall. Failure to do so may result in an inaccurate measure of response. The hearing aid is held in place and sealed using Fun-Tak or a similar material, an interesting "high-tech" coupling solution in this era of high-tech hearing solutions! There also are cases when it might be desirable to assess the function of a behind-the-ear (BTE) hearing aid coupled to the patient's own earmold. In this case, an HA-1 coupler also would be used.

The HA-2 coupler with entrance through a tube is used to measure the acoustic pressure generated by BTE hearing aids. Figure 13–3 shows the basic configuration and standardized dimensions of this coupler. The hearing aid (i.e., ear hook) is attached directly to the tubing

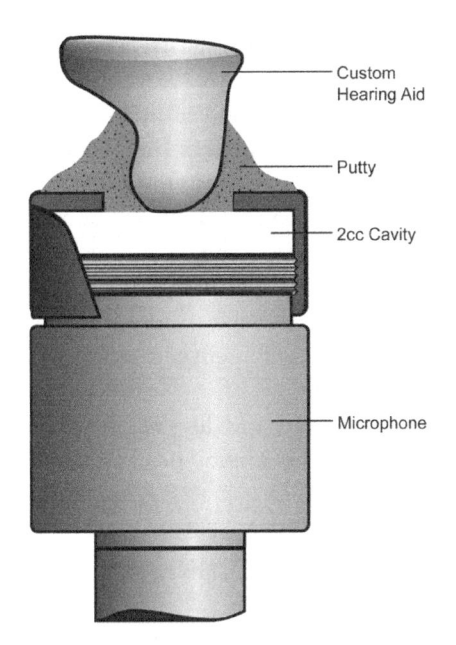

Figure 13–2. HA-1 coupler with basic configuration and standardized dimensions.

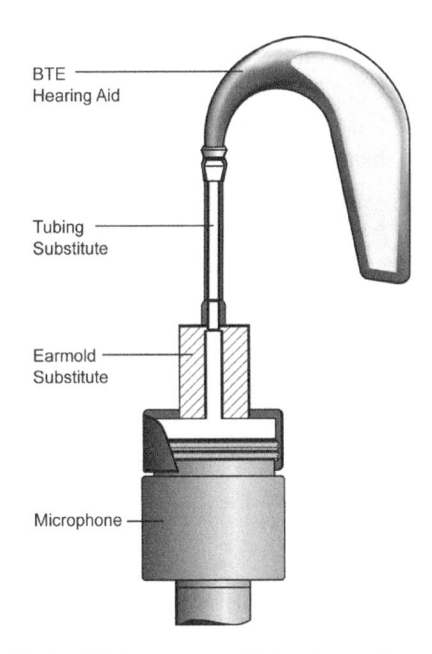

Figure 13–3. HA-2 coupler with basic configuration and standardized dimensions.

for sound entry through the earmold simulator and into the cavity. It should be noted that the earmold simulator of the HA-2 coupler has a 3-mm bore diameter, which can result in a small high-frequency boost in the response compared to an HA-1 coupler. That is, if one evaluated the hearing aid and earmold in an HA-1 coupler, and the actual earmold of the patient used common #13 tubing (I.D. 1.93 mm) to the end of the canal, less high-frequency gain/ output will be realized than measured using an HA-2 coupler. Similarly, a clinician may measure the same high-frequency gain and output for an ITE in a HA-1 coupler and a BTE in and HA-2 coupler, and mistakenly believe the two instruments have equivalent gain.

The HA-3 coupler was designed for use with modular ITE hearing aids and/or nonbutton type receivers. This coupler is rarely used today and is difficult to acquire for current measurement equipment. As is shown in Figure 13–4, the dimensions of the cavity, wall thickness, capillary, and wire are the same as for the HA-1 and HA-2 cavities. The entrance tubing—attached to the metal entrance on top—can be either rigid or flexible.

The HA-4 coupler, not commonly used today, is a variation of the HA-2 and intended for use with either BTE or eyeglass hearing aids. As shown in Figure 13–5, the adaptation of the 2cc coupler is intended for use with hearing aids for which the entire sound path bore from the BTE ear hook or eyeglass sound outlet is assumed

---

TECHNICAL TIP: CALIBRATION OF EARPHONES, TOO!

Our main topic here is to discuss the use of these couplers for the testing of hearing aids, but the HA-1 and HA-2 2cc couplers are also used to calibrate insert earphones, such as the ER-3s. When the HA-1 is used, the ER-3 eartip should be sealed to the top surface of the coupler. With the HA-2, the rigid tube is used. That is, in this case, the sound channel of the coupler is substituted for the sound channel in the eartip. If we compare the reference thresholds for the two different couplers, we see that for all key frequencies between 250 and 8000 Hz the output is within 1.0 dB except for 1500 (2.0 dB), 4000 (5.5 dB) and 8000 Hz (3.5 dB), with all these outputs greater for the HA-1 coupler. Because insert earphones and hearing aids are tested in the same 2cc coupler, this adds convenience for converting from HL to 2cc, which is something you might do when determining the appropriate MPO setting based on the patient's earphone loudness discomfort levels (LDLs).

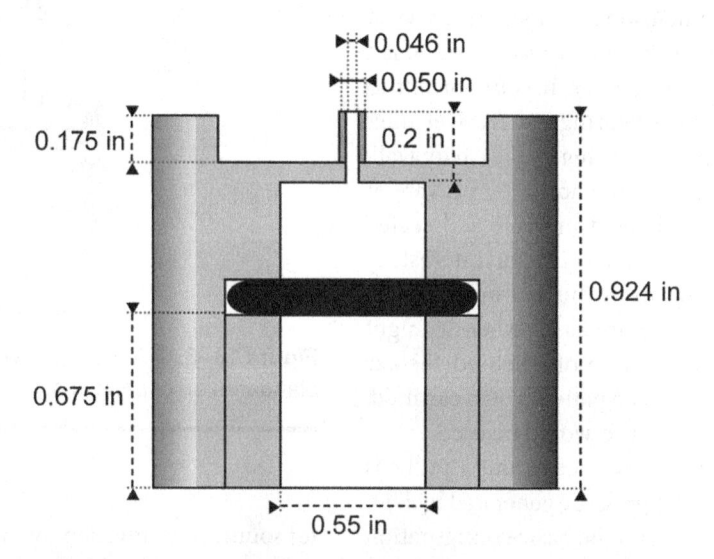

Figure 13–4. Schematic showing dimensions of the HA-3 coupler used with modular ITE hearing aids and/or nonbutton type receivers.

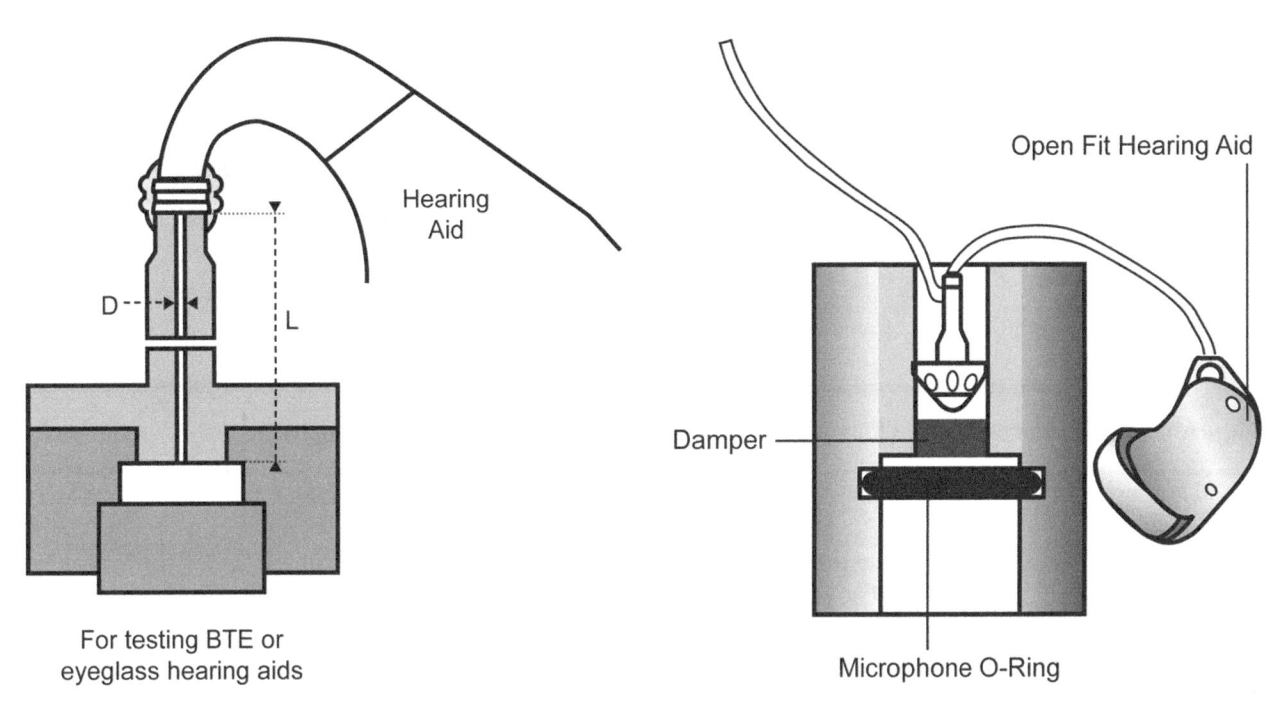

Figure 13–5. Schematic of the HA-4 coupler adapted for intended use with BTE or eyeglass hearing aids. D = 1.93 mm; L = 25 mm.

Figure 13–6. Open-fit or open canal coupler (not a standard 2cc coupler).

to have a uniform diameter (D) of 1.93 mm. That is, the 43 mm length (L) is derived from adding the 25-mm external tube length to the 18-mm earmold simulator length that comprises the two bore diameter sections (g + n) of the HA-2 coupler.

The open-fit coupler (OFC) (Figure 13–6) is not a standard 2cc coupler; that is, there is no ANSI standard to regulate its dimensions. That said, an ANSI working group was working on standardization of the open-fit coupler at the time of this writing and we expect to see this standard soon. The coupler is used for receiver-in-canal (RIC) as well as receiver-in-the-aid (RITA) hearing aid styles with thin tubing. As a result it cannot be used to compare to the manufacturing specifications, but it may provide a more realistic frequency response for the open-fit hearing aids. This type of coupler has an opening designed to fit in the sound outlet portion of the RIC or RITA hearing aid. The sound outlet portion may contain the receiver of the hearing aid or may be the end of a sound delivery tube.

A final coupler that is available for the clinician is the completely-in-the canal (CIC) coupler. Rather than 2cc, this coupler has a volume of 0.4cc. The use of a 0.4cc volume in a coupler was introduced for the Frye 6500 hearing aid analyzer. More recently, a conical 0.4cc-coupler design proposed for standardization was considered by the ANSI S3 Working Group 48 (Gebert & Saltykov, 2013). A similar 0.4cc volume coupler was introduced for the AudioScan hearing aid analyzer (Jonkman, 2015) and by G.R.A.S. for general use. A CIC or any deeply fit custom hearing aid or earmold is intended to fit so closely to the eardrum that the volume of the residual cavity is reduced greatly compared to a standard 2cc coupler. When a CIC hearing aid that is designed to be fitted deeply is tested using a HA-1 coupler—with its 2cc cavity—the frequency response is very misleading. These hearing aids, when placed deeply into the ear canal, provide a great deal more amplification in the patient's ear than is indicated by the 2cc-coupler response. This difference can be 15 dB or greater, as can be seen in Figure 13–7. Some manufacturers provide a CIC coupler option with a much reduced cavity size; others provide one of the standard couplers combined with software correction factors to provide a more realistic picture of what the frequency response will be inside the patient's ear canal. Although real ear measurements are

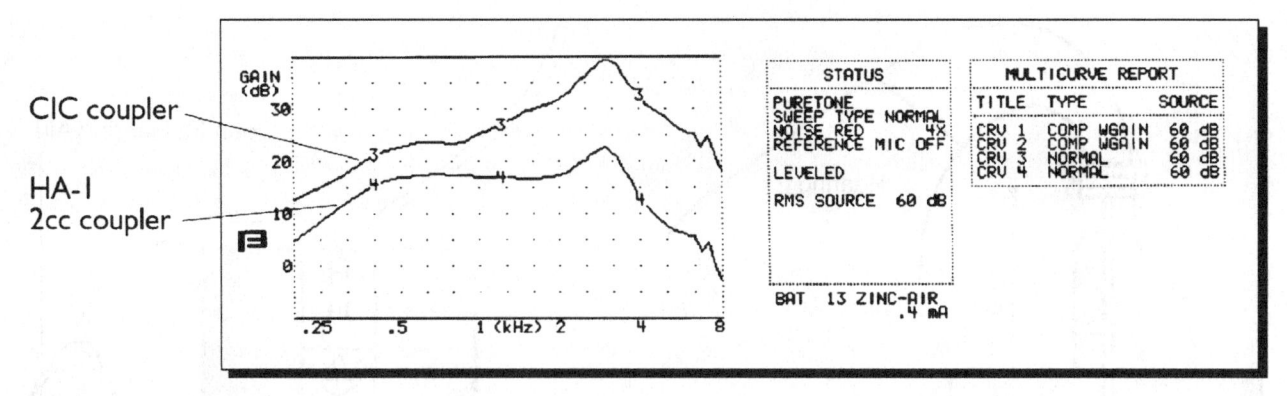

Figure 13–7. An example of error from measuring a CIC hearing aid on the wrong coupler.

the most accurate way of determining the amplification the patient is actually receiving, the CIC-coupler option is the next best thing. When considering measurements in the extended high frequencies, the 0.4cc coupler has some additional advantages compared to a standard 2cc coupler which is one of the reasons it is being considered for standardization. First, the high frequency level increase resulting from decreased volume allows for high frequency measurements at relatively low levels. Common coupler microphones have a noise floor that increases with increasing frequency so the higher levels reduce this noise floor limitation. In addition, with the smaller coupler, the standing wave resonances are increased to frequencies than are generally higher than the measurement range. This helps eliminate contamination from these resonances present in the extended high frequencies when using a 2cc coupler.

Real-Ear Simulators

In some cases, mostly the purview of researchers and engineers, it is of interest not only to have a reliable and repeatable measure but also one that is representative of what would be obtained in the average ear. Measurements made with real-ear simulators are of considerable clinical interest when the goal is to compare or examine the expected function of processing or hearing aid features on average patients, either within or across manufacturers (e.g., compare acoustic directional microphone advantages). The origins of the real-ear simulator/coupler are complex. It was clearly understood as early as 1950 that the 2cc coupler was not a good representation of an occluded human ear canal for a number of reasons:

- The volume of the coupler was (on average) too large when compared with the residual ear canal volume of a typical hearing aid fitting.
- The impedance characteristics of the human ear canal and middle ear were not well represented.
- The plumbing (e.g., earmold) alterations were not accurately represented by the hard-walled cavity.

In addition, even though these couplers were designed to approximate the acoustic load presented by the human ear (ANSI S.7, 1995), none are capable of representing the standing waves found in real ears (ANSI S3.25, 1979). Real-ear simulators can be used for any measurements that assume simulation of the sound transmission characteristics of the human ear (e.g., earphone calibration and hearing aid performance measures). Two standardized real-ear couplers are currently utilized around the world: the Zwislocki coupler and the IEC 711 real-ear simulator. As we note, the Zwislocki coupler is no longer manufactured.

The Zwislocki coupler (Figure 13–8) was developed in the late 1960s by Josef Zwislocki in an effort to circumvent some of the errors apparent in using the hard-walled cylindrical coupler to assess hearing aid function. As shown in the schematic in Figure 13–9, the real-ear effect occurs due to the four branches (V1–V4). Recall that the SPL generated in any cavity is dependent upon the impedance of the cavity, which is dependent upon the

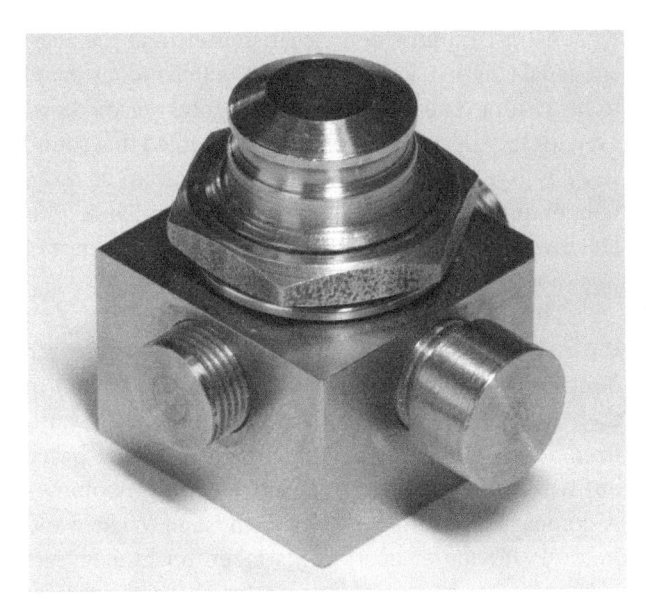

Figure 13–8. Zwislocki coupler, developed in the late 1960s.

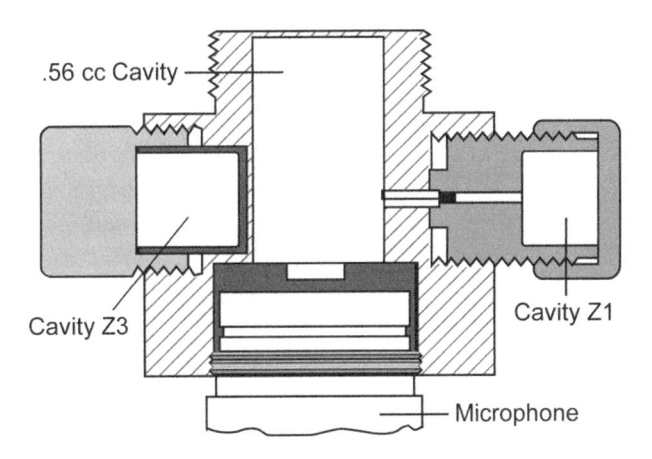

Figure 13–9. Schematic of an original Zwislocki coupler showing the four branches.

volume of the cavity. For an average adult canal, the residual volume is about 0.5cc. Because the canal terminates at the eardrum, with the nearby middle ear cavity and its 0.8cc volume, the combined 1.3cc volume determines the impedance for the low-frequency incoming sounds. As frequency increases, the eardrum and ossicles cause the impedance to rise, whereas the impedance of the residual ear canal volume lowers. This variation is mimicked by the ear simulator. With higher frequencies, the impedance of the cavities (V1–V4) rises until they effectively close off, allowing the total volume to return gradually to 0.6cc.

The same effect occurs using the IEC 711 real-ear simulator, except it has only two cavities. The Zwislocki coupler was standardized by the publication of ANSI S3.25; the 711coupler was introduced in Europe a few years later by Bruel and Kjaer, and is characterized in the IEC 60711 standard. The intent of S3.25-2009 was to make the 711 (now IEC 60318-4) the dominant ear simulator, with the legacy Zwislocki simulator included as a reference design only. In future revisions of S3.25, the Zwislocki will likely disappear from the standard because it is no longer being manufactured or supported by any company. Currently, both the 711/60318-4 design and the Zwislocki design are described (separately) in the ear simulator specifications in S3.25-2009.

The Knowles Electronics Manikin for Acoustic Research (KEMAR)

At about the same time as the real-ear simulator was undergoing development, an acoustic manikin was being developed into which a real-ear simulator could be placed, for a more realistic measure of the head, body, and torso effect on acoustic stimuli. Mahlon Burkard and Rich Sachs, under the direction of Hugh Knowles, developed the Knowles Electronics Manikin for Acoustics Research (KEMAR) which was introduced in 1972. The original KEMAR is shown in Figure 13–10 next to the newer, sleeker-looking version.

The KEMAR has allowed investigators to obtain "real-ear" measurements without the need of human subjects. KEMAR is constructed of fabricated fiberglass reinforced polyester, originally designed to hold one or two Zwislocki couplers with one-half-inch Bruel & Kjer condenser microphones. The dimensions of the manikin were chosen to represent the average human adult using two existing data sets: Churchill and Truett (1957) data for head and face dimensions of Air Force trainees (~80% male), and Dreyfuss (1966) data for average head and torso dimensions for males and females. As many interrelated factors as possible were taken into account in KEMAR's design. For example, the ear canal length of KEMAR is 21.5 mm, somewhat shorter than the average canal length of an adult human, which is considered to be 25 mm. The developers had a good reason, however, for the shorter canal length: They noted that sound velocity is greater at body temperature than at room temperature, and that the microphone compliance adds effective length. Thus, the canal resonance frequency of this shorter ear canal matches the real ear.

The decision to use the Zwislocki coupler for an eardrum simulator was partly due to earlier research done by Bauer, Rosenheck, and Abbagnaro (1967) in their attempts to build an acoustical manikin. They utilized an ear simulator equipped with a coupler based on Zwislocki's measure of "effective eardrum volume." A comparison of their results to those of Wiener and Ross (1946) for measurements taken on human ears indicated that the pressure transfer characteristics of their ear simulator was much like that of a real ear. As

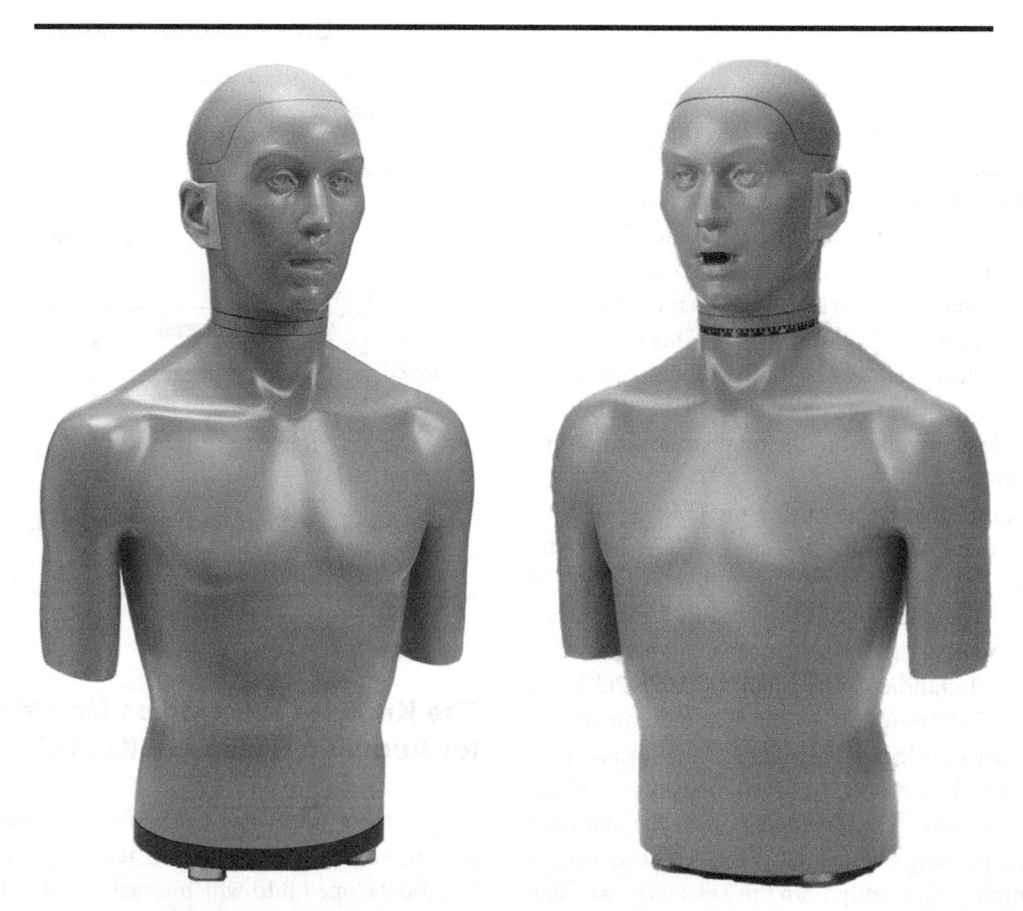

Figure 13–10. Two slightly different versions of the KEMAR. (Reprinted with permission from G.R.A.S. Sound and Vibration.)

> **KEY CONCEPT: DETAILS OF THE KEMAR FABRICATION**
>
> The KEMAR's head and torso are fabricated fiberglass-reinforced polyester; the interior surface is coated with a lead-pellet-filled resin to provide additional mass and reduce the coupling of the manikin to acoustic fields. Another manikin under development at the time by Bauer, Rosenheck, and Abbagnaro (1967) used a plastisol skin covering that is softer than the covering of the KEMAR. The developers of the KEMAR decided to compare the sound pressures at the canal entrance, using the KEMAR's head and a duplicate head composed of a material twice as compressible as human skin. Their results showed no more than 1 dB of difference at any frequency to over 8000 Hz. The developers concluded that the human flesh does not have a low enough impedance to affect the sound coming towards it. Similarly, measures obtained on the KEMAR with and without a wig show only a slight drop in pressure around 10,000 Hz.

noted above, availability and use of the Zwislocki coupler has dwindled in the past decade in favor of the 711 real-ear simulator as KEMAR's internal body part. Shown in Figure 13–11 is the 711 coupler placed in the KEMAR, whose skull conveniently lifts for such arrangement of couplers and cables.

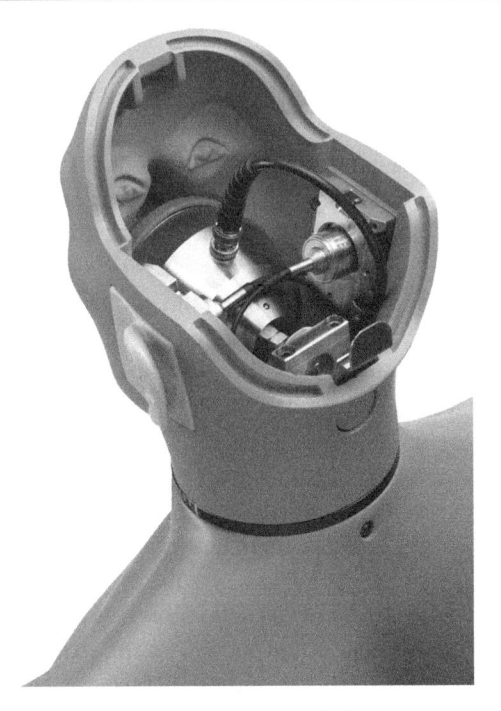

Figure 13–11. KEMAR with open skull. (Reprinted with permission from G.R.A.S. Sound and Vibration.)

The KEMAR was acquired by G.R.A.S. Sound and Vibration in 2005 from Knowles Electronics. At the time of this writing the KEMAR could be obtained through G.R.A.S. either with or without IEC 711 couplers. A range of pinna with different sizes and stiffness are available. Conversion kits are also available to convert the legacy KEMAR from the Zwislocki coupler to IEC 711 compatibility. A number of other head and torso simulators (HATS) are also available from other manufacturers, including B & K. Some of these are also compatible with IEC 711 coupling, whereas others are not.

ANSI Standards Used In Hearing Aid Assessment

The following standards, printed with permission of the Acoustical Society of America Standards Secretary, can be purchased from http://asastore.aip.org/shop

- S3.22-2014—Specification of Hearing Aid Characteristics. This standard describes air-conduction hearing aid measurement methods that are particularly suitable for specification and tolerance purposes. Among the test methods described are output sound pressure level (SPL) with a 90-dB input SPL, full-on gain, frequency response, harmonic distortion, equivalent input noise, current drain, and induction-coil sensitivity. Specific configurations are given for measuring the input SPL to a hearing aid. Allowable tolerances in relation to values specified by the manufacturer are given for certain parameters. Annexes are provided to describe an equivalent substitution method, characteristics of battery simulators, static and dynamic characteristics of automatic gain control (AGC) hearing aids, and additional tests to characterize more completely the electroacoustic performance of hearing aids.

- S3.25-2009 (R2014)—Occluded Ear Simulator. The acoustical performance of an occluded ear simulator is specified. This device is designed to simulate the acoustical behavior of the ear canal between the tip of an earmold and the eardrum, and include the acoustic impedance at the eardrum of a median adult human ear. The occluded ear simulator is intended for transducers that are sensitive to acoustic loading. It is also suitable as the basis for extensions intended to simulate the complete ear canal and the outer ear (e.g., head and torso simulators). Specific physical realizations of the ear simulator are described.

- S3.35-2010—Measurement of Performance Characteristics of Hearing Aids under Simulated Real-Ear Working Conditions. This standard describes techniques for measuring hearing aids under simulated conditions of real-ear use. The need for such a standard arises from the importance of capturing the acoustical variations in the performance data that are caused when hearing aids are worn. For example, the diffraction of the incident sound caused by the body and head of a hearing aid wearer can significantly change the input sound pressure to a hearing aid microphone. For the purpose of these measurements, a suitable manikin and ear simulator are used to represent a typical hearing aid wearer. Acoustical requirements of the test space, as well as how the manikin is positioned with respect to the loudspeaker, are given. Two methods are presented for controlling the level of the incident sound field at the location of the hearing aid on the manikin during the testing. Procedures are provided to obtain the insertion gain, or the amount by which the hearing aid changes the eardrum sound pressure in the ear simulator of the manikin relative to that in the unaided condition. Procedures are also provided to obtain the directional responses of the manikin as a function of azimuth and elevation of the sound source, both with and without the assistance of a hearing aid, and to calculate the directivity index from the directional response. The gains obtained with a hearing aid are distinguished according to whether the unaided manikin frequency response is included in (simulated real-ear gain), or subtracted from (simulated real-ear gain), the aided gain.

- S3.36-2012—Specification for a Manikin for Simulated In Situ Airborne Acoustic Measurements. The present standard describes a manikin for airborne acoustic measurements. It comprises a head with external ears and ear canals, and a torso that simulates a median human adult. It is intended primarily as an instrument for measuring the acoustic gain of hearing aids under simulated in situ conditions. Acoustical performance requirements are given, as are informative geometric descriptors.

- S3.42-1992 Part 1 (R2012)—Testing Hearing Aids with a Broad-Band Noise Signal. This standard describes techniques for characterizing the steady-state performance of hearing aids with a broadband noise signal. The need for such a standard arises from the importance of assessing the performance of hearing aids in environments more nearly representing their real-world use. The noise test signal specified herein has been employed by the National Bureau of Standards for more than 20 years in testing hearing aids. Among the tests described are noise saturation sound pressure level, noise gain, frequency response, family of frequency response curves, and output versus input characteristic. Additionally, the appendix of the standard recommends use of the coherence function to indicate the validity of frequency response measures, and distinguishes between use of random and pseudo-random noise and asynchronous versus synchronous analysis.

- S3.42-2012 Part 2—Testing Hearing Aids Methods for characterizing signal processing in hearing aids with a speech-like signal. This standard describes a recommended speech-like test signal, the International Speech Test Signal (ISTS), and a method for the characterization of hearing aids using this signal with the hearing aid set to actual user settings or to the manufacturer's recommended settings for one of a range of audiograms. For the purposes of this standard, the hearing aid is considered to be a combination of the physical hearing aid and the fitting of software that accompanies it.

- S3.46-2014—Measurement of Real-Ear Performance Characteristics of Hearing Aids. This standard provides definitions for terms used in the measurement of real-ear performance characteristics of hearing aids, provides procedural and reporting guidelines, and identifies essential characteristics to be reported by the manufacturer of equipment used for this purpose. Acceptable tolerances for the control and measurement of sound pressure levels are indicated. Where possible, sources of error have been identified and suggestions provided for their management.

- S3.7-1995 (R2008)—Method for Coupler Calibration of Earphones. The physical configuration and acoustical performance of couplers for calibration of supra-aural and insert earphones are specified. The standard, which is a revision of S3.7-1973, describes a family of 6.0cc and 2.0cc couplers, and provides information on the methods for coupler calibration of the respective supra-aural and insert earphones. The family of 6.0cc couplers includes the NBS 9-A Coupler for testing supra-aural earphones (ANSI S3.6-1989), the Type-1 Earphone coupler for testing supra-aural earphones without cushions, and the IEC Coupler for supra-aural earphones. The family of 2.0cc earphone couplers includes the HA-1 Coupler for earphones mounted in an ear insert or an ear insert connected to an earphone, the HA-2 Coupler for tests in which an acoustic tube connects an earphone to an earmold or ear insert, the HA-3 Coupler for testing the modular portion of a hearing aid, and a HA-4 Coupler for testing postauricular hearing aids or eyeglass hearing aids assumed to have a uniform 1.93-cm diameter sound path.

Hearing Aid Analyzers

In the previous section the development of coupler types was reviewed. Although it has always been understood that the common 2cc couplers (e.g., HA-1, HA-2) could not replicate the gain and/or output obtained from the hearing aid measured in a real ear—due to volume, resistance, and impedance factors—these couplers continue to be an appropriate solution for most clinics for obtaining quality control measures. A primary factor in this occurrence is the cost: The cost of a real-ear simulator such as the IEC 711 that we mentioned earlier (coupler alone) can be as much as 10 times the cost of an HA-1 or HA-2 coupler. With the constant use and changing of users in many clinical settings, the potential for damage to the coupler also exists; replacement of a 711 simulator every year would be prohibitive in many clinical settings. More importantly, the ANSI standard for obtaining all the quality control measures discussed in this chapter calls for the use of a 2cc coupler. The standard also dictates the type of environment in which these measures should be taken. Without them, the realization of electroacoustic measures for quality control purposes would be nearly impossible to achieve in a clinical setting.

General purpose spectrum analyzers were commonly used in clinics and laboratory settings for many years to assess hearing aid performance. In the 1970s, some larger clinics would have a wall of Bruel and Kjaer equipment dedicated to the electroacoustic measurement of hearing aids. Today these have been replaced in large part by much smaller software-based analysis systems. The laboratory calibration protocols are specific to the task at hand, however, and often require manual adjustment of equipment and test conditions. More efficient for the clinician is the automated test sequencing available with any of the currently marketed equipment.

What Equipment Is Needed?

A number of hearing aid analyzers are currently marketed, some by the manufacturers of hearing aids. Suppliers of this type of equipment are well-versed in the rules of the measurement equipment. Still, regular calibration is necessary to ensure the microphones, sound isolation, loudspeakers, and other components are operating as intended by the suppliers. Always refer to the relevant user manual to ensure consistent calibration.

Requirements From the Standard

Referred to as the hearing aid analyzer—or more succinctly, the test box—the requirements for the test space are clearly outlined in the ANSI S3.22-2009 standard:

1. The test space must be isolated so that ambient noise and stray electrical magnetic fields do not affect the results by more than .5 dB; furthermore, the test signal shall exceed the ambient noise at every analysis frequency, or band, by at least 10 dB. The amount of sound isolation provided by the test box varies dramatically across manufacturers and models. We must therefore carefully consider the amount of ambient noise present in the environment where the testing will take place when considering purchase of a test box.

2. The diameter of the control microphone must be 15 mm or smaller, and the center of the sound inlet port of the hearing aid must be 5 +/− 3 mm of the center of the control microphone grid.

3. The sound source must maintain the stated SPL at the hearing aid microphone entrance within +/− 1.5 dB from 200 to 2000 Hz, and within +/− 2.5 dB from 2000 to 5000 Hz. The sound source must be capable of delivering 50 to 90 dB SPL at the position of the sound entrance to the microphone.

4. Total harmonic distortion of the test signal cannot exceed 2%. For harmonic distortion measurements, total harmonic distortion of the acoustic test signal cannot exceed 0.5%.

5. The frequency of the test signal must be accurate within +/− 2%. Frequencies indicated on the chart must be accurate within +/− 5%.

6. The frequency interval between data points on graphs must not exceed 1/12 of an octave or 100 Hz, whichever is greater. If a noise (or broadband) signal is used, the analysis resolution must be 1/12 of an octave or 100 Hz, and must be stated. (Comment: Manufacturers also vary considerably in the frequency resolution of their instruments, from ≤87 Hz up to 1/12 of an octave. For a 5000-Hz center frequency, 1/12 of an octave has a bandwidth of about 288 Hz. Consequently, very narrow peaks

---

KEY CONCEPT: CLINICAL USE OF COUPLER MEASURES

In Chapter 20, we discuss the correction factors for comparing output in a 2cc coupler to output in a human ear (RECD) and gain in a coupler to gain in a real ear (CORFIG). These correction factors are used by manufacturers in fitting algorithms to attempt to achieve the appropriate gain and output for a typical clinical patient. That is, the actual gain and output in a specific patient's ear canal, as a result of the amplification device, can only be known after the probe microphone measurement has been carried out. The standard 2cc couplers are intended only for comparison of hearing aid characteristics to those provided by the hearing aid manufacturer. The real-ear simulators represent a normal ear in terms of volume, resistance, and impedance, but rarely do we see that "average" human in our clinical setting. Thus, there is need for probe microphone equipment and measures in the verification of hearing aid performance (see Chapters 17 and 18).

and valleys in the frequency response may not be visible in the higher frequencies of some measurement equipment.)
7. The appropriate coupler must be in accordance with ANSI S3.7-1995—Method for Coupler Calibration of Earphones. The total harmonic distortion of the acoustic test signal must not exceed 2% for response measures, and 0.5% for total harmonic distortion measures.
8. The standard ambient conditions must be:
   - Temperature of 23° +/− 5°C (73° +/− 9°F)
   - Relative humidity from 0% to 80%
   - Atmospheric pressure of 760 (+35, −150) mm of Hg, or 101.3 (= 5, −10) kPa

Electroacoustic Measures

The ANSI S3.22 standard clearly defines the setup and measurements of a number of parameters of hearing aids. Although the test sequence is typically automated, it is imperative that the clinician understand the measures and their derivations. Each measure has some tolerance level, which, if exceeded, places the hearing aid "out of specs." If a hearing aid does not meet specifications it may require repair. Alternatively, it's sometimes necessary to make a commonsense call. A particular measurement may be slightly different from that which was specified, yet this difference has no impact on the fitting. Is it worth packing up the hearing aid and sending it back? Probably not. Each of the measures is described in detail in the following.

Making the Measurements: A Step-By-Step Guide

Although there are some differences in the exact buttons that are pushed (or clicked on) across manufacturers, the general technique for electroacoustic evaluation of hearing aids remains the same. A walk-through of the general procedures is provided.

1. Attach the hearing aid to the programmer/computer. Each manufacturer has their own strips, boots and/or cables as shown in Figures 13–12 to 13–14. This step can skipped if the primary purpose is to check the hearing aid as it is currently set to function. In that case, the hearing aid will be tested on the coupler (start with Step 3 below) without any other cabling to the computer or programmer.
2. Set the hearing aid to test mode or refer to manufacturer specifications (attached documentation) for required settings prior to measurement. This typically results in the aid being set to omnidirectional mode, the widest frequency response, and the least compression effect. Adaptive features should be disabled (unless checking function of a particular feature). Unfortunately, not all manufacturers make this as clear as it should be, so in some cases you may need to call a manufacturer to obtain

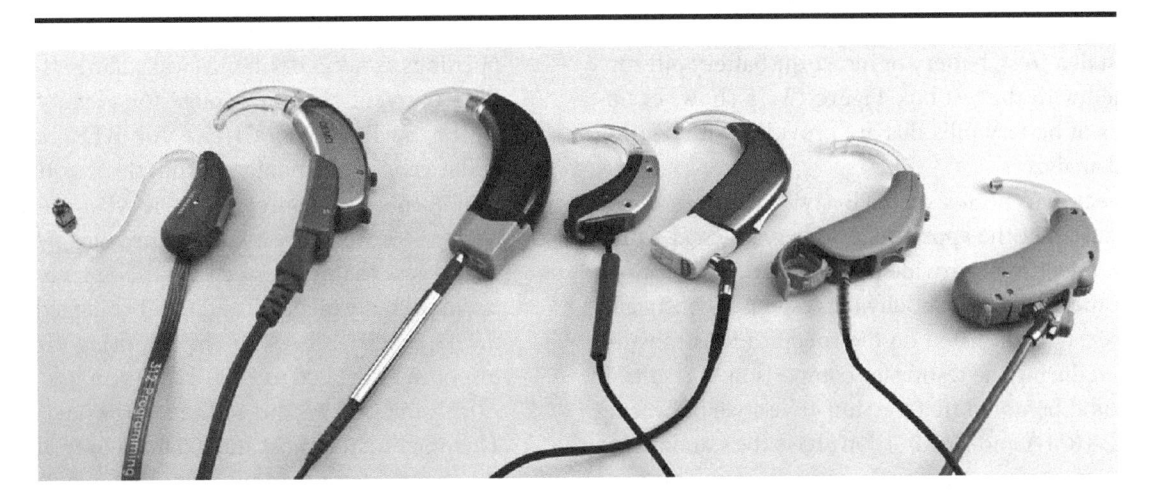

Figure 13–12. Examples of connection options for different manufacturers.

Figure 13–13. Example of a Flex strip.

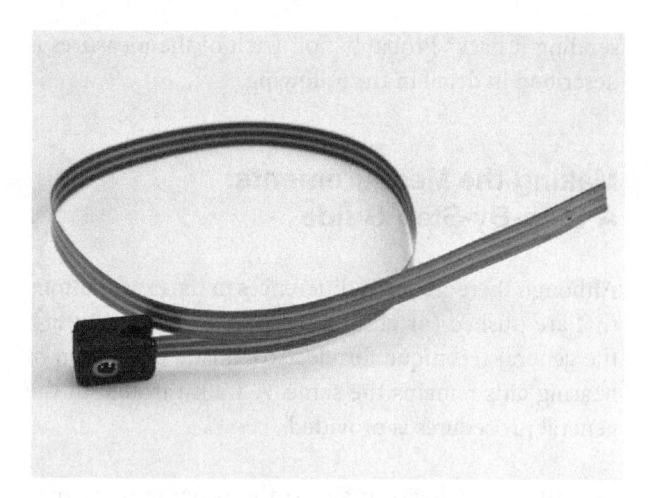

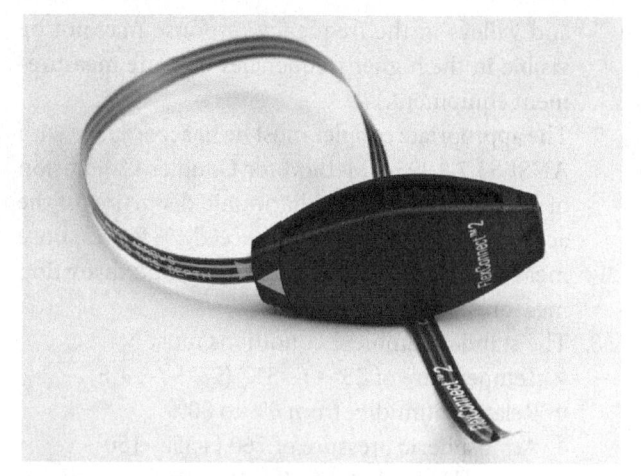

Figure 13–14. Example of a FlexConnect.

> **KEY CONCEPT: WHAT'S THE BEST HEARING AID SETTING?**
>
> For years (including the current standardized approach) the clinician has been instructed to set the hearing aid "to have the widest available frequency response range" as well as the highest available gain and output (ANSI 3.22-2009, p. 8). With the availability of highly flexible, programmable products today, that setting is both hard to achieve and relatively useless to the understanding of the hearing aid's function. As a result, manufacturers provide either a test mode, with specifications provided, or provide specifications for the hearing aid set in the manner it was shipped. In either case, the clinician has some reference for comparison of the measures obtained below. For quality control measures of gain and output, it is still recommended that adaptive features like DNR, feedback management, and/or directional microphone schemes be turned off for the initial quality control measures.

the correct hearing aid settings for electroacoustic evaluation.

3. Install a fresh battery or insert the battery pill supplied with the test box. Figure 13–15 shows examples of battery pills that are provided with hearing aid analyzers.
4. Check ear hooks on BTE style hearing aids to ensure that the appropriate style is attached. Often manufacturers provide damped ear hook options for the clinician to modify the response acoustically. The ear hook listed on the specifications must be used during the testing for comparison of results. It should be noted that the thin-tube style of hearing aids (RITA and/or RIC) don't have the standard ear hooks. For those styles, the open-fit coupler is used (see Figure 13–6).
5. For any style of hearing aid, check microphone ports and receiver tubing for obstruction. Brush openings as needed. Change wax guards as needed.
6. Plug the vent at the faceplate for ITE styles, and at the outside (lateral) end for BTE earmolds. If the vent is not plugged properly, it is likely the vent events will be present in the response. In Figure 13–16, we show a custom hearing aid with a 2-mm vent that was tested with the vent completely open, partially plugged, and totally plugged. Notice the large differences in the resulting frequency response in the 200 to 1000-Hz region.
7. Attach the hearing aid to the appropriate coupler. This may be the most important step in the measurement-taking procedure (see related Technical Tip). For traditional BTE styles of hearing aids,

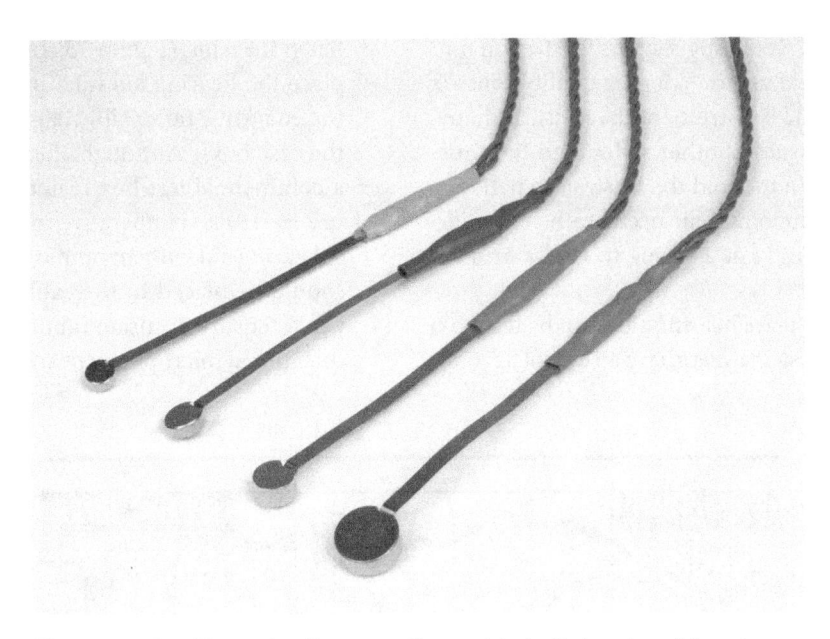

Figure 13–15. Example of battery pills provided with hearing aid analyzers.

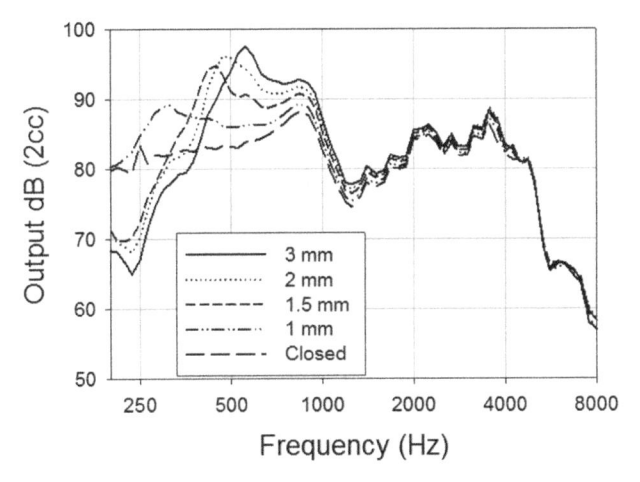

Figure 13–16. Example of vent effect as tested with the vent completely open, partially plugged, and totally plugged.

there is little opportunity for error, in that the ear hook of the hearing aid is securely attached to the 25 mm × 2 mm tubing extending from the coupler (with simulated earpiece). The key here is to use the correct tubing.

8. For the ITE style of hearing aid, placement of the hearing aid so that the canal end is flush with the opening of the coupler is critical to the accuracy (see Figure 13–2). For RIC and RITA instruments, this has presented a challenge because a standard coupler did not exist for mini-BTE hearing aids (although nonstandard adaptors are available), as of this writing. As shown in Figure 13–17, without proper placement, an artifactual low-frequency "dip" in the response is likely to occur. Since it is unlikely that the intended response of any hearing aid is *bimodal*, as indicated in the figure, such a response typically is an indication for the clinician that the aid was not properly placed. Removal of the coupler from the microphone (or the microphone cover) will allow for better visualization of the placement. Once the hearing aid is placed properly the necessary measures can be obtained. In the case of some RITA instruments, the manufacturer recommends removing the thin tube and replacing it with a standard ear hook for quality control measures. Other hearing aid test box manufacturers have either nonstandard couplers or coupler attachments made specifically for the mini-BTE tubing or receiver that can be mounted on a standard coupler. Regardless of the method, it is important that each individual manufacturer is contacted and its recommended method is applied when completing electroacoustic evaluation for quality control purposes. Although the lack of a standard method can

be frustrating, we would suggest this frustration not be used to as an excuse for skipping quality control measures. Mini-BTE instruments have just as many quality control issues as other styles, and the time spent is well worth to avoid the frustration patients feel when their appointment needs to be rescheduled after they arrive at a fitting to find a broken hearing aid.

9. It is important to place hearing aid into the test box appropriately. Most analyzers have an obvious crosshatch marking (Figure 13–18) with instructions to place the hearing aid microphone in the center of the marking (after all, that is why we calibrated the test box). Although the sound source within a commercial test box is not always obvious (Figure 13–19) it is imperative that the clinician find it. A hearing aid with an omnidirectional microphone should be placed in the calibrated circle or crossbar to ensure accurate input level. Placement of a directional microphone hearing aid requires special

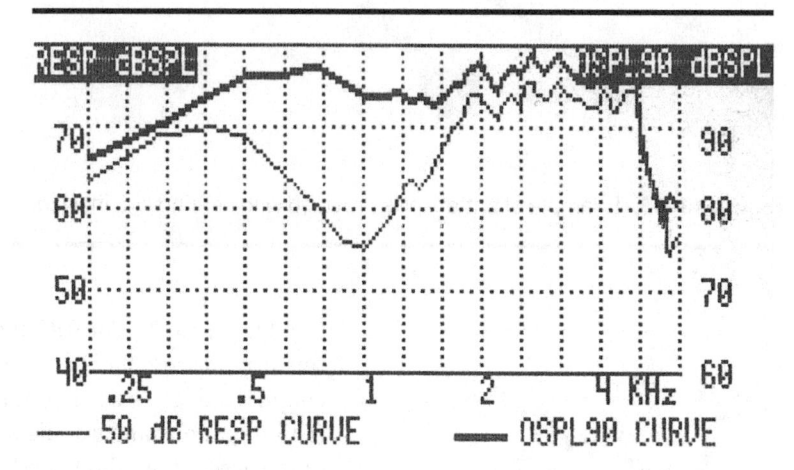

Figure 13–17. Low-frequency dip that occurs without proper placement of the ITE hearing aid.

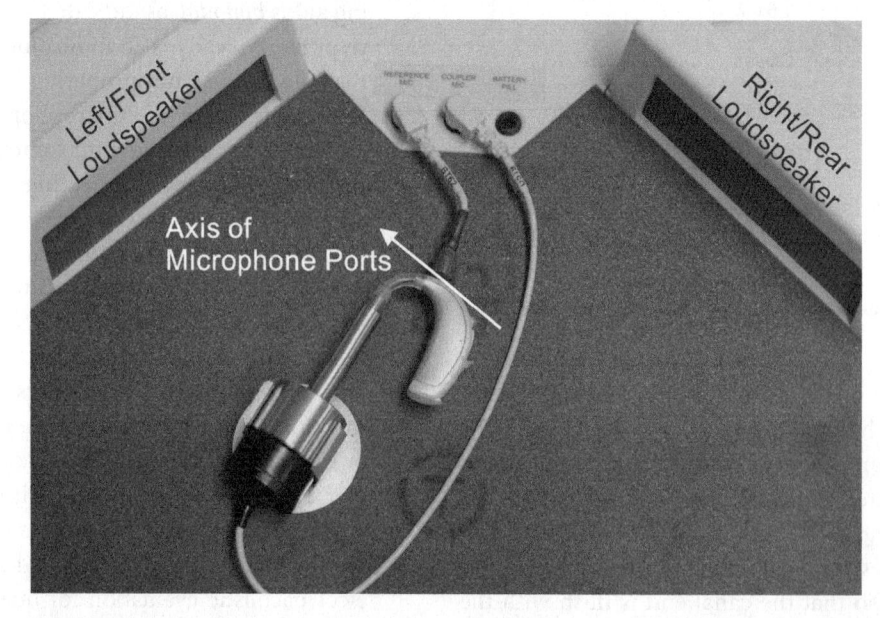

Figure 13–18. An example of appropriate placement of hearing aid in test box.

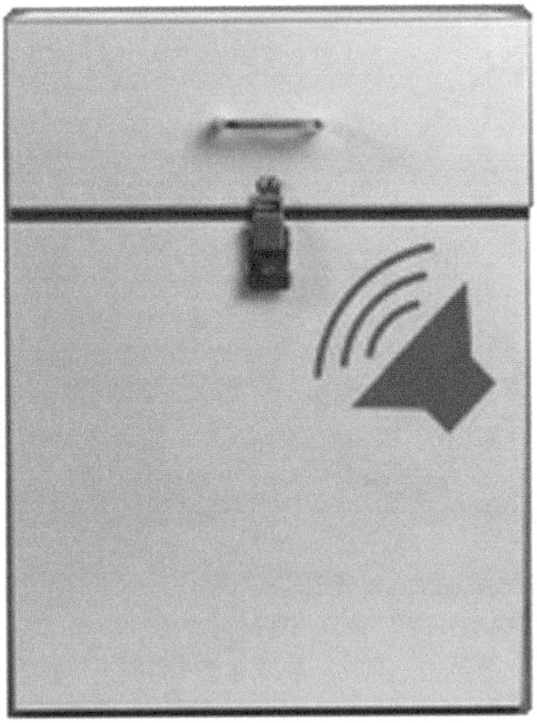

Figure 13–19. An example of a commercial hearing aid analyzer. The sound source is below the felt-like floor on which the hearing aid is placed. (Reprinted with permission from Frye Electronics.)

consideration, and will be further explained later in this chapter.

10. Close the lid securely. Many clinicians are not too concerned with this minor detail, but without a sealed chamber the background noise and clinic conversation may be mistaken as input to the hearing aid under test. Sound isolation is necessary to ensure accuracy of the measures.
11. Obtain measurements according to ANSI S3.22. This step is typically automated by the analyzer's software. As a final check before obtaining and comparing values to those provided by the manufacturer (remember that this is a quality check to determine whether the hearing aid is operating as intended by the manufacturer), be sure that the automated sequence is testing according to the same version of the ANSI standard that the manufacturer used initially.
12. Finally, never consider the quality control step to be complete without *listening* to the hearing aid, a simple step that can supplement (not *replace*) the electroacoustic measures. This check often identifies high internal noise, poor sound quality, and other irregularities. This step is easily implemented in one of two ways:
    - Many clinicians have their own earmolds for attachment to hearing aids. These are ordered with extended tubing (called listening tubes) that can be attached to the tone hook of a BTE instrument.
    - Standard in any audiology clinic is the listening stethoscope (Figure 13–20). For custom products, RIC and RITA hearing aids, a modified listening stethoscope (usually just a wider rubber nubbin at the end) is used.

Output Sound Pressure Level With 90 dB Input (OSPL90)

Previously referred to as saturated sound pressure level with 90 dB input (SSPL90), this measurement term was altered at the time of the 2003 revision of the ANSI S3.32 standard. Saturation refers to the point at which increased input does not result in increased output from the hearing aid. This measurement was changed from SSPL90 to OSPL90 for two reasons: (1) most hearing aids utilize compression limiting in their output stage,

---

THINGS TO REMEMBER: AMPLIFIED STETHOSCOPES

While made to listen to breath sounds and heartbeats instead of hearing aids, we wanted to take this opportunity to let you know there are also amplified stethoscopes for healthcare professionals with hearing loss. These devices can be purchased online and are more costly than the simple clinical device but are essential to good clinical care. Examples of the amplified stethoscope are shown in Figure 13–21.

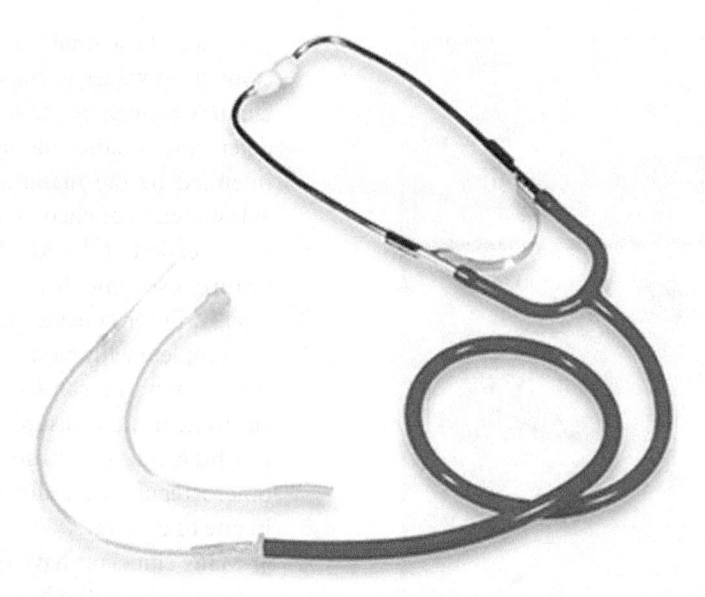

Figure 13–20. An example of a stethoscope used for listening checks of hearing aids. (Reprinted with permission from Westone.)

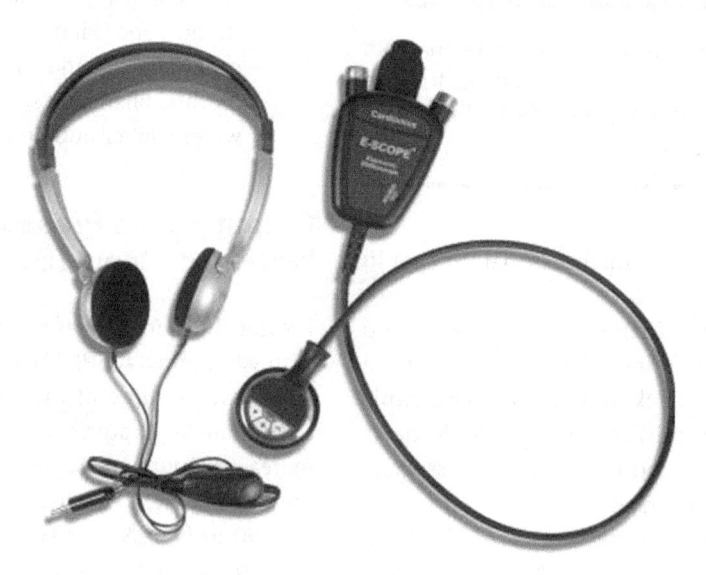

Figure 13–21. Examples of amplified stethoscope. (Reprinted with permission from Westone.)

thus technically eliminating the saturation of the amplifier; and (2) most hearing aids utilize low threshold input compression (AGC-i), which typically precludes the 90 dB input from providing the maximum output available. As shown in Figure 13–22, the maximum output might be achieved only when an input of 95 or 100 is realized. Still commonly referred to at the maximum power output (MPO) of the hearing aid because the usual range of inputs does not often exceed the 90 dB level, the correct terminology for this measurement is OSPL90. We instead use MPO to refer to the clinician software control within the hearing aid that is used to

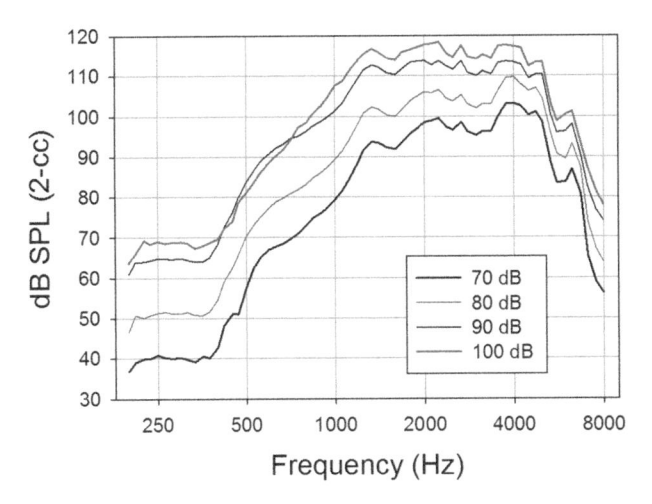

Figure 13–22. Multiple inputs to show where saturation begins. Note that when moving from 90 dB to 100 dB inputs the change of 10 dB in input no longer equals a 10 dB change in output."

affect the maximum output the hearing aid allows. That is, a hearing aid could have an *OSPL90* of 120 dB SPL, but the clinician could have set the *MPO* to 110 dB SPL so that the output did not exceed the patient's LDL. Tolerance is 3 dB for maximum OSPL90.

The HFA-OSPL90

The HFA-OSPL90 refers to the average output at the HFA frequencies. HFA refers to the frequencies of 1000, 1600, and 2500 Hz, unless the manufacturer selects different frequencies for averaging; these are referred to as special purpose average (SPA). Those SPA frequencies might be preferable for hearing aids whose response at 1000, 1600, and/or 2500 Hz is insufficient to result in a meaningful average, for example, a high-frequency emphasis hearing aid. Tolerance is +/− 4dB for HFA-OSPL90.

Full-On Gain (FOG) and High-Frequency Average Full-On Gain (HFA-FOG)

The FOG measures are obtained with an input SPL of 50 dB (ANSI, 2014). As with the OSPL90 measures, the standard HFA frequencies include 1000, 1600, and 2500 Hz, and should be used unless the manufacturer specifies SPA frequencies. Depending upon the reference used for the measure, the volume control should be at maximum. That is, if the manufacturer provides a reference for comparison that requires test mode or some other programmed settings of the hearing aid to which the electroacoustic measures are to be compared, the volume control is assumed to be set to its maximum. Since the acoustic gain is equal to the output minus the input, the measurement equipment can display this information in both output and gain, as shown in Figure 13–23. Tolerance: The value should not deviate from the value provided by the manufacturer by more than +/− 5 dB for FOG.

Reference Test Gain (RTG)

One of the least understood measures (and/or control settings) in hearing aid measurement is that of reference test gain (RTG). The rationale for this measure dates back to the earliest version of the ANSI S3.22 standard, wherein the intent was to set the volume control wheel (VCW) so that any speech input *plus* the gain of the hearing aid would not saturate the hearing aid. In those earlier days of hearing aid technology, saturation of the amplifier typically meant increased distortion due to the peak clipping that would occur with higher inputs. The logic was that, if the average level of speech at 1m is 65 dB SPL, and if the speech peaks are 12 dB greater, then the peak input to the microphone for speech would be 77 dB. Because the goal was to keep the 77 dB input *plus* the gain of the hearing aid from saturating the hearing aid (to preclude the distortion from negatively impacting the perceived sound quality), the gain needed to be carefully set. To achieve that, the hearing aid's volume (i.e., gain/output) could be adjusted to 12 dB below saturation, with the assumption that speech (77 dB at the microphone) would *not* saturate it. As most testing equipment of the time had no 65 SPL input setting available, it was recommended that 60 be used as the input and the VCW be set so that the output was 17 dB below the HFA SSPL90; this would give equivalent results. Clear as mud? Simply stated, the VCW of the hearing aid was set so that gain plus speech input would not allow for the amplifying stage to be saturated. As many hearing aids do not have external VCWs and most implement some type of compression to avoid saturation, the usefulness of this measure has been challenged.

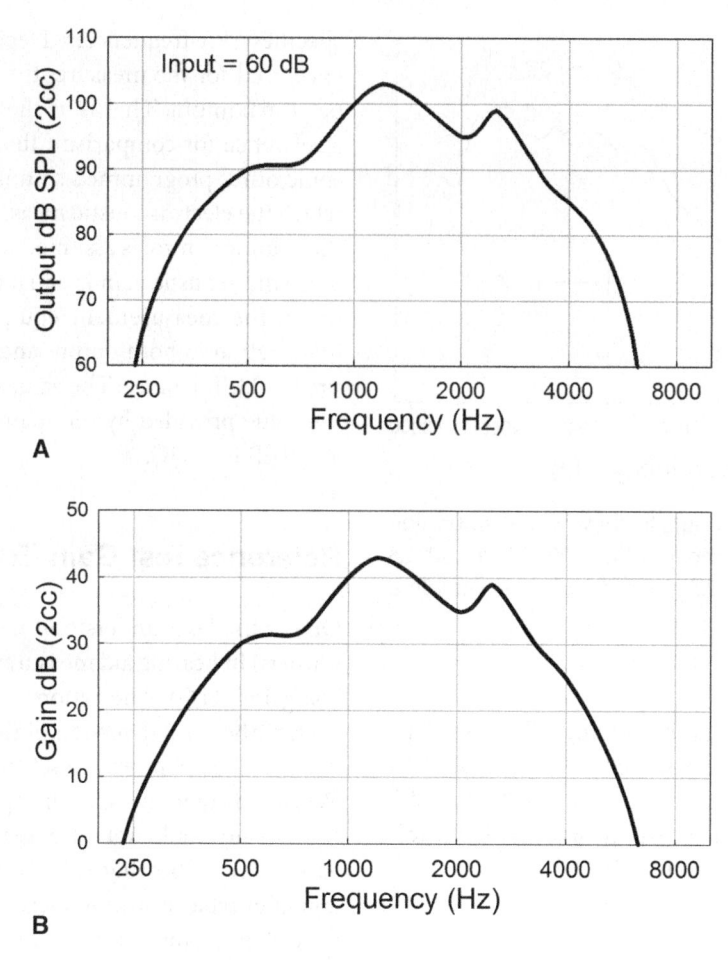

Figure 13–23. Display from measurement equipment. **A.** Acoustic output. **B.** Acoustic gain.

When the hearing aid is connected to the programmer, it is still possible to adjust the volume or gain to achieve the RTG position. RTG refers to the HFA gain from the hearing aid when measured in this manner. RTG is stated for informational purposes only; consequently, no tolerance information is required.

Frequency Response

With the RTG volume (gain) achieved, and using the 60 dB input necessary to achieve it, several other measures are obtained and reported. The frequency response (which is actually more accurately described as the frequency *limits* of the hearing aid's bandwidth) of the hearing aid under test is also derived at this volume setting. Frequency response curves can be displayed in terms of gain or output. To determine the frequency range, the following steps are followed as shown in Figure 13–24 (we will assume an output curve here for the derivation; the same steps are followed with the gain curves):

1. Determine the HFA from the response curve.
2. Subtract 20 dB.
3. Draw a horizontal line on parallel to the X-axis at that reduced dB level that intersects f_1 (lower end of frequency response) and f_2 (upper end of frequency response). These values represent the frequency range of the hearing aid, with the following tolerances allowed for comparison to the spec provided:
   a. $1.25f_1$ or 200 Hz (whichever is higher) +/– 4 dB
   b. $0.8f_2$ or 2000 to 4000 (whichever is lower) +/– 6 dB

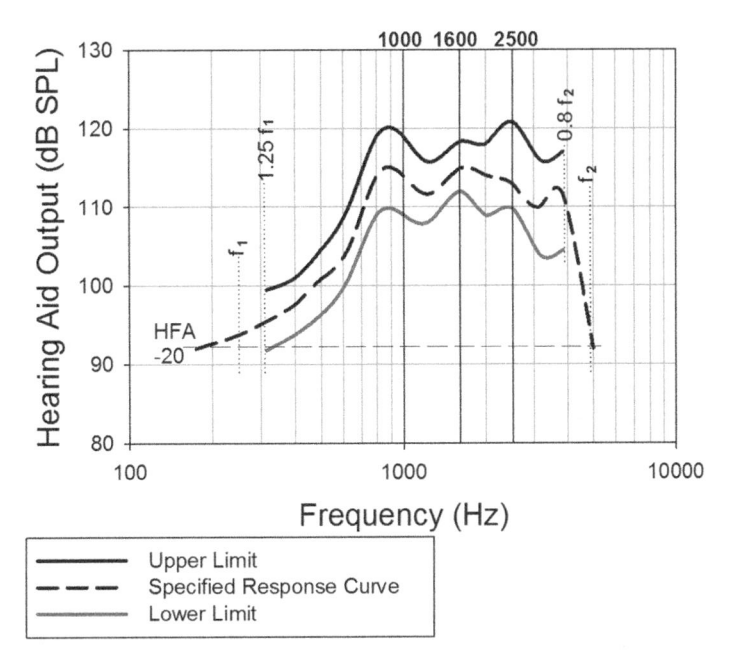

Figure 13–24. Example of frequency response calculation.

Harmonic Distortion Measures

A measurement of high harmonic distortion continues to be a good indication that the hearing aid (often the receiver) may be close to failing. The ANSI S.32 standard calls for measuring and recording the total harmonic distortion from a hearing aid, as measured in its RTG position for the following frequencies and inputs: 70 dB SPL input at 500 and 800 Hz (or at the lower of the two SPA frequencies that corresponds to 0.5 of the special purpose frequencies); 65 dB at 1600 Hz (or at the lower of the two SPA frequencies that corresponds to 0.5 of the special purpose frequencies). The distortion is reported in terms of percentages at the chosen frequencies. If the frequency response curve rises by 12 dB or more per octave between any test frequency and its second harmonic, however, distortion testing at that frequency may be omitted. Total harmonic distortion may be determined using either of the following methods:

$$\% \text{ THD} = 100 \sqrt{(p^2_2 + p^2_3 + p^2_4 + \ldots)/p^2_1}$$

$$\% \text{ THD} = 100 \sqrt{(p^2_2 + p^2_3 + p^2_4 + \ldots)/(p^2_1 + p^2_2 + p^2_3 + p^2_4 + \ldots)}$$

Where p_1 = the sound pressure of the fundamental as measured in the coupler and p_2, p_3, p_4, (and so forth) = the sound pressure of the second, third, fourth (and so forth) harmonics as measured in the coupler.

Tolerance: The total value shall not exceed the value provided by the manufacturer plus 3%. A sample printout of distortion measures is shown in Figure 13–25. In this case, the distortion obviously exceeds the manufacturers specs (no one should allow for distortion levels above 10% at any frequency, we would argue). It can also be seen in the righthand figure that the high levels of distortion have resulted in a "ragged" response from the hearing aid.

Equivalent Input Noise (EIN)

The intended purpose of the EIN is to measure the internal noise of the hearing aid. The formula calls for subtracting the HFAG50 (high-frequency average gain with 50 dB input) from the output measured from the hearing aid when no signal is being delivered to it. Because circuit noise can also be affected by the bandwidth, the measure could be higher than expected for that reason. Additionally, since many manufacturers use expansion to reduce output for low-level inputs, the measurement could be inaccurate. The manufacturer must state whether expansion was used during the measurement.

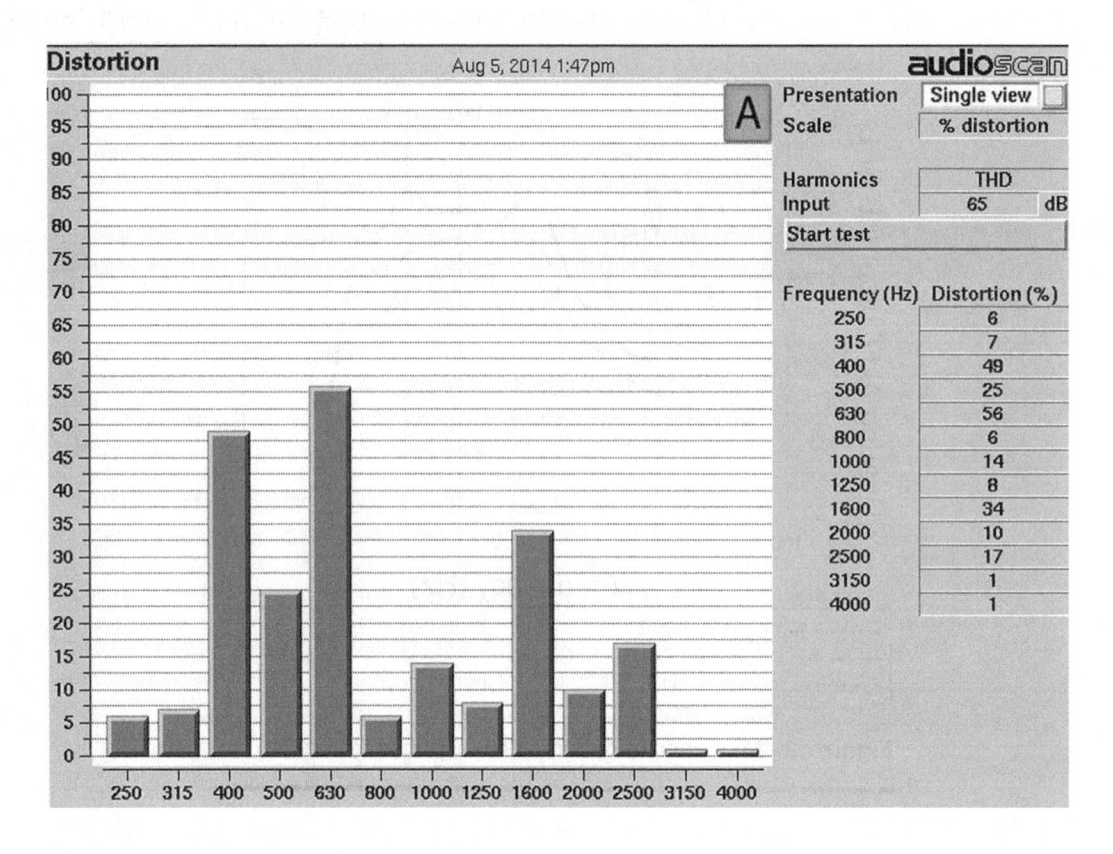

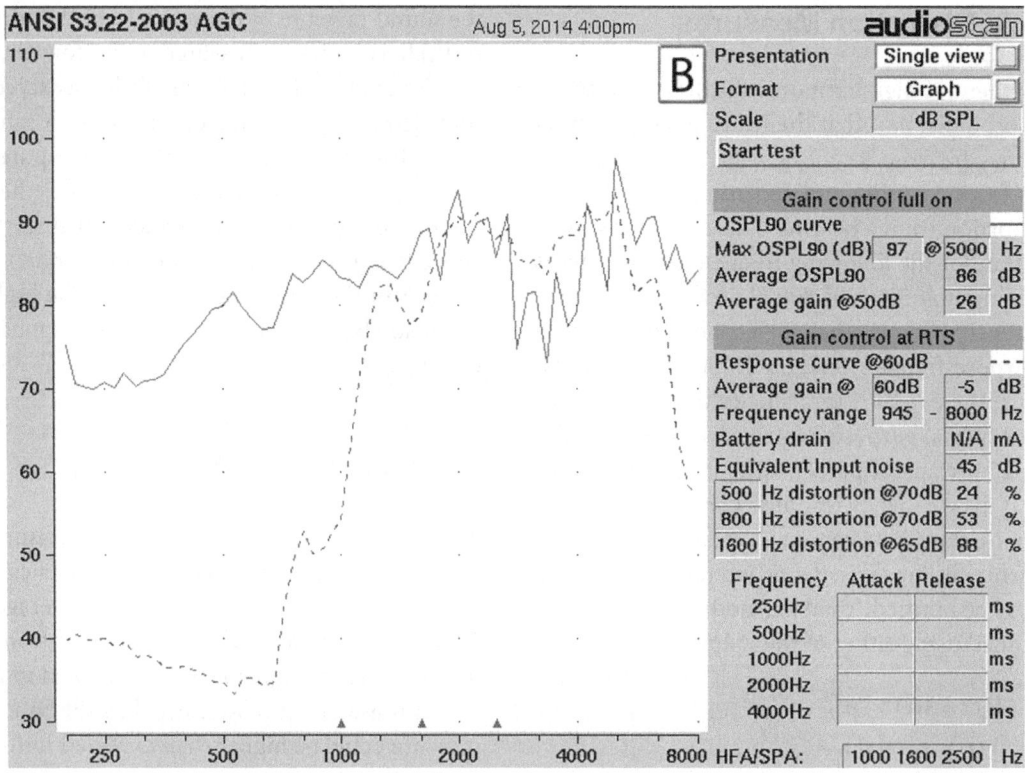

Figure 13–25. A. A sample printout of distortion measures shown in bar graph and numerical values. **B.** The resultant frequency response from the high levels of distortion.

More importantly, however, is the fact the measurement itself assumes that the gain of the hearing aid with a 50 dB input is a valid representation of the gain to be subtracted from the output of the hearing aid with no signal being delivered. Because most hearing aids are nonlinear, and with expansion affecting low-level gain and processing schemes affecting circuit noise, the measure itself may not be valid in its current form as it often does not reflect the noise level generated by the hearing aid under typical listening conditions (Lewis, Goodman, & Bentler, 2010). With this said, this measurement remains an important quality control check to ensure that the noise levels generated by the hearing aid correspond to the levels specified by the manufacturer. Recent work has revealed that some manufacturers' EIN measures are consistently well outside of specifications (Holder, Picou, Gruenwald, & Ricketts, 2016). Although we believe this may not reflect a problem for the patient, it does leave the clinician in a difficult situation regarding whether such instruments need to be returned or if the measure should be ignored. Holder and Colleagues point out, it is imperative that clinicians can easily complete meaningful quality control measures because, in some cases, measures that are out of specifications do reflect a problem with the hearing aid.

Battery Current Drain

In the past, the expected life of a battery was measured fairly easily by considering the battery's capacity (in milliamp hours) divided by the circuit's drain on that battery (in milliamps). For the majority of modern circuitry, battery drain will depend on factors such as the VC position, the signal input level, and the activation and operation of various processing features. Most importantly, unlike the Class A analog amplifiers used in hearing aids of decades past, modern digital amplifiers consume significantly less current when an input is not present than when one is. Consequently, the more time a listener spends in a quiet setting, the longer the battery will last. This can cause conflicting data, as the battery drain for a patient who has an open fitting, and spends all day in background noise—which might have noise reduction, feedback suppression, directional processing, feedback lowering and ear-to-ear data sharing active all the time—will be quite different from how battery drain was measured in the manufacturer's laboratory. Although it is no longer easy to predict battery life in a modern hearing aid, evaluation of battery drain

> **KEY CONCEPT: TOLERANCE**
>
> EIN shall not exceed the maximum value specified by the manufacturer plus 3 dB. A sample EIN measurement display is shown in Figure 13–26.

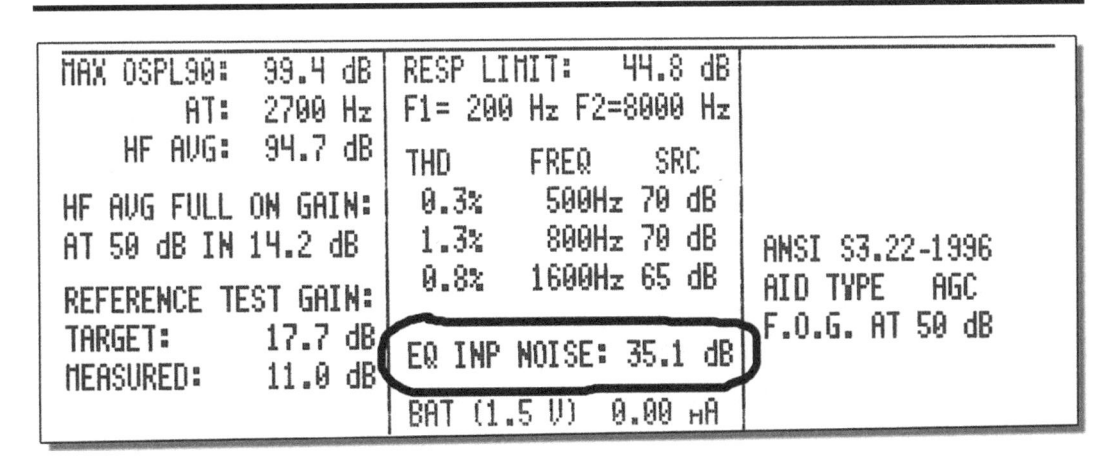

Figure 13–26. This is an example of a test printout showing the equivalent input noise (EIN) value.

is still important as a quality control measure. Higher than expected battery drain is usually indicative of a mechanical failure that has either already occurred or will soon.

To evaluate battery drain, the gain control is placed in the reference test position, and a 1000-Hz input at a level of 65 dB SPL is presented.

Tolerance: The battery drain obtained in this manner shall not exceed the maximum value specified by the manufacturer plus 20%.

Annex C of the S3.22 standard provides guidance for other manners of measurement (for informational purposes only) including:

1. Quiescent battery current refers to the drain with no input signal, obtained with the hearing aid set to RTG.
2. Maximum battery current value can be obtained by setting the hearing aid to produce the highest HFA-OSPL90, and presenting an input of 90 dB at the three HFA test frequencies. The average of these three frequencies is the reported value.
3. The ANSI standard suggests that a reasonable approximation of the current drain in actual use conditions can be expressed as a weighted sum of the quiescent current and the maximum current, for example, I (actual) = 0.8 (quiescent current) + 0.2 (HFA maximum current). As shown in Figure 13–27, it is possible to obtain and display the measures simultaneously on current equipment.

Induction Coil Response

Placing the handset of a telephone (land line or cellular style) near the microphone inlet of the hearing aid

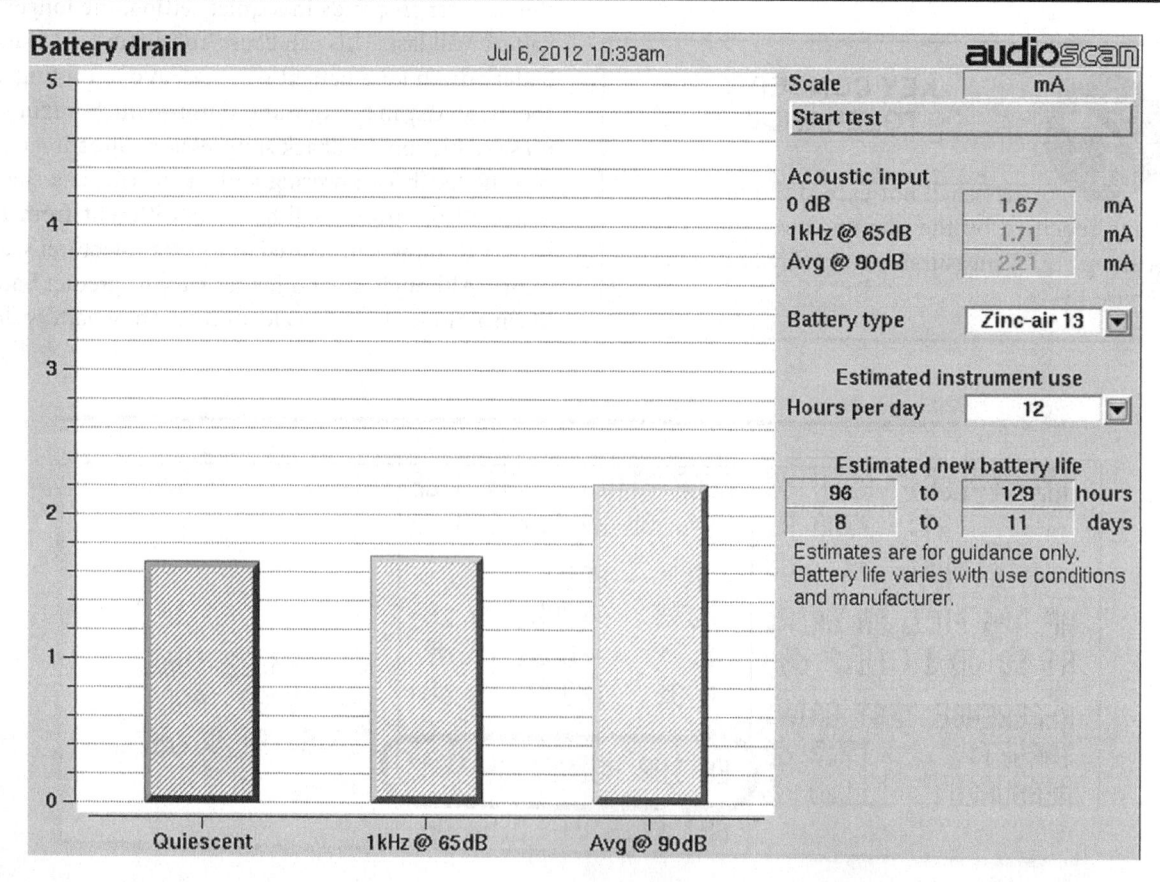

Figure 13–27. Testing equipment results demonstrating the quiescent, maximum, and weighted sum of the battery drain.

> ### TECHNICAL TIP: TOLERANCES, TOLERANCES, AND TOLERANCES
>
> Throughout the S3.22—Standard for Specification of Hearing Aid Characteristics, there are noted tolerances for every measure. These tolerances apply to the hearing aid itself and assume the measurement equipment is accurate. For imperfectly functioning equipment, the hearing aid would have to be even more exact in order to meet the standard's recommendations. It is, therefore, important for the clinician to be confident of the accuracy of the measurement equipment itself. This is typically accomplished with the help of audiological equipment distributors. For example, the microphone sensitivity must be accurate, the seals on the analyzers must be updated every 10 years or so, even the grids that outline the placement of the hearing aid properly tend to wear off and need replacement. Even if the clinician takes the responsibility for calibration of all test equipment, the calibrator (modern version of a piston phone) needs to be calibrated. An ongoing dialogue with the equipment distributors can typically keep these concerns in check.

can cause feedback to occur. To alleviate that problem and provide a more ambient noise-free listening experience for the user, induction coils were used in hearing aids beginning in 1947 (Lybarger, 1947). To measure the induction coil response, the hearing aid is set to the RTG position and "T" (telecoil) setting. The aid must be positioned on the telephone magnetic field simulator (TMFS), as shown in Figure 13–28. This simulator produces a magnetic field of consistent level and geometric shape when driven by a specified current (6/N mA, where N = number of coils). As noted in the ANSI S3.22 standard, the faceplate of the ITE or ITC hearing aid should be parallel with the test surface of the TMFS and as close as possible to it. The SPL from 200 to 5000 Hz is then recorded. The HFA SPL for the induction telephone simulator (HFA-SPLITS) is calculated as the average SPL at 1000, 1600, and 2500 Hz. Another value, the relative simulated equivalent telephone sensitivity (RSETS), is also obtained by subtracting the RTG = 60 dB from the HFA-SPLITS.

Tolerance: The SPLITS value must be within +/− 6 dB of the manufacturer's specified value.

Other Important Quality Control Procedures

Although not part of an ANSI standard, it is also useful to assess the function of several specific hearing aid technologies for quality control purposes. In some cases, this assessment can also provide important information regarding how a technology functions for a particular model, and will provide important insights that can be used in patient counseling—the onset and offset of noise reduction, for example. In most cases, however, this assessment is usually completed to make sure the technology is functioning as expected. Although we suggest that these measures be conducted before the initial fitting, it is as just as important to repeat this testing on repeat visits. As we discuss shortly, directional microphones, for example, easily may become less effective following use.

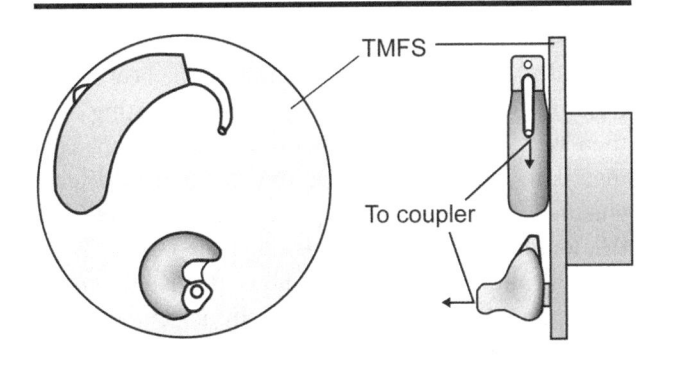

Figure 13–28. Correct placement of the HA on the telephone magnetic field simulator (TMFS).

Directional Microphone Technology

With directional microphone technology, there are many ways industry and independent researchers can assess and represent the intended effect of each design for polar response pattern, directivity index (DI), and even unidirectional index (UDI). Most clinicians do not have the anechoic environment or related software algorithms for taking such measures, nor do they have the time or interest in those details of outcome. For quality control, however, it is necessary for the clinician to make at least cursory measures of the microphone function to confirm that it is, indeed, functioning like a directional microphone.

Assessment of directional microphone function is critical for a variety of reasons. Most importantly, debris and moisture in the hearing aid wearer's environment can act to clog the microphone screens and ports, thus changing relative sensitivity across the two ports.

On occasion, directional products may not be functioning properly when they arrive at your clinic. Although we know of no peer-reviewed studies that have been published to date examining quality control of commercial directional microphone hearing aids, there have been a few unpublished reports. Ricketts (2012) has reported on the directivity of 12 pairs of instruments (24 individual) that were acquired clinically from 2003 to 2006 in both directional and omnidirectional modes. All instruments were commercially available and represented 12 different models of mini-BTE hearing aids from eight different manufacturers. The directivity index (DI) of these hearing aids was measured by comparing hearing aid output, as measured in an anechoic chamber, to that measured in a relatively diffuse reverberation room. In both cases, the test signal was a 70 dB SPL speech-shaped noise of the same total acoustic power. The results of this investigation revealed that three of the 24 hearing aids had directional modes that functioned as omnidirectional (nonfunctioning directional microphones). In five other instances, one hearing aid within a pair had a DI value (averaged across 500, 1000, 2000, and 4000 Hz) that was at least 0.5 dB lower than its matched pair. These data suggest there may be issues with initial quality control in directional hearing aids. This is not something that is normally tested as part of the manufacturing quality control.

Although initial quality control is concerning, there can also be failures that occur over time. The clinical directivity of mini-BTE and ITE hearing aids was assessed in a large group of hearing aids upon initial fitting and after a wear period of two to nine months, using the front-to-back ratio (FBR) method described in the next section (Ricketts, McCardle, Smith, Chisolm, & Bratt, 2011). The initial data reported herein reflect 468 ITEs and 319 BTEs fitted bilaterally to 434 patients fitted at Veterans' Affairs Medical Centers. The hearing aids in question all implemented a single microphone (pressure gradient) approach to directivity. Only three of the 787 instruments evaluated (all mini-BTEs) failed the initial screening, which suggests excellent initial quality control. With this single-microphone style, no microphone matching is necessary and, consistent with the differences seen when comparing this study to the ones presented above, initial quality control is expected to be higher in comparison to dual microphone directional systems. In contrast to the high initial quality control values, between 12 and 15% of instruments failed upon rescreening after being worn in the field. The hearing aids in question were fitted primarily to individuals living in Tennessee and Florida. Not surprisingly, more hearing aids failed during July and August than any other months, consistent with what might be expected given the relatively high humidity at that time of the year.

Altogether, these data are seen as providing strong support for evaluating directivity clinically for quality control purposes both at the initial fitting and during annual or semiannual follow-up visits. Clinical measures can take any of the following forms.

Stethoscope Listening

This five-second test involves pointing the hearing aid towards the mouth while saying, "Testing, testing," and then away from the mouth while saying, "Testing, testing." This simple test allows the clinician to discern whether the backward-facing utterance was softer than the forward-facing utterance. There is obviously no quantification with respect to how effective the directional microphone scheme actually is, but the rare occurrence of a reversed microphone is easily identified.

Measurement of Front-to-Back Ratio (FBR)

Regardless of the measurement equipment at the clinician's disposal (assuming the coupler and test box are standard), the FBR can be measured. The hearing aid is attached to the appropriate coupler and placed in the test box with the front port nearest the sound source—referred to as on-axis (Figure 13–29). An output measure is obtained. The hearing aid is adjusted so that the rear port now is nearest the sound sources, referred to here as off-axis, and the measurement is repeated. As shown in Figure 13–30, the top curve indicates the output from the hearing aid as measured when the front microphone port is closer to the sound source; the bottom curve indicates the output from the hearing aid as measured when the rear microphone port is closer to the sound source. Some call this an FBR; technically, however, the FBR is the difference between these two curves, or more precisely, the output difference on a polar plot between the 0° and 180° inputs. Occasionally the FBR will be reported as a single number: either the difference in the curves at a specified frequency or the average difference between the curves. This version of FBR is more efficient in that it represents the difference in dB across the entire frequency range.

Measurement of the FBR can be complicated by other ongoing hearing aid features. It is important that, in order to obtain reliable FBR measures, the hearing aid be programmed: (1) with a fixed directional mode, (2) with adaptive processing disabled, (3) with DNR disabled if a steady-state test signal is used, and (4) with digital feedback suppression (DFS) disabled if a pure-tone test signal is used. Using speech or speech in noise for FBR measures will alleviate the need to disable DNR and DFS, but requires a bit more test time than using steady state noise, composite noise, tone composites or swept tones. Low-threshold compression will reduce the magnitude of the measured FBR (although it will not affect directivity when operating in the real world as we describe in Chapter 11). For example, if the true FBR is 20 dB at 2000 Hz; application of a 2:1 compression ratio will result in a measured FBR of 10 dB. Therefore, it is important to disable compression consistently or use similar compression parameters within each hearing aid model whenever evaluating FBR for quality control purposes. Let's again assume you generally fit a particular model that has a high frequency FBR of approximately 20 dB. If you typically fit patients with sloping hearing loss, resulting in high frequency compression ratios of between 2:1 and 3:1, you can leave compression active

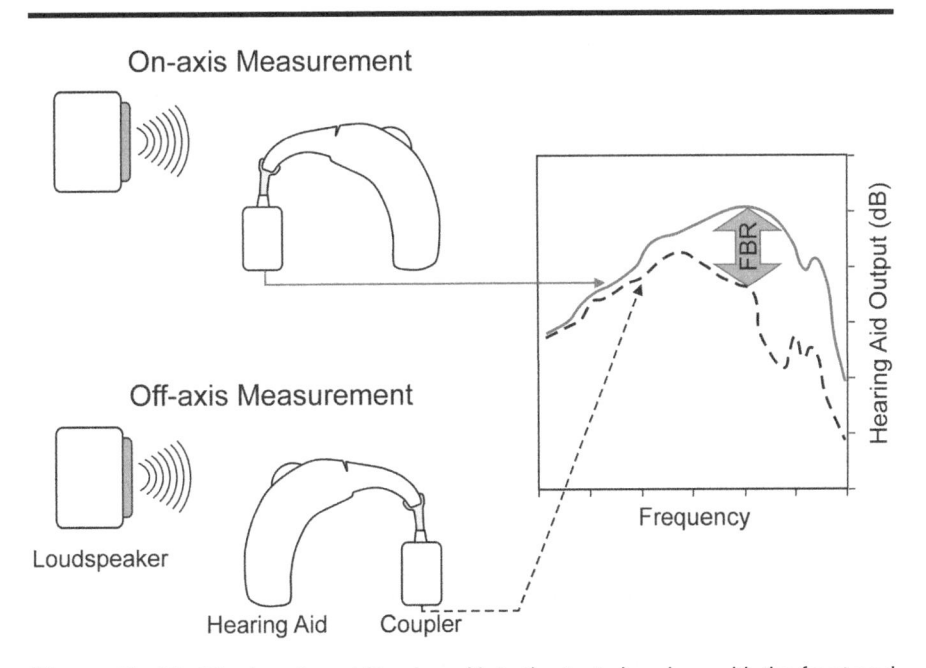

Figure 13–29. The hearing aid is placed into the test chamber, with the front and back ports aligned on the crosshatches, and aiming toward the left (front port) and right (rear port) sound sources. The exact orientation depends on the model of test chamber, so check the user manual to confirm the appropriate orientation.

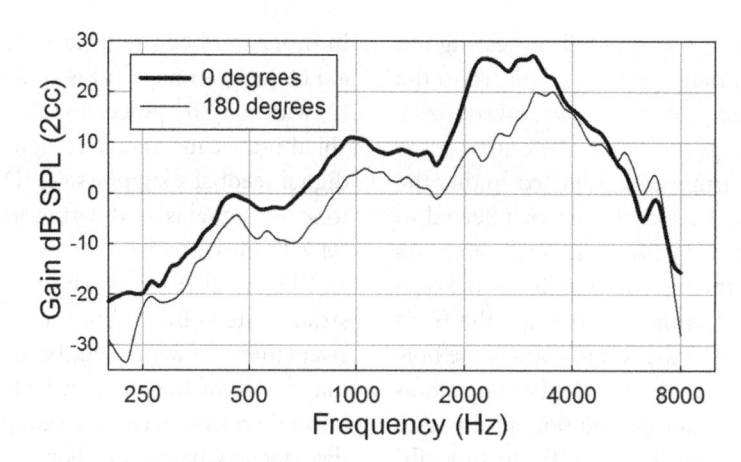

Figure 13–30. Example of a hearing aid test box printout of a front-to-back ratio (FBR). The 0-degree reading corresponds to the front port of the microphone of the hearing aid being aimed toward the sound source, whereas the 180-degree reading refers to the front port being aimed away from the sound source.

and know that the directional microphone is functioning properly if you measure FBRs of approximately 7 to 10 dB (roughly one-third to one-half of 20).

At least one manufacturer markets hearing aid analyzers that allows for both front and back source directions to be taken simultaneously by presenting interleaved pure tones from two speakers oriented in the front and rear facing portion of the hearing aid test chamber. Since the hearing aid analyzer knows which pure tones are presented from which speaker, the relative hearing aid output for sounds arriving from in front and behind the hearing aid can rapidly be assessed. An additional advantage of using the simultaneous presentation is that compression and DNR do not need to be disabled for the measurement. However, since the test signals are tonal, DFS does need to be disabled for accurate measurements in many models.

Polar Response Pattern

A final measurement technique for quality control assessment of the directional microphone is the actual

---

TECHNICAL TIP: ALPHABET SOUP—THE VALUE OF THE FBR

Importantly, the magnitude of the FBR may not be useful for comparisons across hearing aid models or brands because the values will be larger for instruments that place the null at or near 180 degrees, even if there is little attenuation at other angles. Instead, we use the magnitude of FBR as a quality control within individual models to ensure the microphones are operating as intended. Most clinics tend to fit the same products. If you know that Model XYZ hearing aid usually has an FBR of 15 dB when tested in a certain manner, then an FBR measure of only 5 dB for a Model XYZ product is cause for concern. Conversely, model ABC may typically have an FBR of around 5 dB, but provide just as much benefit in the real world as model XYZ. How could this be possible? Consider the theoretical polar patterns we introduced in Chapter 10. Assume the relative FBR for XYZ results from roughly a cardioid design, while the FBR for model ABC results from a supercardioid design. In this case the DI for model ABC may actually be higher, even though the FBR for XYZ is larger.

measurement of the polar response pattern. Previously, polar measures were difficult to obtain outside of an anechoic chamber of fairly significant size. More recently, a small-sized chamber has been marketed for clinicians to obtain their own polar response patterns for comparison to the manufacturer-provided data. Figure 13–31 shows the placement of the hearing aid, which is clipped to the top of the spindle onto a small platform that automatically rotates the hearing aid in a 360-degree circle and takes measurements at angles specified by the user. A special damping configuration is used within the sound chamber to minimize acoustic reflections and provide as much accuracy as possible within the small confines of the desktop chamber.

TECHNICAL TIP: QUICK CHECK OF PRODUCTS

All of these measures take time, of course, and we're happy to go along with faster applications if the final results are as good (or nearly as good). Some clinicians, when testing the directionality of different hearing aids, simply leave the cover of the box open, turn on the test signal, and then while holding the hearing aid in their hand (attached to the coupler, of course), they turn the hearing aid to different positions (front port facing versus rear port facing) and observe the output on the screen. Easy to do and quick, but does this work? Pam Burton, (2006) examined this question with a group of audiologists. Using three different pairs of hearing aids—ITE, ITC, and BTE—one of each pair was programmed to directional, the other to omnidirectional. All directional products previously had been tested to confirm good directionality. Twelve different audiologists conducted the testing and were blinded to the programming. Using the procedure described above, they were asked to rate each product as either directional or omnidirectional, and to state their level of confidence ("definitely" versus "probably"). An "unsure" rating also was an option. All six products were rated correctly by at least 11 of the 12 audiologists (both ITE models were 12/12 correct); the individual ratings that were not correct were "unsure," therefore no product was rated incorrectly using this procedure. Approximately 70% of the correct ratings were rated "definitely."

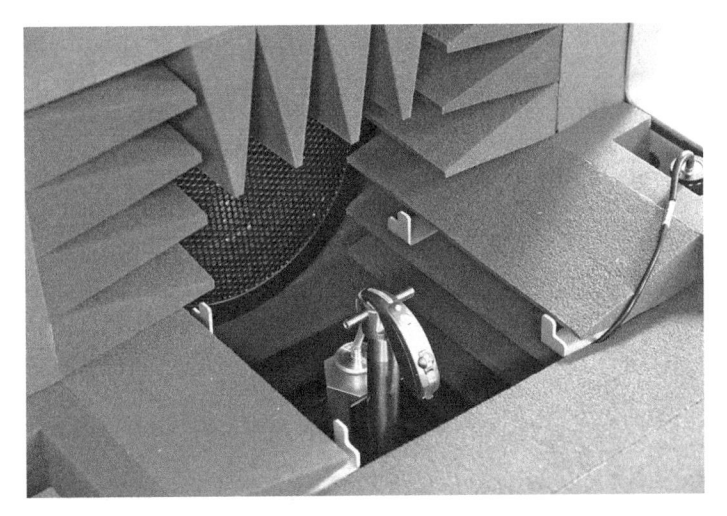

Figure 13–31. In this chamber, the hearing aid is placed onto a small rotating platform and the polar response pattern is derived.

Results are displayed in polar plot format on a screen as shown in Figure 13–32. Since these measures are collected one at a time, all test precautions that are applied for FBR testing—including using a fixed, nonadaptive directional mode, and disabling DNR—must be applied.

Quality Control Measures Assessing Digital Noise Reduction (DNR)

There is no standardized measurement protocol for assessing the function of noise reduction algorithms. Most manufacturers have several overlapping algorithms in their DNR scheme, and it often is not possible to test them separately. Any quality control measurement of that function is likely to evaluate more than one algorithm (e.g., slower modulation-based gain reduction, faster Wiener-like filtering, transient noise reduction, wind-noise reduction). Coupler measures, however, still can be used to assess such aspects as the onset time of the overall feature, as well as the impact of the resultant gain reduction across frequency for a variety of stimuli, although a random noise will typically produce the greatest effect. Although not exactly quality control, it is useful to know the behavior of the DNR clinically for counseling and fitting purposes.

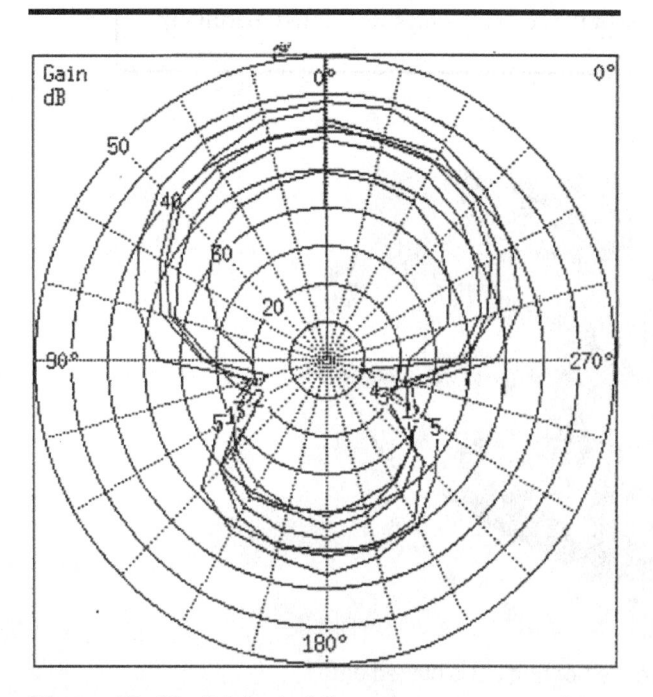

Figure 13–32. Printout of the polar response patterns at multiple frequencies.

Importantly, DNR typically functions the same regardless of gain settings (assuming there is substantial gain) and rarely stops functioning over time. It may be useful to evaluate all the DNR settings, however, to obtain a complete picture of the range of function and the operating characteristics. The magnitude of the DNR may also change as a function of the input intensity of the noise signal, so it may be useful to test at a couple different inputs (e.g., 60 and 80 dB SPL).

For these measures, the hearing aid is placed onto the appropriate coupler. The sound source must be a random noise of some sort (pink, white), or some noise of choice, to determine effectiveness. Manufacturers of hearing aid test box equipment have introduced into their software other environmental noises that can be used as the input for this testing as well. As soon as the noise source is turned on, the clinician can watch the screen to determine the time and effect of the algorithm. As shown in Figure 13–33, visual inspection indicates the overall output reduction provided by the DNR algorithm. In terms of capturing the time it takes for the hearing aid to react to or reduce the output (which can range from one to 30 seconds across products), the clinician can simply watch the screen.

Quality Control of Feedback Management Scheme

Audible feedback has been a significant problem for hearing aid users in the past. In fact, in a 2002 MarkeTrak survey, it was listed among the most prominent problems for hearing aid users and their families (Kochkin, 2002). In some instances the annoyance of the squeal negated the usefulness of the hearing aid, as well as the enjoyment of many communication partners. Many hearing aids employ a feedback management algorithm, although the effectiveness can vary considerably among manufacturers as we discuss in Chapter 12. Good practice protocol dictates that the clinician evaluate the quality of the feedback reduction algorithm for different products. The effectiveness does not vary significantly within different models of the same product but may be quite different for different models from the same manufacturer (e.g., entry level versus premier).

Assessment of the feedback management scheme employed by the hearing aid at hand can be done both crudely and with great sophistication. The sophisticated manner should probably come first in this quality check process. Figure 13–34 shows one example of assessment

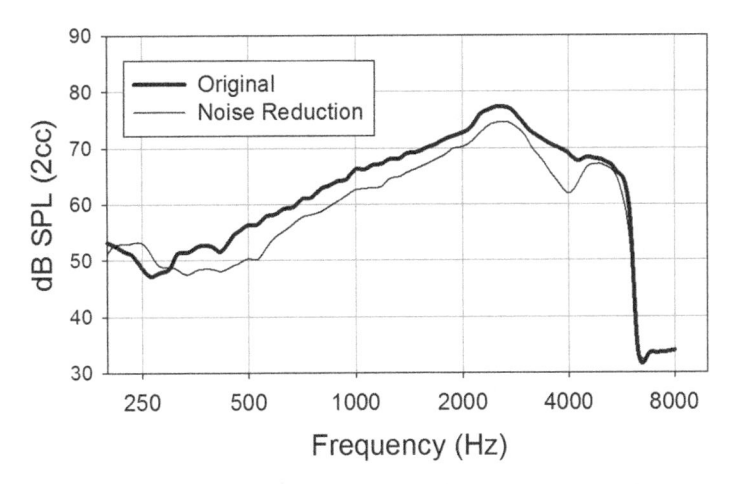

Figure 13–33. An example of the effect of DNR in a hearing aid. Using a steady-state noise, an output response is recorded (original) and compared to the output response with DNR engaged.

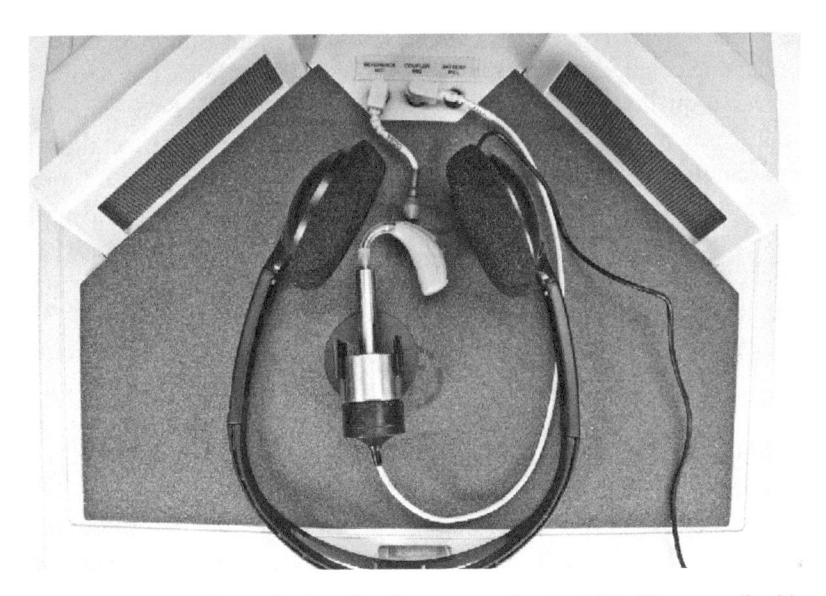

Figure 13–34. Setup for feedback suppression test (Verifit manual) with a BTE hearing aid. Directionality does not use headphones.

as recommended by the test box manufacturer. The setup requires the use of headphones that allow for generating a feedback signal. The result of the FBR algorithm turned *OFF* versus *ON* is shown in Figure 13–35, indicating that the feedback manager in this hearing aid reduced gain by over 25 dB in the high frequencies in order to eliminate feedback. This is not good. With these methods, however, is that DFS is greatly affected by the specific coupling used, and different hearing aid modes show dramatically different behaviors at the onset of feedback, ranging from gain reduction to strong cancellation. Therefore we recommend the probe microphone techniques discussed in Chapters 16 and 17 to obtain the best estimate of DFS behavior.

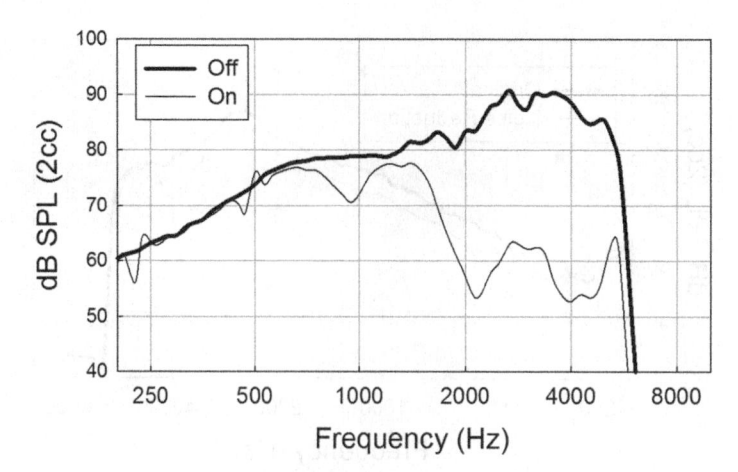

Figure 13–35. Feedback manager and result of the FBR algorithm being turned *OFF* versus *ON*.

What Can Go Wrong?

As we've described, conducting coupler measures is an important part of the overall quality control process. For the most part, the instrumentation is easy to use and provides the most accurate and reliable information. We hesitate to say this, but probably the weakest links are the technical skills or attention to detail of the audiologist conducting the measures. For that reason, we thought we'd include, in no particular order, the 10 most common errors in coupler measurement of hearing aid performance:

1. Failure to set the hearing aid to its "test mode." Since the primary purpose of most (if not all) coupler measures is to see that the hearing aid is working according to the manufacturer's intent, the hearing aid must be set to the same settings as applied prior to shipping.
2. Failure to calibrate. Although most commercially available test boxes provide for a calibration stage—either daily, weekly, or with each measurement—that calibration can only be effective if the test microphone and reference microphone are also shown to be accurate. Calibration of these microphones should be conducted on a monthly basis.
3. Incorrect HA-2 tubing used. This is a calibration issue as well, but often in the clinical setting the tubing hardens and requires replacement at inopportune times. Simply attaching another piece of the most convenient tubing will cause error in subsequent measurements.
4. Failure to latch the door tightly. Ambient noise, especially in a busy clinic with intermittent voices and activity, will affect the accuracy of the intended input to the hearing aid microphone. On a related note, some hearing aid test boxes simply do not attenuate ambient noise very well. When using these models a relatively quiet test room may also be necessary.
5. Not closing the vent for custom products or BTEs assessed with earmold on the HA-1. Failure to "putty" the vent can result in a Helmholtz resonator effect (increased gain in the 250 to 1000 Hz; see Figure 13–16).
6. Not orienting the custom product appropriately on the HA-1 coupler. Failure to do so can also result in the Helmholtz resonator effect.
7. Not placing the hearing aid microphone close enough to the reference microphone in the test box. Failure to do so can invalidate the calibration and will typically suggest less output than is realized.
8. Not orienting the hearing aid for maximum induction coil sensitivity. As discussed earlier in this chapter, this measurement is easily influenced by orientation of the induction coil.
9. Using too few input levels. Multiple input levels give much more information relative to high- and low-level speech.

10. Using the wrong standard. Most manufacturers of a hearing aid test box will provide the software for an updated test sequence as the ANSI S3.22 standard undergoes change. Because the purpose of the coupler measures is to compare to the manufacturer's measures, both entities must use the same protocol (inputs, couplers, etc.) to obtain those measures.

In Closing

The listing of each measurement, as well as the hearing aid setting and input requirements, may seem overwhelming to the new clinician. The whole "ANSI run," as it has been affectionately named, takes less than two minutes using currently marketed equipment, however. Best practice (AAA, 2006; ASHA, 1998) mandates electroacoustic measures upon arrival of the hearing aid to determine whether the hearing aid meets its design parameters. Indeed, recent research indicates that current, new hearing aids may exhibit unsystematic errors, indicating occasional quality control issues (Holder, Picou, Gruenwald, & Ricketts, 2016). Many clinicians are concerned about the value of testing the hearing aid while all the bells and whistles are going on/off. As hearing aids today have maximum flexibility in terms of their gain/output, in addition to all of the possible feature activation, most manufacturers provide what they refer to as a test mode. The specification sheet or "strip" provided by the manufacturer allows for a quick comparison to how the manufacturer expects the hearing aid to perform in that test mode.

There are several ways to accomplish this test run and any one of them is acceptable—if you understand the purpose:

- Run the hearing aid as it arrives into the clinic and compare these findings to the printout that accompanied it from the manufacturer.
- Set the hearing aid to its broadest/maximum response and compare to the manufacturer's specifications or spec sheet.
- Run the hearing aid as it arrives *back* in the clinic with the patient on post-fitting visits, and compare these findings to the results from the day of the fitting.

Any of these uses can improve clinical outcomes. If the clinician knows—even before the patient is scheduled to return for the fitting—that the hearing aid is not functioning as intended, then steps can be taken to get it replaced or repaired. In the end, this all will lead to more efficient fittings and more satisfied patients.

14
Prescriptive Formulas and Programming

As recently as 30 years ago we were often faced with fitting a patient with an analog hearing aid that had, at best, one screwdriver potentiometer that allowed us to vary gain in the 500 Hz region by 5 to 10 dB. There was only one channel, no input or output compression, and very little control of the frequency response. Much has changed. It is clear that, with today's highly adjustable digital products with multiple channels of gain and compression, and more flexible venting options in part due to effective digital feedback suppression, we have the capability to select almost any frequency response and output characteristics desired for a given patient. And, as we discuss in earlier chapters, through careful pretesting and patient needs assessments we are also equipped to include patient-specific factors in our decision process. Now that we have the capability to craft almost any frequency response and input/output function characteristics that we desire, how do we know what is best?

Most would agree that a *good* hearing aid fitting must be a combination of optimizing audibility and speech recognition, matching preferred loudness levels for different input levels, avoiding loudness discomfort, and providing good sound quality. For a reluctant new hearing aid user, we might also want to consider using an algorithm that would be rated *highly acceptable* during initial use, something we would typically assume to be true if all of our other goals are met. These goals have led to the development of several prescriptive gain/output methods over the years including the original methods that were developed more than 80 years ago, and the resurgence of newer prescriptive methods aimed at fitting amplitude compression that have been proposed in the past 25 years or so.

Let's consider your Monday morning patient. She has a relatively flat bilateral 60 dB HL sensorineural hearing loss. Not surprisingly, she is having significant problems understanding speech, even in quiet, and is anxious to purchase hearing aids from you. You are ready to program channel-specific gain for her for average-level speech inputs. How much gain is enough? How much is too much? Your knowledge of average-level speech—the LTASSs you read about in this book and others—tells you that 10 dB of gain isn't enough and 50 dB of gain certainly seems like too much, but you still have a 40 dB range to choose from. We need to narrow the range and try to define an optimal starting point given the specific hearing loss, and that is exactly the purpose of prescriptive fitting approaches.

In general, prescriptive methods are based on the assumption that using the patient's pure-tone thresholds, and perhaps some supra-threshold measures, hearing aid gain and/or output can be *prescribed* that will result in the best fitting for the average patient for the desired attributes (e.g., intelligibility, sound quality, listening comfort). With modern hearing aids the intent is also to accomplish these goals for a wide range of sound input levels and listening environments. There are a number of variables to consider, and no single procedure is going to get it perfect for all patients all the time. But we need a starting point, and research studies have shown that the chances for success will be maximized when we use validated procedures.

The moment that one attempts something as simple as selecting the maximum gain or what instrument to fit to a given patient, at least some rudimentary form of a prescriptive method is being used. This is true even if the fitter doesn't actually know it. Denis Byrne (1982, p. 176) said it best: "The only choices are whether we admit to using a theoretical procedure, or even realize that we are doing so, and whether we are prepared to say what procedure we are using . . . The only problem with confessing to using a theoretical procedure is that it inevitably exposes our inadequacies."

If you are new to fitting hearing aids, Byrne's statement might not make much sense. Consider that if you didn't know that the aided output at 4000 Hz should be 90 dB SPL (ear canal sound pressure level) for a 55 dB speech signal input; it probably wouldn't bother you at all when the ear canal output for this signal was only 80 dB. Or maybe you wouldn't even measure it.

Overview of Fitting Eras

Today, most audiologists take it for granted that, when they are fitting hearing aids, a computerized algorithm will do some number crunching and desired gain and output values will appear; then in most cases with a single mouse click, the hearing aid will be programmed automatically to these desired values. But it wasn't always like this, and we're not just referring to the automation aspect. The underlying philosophical issues regarding how hearing aids should be fitted have also evolved over the years.

The Very Early Years

In the 1930s and 1940s, the term *selective amplification* was often used, which meant that the frequency response of the hearing aid would be tailored from the audiogram, similar to what we now call *prescriptive fitting*. As today, approaches varied then, although often the general notion was to restore normal hearing; in fact, one method suggested was to mirror the audiogram (gain = amount of hearing loss). Several early pioneers of this time, however, did point out the importance of considering the range of comfort, equal loudness curves, and uncomfortable loudness level (Watson & Tolan, 1949). The Harvard Report (Davis et al., 1946), however, concluded that patient-specific information might not be that critical, as they concluded that even for people with different audiometric configurations, the best performance was with a frequency response that was relatively flat or gradually upward sloping (+6 dB/octave). In general, during this period, audiometric data were used for hearing aid selection, although no specific prescriptive method emerged other than the general recommendations of the Harvard Report.

One method of setting the gain/frequency from this period is what has now become known as the "Lybarger half-gain rule." The method which was proposed by Samuel Lybarger, an engineer with Radioear (then a hearing aid manufacturer) as part of a 1944 patent application, was published in Radioear fitting manuals in the 1950s. Lybarger did present his procedure at the 1957 ASHA convention; however, there was little acceptance among the audiology community (see the following discussion on the popularity of speech testing). A revision of the procedure was published in 1963, but even then it was little known, as this also was an internal publication of the Radioear Company. It was not until later years, when other prescriptive procedures emerged using a similar 50% gain rule, that Lybarger's pioneering work was more widely acknowledged. In general, the goal of this half-gain rule and many rules to follow was to amplify average speech inputs so they were somewhat near the patient's most comfortable loudness (MCL) level.

The Speech Recognition Years

In the mid-1940s, Army Rehabilitation Centers were established to fit hearing aids and conduct aural rehabilitation for returning World War II veterans. One such center was at Deshon Army Hospital in Butler, Pennsylvania where the director of the Acoustics Section was Captain Raymond Carhart, now often referred to as "the father of audiology." During this time, Carhart

> **KEY CONCEPT: HAVE THINGS REALLY CHANGED THAT MUCH?**
>
> Watson and Tolan (1949) describe audiometric measures that would be helpful in the selection and fitting of hearing aids. Although the guidelines were written more than 65 years ago as assistance for fitting vacuum tube body-worn instruments, they serve as a reasonably good method of hearing aid selection today. Listed below is a paraphrasing of some of their suggestions:
>
> - Threshold determination, and in particular the relationship of the curve above and below the pivot frequency of 1000 Hz.
> - Determine range of comfortable loudness (RCL). They note that if this range is narrow this is an indication of "sharp" recruitment.
> - Determine equal loudness curve or curve of comfortable loudness.
> - Determine whether there is a low uncomfortable loudness level. If so, this is an indication of the need for "strong suppressive action" in the amplifier.
> - The authors also published one of the first formulas for the prescriptive fitting of a hearing aid: $Gf = HLf - (Drf - Df) + K$. Where Gf is the desired gain at a given frequency, HLf is the hearing level at the frequency, Drf is the difference between MCL and the HL at a reference frequency, Df is the difference between MCL and HL at the test frequency, and K is a constant.

developed an extensive 12-step test protocol for selecting appropriate amplification (Carhart, 1946a). In one respect, this procedure could be considered *prescriptive*, in that the selection process included an extensive preselection procedure, at which time the only included hearing aids were those subjectively rated as superior. The selection was narrowed down to three or four hearing aids, which were then comparatively tested using different speech tests over several weeks. Ultimately, the patient would receive the hearing aid that provided the best performance on aided speech recognition tests. We say hearing *aid* in the singular, as at that time everyone was fitted monaurally.

In the 1950s, 1960s, and through the mid-1970s, audiologists shortened the three- to four-week comparative procedure of Carhart to one or maybe two hours in university settings. In addition, rather than conduct a battery of speech tests, often, no more than a 25-word list of live-voice monosyllables in quiet was delivered. It was still common to test three different hearing aids, and the hearing aid that resulted in the best percentage correct score usually was recommended (even though it often was only 2 to 4% superior to another—so not actually statistically different at all). Audiologists using these procedures tended to report that they were using the Carhart fitting method. Surveys taken during this time indicated that this fitting approach was used by 80% to 85% of audiologists (Burney, 1972).

Indirectly, this fitting method (philosophy) discouraged the use of a prescriptive gain fitting, as the best hearing aid was determined by a percentage correct score and not any type of gain or output match based on the patient's hearing loss. This takes us back to the earlier quote from Byrne, however, in that the selection of the three hearing aids used for comparison was no doubt based on a reasonable hunch of what might work the best. That is, if the patient had a significant low-frequency loss, the only hearing aids used for comparison were those with low-frequency gain. Hence, the *comparative* approach was much more a *prescriptive gain* approach than audiologists realized.

The 1970s and Early 1980s

The move toward the current routine use of prescriptive fitting methods for hearing aid selection began in the mid- to late-1970s. There may be several converging reasons why audiologists began to abandon their repeated speech testing and began to measure aided gain in order to determine if it met some predetermined desired value. Factors that probably influenced this transformation included the following:

- Opinion leaders were presenting new data at national meetings that revealed the poor reliability and validity of using monosyllabic word lists to select the best hearing aid.
- Audiologists were going into private practice, and it was now ethical for them to sell hearing aids. This increased the interest level in finding an efficient and effective method to select the appropriate hearing aid. The traditional two-hour university fitting method did not lend itself to a busy private practice.
- Custom hearing aids were becoming popular. Unlike their behind-the-ear (BTE) counterparts, there was not a stock of hearing aids to use for comparative testing.
- New prescriptive methods were emerging and audiologists like Kenneth Berger were presenting workshops on prescriptive fittings and the use of functional gain testing for verification.

The Recent Past

Prescriptive formulas continued to proliferate after the 1980s. This was due, in part, to the emergence of the first multichannel programmable hearing aids in the late 1980s and the introduction of the first commercially viable digital hearing aids in the United States in the mid-1990s. Prior to this time only rough changes in hearing aid frequency response were possible via analog potentiometers (trim pots) or through the plumbing modifications we discussed in Chapter 9. In addition, there was a surge of software and tools to ensure the fittings were "accurate." For example, probe microphone systems (see Chapters 16 and 17) allowed for easier visualization of the hearing aid gain targets and the actual gain and output present in the patient's ears. More than any era before, using prescriptive hearing aid fittings methods was actually defensible because frequency-specific hearing aid gain and output could be precisely adjusted and verified.

We are not certain what the next "fitting era" will be or if there even will be one. It's now been more than 30 years since computerized prescriptive approaches and probe microphone verification have married up, and this general fitting philosophy continues to be well accepted with associated real-world supporting evidence. As technology becomes more complex, it is even more necessary to have an underlying, well-researched mathematical model to assist in controlling the myriad of different settings.

The focus of this chapter is the application of prescriptive fitting methods, but before we get to that point, we'd like to review various correction factors that are used with these methods and how these factors relate to hearing aid selection.

Correction Factors Associated With Prescriptive Methods

Later in this chapter, we discuss in some detail regarding the two prescriptive fitting procedures that are most commonly used today: the DSL v5.0 and the NAL-NL2. As we do so, you will notice that there are some transformations that occur, in which values that once were in HL are now in ear canal SPL, or values that once were in 2cc-coupler gain have been transformed to real-ear gain. This is not new; as you will also see, some examples of these conversions in formulas that we present are from prescriptive methods of 30 to 40 years ago that used similar corrections.

The fitting of hearing aids is dependent upon calculations which convert measures obtained in a 2cc coupler to gain in the real ear, or absolute ear canal SPL, or in other cases convert hearing thresholds in dB HL to 2cc coupler or ear canal SPL. This is true whether you use a validated prescriptive method (in which case the calculations are part of the method itself), a manufacturer's proprietary fitting algorithm (in which case the manufacturer has made these corrections), or if you simply view simulated gain on the fitting screen and "ballpark" a good fit (again, the manufacturer used correction factors to develop this display). These correction factors also are part of the verification procedures, as they are used by the manufacturers of probe microphone equipment to display thresholds, LDLs, and fitting targets.

We often use mathematical conversions in our daily lives, especially when we travel; for example, converting temperatures from Fahrenheit to Celsius or vice versa. Conveniently and appropriately, the same temperature conversion factors are used when the Sivantos Audiologische Technik people from Germany visit the SPAMfest in Minnesota, as when the Starkey Laboratories people of Minnesota take in the Oktoberfest in Munich. That is, 80°F is equal to 26.7°C regardless of where you live in the world. Unfortunately, this is not true for coupler-to-real-ear conversions. Different prescriptive methods use different correction factors, different hearing aid manufacturers use different correction factors, and different manufacturers of probe microphone equipment use even different correction factors! There is even some confusion as to whether some factors should be expressed with a "−" or a "+", which then determines if they should be added or subtracted (consider that adding "5 dB" versus subtracting "5 dB" results in a 10 dB mistake—a significant programming or display error). This lack of exactness is sometimes frustrating for audiologists when different data sets are compared during a hearing aid fitting (e.g., real-ear fitting targets on the probe microphone fitting screen versus the targets displayed in the manufacturer's fitting software). This also tends to be very frustrating to students who like preciseness and can't quite understand why someone hasn't figured out the correct numbers to use. Indeed, the two most popular prescriptive methods today, the DSL v5 and the NAL-NL2, use somewhat different correction factors.

In this section, we will briefly discuss four different correction factors that are used with prescriptive fitting approaches. We don't have the universally applicable answers either, but we will provide examples of how these methods are used. At the end of this book, we have included several tables and charts in Chapter 20 where you can view more precise data regarding these conversions.

In some cases as a clinician, you will be using these average values (and may not even know that you are), and the conversions will be seamless. In other cases, especially when fitting the pediatric patient, you will want to conduct some measurements to individualize the conversion process. Even when average values are used, however, it is still useful to understand how the values were derived, as this will help explain things when one set of numbers doesn't match another.

Reference Equivalent Threshold in SPL (RETSPL)

The RETSPL is the difference in dB between HL and the reference coupler used for calibrating the audiometer/earphones (usually a 2cc coupler, which is used for insert earphones). That is, if 70 dB HL at 2000 Hz equals 73 dB SPL in the 2cc coupler, the RETSPL for 2000 Hz would be 3 dB. Because audiometers are calibrated to ANSI standards, we would expect all to have the same RETSPLs for a given frequency and earphone style style—and they do. The RETSPL, therefore, is usually not equipment specific, but it is earphone specific. It is not patient specific because RETSPLs have nothing to do with actual patients. An example of RETSPLs for different earphones is shown in Chapter 20. When using prescriptive fitting methods, the RETSPL is commonly used under various conditions:

- For converting HL values to 2cc-coupler values (e.g., if a patient has an LDL of 105 dB at 2000 Hz, we could add the RETSPL for that frequency to approximate the 2000 Hz 2cc-coupler MPO).
- With the real-ear coupler difference (RECD), RETSPL is used to convert HL values to ear canal SPL values and convert fitting targets to ear canal SPL; a component of the real-ear dial difference (REDD).

Real-Ear Coupler Difference (RECD)

The RECD is the difference (in dB) between the outputs of the hearing aid measured in the 2cc coupler versus the real ear. The RECD is calculated by subtracting the coupler value from the real-ear value. Typically, the real-ear output is the largest, so usually the RECD is a positive number (particularly for the higher frequencies). The smaller the residual ear canal, the larger the real-ear output, and the larger the RECD. With prescriptive methods, applications of the RECD are as follows:

- It can be added to the 2cc-coupler values to obtain predicted ear canal output values. This is a common application when fitting hearing aids to young children and other difficult-to-fit patients using a procedure commonly referred to as "simulated REAR."

- It can be subtracted to obtain a desired 2cc-coupler output, if a desired real-ear output is known.
- It can be used with the RETSPL to convert HL values to ear canal SPL values, and convert fitting targets to ear canal SPL; it is a component of the real-ear dial difference (REDD).

Real-Ear Dial Difference (REDD)

The REDD is the difference between dB HL (e.g., the patient's hearing threshold measured with standard audiometric equipment) and the output in SPL in the ear canal. It can be measured directly using probe microphone equipment or calculated by adding the RECD (either measured or average values) and the RETSPL. The REDD is nearly always a positive number. With prescriptive methods it can be used as follows:

- Added to the dB HL audiogram and LDLs to obtain ear canal SPL values that are displayed on the fitting screen.
- Added to the prescriptive target values to obtain targets expressed in ear canal SPL.

Coupler Response for Flat Insertion Gain (CORFIG)

The CORFIG is the difference between *gain* in the 2cc coupler versus gain in the real ear (in contrast to the RECD, which relates to differences in *output*). It is derived by subtracting the sum of the microphone location effect (MLE) and the RECD from the REUG. In the lower frequencies, the CORFIG often is about 0 dB because there usually is not a large positive or negative value for the MLE, RECD, or the REUG in this frequency range. In the higher frequencies, the CORFIG is influenced significantly by the MLE: it will be positive when the MLE is small and negative when the MLE is large (e.g., a CIC fitting). The CORFIG can be manipulated in two distinctive ways:

- Subtracted from the 2cc-coupler gain to derive predicted REIG, which is often used in simulated REIG displays in the fitting software.
- Added to REIG prescriptive target values to obtain desired REIG re: 2cc coupler.

This has been a brief overview of the common correction factors used in conjunction with prescriptive fittings—see Chapter 20 for specific values. In Chapter 16, we go into more detail regarding how some of these corrections are derived and how they can be individualized. You will see, both directly and indirectly, examples of all of these factors as we go through the different fitting procedures and the programming of hearing aids.

History of Prescriptive Approaches

In the following, we briefly review the thinking, research, and ideas that have been advocated as the *best* way to prescribe hearing aid gain. Although most of these procedures are no longer used, we review them from the standpoint of evidence-based practice. Our modern fitting methods have built on this past work, continually trying to define the best starting point when providing optimal individualized gain prescription. In past years, when opinion-based practice was the norm, clinical practice was often based on ideas that seemed completely logical in theory, but for a number of reasons were not optimal in practice. We therefore believe (to paraphrase the Italian philosopher George Santayana): "It is highly important that we do not forget about the past and become doomed to repeat it." That is, even though researchers and clinicians are constantly working to improve hearing aid fittings, we do not want to retry old ideas that have already been proven not to work.

Watson and Knudsen (1940) Selective Amplification

The goal of this prescriptive formula was to provide an amplified signal that was both equally loud across frequency and consistent with the individual's *most comfortable equal loudness curve*. This would be accomplished by prescribing different amounts of gain for the different speech frequency bands based on the individual's most comfortable loudness (MCL) levels. The MCL was measured at one frequency (1000 Hz) and that measurement was then used to infer the level of gain needed at each additional frequency while maintaining equal loudness across the bands. Thus this method could be described as mirroring the MCL curve as opposed to the threshold curve.

To prescribe gain using this method, first air conduction thresholds were established, followed by MCL level measurement for 1000 Hz. Then monaural loudness balancing was conducted across frequency (referencing 1000 Hz).

Formula: $AF = (HL_F - (DRF - DF) + K)$

where, DRF = difference at 1000 Hz between air conduction threshold and MCL

D_F = difference at test frequency between air conduction and MCL

K = no clear definition

HL_F = hearing loss at that frequency

The authors concluded that their method of prescribing gain resulted in better speech discrimination scores than traditional "mirroring the audiogram" techniques (flat response). However, these differences in scores were later determined not to be statistically significant.

Lybarger Half-Gain Rule (1944, 1953, 1963)

Samuel Lybarger first proposed that gain should be "equal to one half of the hearing loss." This is now referred to as the half-gain rule, indicating that the gain at each frequency should be equal to one-half of the hearing threshold at that frequency. These values were defined as user gain, not full-on gain. To establish full-on gain, 10 to 15 dB of reserve needed to be added to each result from the formula. Additional gain was also to be added to compensate for conductive or mixed losses. It should be mentioned that this formula had no specific rationale or data examining its effectiveness. Because Lybarger worked for a major hearing aid company (RadioEar), however, one might assume that the formula was based on experience with patients and was consistent with placing average speech inputs near expected MCL.

Formula: Operating gain (dB) = AC Loss/2 + AC Loss – BC Loss/4 + 5

Where air-conduction (AC) loss and bone-conduction (BC) loss refer to the mean thresholds (of 500, 1000, and 2000 Hz). An additional formula emerged in later years to reflect the specific gain per frequency:

Gain = HL × .5 >1000 Hz; HL × .33 at 500 Hz

As you can see, this final version suggests a smaller percentage (less gain for the same hearing loss) for the low frequencies than the high frequencies. This philosophy is still applied in modern hearing aid prescriptive methods.

Pascoe (1975)

This method has its foundation in David Pascoe's dissertation at the Central Institute for the Deaf (CID). In that dissertation he studied eight subjects who had mild-to-moderate sloping sensorineural hearing losses. The subjects were evaluated using various frequency responses and it was determined that a flat response (called uniform hearing level) resulted in highest performance. This essentially meant that a flat *aided* audiogram would yield best scores. This method essentially re-establishes the normal audibility curve shape (not the thresholds) for hearing-impaired individuals. That is, while similar to other one-half gain type rules, Pascoe's method explicitly attempts to amplify average speech input levels to the same shape as the average MCL levels for a given amount of hearing loss. There is no discussion regarding the relative loudness of this frequency response. Figure 14–1 shows the resulting MCL and UCL values that were obtained in the data-collection phase of Pascoe's dissertation. These values have been used, albeit sometimes modified, for calculation of target gain and output by multiple commercially available programs, even in relatively recent years. Despite its widespread appeal

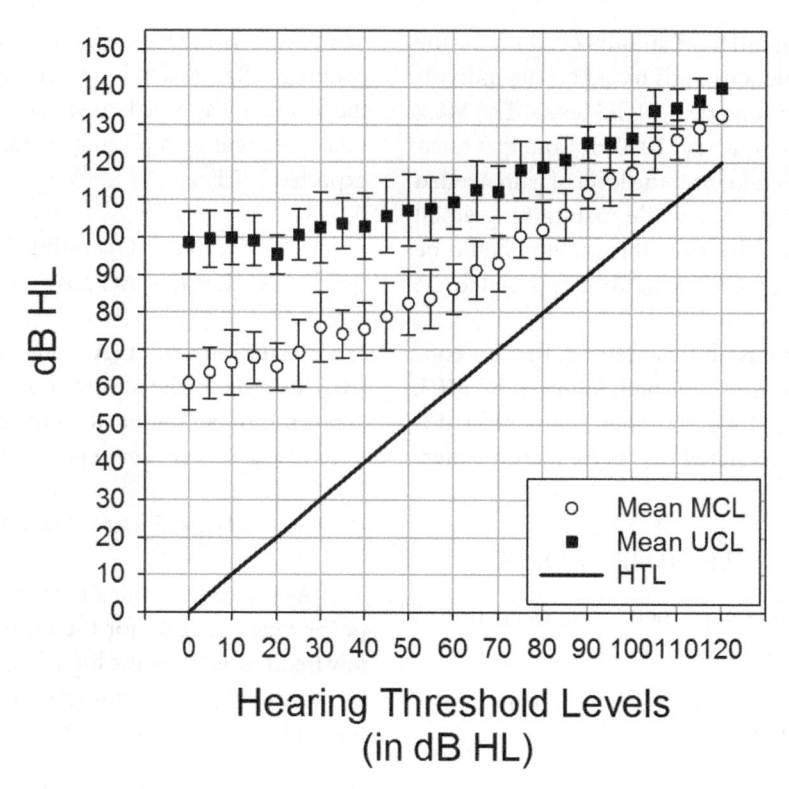

Figure 14–1. Average most comfortable loudness (MCL) and uncomfortable loudness (UCL) levels for various degrees of hearing loss. The values were the basis of the Pascoe prescription of hearing aid gain and output. (Adapted from Jensen, 1988.)

and focus on MCL, the development of this method and the use of these MCL data are limited because it was based on a study with a small number of subjects and therefore has questionable generalizability.

Berger (1976 and 1984)

This prescriptive method was the first to consider prescription of both frequency-specific gain and the hearing aid's maximum power output (MPO). Additionally, this prescription included gain modifications for monaural or binaural fittings, as well as for conductive hearing loss components. This method only required measurement of pure tone thresholds and all suprathreshold data were interpolated, as Berger believed that MCL measurements were too variable (and we agree on this point).

The Berger formulas were derived to produce full-on gain. In other words, use gain would be expected to be approximately 10 dB below the values that can be derived by the following formulas.

BTE Full-On 2cc Gain for Sensorineural Hearing Loss

*500 Hz = HL at 500/2 + 10   1000 Hz = HL at 1000/1.6 + 10

2000 Hz = HL at 2000/1.5 + 12

3000 Hz = HL at 3000/1.7 + 13

4000 Hz = HL at 4000/1.9 + 10

6000 Hz = HL at 6000/2 + 10

*When the hearing loss at 500 Hz is below 50 dB HL the gain at 500Hz should be reduced.

> **THINGS TO REMEMBER: SEVERAL PROBLEMS WITH THE BERGER METHOD**
>
> There were several assumptions under which the Berger prescription method was developed. We now know that some of these assumptions were at least partially in error. Here are three that fall into that category:
>
> - The intensity of average speech falls between 55 and 75 dB SPL. Problem: As we discuss throughout, the dynamic range of speech (across vocal efforts) is much wider than the 20 dB suggested by Berger.
> - The *desired* gain is set to a level just above one-half of the hearing loss. Problem: We know that this is considerably higher than preferred listening levels for most hearing losses and frequencies.
> - The ambient noise (low-frequency noise) should be avoided if possible by providing little or no amplification in the lowest frequencies. Problem: Unless the hearing loss is very mild in the low frequencies, listeners prefer to have some gain in the low-frequency region to maintain good sound quality.

ITE Full-On Gain for Sensorineural Hearing Loss

500 Hz = HL at 500/2 + 10

1000 Hz = HL at 1000/1.6 + 10

2000 Hz = HL at 2000/1.5 + 10

3000 Hz = HL at 3000/1.7 + 10

4000 Hz = HL at 4000/1.9 + 10

6000 Hz = HL at 6000/2 + 10

Body Aid Full-On Gain for Sensorineural Hearing Loss

500 Hz = HL at 500/2.2 + 10

1000 Hz = HL at 1000/1.6 + 10

2000 Hz = HL at 2000/1.4 + 12

3000 Hz = HL at 3000/1.7 + 13

4000 Hz = HL at 4000/1.9 + 10

6000 Hz = HL at 6000/2 + 10

As you can see, the 2cc-coupler formulas differed slightly as a function of hearing aid style to account for body baffle effects. In addition, the formulas were specific to unilateral fittings; however, a 3 dB bilateral correctional was subtracted from the gain at each specific frequency to account for binaural loudness summation. Also, if an individual had a mixed or conductive loss, additional gain was recommended using the equation AC-BC/5 at any frequency of air-bone gap, up to a maximum of 8 dB of additional gain. That is, if a person had a 20 dB air-bone gap, a 4 dB increase in gain would be applied—a very conservative approach for a conductive loss.

Note that the Berger procedure provides the most gain for 1500 and 2000 Hz—this is where the divisor is the smallest, and where recommended gain will be over 50% of the hearing loss. Consider that if someone had a 60 dB loss at 2000 Hz, the desired gain would be 40 dB, or 66% of the hearing loss (60 divided by 1.5). The basis for this was, in part, a function of the actual measurements of functional gain for satisfied BTE hearing aid users. We must point out, however, that at the time this research was conducted, it was very common that BTE hearing aids had peak gain around 1500 to 2000 Hz, partially because of the resonance of the tone hook. So, yes, this was the gain that people were using, but in many cases it was not necessarily because it had been determined to be the best for them. It was just a natural occurrence of fitting a BTE instrument of that time; there were no controls on the hearing aid that would allow an audiologist to alter gain in a frequency-specific manner.

Berger also provided a procedure to determine if the prescription had achieved the desired targets (i.e., determines if the hearing aid is truly reaching the gain values established using the formula, not if the hearing aid is successfully fit to the patient):

1. Subtract "operating gain" from the unaided thresholds to establish "predicted aided thresholds" based on the assumption that 2cc-coupler gain = functional gain. Clearly this is one problem with the development of this formula since this assumption is incorrect—see our earlier discussion of the CORFIG.
2. Measure aided soundfield thresholds.
3. The prescription is considered successful if the aided thresholds are within 9 dB at all frequencies (except 500 and 2000 Hz).
   a. At 500 Hz gain cannot be more than 5 dB better than the predicted gain.
   b. At 2000 Hz gain cannot be more than 5 dB worse than predicted.

"CID procedure" (1982)

Building on previous prescriptive methods, this procedure was developed by Skinner, Karstaedt, and Miller (1982) under the assumption that speech should be amplified over the range of 250 to 6000 Hz, and present at a level just below the patient's MCL while maintaining equal loudness across the frequency spectrum and without reaching loudness discomfort levels. "Just below MCL" was defined as MCL *minus* 3 dB.

The procedure was based on first establishing the individual's "auditory areas," which required measurement in octave bands from 250 to 6000 Hz, the individual's auditory thresholds, MCLs, and LDLs under headphones. To determine MCL and LDL at each frequency, a 10-point loudness scale was utilized (1 = no sound; 10 = too loud) with 4 to 6 indicating MCL range. Then the unaided thresholds were established in the soundfield. MCL and LDL were assumed to remain constant from headphones to soundfield measurements. The next portion of the procedure was based on determining "desired functional gain." The long-term speech spectrum in each frequency region was subtracted from the soundfield MCL, which yielded desired functional gain except at 250 Hz, where the authors indicated that the aided speech spectrum should fall half-way between threshold and MCL to avoid low-frequency spread of masking.

The next part of the procedure involved establishing the individual's "function gain—2cc-coupler gain difference values." That is, a hearing aid was selected that had approximate gain so that aided speech spectrum = MCL. The patient was asked to adjust the volume so that a 65 dB SPL speech signal was at a comfortable level. Soundfield thresholds were then determined using the hearing aid to calculate functional gain. The aids were then removed and measured in the test box. Finally, functional gain and 2cc-coupler gain were subtracted to determine the individual's functional gain-2cc-coupler gain difference.

The last portion of the procedure was to establish desired coupler gain, which involved adding the functional gain-2cc-coupler differences to the coupler gain. This yielded desired 2cc-coupler gain, which was expected to also provide the desired functional gain. A hearing aid was then selected based on its coupler gain and how close it was to "desired" coupler gain. One problem with this procedure was that it required MCL measurements, which as mentioned previously, can be difficult to establish reliably. Clinical adoption of this procedure was also a challenge because, at the time, most clinical audiologists did not have computers handy to assist with the many calculations.

Prescription of Gain and Output—POGO (1983)

This prescriptive approach for selection of gain and OSPL90 was developed by McCandless and Lyregaard (1983) and was based on two main objectives:

- The procedure should be simple, practical, and based on information known about previous hearing aid users and their overall preferences regarding gain.
- The method should be used for individuals with sensorineural hearing losses less than 80 dB HL.

POGO could generally be described as very similar to the Lybarger half-gain rule, except it also provided real-ear insertion gain (REIG) targets. Table 14–1 shows the formula for desired insertion gain.

Given that hearing aids of that time were often ordered based on desired 2cc-coupler gain (by reviewing gain curves in specification sheets) hearing aid style-specific formulas for these calculations also were needed (Table 14–2).

The formulas were designed to yield appropriate gain at the use VCW position, with 10 dB reserve gain added to obtain full-on gain values. According to the authors, OSPL was of even greater importance than the frequency response and should never exceed the UCL. UCL was measured in dB HL, averaged, and then converted to dB SPL by adding 3 dB to approximate the average three-frequency HL to SPL (re: 2cc coupler) conversion.

Table 14–1. Formula for Desired Insertion Gain for the POGO Formula

Frequency	Formulas (Insertion Gain)
250	½ HL − 10
500	½ HL − 5
1000	½ HL
2000	½ HL
3000	½ HL
4000	½ HL

$$OSPL90 = (UCL\,[500] + UCL\,[1000] + UCL\,[2000])/3 + 3$$

Consider that in the early 1980s, the MPO for most hearing aids was controlled by single-channel peak clipping, so a single MPO value was all that was needed, as frequency-specific control of maximum output was not possible. Unfortunately, for most products it was not possible to control the level of peak-clipping activation either, which placed an emphasis on ordering a hearing aid with an appropriate OSPL90 initially.

Audiologists were eager to adopt the POGO method as a fitting guide for prescriptive gain, as even the math-challenged were able to divide by 2 without the use of calculator (dividing by 1.6 for the Berger method presented some concern). Interestingly, the portion of the method used for calculating maximum output was largely ignored. For most, the prescription method actually was "POG," not "POGO."

The Birth of POGO II

In 1988, modifications were made to the original POGO formula to extend it to listeners with severe hearing loss (i.e., when hearing loss was greater than 65 dB HL). POGO II prescribed the same gain as POGO for losses equal to or less than 65 dB HL; however, for greater losses, gain was increased by 1 dB for every 2 dB increase in hearing loss (Table 14–3). This change was based on the finding that people with severe/profound losses are more comfortable listening to speech at an increased sensation level (Schwartz, Lyregaard, & Lundh, 1988).

Table 14–2. Full-on 2cc-Coupler Gain Formulas for the POGO Formula

		Hearing Aid Style		
Frequency	Formulas	ITE	BTE	Body
250	½ HL − 10 +	7	7	3
500	½ HL − 5 +	9	9	3
1000	½ HL +	8	10	0
2000	½ HL +	16	12	21
3000	½ HL +	16	21	23
4000	½ HL +	15	19	23

Table 14–3. POGO II Method for Selecting Real-Ear Gain (if hearing loss >65 dB)

Frequency	Formulas
250	½ HL + ½ (HL − 65) − 10
500	½ HL + ½ (HL − 65) − 5
1000	½ HL + ½ (HL − 65)
2000	½ HL + ½ (HL − 65)
3000	½ HL + ½ (HL − 65)
4000	½ HL + ½ (HL − 65)

MSU (Memphis State University) 1983, 1985

Robyn Cox developed the MSU procedure with inspiration from procedures developed by Watson and Knudsen (1940) as well as the Byrne and Tonisson (1976) NAL procedure to be discussed later. The main assumption for this fitting approach was that a hearing aid should be amplifying the long-term speech spectrum to a level which is equal to the halfway point between the individual's threshold and upper limit of comfortable loudness (ULCL). The ULCL was measured using narrow-band noise; and was established by having the individual determine the point at which the noise was loud but comfortable to listen to over a length of time using a "bracketing" method. In 1989, because of common confusion with the UCL, the ULCL term was replaced by highest comfortable loudness (HCL), and the difference between the individual's threshold and the HCL became known as the long-term listening range (which can be thought of as a residual dynamic range).

The original version of the MSU method required the measurement of both the individual's threshold and HCL; however, with version 3, HCL could be predicted based upon threshold measurements. Additionally, the original version required HCL and threshold measurements to be obtained using an insert receiver calibrated in a 2cc coupler; however, version 3 also allowed for standardized supra-aural earphones to be used instead (Cox, 1988).

Using the MSU procedure, gain was established by determining the halfway point between the bisected long-term listening range and the level of the long-term speech spectrum at each frequency. Threshold and HCL measurements could also be used to calculate gain for full-on 2cc-coupler gain by adding 10 dB of reserve gain. Additionally, if HCL measurements could not be obtained, it was recommended that the correction factors in Table 14–4 be used to establish predicted HCL levels.

Verification of the MSU method was REAR-based in that the hearing aid was adjusted until the root mean square (RMS) output spectrum in the ear canal for the presented speech-shaped test signal was closely matched to the targets at each frequency. OSPL90 targets were also accounted for in this prescriptive method and defined as ULCL +12 dB. If the patient could not complete loudness judgments, the authors recommended estimating OSPL90 as 100 + one-quarter the hearing threshold in HL at each frequency (Tables 14–5 and 14–6).

The MSU procedure was certainly one of the more clearly thought-out algorithms of the day. Unfor-

---

TECHNICAL TIP: UNCOMFORTABLE LOUDNESS—ALPHABET SOUP?

As you're reading about the MSU procedure, you see we mention the ULCL, which was later changed to the HCL. Earlier we talked about the UCL and the LDL. And of course, there is also the TD. Confusing? We discuss this in detail in Chapter 5, but here is a general way to categorize things. If we want to know the point that loud sounds are uncomfortable (which is what many prescriptive methods call for), we would be talking about the UCL, ULL, LDL or TD—Loudness anchor #7 on the Cox Contour Chart (see Chapter 5). One could argue, of course, that we would never want the output to be uncomfortable, and therefore, the value we should be calculating in our prescriptive methods is the ULC or HCL—Loudness anchor #6 on the Cox Contour Chart. For adults with hearing loss with a typical residual dynamic range, the difference between #6 and #7 is usually around 5 dB.

Table 14–4. Memphis State University Procedure for Full-On 2cc Gain Formulas for BTE Hearing Aid

Frequency	Formula 1*	Formula 2
250	½ HCL (dB SPL) + ½ HL (dB SPL) − 62	HCL (dB SPL) − 77
500	½ HCL (dB SPL) + ½ HL (dB SPL) − 55	HCL (dB SPL) − 70
800	½ HCL (dB SPL) + ½ HL (dB SPL) − 49	HCL (dB SPL) − 64
1000	½ HCL (dB SPL) + ½ HL (dB SPL) − 47	HCL (dB SPL) − 62
1600	½ HCL (dB SPL) + ½ HL (dB SPL) − 47	HCL (dB SPL) − 62
2500	½ HCL (dB SPL) + ½ HL (dB SPL) − 42	HCL (dB SPL) − 57
4000	½ HCL (dB SPL) + ½ HL (dB SPL) − 46	HCL (dB SPL) − 61
6300	½ HCL (dB SPL) + ½ HL (dB SPL) − 47	HCL (dB SPL) − 62

Note. *Choose the formula that yields the lowest gain value at each frequency. HCL = highest comfortable loudness.

Table 14–5. Corrections to Table 14–4 Values for Full-On 2cc Gain for ITE Hearing Aids

Frequency	Correction
250	−1.0
500	−1.0
800	−1.5
1000	−1.0
1600	−1.0
2500	−4.5
4000	−6.0
6300	−3.0

Table 14–6. Formulas to Predict Highest Comfortable Loudness (HCL) from Auditory Thresholds (MSU Procedure)

Frequency	Formula
250	.37 (HL in dB SPL) + 85
500	.25 (HL in dB SPL) + 83
800	.45 (HL in dB SPL) + 73
1000	.44 (HL in dB SPL) + 71
1600	.41 (HL in dB SPL) + 69
2500	.37 (HL in dB SPL) + 69
4000	.39 (HL in dB SPL) + 68
6300	.39 (HL in dB SPL) + 68

tunately, the real-world success of this prescription method was never really assessed, as it never gained any traction among clinical audiologists. There were several reasons for this, one being that it called for threshold measures using insert earphones. Although these were readily available in the mid 1980s, most audiologists were still using supra-aural earphones. Another factor was that the fitting targets were in SPL, and at that time audiologists liked to think in terms of gain. Verification required the use of REAR measures; again, audiologists were accustomed to functional gain, which then translated to insertion gain, not aided output, when probe microphone measures came along. The simple alternative to the MSU procedure at that time was POGO, which required nothing more than dividing by two and verifying in gain. Interestingly, the factors that prevented the MSU procedure from gaining clinical acceptance (insert earphones and verification via REAR) are commonplace today—it may have just been 30 years ahead of its time.

Libby (1986)

This prescription was very similar to the POGO procedure except, based on his own experiences using probe microphone measures fitting hearing aids, E. Robert "Cy" Libby concluded that people with mild or moderate hearing losses prefer gain which is equal to one-third (rather than one-half) of their hearing loss and there was less gain reduction in the low frequencies (250 and 500 Hz). Furthermore, he concluded that the proportion of hearing loss used for calculation of gain should increase with increasing degrees of hearing loss. Specifically, for moderate-to-severe hearing loss, one-half of the hearing loss was used to establish gain, whereas two-thirds of the hearing loss was used for severe hearing loss. Unfortunately, no clear values were suggested as to when to alter the formula from one-third to one-half to two-thirds except for "when the hearing loss changes categories."

The values calculated by this method were insertion gain values. In addition, gain was reduced by 3 dB when the fitting was bilateral; and gain, which was equal to one-fourth the air-bone difference (maximum 8 dB), was added for conductive components (Tables 14–7 and 14–8).

The Australian National Acoustic Laboratories Family of Prescriptive Methods

Over the years, the research from the Australian National Acoustic Laboratories (NAL) has significantly shaped the way we select and fit hearing aids. The early work in this area was led by audiologist Denis Byrne. Byrne's rational thinking in this area was summarized in an article by Harvey Dillon (2001), which he based on his Denis Byrne Memorial address:

> From time to time, Denis encountered critics of his work who claimed they selected and adjusted hearing aids using their considerable "clinical experience." Furthermore, they claimed, such methods were more effective than anything based on a formula could ever be, as they took many more aspects of the patient into account than did any prescriptive approach. While Denis readily agreed that there was more to a patient than an audiogram, he was scathing of "experience" as a scientific approach to audiology. His attitude can be summarized in the following

Table 14–7. Libby Procedure Real-Ear Insertion Gain Formulas for Use VCW Position (mild to moderate losses)

Frequency	Formulas
250	1/3 HL – 5
500	1/3 HL – 3
1000	1/3 HL
2000	1/3 HL
3000	1/3 HL
4000	1/3 HL
6000	1/3 HL – 5

Note. The multiplier is simply increased from 1/3 to 1/2 or 2/3 with increasing hearing loss.

Table 14–8. Libby Procedure on Full-On 2cc Gain Formulas (+15 dB of Reserve Gain)

		Hearing Aid Style		
Frequency	Formulas	ITE	BTE	Body
250	1/3 HL +	6	6	3
500	1/3 HL +	8	8	5
1000	1/3 HL +	11	12	5
2000	1/3 HL +	16	21	26
3000	1/3 HL +	18	25	28
4000	1/3 HL +	12	20	28
6000	1/3 HL +	2	13	10

paraphrases: (1) If you can't write down the rules you use, you probably don't understand what you do; (2) If it's not written down, no one else can do it, and no one can test whether it's better or worse than some alternative approach; (3) If you can't evaluate your procedure you can't improve it.

Regarding the final point Harvey makes, the NAL methods indeed have been evaluated many times by the NAL researchers, and, as a result, changes have been made over the years. We will briefly review some of the earlier milestones that have taken us to the first nonlinear version of the NAL, which we will discuss later.

Original National Acoustic Laboratories (NAL) Method

The first version of NAL was published by Byrne & Tonisson (1976). In the United States, the procedure was not commonly referred to as the *NAL procedure* but, rather, identified by the authors as the *Byrne and Tonisson method*. Because this prescriptive approach was competing with the much simpler methods developed in the United States (e.g., Berger, POGO, Libby) it received little attention.

The rationale, which guided the first NAL method and the decades-long development of this prescription, was that it is necessary to amplify the long-term spectrum of speech so that it is equally loud across all frequencies and remains at a comfortable listening level. To meet this goal, frequency-specific gain was provided so that each frequency band plays an equal part in contributing to the overall loudness. Instead of attempting to return loudness to "normal," the authors advocated equal loudness across frequency bands as a possible way to optimize speech intelligibility while keeping speech from becoming too loud. They rationalized equal loudness by noting that if one band was deemed "too loud," it may cause hearing aid users to turn down their overall gain, which may then make other bands too soft.

It is important to note that, because the LTASS does not have the same shape as an equal loudness contour, speech is *not* equally loud across all frequencies for listeners with normal hearing. Consequently, the philosophy of equal loudness will result in greater than normal relative loudness for higher frequency speech sounds compared to the lower frequencies than is present in normal-hearing listeners. The concepts of loudness normalization versus loudness equalization are discussed in a related Points to Ponder later in this chapter.

POINTS TO PONDER: DID THEY REALLY *PREFER* ONE-THIRD GAIN?

As we discuss, the "Libby one-third method" was based on observations made by Libby, an optometrist in Philadelphia who sold audiologic equipment and dispensed hearing aids. Libby was one of the first in the United States to distribute the Rastronics probe-microphone system (ca. 1984), and was an early adopter of routinely conducting probe-microphone measures when fitting hearing aids. He observed, upon testing hundreds of individuals, that even though he was attempting to fit his patients to the POGO prescription (~one-half gain), when they returned for follow-up, many patients tended to use and prefer something closer to one-third gain (based on their use-gain VC adjustments). Consider, however, that these were linear instruments, with relatively high OSPL90s (common at the time), and, in most cases, there was no maximum power output (MPO) control on the hearing aid. We suspect that for many of these individuals, one-half gain caused loud sounds to be too loud and/or distorted, and they turned down gain to closer to one-third of their hearing loss because that was what was required to keep loud sounds below their LDLs. Consider that a hearing loss of 50 dB HL would result in a POGO gain prescription of 25 dB, which might be just fine for average inputs but would most often be too much gain for inputs of 75 to 80 dB SPL, as these individuals typically have LDLs similar to people with normal hearing. Today, of course, we have adjustable WDRC and MPO, so that the patient's preferred listening level for one input level is not influenced by inputs of other intensity levels.

The original NAL method required clinicians to measure the MCL threshold, which was referred to at the time as the *preferred sensation level* (PSL). Early data revealed that for every 10 dB increase in hearing loss, the PSL decreased by 5.4 dB. Therefore, the authors concluded it was necessary to increase real-ear gain by 4.6 dB for each 10 dB of hearing loss. As you can see, this is fairly close to a traditional half-gain rule. From this start, Byrne and Tonisson (1976) report that three modifications were applied that altered the PSL values:

- First, it was necessary to compensate for the loudness differences across the frequency range to ensure that aided thresholds were equally loud across the spectrum (Table 14–9).
- Then the values were modified further to compensate for the shape of the assumed LTASS (Table 14–10).
- Finally, the 2cc coupler/functional gain differences were calculated and correction factors applied, and 15 dB of reserve gain was added to arrive at full-on 2cc-coupler target values.

Table 14–9. Original NAL Modification A: Equal Loudness Corrections Based on the 60-Phon Equal Loudness Contour Line

250 Hz	−2
500 Hz	−4
2000 Hz	−2
3000 Hz	−7
4000 Hz	−8

Table 14–10. Original NAL Modification B: LTASS Shape Adjustment Assuming No Change at 1000 Hz

250 Hz	−13
500 Hz	−9
2000 Hz	5
3000 Hz	5
4000 Hz	2

NAL-Revised (NAL-R)

Approximately 10 years after the introduction of the first NAL method, a revised prescription was published (NAL-R; Byrne and Dillon, 1986). The authors, consistent with the original NAL, continued to advocate for equal loudness across frequencies; however, they corrected the original formula after deciding their original method for arriving at equal loudness was incorrect, particularly for sloping hearing loss. The authors reported that the NAL-R prescribed frequency response was seldom inferior to, and usually better than, any of several variations having more or less low and/or high-frequency amplification, and on the average, use-gain was approximately equal to prescribed gain.

The basis of this revision was the findings from a study by Byrne and Murray (1986) that sought to determine the relationship between audiometric slope and required frequency response slope. Their research revealed that there was a good relationship between the slope of the patient's audiogram and the optimal frequency slope of the hearing aid's amplification characteristics, suggesting that the frequency response of a hearing aid could be fairly accurately predicted from the audiogram. The mean value of 0.31 was applied to all frequencies, based on the frequency response required for a 0 dB/octave slope audiogram.

To calculate desired real-ear gain using this formula, an X value is first calculated. This constant is the same for all frequencies and is determined by multiplying 0.05 by the sum of the hearing loss at 500, 1000, and 2000 Hz. This value is then added to the frequency response slope value (0.31 multiplied by the hearing loss at each frequency). Finally, a frequency-dependent constant is added to account for the variation in required slope across the frequency range (Tables 14–11 and 14–12). The NAL authors were quite optimistic regarding this new fitting method, as stated in the final line of their abstract (Byrne & Dillon, 1986): "It is concluded that the new formula should prescribe a near optimal frequency response with few exceptions."

As you can see in the formulas, the real-ear insertion gain calculation is the same regardless of hearing aid style; however, different coupler gain calculations are necessary for different styles to arrive at the same REIG due to differences in CORFIG (Byrne & Dillon, 1986). The final numbers added for the 2cc-coupler tar-

Table 14–11. NAL-R Calculation of Real-Ear Insertion Gain at User Volume

250 Hz	X + .31 HL$_{250}$ – 17
500 Hz	X + .31 HL$_{500}$ – 8
750 Hz	X + .31 HL$_{750}$ – 3
1000 Hz	X + .31 HL$_{1000}$ +1
1500 Hz	X + .31 HL$_{1500}$ + 1
2000 Hz	X + .31 HL$_{2000}$ – 1
3000 Hz	X + .31 HL$_{3000}$ – 2
4000 Hz	X + .31 HL$_{4000}$ – 2
6000 Hz	X + .31 HL$_{6000}$ – 2

Note. X = .05 (HL$_{500}$ + HL$_{1000}$ + HL$_{2000}$).

Table 14–12. NAL-R Calculation of Full-On 2cc Gain

		BTE	ITE
250 Hz	X + .31 HL$_{250}$	+1	–1
500 Hz	X + .31 HL$_{500}$	+9	+9
750 Hz	X + .31 HL$_{750}$	+12	+13
1000 Hz	X + .31 HL$_{1000}$	+16	+16
1500 Hz	X + .31 HL$_{1500}$	+13	+14
2000 Hz	X + .31 HL$_{2000}$	+15	+14
3000 Hz	X + .31 HL$_{3000}$	+22	+15
4000 Hz	X + .31 HL$_{4000}$	+18	+13
6000 Hz	X + .31 HL$_{6000}$	+12	+4

Note. X = .05 (HL$_{500}$ + HL$_{1000}$ + HL$_{2000}$).

gets for both the BTEs and ITEs are a combination of three corrections: the slope correction values shown on the desired REIG table, the CORFIG, and the reserve gain (15 dB for all frequencies).

Validation of the NAL-R. Following the introduction of the NAL-R, several research studies compared it to other prescriptive methods in one way or another (see Mueller, 2005, for evidenced-based review). The primary clinical trial, however, was conducted by Byrne and Cotton (1988). In this research the NAL-R prescribed frequency response was compared with four alternative responses with varying high and low-frequency slopes, using both new and experienced subjects. The subject's preferred use gain was assessed after hearing aid use and, in the laboratory, the subjects evaluated each hearing aid response by judging the intelligibility of speech in quiet and the pleasantness of speech in noise using a paired-comparison procedure. It was found that the subjects' use gain was very similar to that prescribed by the NAL-R, and, on average, the NAL-R formula prescribed the frequency response that was judged to be most pleasant and provided the best speech intelligibility.

NAL-Revised for Severe and Profound Losses (NAL-RP)

In 1990, Bryne, Parkinson, and Newall further revised the NAL-R procedure to address gain prescription for severe-to-profound hearing losses. Two modifications were proposed. Specifically, if the PTA was greater than 60 dB, this requires that the X factor be increased by the following amount:

$$.116 (X - 180)$$

Where X = sum of 500, 1000, and 2000 Hz

For hearing loss greater than 90 dB HL at 2000 Hz an additional correction, which the authors referred to as the Profound Correction (PC) factor, was added (Table 14–13). This formula for fitting severe-to-profound losses became known as NAL-RP.

Desired Sensation Level (DSL)

We mentioned earlier that the work from the NAL has helped guide us in the programming and fitting of hearing aids for decades. Much of the same can be said for the work from the University of Western Ontario. Richard Seewald and his colleagues published the original Desired Sensation Level (DSL) method in 1985 (Seewald, Ross, & Spiro, 1985), although the conceptual work on this fitting method actually started when Seewald began his studies with Mark Ross in 1976. The first algorithms were being studied around 1982. As stated by Seewald, Moodie, Scollie, and Bagatto (2005, p. 145):

Table 14–13. Correction Factors to Be Added for NAL-RP when Losses Exceeds 90 dB HL at Any Frequency

If HTL_{2000} = 95 dB, add the following:

HTL_{2000}	250	500	750	1000	1500	2000	3000	4000	6000
95	4	3	1	0	−1	−2	−2	−2	−2
100	6	4	2	0	−2	−3	−3	−3	−3
105	8	5	2	0	−3	−5	−5	−5	−5
110	11	7	3	0	−3	−6	−6	−6	−6
115	13	8	4	0	−4	−8	−8	−8	−8
120	15	9	4	0	−5	−9	−9	−9	−9

"The DSL method was originally developed to provide clinicians with a systematic, science-based approach to pediatric hearing instrument fitting that ensures audibility of amplified speech by accounting for factors that are uniquely associated with the provision of amplification to infants and young children who have hearing loss."

The basic philosophy driving the development of the algorithm focused on optimizing speech recognition for children with hearing loss, given acknowledgment that speech must be amplified to a certain sensation level (SL) to maximize intelligibility (Kamm, Dirks, & Mickey, 1977; Pascoe, 1978, 1988; Erber & Witt, 1977; Macrae, 1986). Furthermore, they argued that, based on the work of Erber and Witt, the SL for maximum speech intelligibility in children needed to be quite high. The findings from these studies were then used to define target SLs for amplified speech for children with hearing loss (Seewald, Ross, & Spiro, 1985) as a function of degree of hearing loss. According to the developers, a longstanding goal of this prescriptive method is to amplify speech to the DSLs across as broad a frequency range as possible to support auditory learning via audibility of speech cues. Another goal of the DSL method has been to provide targets that limit the maximum output while still providing appropriate headroom and comfort for loud sounds.

The original versions of this procedure required some time to calculate on paper and pencil worksheets. The DSL has been revised several times since those early days. As the authors have already applied what they have

KEY CONCEPT: THE NAL BECOMES KNOWN

We mentioned that the first NAL method was not commonly known in the United States. That changed with the NAL-R. Audiologists were now using probe-microphone systems for verification, which displayed insertion gain targets for a variety of methods, and one of them was the new NAL-R. As more publications about this fitting procedure emerged, it was clear that this method was more evidence-based than most of the other algorithms currently in use for fitting adults (the DSL was considered an algorithm for children at the time). The emergence of the NAL-R fitting method coincided with the increased popularity of custom instruments, which at the time were not programmable and were ordered by specifying desired 2cc coupler—or, the cavalier audiologist could just mail an audiogram to the manufacturer. The probe systems of the day did not calculate 2cc-coupler targets, and therefore, it was necessary to use a set of slide rules (one each for BTEs, ITEs, and body aids) that could be ordered from the NAL.

learned in subsequent versions, we will not detail the earliest versions here but instead spend more time on the later iterations.

Early Nonlinear Years (1990s)

In response to the advent of WDRC and the increased control over the compression parameters in the digitally programmable hearing aids of the 1990s, several additional fitting methods were developed that provided gain targets which varied as a function of input level. Most of these procedures were rooted in the philosophy of loudness normalization (Allen, Hall, & Jeng, 1990; Cornelisse, Seewald, & Jamieson, 1994; Cox, Taylor, Gray, & Brainerd, 1994; Valente & Van Vliet, 1997; Killion, 1994) or some combination of loudness normalization and loudness equalization (Ricketts, 1996). In fact, several of these procedures required quantification of individual listener's frequency-specific loudness growth patterns as a first step to assign prescriptive gain targets.

Loudness Growth in One-Half Octave Bands (LGOB)

One of the earliest loudness-growth quantification-based fitting procedures was the LGOB method, which was implemented in ReSound hearing aids beginning in the late 1980s. The ReSound product was one of the first to use multichannel AGCi with a low compression kneepoint, referred to as wide dynamic range compression (WDRC), and consequently, input-specific targets were needed. A device was provided for patients to record their frequency-specific loudness ratings, which were taken for seven loudness levels and then electronically transferred to the programmer to be used for programming the hearing aids.

Visual Input/Output Locater Algorithm (VIOLA)

In 1992, a group of 12 audiologists formed the Independent Hearing Aid Fitting Forum (IHAFF), with the primary goal of developing a prescriptive method for fitting the new nonlinear hearing aids that were being introduced. The method that evolved from this group, sometimes referred to as the IHAFF method, is the VIOLA. Robyn Cox, a member of the IHAFF, was largely responsible for developing this method.

The VIOLA strategy (Cox et al., 1994) attempted to restore "normal" loudness growth of speech by restoring the relationship between the loudness perception of soft, comfortable, and loud warble tone stimuli, and the corresponding levels of unfiltered, wide-band speech observed in normal-hearing listeners. Normal levels

---

KEY CONCEPT: THEY EVEN HAD THE AUDIOGRAM UPSIDE DOWN!

Consider that when the first DSL method was introduced, audiologists were living in a pretty simple gain-based world for fitting hearing aids. The patient has a 50 dB loss at 2000 Hz? Okay—he needs 25 dB of gain. Compared to this simplistic way of selecting amplification characteristics, the early calculation of the DSL targets by hand was a bit overwhelming for some. Worksheets, workbooks, and workshops were provided to facilitate the use of this method. Adding to the confusion was that the common audiogram was now upside down and called an SPL-O-Gram. This had been advocated by Norm Erber and others years earlier, but was still foreign to most. As time went on, however, dedicated pediatric audiologists realized that there was a payoff for the extra math as they began fitting their hearing aids differently. The computerized version, introduced a few years later, nevertheless, was still warmly welcomed. Today, of course, looking at a patient's audiogram and an average speech signal referenced to ear canal SPL, and then attempting to obtain appropriate audibility with amplification, is common place.

> **POINTS TO PONDER: LOUDNESS NORMALIZATION VERSUS LOUDNESS EQUALIZATION**
>
> A reasonable question when selecting a prescriptive fitting approach is whether your goal is to *normalize* or *equalize* loudness and yes, there is a difference—and different approaches will result in different gain prescriptions (most of the time).
>
> *Loudness normalization* intends to restore, usually for certain frequency bands, the loudness perception of the listener with hearing impairment to the same loudness perceived by a listener with normal hearing. Loudness normalization can also mean that soft, medium, and loud speech as heard by a normal hearer are appropriately amplified to the categorical rating descriptor of *soft, average*, and *loud* by an individual with hearing impairment. In other words, soft sounds are soft and loud sounds are loud. Because the specific loudness patterns differ in individuals with the same hearing loss, trying to normalize loudness precisely would require consideration of individual loudness growth patterns. Furthermore, in order to control the loudness of all segments of sound precisely, gain changes in hearing aids would need to be very rapid. Fortunately, evidence does not support the assumption that precise loudness normalization leads to better outcomes. More generally accurate, frequency-specific loudness normalization provides much more gain in the low frequencies and much higher compression ratios than provided by current, validated prescriptive methods such as DSL v5 and NAL-NL2. Consequently, whereas the general concept of loudness normalization makes intuitive sense, evidence suggests precise loudness normalization is probably not an appropriate hearing aid fitting goal. There also was a critical flaw inherent to strict loudness normalization procedures. They did not account for the fact that all speech frequencies are not equally important, and we have only have so much loudness to work with before patients find amplified sounds too loud. Wisely allocating loudness to optimize audibility for the most important frequency ranges of speech as an alternative to strict loudness normalization now seems somewhat intuitive. Consequently, it is not surprising that the majority of the loudness normalization fitting methods of the 1990s have since been abandoned.
>
> In contrast to loudness normalization, *loudness equalization* aims to equalize the perception of loudness over a range of frequencies instead of having lower frequencies dominate loudness, as is the case for listeners with normal hearing. For example, the frequency range of 500 to 4000 Hz can be amplified such that the loudness perception of 500 Hz and 4000 Hz, as well as the various narrow bands in between, are equivalent in the unit of sones. This process was explicit in the earlier years of linear NAL prescriptions and carries forward in the current iterations as well. The assumption made by the authors of the NAL procedure was that loudness equalization would better distribute loudness to the speech frequencies that were most important for speech understanding when compared to loudness normalization.

for soft, comfortable, and loud speech were assumed to reflect the corresponding levels of long-term average speech. The speech inputs assumed for the "preferred listening range" reflect these levels of vocal effort and correspond to a dynamic range of approximately 35 dB.

In the development of the VIOLA strategy, the categorical scaling of loudness of both warble tones and 5s samples of wide-band speech obtained from the Connected Speech Test (CST) were measured and compared across individuals with normal hearing. Results indicated that speech was rated as louder than warble tones when matched for intensity level. Additionally, the loudness of speech appeared to increase more quickly than the loudness of warble tones at low intensities

(Cox et al., 1994a). Based on the established relationship between the level of warble tones and corresponding long-term average speech spectrum (LTASS) levels, Cox et al. (1994) suggested that restoration of "normal" loudness growth for speech could be accomplished through measurement of individual loudness growth patterns for warble tones. Measurement of loudness was completed using the Contour Test, one of the only clinically based loudness procedures that is still in use by clinicians. The forms for the Contour Test are available the University of Memphis HARL website.

The VIOLA method provided 2cc targets, not REIG or REAR targets. This limited its use, as many audiologists were not prepared to run coupler measures just for this purpose. It was also discovered early on that most audiologists did not want to take the time to conduct the seven-point loudness contour. The software did provide the option, however, to simply enter the thresholds and the LDLs for each frequency, and the intermediate values would be predicted. Although the VIOLA was never widely accepted as a fitting method, the software provided by Cox and colleagues was extremely valuable in helping audiologists understand WDRC, as input/output functions could be observed by inserting a wide range of gain values, output levels, compression kneepoints, and ratios.

Ricketts and Bentler (RAB)

Two of the authors of this book (Ricketts and Bentler) also took a stab at developing an automated individualized loudness growth based fitting method (Ricketts, 1996). The main differences between this method and the VIOLA were the exact method for measuring loudness growth (a magnitude estimation procedure instead of the categorical scaling used in the VIOLA method) and the calculation of gain for average speech inputs, which was based on a loudness equalization procedure (the NAL-R). Therefore, the loudness growth data were used only to assign compression parameters and not for frequency shaping. Perhaps not surprisingly, given the similar philosophies present in their development, the gain and compression parameters assigned by the RAB method for an average patient were relatively similar to those prescribed by the NAL-NL procedure described later in this chapter.

FIG6

The most popular WDRC circuit of early 1990s was the K-Amp, developed by Mead Killion. Not surprisingly, therefore, Killion and his staff were interested in developing a fitting method that could be used with this compression strategy. As an alternative to methods that measured individual loudness growth, Killion (1994) proposed that normal loudness impressions for a *preferred dynamic range* could be restored based on average loudness growth data. The FIG6 strategy (Killion, 1994) utilized previously collected cross-modality loudness matching data categorized by average threshold (Hellman & Meiselman, 1990; 1993). Hearing aid gain was then calculated at octave frequencies based on differences between average normal and impaired loudness growth, given a particular hearing loss. This gain calculation was made at three different inputs that were assumed to reflect the preferred listening range of speech inputs (40, 65, 90 dB SPL). This is a wider range of speech inputs than is assumed by the VIOLA but identical to the range assumed by the RAB (40, 65, 90 dB SPL). The gain targets for the FIG6 were as follows:

1. For low-level sounds (40 dB input):

    0–20 dB HL loss   Gain = 0

    20–60 dB HL loss   Gain = HL – 0

    60 db HL loss   Gain = (HL – 20) – 0.5 (HL – 60)

2. For conversational level sounds (65 dB input):

    0–20 dB HL loss   Gain = 0

    20–60 dB HL loss   Gain = 0.6 (HL – 20)

    60 db HL loss   Gain = (0.8 * HL) – 23

3. For high level sounds (95 dB input):

    0–40 dB HL loss   Gain = 0

    40 HL loss   Gain = (0.1 * HL) – 40 ^ 1.4

It should be noted that the 40 dB SPL input gain calculation was based on audibility considerations rather than loudness. Specifically, Killion suggested that gain sufficient to bring aided soundfield thresholds to

20 dB hearing level was necessary in order to ensure the audibility of the lowest intensity elements of speech.

National Acoustic Laboratories-Nonlinear 1 (NAL-NL1)

You've already heard about the early work from the NAL, but as time went on these researchers also developed a fitting method for nonlinear hearing aids, the NAL-NL1, which became available for clinical use around 1998. As stated by Dillon (1999), the aim of the NAL-NL1 was to provide the gain-frequency response that maximizes speech intelligibility while keeping overall loudness at a level no greater than that perceived by a normal-hearing person listening to the same sound. This is then a nonlinear method, as the gain-frequency response that achieves this varies with input level. The principle of the NAL-NL1 includes the idea of normalizing loudness; however, this notion applies to the total or overall loudness, not the relative loudness at each frequency.

Dillon (1999, 2001) described the development of the NAL-NL1 which we summarize here:

- One theoretical model used was a modification of the speech intelligibility index (SII) method, with allowance for desensitization (see related Technical Tip) and for listening at high input levels.
- A second model was a method for calculating loudness, allowing for the effects of a sensorineural hearing loss.
- Using a high-speed computer, the loudness and intelligibility programs were linked using data that were generated using a method known as a "constrained numerical optimizer." That is, a best fit for the two models was determined for 50 to 90 dB SPL inputs (see related Things to Remember).
- So that the findings of this analysis could be easily used clinically for any audiogram and speech level in order to predict gain for all frequencies, a formula was constructed based on the following factors:
  - Hearing threshold at that frequency.
  - Three-frequency average hearing threshold (500 Hz, 1000 Hz, and 2000 Hz).
  - Slope of the audiogram from 500 to 2000 Hz.
  - Overall level of the speech input signal.
- Dillon adds that the gain at any frequency ended up depending on the hearing loss

---

TECHNICAL TIP: CONSIDERING *DESENSITIZATION* IN PRESCRIBING GAIN

It has been shown that as hearing thresholds increase above 60 dB, particularly in downward sloping hearing losses, the usefulness of high-frequency speech information is reduced significantly. That is, there is a range of effective audibility, and beyond that point, increased audibility does not provide the benefit that might be predicted. In some individuals, increased audibility may even cause a reduction in speech understanding. This has been referred to as hearing loss *desensitization* (see Pavlovic, Studebaker, & Sherbecoe, 1986; Ching, Dillon, & Byrne, 1998). Accordingly, methods such as the SII may overestimate intelligibility when the hearing loss is severe to profound. Some prescriptive methods, in particular those of the NAL, have taken desensitization into account when prescribing gain. As we discuss in Chapter 17, this factor often causes concern among audiologists when fitting a downward sloping hearing loss, as they see real-ear target NAL-NL2 values in the high frequencies that appear to provide insufficient audibility. The issue is that increasing audibility to where it will be of questionable use will increase overall loudness, which may prompt the patient to turn down gain, losing audibility for other frequencies where it is of much greater value.

> **THINGS TO REMEMBER:**
> **CONSTRAINED NUMERICAL OPTIMIZER?**
>
> When using prescriptive fitting methods, audiologists often ask, where did those target values come from? Ever since we stopped taking about using one-half the hearing loss to determine gain for an analog, single-channel linear hearing aid fitting, there has never been a short or simple answer. Note that, when describing the generation of the NAL-NL1 targets, we mentioned that the NAL-NL1 had used a constrained numerical optimizer. In his 1999 article, Dillon stated that the researchers obtained the fastest computer they could afford, and he then provided this explanation of their procedure:
>
> It works like this: We input the first audiogram, chose an overall speech level of 40 dB SPL, and let the computer loose. Essentially, it semirandomly altered the gain at each one-third-octave frequency and computed the total loudness and speech intelligibility index (SII) that resulted. Over the next hour or so, it kept altering the gain characteristic until it found the characteristic that maximized the calculated speech intelligibility without exceeding the normal loudness for 40 dB SPL speech. We then repeated this for five more speech levels from 50 to 90 dB SPL. Then we repeated all of this for the other 51 audiograms. The result of this long process was a set of 312 gain curves that we believed were appropriate for these audiograms and input levels.

at several frequencies rather than only the frequency in question, just as with its NAL-RP predecessor. For a speech input level of 65 to 70 dB SPL, the NAL-NL1 prescribes a gain-frequency response similar to that prescribed by NAL-RP.

The NAL-NL1 was available as stand-alone software with which clinicians could enter audiometric data and then view the gain and channel-specific compression parameters. This procedure also was quickly adapted by both hearing aid and probe microphone equipment manufacturers. Although the NAL-NL1 was somewhat of a latecomer to the nonlinear prescriptive party, it quickly became the method of choice for both clinicians and researchers. One factor that led to its popularity was that the software calculated targets in just about any form one might want. Gain could be expressed as REIG, REAG, 2cc-coupler gain, or ear-simulator gain, with test signals being pure tones or broadband speech-shaped noises (different targets for the different test signals). The availability of REAG targets encouraged verification using ear canal SPL values, rather than REIG, making the NAL verification process similar to what previously had been used only for the DSL.

Desired Sensation Level Input/Output (DSL [i/o])

An updated version of the DSL method was also developed to address the fitting of WDRC instruments. In 1995, Cornelisse and colleagues designed the *input/output formula* (DSL [i/o]) by using Steven's power law to map a wide range of input levels to target hearing aid output levels across various frequencies. The DSL [i/o] method version 4.1 prescribed targets for gain, output limiting, and compression ratios. The average speech SLs were approximately equivalent to those recommended by earlier versions of the DSL (Cornelisse, Seewald, & Jamieson, 1995); however, the listener's residual dynamic range (from frequency-specific threshold to predicted LDL) was used to assign compression parameters. This was labeled a *loudness normalization* procedure at the time, although restoration of the normal dynamic range may be a more accurate description of the goal of the calculations for compression parameters. The DSL [i/o] v4.1 prescription was calculated using the following set of formulas:

For the region of linear gain:

$$O = TH_{hi} - ([TH_n - SF_t] - I)$$

For the region of compression:

$$O = ([\{I + SF_t\} - TH_n]/[UL_{hi} - TH_n]) \times (UL_{hi} - TH_{hi}) + TH_{hi}$$

For output limiting:

$$O = UL_{hi}$$

Where O is output, TH_{hi} is the hearing-impaired threshold, TH_n is the normal threshold, UL_{hi} is the hearing-impaired threshold of discomfort, SF_t is the threshold in the soundfield, and I is the input. It is evident that the compression ratio was determined by simply dividing the dynamic range of the impaired ear by that obtained for a normal ear at that same frequency.

A key feature of the original DSL method was to display the characteristics of the hearing aid output together with the child's auditory characteristics in an SPL-O-Gram format. The SPL-O-Gram uses a real-ear SPL reference scale across frequencies to permit direct comparison of the output levels of the hearing aid for known input levels with the listener's thresholds and LDLs. Clearly this had considerable influence on hearing aid fitting, as this approach has been adopted, at least as an option, in nearly all current probe microphone equipment.

Several validation studies of the DSL [i/o] v4.1 algorithm were conducted in the late 1990s. The work showed that the preferred listening levels (PLLs) of children were 2 dB higher than the listening levels recommended by DSL, with about 70% of the PLLs falling within 5 dB of the DSL target (Scollie, Seewald, Moodie, & Dekok, 2000). In addition, WDRC hearing aids fitted to DSL [i/o] targets achieved comfort, intelligibility, and the perception of normal loudness of speech across a range of speech input levels (Jenstad, Pumford, Seewald, & Cornelisse., 2000; Lindley & Palmer, 1997).

Current Prescriptive Approaches

Our history lesson is over. We are now to the point of talking about the prescriptive methods that we currently use. The good news is that there are only two survivors! Both have been modified in the fairly recent past, are available from all or nearly all manufacturers, and have been incorporated into all probe microphone equipment. We are talking about the NAL-NL2 (a revision of the NAL-NL1) and the DSL v5.0 (a revision of the DSL 4.1 [i/o]). The DSL v5.0 has been out the longest, so we will talk about that first.

DSL v5.0

In 2005, the DSL Multistage Input/Output v5.0a—or simply the DSL v5.0—was first released. The authors reported that the fitting targets were now more flex-

---

TECHNICAL TIP: YOU HAVE TO START SOMEWHERE!

We often hear people question the value of prescriptive fitting methods, often suggesting that they have a better way to fit hearing aids. Maybe that's true, but as we've said a couple times in this chapter—you have to start some place. Earl Johnson made that point nicely in one of his articles (Johnson, 2012). His example was that of an experienced clinician, who was skillful enough to narrow down the possible choices to a 20 dB range/frequency for a given patient, simply based on the patient's audiogram. The clinician was fitting a 16-channel hearing aid. Johnson's calculations show that there still are 1,430 possible frequency responses to choose from (see the article for the formula he used). And that was just for one input level! So as we said, you have to start someplace, so why not use a validated fitting method?

ible than they had been in past versions. There was no longer a single DSL target but rather a family of targets that vary based on the type of fitting. Another obvious outcome of this change was the introduction of targets that differ as a function of age. These changes were based on data demonstrating clear differences in the preferred listening levels for adults and children (Figure 14–2). Although the habilitative audibility goals are the same as previous versions of the DSL Method, DSL v5.0a provides compatibility with frequency specific ABR threshold estimates (nHL), updated RECD normative data for infants and children, infant-friendly RECD measurement techniques, targets for quiet and noisy environments, adjustments for conductive losses and bilateral fittings, and accounts for multichannel compression characteristics of modern hearing aids. Detailed descriptions of these modifications and additions can be found in Scollie et al. (2005) and Bagatto et al. (2005). This version of DSL is widely implemented in hearing aid fitting and verification systems.

Scollie (2007) provides a comprehensive review of the different areas where DSL v5.0 varies from the previous DSL 4.1 [i/o], based on the Scollie et al. 2005 publication. A revision of DSL v5.0 (v5.0b) added conversions from nHL to eHL to further enhance implementation of ABR estimates of threshold, and also provided new corrections for mixed hearing loss and conductive components. A summary of Scollie (2007) is provided here and in Table 14–14:

- Age and Etiology. A fairly significant modification to DSL v4.1 is the change in fitting targets based on the patient's age and etiology of the hearing loss. DSL v5.0 was adjusted to recommend a higher listening level for pediatric patients (presumably with congenital hearing losses) than for adult patients (presumably with acquired hearing losses). Clinically, this is selected by the clinician rather than automatically based on birthdate, so that either target type can be chosen. For example, for adults who have congenital hearing losses or who prefer a setting that provides maximal audibility of speech, the higher listening levels would be chosen. As reviewed in Scollie et al. (2005), the size of this difference appears to be greater than 5 dB and likely less than 10 dB, where

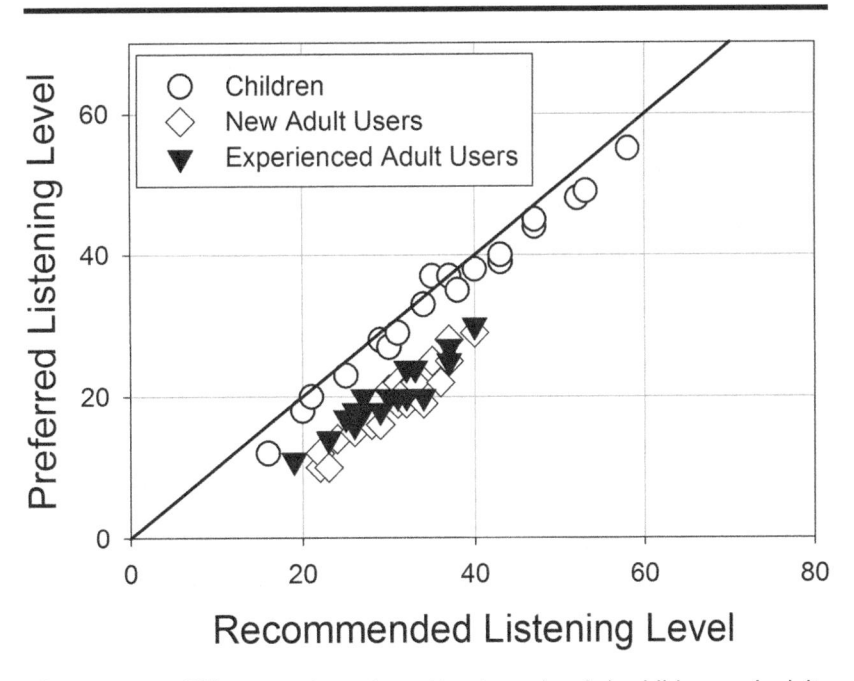

Figure 14–2. Differences in preferred loudness levels in children and adults with two levels of experience plotted against DSL v4.1 recommended listening levels. (Adapted from Scollie et al., 2005, with permission.)

Table 14–14. Summary of Changes in DSL v5.0

Change Description	Change Amount and Direction
Adult/acquired versus pediatric/congenital target	7 dB reduction for moderate losses, 3 dB for severe losses.
Interpolation	Greater number of target values across frequencies when working with partial audiograms.
Compression threshold	Less gain and output for low-level inputs due to prescribed compression threshold. Inputs of 70 dB and above are not affected.
Output limiting	Narrow-band output limiting targets largely unaffected. Output limiting for speech may cause target reductions of 5 to 10 dB if hearing loss is severe or test level is high.
Quiet versus noisy environment	Compression threshold raised by 10 dB and gain reduced at low-importance speech frequencies by about 5 dB.
Bilateral fittings	Optional. Will reduce targets for speech by 3 dB. Output limiting targets are not affected.
Conductive or mixed hearing loss	Increases gain by up to 9 dB for mild losses, 5 dB for severe losses, depending on magnitude of air-bone gap.

Source: From Scollie (2007).

children both require and prefer greater gain than do adults. DSL v5.0 accommodates this difference by reducing the gain recommended for adults by 7 dB for a 50 dB HL audiogram and a 60 dB SPL speech input. As hearing levels increase, the method uses a gradually decreasing adult-child difference in order to maintain audibility of the speech signal for both populations. For hearing losses greater than about 80 dB HL, the age-related difference in target is very small. A general guideline is that the DSL v5.0 targets are most similar to DSL v4.1 targets with the age variable set to "child" and with the bilateral correction disabled.

- Treatment of Missing Data. With pediatric fittings, it is common that thresholds are not available for all frequencies of interest. DSL v5.0 includes an interpolation routine to derive a full spectrum of targets for any audiogram from two or more thresholds. This interpolation may not be shown in the fitting screens of all systems but will be implemented whenever a manufacturer chooses to provide interpolation.

- Compression Characteristics. Version 5.0 of DSL uses a new input/output algorithm that is based on DSL v4.1. It was modified so that the target input/output functions can be clustered according to the channels of the hearing aid so that compression targets per channel are computed. It also allows for appropriate calculation for hearing aids with expansion. Scollie (2007) notes that the matching of channel structures between the prescription and the hearing aid will be done within hearing aid fitting software and is not something the audiologist must do. Also, probe microphone systems using speech as a test signal can derive DSL v5.0 targets without adjustments for channel structure because the effects of channel structure are minimized by testing with speech. Compression thresholds (CTs) are also revised in DSL v5.0; a channel-specific CT prescription recommends a low compression threshold for milder hearing

losses. The prescribed CT is about 50 dB SPL for moderate hearing losses, and is gradually raised as hearing loss increases, to about 70 dB SPL for severe to profound losses. The prescribed CT may be overridden by the clinician or by fitting software.
- Limits to High-Level Speech. Scollie et al. (2005) report that experimental evidence with today's hearing aids with multichannel processing show that high-level speech exhibits at least 9 dB of crest factor. That is, the speech peaks fall about 9 dB above the LTASS. In DSL v5.0, the targets for aided speech are limited so that speech peaks do not exceed the listener's upper limit of comfort (ULC—as a reminder, #6 on the Cox Contour Test). This can have the effect of limiting the LTASS target values through a target variable called the Broadband Output Limiting Thresholds, or BOLT. This makes targets appear somewhat lower than they were in DSL v4.1 for the same audiogram. BOLT-limited targets are most likely to occur for higher input levels and/or severe hearing losses, and can be identified by a target LTASS that parallels the ULC contour and is exactly 13 dB below the ULC.
- Listening Environments. DSL targets for speech are computed with the assumption that spoken communication is taking place in a quiet environment, and therefore aims to provide full, or nearly full, audibility of speech. Scollie (2007) notes that in noisy environments, this degree of audibility may decrease comfort without improving intelligibility. DSL v5.0 provides targets for a noise program that combine less gain at speech frequencies of lower importance with a raised CT.
- Bilateral Fittings. DSL v5.0 includes an optional bilateral correction that reduces speech targets by 3 dB. Sloping losses receive a small adjustment that provides more mid-frequency and less high-frequency gain.

There also are a few other features of the DSL fitting method, which we will discuss later when we compare this method to the NAL-NL2. As we mentioned, the DSL v5.0 software has been implemented by nearly all major manufacturers and is a verification option in most probe microphone equipment. There is not stand-alone software, however, to purchase for clinical use.

NAL-NL2

In 2011, the current version of the NAL prescriptive formula was released. It is referred to as the NAL-NL2. The rationale behind this newest version of NAL is consistent with previous versions focusing on optimizing speech intelligibility and loudness comfort. The aim is to maximize intelligibility by increased gain in the frequency response, while modifying the gain so that the loudness is not greater than that perceived by normal-hearing listeners. The newest NAL makes use of a neural network to calculate the gain based on the audiogram. The authors state that they now have available more extensive data on how much information people with hearing loss can extract from speech once it has been made audible, which has enabled the development of an improved method for predicting speech intelligibility.

Following the release of NAL-NL1, there was some concern, from both audiologists using the method and patients being fitting with hearing aids programmed to the method, that the NAL-NL1 called for a little too much gain. Specifically, Dillon reported the findings from several studies involving 187 adult hearing aid users who had their hearing aids fitted and fine-tuned to preferred gain. The findings revealed that the NAL-NL1 prescription was "just right," for 49%, "too soft" for only 5%, and for 46% of the sample, the NAL-NL1 gain was "too loud" (Dillon, 2007). Dispensers using the NAL-NL1 had similar opinions, especially when fitting new users. One change that was applied in the NAL-NL2, therefore, was gain changes that result in an overall reduction in loudness.

Figure 14–3 shows the average selected overall gain relative to that prescribed by NAL-NL1. The gain variations are shown separately for females and males, for both new hearing aid users and experienced hearing aid users with a mild, moderate, or severe hearing loss. Negative values indicate that the subjects preferred less gain than prescribed. Notice that, on average, these hearing aid users preferred about 3 dB less gain than that prescribed by the NAL-NL1.

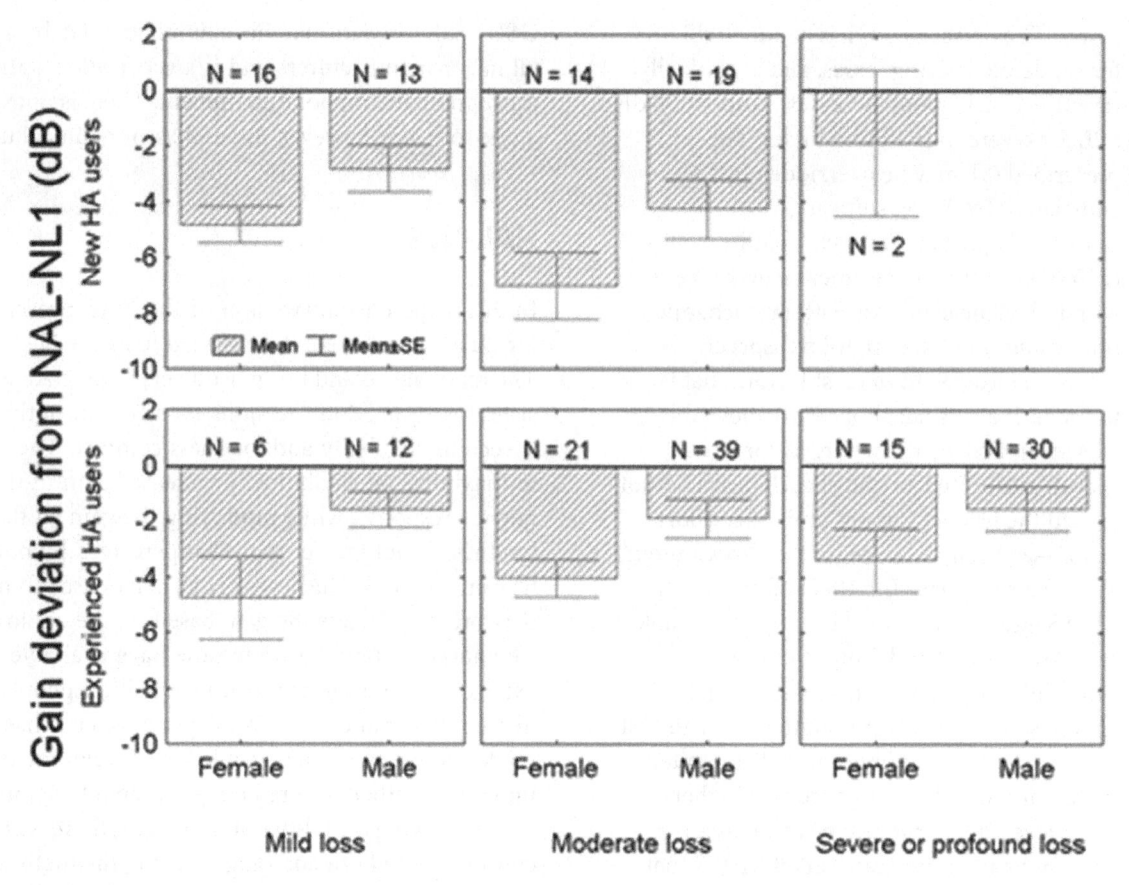

Figure 14–3. Average selected overall gain relative to that prescribed by NAL-NL1. The gain variations are shown separately for females and males, and for both new and experienced hearing aid users with a mild, moderate, or severe hearing loss. (Reprinted from Keidser and Dillon, 2012, with permission.)

There are specific modifications that have been made to the earlier formulas based on data gathered from previous NAL prescriptions users. Some general findings, based on research from the NAL laboratories and the experience gained from using NAL-NL1, and which resulted in prescriptive changes for NAL-NL2 include the following:

1. Males prefer slightly more gain than females.
2. Individuals who are experienced hearing aid users and have a moderate/severe loss prefer more gain than new users with a similar hearing loss (Figure 14–4).
3. Hearing aid users prefer slightly higher compression ratios than what was prescribed using NAL-NL1.
4. There should be less gain for bilateral fittings (especially at high input levels) than for unilateral fittings to account for loudness summation.
5. Children prefer more gain than adults, particularly at low input levels. Although the measured differences in preferred level were smaller than those reported by the DSL group, this finding led to different prescriptions for adults and children within NAL-NL2. Specifically, NAL-NL2 provides more gain for low inputs for children, but less gain at high input levels for adults than NAL-NL1. As a result, higher compression ratios are prescribed for children than adults.

There are also currently two versions of NAL-NL2 focused on tonal and non-tonal languages. This is necessary because low frequencies are more important in tonal languages; therefore, the version targeting tonal language is designed to give slightly more gain at low frequencies. The NAL-NL2 has been implemented by

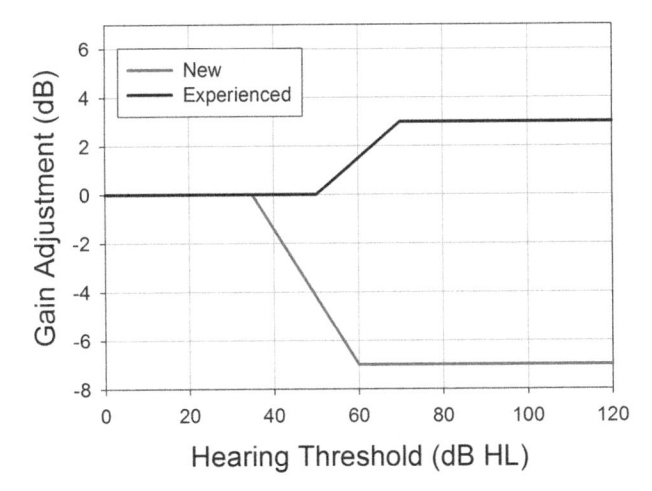

Figure 14–4. Adjustments to default NAL-NL2 prescribed gain derivations based on the hearing aid experience and pure-tone average hearing threshold level of the patient.

most manufactures of hearing aids and probe microphone equipment, and also is available as stand-alone software from the NAL Shop (http://www.nal.gov.au/online-shop.shtml)

Comparing the Current Approaches

As we've previously stated, it is considered best practice to start a hearing aid fitting with a validated prescriptive approach for estimating optimal gain and output. We believe that either of the current NAL or DSL prescriptions are good starting points, at least for our adult patients. If we consider adults only, just how different are the prescriptions from NAL-NL2 and DSL v.5.0? We compare them based on several different criteria:

Experience:

- DSL v5.0 does not incorporate a correction for gain based on new or experienced hearing aid user status (Scollie et al., 2005).
- NAL-NL2 incorporates adjustments that not only differ as a function of hearing loss but include an increase for experienced users and a decrease for new users (see Figure 14–4). It is important to note that in new users this correction could not be accounted for during the initial hearing aid fitting and verification; instead, it would need to be implemented over time by either the fitting clinician or automatically through the hearing aid. See Chapter 8 for a more detailed discussion of automatic gain increase (AGI) algorithms in hearing aids.

Gender:

- DSL v5.0 does not include an adjustment for gender, whereas NAL-NL2 includes a 1 dB increase in gain for male wearers and a 1 dB decrease in gain for female wearers.
- The NAL-NL2 adjustment was based on an analysis, irrespective of degree of hearing loss and experience with amplification, that females preferred 2 dB, on average, less gain than males (Keidser & Dillon, 2006; Keidser, Yeend, O'Brien, & Hartley, 2011).

Bilateral fittings:

- DSL v5.0 targets for speech are reduced by 3 dB across input levels for bilateral fittings re: unilateral fittings (Scollie et al., 2005).
- NAL-NL2 has a bilateral gain correction that increases with input level. The correction for binaural summation is 2 dB at low-input levels and up to 6 dB at high-input levels for symmetric losses, and less for asymmetric losses (Figure 14–5).

Listening in noise:

- DSL v5.0 targets for speech are reduced by 3 to 5 dB for low-importance frequencies for listening in noise. It is important to note that actually applying this difference would require the hearing aid to change gain depending on whether noise was present or not. For clinical fitting and verification, the probe microphone manufacturer must either allow the fitter to choose between these two prescriptions or default to a single choice (typically the listening in noise prescription).
- The NAL-NL2 does not have corrections for listening in noise.

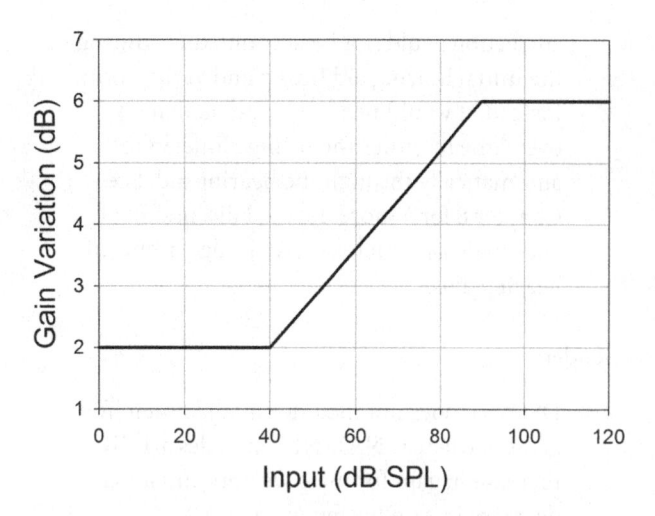

Figure 14–5. Adjustments to default NAL-NL 2 prescribed gain derivations based on the binaural fitting of hearing aids. The correction for binaural summation is 2 dB at low-input levels and up to 6 dB at high-input levels for symmetric losses (but less for asymmetric losses).

Correction for A/B gap:

- The NAL-NL2 first applies prescribed gain for the sensorineural component of the hearing loss, then adds 75% of the air-bone gap to this value.
- DSL v5.0 raises the predicted ULC by 25% of the average air-bone gap, which raises the upper limit of the target input/output curve, resulting in small corrections for gain for most audiograms. For a maximal air-bone gap, the correction adds 5 to 9 dB of gain and output to the aided speech targets, depending upon the hearing level.

Loudness discomfort measures:

- NAL-NL2 does not alter its prescription of gain and output at any input level based on LDLs or uncomfortable listening levels (ULLs). In fact, an entry for patient-specific loudness discomfort measures is not an option.
- DSL v5.0 will accept patient-specific loudness discomfort measures; subsequently, it will alter its prescription of gain and output for not only high-input levels that approximate the loudness discomfort measure but also the desired output for average and soft input levels as well.

One other difference is that NAL-NL2 includes a slight adjustment for less gain with an increasing number of channels (a channel summation effect). To illustrate how the differences we've discussed can impact

---

POINTS TO PONDER: SHOULD EXPERIENCED USERS BE PRESCRIBED MORE GAIN?

There is a general thought among clinicians that experienced users should be prescribed more gain than new users. This certainly makes sense, as one would think that there would be some sort of adaptation to gain over time. Shortly after programmable instruments were introduced, manufacturers entered a box in the software to indicate if the user was new or experienced, and increased gain (usually around 3 dB) was added for he experienced user. But is there research to support that this is true? The NAL group believes there is. Keidser, Dillon, & Convery (2008) reported on adaptation to hearing aid gain prescriptions based on the NAL-NL1 fitting algorithm. The researchers studied 50 new and 26 experienced hearing aid wearers. Gain preferences and comfortable loudness measures were obtained at one, four, and 13 months post-fitting for new wearers, and at one month post-fitting for experienced wearers. New wearers preferred progressively less gain (as hearing loss increased). The researchers concluded for new users with a 4FA HTL of 25 dB HL, gain reduction from NAL-NL1 was approximately −2 dB; whereas for those with a 4FA HTL of 55 dB HL, gain reduction preference was −9 dB. A literature review by Convery, Keidser, and Dillon (2005) found little evidence to support a gain adjustment for new users of hearing aids, at least no more than 2 dB, which was not deemed to be statistically significant. Until recently, prescriptive fitting methods did not even consider a correction for experience, and the DSL v5.0 still doesn't.

prescribed gain, we show examples of what a clinician can expect for the current prescriptions, NAL-NL2 and DSL v5.0 in Figures 14-6 and 14-7. The examples for three different input levels are for a gradual downward-sloping and a flat hearing loss, respectively. It is clear that the difference in prescribed output depends on input level, and as expected, differ for children and adults.

Comparison of Outcomes?

We are not aware of clinical studies in which a group of subjects have been fitted with both the DSL v5.0 and NAL-NL2 in some kind of real-world trial. There was a comprehensive comparison conducted by Johnson and Dillon (2011) that didn't involve real people but did involve a lot of math. They reported the differences observed in prescribed insertion gain for seven different audiometric types (five sensorineural), and conducted an analysis of predicted specific loudness, overall loudness, bandwidth of cochlear excitation, and effective audibility, as well as speech intelligibility using the international long-term average speech spectrum (ILT-ASS) at an average conversational input level. In general, they found that the NAL-NL2 and DSL v5.0 provided comparable overall loudness (~8 sones). The two prescriptive methods also provided comparable predicted speech intelligibility in quiet and in background noise.

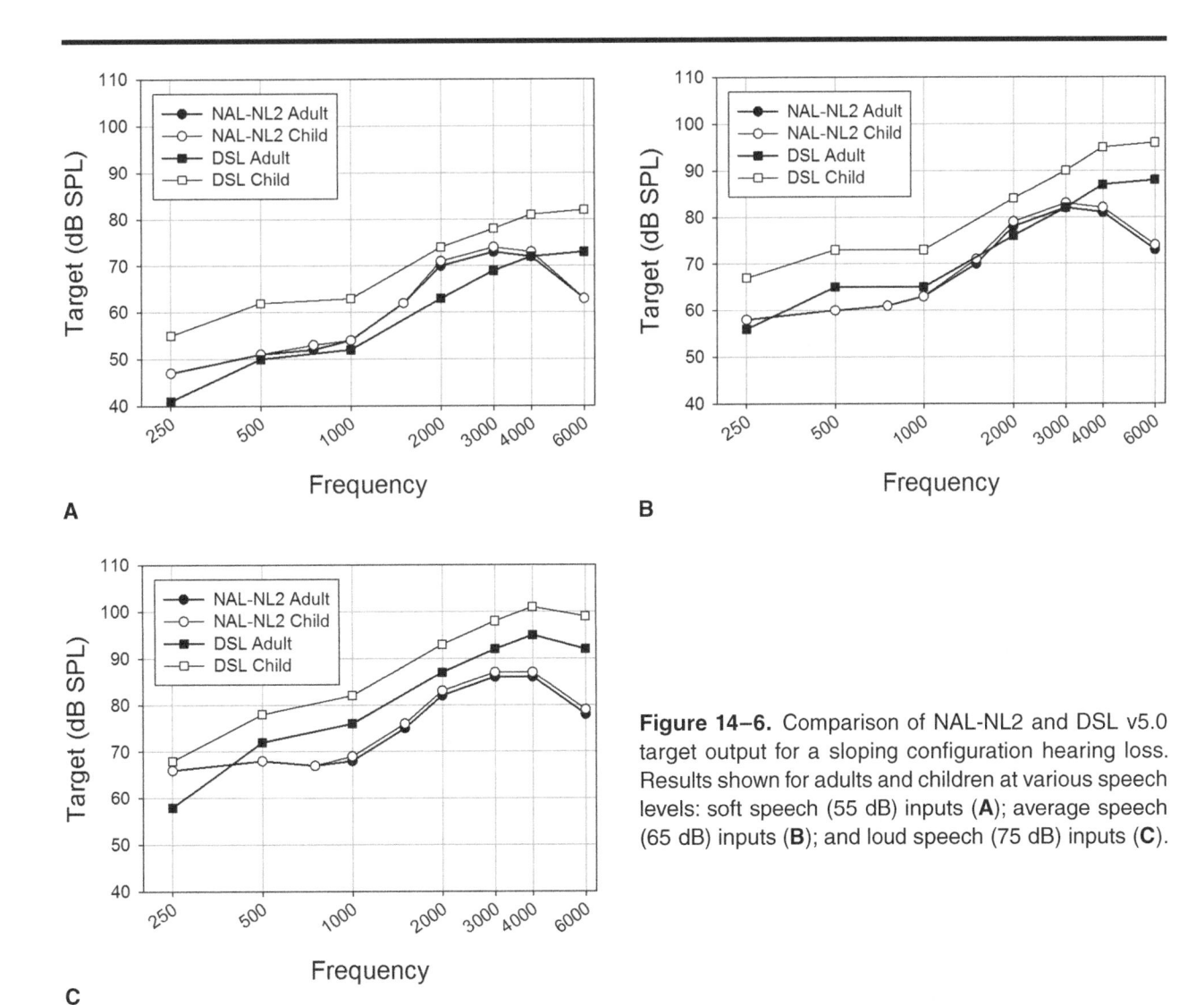

Figure 14–6. Comparison of NAL-NL2 and DSL v5.0 target output for a sloping configuration hearing loss. Results shown for adults and children at various speech levels: soft speech (55 dB) inputs (**A**); average speech (65 dB) inputs (**B**); and loud speech (75 dB) inputs (**C**).

Figure 14–7. Comparison of NAL-NL2 and DSL v5.0 target output for a flat configuration hearing loss. Results shown for adults and children at various speech levels: soft speech (55 dB) inputs (**A**); average speech (65 dB) inputs (**B**); and loud speech (75 dB) inputs (**C**).

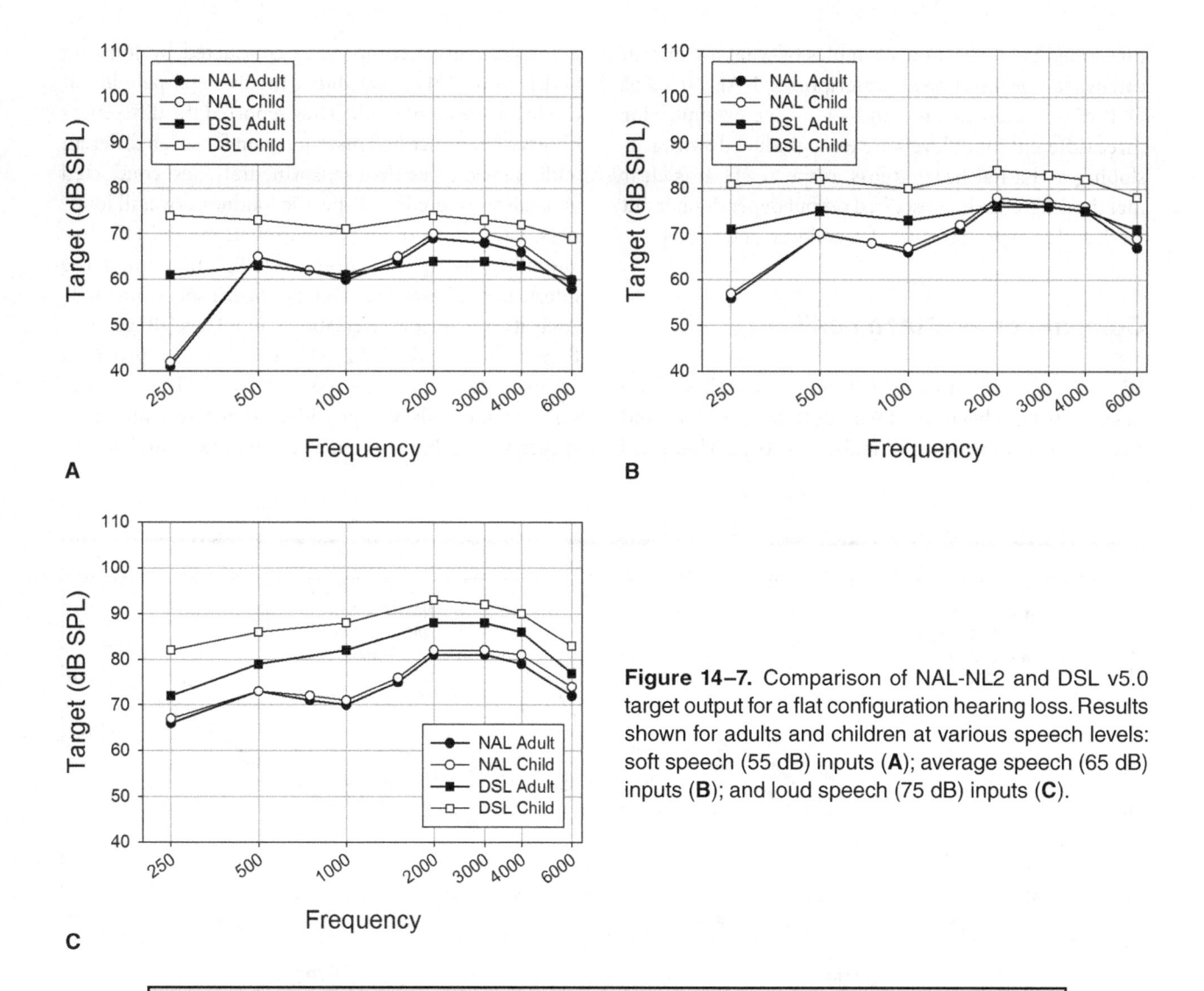

TECHNICAL TIP: DO NAL-NL2 CORRECTIONS FOR GENDER AND EXPERIENCE REALLY MATTER?

As we have mentioned, the NL2 added some corrections that hadn't been used in NL1. Two of these are for gender and experience. For the most part, the corrections are fairly small, and one might ask if they really matter. They do. Here is an example from Johnson (2012) to illustrate this point: We start with two different patients with the same hearing loss, 20–30 dB HL in the low frequencies sloping down to 70 dB HL at 2000 Hz and above. One is a woman obtaining her first set of hearing aids, and the other an experienced male user, obtaining a new set of hearing aids. Even though they have the same hearing loss, the prescribed insertion gain at 2000 Hz for the female for a 65 dB SPL speech input would be 16 dB, whereas for the male it would be 21 dB. At 4000 Hz, the respective insertion gains would be 23 and 29 dB. Would gain differences of 5 to 6 dB make a difference? Probably, when you consider we are typically balancing provision of as much audibility as possible while ensuring sounds are not too loud. This also points out why it is important to enter this information into the probe microphone equipment in order that appropriate fitting targets can be displayed.

There were some interesting differences, however, in the gain prescribed as a function of the audiometric configuration. Shown in Figure 14–8 are the five different sensorineural hearing losses used in the study, and Figure 14–9 shows the differences in the gain provided by the two methods. Values above the zero-line mean that more gain was prescribed by the DSL 5.0. Values below the zero-line mean that more gain was prescribed by the NAL-NL2.

At first glance at Figure 14–9, it appears that there are large differences between these two methods. Closer examination of the frequency scale, however, will reveal that the largest differences, at the low and high extremes, are at frequencies that we are not concerned with for the typical hearing aid fitting (or ranges where many hearing aids are unable to provide enough amplification to match targets). In fact, if we limit our observation to 500 to 4000 Hz and use a +/− 5 dB criterion, we see that the two methods are within these boundaries for nearly all frequencies for all audiogram types. For two of the audiograms (A-1 and A-3, which are flat and gently sloping) the two methods are essentially identical. Where they differ the most are for either rising configurations or very steeply sloping audiograms.

The bottom line is that we have two well-researched prescriptive methods to guide us in our hearing aid fittings. Their similarities seem to be greater than their differences. When differences do exist, the best method will probably depend on patient characteristics that would be difficult to predict prior to the fitting. We are quite certain, however, that using either of these methods places you far ahead of clinical experience or other approaches that have not been validated.

Modern Programming of Hearing Aids

We have reviewed the prescriptive fitting approaches that are available, so now it is time to program some hearing aids. A lot has changed relative to our fitting process since we had one or two potentiometers, and

---

THINGS TO REMEMBER: CAMFIT ALGORITHMS

Although the focus of this section is on the NAL-NL2 and the DSL v5.0, we do want to mention one other fitting algorithm that has been extensively developed and researched, as well as being revised in recent years. The method referred to as *Camfit* was developed at the University of Cambridge, England, by Brian Moore and his colleagues. Although it is seldom used by clinicians in the United States, there is considerable research supporting not only its development but also its clinical effectiveness. Similar to the other methods we're discussing, this algorithm determines gain and compression ratios that should be applied across frequency channels based on audiometric data.

In the software, one of two different theoretical rationales can be selected for programming a hearing aid using Camfit. As described by the authors, one is based on the idea of giving a flat, specific loudness pattern over the frequency range important for speech when the input is speech with a level of 65 or 85 dB SPL. The procedure also aims to give about the same overall loudness as normal for speech at 65 or 85 dB SPL. This procedure is called *Equalization* or *CamEQ* and is similar to the NAL-NL1, at least for average inputs. The second procedure determines the gains needed to give "normal" specific loudness patterns for speech-shaped noise at 65 and 85 dB SPL. This fitting rationale is called *Restoration* or *CamREST* (more similar to the DSL rationale). The most commonly used of the Camfit methods is the revised Cambridge method for loudness equalization 2-high-frequency (CAMEQ2-HF). This newest method was included in the Johnson and Dillon study mentioned earlier, where it was compared to the DSL v5.0 and the NAL-NL2.

This software is commercially available. For more information, including references of background theory and clinical verification, go to: http://hearing.psychol.cam.ac.uk/Demos/camfit.html

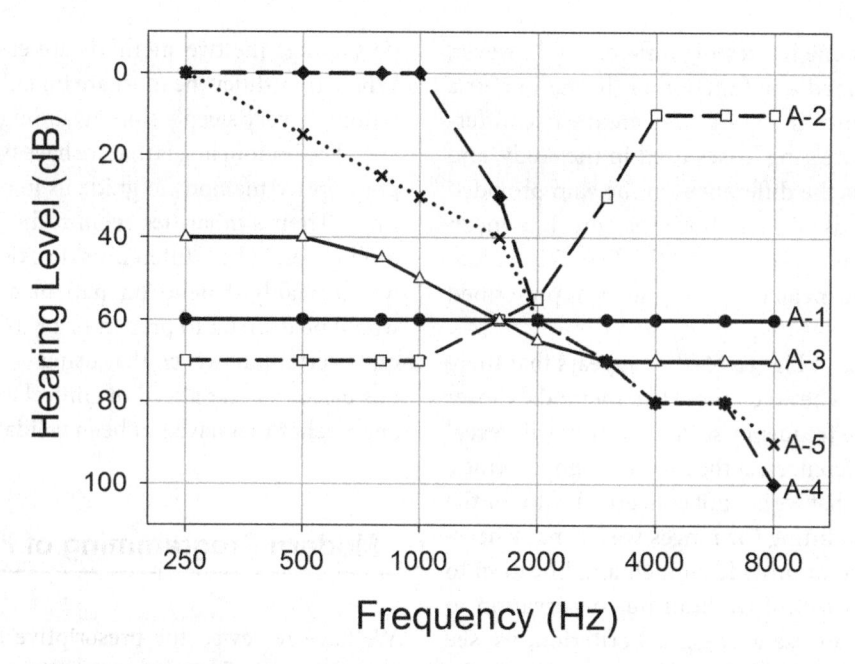

Figure 14–8. Five configurations of hearing loss used by Johnson and Dillon to determine differences in prescribed gain by NAL-NL2 and DSL v5.0 shown in Figure 14–9.

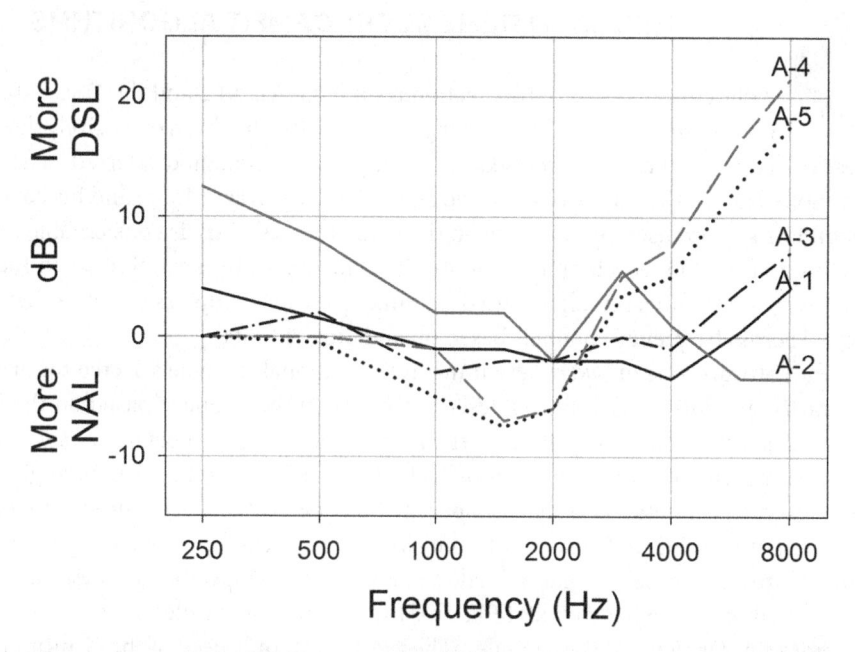

Figure 14–9. Differences in prescribed gain by NAL-NL2 and DSL v5.0 across the five configurations of hearing loss. Values above the zero-line mean that more gain was prescribed by the DSL 5.0. Values below the zero-line mean that more gain was prescribed by the NAL-NL2.

used a screwdriver to control gain and output. We are not talking about changes in signal processing; we cover those in detail in earlier chapters. Instead, we are referring to the actual process of adjusting how a hearing aid works in an attempt to optimally fit a patient.

A lot has changed even since computerized programming was introduced in the late 1980s. For a decade or so, hearing aid programming devolved into a bit of chaos with most manufacturers introducing proprietary programming systems. Fortunately, manufacturers realized they were all in the same boat, and for the good of all, a standard programming system would benefit the industry as a whole. This realization lead to the development of the Noah system described below. Let's start by reviewing some of the terms and equipment that play a part in the modern hearing aid fitting process.

What Is HIMSA

The Hearing Instrument Manufacturers' Software Association (HIMSA) was founded at the beginning of 1993 with the objective of developing, marketing, and supporting Noah, a single standard for integrated hearing care software. HIMSA is a privately owned company, but it operates much like a consortium—all suppliers within the hearing care industry who are HIMSA members have a significant say in the running of HIMSA and in how the standard evolves. Today, HIMSA is privately owned by six hearing instrument manufacturers: ReSound, Oticon, Sonova (Phonak), Sivantos (Signia), Starkey, and Widex. All suppliers who provide Noah-compatible products have a significant say in how the standard evolves. Today, over 130 companies support the Noah software standard. The largest portion of these companies are hearing instrument manufacturers, representing a market share of approximately 90 percent. HIMSA is based in Copenhagen, Denmark. HIMSA's single largest market is served by its U.S. subsidiary in Minneapolis, Minnesota.

Noah

The Noah software system is designed specifically for the hearing care industry, providing professionals with a single system for performing patient-related tasks. Noah is the "integration framework" that allows hearing instrument fitting, audiologic measurement, and office management systems to share a common database. Noah provides a de facto standard for controlling the exchange of data between these applications and systems. Noah has undergone a series up updates since its inception. Currently, we are at Noah System 4. Over 14,000 copies of Noah have been registered in the United States, with more than 35,000 units registered worldwide. In fact, nearly 70% of hearing health care professionals in the United States are Noah users.

Programming Hardware for Use With Noah

To use the software requires an interface to the hearing aid. In October 1993, the first HI-PRO interface box was introduced by Madsen (Figure 14–10). This box was first introduced with a serial (RS-232) interface, which it held onto for a very long time. HIMSA explained that, although this interface was limited by rather slow transfer speeds, it had the goal of working well with computer hardware that was up to five-years-old or more. The focus on being backward-compatible, combined with increasing amounts of data to be transferred, made programming rather slow on some devices, prompting a "back to the past" reaction from some manufacturers who again introduced proprietary, but higher speed, programmers. Eventually, the mini-HI-PRO (HI-PRO-2), which implemented a USB2.0 interface, was introduced and offered greatly improved data transfer speeds. Manufactured according to HIMSA's specifications, the Hi-PRO found its way into just about every hearing aid dispenser's shop or clinic in the world. Progress to higher speeds and wireless transfers continued with the NOAHlink.

NOAHlink and Noahlink™ Wireless

In 2002, HIMSA released NOAHlink, a hardware interface for programming hearing instruments, as shown in Figure 14–11. To date, over 65,000 NOAHlink units have been sold. Noahlink was designed to replace HI-PRO for programming advanced hearing instruments. It provides faster data communication and greater throughput between Noah and the hearing instrument. The NOAHlink receiver is designed for the patient to wear around the neck with a wired connection to the hearing

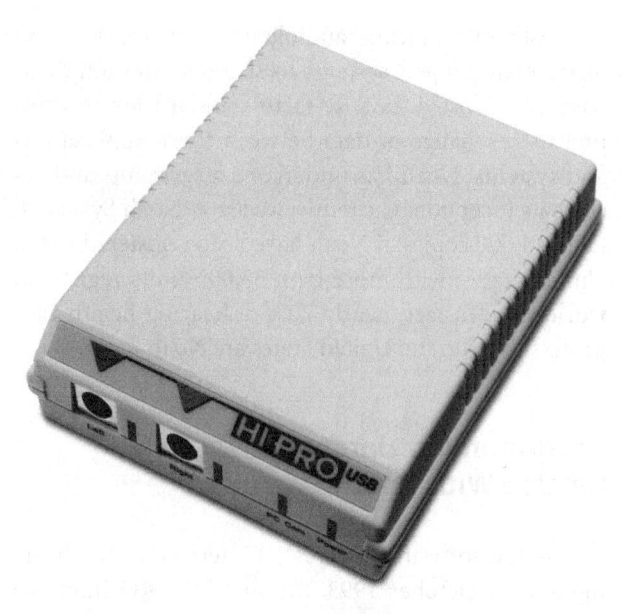

Figure 14–10. HI-PRO USB interface box.

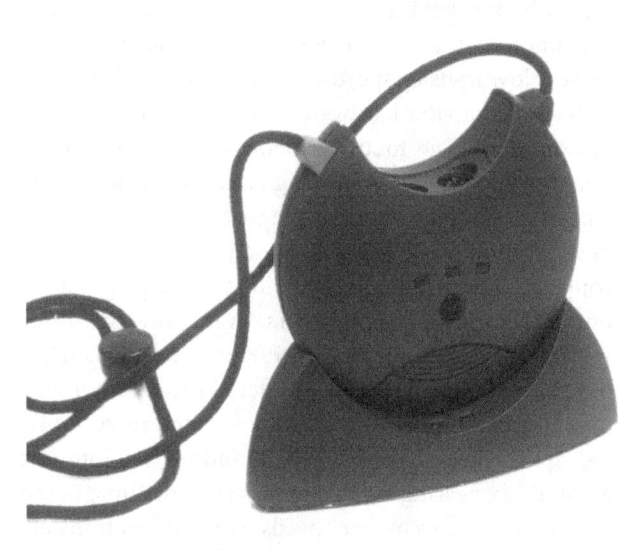

Figure 14–11. NOAHlink.

aids during programming. Wireless transmission is used for sending signals from the PC to the Noahlink enabling flexibility and freedom of movement during the fitting process.

HIMSA's latest programming device, the Noahlink™ Wireless, incorporates a wireless programming standard for programming Bluetooth Low Energy (BLE) enabled hearing aids. Specifically, this device plugs into the hearing professional's computer via USB and allows for a completely wireless programming interface. That is, unlike the NOAHlink, the patient does not have to wear any programming device other than the hearing aids themselves. This programming device was created with guidance and cooperation of major hearing aid manufacturers including ReSound, Phonak, Oticon, Signia, Widex, and Starkey.

Noah Modules

Although Noah includes modules that allow for performing basic fitting, measurement, and office management functions, as we note above, its greatest benefit is serving as an integration framework for more advanced software modules. Early versions of Noah included very simple office management functions but primarily served as a common interface for manufacturer-specific hearing aid programming and fitting modules. Over time, the sophistication and security of the included business management functions increased dramatically. That said, third-party, "Noah-Certified" management systems have also been developed to provide more focused business management solutions. In addition to this functionality, Noah matured to include an increasing number of modules for cochlear implants, various probe microphone and hearing aid test box manufacturers, as well as audiometers and other diagnostic test equipment. This integration allows Noah to serve as a central database for a large range of patient information, from diagnostics, to hearing aid fitting, to verification and validation, to billing information.

Noah Management Systems

As electronic patient records become increasingly important, HIMSA reported continuing to receive many requests from Noah users regarding integrating Noah data with other systems. Based on feedback from user groups, individuals, and organizations, HIMSA devised two management system methods for companies to integrate Noah data to meet these users' needs: Noah-compatible business systems and web service integration (WSI). The Noah business system method implements a single user interface for completing both business and Noah system related tasks. All Noah tasks are integrated in the third-party business systems software. Using this method, third party software developers are able to implement the same core features as Noah System software, run Noah fitting and measurement modules, and store the resulting data in the third-party software database. In contrast, the WSI method is aimed at users with an existing electronic management system. The Noah and management systems continue to operate as separate systems, but the WSI solution allows for data exchange between the systems. Diagnostic data can be exported to the management system, and patient information and demographic data can be exported from the management system to Noah. In addition to integration and data exchange, these third-party business solutions often include a range of additional useful features that are not limited to scheduling and billing functionality, accounting tools, purchase management, and advanced security compliance.

Programming the Hearing Aid

The software for programming hearing aids comes in the form of either a Noah programming module or standalone software. All major hearing aid manufacturers offer Noah programming modules, meanwhile some manufacturers also offer stand-alone versions of their programming software, in addition to their Noah modules for those clinicians who wish to program hearing aids outside the structure of Noah.

Although the intent of programming is to set the hearing aid in the manner that is desired for a given patient, there are several means to that end. For example, the clinician can hook the hearing aid up to the programming hardware (e.g., NOAHlink) directly through cables terminating in a plug connector; otherwise, this cable may be connected to the hearing aid using battery pill programming tips, flex strips, or boots. More recently, many hearing aids can be programmed without the need for wired connection to the hearing aid. Instead, a wireless programming interface is connected to the computer, typically via USB, and this interface communicates wirelessly with the hearing aids. Proprietary wireless programming has been available for some time, but standardization continues to be implemented across manufacturers. Currently there are differences in how far the wireless programming interface can be placed from the hearing aid. Specifically, some require the programmer to be worn around the patient's neck, whereas others can be placed several feet away. In the relatively near future we expect true wireless programming through a programming interface placed some distance from the patient to be implemented by all major manufacturers for most, if not all, of their hearing aid models.

Various cable connections are available, differing among and within manufacturers. Some require battery insertion, meanwhile others provide power to the hearing aid through the programing cable connection. The plugs on these cables that connect directly to the hearing aid or other connector vary in the number of connector pins from three to five, with four being the most common. Flex strips, likewise, vary slightly from manufacturer to manufacturer; these flat plastic connections have metal threads that serve as the contacts for the programming. Boots, or plastic covers that couple to the hearing aids, are also a programming option for some manufacturers. Direct cable connections are pretty straightforward as long as you have the correct cable. One end is plugged into a jack on the hearing aid (typically hidden either inside the battery door or under a small door on the instrument case) and the other end is plugged into the Noahlink or other programming interface. The other types of connections can be a little trickier. Due in part to advances in technology, the programming connections are not even standardized within most manufacturers, let alone across manufacturers. Consequently, we will generally discuss each of the other types of connections and then step through the fitting process.

Connecting Programming Boots

1. Choose the appropriate boot for the hearing aid at hand. Each manufacturer has varying sizes of boots for behind-the-ear (BTE) and mini-BTE receiver-in-canal (RIC) style hearing aids with boot size typically associated with different battery sizes. Each boot has metal contacts located on the body of the boot.
2. Find the metal programming contacts on the hearing aid. For some hearing aids these contacts may be located on the bottom of the battery door or on the back of the body of the hearing aid.
3. Attach the boot onto the lower body of the hearing aid. The metal contacts on the programming boot

should line up with the metal contacts on the hearing aid. The boot will click in place if it is correctly oriented with the hearing aid. For some manufacturers, the battery door should be opened to allow the boot to slide onto the hearing aid, and the battery door should be closed to allow the boot to be locked in place. Fortunately, manufacturers generally no longer require removal of the battery door to connect the programming boot. *Note:* Depending on the manufacturer and hearing aid model, some hearing aids may need a zinc-air battery inserted in the battery door to allow for connection of the hearing aid to the manufacturer software.
4. Located on the programming boot is a cable port. Choose the appropriate cable. The cable will connect to the boot with prongs that are located on the programming boot. Insert the cable into the cable port on the programming boot.
5. On the opposite end of the cable is the connector to be used with either the NoahLink or other programming interface.

Connecting FlexConnect Flex Strips

1. Flex strips are commonly used with mini-BTE and custom hearing aids. At the end of some flex strips is a plastic adapter piece that contains a cable port. Other flex strips require a FlexConnect2 adapter.
2. Open the battery door of the hearing aid to ensure that metal contacts are located within the battery compartment.
3. Located at one end of the flex strip are metal contacts (typically three or four). At the top of the battery door on the back body of the hearing aid, with the metal contacts facing upward, insert the flex strip into the top of the battery door. A black, raised dot on the flex strip indicates how deeply the flex strip should be inserted into the battery door compartment.
4. Close the battery door. This will lock the flex strip in place and allow the metal contacts to communicate with one another. A zinc air battery is required for most hearing aid models to allow for communication between the hearing aid and the manufacturer software.
5. Connect the appropriate cable to the cable port located at either the end of the flex strip or on the FlexConnect2 adapter.

6. On the opposite end of the cable is the connector to be used with the NOAHlink or other programming interface.

Connecting for Wireless Programming

1. The wireless programmer must first be installed on the computer. Typically this simply requires plugging the programmer into an available USB port on the computer during installation of the programming software or Noah module. The programmer will then need to be selected either within the Noah module or in the manufacturer's standalone software.
2. The largest current difference across manufacturers is where the programmer is placed. In many cases the hearing aids must be within close range to connect. In some cases a wireless loop must be oriented so that it completely surrounds the hearing aid. In other cases, the programmer is simply hung around the patient's neck. In still other cases, including manufacturer-specific devices and the Noahlink Wireless™, the programmer can be left on a desk some distance away from the patient. In all cases the hearing aids should be placed on the patient's ear. To connect the hearing aid with the programming software, the hearing aid must be turned on with a battery inserted in the battery compartment.

Programming the Hearing Aids

1. Open the manufacturer fitting software.
2. Click "connect" button to initiate communication between the hearing aids and software. In the case of wireless programming the hearing aid must still be detected in the programming software. Usually this is done by clicking on some type of "Detect Wireless" icon. The software will then search for the hearing aid.
3. Once detected, the software will ask to choose the ear to which the hearing aid is to be configured and will ask to set the acoustic parameters of the hearing aid. Set individual hearing aid characteristics such as tubing type or diameter, earmold and vent parameters, and patient characteristics including new user, experienced user, and so forth. Note

that different manufacturers may provide different options for these types of pre-fitting decisions.
4. Following the programming to the selected NAL or DSL prescriptive algorithm, conduct probe microphone verification measures to determine whether the selected algorithm meets preferred targets.
5. Select the fitting tab or fine-tuning tab; to make changes, select one or more channels (preferably for all input levels) and click the up or down arrows (see Figure 14–12 for example from one manufacturer). A detailed discussion of the changes you will make and suggested steps are in the verification section of Chapter 16.
6. If necessary, adjust for patient preference/comfort.
7. Add and modify the settings for any desired additional programs.

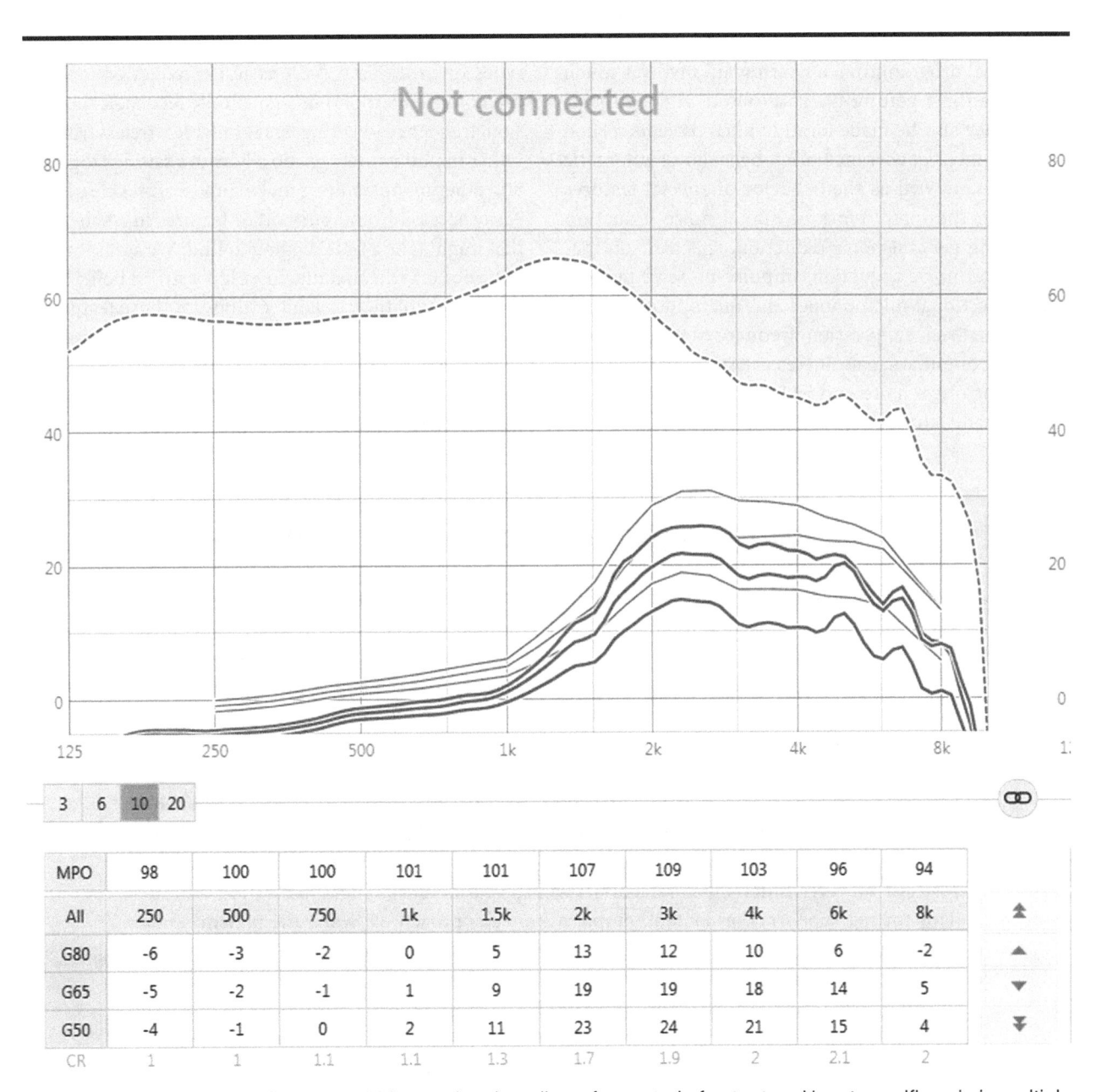

MPO	98	100	100	101	101	107	109	103	96	94
All	250	500	750	1k	1.5k	2k	3k	4k	6k	8k
G80	-6	-3	-2	0	5	13	12	10	6	-2
G65	-5	-2	-1	1	9	19	19	18	14	5
G50	-4	-1	0	2	11	23	24	21	15	4
CR	1	1	1.1	1.1	1.3	1.7	1.9	2	2.1	2

Figure 14–12. Example of hearing aid fine tuning that allows for control of output and input specific gain in multiple frequency ranges.

8. Confirm or modify the volume control/program button settings.
9. Save the settings to the hearing aids as well as the programming software or Noah database.
10. Disconnect the hearing aids within the software.
11. Disconnect the cables if applicable.

Programming Features and Options

Of course, programming a hearing aid involves much more than just getting the gain/output right. Adjustments may also be made for individual patients related to the number of user memories, behavior of automatic programs, as well as the behavior of special features including the many types of digital noise reduction (including general noise reduction, spectral subtraction, wind noise reduction, impulse noise reduction, etc.), directional microphones and microphone arrays, digital feedback suppression, frequency lowering technologies, automatic gain increase (AGI), learning volume controls, remote and FM microphones, wireless features, and a host of other types of processing.

Manufacturers' programming interfaces vary greatly. One common scheme, however, is to have a tab or page for hearing aid fine tuning that allows for control of output and input specific gain typically in multiple frequency ranges (Figure 14–12). Most manufacturers also include some sort of "automatic fine tuning" page or control that automatically makes a variety of programming changes in response to specific patient complaints.

A separate page(s) or tab(s) is also typically available for programming advanced hearing aid features. Sometimes there are many separate pages for different types of processing such as noise reduction, various directional microphone algorithms, feedback suppression, frequency lowering, and available wireless features. Other manufacturers group all feature settings together. Still other manufacturers make some features clearly and easily accessible and bury other features in a sub-menu that might take a little digging to find. We assume this is done because the manufacturer has a strong belief in the correctness of their default settings for those features or there is concern that we may *mis*-program, leading to a setting that is commonly rejected by patients.

In some cases the choice is simply to activate the feature or not, meanwhile in other cases a large range

---

POINTS TO PONDER: AUTOMATIC FINE TUNING

Most fitting software has a feature that allows the clinician to select a particular patient complaint—e.g., soft sounds too loud—and then the software makes an automatic adjustment. Perhaps it is just our controlling nature, but we tend not to simply trust the manufacturer to always make the right set of adjustments corresponding to complaints. It is not that we assume the manufacturers are wrong; rather, there are just too many differences in individual patients and the language they use to describe a problem. For example, does the complaint of an echo refer to too much low-frequency gain, frequency lowering that is too aggressive, occlusion effect problems, or some other problem? All are possible. For some simple complaints (e.g., fire trucks are too loud) the fix can be rather straightforward. When you push the "fix-it" button in response to some specific patient complaints that are a bit less straightforward, however, different manufacturers will apply different changes to the programming. This further supports our contention that a simple approach of "when the patient reports complaint X, always make change Y" approach is probably less than satisfactory. Therefore, we prefer to make fine-tuning adjustments ourselves by directly controlling the gain, compression, output, and features rather than simply trusting automatic fine tuning. Moreover, in the current climate of Internet sales, mail-order PSAPs, over-the-counter products, and the like, is it not the savvy of the trained audiologist that separates us from the rest of the pack? A clerk at Walmart can click the "automatic fine tuning" button!

of fine-tuning adjustments can be made. We discuss troubleshooting of features in Chapter 18 of this book; we will take some time to discuss basic decision-making and programming features here.

User Memories

Most modern hearing aids default to a master automatic program that automatically switches between multiple subprograms depending on how the hearing aid classifies the sound environment (see Chapter 12). For example, a hearing aid may have default programs that assign special features differently for listening in quiet, speech in noise, noise, and music. The number of subprograms within the master automatic program varies quite a bit within and across manufacturers, but three to five general listening environment programs are common. Depending on the specific manufacturer and model, the master program may switch between fixed settings for each of these subprograms or the settings in the subprograms may not be fixed and instead adapt further based on environmental factors (e.g., setting may change when the environment changes from speech in noise with a lower overall level to a higher overall level). Conversely, rather than implementing subprograms at all, the master program may include a complex algorithm that shifts the settings of all features in a multidimensional fashion based on specified criteria as a function of the sound environment. When we program hearing aids, the subprograms are typically all linked together under the master program, so any changes in gain and output made affect all of the subprograms as well. Consequently, if for any reason we wish to change gain in any of the individual subprograms without affecting others, the subprograms must first be unlinked. One common reason to unlink programs occurs when the manufacturer does not automatically make up for the reduced low-frequency sensitivity in the directional microphone setting and we want to equalize the frequency response for directional and omnidirectional settings.

Although the automatic programs may work well for many patients, they are not perfect and often satisfaction and/or benefit can be enhanced from individualization because of large differences across patients' hearing and cognitive abilities and the sound environments that are important to them. One common programming change is to add a separate user program for a specified listening situation. For example, a program like the default automatic program can be specified as the start-up program, and additional programs may be assigned to additional user memories. Common examples of specific listening environments that a patient may want to have a specific setting include (1) patients in very high noise environments who may find remote microphone, FM, or bilateral beamformer program useful; (2) a special music program for patients unhappy with the default programming when listening to music; (3) an omnidirectional program for overhearing for patients unsatisfied with the default programming when trying to listen to talkers who are not in the field of vision in noisy environments; and (4) a reverse directional program for listening to talkers in the back seat of a car while driving. It is common for hearing aids to allow up to three or four user-selectable programs, but in practice we find most users prefer either fully automatic or no more than two user-selectable programs.

Adjusting or Activating Specific Features

Regardless of whether it is the master automatic program, a separate user-selectable program, or a subprogram integrated into the master automatic program, some adjustments to individual hearing aid features are often necessary to optimize the hearing aid fitting. Some settings affect how the patient is able to interact with the hearing aid, and so greatly depend on whether that interaction is desirable. The decision to activate these features is typically based on patient preferences, patient ability, and the overall need for the feature; activation typically affects operation regardless of the hearing aid program. This includes features that can activate any number of operations like (1) audioalerts for program changes, low battery, and so forth; (2) manual volume control, perhaps including start volume, range, step size, and any learning VC parameters; and (3) a remote control.

The second type of feature programming is control and adjustment of specific sound processing features of the hearing aid such as feedback suppression, tinnitus masking, activation of gain expansion (when not controlled by the gain adjustments), various types of noise reduction, microphone type, operation, and frequency lowering. Such programming can also activate an external device interface such as direct audio input, remote microphone, wireless streaming, and so forth. For most manufacturers, changes to the settings for these features can be completed within specific subprograms that exist within the master program or as stand-alone user programs. Changes in default programming for these features may be in response to specific patient complaints, an attempt to address specific listening situations for a patient, or an attempt to optimize a features for individual patient differences, as we discuss in Chapter 18.

The fact that controls, settings, ranges, and underlying operation of these features vary dramatically across manufacturers can make adjustments somewhat challenging, particularly if it is a hearing aid brand with which we are less familiar. A few of the differences that may be encountered are (1) Manufacturer A for one model may have digital noise reduction settings that include on and off; (2) Manufacturer B for a different model may have a single noise reduction control including settings of weak, moderate, strong; and (3) Manufacturer C, for yet a different model, may have three separate continuous adjustments for three different types of noise reduction that range from off to maximum. The type of noise reduction in each case may be different, as may the range in the amount of gain reduction for noise and the timing of changes; even the operation for a specific setting such as "moderate" may vary dramatically across manufacturers. Therefore, we strongly believe that it is critical that we get to know the settings within each new model and the effects they have before attempting to make adjustments on real patients. In many cases this is as simple as completing a coupler fitting in a hearing aid test box, adjusting the settings, and looking at the effects on various input signal types and levels.

A final type of feature programming relates specifically to digital feedback suppression. Many manufacturers suggest or require an initialization procedure prior to activation of feedback suppression. In many cases this occurs very early in the fitting, often even prior to assignment and adjustment of gain and output. Depending on the manufacturer, the initialization phase may be used to measure and limit the maximum gain before feedback for the specific patient and coupling, to measure the acoustics of the specific feedback pathway to enhance the operation of the feedback suppressor, or both. In some cases we find the initialization process only serves to lock the gain settings within each channel to ensure the gain cannot be increased to a point where feedback will occur. Although this gain limiting works well for some models, it is overly aggressive for other models. Therefore, as a general rule of thumb, we tend to skip the initialization phase if it is not also used to improve the operation of the DFS processing and instead use traditional clinical gain adjustments to ensure the hearing aid does not produce unwanted feedback. Specifically, in some users and fittings, greater susceptibility to occasional low-level feedback is worth it to provide more gain and better audibility for important high-frequency sounds.

In Closing

We have come a long way from placing various hearing aids on a patient and attempting to choose the best based on word recognition results. After decades of building an evidence base, we are left with a few converging methods for prescribing gain and output and a myriad of tools for precisely programming hearing aid function. Despite how far we have come, the use of proper correction factors when calculating prescribed gain and output is still critical. We hope this chapter provides some appreciation for the long road that was travelled to arrive at modern hearing aid programming, as well as greater understanding about the nuts and bolts of programming a hearing aid, in addition to the great number of differences you can see across models and manufacturers when applying changes to programming. Of course these are just the basic tools. The true art (and *applied* science) of modern hearing aid fittings is applying what we learned during the hearing aid selection process about the patient's listening needs and hearing abilities, considering patient feedback after being fitted, and adjusting and optimizing the hearing aid fitting for each individual patient, not just each individual hearing loss. We focus on the challenges in attempting to achieve an optimized and individualized fit in much of the rest of this book.

15
Behavioral Assessment During Clinical Fittings

In Chapter 14, we review how to assign prescriptive targets and program hearing aids, and in Chapters 16 and 17 we discuss techniques for verification of hearing aid gain and output using probe microphone measures. These areas are the cornerstones of hearing aid fitting and verification related to determining the optimal amount of gain and output for each individual. In later chapters, we discuss validation of the hearing aid fitting using various outcome measures, primarily self-assessment inventories. There are other tests of aided performance, however, that often are conducted on the day of the fitting. In this chapter, we discuss a variety of behavioral measures that are sometimes used as part of the overall hearing aid fitting process.

Verification Versus Validation

If you look up dictionary definitions of *verification* and *validation*, you may be hard pressed to discriminate between the two words, which are often used to mean essentially the same thing. In the world of quality control, there has been a great deal of discussion on the topic, however, and several industries have provided definitions for these two words that are specific to their work. In most cases, verification is used when discussing whether specific goals, often design or manufacturing goals, were met. For example, does specific graphing software actually produce the intended graphs in the intended way? In contrast, validation is used to describe whether the end user/target audience obtains what is wanted or needed. For example, does the user think the graphing software actually meets his or her needs? Stated simply:

- Verification: Are we building the system right?
- Validation: Are we building the right system?

Applied to the selection and fitting of hearing aids, hearing aid verification is often used to refer to the process of ensuring that the hearing aid meets specific criteria (are we building the system right?). For example, we verify that we achieve our target prescriptive gain and output, we verify that aided loudness does not exceed threshold of discomfort, or we verify that aided thresholds meet expected levels. In contrast, hearing aid validation is the process of ensuring we meet the goals set forth in the communication needs assessment (are we building the right system?). For example, we demonstrate that patient goals were met through subjective assessment.

The verification-validation differentiation becomes somewhat blurred when we think of the clinical behavioral measures described in this chapter. For example, is aided speech recognition verification or validation? This question generated a lively discussion between the three authors: Is it verification (e.g., it is our fitting goal is to improve speech recognition by X%) or validation (e.g., it is the hearing aid wearer's goal to have better speech recognition). Another interpretation would be to consider the testing conducted on the day of the fitting as verification, and all testing following that as validation (assuming that use in the real world is needed to determine if it meets the patient's needs).

The final vote regarding the material here was two to one, so we never did reach a consensus. Therefore, for our purposes, this chapter considers many behavioral measures as *verification* of the hearing aid fitting; however, this debate could continue for years!

The Role of Behavioral Outcomes

Although it is obviously of interest to determine whether a hearing aid fitting is a successful one, why do we sometimes go to the extra effort of examining specific changes in behavioral outcomes? Certainly, there are differences in the fitting goals of individual patients. In some cases the prescribed gain and output, the specific style chosen, and the importance and activation of certain hearing aid features represent a compromise among different factors that determine a successful fitting. These factors may include such things as obtaining appropriate audibility, physical comfort, cosmetics, optimizing speech intelligibility (for both listening in quiet and in noise), and presenting good sound quality. The prescribed fitting also must be acceptable to the user, at least acceptable enough that the patient will wear the hearing aids during the initial adjustment period and beyond. Because there are tradeoffs, the measures described in this chapter can help us identify whether we have met specific fitting goals, and help identify areas where changes or additional counseling may be necessary.

To some extent, the measures that are taken on the day of the fitting reflect the audiologist's gold standard regarding what is a "good" fitting or, at the least, what is an "acceptable" fitting. For example, if the audiologist believes that the most important aspect of the fitting is

---

SOAPBOX: ARE ALL MEASURES "GOOD" MEASURES?

In this chapter, we will discuss several different measures that are used clinically as part of the hearing aid fitting by at least some audiologists. We want to make it very clear, however, that we are not in any way suggesting that all these measures are necessarily "good" or appropriate things to do routinely, even on a very small subset of patients. Some of these measures are included only because they are used in some clinics. We include them for two main reasons:

- If an audiologist does choose to use them, we want to at least provide what we believe is the best clinical method for administration, scoring, and interpretation.
- Rather than simply labeling them as inappropriate or ignoring them, we believe it is important to discuss why they may lead to erroneous or misleading conclusions.

Consequently, we have rated the various measures (based on our obviously biased opinions) into three categories (*Note*: Although biased, these opinions certainly have considerable basis in science). The categories we have used to rate each procedure are:

- Rarely useful—use considerable caution when interpreting results.
- Useful for some patients.
- Useful for most patients.
- Newer, but potentially useful—methods to watch.

the patient's opinion of sound quality, then some type of formal sound quality judgments would be implemented. We have summarized the association between various fitting goals and selected behavioral verification measures in Table 15–1. Note that we say *behavioral measures*, and therefore probe microphone verification is not included (see Chapters 16 and 17 for this essential part of the fitting protocol).

The measures that we discuss in this chapter should not be considered a substitute for the outcome measures discussed in Chapter 19 because clinical testing is a poor predictor of real-world benefit (e.g., Humes, Halling, & Coughlin, 1996; Wu & Bentler, 2012). The poor relationship between these laboratory measures and real world benefit is the crux of the argument for labeling the measures verification rather than validation. In Chapter 19,

Table 15–1. Examples of Possible Fitting Goals and Corresponding Behavioral Measure

Fitting Goal	Behavioral Measure
Meet prescriptive target for soft inputs	Functional Gain: Using frequency-specific signals, the patient's hearing thresholds are determined, both unaided and aided in the soundfield; the difference of these thresholds is calculated, which is *functional gain*.
Audibility of soft sounds	Using frequency-specific signals, the patient's aided hearing thresholds are determined in the soundfield. The aided thresholds are compared to desired threshold levels (although the general verification is to determine if soft speech is audible, desired levels may vary as the hearing loss becomes more severe).
Optimal speech recognition	While aided in the soundfield (or mildly reverberant room), the patient is presented one or more standardized speech tests (in quiet and/or in noise), typically at a level ~45–50 dB HL; 60–65 dB SPL. The patient's scores are compared to that of normal-hearing individuals, or a predetermined value believed to be optimal for someone with a similar degree of hearing loss. Alternatively, because hearing aid benefit for speech recognition is highly dependent on changes in audibility, some clinicians test at lower presentation levels (e.g., 40 HL; 53 dB SPL) to examine changes for soft vocal efforts.
Optimal subjective speech recognition	While aided in the soundfield (or mildly reverberant room), the patient is presented speech materials (in quiet and/or in noise), typically at a level ~45–50 dB HL; 60–65 dB SPL. Ratings could be obtained using bounded category scaling, or other standard speech recognition rating scale. The patient's scores are compared to that of normal-hearing individuals, or a predetermined value believed to be optimal for someone with a similar degree of hearing loss.
Optimal sound quality	While aided in the soundfield (or mildly reverberant room), the patient is presented speech materials (in quiet and/or in noise), typically at a level ~45–50 dB HL; 60–65 dB SPL. Sound quality ratings could be obtained using bounded category scaling, or other standard sound quality rating scale. The patient's scores are compared to that of normal-hearing individuals, or a predetermined value believed to be optimal for someone with a similar degree of hearing loss.
Appropriate loudness perceptions	Using the Cox Loudness Anchors for the response, the patient performs loudness judgments for speech discourse. The patient rates the loudness of different input levels (e.g., ~45 dB SPL should be rated *Soft*; ~65 dB SPL should be rated *Comfortable*; ~85 dB SPL should be rated *Loud, But Okay*.)
Loud sounds *Loud, But Okay*	Using the Cox Loudness Anchors for the response, the patient performs loudness judgments for different obnoxious noise signals presented at 85 dB SPL. The target response is #6—*Loud, But Okay*.

we discuss how self-assessment inventories like the COSI, APHAB, or IOI-HA—all of which have the patient rate his or her benefit for different real-world listening situations—can be useful for validating general hearing aid outcomes. It is possible for a patient's hearing aids to meet the audiologist's fitting standards, yet not meet a patient's real-world validation standards. We know this is true, as around 5 to 8% of hearing aid owners never use their hearing aids, even though we presume they met someone's verification and validation standards when they were purchased.

Functional Gain Verification

Rating: Rarely Useful—Use considerable caution when interpreting results.

As we describe in Chapter 16, the preferred method of determining the real-ear gain and output of hearing aids is to conduct probe microphone measures. An alternative method, which can provide some limited information, is to conduct unaided and aided threshold measures in the sound field and calculate the difference; this will provide a "functional gain" value.

The popularity of gain-based prescriptive fitting began in the 1970s, fueled by the original NAL and the many publications and workshops of Lybarger, Mac-Candless, and Berger. As clinicians gradually started abandoning the time-honored method of using speech testing to select the best hearing aid, they needed a replacement method to go along with these new prescriptive approaches. Given that the method prescribed gain, soundfield functional gain measurement was the logical verification strategy (clinically-friendly; probe microphone insertion gain measures did not routinely become available until the mid-1980s).

The measurement protocol for functional gain is quite simple (until one considers potential pitfalls). The patient is first seated in an audiometric test booth, positioned at a calibrated spot, usually one meter from a loudspeaker located at 0 degrees azimuth. The patients are instructed to not lean forward or back, nor turn their heads (although they nearly always do anyway). Masking is applied via earphone to the non-test ear. Using pulsed pure tones, thresholds are obtained for the key octave or one-half octave test frequencies (e.g., usually 250 Hz through 4000 Hz) using a conventional threshold determination procedure. Following this testing, the hearing aid is placed on the ear, presumably set to the patient's use-gain, and threshold testing is repeated. The aided thresholds are subtracted from the unaided, and this is the frequency-specific functional gain.

On the surface, functional gain testing sounds like a simple substitute for the insertion gain measures described in Chapter 16. In one way it is even simpler, in that extra equipment is not required. When done correctly, similar results can be obtained for functional gain as for probe microphone insertion gain, but only with linear hearing aids that use no special processing—and if low-level inputs are used for the latter. There are many issues/limitations with functional gain, however, that must be considered whenever this procedure is attempted or when it is compared to insertion gain testing. These issues/limitations include the following:

- **Eliminating the non-test ear.** Most people being fit with hearing aids have fairly symmetrical hearing loss and, therefore, when soundfield testing is conducted, it is important to ensure that the non-test ear is eliminated. Whereas it is tempting to simply use an E-A-R foam earplug in the non-test ear, this usually is not enough attenuation. Rather, narrow-band noise via an earphone must be used. This often is a logistically daunting task (earphone cords stretched to the middle of the test booth), and adds to patient confusion.
- **Room masking effects.** Most of today's hearing aids use low-threshold compression and provide the most gain for lower level inputs. One of these inputs is the ambient noise of audiometric test rooms. This seemingly low-level background noise will be amplified by 30 to 40 dB in some cases, which will then prevent the patient from hearing the target pure-tone signal for the aided testing. In some cases this will then result in a *negative* functional gain value, when in fact the hearing aid may provide 10 to 15 dB of gain for soft speech in the frequency region. This is a particular problem for patients with normal hearing in the low and mid frequencies.
- **Low-level expansion.** Nearly all hearing aids have low-level expansion, processing designed to reduce gain for low-level signals. If the patient has only a mild hearing loss, and aided thresholds are expected to be in the 20 dB

HL range, expansion may reduce the input of these signals, which would make aided thresholds appear worse than they actually are.
- Feedback suppression. Most hearing aids have an automatic feedback suppression system. In some cases, the signal classification system will interpret the pure-tone signal as hearing aid feedback (rather than an external signal) and attempt to reduce or eliminate it. This would have the effect of making aided thresholds appear worse than they actually are.
- Gain information provided. With wide dynamic range compression (WDRC) instruments, it is important to verify gain for a variety of inputs ranging from soft to loud. Functional gain (even when all contaminating variables are eliminated) only provides information for low-level inputs, as threshold measures are used. It is very difficult to interpolate gain for higher input levels with only this information. Even if you trust the manufacturers' reported compression ratios and thresholds, calculating expected frequency specific gain for speech signals for higher level inputs would require a fair bit of cumbersome calculation.
- Frequency information provided. Although it would be possible to conduct some type of frequency sweep and use a Bekesy tracking procedure for functional gain measurements, this isn't done. Rather, only key frequencies are tested. Many important aspects of the hearing aid fitting involve peaks and dips in the gain and output, which often are not revealed with functional gain measures at discrete frequencies. A narrow peak or dip at the tested frequency can give us a much distorted view of the actual gain provided over a broader frequency range.
- Efficiency. Once the patient is set up, a probe microphone assessment of gain can be accomplished in 5 to 10 seconds. During the hearing aid fitting process, it often is necessary to repeat this measure 10 or more times as the frequency response and compression are tweaked to obtain the best fitting. It is unlikely that either the audiologist or the patient would have the endurance for 10 or more repeats of functional gain measures.
- Reliability. As we discuss in Chapter 16, the test–retest reliability for probe microphone measures is approximately 2 dB. A number of studies have shown that reliability is considerably worse for functional gain. This is because of room calibration problems, room reflections, patient positioning, patient movements, threshold test procedures, and other factors. One study of functional gain reliability was conducted by Hawkins, Montgomery, Prosek, and Walden (1987); their results are shown in Table 15–2. Observe that even at the conservative 0.2 (which equates to a 80% confidence interval) p value critical differences are around 10 dB, meaning that if you want to be 80% confident that your difference is real—and not a result of chance—you will need a difference of at least 10 dB in your functional gain measures.
- Behavioral requirements. Unlike probe microphone measures, functional gain

Table 15–2. Critical Differences in dB for Aided Soundfield Thresholds for Four Probability Levels

	Frequency (Hz)					
p	250	500	1000	2000	3000	4000
.05	11.9	15.7	15.1	15.1	16.1	16.5
.1	10.0	13.2	12.7	12.7	13.5	13.8
.2	7.8	10.2	9.9	9.9	10.7	10.8
.3	6.3	8.3	8.0	8.0	8.5	8.7

Source: Adapted from Hawkins, Walden, Montgomery, & Prosek (1987).

> ### TECHNICAL TIP: COMPARE APPLES TO APPLES
>
> As we mention, there may be some isolated cases when it is necessary to conduct functional gain to determine real-ear hearing aid performance. Although it might be a tempting time-saver to use the earphone thresholds as the unaided reference, this is risky practice for two reasons. First, it's simply good science to use the same setting for the unaided and aided so that all test conditions are the same; moreover, earphone thresholds were probably obtained at an earlier date and the patient's hearing could have changed. Second, soundfield calibration may not match earphone calibration—in some clinics, differences are 10 dB or more between these presentation modes. If both measures, however, are taken in the sound field, these errors will not matter, as we are only looking at difference values (gain), not absolute thresholds.

requires a cooperative, alert patient who is mentally capable of providing reliable thresholds. This may be particularly problematic for young children and some older adults.

As described, there are many pitfalls and limitations associated with functional gain. So much so that we might ask, "When would it ever be appropriate to conduct these measures?" There are some instances when it might be considered:

- When the validity of the unaided thresholds is in question, such as in young children or difficult to test adults. In contrast to probe microphone measures, functional gain can serve as a cross-check for the conventional threshold test results. For example, if a hearing aid is expected to provide around 30 dB of gain for a given VC setting (based on the simulated response of the manufacturer), and thresholds go from 60 dB (unaided) to 30 dB (aided), all is well. If the aided threshold for that setting is only 55 dB, however, it might be questioned whether the unaided thresholds are correct (assuming you remembered to turn on the hearing aid).
- Current fitting systems that deliver sound through bone conduction, including implantable osseo-integrated devices, present a very real challenge to verification. The same challenge is present for middle ear implants. We cannot simply measure the level in the ear canal for these products because the sound is delivered to the middle ear or through bone conduction (although some methods of plugging the ear and measuring sound in the ear canal hold promise for bone conduction devices). This challenge is further heightened by the introduction of modern hearing aid processing including multichannel low-threshold compression, noise reduction, feedback suppression, and other processing. Consequently, verification of these devices is commonly accomplished through functional gain. All of the problems and cautions related to procedure exist for this class of devices as well; however, functional gain can at least provide some indication if gain for low-level inputs is appropriate. Some manufacturers assist us further by providing software which approximates gain for high-level inputs based on these measures and the device settings.
- When there is excessive cerumen in the ear canal that plugs the probe tip (preventing probe microphone measures) but does not occlude the canal, soundfield threshold measures would probably still be valid. Best clinical practice would have this patient return for the probe microphone verification after an ear cleaning, but sometimes patients come from 100 miles away and this is not as simple as it sounds. Functional gain (conducted carefully) would at least provide some indication of whether gain for low-level inputs was appropriate. If not, programming changes could be made and key frequencies retested.

In this way, patients might be able to go home with hearing aids that are likely to have gain that is at least in the ballpark of appropriate values while they are waiting to have their ears cleaned. Having the patient return for complete probe microphone verification after the cleaning is highly recommended, of course.

■ Unfortunately, some federal and state government agencies and third party payers will not accept probe microphone data and still require aided soundfield documentation before determining fitness for duty or approving funding. In such cases it is necessary to conduct functional gain, but we would recommend that this be done in addition to (and after) probe microphone verification. There is a way to generate pseudo aided thresholds using probe microphone insertion gain data, however, which we explain in Chapter 17.

When functional gain is conducted, the unaided and aided thresholds are normally plotted on the audiogram, and then the calculated difference is recorded. Figure 15–1 shows the unaided and aided testing for an individual who was not able to have probe microphone testing (wet cerumen in ear canal). We recommend plotting the results on the count-the-dot audiogram, as this facilitates counseling regarding aided speech audibility.

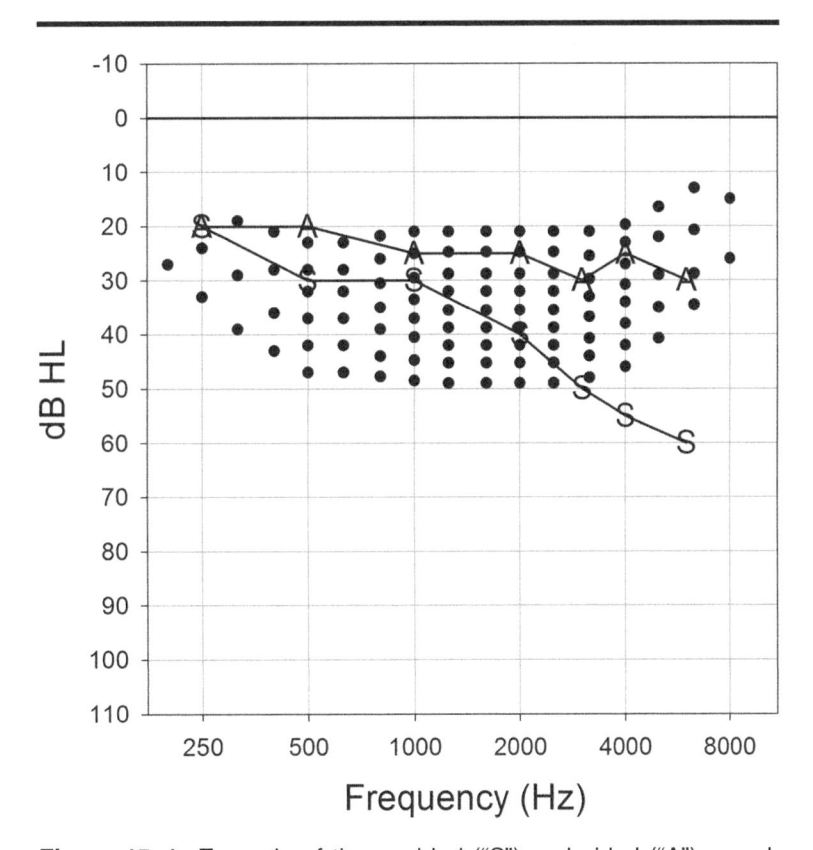

Figure 15–1. Example of the unaided ("S") and aided ("A") soundfield thresholds obtained from a patient who was not able to have probe microphone testing due to wet cerumen in the ear canal. The difference between these threshold estimates is considered to be a measure of functional gain. For example, at 4000 Hz we see sound field thresholds going from 55 dB HL unaided to 25 dB HL aided, which would then be interpreted as 30 dB of functional gain (see text for cautionary considerations relative to the use of functional gain).

> ### POINTS TO PONDER: TERMINOLOGY USED TO DEFINE *GAIN*
>
> In this chapter and Chapters 16 and 17, we discuss different types of gain measures that can be used to verify the hearing aid fitting. There have been at least eight different terms used to describe hearing aid gain at one time or another. Here is a brief summary (modified from Mueller & Hall, 1998). Don't worry if some of the terms related to probe microphone measures are unfamiliar to you; these will be described in detail in Chapter 16.
>
> - Coupler Gain. A term that has withstood the test of time is coupler gain, with the most noted reference the classic JASA article of Romanow in 1942. Coupler gain usually refers to the gain measured in the 2cc coupler as described in ANSI Standard S3.22, although there are other special purpose couplers of different sizes. In general, coupler gain is the difference between the output measured in the coupler and the input signal (usually 50 or 60 dB SPL), and is commonly used as part of the hearing aid quality control measures discussed in Chapter 13.
> - Orthotelephonic Gain. This term was devised in telephone communication research in the 1930s to relate the fidelity of sound reproduction by the telephone to face-to-face communication between a talker and a listener, separated by one meter in an anechoic chamber. In the early days of the Knowles Electronics Manikin for Acoustic Research (KEMAR), the term was used to describe hearing aid gain measured using this manikin.
> - Etymotic Gain. The term, inspired by the Greek word *etymom* meaning *true ear* or *real ear*, was coined in the 1970s by a linguist friend of Mead Killion's. Etymotic was meant to describe gain measured using the KEMAR. The reference for etymotic gain is the open-ear response; hence, this is the value now known as *insertion gain*.
> - Simulated Gain. A term used to describe the gain measured on the KEMAR with the open ear as the reference. Because the KEMAR is not an individual's *real* ear and uses an ear simulator, the term has been suggested to make this point (in this case, simulated gain would be the same as insertion gain). The term, however, also is used in the fitting software of most manufacturers when corrections are made to the 2cc-coupler response and *simulated* real-ear gain is plotted. In this case, the simulated gain could be either real-ear insertion gain (REIG) or real-ear aided gain (REAG). Some probe microphone systems also plot simulated REAG by adding the real-ear coupler difference (RECD) (average or measured) to the 2cc-coupler response.
> - Insertion Gain. When the open-ear response (either real-ear or KEMAR) is subtracted from the aided response, this is referred to as insertion gain. That is, the net gain that resulted from inserting the hearing aid. This term was used as early as 1972 in an IEEE standard. Historically, the REIG was been the most common calculation used to verify a prescriptive fitting approach.
> - *In Situ* Gain. *In situ* is a Latin term meaning *in place* or *in the natural or original position*. The term primarily has been used to describe measures taken on the real ear (or in some cases the KEMAR ear) to differentiate from conventional coupler measures (e.g., ANSI Standard S3.22). Also, for the traditional calculation of in situ gain, the term gain is used to mean that the input signal is subtracted rather

than the open-ear response as is the case with insertion gain. In this case, in situ gain would be the same as REAG. Because "in place" could refer to almost any type of gain measured on the ear, in situ gain has been used to refer to insertion gain or the use of hearing aid generated signals to measure gain. Clearly, other than ANSI standards, there does not seem to be a consistent measure associated with this term.
- Aided Gain. This term refers to the REAG, which is the output of the hearing aid measured in the real ear (REAR) with the input level subtracted. The difference between the REAG and insertion gain is the real-ear unaided gain (REUG). Aided gain is used for verification of prescriptive methods that specify targets in real-ear SPL, most notably DSL v5.0.
- Functional Gain. This gain term is the only one that requires a behavioral response. It is the difference between soundfield open-ear unaided thresholds and aided thresholds. These two measures are the corollary of the REUR and the REAR, and therefore—not surprisingly—functional gain should be fairly similar to the REIG for low-level inputs (when testing is conducted carefully).

Aided Soundfield Threshold Verification

Rating: Rarely Useful—Use considerable caution when interpreting results.

Aided soundfield thresholds were described in the previous section as one-half of the data needed to calculate functional gain. Although we have indirectly already talked about this, in practice, aided soundfield thresholds on their own are measured for different reasons than functional gain. Specifically, we are not directly interested in the gain of the hearing aid or if the hearing aid's gain meets a prescriptive target. Rather, a soundfield threshold is a measure of aided audibility that tells us the softest sound a patient can hear at a specific frequency.

An example of this is shown in Figure 15–2. The patient was fitted with a Baha device (see Chapter 8) for his right ear and, therefore, probe microphone measures were not a verification option. The "A" symbols are his soundfield thresholds after the implant. As shown, with the Baha device, nearly all of the average speech spectrum is audible.

Essentially, all the pitfalls that accompany the functional gain verification procedure also exist for aided audibility measures. In particular, the sound field must be calibrated, the patient must sit in the calibrated spot with minimal head movements, and the non-test ear must be eliminated from the test. It is also possible or even probable that amplifier noise and amplified room noise may prevent the measurement of true aided thresholds.

Cautions When Interpreting Aided Results

Testing aided audibility in the sound field has been popular over the years when evaluating pediatric patients. Although the limitations have been spelled out in hearing aid fitting guidelines (e.g., those of the American Academy of Audiology), many pediatric audiologists continue to consider this a preferred verification method. In some cases, this approach is used to determine the best product by testing aided thresholds for different models from different manufacturers. The "winner" is the product that provides the best aided thresholds (e.g., a 10 dB HL aided threshold is considered better than a threshold of 20 dB HL). On the surface, this thinking might seem reasonable; however, there are at least two problems with applying this strategy. First, when the threshold numbers are this low, the measured threshold has little relevance to real-world hearing aid use because the world is not as quiet as an audiometric test booth. Ambient noise masks out low-level sounds as experienced by people with normal

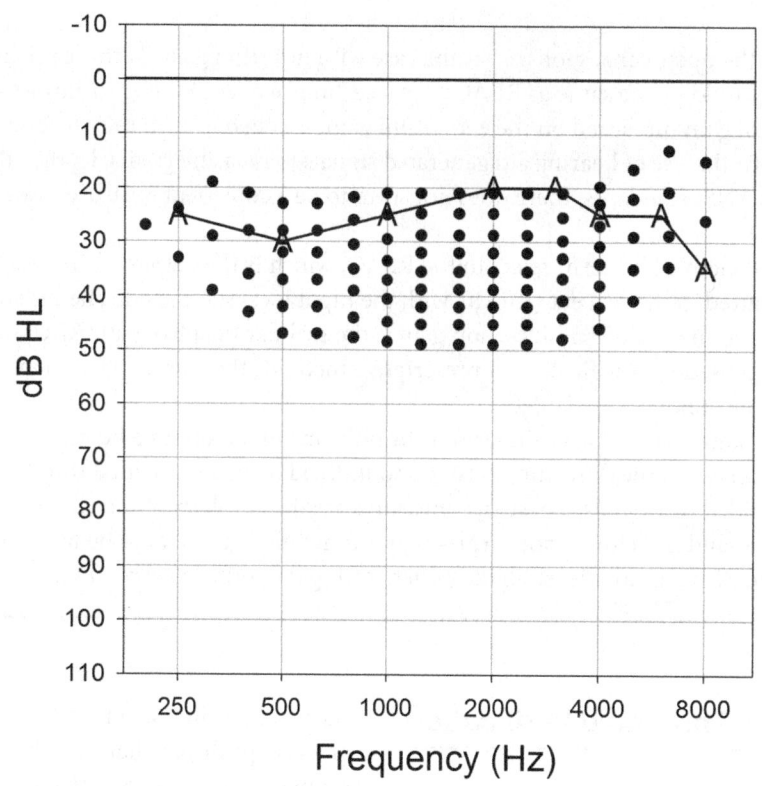

Figure 15–2. Aided sound field thresholds for a Baha user, plotted on the count-the dots audiogram.

KEY CONCEPT: SOUNDFIELD CALIBRATION

When aided soundfield testing is conducted, it is important to ensure that the loudspeakers have been appropriately calibrated. A setting of 60 dB HL that has been calibrated for insert earphones will likely not equate to 60 dB HL in the sound field. This isn't as much of a problem for functional gain calculation (where two incorrect thresholds could still result in a correct gain value), but is an important issue when soundfield thresholds alone are used, especially when measuring aided audibility for young children. This is one reason that we advocate for discussing levels in the sound field in dBA (A-weighted dB SPL) for broadband signals and dB SPL for narrow-band signals when we are discussing signal level in the sound field. This is a reference to a known standard level and is also consistent with the SPL-O-Gram or REAR in dB SPL probe microphone approaches to fitting hearing aids that are increasingly popular and discussed in Chapters 16 and 17.

Unfortunately, based on a survey of more than 400 audiologists, Rochlin (1993) reports that although over 80% of the respondents conducted some type of soundfield testing, only a small percentage knew how the sound field was calibrated. Moreover, the survey findings showed a lack of standardization among soundfield test rooms, great diversity in the stimuli used for soundfield testing, and inconsistent calibration methods. The bottom line is that soundfield calibration requires a sound level meter (SLM), preferably one that has octave filters in order to gather frequency-specific information.

hearing and hearing aid users alike. The average quiet living room has an ambient noise level of 42 dBA; most real-world situations have even higher levels of ambient noise. Hence, aided soundfield thresholds lower than these levels are probably not very meaningful in many real-world listening situations. The conversion from dBA to HL varies from frequency to frequency; we consider 20 dB HL roughly the cutoff value. That is, a hearing aid that provides an aided soundfield threshold of 5 dB in a test booth would probably provide no more audibility in the real world than a hearing aid that provides a 20 dB soundfield threshold.

Second, and perhaps more important, are the effects that compression threshold can have on these measures. As reviewed in Chapter 10, low-threshold compression fittings lead to more gain for low-level sounds and less gain for high-level sounds when compared to linear fittings. When the compression threshold is lowered, the softest sounds are provided even more gain, which can lead to misleading finding when soundfield threshold testing is conducted. The same principles would apply when soundfield aided thresholds are used for verification of implantable hearing aids, so considerable caution is warranted there as well—see Chapter 10 for detailed explanation.

Aided Speech Recognition Benefit

Rating: Perhaps useful for specific patients.

The pros and cons of using speech testing to quantify the success of a hearing aid fitting has been debated since about as long as hearing aids have been fitted by someone with the professional title of audiologist. The term *enigma* is defined as "something hard to understand or explain," and this term often has been applied to the relationship between aided speech testing and determining the best hearing aid fitting.

Consider that many, if not most, individuals purchase hearing aids because they have problems understanding speech, most commonly speech in background noise. As professionals we sell them a device (usually two) designed to solve their problems and hopefully meet their expectations. Isn't it reasonable then, for a new hearing aid user to expect that during the fitting process a test would be conducted that assesses the improvement the hearing aids provide for understanding speech, the primary problem that triggered their purchase decision? To state the obvious corollary, a nearsighted person fitted with contact lenses would expect that part of the fitting would be a before and after reading of the Snellen chart to ensure that an appropriate improvement in vision had occurred.

Speech recognition, when used for hearing aid selection or verification, has been fraught with reliability issues (see related Things to Remember), but there are several other issues that also limit the usefulness of this tool. Typical speech recognition in noise tests used in the clinic often do not reflect real-world conditions. Specifically, for testing in the clinic, reverberation is more limited, visual cues are typically not present, talkers have clear speaking voices, speech is usually presented at conversational levels (even though softer levels would be more challenging), and conditions tend to represent one-on-one conversations with very small speaker-to-listener distance (typically ~ one meter). In fact, the test conditions are so easy for listeners with mild and moderate hearing loss that there is little or no room to demonstrate hearing aid benefit. That is, we do not expect the speech recognition to improve with amplification based on calculated changes in audibility. Moreover, even if all these factors could be overcome, if you were using speech testing on the day of the fitting to determine the appropriateness of the fitting, you would still be left with the following practical questions for a given patient:

- How good does this patient's speech recognition have to be to be "good enough"?
- How do you know when you've reached the patient's optimal level of speech recognition?
- How do you know when one more change of programming won't make recognition better?
- How do you know when a different pair of instruments with slightly different signal processing won't make speech recognition better?

As we go through these challenges, it becomes clear that clinical speech testing has many limitations for validating or selecting the *best* amplification strategy. Furthermore, only one specific listening condition typically is evaluated. In addition, we haven't even addressed the clinical time investment that would be required.

> **THINGS TO REMEMBER: HISTORICAL PERSPECTIVE**
>
> From the very beginning of audiology, the use of speech audiometry to differentiate one hearing aid from another has been the basis of most speech testing in the hearing aid evaluation. For example, in 1946, Wiener and Miller published a fitting protocol using speech testing that was designed to compare carbon versus vacuum tube hearing aids. (This article was published in the monograph *Combat Instrumentation*, so you know they were serious about their procedure!)
>
> The publications of Carhart and others in the late 1940s helped promote speech testing in the evaluation and differentiation of hearing aids, and speech audiometry quickly became the preferred method to evaluate real-ear hearing aid performance—a position it would hold for more than 30 years. While serving in the U.S. Army, Captain Carhart developed a protocol for fitting hearing aids for returning World War II veterans. It was a lengthy procedure spanning several weeks and different tests, but an important component was speech intelligibility testing with different hearing aids. When summarizing the procedure Carhart (1946a) states: "Obviously, the final criterion of hearing excellence is the success with which the instrument functions in everyday situations; thus, selection procedures need to be chosen so as to yield estimates of the future usefulness promised by each hearing aid" (p. 780).
>
> Even in these early years, however, not everyone believed that speech audiometry was a worthwhile tool for comparative hearing aid evaluation. For example, in 1960, researchers Shore, Bilger, and Hirsh, who conducted comparative testing of hearing aids using speech reception thresholds and monosyllabic word recognition in quiet and in noise, concluded: "The reliability of these measures is not good enough to warrant the investment of a large amount of clinical time with them in selecting hearing aids." Dave Resnick and Marshall Becker (1963) reached the same conclusions three years later when they announced in *ASHA* magazine the discontinuation of comparative speech testing at Washington Hospital Center (Resnick & Becker, 1963). In general, these negative reports were not well received by the audiological community and were considered by some to be Carhart bashing. Speech audiometry, therefore, continued to be the cornerstone of hearing aid selection, as surveys conducted in the 1960s and 1970s revealed that about 85% of audiologists used speech testing for hearing aid differentiation (Burney, 1972). However, things have changed significantly in the past few decades.

Despite these considerable limitations, we believe it is sometimes useful to measure speech recognition benefit as a supplemental measure. Because it's not possible to have a specific aim (X% improvement in speech recognition, or an aided score of X%) it is not really a verification procedure either. In addition, because it is somewhat unreliable and the listening conditions don't really reflect those commonly experienced in the real world, it is not really a validation procedure. Instead, its clinical value (when there is one) most often relates to counseling or demonstration, so we will refer to it as a *supplemental measure*. We also can't forget that simply using this measure in the fitting process seems to increase patient satisfaction with amplification (see related Points to Ponder).

As we already mention, it may not be necessary in many cases to perform aided speech recognition testing. If you have the clinical time available and you have a patient for whom this testing will enhance the fitting procedure through changes in counseling, counseling reinforcement, or other reasons, we encourage you to obtain as much information, or as specific information, as possible. Rather than simply describe the speech tests you might use, in the following section we describe four general situations for which you may consider measuring speech recognition performance. We then

> **POINTS TO PONDER: CAN MORE TESTING INCREASE SATISFACTION**
>
> We propose that hearing aid fitting should include probe microphone verification to a validated prescriptive method and validation of the fitting with appropriate outcome measures. It is reasonable then to question if aided speech recognition testing is really necessary. A point to consider, however, is that patients seem to embrace the speech testing component of the overall fitting process, and we suspect that conducting some type of speech verification might lead to improved satisfaction with amplification, even if you change nothing based on the results. The MarkeTrak VIII survey would suggest that this is true (Kochkin et al., 2010). As part of this survey, hearing aid users were asked several questions regarding hearing aid benefit and satisfaction. Kochkin then developed a composite "satisfaction with benefit" score. Seventy-nine percent of individuals who were more than one standard deviation above average in satisfaction with benefit received an objective test to measure benefit at the time of their fitting. On the other hand, only 53% of individuals who were more than one standard deviation below average had such a test. There were other factors that contributed to these individuals' satisfaction ratings, but overall the MarkeTrak VIII data show that there is a payoff for more testing—greater satisfaction with hearing aids.

describe our favorite tests for completing this testing as well as an example of specific procedures we might use and how we would interpret the findings. The general purposes for completing speech recognition testing include the following:

- Demonstrate that the hearing aids improve audibility leading to improved speech recognition.
- Demonstrate that a technology aimed at improving SNR (directional microphones, beamformers, FM systems, remote microphones, etc.) can lead to improved speech recognition in noise.
- Demonstrate the limitations of performance in noise (even with SNR improving technologies) to aid in counseling-related to realistic expectations.
- Demonstrate that hearing aids can improve speech recognition performance when visual cues are present for listeners with severe-to-profound hearing loss.

Considerations for Soundfield Aided Testing

Before describing the speech tests we will be using for the different cases, we first need to remind you of some preliminary considerations that need to be made for this type of testing. The checklist for preparation includes several steps:

- Ensure that the sound field is calibrated.
- Determine the best presentation level.
- Decide to use either an adaptive or fixed presentation of the background noise.

We reviewed these three factors in Chapter 6 regarding pre-fitting speech testing, and the same general rules and considerations apply for aided speech testing (see Chapter 6 for important guidance).

Clinical Case 1A: Demonstrating That the Hearing Aids Improve Audibility Leading to Improved Speech Recognition

Occasionally, it is of interest to demonstrate that speech recognition is improved by the hearing aids. Commonly, we want to do this for the listener with less severe hearing loss, which is the typical new user. These patients often have a mild loss in the low frequencies, sloping to moderate or worse in the high frequencies. This is the patient with the common complaint, "I hear okay, but people seem to mumble," or the classic, "I can hear but I can't understand." In this case, the patient may benefit from a little extra demonstration of how the hearing aids can help them. The patient may also end up more satisfied with the benefit received as discussed in the associated Points to Ponder.

This type of patient may have quite good speech recognition in non-reverberant environments as long as everything is loud enough. Consequently, it may be very difficult to demonstrate aided benefit in a sound booth, even using speech presented at a level equivalent to average vocal effort (62 dBA). In such cases, demonstrating the benefits of improved audibility may be easier if a lower speech level is used, which is what we recommend. We don't view this as "contrived", because there are a variety of listening conditions in the real world which may reduce performance, in which similar benefits from improved audibility will result. These listening situations include increased reverberation, increased talker-to-listener distance, listening to talkers with soft voices or who are difficult to understand, and so forth. Furthermore, the purpose of conducting this testing is a demonstration for counseling purposes rather than an attempt to predict accurately maximum aided speech recognition or real-world benefits. In addition to a lower presentation level, we also prefer to use sentence materials for this purpose because they have better face validity for patients than words or nonsense syllables.

Really, almost any speech recognition test could be used for this purpose, but we chose the CST that was developed in the Hearing Aid Research Laboratory at the University of Memphis for this example (see Chapter 6 for detailed background information on the CST). Although we find the CST, which includes testing each ear individually, a little long for routine clinical uses, when there are only two conditions (unaided and aided) we view it of reasonable length if you are going to the effort of quantifying the potential benefits of improved audibility. For situations in which you want this aided information but are a bit more time pressured, there are other tests that take less time to administer.

Testing the Patient

So how can we use a speech-in-noise test to assess changes in speech recognition primarily due to changes in audibility? Even though noise is present, if we administer these tests in the sound field with a maximum speech level of 50 dBA (note: this is typically *not* 50 dB HL) to an unaided listener with relatively good speech understanding in noise, it will typically be audibility (at least mostly) that limits performance. That is, it will likely be the individual's hearing thresholds, rather than the masking effects of noise, that limit audibility (assuming that a reasonable noise level was applied). Of course, we may not see a difference between aided and unaided performance in individuals with less than a moderate hearing loss if noise, rather than hearing thresholds, limits performance.

Let's consider EMP, a 58-year old lawyer who is not sure she needs hearing aids but is worried she may be missing some things said during court cases. She shares with us that she is concerned that hearing aids will make her look old, less intelligent, and maybe vulnerable. Her audiogram is shown in Figure 15–3. During the initial pre-fitting evaluation, we found that her unaided score for the BKB-SIN was +0.4 to +1.0 dB for both ears when presented under headphones at 70 dB HL, indicating she understands speech well, even in noise, as long as it is presented at a high enough level (suggesting relatively good cochlear function once the loss of audibility is overcome). We chose to fit her bilaterally with mini-BTE hearing aids with non-custom open eartips. Probe microphone results revealed an excellent fit to NAL-NL2 prescriptive targets bilaterally. In order to demonstrate the potential for hearing aid benefit related to improved audibility, we tested her unaided and then aided using the CST.

Since we are simply trying to show the effects of audibility, we used speech in quiet, but presented it at 50 dBA (soft vocal effort) in the sound field. Her unaided scores are pretty high at 72%, but her aided performance (aided bilaterally) was 98%, revealing a 26% hearing aid benefit. As there are no published normative data for the CST (too many options of level, SNR, and hearing loss) we can't actually compare those scores to any other groups. We can use these data, however, to counsel EMP that it appears she does have some difficulty, particularly when speech is at a low level, but that she exhibits excellent performance once we make speech loud enough. For most patients, it is not even necessary to tell them this, as they will notice the benefit themselves.

Clinical Case 1B: Demonstrating That the Hearing Aids Improve Audibility Leading to Improved Speech Recognition

We again consider EMP, the 58-year-old lawyer we described in Case 1A, who was not sure she needed hearing aids. Because it is a very busy day in the clinic

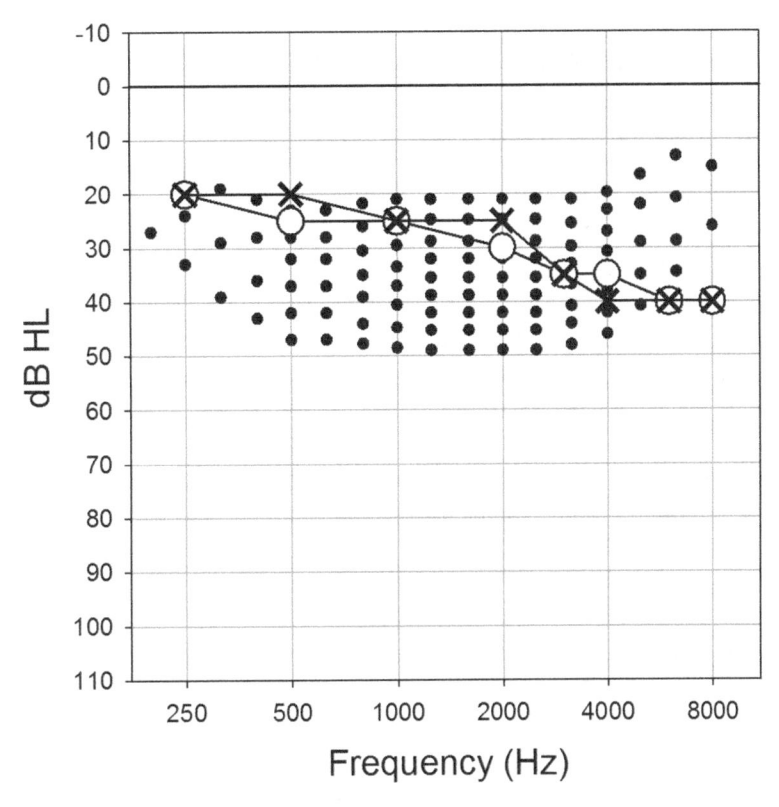

Figure 15–3. Audiometric results for EMP, a 58-year-old lawyer who is not certain that she needs hearing aids. Her unaided thresholds are sufficient to hear a good portion of the speech signal when presented at an average level, as is indicated on the typical count-the-dot audiogram.

you need to save as much time as possible, so you decide to use the Words in Noise (WIN) test (see Chapter 6 for a complete description of this test). As with the CST example, we are really just trying to show the effects of audibility, so we again use a presentation level of 50 dBA (soft vocal effort) in the sound field. Both the noise and the speech are presented from a single loudspeaker directly in front of her and about three feet away in the sound booth. Using the WIN test, her unaided scores show good speech recognition in noise of +5.2 dB, but her aided performance was even better at −1.2 dB, revealing a +6.4 dB hearing aid benefit. As described in more detail later in this section, we first use these data to counsel EMP that it appears she does have some difficulty, particularly when speech is low level. We then point out that she exhibits excellent performance, however, once we make speech loud enough. And perhaps, most importantly, we emphasize that this improvement is noted in the presence of background noise (multitalker babble for the WIN test, a commonly encountered background noise in the real world).

There are limitations, of course, to both of the approaches we presented in Case 1A and Case 1B. With the first approach, as we have discussed, unless the patient performs at or near the level of someone with normal hearing, it is difficult to know if the fitting has been optimized. With the second approach, one might say that the test situation is contrived. It is. But this is okay. It is simply designed to show the patient that, indeed, hearing aids work, and hearing aids tend to provide the most benefit for most people when the speech signal is somewhat softer than average, which is why we recommend a lower presentation level. This is not meant to be science—just a way to demonstrate the benefits of hearing aids, something that is not readily obvious during probe microphone verification.

> ### TECHNICAL TIP: SNRS AND AUDIBILITY
>
> We know that if audibility is not changed from the unaided to the aided presentation of the adaptive SNR test, it is unlikely that we will see an improvement between the aided and unaided scores. For example, if the sentences are presented at a level where most cues are audible (refer back to our lawyer patient), we don't expect to see much change in performance across SNRs between the unaided and aided conditions. Data shown in Figure 15–4 were obtained across 25 subjects using various amplification schemes (the *infamous* ear trumpet study). What is apparent in that figure is that there was no significant difference between performance in the unaided condition and any of the more modern hearing aids. Why? Audibility was sufficient in the unaided condition; adding the hearing aids did not change that fact, although they may have provided more loudness for the subjects. Also note from the figure that the SNR-50 decreased for the body-style hearing aid. Why again? That aid had so much distortion in its signal processing that the SNR-50 actually got worse. All of this is explained to highlight how important it is for us to always consider the purpose of the test and the logical outcomes. Alternately, had the speech and noise been presented from spatially separated speakers and the purpose was to determine the improvement in SNR with a directional microphone scheme, then we could expect an actual difference in the scores. In our example of Case study 1B, the improvement in the SNR-50 was due to an improvement in the audibility afforded by the hearing aids when the presentation level was low (50 dBA) rather than at higher presentation levels.

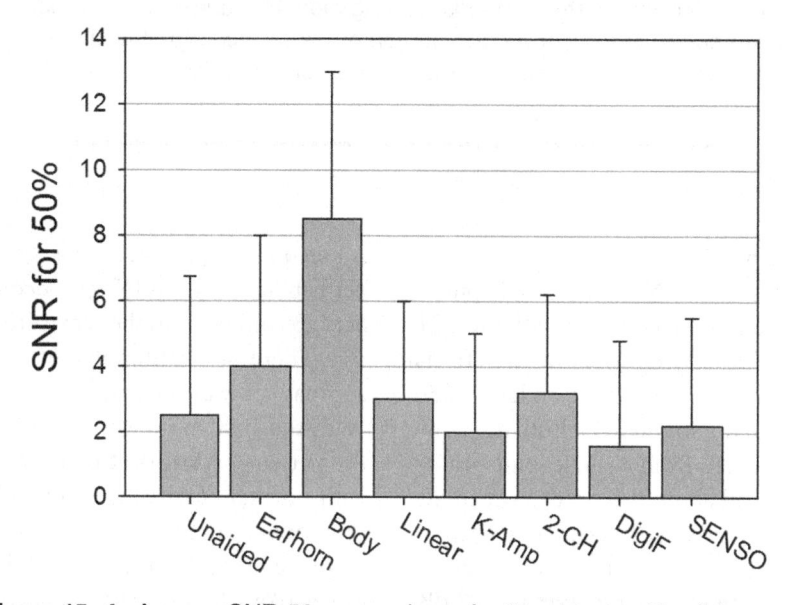

Figure 15–4. Average SNR-50 scores shown for 25 subjects with mild-to-moderate hearing loss across unaided and seven amplification strategies. Because the adaptive speech level was relative to a fixed noise level of 65 dBA (HINT), the speech cues were audible enough even in the unaided condition. With the addition of amplification, these scores did not change significantly except when the signal processor reduced the bandwidth (ear trumpet) or introduced distortion (body aid). (Adapted from Bentler and Duve, 2000, with permission.)

POINTS TO PONDER: HOW NOISY ARE VARIOUS ENVIRONMENTS?

We all know that different environments carry different speech recognition challenges for our patients. For years we have relied on the data of Pearsons, Bennett, and Fidell (1977) to help us understand those environmental levels and the concomitant SNRs. Recently, Karolina Smeds (2015) and colleagues conducted related research; some of her findings are shown in Figures 15–5 and 15–6. Her intent was to inform the clinician (and researcher) better as to typical sound and noise levels in environments encountered by persons with hearing loss. Her results indicated that these potential hearing aid users rarely encounter environmental SNRs worse than 0 dB. This is in striking contrast to the SNRs that have been assumed from the earlier work of Pearsons et al. (1977). Smeds explains that in her analysis methodology, fairly short excerpts of noise and noisy speech were analyzed (typically one or a couple of sentences of the noisy speech) for each environment to create estimates of the speech and the noise signal. This estimation method might have led to higher/better estimated SNRs than if longer stretches of speech with more natural pauses had been used. In the Pearsons et al. data, recordings were made of "normal conversation" of at least 10 seconds in length. It is difficult to know how long the speech pauses could have been in these 10 seconds of speech. These investigators note that if two of the 10 seconds of speech contained pauses, their SNR estimation method would result in an SNR that was 1 dB higher than was actually encountered.

KEY CONCEPT: HOW BIG DOES AN SNR DIFFERENCE NEED TO BE TO BE MEANINGFUL?

As we provide examples of using speech recognition for hearing aid verification, we often talk about an aided improvement in the patient's SNR-50 (the point where they can recognize ~50% of the target speech signal). This improvement could simply be because we made speech (and noise) more audible, or it could be because directional technology or some other noise reduction strategy was employed. In research, if the sample size is fairly large, and the group variance is fairly small, it's possible that an SNR as small as 1 dB can be significant. That is, a manufacturer could claim that its new DNR system was significantly better than that of competitors if the group average improved from SNR = 4.0 dB to SNR = 3.0 dB. But how much difference really is necessary for an individual patient to notice? This recently was studied by McShefferty, Whitmer, and Akeroyd (2015) who found that, in the laboratory, the just-noticeable-difference (JND) for SNR tended to be about 3 dB and this value was not correlated with hearing loss level. In further study they looked at what size the SNR change would need to be for a patient to seek out such a product or to swap one device for another—in other words, big enough to prompt action. Their findings revealed . . . a 6-dB change! So although as audiologists we sometimes get excited about products that provide a 1 to 2 dB SNR benefit, it appears that our patients require something considerably more substantial. In the authors' words: "While an SNR increase of 3 dB may have relevance to speech-recognition performance, it may not be enough of an SNR improvement to be reliably recognized and, furthermore, may be too little increase to motivate potential (hearing aid) users."

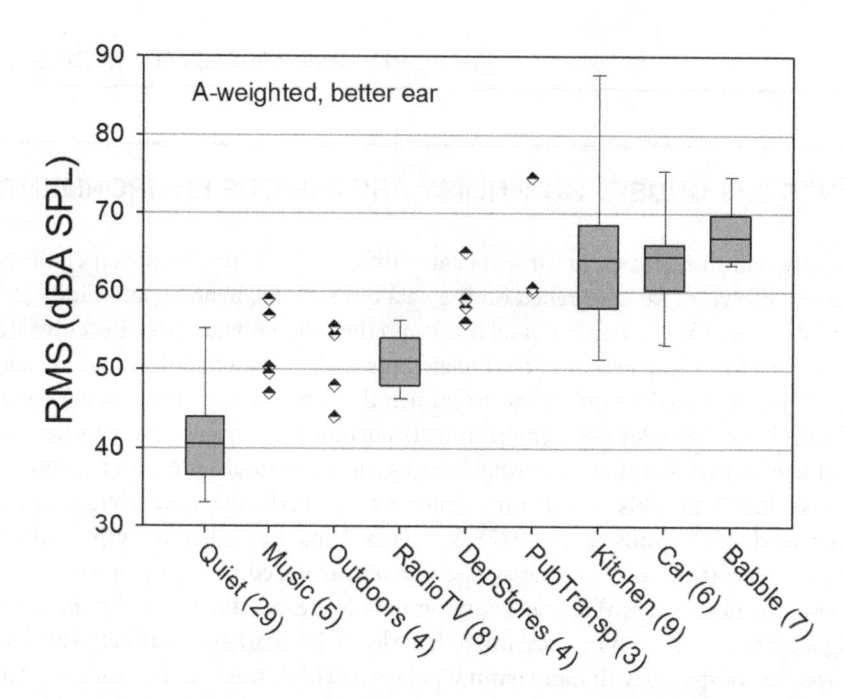

Figure 15–5. Long-term average RMS levels of the background noise at the better ear for each category of listening environment. For categories with five recordings or fewer, the actual RMS estimates are presented (*diamonds*), whereas boxplots are used for the categories with more than five recordings. The central mark in each boxplot shows the median across the recordings, the box the interquartile range, and the whiskers extend to the most extreme data points. The number in brackets after the category name gives the number of recordings in that category. (Adapted from Smeds, Wolters, and Rung, 2015.)

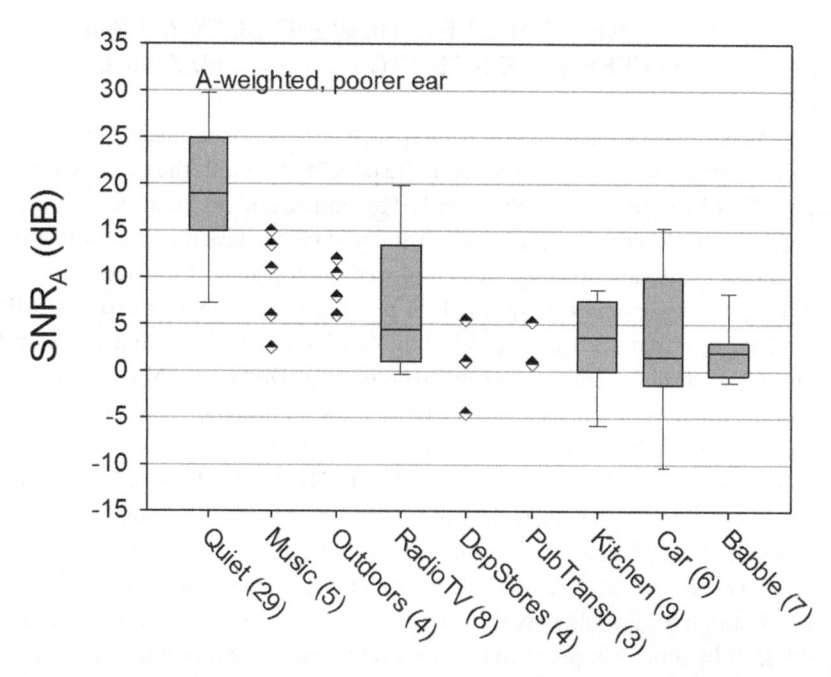

Figure 15–6. SNRs for the poorer ear for each of the noise categories. For noise categories with five recordings or fewer, the actual SNR estimates are plotted. For noise categories with more than five recordings, box plots are shown. The central mark in each boxplot shows the median across the recordings, the box the interquartile range, and the whiskers extend to the most extreme data points. The number in brackets after each noise category name gives the number of recordings in that category. (Adapted from Smeds, Wolters, and Rung, 2015.)

Telling a patient that a hearing aid provides a 6.4 dB SNR benefit is likely not very meaningful. Instead, for this application we ignore the recommended WIN scoring method and use the number correct to calculate a percentage for aided and unaided performance. We can then counsel EMP that her performance moved from 74% (26 of 35 correct) unaided to 97% (34 of 35 correct) aided, a hearing aid benefit of 23%.

Clinical Case 2A: Demonstrating Technology Aimed at Improving SNR

In some cases we might want to demonstrate that a technology aimed at improving SNR (directional microphones, beamformers, FM systems, companion microphones, etc.) can lead to improved speech recognition in noise. Many patients appreciate demonstrations of how a technology they have not used before may work for them. In addition, this demonstration can serve as a springboard to discuss the benefits and limitations of the technology in the real world, and strategies a patient can use to optimize benefit across all the different listening situations they are in.

This demonstration can be particularly useful with technologies such as directional microphones because we know this feature may be beneficial in some listening situations and provide little or no benefit in others. As it is for demonstration purposes only, we can perform a speech recognition test where speech is presented from the front and noise from a second loudspeaker placed behind the listener. It is important to note that there is not strong evidence that the magnitude of directional benefit measured in this manner relates to the magnitude of benefit in the real world; therefore, we do not suggest using this method to make decisions about directional microphone candidacy. Instead, this method can be useful for expectations counseling, as well as demonstrating feature success to patients. If a benefit is obtained, it is also efficacy documentation of the technology for that particular product.

A number of standardized tests that allow for the speech and noise to be separated can be used for this demonstration including the CST or the BKB-SIN (described in a later clinical case). Even the HINT described in the second example of this case could be used; however, we decided to use the QuickSIN, as it is efficient, well-researched, and probably the most popular standardized speech in noise test used among audiologists (see Chapter 6 for a complete description of this test and its use).

CMC is a 67-year-old male, a recent retiree, and a first-time hearing aid user. He arrived at the clinic with goals primarily related to understanding speech in noise. For example, one of his goals on the Client Oriented Scale of Improvement (COSI) was to understand his wife more clearly when they are at a noisy restaurant. His audiogram is shown in Figure 15–7. We decided to fit him with bilateral mini-BTE hearing aids with non-custom dome ear tips. Probe microphone results revealed that the outputs for real-speech signals were matched within 3 to 5 dB of desired prescriptive targets bilaterally.

In order to demonstrate the potential for directional benefit, speech recognition in noise testing was completed for omnidirectional and directional microphone modes using sentences presented in noise. We do this in a sound booth with the patient facing the speech loudspeaker directly (about 3–4 feet is a good distance) and a competing noise loudspeaker speaker about the same distance away, placed somewhere behind the listener (directly behind works fine, but some clinicians like to place the noise loudspeaker in the directional "null" to show as much benefit as possible, which may not be directly at 180 degrees). Since this is just a demonstration, and in no way predictive or representative of speech recognition benefits in the real world (either on average or on a single patient), the exact speaker configuration is not crucial. Using the QuickSIN, we present speech at 65 dBA to provide a level that is near conversational speech levels. We find that his score suggests an SNR loss of +6.5 dB in omnidirectional mode and +0.5 dB in directional mode (for this testing we recommend using the fixed directional mode, not the "automatic" setting). As described later in this section, if we instead score this as percentage correct (following administration of two lists; 60 key words), performance corresponds to 63% (38 of 60) and 83% (50 of 60) for the omnidirectional and directional modes, respectively. We use this percent correct data to counsel CMC that it appears he can benefit from the directional setting in noise.

We further counsel CMC that, even though he performs well in noise with his hearing aids, performance will be best if he applies a few strategies. For example, we inform him that he will maximize benefits from

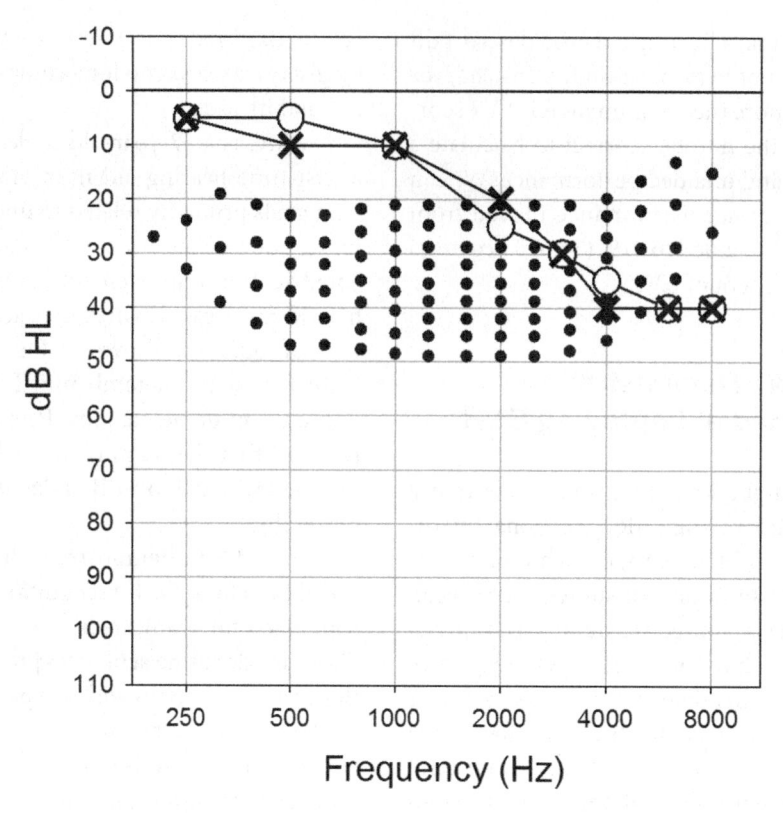

Figure 15–7. Audiogram for clinical case study of CMC.

directional hearing aids if he is able to face the talker of interest and position himself as close as possible. Finally, we let him know that the specific hearing aid he is fitted with will go into the directional mode automatically in noisy environments even if the talker of interest is behind him, but that in some specific cases, he may perform more poorly if he is unable to turn and face the talker. For these situations where understanding speech from a variety of azimuths is important, we provide him the ability to manually switch to a different program (perhaps using a smartphone app), which is a dedicated omnidirectional mode.

Graphing the QuickSIN for Patient Counseling

As we discussed with case study CMC, although patients usually notice improved performance with hearing aids when tested with the QuickSIN, the standard scoring does not lend itself to effective counseling. That is, telling someone that his QuickSIN score was lowered by 6 dB with his new (and expensive) hearing aids has little meaning to the average patient. Patients are accustomed to dealing with percent correct and percent change, so we find it helpful to score (and graph) the QuickSIN in percent for counseling purposes. We always use two lists, which means there are 10 key words presented at each of the six SNR levels, resulting in easy calculation of percent correct (no calculator required!).

We told you earlier that our patient had 63% correct for the unaided and 83% correct for the aided. Although this is meaningful to the patient, it is even more meaningful to graph out the scores for each of the six SNRs. We prefer to do this on a white board in the office, but it works just fine using paper and pen sitting knee-to-knee at your desk. Or, the more enterprising audiologist might use a simple computer program and display the findings on a 55-inch flat screen wall-mounted monitor. This patient's results for unaided and aided are displayed in Figure 15–8.

Having the performance distributed as a function of SNR allows us to relate these findings to the real

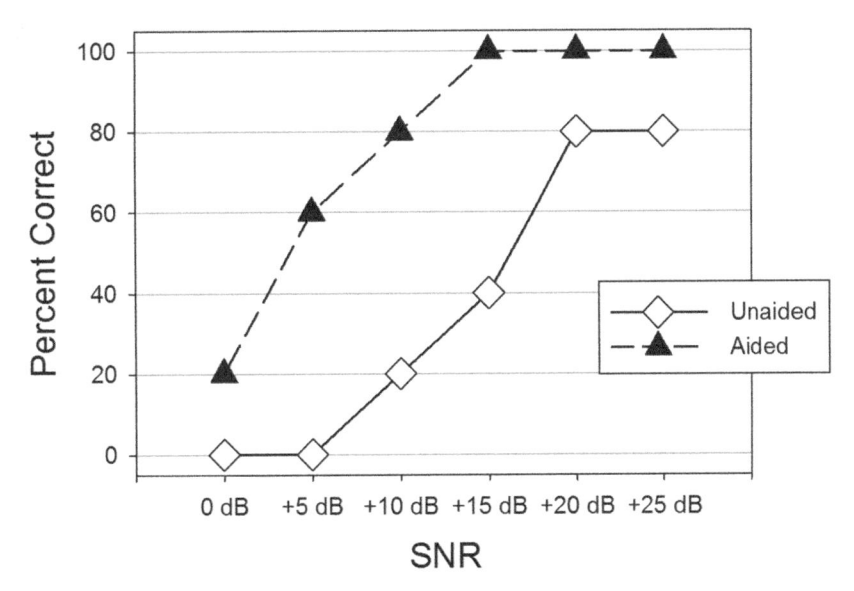

Figure 15-8. Worksheet showing patient scores as a function of the SNR for both the aided and the unaided conditions. Recall that testing was done with a soft speech level, so even if the scoring for the QuickSin is represented as SNR-loss, it is possible to see the percent correct across the various SNRs to show the result of increased audibility.

world. For example, notice that for the SNRs of +20, and +25 dB, directional technology didn't provide as much benefit as at poorer SNRs, as the patient was doing reasonably well for unaided (recall that we were using a 65 dB SPL input—loud enough to compensate for some audibility issues, at least enough for sentence recognition). Also note that the directional technology provided less benefit at 0 dB SNR. Why was this? Because the SNR improvement was not enough to overcome the SNR loss associated with cochlear pathology, and moreover, we are approaching the SNR when even normal-hearing individuals do not understand 100% for this listening condition. What we want to focus on in our counseling, however, is the improvement noted at the SNRs of +5, +10 and +15 dB. It may be useful to point out to the patient real-world situations where this SNR might be expected (see Figure 15-6 for examples).

Clinical Case 2B: Demonstrating Technology Aimed at Improving SNR

Another technology that improves SNR, and for which a demonstration using speech recognition testing can help with counseling, is wireless microphones, including FM systems. As with a directional microphone, the FM system may be very beneficial in some listening situations and provide little benefit in others. Furthermore, these systems are often fitted to children and the parents may appreciate a demonstration of potential benefits. We would not expect that the laboratory-measured FM benefit will directly relate to real-world performance, so we again perform this testing for demonstration purposes rather than for making candidacy decisions. Even though there are a variety of speech recognition in noise tests, the Pediatric Hearing in Noise Test (described for this example) and the BKB-SIN (described as part of a later case) are unique in that both avoid ceiling and floor effects due to their adaptive nature, can be presented with the target and competing sources sent to either the same or two different loudspeakers, and can also be used with patients who are children.

GPB is a 7-year-old boy with a bilateral, congenital, flat, moderate, sensorineural hearing loss. He is entering first grade and resources have just become available so that he may be fitted with an FM system to be used with his bilateral BTE hearing aids for the first time. His mother is very happy that a technology may help GPB understand the teacher better, but she does not want him to stand out more and does not understand when and how the technology works.

In order to demonstrate the potential for FM benefit, speech recognition in noise testing was completed for the hearing aids only (HA) and the hearing aids plus FM fittings (HA+FM) using sentences presented in noise. We do this in a sound booth with GPB facing the speech loudspeaker directly (about 3–4 feet is probably far enough away) and a competing noise loudspeaker directly behind him. Since this is just a demonstration, and not expected to be representative of speech recognition benefits in the real world (either on average or on a single patient), the exact speaker configuration is not crucial, but pointing out similarities to realistic environments can help patients with face validity.

In this case, we describe the situation to both GPB and his mother as roughly simulating a teacher in front of the class with noisy classmates behind. We let them know we will find the highest noise level for which GPB can still understand about half the sentences he will hear, which will be presented at a conversational speech level. We place the FM microphone seven inches from the speech presentation speaker and explain that this is approximately the distance the teacher will be from the microphone when worn around the neck. One list is usually adequate per condition, especially when used simply for demonstration purposes, as in this case. GPB is a little less reliable than many kids, however, so we decide to use two lists for both the HA and HA+FM fittings. Note that using two lists for the HINT-C works a bit differently than some other tests. Specifically, rather than repeating the same procedure twice and averaging the results, we simply continue testing using 20 sentences instead of 10.

After testing we see that GPB's RTS is +11 dB with his hearing aids and −2 dB when using the FM system, corresponding to a 13 dB FM benefit. We use these data to counsel the patient and his mother that it appears he can benefit greatly from the FM system in background noise. Furthermore, we continue counseling, emphasizing the point that since the teacher or other talker will wear the microphone around their neck, benefits will be present even when the teacher walks around. We point out that it is like moving the talker right next to GPB's ear, helping tremendously in noise. We continue by discussing how to best use, operate, and care for the FM system.

A Little About the Pediatric HINT

The Pediatric HINT was based on the development of the HINT test for adult listeners (see Chapter 6 for a review of the HINT and its use) and it is very similar to the original HINT. It was derived from the same base materials and even includes some very similar lists. This version ensures more limited language and can be used for children as young as five years of age. It includes 13 lists (plus three practice lists), considerably fewer than the 25 available HINT lists (Gelnett, Sumida, Nilsson, & Soli, 1995). The administration and scoring of the pediatric HINT is the same as for the HINT (see Chapter 6 for detailed guidelines). List 5 shown below is a sample of a 10-item word list from the HINT-C. Adapted from *HINT Manual Two*, from the House Ear Institute, are 10 sample sentences:

1. (A/The) boy did (a/the) handstand.
2. They took some food outside.
3. The young people (are/were) dancing.
4. (A/The) grocer sells butter.
5. The shirts (are/were) in (a/the) closet.
6. They watched (a/the) scary movie.
7. A tree fell on the house.
8. They went on vacation.
9. (A/The) girl (is/was) fixing her dress.
10. (A/The) baby broke the cup.

Clinical Case 3A: Demonstrating the Limitations of Performance in Noise

We find that information regarding the aided SNR threshold can be quite useful when counseling about realistic expectations for real-world hearing aid use. Often, this use may be in conjunction with demonstrating the benefits of SNR improvement technologies as described in the previous two cases and illustrated in the graphing of sample QuickSIN performance (see Figure 15–8). Sometimes, however, the information can be used to demonstrate limitations or even to help show a patient that additional assistive technologies may be necessary in order to achieve their communication goals. As we already described as part of Case 2A, counseling can be enhanced by examining performance while also considering the pre- and post-fitting completion of the COSI, which we discuss in detail in Chapter 19.

NTL is a 52-year-old first-time hearing aid user. He is an active hunter and has a long history of noise exposure. His audiogram is consistent with his history of prolonged noise exposure and is shown in Figure 15–9. Bilateral mini-BTE hearing aids with custom non-occluding eartips were selected. Probe microphone results revealed that target gain was matched within 3 to 5 dB to NAL-NL2 prescriptive targets through 2000 Hz. NTL expressed a strong interest in better understanding speech in background noise. His COSI listed as communication goals better understanding of his friends at work and being able to understand his wife at their favorite tavern. After probing these situations more, we estimated the SNR at his work setting to be approximately +10 dB and at the tavern to be approximately +0 to 2 dB. We fitted him with advanced directional microphone technology, and selected hearing aids that had the option of a wireless microphone input.

In order to demonstrate the potential benefits and limitations of his hearing aids, sentence recognition in noise testing was completed for the omnidirectional and directional microphone modes. Many adaptive tests, including the previously discussed QuickSIN, would be appropriate for this testing, but in this case we chose the BKB-SIN (see Chapter 6 for complete description of this test and its use). Similar to our previous cases, we completed this testing in a sound booth with the patient facing the speech loudspeaker and a competing noise loudspeaker directly behind him. Although we are trying to estimate potential benefits, we know we will only obtain a very rough estimate of real-world performance, which we plan to use for counseling.

In this case, we present speech at 65 dBA to provide a level that is near conversational speech levels for the situations of interest to the patient. NTL scores an SNR-50 of +12.5 dB in omnidirectional mode and +8.5 dB in directional mode, showing us a 4 dB advantage using the directional microphone technology. We could

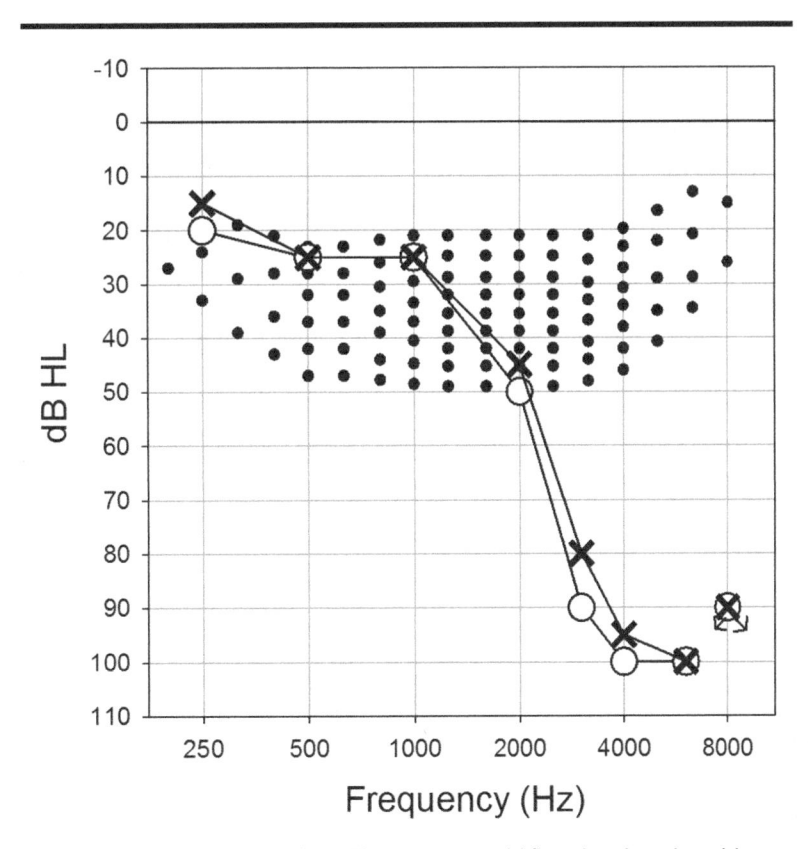

Figure 15–9. Audiogram for NTL, a 52-year-old first-time hearing aid user.

also calculate the percent correct for this patient using a method very similar to that described for the QuickSIN. Unlike the QuickSIN, however, the number of words in a BKB-SIN list will depend on the list number. Similar to Case #2A described earlier, we also use these data to point out limitations and suggest additional strategies.

In this example, we caution NTL that even with his directional hearing aids, he does not perform as well as a person with normal hearing (Table 15–3). When things get noisy enough, he will still have considerable difficulty understanding. We point out that, even with his directional hearing aids, he needs a much lower noise level relative to the level of the speech to even recognize 50% of the words. Moreover, the level at which he is scoring 50% correct here in the clinic, where the conditions are relatively controlled, is not nearly as adverse as he likely will experience in the tavern, where additional reverberation will make things even worse. We reinforce our previous counseling that he should try his hearing aids in a variety of noisy settings, but if he still has too much difficulty, a discreet wireless microphone that his wife can wear may improve things considerably, and allow him to better achieve his communication goals.

Clinical Case 3B: Demonstrating the Limitations of Hearing Aid Performance

Let's consider MNL, an 18-year-old college freshman with congenital severe-to-profound hearing loss. Her audiogram is shown in Figure 15–10. MNL primarily uses oral communication, and has decided against pursuing a cochlear implant at this time due to other medical complications. She is particularly interested in the newest hearing aid technologies and hopes they will help her even more with oral communication than her old power hearing aids that she wore for nearly eight years. She is entering college soon and is hopeful that the new technologies will help her understand instructors better in her college classrooms. Although she can communicate reasonably well one-on-one, visual cues are crucial and her aided speech recognition scores on the NU-6 presented at conversational levels are near 0%. We decided to fit her with super power BTE hearing aids with custom earmolds. Probe microphone results revealed a good fit to NAL-NL2 targets. In order to demonstrate the potential for hearing aid benefit related to improved audibility for at least some speech sounds, we test her aided and unaided hearing using the AV version of the CST. Because we know audibility will be very limited and speech recognition will be very challenging in general, we present the CST in quiet at 65 dBA (approximately average vocal effort) in the sound field. In this case the CST is calibrated as discussed for Case 1A; however, the CST DVD is presented using a DVD player and the video output is routed to a video monitor that is placed on top of the loudspeaker used to present the audio stimuli.

Even with the visual cues and knowledge of the topic, as is always the case when presenting the CST, MNL's unaided scores were fairly low at 24%. Her aided performance was significantly better at 84%. We used these data to counsel MNL that it appears the hearing aids really do provide considerable benefit to her speech reading abilities. We further counsel, however, that even with visual cues and clearly seeing the speakers face, she is unable to obtain all of the speech information in quiet. We therefore suggest that in addition to the hearing aids and a wireless microphone for the instructor, additional interventions will likely be required for her to achieve the best success possible in the classroom. Specifically, note taking or captioning-in-real-time (CART) services are recommended.

Table 15–3. BKB-SIN Test Norms

	Adults		Children by Age		
	Normal Hearing	CI Users	Ages 5–6	Ages 7–10	Ages 11–14
Mean SNR-50	–2.5	*	3.5	0.8	–0.9
Standard Deviation	0.8	1.6	2.0	1.2	1.1

Note. *Compare to normal-hearing adult value to determine SNR loss.
Source: From the BKB-SIN manual.

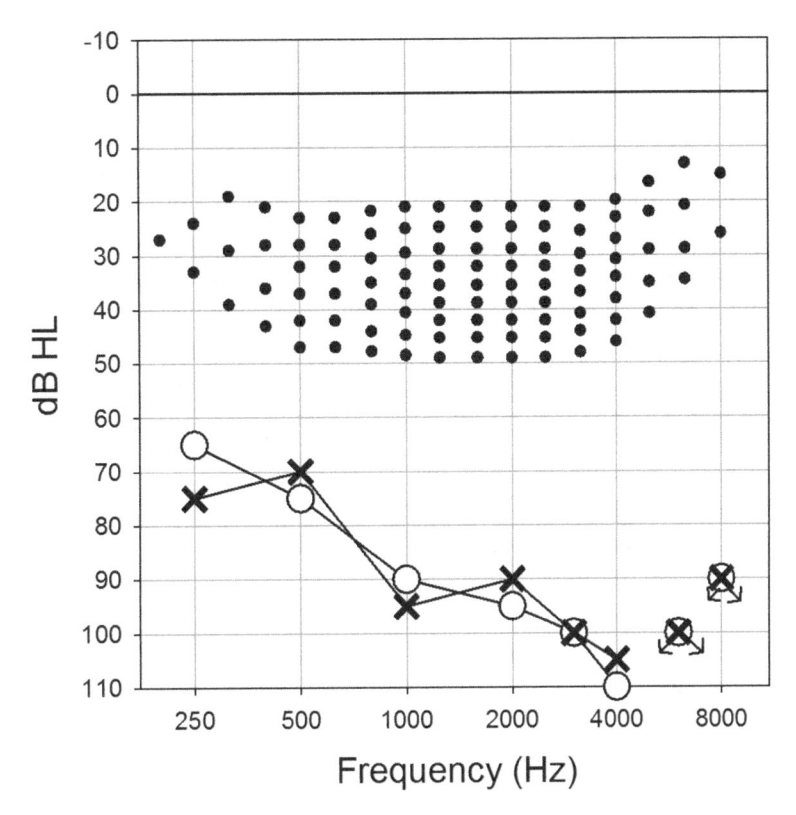

Figure 15–10. Audiogram for case study of MNL.

KEY CONCEPT: ARE TEST BOOTHS REQUIRED?

For most of the examples here, we have discussed doing the testing in an audiometric sound room. But recall that we are doing these aided speech recognition tests to demonstrate that hearing aids indeed do work and to assist us in counseling, which sometimes includes talking about situations in which hearing aids might not work very well for specific patients. Our point is that we are not doing this testing to determine whether an MRI is needed, determine fitness for duty, determine compensation, or anything else that might involve a medical-legal issue down the road. You probably won't enter these results into the patient's chart. Hence, it's just fine to conduct the testing in the hearing aid fitting room, assuming that some basic calibration is performed. In fact, this would add some face validity to the measures. It might be difficult to add a second loudspeaker to place behind the patient for directional demos, but you certainly could conduct most of these tests simply by presenting the speech and noise from the same loudspeaker located in front of the patient. This works well for aided versus unaided benefit, and for comparing aided performance to earphones scores and the performance of people with normal hearing.

Subjective Ratings of Intelligibility and Quality

Rating: Perhaps useful for specific patients.

We're moving on to yet another form of clinical verification that typically involves the use of speech material. It's something practiced by all audiologists fitting hearing aids—eliciting a response from the patient regarding the sound quality while indirectly measuring the patient's speech intelligibility when using the hearing instruments. The simple question, "How does that sound?" can produce a diverse range of responses: "great," "a little distorted," "rather tinny," "it's whistling," "what did you say?" We encourage communication with the patient during the fitting process, and talking about the sound quality and function of the hearing aids being fitted is certainly an excellent topic. And in fact, sometimes these casual conversations can lead to fitting improvements. What we are talking about in this section, however, is adding a bit of science and structure to the procedure, so that the patient's subjective comments potentially can be used to alter the fitting or to verify that the fitting doesn't need any changes.

If you choose to use some type of structured subjective ratings as verification, or as a supplement to other test procedures in your protocol, there are some things to think about. Here are three such considerations:

- If categorical scaling is used as the metric, and it often is, how do you know that the fitting is good enough (same issues we raised regarding speech recognition testing)? For example, when fitted to NAL-NL2 targets, the patient rates his speech understanding in noise a 7.5 (0 to 10 scale; 10= "understand everything"). Is this good? What if you increased gain the high frequencies by 5 dB? Might he then rate it an 8.0? Is 8.0 significantly different from 7.5 for this task? What rating is good enough for this patient? What rating do young normal-hearing individuals give for this speech-in-noise signal?
- The starting point—how the hearing aids are programmed—is important for all subjective ratings tasks for at least two reasons. First, if patients do not start off somewhat close to the "best" ending point, it may take a long time to find it or they may never settle at a good setting. For most hearing aid fittings, we have a reasonable idea about the acceptable boundaries for a given a patient. It would not be reasonable to take a person with a 40 dB to 80 dB downward sloping hearing loss and conduct judgments with the hearing aids set at 5 dB of gain. This takes us to the second point. If the purpose of the subjective judgments is to find the best settings, it will take some time, maybe more than typically allocated for a fitting in a busy clinic. Today's hearing aids are not like those of the 1980s (and before) when the only two listening options were putting the screwdriver controlled tone-control potentiometer on either "N" or "H." Starting with the programming close to the predicted end point (e.g., that prescribed by a prescriptive fitting algorithm) will speed up the process.
- Do the patients know what is best for them? Will they select what is best for them? This relates to our discussion in Chapter 12 regarding trainable hearing aids, which indirectly is a series of on-going subjective ratings conducted in the real world. So again, if indeed your verification procedure includes subjective ratings, and you alter the patient's fitting based on the results, then you must ask the question whether the patient is best served by allowing him or her to pick the amplification characteristics. This particularly can be a problem for new users when the task is "speech quality" ratings. We have found many cases in which, if you allow these patients to "drive" the fitting, they will select an amplification output that is not much greater than their own open ear canal response! And of course, they report that it sounds *normal*.

Conducting Meaningful Subjective Judgments

We've already mentioned some of the many limitations associated with relying on subjective judgments as a clinical validation tool, and our rating for this testing was no higher than "Perhaps useful for specific patients." With that said, we also must recognize that the average audiologist is fond of subjective ratings, to the extent

> **KEY CONCEPT: CLINICAL SUBJECTIVE RATINGS**
>
> If you believe that the patient's subjective ratings of speech material should be used to verify the fitting or assist in post-fitting adjustments, there are three general procedures that can be used. These ratings could be used for intelligibility, ease of listening, or speech/sound quality.
>
> - Magnitude Estimation. The patient assigns a given value to a speech stimulus which reflects the "goodness" of the signal based on the task assigned (e.g., intelligibility, quality).
> - Category Scaling. The patient is given a bounded scale (e.g., 0 = very unclear, 100 = very clear); multiple sequential categories (e.g. very soft, soft, OK, loud, too loud); or a bipolar rating (full versus thin) and makes a judgment at some point at or between the two extremes.
> - Paired Comparisons. Two different programmed settings (or hearing aids) are compared directly. The patient must choose one or the other based on some qualitative dimension (e.g., speech understanding, sound quality). Usually a forced-choice paradigm is preferred, but adding the optional response of "no difference" is also sometimes used.

that they are the only validation method used by many audiologists. So it is probably worthwhile to provide a few examples of how these judgments could be used to obtain at least somewhat meaningful information.

Before we get started, we will remind you of one more caution which we discussed earlier in this text—the placebo effect. That is, your patients can be influenced very easily by how you present the hearing aids or features that are being compared. Specifically, a number of studies have shown just labeling something "new" or "digital" or "advanced" can have a strong effect on subjective preference, even if the exact same intervention is used. Keep this in mind when conducting any type of subjective comparative testing.

Categorical, Ordinal, or Interval Scale?

For purposes of clinical demonstration, most audiologists have not concerned themselves with the statistics of scaling tools. There is no real reason to start now unless the "data" obtained in the clinical setting end up being analyzed. This might be done for a variety of reasons including comparing a new feature against an older design or comparing sound quality with different signal processing schemes. A *categorical* variable (sometimes called a nominal variable) is one that has two or more categories, but there is no intrinsic ordering to the categories. For example, hair color is a categorical variable with a number of categories (blonde, brown, brunette, red, etc.), and there is no agreed way to order these from highest to lowest. A pure categorical variable is one that simply allows you to assign categories, but you cannot clearly order the variables. If the variable has a clear ordering, then that variable would be an ordinal variable, as described below. An ordinal variable is similar to a categorical variable. The difference between the two is that there is a clear ordering of the variables with ordinal variables.

In the world of hearing aids—particularly when attempting to assess sound quality, loudness, or even overall goodness of a hearing aid fitting scheme—we often ask our patients to rate the hearing aid on one of these variables. That rating scale could be from 1 to 7, 1 to 10, 0 to 100, and so on. Assigning anchors—or categories—to the end points of those numbers often carries more meaning to the patient completing the task. As a result, there are many examples of categorical scaling tools being used in labs and clinics.

The advantage of categorical scaling is that you can add different terms to the end points, which allows for testing several different factors: speech understanding, quality, own voice, background noise, music, and so forth. One tool that we have used in both our clinic and laboratory settings is derived from the early work of Alf Gabrielsson in Sweden (Figure 15–11). The actual definitions of the attributes we are assessing (e.g., fullness or spaciousness) can be left to the patient or described and defined prior to the testing. Remember, we want to *know how our current patient is reacting to our fitting decisions*—we are not collecting data for later analysis. The instructions for the assessment process are captured below (Gabrielsson, Schenkman, & Hagerman, 1988):

> Your task is to judge the sound quality. You shall now try to describe sounds by means of scales that you see on the response form. The scales refer to various properties of the sound reproduction. They are graded from 10 (maximum) to 0 (minimum). You decide on the accuracy that you consider necessary. The integers 9, 7, 5, 3, and 1 on the response form are defined. For instance in the scale for clarity, 10 means maximum (highest possible) clarity, 9 means very clear, and 0 minimum clarity.
>
> The scales are described as follows:
>
> - Softness. The reproduction sounds soft and gentle, in opposition to sharp, hard, keen, and shrill.
> - Brightness. The reproduction sounds bright, in opposition to dull and dark.
> - Clarity. The reproduction sounds clear, distinct, and pure. The opposite is that the sound is diffuse, blurred, thick, and the like.
> - Fullness. The reproduction sounds full, in opposition to thin.
> - Nearness. The sound seems to be close to you, in opposition to at a distance.
> - Loudness. The sound is loud, in opposition to soft (faint).
> - Spaciousness. The reproduction sounds open and spacious, in opposition to closed and shut up.
> - Total impression. An overall judgment of how good you think the reproduction is.

The patient is placed in the sound field and the chosen stimuli presented from the speaker or speakers. You will want to select a couple speech passages—speech in quiet and speech in background noise. We would use a speech babble with a 5 to 10 dB SNR. It is possible that you might want to develop some sort of clinic norms from satisfied hearing aid users for your material using this scale. Let's say that your norms are 8.5 for speech in quiet and 7.5 for speech in background noise. If you receive ratings at or near these levels you could grade your fitting as "okay." What if you had a patient who gave a "4" rating for speech in background noise? Not good, but why did it happen? You first would have to determine this patient's expected performance for this SNR. You could base this somewhat from his audiogram, but the best comparison would be to look at his QuickSIN or WIN score (or whatever test you used) under earphones. If earphone testing indicated he should be performing fairly well at this level, then reprogramming of the hearing aids would be the reasonable course of action.

Another method of assessing sound quality is to use what are called bipolar scales. The classic scales of this type were bipolar adjective pairs, first published by Alf Gabriellson in 1979. Again, you would want to have clinic norms for this scale from satisfied hearing aid users. In general, it would seem that a "good" fitting would be ratings at the midpoint, although this may not always be true. For example, in Figure 15–12, it is possible that there is no right answer for some of the pairs like loud/soft or near/far.

A similar type of scaling could be conducted using a chart labeling "0" as the midpoint with the values going to the left and right representing degree of superiority (Figure 15–13). A chart like this could also be used for clinical paired-comparison testing, and the end points could be labeled "A" and "B" to reflect two different fitting possibilities for our patient (in this case you would have positive numbers on both sides of the zero midpoint). For example, consider a fitting for a patient with a steeply sloping hearing loss whose audiogram drops to a severe loss at 3000 Hz and above. Some audiologists might fit hearing aids with frequency lowering for this patient. After using your probe microphone equipment to optimize audibility for the lowered speech signals, you might want to conduct some subjective measures. In this case, we would place the frequency-lowered settings in Program 2 and the standard NL2 fitting in Program 1. We would label the two programs A and B, and switch back and forth while the patient is judging the clarity of speech, the background noise, and his or her overall listening satisfaction. For each stimulus the patient could rate his or her preference for either A or B. (*Hint*: Do not consistently label one of the programs A or B but randomly switch the labeling).

Example

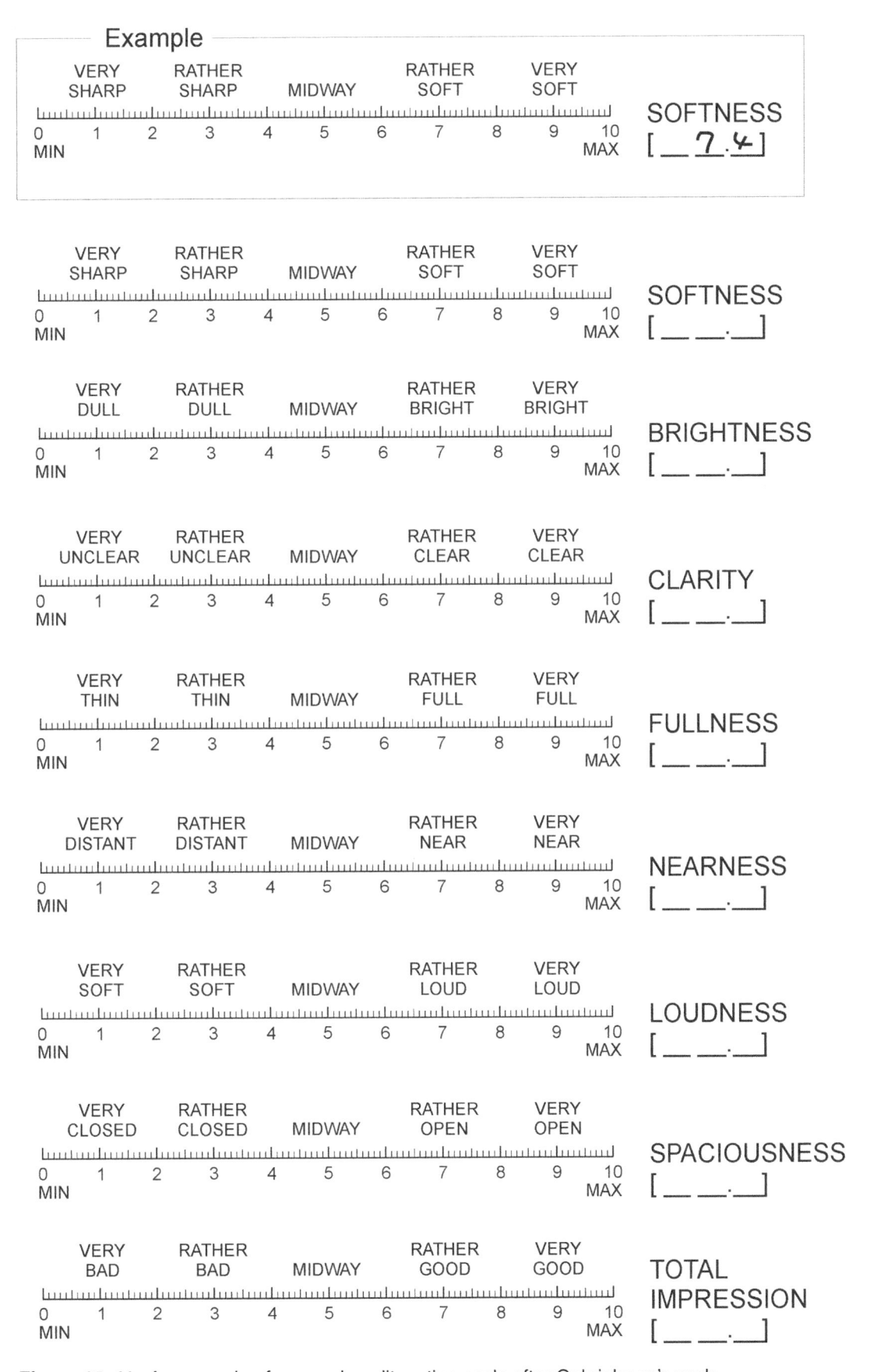

VERY SHARP	RATHER SHARP	MIDWAY	RATHER SOFT	VERY SOFT	
0　1　2　3　4　5　6　7　8　9　10 MIN　　　　　　　　　　　　　　　　　　MAX					SOFTNESS [_7.4_]

| VERY SHARP | RATHER SHARP | MIDWAY | RATHER SOFT | VERY SOFT | SOFTNESS [__.__] |

| VERY DULL | RATHER DULL | MIDWAY | RATHER BRIGHT | VERY BRIGHT | BRIGHTNESS [__.__] |

| VERY UNCLEAR | RATHER UNCLEAR | MIDWAY | RATHER CLEAR | VERY CLEAR | CLARITY [__.__] |

| VERY THIN | RATHER THIN | MIDWAY | RATHER FULL | VERY FULL | FULLNESS [__.__] |

| VERY DISTANT | RATHER DISTANT | MIDWAY | RATHER NEAR | VERY NEAR | NEARNESS [__.__] |

| VERY SOFT | RATHER SOFT | MIDWAY | RATHER LOUD | VERY LOUD | LOUDNESS [__.__] |

| VERY CLOSED | RATHER CLOSED | MIDWAY | RATHER OPEN | VERY OPEN | SPACIOUSNESS [__.__] |

| VERY BAD | RATHER BAD | MIDWAY | RATHER GOOD | VERY GOOD | TOTAL IMPRESSION [__.__] |

Figure 15–11. An example of a sound quality rating scale after Gabrielsson's work.

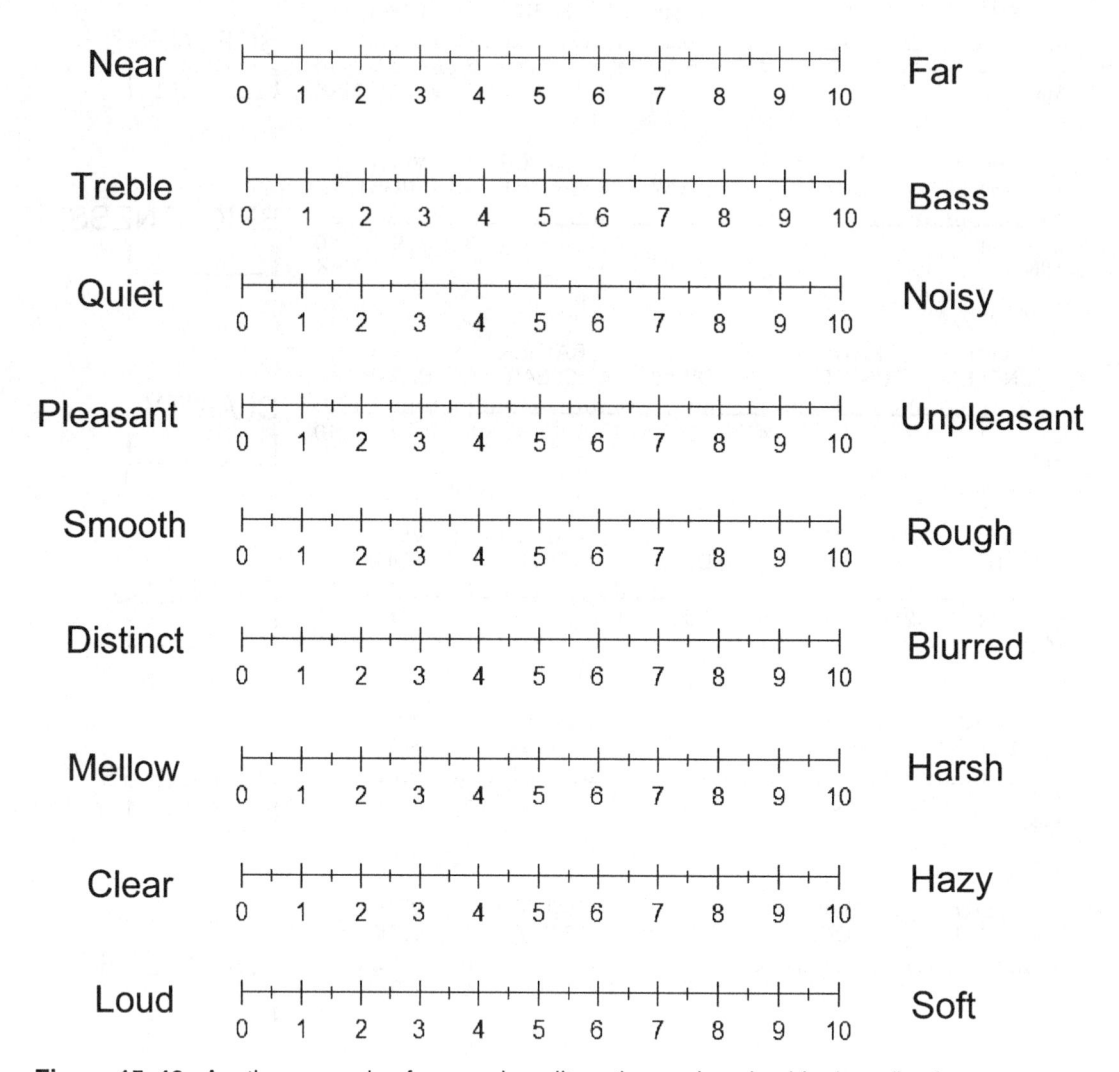

Near	0 1 2 3 4 5 6 7 8 9 10	Far
Treble	0 1 2 3 4 5 6 7 8 9 10	Bass
Quiet	0 1 2 3 4 5 6 7 8 9 10	Noisy
Pleasant	0 1 2 3 4 5 6 7 8 9 10	Unpleasant
Smooth	0 1 2 3 4 5 6 7 8 9 10	Rough
Distinct	0 1 2 3 4 5 6 7 8 9 10	Blurred
Mellow	0 1 2 3 4 5 6 7 8 9 10	Harsh
Clear	0 1 2 3 4 5 6 7 8 9 10	Hazy
Loud	0 1 2 3 4 5 6 7 8 9 10	Soft

Figure 15–12. Another example of a sound-quality rating scale using bipolar adjectives.

Clarity of Speech

|—+—+—+—+—+—+—+—+—+—+—+—+—+—+—+—+—+—+—+—|
-5   -4   -3   -2   -1   0   1   2   3   4   5

Extremely Unclear   Extremely Clear

Background Noise

|—+—+—+—+—+—+—+—+—+—+—+—+—+—+—+—+—+—+—+—|
-5   -4   -3   -2   -1   0   1   2   3   4   5

Significant Noise   Minimal Noise

Overall Satisfaction

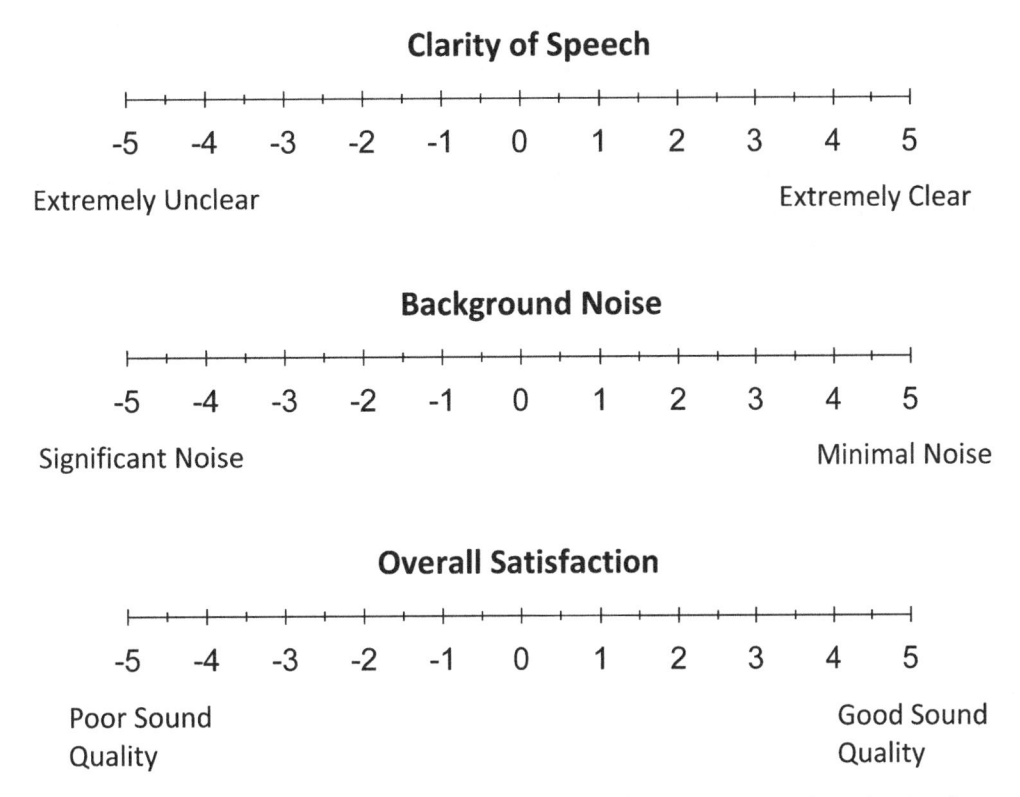

|—+—+—+—+—+—+—+—+—+—+—+—+—+—+—+—+—+—+—+—|
-5   -4   -3   -2   -1   0   1   2   3   4   5

Poor Sound   Good Sound
Quality   Quality

Figure 15–13. An example of a scaling score sheet for testing speech understanding, sound quality, and/or overall satisfaction.

POINTS TO PONDER: NORMATIVE DATA APPLIED TO CATEGORICAL SCALING

The importance of understanding the "norms" for a categorical scaling task was illustrated in a study by Palmer, Bentler, and Mueller (2006b). These authors, in evaluating a new DNR algorithm, used a Noise Annoyance scale with 10 being "not annoying at all" and 0 being "very annoying." The stimuli were traffic and dinner noise. Unaided, the 49 hearing-impaired participants had a mean annoyance rating of 7.0 to 7.4 for the two signals. When fitted bilaterally with the hearing aids and DNR set to "max," the annoyance ratings dropped (got worse) and were now averaging around 4.5. On the surface, not a good omen for the new DNR algorithm. The authors, however, also had a group of young normal-hearing individuals perform the same task. Their ratings? The same as for the hearing-impaired group when they were aided and using DNR—in other words, the hearing-impaired group were actually hearing like normal-hearing individuals. Having data such as this to calibrate the scale altered the interpretation of the findings. All clinical scales need some type of calibration or norming so that ratings provided by an individual patient are meaningful.

> **TECHNICAL TIP: AUDITORY MEMORY MATTERS**
>
> It often is tempting to allow the patient to become involved in the fitting process, and have them informally provide their opinions about the changes that you are making to the fitting. This is especially true on a post-fitting visit when things aren't going too well. After making an alteration in the software, audiologists frequently ask the question: Does this sound better? It is important to remember, however, that unless you switch rapidly between two different programmed settings (e.g., within 2–3 seconds), the patient's auditory memory will not be sufficient to make a reliable judgment.

Aided Loudness Judgments

Rating: Useful for most patients.

A general goal of almost all hearing aid fittings is to restore normal or near-normal loudness perceptions for the hearing-impaired patient. That is, when the patients are wearing their hearing aids, soft sounds should be audible, average sounds should be comfortable, and loud sounds should be loud but not too loud (see Mueller, 1999, for review). In Chapter 10 we discuss the popularity of low-threshold compression, and how it is related to this general fitting goal. In most hearing aid wearers, it would be impossible to accomplish the remapping of different inputs with linear amplification. We also discuss in Chapter 14 that, to some extent, prescriptive fitting algorithms are geared toward loudness normalization, although a *true* loudness normalization approach tends to result in too much gain in the low frequencies for most patients, and compression ratios that are too high. In general, our initial approach for providing appropriate loudness for speech is to measure hearing thresholds and then program the hearing aids based on these thresholds to a validated prescriptive method. Verification is probe microphone measures—but these values are not directly related to the patient's loudness perceptions.

A related, and perhaps more important issue regarding loudness, is testing to ensure that the frequency-specific hearing aid MPO is set correctly and that outputs do not exceed the individual patient's LDLs. In general, our approach to accomplish this is to first measure frequency-specific LDLs, and then use these values to set the MPO accordingly (via adjusting AGCo kneepoints) for the different frequency channels (see Chapter 5). As we describe in Chapter 17, verification is through probe microphone measures, by comparing the REAR-85 for a swept tone to the patient's LDLs—but again, these values are not directly linked to loudness perceptions.

The Need for Behavioral Aided Loudness Measures

If prescriptive gain has been achieved and verified with probe microphone measures, and the MPO has been set correctly based on the patient's LDLs and REAR-85 testing, one might question why it is still necessary to include aided loudness testing as part of the hearing aid verification process. There are several reasons for this additional testing:

- Average values. Regarding soft and average inputs, prescriptive gain targets are for the average patient. Even though these values typically place the amplified speech signal at or near the patient's preferred loudness levels, adjustments are needed for some patients.
- Measurement errors. Regarding the MPO settings, errors in the earphone LDL assessment are possible, which would influence AGCo settings. If the manufacturer's default MPO settings were used, or if earphone LDLs were not obtained, then the need for behavioral aided LDL testing is even more critical.
- Monaural summation. Previous testing involved pure-tone stimuli. The monaural summing of broadband signals such as speech varies from individual to individual.

- Binaural (bilateral) summation. At this point in the overall fitting process, behavioral testing only has been conducted monaurally. Summation has been accounted for in the prescriptive method (see Chapter 14), but again, these are average values and summation could vary by 5 dB or more among different individuals. The bilateral LDL may not be too different from the unilateral one, but it remains important to account for this.
- Channel summation. There is a summing of the signal when multiple channels are used in the processing that occurs with all modern instruments. The exact degree varies depending on the number of channels, how much they overlap, and the settings of the instrument; therefore, this also is difficult to predict.

All of these factors have the potential to affect loudness perceptions with hearing aids, or to cause bilateral aided judgments for speech to differ from what would be predicted based on unilateral earphone testing using pure tones. We know that nearly 50% of patients are not satisfied with the loudness of their hearing aids (Kochkin, 2010). This tells us that aided loudness testing and related MPO adjustment are well worth the clinical time investment.

Conducting Aided Loudness Testing

Before conducting the aided loudness testing you will need two tools discussed in Chapter 5 that were used for the unaided earphone LDL measures: the Cox Contour Anchors (see Figure 5–6) and the written instructions for the loudness rating task (see Figure 5–7). The next step is to ensure that your equipment is calibrated—consider that for this testing we will be focusing on SPL values, not HL values. Loudness verification can be conducted in an audiometric test booth via the soundfield speakers, or in the hearing aid fitting room using some other sound source. We will start off with a protocol for conducting the testing in a test booth (adapted from Mueller and Hall, 1998):

- Obtain an SLM (inexpensive models will work just fine for this measure).
- Set the audiometer dial to a fixed HL value (e.g., 50 dB HL) and present speech via the loudspeaker. Almost any recorded, calibrated speech signal will likely work, but we recommend a continuous discourse passage—CD recordings are available from Auditec of St. Louis, Missouri.
- Place the SLM at the presumed location of the patient's head. Observe the average levels of the peaks of speech with the SLM set to "linear" weighting (e.g., for the 50 dB HL signal, the peaks of speech might be measured to be in the 66–68 SPL range).
- The correction values for "average speech" will be 2 to 3 dB below the noted peak level. If the peaks were 68 dB SPL, we would then predict the average speech signal to be around 65 dB SPL.
- Subtract the HL value from the soundfield SPL value and you will have a correction factor for all presentation levels: 65 minus 50 = 15. Therefore, for this example, for loudness testing you know that you would use 30 dB HL (45 dB SPL; soft), 50 dB HL (65 dB SPL; average), and 70 dB HL (85 dB HL; loud). These corrections would be easy to remember, but usually the numbers don't work out quite as well—if you had measured peaks of 72 dB SPL, which would give you an overall level of 69 dB SPL, the correction factor would have been 19 dB, and the presentation levels would be 26, 46, and 66 dB HL.
- Fit the hearing aids to the patient and set at projected "use gain." Provide the patient with the Loudness Anchors and read the Cox instructions. Most patients will remember the procedure from the previous unaided loudness testing.
- Present the soft speech signal (45 dB SPL)
  - Desired rating: #2 (Soft)
  - Acceptable ratings: #1 (Very Soft) or #3 (Comfortable, But Slightly Soft)
- Present the average speech signal (65 dB SPL)
  - Desired rating: #4 (Average)
  - Acceptable ratings: #3 (Comfortable, But Slightly Soft) or #5 (Comfortable, But Slightly Loud).

- Present the loud speech signal (85 dB SPL)
  - Desired rating: #6 (Loud, But Okay)
  - Acceptable rating: #5 (Comfortable, But Slightly Loud).
- For any judgments that do not fall into the acceptable range, conduct intuitive tweaking and repeat judgment. Most manufacturers provide easy-to-use tabs in the fitting software for this purpose. Our experience has been that many patients, especially new users, tend to be a little startled by the 85 dB SPL input, which prompts them to assign it a #7 rating. We suggest that before making programming changes, repeat the testing for this level a couple times after providing a little more instruction: Was it truly uncomfortable or was it just startling or annoying? Many times, once the patient is aware the signal will be produced and are prepared, the rating is a #6—Loud, But Okay.

Conducting Loudness Judgments Outside of the Test Booth

In our previous example, we discussed how you would use an audiometer to conduct aided loudness testing in your audiometric test booth. This setting is efficient for producing the different signals at desired levels in a controlled setting, but it is not very practical. It is possible that the results of this testing will indicate that programming changes must be made, and this needs to be done efficiently. What works best, therefore, is to conduct this testing at the fitting site with the patient's hearing aids attached to the programming cables, so that immediate changes and retesting can be conducted. This means that the patient must be sitting in the fitting area, not the test booth, and a different sound source must be used. Here are three ways to evaluate aided loudness outside the test booth:

1. Use probe microphone equipment. Probe microphone equipment produces real speech and/or speech-like sounds that work well for loudness judgments. Moreover, the monitor microphone of the probe microphone system can then be used to calibrate each signal at the ear to the desired presentation level. Some probe microphone systems also have environmental sounds that can be used or, if PC-based, allow for different wave files to be added.
2. Use the fitting software. Most fitting software from the manufacturer also will have signals that can be used for loudness measures using external speakers attached to the laptop. A sound-level meter can be used to ensure that the signals are presented at the desired intensity. Or, if this is conducted during probe microphone testing, the probe microphone equipment can be configured (at least in most systems) to act as a SLM by placing the tip of the probe tube near the inlet for the monitor microphone, as one would do for probe tube calibration.
3. Use a portable music player/CD player. Another method that easily can be used to conduct aided loudness measures outside of the test booth is to

---

TECHNICAL TIP: UNILATERAL OR BILATERAL LOUDNESS TESTING?

In a perfect world, we would first do aided behavioral loudness testing for each ear individually, make gain and output changes if necessary, and then conduct the testing again with the patient aided bilaterally. In this way we could first correct for any measurement errors, and address issues related to the patient being different from the average for monaural summation and preferred gain. The impact of binaural summation could then subsequently be assessed. Although this approach is ideal, it does require more time; therefore unilateral loudness testing is usually skipped and only aided bilateral measures are conducted. This does have some face validity, as we assume the patient will most commonly be using both hearing aids. The downside is that if there is a problem, how do you know if it's being caused by the right hearing aid, the left hearing aid, or both? The patient can sometimes help with this, but not always.

> **KEY CONCEPT: OPEN FITTINGS AND LOUDNESS MEASURES**
>
> We are reminded of an interesting case regarding aided loudness judgments for a patient fitted with open earmolds. The student clinician was dutifully conducting aided LDL testing using the Cox Contour Anchors (she had not conducted REAR-85 measures when she conducted the probe microphone prescriptive verification—more on that in a moment). When the 85dB-SPL "obnoxious noise" signal was presented, the patient indicated it was a #7 on the loudness chart (Uncomfortably Loud), meaning that an MPO programming change was warranted. The student appropriately reduced the MPO (AGCo kneepoints) for the peak frequency of the stimulus by 5 dB (this is why knowing the location of the peaks of different noise stimuli is important), and repeated the testing. The rating was still a #7. Another 5 dB reduction took the AGCo kneepoints to their lowest level. Again, a #7 rating from the patient. At this point, the fitting screen showed that the kneepoint was lower than the input signal, yet the patient's loudness perceptions were not changing. What was going on? This prompted a move back to the probe microphone equipment to see what was happening regarding ear canal SPL. Even though the fitting screen was showing a lowering of the AGO kneepoints, maybe this wasn't really happening? The REAR-85 for this noise signal showed a peak around 103 dB SPL, which indeed exceeded this patient's lower-than-average LDL for this frequency. But the AGCo setting should have kept the output around 95 dB SPL. It was then that we had an "aha!" moment. We turned the hearing aid off and conducted another REAR-85: exactly the same as the previous one with the hearing aid turned on. So what we were seeing was the patient's REUG (which was larger than average) added to the input signal. Lesson learned: When conducting behavioral loudness testing don't forget about the signal going through the open ear canal—a quick REOR will tell the true story!

use a portable music player (MP3, iPod, or even a cell phone) or CD player with an external speaker system. This easily can be set up in any clinic, and often is used when probe microphone equipment isn't available. With this system you will need tracks containing continuous discourse and a variety of everyday environmental noises (see related Technical Tip). CDs containing the necessary material are available from Auditec of St. Louis, Missouri, and there are various online resources for obtaining digital materials. An inexpensive SLM is needed to assure the correct levels at the ear of the patient.

Verification of MPO

We have discussed the aided verification procedures for assessing loudness perceptions for soft, average, and loud inputs. This usually is accomplished using speech or speech-like materials. For some patients, however, the primary interest simply is to ensure that loud sounds are not uncomfortably loud. For this testing, we suggest the use of loud obnoxious noises. By obnoxious noises we mean everyday sounds such as a door slamming, toilet flushing, baby crying, dog yapping, dishes clattering, and so forth. There are two reasons for using these types of signals. First, some of the noises are composed of relatively narrow bands—this will drive the hearing aid to a higher MPO than a broadband signal such as speech. Secondly, the quality of the signal can impact the LDL; LDLs tend to be lower for noises that are not pleasant to listen to (see review in Chapter 5). In the clinic, on the day of the fitting and verification, we typically want to create a worst case scenario so that the patient has no unpleasant surprises when he or she starts using the hearing aids in everyday settings.

The following is a step-by-step procedure for conducting this testing. The example we describe below is using a portable sound delivery system; signal calibration is, of course, even easier when using your probe microphone equipment.

> ### TECHNICAL TIP: SPECIAL CD FOR LOUDNESS VERIFICATION
>
> As we've discussed, using speech signals presented from the probe microphone system is the most efficient method to verify aided loudness perceptions. For a variety of reasons, this is not always possible, and some clinicians, therefore, use a portable music player to produce the required signals. If indeed the goal is to ensure that soft, average, and loud sounds are appropriate, this requires considerable repeated soundfield measures and adjustments to assure that the signals are 45, 65, and 85 dB at the ear of the patient. But there is a much easier way to do this—order a CD from Auditec of Saint Louis, Missouri, and ask for the following:
>
> - Track 1: Calibration tone.
> - Track 2: Continuous discourse recorded 20 dB below the level of the calibration tone.
> - Track 3: Continuous discourse at the level of the calibration tone.
> - Track 4: Continuous discourse recorded 20 dB above the level of the calibration tone.
> - Tracks 5–10: Obnoxious noises recorded 20 dB above the level of the calibrations tone.
>
> Using a CD configured such as this then only requires one soundfield measure—setting the calibration tone to 65 dB SPL. If the portable system is only used for this purpose, and the volume control is not changed, then it's a simple matter of turning it on and selecting the appropriate tracks for each patient. To save some desk space you can rip these tracks to your computer or personal music player for presentation instead.
>
> *Source:* Auditec of St. Louis, Missouri; (314) 781-8890

Step 1. Before conducting the test, calibrate the test signal. This is done by placing the SLM approximately 1 m from the speaker (at the place of the patient's head) and setting the volume of the system so that the reading on the SLM reaches 85 dBA (peaks around 88 dB for linear setting).

Step 2. Place the patient 1 m from the speaker while wearing the hearing aids (fitted bilaterally) with the gain adjusted a little higher than his or her "average use level"—we want to account for the possibility that the patient will tend to use slightly more gain as he or she becomes accustomed to the amplification.

Step 3. Provide the patient with the Cox Loudness Anchors and read the patient the instructions. We typically emphasize the fact that the signals will be loud and annoying, but that he or she should decide when they are "okay" or if they indeed are "uncomfortable."

Step 4. One by one, present several obnoxious noises to the patient, and have him or her rate the loudness level on the Cox scale. Patients should rate the noise as #6 on the chart. If the patient rates a given noise as #7 (and this is verified on retest), the output (AGCo kneepoint) of the hearing aids (or at least one hearing aid) needs to be adjusted downward. If the peak of the noise signal is known, adjust only the AGCo for this frequency region.

Step 5. Following the AGCo adjustment, repeat testing until a consistent #6 rating is obtained. If this cannot be obtained using the AGCo setting, it might be necessary to make the compression ratio larger for the WDRC—this is termed "gain for loud sounds" in most fitting software.

Here are a few caveats:

- We mention using different noise signals. These noise signals will have different spectra, and it is useful to use signals that differ in spectrum. How do you know the spectrum?

A simple procedure is to simply configure your probe microphone signal to act as a spectrum analyzer (e.g., Live Voice for many systems). Grab a colleague over lunch, place the probe assembly on the ear with the probe tip at the regulating microphone, and play the different noise signals to the individual with the equipment set in the appropriate measurement mode. You will see on the monitor a graphic representation of the spectrum of each noise, which can be printed and used for future reference.

- As discussed in the associated Technical Tip, for open fittings, when a #7 rating persists after lowering the MPO, it is important to assure that the *unaided signal* is not uncomfortably loud—simply conduct testing with the hearing aid turned off to check for this.
- Whereas we normally are concerned that loud sounds are too loud, you might also consider changing the programming for the patient who has a #5 rating for the 85 dB SPL input signals that should be perceived as #6. While "loud sounds too soft" does not seem to lead to the same rate of hearing aid rejection as "loud sounds too loud," there is little reason not to use all of the patient's residual dynamic range. In our experience, when the patient has lower-than-average ratings, it is usually because of an aggressive WDRC setting and is unrelated to the AGCo. A few mouse clicks and probe measures will quickly tell you if it is the input or output compression that is controlling the MPO.

Listening Effort and Fatigue

Rating: Newer, but potentially useful—Methods to Watch.

Speech recognition abilities are typically viewed as paramount when considering receptive communication

---

KEY CONCEPT: MPO VERIFICATION— NUTS, BOLTS, AND MARBLES!

Every now and then we hear someone say: "I'd really like to do that testing, but I don't have the equipment." If the testing in question is MPO verification, Robyn Cox has the low-tech solution, which she outlined in her 2009 paper titled: "Verification and What to Do Until Your Probe Microphone System Arrives."

To try out this low-tech approach, you need to collect a few materials that will allow you to generate loud sounds of different types. Cox calls hers the HARL obnoxious noise kit or HONK, which consists of two noisemakers that are easy to construct and probably costs no more than $20.00. The first is a 12-ounce metal coffee can with a plastic lid containing three ¾-inch × 1½-inch hex-head bolts and four ⅝-inch hex nuts. You hold the coffee can by the ends and shake it. According to Cox, this makes a flat-spectrum, broadband noise of about 80 dB SPL with peaks about 100 dB SPL.

The second noisemaker is a pair of 16-ounce glass jars (canning jars work well) and about two dozen small glass marbles. You hold the glass jars around the tops and pour the marbles back and forth between them in a stream. Cox reports that this makes a high frequency noise with spectral peaks in the range of 5000 to 10,000 Hz, and a level around 100 dB SPL with peaks up to about 115 dB SPL.

The verification procedure is simple: Stand in front of the patient and activate the given noisemaker for about 10 to 15 seconds. Ask the patient to choose the appropriate loudness level from the Cox Loudness Anchors. The goal is for the patient to pick #6. If he or she finds either of the noisemakers seriously uncomfortable, adjust the programming to reduce the MPO.

and, consequently, considerable research has focused in this area. More recently, investigators have become increasingly interested in how extra-perceptual factors like listening effort affect the total communication experience (e.g., Picou & Ricketts, 2014a, 2014b). Defining *listening effort* can be difficult, and the definition might be different depending on who is defining the term. We all have this general idea that effort is probably related to that feeling of being tired when you have to work really hard to understand what is being said. Even listeners with normal hearing might experience this in a crowded restaurant, over a poor cell phone connection, in a big lecture hall, or in any listening environment where there is noise or multiple talkers. A more formal definition that has been recently used is "the mental exertion required to attend to, and understand, an auditory message" (McGarrigle et al., 2014). Conceptually this is described in detail by the ease of language understanding (ELU) model (Rönnberg, 2003; Rönnberg, Rudner, Foo, & Lunner, 2008; Rönnberg et al., 2013). The model suggests that language information is automatically and rapidly bound together and then compared to long-term language memory stores. A match between the language input and the long-term memory stores results in speech recognition. Listening effort increases when there is a mismatch between the language input and memory stores and cognitive resources are necessary to achieve understanding, as can be the case if the language input is degraded. Although this model explains many research findings, it does not account for other cognitive factors like a listener's motivation, which has been shown to affect listening effort (Picou & Ricketts, 2014). Consequently, more comprehensive models have been introduced to account for the effects of higher level cognitive processes, such as motivation, on listening effort (e.g., Pichora-Fuller et al., 2016).

Not surprisingly, several studies, using a wide range of methodologies, have shown that the presence of background noise increases listening effort. In addition, people with hearing loss demonstrate more listening effort than those with normal hearing. It doesn't take much hearing loss either. Several researchers have reported that even mild hearing loss causes increased listening effort. This means that most of our patients are experiencing more listening effort than people with normal hearing. The consequences of continued expenditure of high levels of listening effort may be substantial and can include mental fatigue (Hornsby, 2013), communicative disengagement (Hétu, Jones, & Getty, 1993; Hétu. Riverin, Laland, Getty, & St-Cyr, 1988), decreased physical wellbeing (Hua, Karlsson, Widén, Möller, & Lyxell, 2013), reduced academic involvement (Kramer, Kapteyn, & Houtgast, 2006), and even absenteeism at work (Nachtegaal et al., 2009).

Clinical Application?

Clearly, listening effort has some direct relevance to our patients—so should we measure it clinically? At this

---

POINTS TO PONDER: DOES LISTENING EFFORT LEAD TO FATIGUE?

Working hard to hear in noise can add up over time, leading patients to feel tired all day long or, at the least, at the end of the day. Many believe it is this use of additional cognitive resources that leads to the feelings of fatigue, mental tiredness, or being drained after a period of trying to understand degraded speech. Indeed, researchers have found that people with hearing loss may need more time at the end of the day to rest and recover from working so hard to hear (Nachtegaal et al., 2009). Many studies have shown that increases in listening effort, however, often do not directly lead to increased fatigue. Why this is the case remains unclear, but some speculate that increased effort can lead to increased attention on the task, which can offset the effects of fatigue. The complex relationship between listening effort and fatigue continues to be a focus of considerable research (e.g., Pichora-Fuller et al., 2016).

point, we do not believe there is enough information or support to warrant clinical measures of listening effort or fatigue. Nevertheless, there are certainly some possible scenarios that could lead us to consider their measurement in the future:

- Current evidence already supports that hearing aid use may reduce listening effort. If, in the future, we are able to clearly define the relationship between listening effort and fatigue, there may be utility in measuring listening effort as a hearing aid outcome measure. Specifically, we could use this as another way to quantify the benefit of hearing aids and whether they achieve an individual patient's goal of reducing listening effort. If the relationship between listening effort and fatigue remains too complex to define, it may still be worthwhile to apply clinical outcome measures of fatigue. As of this writing, however, the procedures for quantifying listening effort were considerably more robust and mature than those quantifying auditory fatigue.
- If hearing aid technologies are developed or identified that affect listening effort in a way that is not directly related to changes in speech recognition, it may be of interest to validate benefit from these specific technologies. Some investigators have reported that specific hearing aid features, such as digital noise reduction, may reduce listening effort without concomitant changes in speech recognition (e.g., Desjardins & Doherty, 2014; Ng, Rudner, Lunner, Pedersen, & Rönnberg, 2013; Sarampalis, Kalluri, Edwards, & Hafter, 2009). Studies of this type have shown mixed results, however, and more work is needed in this area.

Measurement Procedures

If we do decide that clinical measurement of listening effort is worthwhile sometime in the future, what tools might we use for quantification? Generally, there are four kinds of approaches: subjective, physiologic, recall, and reaction time-based paradigms; we briefly review them here.

Subjective Measures of Listening Effort and Fatigue. One way to assess listening effort is simply to ask someone how much effort they put in or how tired they feel, resulting in a subjective rating of listening effort. For example, we might use informal questions like, "How tired do you feel now" or "How much effort did you put into listening," and then have the patients rate their responses on a Likert scale. Some use questionnaires that have been developed especially with listening effort in mind. For example, the speech, spatial, and qualities of hearing scale (SSQ; Gatehouse & Noble, 2004) includes some questions about listening effort (see Chapter 7). The most relevant question is, "Do you have to put in a lot of effort to hear what is being said in conversation with others?" A patient would rate his or her effort on a scale of 0 to 10, where 0 is *lots of effort* and 10 is *no effort*. Finally, there are more general scales of the physical effort or work that have been applied to listening effort. For example, Borg's CR-10 scales of physical exertion (Borg, 1990; Table 15–4) are used to quantify listening effort (Hallgren, Larsby, Lyxell, & Arlinger, 2005; Larsby, Hallgren, & Lyxell, 2005). In this case, patients rate their perceived mental exertion on a scale of 0 to 10, where 0 is *nothing at all* and 10 is *maximum exertion*. A rating of 10 would indicate the most effort or exertion a person has ever experienced.

Table 15–4. Example of a Borg CR-10 Scale

Rating	Description
0	Nothing at all
0.5	Very, very light
1	Very light
2	Fairly light
3	Moderate
4	Somewhat hard
5	Hard
6	
7	Very hard
8	
9	
10	Very, very hard (maximal)

Objective Measures of Listening Effort: Physiologic. Physiologic paradigms rely on the bodily responses that are thought to occur when listening is tough. Briefly, the body's response and how it changes when listening is more difficult to measure. Common research techniques include pupil dilation (e.g., Zekveld, Kramer, & Festen, 2010), heart rate and skin conductance (e.g., Mackersie & Cones, 2011). Some recent research has used the phase distribution of the ongoing oscillatory EEG activity to study the relationship between listening effort and hearing aid features (e.g., Bernarding, Strauss, Hannemann, Seidler, & Corona-Strauss, 2014).

Physiologic measures have upsides and downsides. On the plus side, they measure something involuntary, so we don't have to trust that the patient is being honest or is trying as hard as possible. One downside is it is not clear what role other factors like emotions play in these responses. We know that responses to emotional stimuli may influence these involuntary responses. For example, emotional stimuli have been shown to increase pupil size (Partala & Surakka, 2003) and skin conductance (Bradley, Greenwald, Petry, & Lang, 1992; Meyers & Smith, 1986), which are the same expected effects of increased listening effort (Mackersie & Cones, 2011; Zekveld et al., 2010). There may also be interactions with aging. For example, pupil size generally decreases with advanced age. Therefore, it may be more difficult to measure changes in pupil size. Measures of skin conductance may also be more difficult with the elderly because their skin may be more dry or wrinkled. A final and important downside is that it takes considerable expertise and specialized equipment to make these measurements—therefore, these are really research tools and we are doubtful they will be applied clinically.

Behavioral Measures of Listening Effort: Recall Tasks. Both recall and reaction time-based paradigms capitalize on the fact that human cognitive capacity is fixed; that is, each individual has a finite amount of cognitive resources (Kahneman, 1973). So, if you have to use more resources to understand speech, there are fewer resources available to do other things. It is then reasonable to assume that if cognitive resources have been diverted *toward* speech understanding, they must have been directed *away* from something else.

In the case of a recall paradigm, resources are directed away from rehearsal and recall. During a recall paradigm, participants listen to speech (e.g., words, sentences, or numbers) and are asked to recall what they heard. Recalling fewer items is interpreted as increased listening effort. For example, during one commonly used paradigm, the patient listens to sentences and is instructed to repeat the last word in each sentence (Pichora-Fuller, Schneider, & Daneman, 1995). After a certain number of sentences have been presented (e.g., eight sentences), the patient's task is to recall all of the last words in that block (e.g., eight final words). Recall tasks seem to have solid face validity since people in daily life are often confronted with the task of listening to speech and remembering what they heard. It makes some sense to ask people to do something with the speech they heard in order to get an idea of how much brain power they are using. Also, recall tasks are easy to administer with standard audiometric equipment.

Recall paradigms may also be susceptible to the effects of aging. Older adults may have more difficulty remembering, in general, even in the absence of hearing loss. This increased difficulty with memory may lead to floor effects if the recall task is too difficult. Making the task easier to avoid floor effects for older adults may make the task too easy for patients who are younger or have normal hearing, however, leading to ceiling effects in this population. Thus, it is a balancing act to find a task difficulty level that would be appropriate for comparing adults with normal hearing to adults with hearing loss when using a recall paradigm.

Behavioral Measures of Listening Effort: Reaction Time Tasks. As with recall tasks, the assumption with reaction time-based tasks is that during situations of increased listening effort fewer resources will be available for other things. In this case, the "other things" involve a physical response. The simplest form of this kind of task is to measure how long it takes to begin repeating a word or sentence. More complicated tasks involve pressing a button whenever a light appears or asking a listener to trace a circle on a computer screen while simultaneously performing the speech recognition tasks. Reaction time tasks have the advantage of being relatively easy to implement, although a reliable method to measure response time is needed. Given the high use of computers clinically, however, this may be less of a challenge clinically in the future than it might have been in decades past.

> **POINTS TO PONDER: DO SUBJECTIVE, BEHAVIORAL AND OBJECTIVE MEASURES OF LISTENING EFFORT QUANTIFY THE SAME UNDERLYING FACTORS?**
>
> It's very easy to ask someone to rate his or her subjective perception of listening effort. Clinically, this is quick, easy, and seems to be directly related to what we're after. Subjective measures may not be the most reflective of "increased cognitive resources used," however. There is emerging evidence from several laboratories that the subjective ratings of effort are not correlated with behavioral or objective measures of effort (e.g., Fraser et al., 2010; Mackersie & Cones, 2011; Sarampalis et al., 2009). There are many potential explanations for why these measures aren't strongly related. For example, patients may have trouble being introspective and unbiased. Specifically, you might ask your patient how much effort they exerted while listening to some sentences in quiet. They might reply that they exerted a lot of effort, even though it's early in the test session and the sentences should be relatively easy to hear. The reason for this response may be that the patient was tired because of something unrelated to listening, like a restless night's sleep. In addition, the patient may not have yet experienced a difficult listening condition in your office, and has to recalibrate his or her response after listening to something more challenging. Similarly, patients may have trouble remembering perceived effort over the course of the test session. Finally, patients may be rating their perceived performance and not perceived effort. Furthermore, researchers have identified that some questions may do a better job of assessing effort than others. For example, Picou, Moore, and Ricketts (2017) found that asking patients "How likely are you to do something different, like move to a quiet room?" was more closely related to an objective measure of effort. Conversely, asking patients "How much effort did you need to understand those words?" resulted in answers that more closely aligned with speech recognition performance than listening effort. In total, research from recent studies suggest that asking people to rate effort directly may not be a valid measure of effort because patients may not always be able to differentiate it from their performance. Nonetheless, we certainly shouldn't discount subjective measures completely. After all, they successfully elicit the patient's conscious perception. We just need to be aware that subjective and objective measurements may give us different results.

Even though there are many positives, reaction time tasks lack some face validity. The patient might, for example, wonder what pressing a button tells us about their hearing. Wu and colleagues found that listening measured by dual-task paradigms using a simulated real-world driving task and a conventional laboratory-style reaction-time task showed generally consistent results (Wu, Stangl, & Perkins, 2014). In addition, reaction time measures may be pretty variable within and across patients. Also, they tend to be sensitive to learning and fatigue effects. That is, people are a little slow at first, get better at the task over time so they get faster, and then slow down again as they get tired of being tested.

Reaction time paradigms also require consideration when testing adults who are older. In addition to the reduction in memory ability with age, older adults' reaction times tend to be generally slower than younger listeners', regardless of hearing status. One way to get around this is to use a baseline measure and subtract this baseline from performance during the reaction time task.

In addition to the aforementioned challenges to implementing reaction time based paradigms to measure listening effort, methodological considerations become critically important when using these paradigms to make judgements about listening effort. Three of these considerations are the nature of the secondary task, test environment, and the SNR used for testing. First, the secondary task needs to be the right level of difficulty to be maximally sensitive to factors that affect effort. A critical assumption using dual-task paradigms is that the secondary task competes with the primary task (speech recognition) for cognitive resources. If the secondary task is too easy, listeners can do it automatically and the measures will not tell us anything about cognitive effort. If the secondary task is too hard, listeners will put too much brain power toward it and not focus on speech recognition, so their speech recognition performance will decline. For adults, one task that has been shown to be sensitive to the effects of noise is to ask listeners to think about the speech they heard, specifically to decide if the word they heard was a noun and to press a button as quickly as possible if it was. This secondary task seemed to be better than other, visual secondary tasks (e.g., press a button as soon as a red box appears).

For children, investigators have used secondary tasks that range from simple responses to a light to playing a dot-to-dot game. Use of the simple tasks did not interfere with speech recognition but also did not reveal expected effects of background noise on listening effort (e.g., Hicks & Tharpe, 2002). Conversely, use of the dot-to-dot game may have been too engaging because the game interfered with speech recognition and was also insensitive to the effects of background noise (McFadden & Pittman, 2008). Research into identifying secondary tasks at the right level of difficulty for children is still ongoing.

Second, the test environment seems to interact with listening effort. For example, Picou, Moore, and Ricketts (2017) investigated the potential for using directional microphones to improve listening effort. Adults with acquired hearing loss were tested using a dual-task paradigm in a sound booth and a moderately reverberant environment. Their results suggest that, although directional microphones improved speech recognition performance in both environments, benefits for listening effort were only seen in the reverberant environment. If this finding is confirmed by additional research, it would suggest that clinical measures of effort in sound-treated booths may not reflect effort in the real world, which tends to be more reverberant.

Finally, the choice of SNR for testing with reaction-time based measures is important. Wu et al. (2014) investigated the effect of changing the SNR on listening effort. He had two significant findings. First, reaction time (RT) does not increase asymptotically at less favorable SNRs even though speech performance became worse. Instead, the psychometric functions of the secondary task were peaked. As noise level increased, the RT initially increased and then decreased with the peak falling around 0 dB (Re: SNR50). Second, at very difficult SNR conditions, speech cues are very limited. Because in this case allocating more cognitive resources to speech understanding will not improve speech performance, subjects (consciously or unconsciously) allocate less cognitive resource to speech understanding, resulting in short RTs. These data suggest that SNRs that are too easy or too challenging will not be sensitive to changes in effort.

The preceding discussion highlights the variability in the research approaches used to measure listening effort and also that the field of study is in its infancy. The newness of effort as a hearing aid outcome, combined with the challenges associated with applying research methodologies in the clinic, makes this topic exciting to watch for potential future clinical verification applications. In the meantime, we believe an understanding of the concepts of effort and fatigue may assist with counseling and with understanding patients. The patient reports of being tired of listening are backed by research. Fortunately, hearing aids and hearing aid technologies can reduce this effort.

In Closing

Going back to our opening comments, we believe that the primary verification procedure for fitting hearing aids is the careful assessment of gain and output using probe microphone measures. We recognize, however, that behavioral testing is popular and does have an appeal, as the patient is often actively involved. But simply doing the testing because it makes us feel good or makes the patient feel good probably isn't reason enough to continue using such an approach. For that reason, we have attempted to review critically the different behavioral methods of verification/validation—limited to tests typically conducted on the day of the fitting—and provide how they can be used in a meaningful way. For the most part, this relates to more effective counseling, rather than how to program the hearing aids.

The bottom line regarding this testing, therefore, is don't try to make it a bigger deal than what it is. Think of it as a "demonstration." Other than the aided loudness measures, these tests are very poor predictors of subsequent benefit and satisfaction with hearing aids. Yes, there is some evidence to suggest that patients are more satisfied when we do more testing. That seems like a good thing, and may be reason enough to continue doing it—but let's not pretend it is *science*.

16
Probe Microphone Measures: Rationale and Procedures

We want all of our hearing aid patients to be happy when they leave our offices, right? And, although it is nice to see them smile, we believe this *verification* approach isn't quite good enough, and that a *validated* prescriptive fitting method should be used as a starting point for *verification*. As we discuss in Chapter 14, when we have verification of a validated prescriptive method, we then have a good understanding of the tradeoffs between audibility, speech understanding, sound quality, comfort, and other factors in the fitting of the typical patient. This may not be the end point for all patients, however, and gain adjustments may be necessary. If we start with ear canal sound pressure level (SPL) reference information relative to the individual patient's dynamic range, we then know what effect we are having on audibility when we make changes from a validated method, and the potential impact of the changes.

We all know of cases in which a patient was fitted without real-ear verification: Several patient-driven adjustments had to be made, and the patient ended up with little or no gain. For instance, we recall one case of a hearing aid wearer—who also happened to be an audiologist—using new instruments he had fitted to himself through careful listening. After volunteering to be a demonstration patient at a probe microphone workshop, he and the rest of the audience discovered that he had simply programmed the hearing aids to match his unaided open-ear canal resonance—the hearing aids had no real-ear gain above 1500 Hz.

Although behavioral measures, discussed in Chapter 15, are helpful, they are complementary and not a substitute for the objective assessment of hearing aid output in the ear canal. Understanding that a *prescriptive fitting* is ultimately based on the desired amplified signal level in the ear canal, not a 2cc-coupler measure (at least not without correcting for differences between the ear and the coupler), a KEMAR measure, or a computer simulation in the fitting software, *probe microphone measures* of hearing aid performance *(or individual real-ear corrections to the coupler these provide)* are therefore needed for verification of our chosen prescriptive method.

Probe microphone verification procedures are the primary focus of this chapter. The importance of these procedures has been emphasized and recommended in every hearing aid fitting guideline published in the past

20 years (see Chapter 2). As an example, the following excerpt is taken from the 2007 fitting guidelines of the American Academy of Audiology (p. 25):

> The objective of this segment of the fitting process is to ensure that the fitting and verification procedure is viewed as a process, rather than an event, that culminates in the optimal fitting for the patient. Verification procedures also serve as a benchmark against which future hearing aid changes can be compared. Specific goals and rationales underlie all hearing aid fittings. Verification procedures should be based on validated hearing aid fitting rationales.

What hopefully is obvious from the preceding statement is that you are using a validated method only when that method's prescribed gain and/or output are referenced to what is required in the ear canal. We mention this again as this concept might not be obvious to all clinicians. For example, Mueller (2006) reported that, in a survey of audiologists fitting hearing aids, 78% stated that they routinely were using a validated prescriptive fitting approach (i.e., either the NAL or the DSL). Interestingly, however, is that of this 78%, only 44% reported routinely using probe microphone measures. Question of the day: How do the remaining 56% know what method they are using or whether they are using any method at all?

Mueller and Picou (2010) identified a similar disconnect in their survey findings. From their sample, 79% of audiologists reported using a validated prescriptive fitting approach, and yet only 59% of this group routinely used probe microphone verification. Another peculiar finding from this survey was that of the respondents who said they used prescriptive methods routinely *and* also reported conducting probe microphone testing routinely, only 37% said that their primary reason for using probe microphone testing was to verify these targets.

Real Ear Versus Probe Microphone Versus Speech Mapping

There are a few different terms that refer to the act of putting a tube in the ear canal and measuring the output from the hearing aid in the real ear. As we discuss in Chapter 15, an early term that was used for this was *in situ* measurement, meaning in position—a reasonable term, as indeed the hearing aid is measured in the *use position*. In early marketing efforts of probe microphone equipment, however, it was important to make the distinction that the testing was conducted on the *real ear* and not in a 2cc coupler. In situ did not have much meaning to most audiologists, so it made more sense to refer to the testing as *real-ear measurements* (REM). The term REM is sometimes used today by manufacturers and audiologists.

Whereas testing during the first 20 years of probe microphone assessment mostly involved swept pure tones and composite noise as the input signal, in the past decade speech-shaped signals or real-speech inputs have become routine. The use of these signals in combination with plotting the patient's dynamic range in SPL has prompted audiologists to refer to the testing as *speech mapping*. This term was first used in the early 1990s when Bill Cole and his colleagues introduced this feature, trademarked as Speechmap™ on the Audioscan coupler/probe microphone unit at his company, Etymonic Design Incorporated. This equipment did not produce a shaped-speech signal all at once but rather as a series of tone pips/bursts whose levels reflected the frequency-specific long-term average speech spectrum (LTASS) levels. Most audiologists today use a speech-shaped/shaped-speech input signal, and if different input levels are used and they are plotted relative to the patient's residual range of hearing, they are conducting speech mapping. That is, if it's not plotted for different input levels, it's not really a map of the ear canal output. Of course, you can't do REM or speech mapping without a probe microphone, so that too is a reasonable term.

Which term is correct? Or better yet, which term will cause the least confusion? We believe there is a clear choice, and that choice is probe microphone measures for several reasons. First, recall that in Chapter 15 we describe procedures for conducting aided soundfield testing, and functional gain. The last time we checked, these are real-ear measures of hearing aid performance. There are government forms that very specifically require the real-ear measure of hearing aid performance with the patient wearing one versus two hearing aids. They are referring to aided soundfield testing. If you believe that the term real ear relates only to probe microphone measures, this request would be

> **KEY CONCEPT: YOU DON'T FIT HEARING AIDS BY *PROBE***
>
> We often overhear at audiology meetings, perhaps around a cocktail table, one audiologist asking another: "So do you fit your aids by probe?" There seems to be a common belief that probe microphone measures are a way to fit hearing aids. They are not. They are simply a way to verify your way of fitting hearing aids. We know of large clinics where the audiologists are required by their supervisor to do probe microphone measures. What audiologists may do is push the magic button that provides a fit to the manufacturer's default fitting, then conduct probe microphone testing for inputs of 55, 65, and 75 dB SPL, print the results, and put them in the patient's chart. Not one hearing aid adjustment involved! Did they fit by probe? Some might say they do. Are they fitting by a validated rationale? Not likely, as we describe in detail later in this chapter. Again, the act of conducting probe microphone testing is not a way of fitting hearing aids—the validated rationale is the way—which needs to be verified.
>
> To iterate this point, we use a weekend construction project as analogous to the fitting of a hearing aid. Let's say you are going to build a dog house. You start with a general design (type of roof, door size, etc.—just as you start with selection of a validated fitting rationale). You then go online and find a blueprint for building the dog house that fits your design (exact dimensions for all the pieces that will need to be assembled—just as you obtain desired gain and output values for your fitting method). Now, while cutting the pieces for this dog house you might use a tape measure to verify that all the pieces fit your blueprint. (Remember the adage: Measure twice, cut once.) Would you tell your wood-working colleagues that a tape measure is a way to build a dog house? Not likely. But could you build a sturdy and nice-looking dog house without using a tape measure? Probably not!

quite puzzling, as there is no probe microphone measure that would assess the summation effects of two instruments.

On a 2015 audiology Listserv we saw this posting: "I'm going to buy some real-ear equipment, but I can't decide if I should purchase probe microphone or speech mapping." This posting highlights our second point. Probe microphone testing nearly always *is* speech mapping; speech mapping nearly always *is* a component of the probe microphone assessment of a hearing aid. They are not two different things. Therefore, it is much simpler to call the entire process *probe microphone measures* as, although it is likely that this will include speech mapping, it is also very possible that some of the testing will not be speech mapping. For example, testing can include a swept-tone MPO measure, the measure of the occlusion effect, and so forth. We use the term probe microphone measures to describe this type of real-ear testing of hearing aid performance.

Compliance With Best Practice Guidelines

The use of probe microphone measures for hearing aid verification has always been assumed when best practice guidelines were written. Going back to the recommendations of the Vanderbilt Report II in 1991, probe microphone assessment has been mentioned as either the preferred method or one of the preferred methods for verification. Over the years, published guidelines from the Independent Hearing Aid Fitting Forum (IHAFF), the ASHA, and the AAA have recommended the use of probe microphone verification. The statement on this topic from the 2006 AAA document is unambiguous (p. 26): Prescribed gain (output) from a validated prescriptive method should be verified using a probe microphone approach that is referenced to ear canal SPL.

In case you think this is only a U.S. recommendation, the International Society of Audiology document, Good Practice Guidance for Adult Hearing Aid Fittings and Services states the fitting tolerances that are acceptable internationally:

> Where a fitting rationale contains an acoustical target, each hearing aid fitting should be verified by real-ear measurement using an input stimulus appropriate for the hearing aid under test prior to any fine-tuning. Tolerances to the prescription rationale of ±5 dB at frequencies of 250 Hz, 500 Hz, 1000 Hz, and 2000 Hz, and of ±8 dB at 3000 and 4000 Hz should be achieved in all cases. In addition, the slope in each octave should be within ±5 dB/octave of the target. Where it is not desirable or possible to achieve a prescriptive target (e.g., because of feedback issues) or where the measurement is not technically feasible, the clinical record should contain an explicit statement to this effect. (International Society of Audiology, 2005, p. 5)

We know, however, that what is supported by research evidence, recommended by opinion leaders, and published in best practice documents, does not always find its way into routine clinical audiology use. The best example of this might be the persistent use of live-voice speech recognition testing despite the abundance of literature showing the many shortcomings of this practice (see Hornsby & Mueller, 2013; Mueller, Ricketts, & Bentler, 2014). But what about probe microphone measures? The clinically-friendly equipment for this testing has been available for more than 30 years. Are these measures a routine part of the hearing aid fitting protocol for all or most audiologists? The topic has generated a number of surveys, so we do have a pretty good idea of compliance. In the following four surveys, the audiologists responding were actively engaged in the fitting of hearing aids, and *routine use* was defined as using probe microphone measures with at least 50% of adult patients:

- In 1995, Mueller and Strouse reported that the routine use of probe microphone measures was 54% for audiologists ($n = 134$) and 18% for hearing instrument specialists (HISs; $n = 108$), with an overall average use rate of 39%.
- In 1999, Mueller again examined use rates for both audiologists and HISs, but this time limited the survey to those who owned or had access to the equipment. When the two professional groups were combined, 42% reported routine use.
- In 2003, a survey by Mueller of primarily audiologists ($n = 558$ audiologists, 49 HISs) showed an overall routine use rate of 37%.
- In 2005, Mueller again examined the popularity of these measures, this time among audiologists only. The overall use rate was 34%. It was slightly higher (~ 40%) for recent graduates (either master's level or AuDs) and for experienced audiologists who had obtained their AuD through distance learning.

The results of these surveys are surprisingly similar, and show, in general, routine use of probe microphone verification by about 35% to 40% of responding practitioners. This takes us to the most recent and extensive survey on the topic by Mueller and Picou (2010). This online survey used data only from U.S. practitioners who dispense hearing aids and included a total of 420 respondents: 309 audiologists (74%) and 111 (26%) HISs. One of the questions asked in the survey related to the routine use of the equipment on the day of the fitting. The results are shown in Figure 16–1.

If we first look at the left portion of Figure 16–1, we see use rates that are quite similar to what has been found in other surveys: about 45% for audiologists and 36% for HISs, with an overall use rate of 41%. These data are for the total sample. The data on the right portion of the chart are only for the individuals who have the equipment available. As we would predict, this increases the use of this testing (more so for HISs) but not by nearly the amount that would be expected. Consider that for, both groups, about 45% of the audiologists and HISs who have the equipment don't use it routinely. These data are nearly as low as surveys regarding use rates for people who own treadmills! Of course, people completing this survey knew what the correct answer was; using the findings from some lie detector questions, Mueller and Picou (2010) suggest that the actual use rate is not even as high as their results indicated.

One finding we find interesting is that in 1995, probe microphone use for audiologists versus hearing instrument specialists (HISs) was 54 to 18%. Today, or

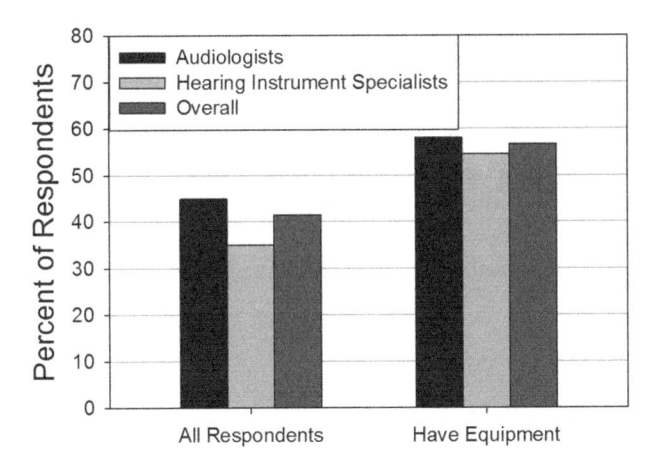

Figure 16–1. Survey results comparing routine use of probe microphone measures that indicate about 41% use across all respondents, and about 55% use across practitioners who have the equipment. (Adapted from Mueller and Picou, 2010, with permission.)

at least in the 2010 survey, the use rate is essentially the same between these two groups, due to a considerable uptake by the HISs. Why is this? Although we have little data on the topic, we do have some opinions, formed from discussions with individuals from both groups, as well as manufacturer's sales reps, who probably know the straight scoop the best. Here are our thoughts:

- There are fewer mom and pop HISs today than there were 20 years ago. Currently, HISs are younger and more tech savvy.
- Many HISs in private practice are no longer with a franchise company but now are selling the same hearing aids as the audiology practice down the street. This places a greater emphasis on the quality of the fitting, using the right equipment, and a contemporary fitting protocol.
- More and more, the fitting is driven by consumers as they become better educated regarding the right and wrong way to fit a hearing aid. In July, 2009, *Consumer Reports* reported that according to its sampling, about two-thirds of hearing aids sold were fitted incorrectly. The article concluded: The provider should do several tests to verify that they (hearing aids) are working optimally. Of that battery of tests, one stands out as a must-have: the real-ear test.

- Finally, in recent years the hearing aid distribution system has changed, with many chains and big-box stores dispensing hearing aids. These are common employment sites for HISs and many, if not most, of these stores make an effort to follow best practice guidelines; sadly, perhaps more so than some audiology practices. Individuals working at these sites are strongly encouraged to follow the established best practice protocols.

As discussed in Chapter 1, much of the Marke-Trak VIII report focused on verification including the administration of tests such as probe microphone measurements (e.g., Kochkin et al., 2010; Kochkin, 2011a). The approach taken by MarkeTrak VIII was different from that used in the other surveys we have reported. Rather than asking audiologists and HISs whether they conducted the testing, individuals purchasing hearing aids were queried about whether they had received the testing. Survey findings reported that 42% of the respondents stated that they received the testing; there was not a significant difference in the frequency whether the patient had been fitted by an audiologist or an HIS.

Possible Ethics Violation?

Ever since it became obvious that audiologists were not adopting the use of probe microphone measures at the rate that everyone expected, many of us have publicly commented that not doing probe microphone assessment when hearing aids are fitted is clearly poor clinical practice. In a 2009 article in *Audiology Today* entitled, "It's a Matter of Ethics", Catherine Palmer took it to a different level. She questioned whether not doing probe microphone testing is a violation of the code of ethics of our major audiology professional organizations. She specifically stated, "If we talk about ethical practice, then we have to be comfortable saying that there are hearing health care providers (audiologists) who are not practicing ethically" (p. 32).

Most of us think of unethical practice related to the fitting of hearing aids as things like trips to Hawaii or kick-backs given to referral sources. But the Code of Ethics also includes items related to how we perform clinical audiology. For example, Principle 2 of the AAA Code of Ethics states that Members shall maintain high standards of professional competence in rendering services. Principle 4 states that Members shall provide only services and products that are in the best interest of those served. Principle of Ethics II from the ASHA *Code of Ethics* states that Individuals shall honor their responsibility to achieve and maintain the highest level of professional competence.

Consider this example: If you don't use probe microphone measures, how would you know if you had even made soft sounds audible—one of the most basic components of the hearing aid fitting? If you actually sold a pair of hearing aids and didn't make soft sounds audible (simply because the necessary software adjustments were not made), would this be a high standard of professional competence? Would it be providing services that are in the best interests of those served? Not really.

Palmer concludes her article with the following hope for the future:

> I hope we can continue to discuss the reasons that hearing aid acceptance is not higher in the hearing-impaired population. The fact that a doctoral profession is arguing about whether or not to individually verify the gain and output of a hearing aid in a patient's ear that takes less than five minutes might just be a good place to start. If you are wondering if providing this level of verification will establish you as an expert and set you apart from other providers, keep in mind that it does not require any particular expertise to attach cords to a HIPRO Box, double click on NOAH, enter a patient name, click hearing thresholds on a graph, double click on a manufacturer icon, and click first fit. This level of expertise does not require a doctoral degree. As a profession, it is time to be an expert. An expert knows exactly what levels of sound are being produced in an individual's ear canal and how those levels correspond to the listener's residual dynamic range of hearing. (*Audiology Today*, 2009, p. 34)

Reasons for Not Conducting Probe Microphone Measures

More important than the recommendations from best fitting practices and experts is that the research evidence that we detail in the following discussion clearly demonstrates the importance of completing probe microphone measurements. Despite being the intuitive thing to do, the right thing to do, the evidence-based thing to do, and therefore we think the ethical thing to do, probe microphone testing is not conducted by most audiologists when they fit hearing aids. Over the years, there have been many reasons postulated regarding why this is true, as well as articles written on the topic (Mueller, 2005b). We review several of those reasons here.

Equipment Isn't Available

Why would one choose to set up a practice without the necessary equipment? Certainly, the overall cost of essential equipment must be considered, but used systems in good working condition are available for a few thousand dollars; more basic new systems sell for only a little more. Lease-to-buy deals are available for around $100 per month. Given that many clinics and offices will have gross annual hearing aid sales of $300,000 to $500,000, a $5000 equipment purchase that leads to improved patient satisfaction and benefit does not seem very unreasonable. Would an audiologist open a clinical practice without an audiometer?

Not Enough Time

Indirectly, the time issue takes us back to our bundle versus unbundle discussion in Chapter 2. What percentage of the total cost of a pair of hearing aids is for the hearing aids themselves, and what portion is for our services? But even when the price of hearing aids is bundled, we know that a good share of the money paid by the patient is for our professional services. These professional services include optimizing gain to provide as much hearing aid benefit as possible while ensuring satisfaction and comfort. This is the very goal of many of the validated prescriptive gain and output procedures we are verifying through probe microphone testing. As professionals, we take as much time as necessary to get the job done right.

Not Valid With Today's Technology

Those of us fitting hearing aids for several years have heard a lot of what you can't do. It started with you can't

> ## SOAPBOX: LEO TOLSTOY AND PROBE MICROPHONE MEASURES
>
> As we've reviewed in this chapter, there is an unexplainable reluctance among audiologists to conduct probe microphone measures; as a result, most audiologists fitting hearing aids do not use this measure routinely. To make our first Soapbox point, we quote Leo Tolstoy: "Wrong does not cease to be wrong because the majority share in it". You're the only student who refuses to go to a placement because they don't use probe microphone verification for fitting hearing aids? Good for you. You're a practicing audiologist and you're the only one in the clinic doing probe microphone? Good for you. The place where you work doesn't have probe microphone equipment? Buy it yourself. Your employer tells you that there isn't time to do probe microphone testing for your hearing aid fittings? Find a new job!
>
> There is considerable evidence to show that the use of hearing aids will improve individual's lives. There is also evidence to show that well-fitted hearing aids will have an even greater impact.

do probe microphone testing with wide dynamic range compression (WDRC) hearing aids. Then we heard you can't do probe microphone testing with programmable hearing aids, which then led to you can't do probe microphone testing with digital processing hearing aids (Mueller, 2001). Even today we often hear clinicians say: I was told by my rep that probe microphone testing really doesn't tell you much with the product. All this simply is not true. In fact in many cases, the more sophisticated the processing, the more things that you can verify—and the more important it is to verify. With today's real-speech inputs, the probe microphone findings provide a very reasonable estimate of real-world audibility for speech. Sure, there are a few caveats to this, but they are easy to overcome. We will discuss those in Chapter 17. The bottom line is, if one of our primary goals is achieving the right amount of audibility for speech, it seems to make good sense to measure it in the real ear.

Poor Training?

Could it be that AuD students simply are not trained properly regarding the importance and use of probe microphone measures? This has been suggested by some. We find it unlikely that an accredited AuD program would not teach the verification procedures recommended in best practices guidelines. Nonetheless, there are sometimes disconnects between academic training and clinical practice and mentoring. Here is a comment on the topic from Mike Valente, certainly one of the strongest advocates of probe microphone testing that you will find in an AuD training program:

> According to the clinic coordinator at one graduate program, in 16 of 20 external clinical sites where she sends her students for clinical experience, probe microphone equipment is never used or used only in special cases. Therefore, some students wonder if probe microphone verification really is necessary if seasoned audiologists with successful practices do not use it. Also, I believe a majority of students graduate understanding the need for probe microphone measures to implement a best practice, but the facility in which they are then employed either does not have the equipment and/or has staff who do not promote its routine use. It is very difficult, if not impossible, for new graduates to arrive at their first job and change the method of practice. (Comments of Valente, taken from Mueller, 2005)

We agree with Mike's comments—we have heard the same thing from others. You would think that doctoral students in audiology only would be allowed to do practicum at sites that follow best practices, but for some reason that doesn't always seem to be possible. The critical need to change the culture in the workplace is probably related to the reason we discuss next.

The Fitting Software Gets It Right

The biggest factor in the failure to use probe microphone verification is probably the general belief of many audiologists that the fitting software will somehow get things right. That is, if you click the default button in the fitting software, the patient will most likely have the best fitting. If you click the NAL-NL2 button, the patient will most likely be fitted to NAL-NL2. Or, if you look at the simulated gain or output displayed by the fitting software, you actually see a true representation of the actual gain or SPL levels in the real ear. Unfortunately, research has shown that none of these assumptions is true, as we detail in the following sections.

Of course we would not expect the software fitting to be perfectly accurate for individual patients, as average correction values are used and there are differences in individual ears. We already address this in Chapter 5. What we are talking about here, however, is something different: variances that have a greater impact than the usual 3 to 4 dB differences in RECDs or CORFIGs. In general, the issues surround both the manufacturer's proprietary fitting (what actually happens in the ear when you activate the default fitting for a specific hearing loss) and the manufacturer's software implementation of a validated prescriptive method such as the NAL-NL2. We will address each of these issues separately.

Proprietary Fittings Are Best?

As discussed in Chapter 14, all major manufacturers have a proprietary fitting. How this fitting was developed probably varies from manufacturer to manufacturer. To some extent, this fitting relates to specific processing of a given manufacture's product, but for the most part it is based on two types of data from research studies and/or patient or clinician complaints compiled by the manufacturer: (1) preferred sound quality including naturalness, and (2) initial acceptance data (e.g., return for credit rates). Sometimes, these proprietary fittings have been simply employed to compensate for past problems or perceived problems. Examples include the following: (1) patients say our first fit sounds tinny, let's roll off the highs; (2) patients (or audiologists buying our instruments) say our first fit results in feedback, let's roll off the highs; and (3) patients (or audiologists buying our instruments) say the first fit of Brand X sounds better than ours, so let's make ours just like Brand X.

How this relates back to the non-use of probe microphone assessment is that it is very difficult to verify a proprietary fit in the real ear, starting with the term *proprietary*. If you want to verify to the NAL-NL2 or DSL v5, you simply select this in the software of your probe microphone system and the prescriptive targets will appear on the screen. But if you want to verify to Starkey Fit, or Signia Fit or Phonak Fit . . . there are no real-ear targets in your probe microphone system. Now it could be that there are some simulated curves in the fitting software; you could maybe print these out and then maybe eyeball them while conducting probe microphone testing, but this is more trouble than most audiologists want to go through. And, even if you went through the trouble of trying this, your results only would be valid if the LTASS used to construct the proprietary gain and output curves was the same as the LTASS of the input signal with your probe microphone equipment when the real-ear measure is performed. This is probably unlikely, and ensuring that the same LTASS is used is sometimes difficult to even determine.

So maybe the first question should be: Are proprietary fittings a reasonable starting point for the fitting? If so, then maybe you really don't need to do probe microphone testing. Experts have commented on the use of proprietary fittings for some time. Denis Byrne, for example, expressed his concerns in 1996:

> Scientifically, the concern is that amplification may become prescribed by a wide variety of proprietary formulae of which few, if any, are validated by published research. A possible philosophical problem is that control of the fitting process is taken away from the fitter, who is responsible for the care of the client. (p. 378)

The concerns of Byrne (1996) appear to be well-founded. Here is a brief summary of research, adapted from Mueller (2006), that has looked at how these strategies compare to validated approaches:

- Keidser, Brew, and Peck (2003), in a study examining the recommended algorithms of five different major manufacturers, showed that it is common for prescribed gain to differ

by 10 dB or more from the NAL-NL1 targets in the high frequencies for average-level input signals.
- Bentler (2004) examined the default algorithm of the premier product from six leading hearing aid manufacturers using a real-speech input (long-term 65 dB SPL input). In general, all algorithms prescribed gain below the NAL-NL1 target levels. Of particular concern was that for key frequencies such as 2000 Hz, the difference in prescribed gain was as much as 15 to 20 dB, with some algorithms only prescribing 5 dB of gain for the sample patient with a 50 dB hearing loss at that frequency.
- Bentler, Wu, and Jeon (2006) calculated the real-ear insertion gain (REIG) for four different open canal (OC) products based on the manufacturers' recommended fitting. The hearing aids were programmed for an individual with a high-frequency hearing loss (50 dB at 2000 Hz, 60 dB at 3000–6000 Hz). They observed about a 5 dB difference among manufacturers but, in general, the average recommended gain fell 10 to 15 dB below NAL-NL1 targets in the 2000 to 4000 range. Two of the four products provided no more than 7 dB of gain at 4000 Hz for this sample patient with a 60 dB hearing loss at that frequency.

These studies suggest that the default proprietary fittings fall seriously short on providing appropriate audibility. Even if you are not a believer in validated fitting methods such as the NAL and *Hearing Aids 101*, a little horse sense tells us that a patient needs more than 5 dB of gain when they have a 50 dB hearing loss. It's true, however, that the studies we cited are somewhat dated, but we have evidence that things haven't gotten any better.

In a unique and eye-opening study, Leavitt and Flexer (2012) reported how modern-day default fittings actually influence speech recognition in background noise. They compared the premier 2012 product of the six major manufacturers to a single-channel analog product from 2002. Subjects were fitted bilaterally and tested using the QuickSIN, presented at 57 dB SPL—slightly below average speech. The old analog hearing aids were programmed (and verified) to NAL-NL1 for each subject. Two different settings were used for the six pairs of premier hearing aids: The hearing aids were tested while programmed to the manufacturer's default setting, and also when programmed to NAL-NL1. The old hearing aids did not have directional technology or digital noise reduction. The new hearing aids did, and these features were activated at the levels suggested in the default software. The mean results of QuickSIN speech recognition testing are shown in Figure 16–2.

As described in Chapter 6, the QuickSIN is scored as signal-to-noise (SNR) loss, and therefore the graph indicates worsening performance as the bar extends downward in Figure 16–2. Note that the average SNR-Loss for the old hearing aid was about 8.5 dB. What stands out, however, is the poor performance for all the modern-day hearing aids when fitted to the manufacturer's proprietary fitting. Note that for HA-3, HA-4, and HA-5, the SNR loss is greater than 15 dB, about a 7 dB drop from the mean performance obtained with the old analog hearing aids.

Let's put the Leavitt and Flexer (2012) findings into practical terms—we'll say that an audiologist has fit someone with a pair of new, high-end hearing aids, programmed to the manufacturer's default settings. The

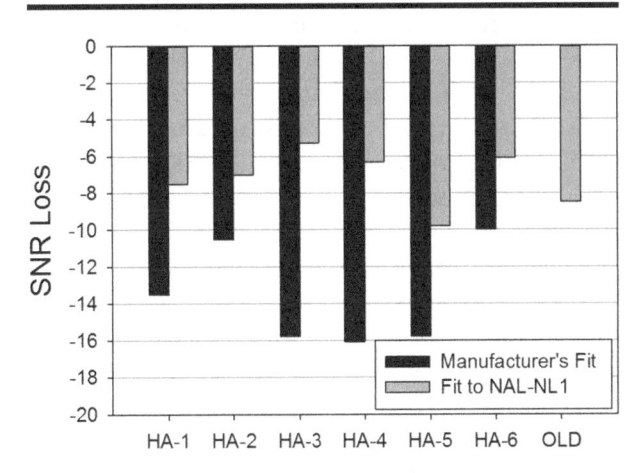

Figure 16–2. SNR loss is shown across five premiere hearing aids and one older style analog hearing aid as a function of the manufacturer's default setting and the NAL-NL-1 fitting. Lower numbers show better QuickSin performance. (Adapted from Leavitt and Flexer, 2012, with permission.)

patient was a previous user of old analog hearing aids programmed to the NAL-NL1. The audiologist's counseling would have to go something like this: Bob, thanks again for the $5000, but I do have to tell you that when you go back to your favorite restaurant this weekend, you'll somehow have to convince management to reduce the background noise level by 7 dB if you want to understand speech as well as you did with your old hearing aids. Why would an audiologist ever do that to a patient?

Notice, referring back to Figure 16-2, that by simply programming the hearing aids to the NAL-NL1 prescriptive targets, average SNR loss improved significantly for all models, and 9 to 10 dB for HA-3 and HA-4. When programmed to NAL-NL1, all products except HA-5 had performance better than the old hearing aids. Patients often walk in the door looking for the best and latest technology. These findings clearly show that's it is not just the technology. Simple technology programmed well will outperform fancy technology programmed poorly almost every day.

In a recent study examining today's proprietary fittings, Sanders, Stoody, Weber, and Mueller (2015) conducted probe microphone measures for the premier hearing aids of the five leading manufacturers, using products and software current in 2015. The hearing aids were all programmed to the respective proprietary fitting for a common, gradually downward sloping hearing loss (e.g., 25 dB in the lows, dropping to 75 dB in the high frequencies); real-ear output was obtained (16 ears) for inputs of 55, 65, and 75 SPL. The testing was conducted with the Audioscan Verifit®, which calculates the SII, and these values were used for comparison. The findings from Sanders et al. (2015) are shown in Figure 16-3. The SII values reflect a familiar theme—reduced audibility. It appears, however, that the differences among manufacturers, and the variance from the NAL-NL2, become smaller as the input signal increases (most probably because the proprietary methods are more linear than what would be prescribed by NL2). For example, for the 55 dB SPL input, SIIs among manufacturers vary from a low of 0.25 to 0.40 compared to a 0.47 values for a NL2 fitting. For average inputs, the different products vary from 0.46 to 0.57 compared to 0.65 for the NALNL2. For the 75 dB SPL input, the products were similar, and were only 0.1 to 0.5 below the NAL-NL2 SII. The authors did not measure speech recognition directly and it is somewhat difficult to predict speech recognition from SII values; still, if we look at the 55 dB

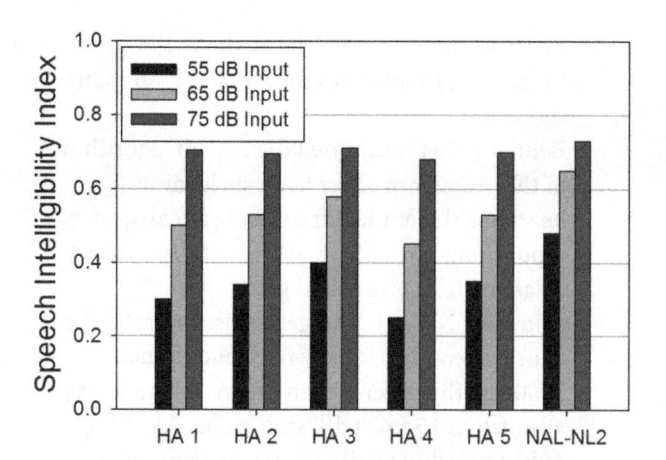

Figure 16-3. Derived Speech Intelligibility Index (SII) values (ANSI, 1997a) across five premier hearing aids and compared to the NAL-NL2 prescriptive gain as a function of the input level. (Adapted from Sanders, Stoody, Weber, and Mueller, 2015, with permission.)

SPL input, we would expect that the lower SIIs from some instruments would results in 20 to 50% poorer speech recognition than if the patient had been fitted to the NAL-NL2 (e.g., based on the SII conversion chart of Killion and Mueller (2010), as shown in Figure 16-4).

Of course, the most critical factor when comparing default fittings to validated methods is the patient-reported outcome. The laboratory data of Leavitt and Flexer (2012) are quite compelling—improvements in the average SNR of 6 to 10 dB for most manufacturers. If we look at real-world outcomes, however, it should be noted that the sensitivity of these measures is limited, so one might not expect significant differences in self-reported patient outcomes, even in cases where there are clear differences in audibility and speech recognition performance. Is there any evidence that sending the patient out the door with a verified prescriptive method instead of using manufacturer defaults leads to better outcomes? We certainly would view such data as convincing reason to conduct verification measures.

This was conducted indirectly by Cox, Johnson, and Alexander (2012). We say indirectly, as these authors did not specifically use the proprietary algorithm of a given manufacturer, but rather programmed the hearing aids to mimic the typical proprietary real-ear output as shown in Figure 1-3. Making this research even more intriguing, the authors also studied the NAL-NL2 vs. proprietary fitting with individuals with cochlear dead regions.

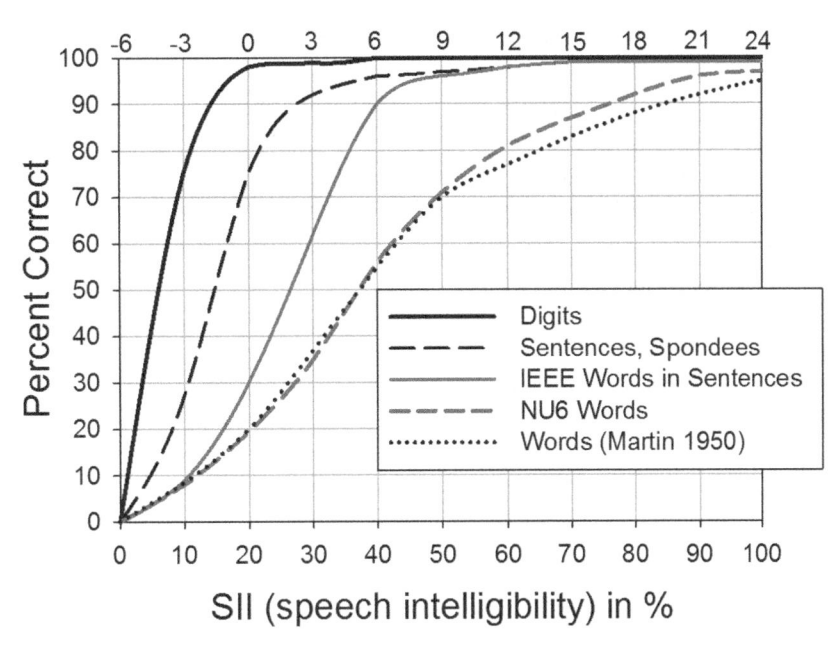

Figure 16–4. Predicted speech recognition performance as a function of SII for different types of speech materials. As contextual content increases, a lower SII will result in higher speech recognition performance. (Adapted from Killion and Mueller, 2010.)

The study was a double-blinded, nonrandomized intervention design with 18 matched pairs of adult subjects. In each pair, one subject had high-frequency cochlear dead regions and the other subject did not. Each subject was fitted with two active programs: the NAL and the mimic of a typical proprietary fitting (gain roll-off in the high frequencies). Outcomes included aided speech recognition in quiet and noise measured in the laboratory, real-world ratings of speech understanding in daily life, and final preference for the NAL or LP program.

The results were as follows:

- In laboratory testing, speech recognition in quiet was significantly better when using the NAL program. This result was observed for subjects with dead regions and without.
- When listening in noise, speech recognition was significantly better when using the NAL program for subjects without dead regions. For subjects with dead regions, results were equivalent for the two programs.
- In daily life, the NAL program received significantly higher ratings for speech understanding, and this result was observed for subjects with and without dead regions.
- Regarding final preference for listening in daily life, roughly 2/3 of the participants preferred to NAL fitting. The reason most frequently given for preferring the default program was that the NAL fitting was too loud.

Overall, adult hearing aid wearers with mild to moderately severe hearing loss benefitted from the additional high-frequency gain provided by the NAL algorithm, whether or not they had dead regions.

Abrams, Chisolm, McManus, & McArdle, (2012), in a crossover design, compared manufacturers' first fit to a verified prescriptive NAL-NL1 fitting across 22 subjects. It is often a challenge in clinical research to weigh clinical reality with complete control. In this study the authors began with verification of a validated prescriptive target (NAL-NL1) and the manufacturers' default. Several manufacturers and models were used, so there was a sampling of different manufacturer default fittings. The authors then chose to lean toward clinical reality, and for both types of fittings made minor gain modifications based on patient input. This is a compelling study design, in part because clinicians will sometimes argue that it is not worth beginning with verification of a validated prescriptive method if you plan to modify the fitting based on patient feedback anyway.

The results of this study revealed that even though the verified fitting was still somewhat below the NAL-NL1 prescribed targets, it was significantly closer than what was obtained with the manufacturers' recommended fitting (as you would predict from our earlier discussion). The participants used the hearing aids with the two different fittings in the real world and, following each trial, completed the Abbreviated Profile of Hearing Aid Benefit (APHAB). After using both prescriptive methods, the participants selected their preferred fitting.

The APHAB mean group results showed significant self-perceived hearing aid benefit with the verified NAL-NL1 fitting for the speech in quiet, reverberation, and listening in background noise subscales. Of the 22 participants, 17 selected the verified NAL as their preferred fitting. For some of the participants, the verified NAL and the initial fit were not significantly different after modification was made based on patient input. In total, the RMS error was significantly closer to the prescribed NAL-NL1 target for the modified NAL-NL1 fit than for the modified initial-fit approach for 13 participants. Of those 13 listeners, 11 preferred the verified fit at the conclusion of the study. In other words, beginning with the NAL-NL1 fit did not lead to a different fitting for everyone, but in those that it did, there was a clear preference for the NAL-NL1 fit over the manufacturer's first fit as a starting point—and there was a significant real-world outcome advantage for the entire group.

A similar study to that of Abrams et al. (2012) was recently conducted by Valente, Oeding, Brockmeyer, Smith, & Kallogieri (2017). These researchers used a randomized controlled design to compare the manufacturers' default fitting to the NAL-NL2. Comparisons were made using three different metrics: clinic performance for speech recognition, real-world self-assessment scales, and final user preference for one algorithm versus the other. In all three areas, the NAL-NL2 was the superior algorithm. When this fitting was employed, the results showed that there was significantly improved speech understanding for the clinical setting, and the participants rated this fitting significantly higher on the APHAB self-assessment scales compared to the proprietary fitting—by about 10% for both the background noise and reverberation sub-scales. At the completion of the field trial, 19 of the 24 participants preferred the NAL-NL2 fitting.

These data certainly do suggest that, on average, fittings approaching NAL-NL targets will provide more real-world benefit, at least when compared to beginning with a manufacturer's default.

NAL-NL2 on the Screen Is NAL-NL2 in the Ear (NOT)

A final area that we believe is one of the leading reasons that audiologists do not conduct probe microphone measures is the misconception that selecting NAL-NL2 or DSL v5 in the fitting software will result in the output in the real ear that corresponds to these fitting targets. This is different from what we discussed in the previous section. In this case, the audiologist indeed does want to use a validated prescriptive method rather than the manufacturer's proprietary method, but incorrectly assumes this only requires a couple of mouse clicks.

There are at least two good reasons why real-ear verification is needed even when a validated prescriptive method is selected in the fitting software. First, as we discuss in Chapter 14, when real-ear gain and output curves are software-simulated based on 2cc-coupler data, there are several factors that must be considered, such as the individual's RECD and REUG, and also microphone location and vent effects. So, even in the best case, we would only expect the fitting to be correct if (1) all the correction factors were applied appropriately, (2) the patient has an average ear, (3) the hearing aid or earmold is at average depth in the ear canal, (4) the microphone is at the average location, and (5) the clinician's description of the tightness of the fit agrees with the manufacturer's definition. Even though some of these variables only amount to a few dB, when added up the effect can be considerable and noticeable to the patient. If we look at the patient and fitting factors we just mentioned, given that most patients are not average we would expect to see real-ear differences from the prescribed targets, with the variances expected to be both above and below the desired levels.

A second problem that has been commonly observed relates to the manufacturer's calculation of prescriptive targets. Specifically, the average fitting does not actually reflect prescribed targets but rather falls below them, especially for the higher frequencies. This suggests there are errors or intentional alterations other than patient variability when applying a manufacturer's version of a validated prescriptive method. Mueller (2014a) illustrated this with examples of real-ear measures from three different leading manufacturers. The hearing aids were programmed to the manufacturers' NAL-NL2 algorithm but when compared to the NAL-NL2 targets in the real ear, output in the high frequencies fell below target by 10 dB or more for all three manufacturers—despite the fact that the on-screen display in the fitting software showed a perfect match to target.

Past research has suggested that the mismatch to target reported by Mueller (2014a) has been common for many years, as illustrated in the following examples:

- Aazh and Moore (2007b) tested four different products, all programmed to the manufacturers' NAL-NL1, from major manufacturers. Probe microphone measurements on 42 ears revealed that 64% of cases failed to come within +/−10 dB of the target at one or more of the key frequencies from 250 to 4000 Hz. After adjusting the frequency-gain response of the hearing aids, 83% of cases came within +/−10 dB of the target, and the fit rate was 100% for the hearing aids with four or more software handles. This shows that it was not that the aids were incapable of matching the prescriptive target, but that the fitting software did not apply the correct gain. And, note that the window of acceptance was 10 dB, which is pretty generous and larger than we would normally use clinically.
- In 2012 Aazh, Moore, and Prasher conducted a similar study, although this time they examined fittings for open-canal (OC) fittings. As before, the hearing aids were all programmed to NAL-NL1 and then tested in the real ear (30 individuals, 51 ears). Fittings were considered acceptable if the real-ear gain was within +/− 10 dB of prescribed target; only 29% met this rather lax criterion, however. After adjustment, 82% were fitted to within 10 dB; for the remaining 18% the primary factor was gain for 4000 Hz, where feedback was an issue (recall that these were OC fittings).

To put these latter findings in simple clinical terms: Without conducting probe microphone testing for your OC fittings, you would expect that when you click on NAL in the fitting software, only 29% of cases will be fitted close to the NAL target. In contrast, by taking a few minutes to conduct probe microphone testing and making appropriate adjustments, you would expect that 82% of your fittings will be close to the NAL target (and this could be even higher if feedback can be resolved). That's more than a 50% improvement in fitting accuracy!

These data suggest that trusting the manufacturer's NAL algorithm to be the true NAL algorithm is risky practice. The Aazh and Moore (2007) findings are somewhat dated, however. The research performed by Aazh et al. (2012) only included one manufacturer, and the Mueller (2014a) data showed only isolated examples. Fortunately, however, we have relatively current findings that address this issue; for the most part they reveal the long-standing software/real-ear mismatch continues to be common. We are referring to the previously mentioned Sanders et al. (2015) research that used hearing aids and software current for 2015. In this study, the authors selected the premier model hearing aid from the five leading companies, and programmed each instrument to the NAL-NL2 using the respective manufacturer's software. Probe microphone measures were then conducted (16 ears; 8 male and 8 female) and the hearing aid output was compared to the NAL-NL2 targets generated by the Audioscan Verifit® (factors such as experience, bilateral fitting, and so forth were matched between the software and the probe microphone equipment). The hearing loss used for the comparison was a typical downward sloping configuration, 30 dB in the lows to 70 dB in the high frequencies. The input signal was the Verifit® male speaker (carrot passage); inputs of 55, 65, and 75 dB SPL were used.

Figure 16–5 shows the deviation from NAL-NL2 targets for the average of the 16 ears. Panels A, B, and C are the inputs of 55 dB, 65 dB, and 75 dB SPL respectively. It appears that only one of the five manufacturers has used an algorithm that is reasonably close to the NAL-NL2 for all inputs (HA5). The greatest variation from target is for the 55 dB input signal—observe that at 3000 Hz, the average output for four of the five products is 10 dB or more below prescribed target. But even for the 65 dB input, the measured output falls 7 to 10 dB below target in the high frequencies for the majority of products. In general, these data add to the body

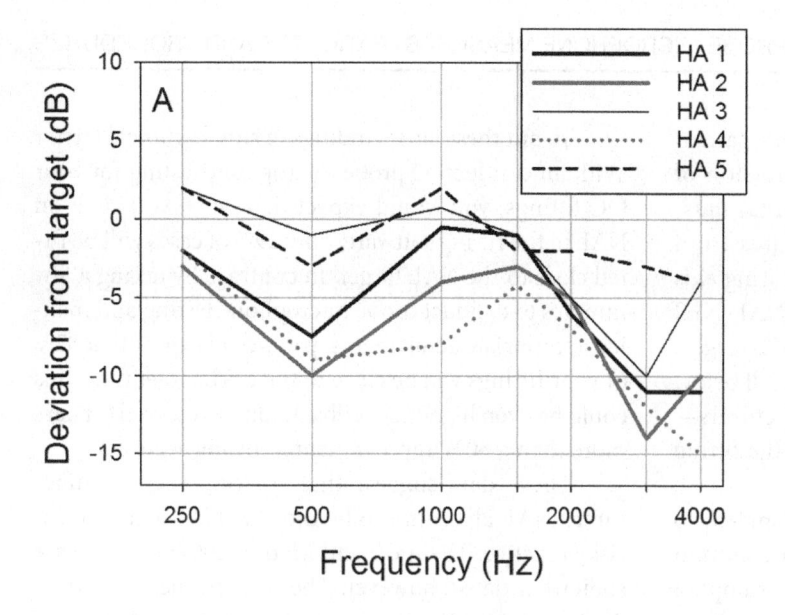

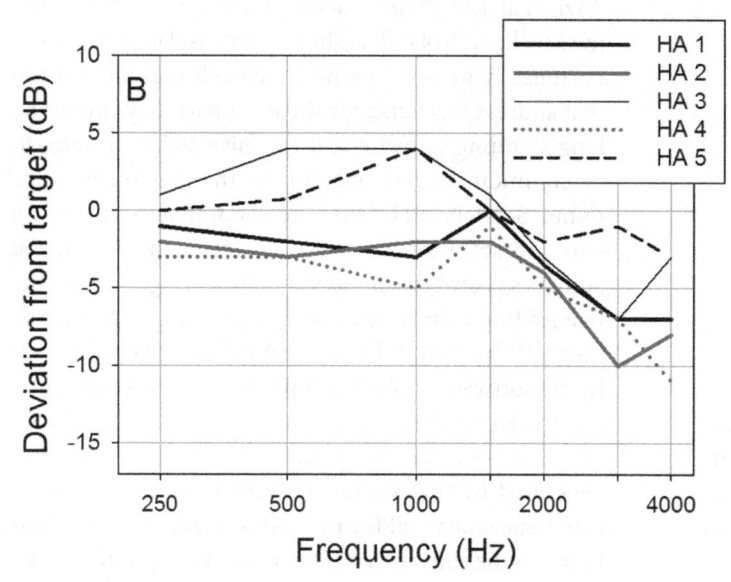

Figure 16–5. Actual deviation from prescribed NAL-NL2 gain is shown for the soft (**A**), average (**B**), and loud (**C**) inputs for each of the five premier hearing aids. (Adapted from Sanders et al., 2015, with permission.)

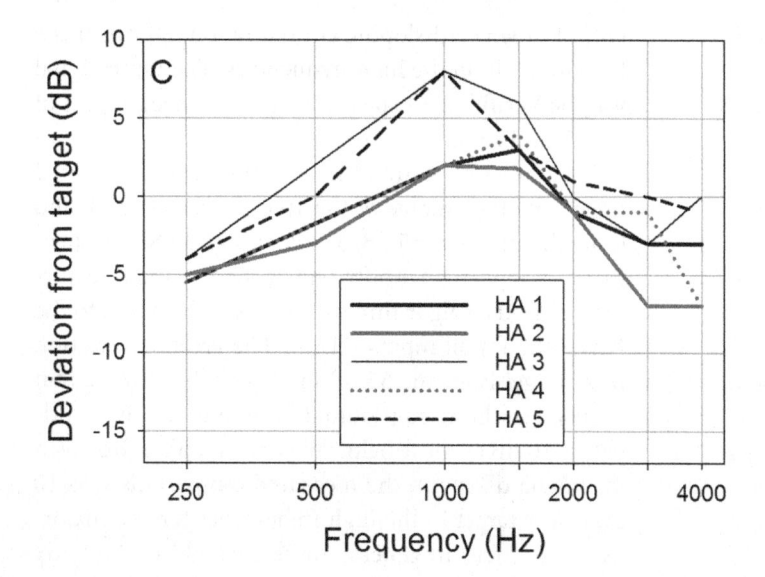

of literature showing that most manufacturers are using a NAL-NL1 or NAL-NL2 fitting that has been modified from the validated version. This is not an issue, of course, if probe microphone verification is conducted and appropriate gain corrections are made.

Accuracy of Software Display. A related issue is the accuracy of the gain and output values displayed in the fitting software. Going back to our previous discussion, if you knew that the NAL-NL2 prescribed output for your patient for a 65-dB-SPL LTASS signal was 90 dB at 3000 Hz (reference ear canal SPL; you could obtain this target from your NAL-NL2 stand-alone software), and after clicking the NAL-NL2 button of your favorite manufacturer's software, their fitting screen showed an output of 80 dB SPL at 3000 Hz, you would assume that you needed to turn up gain by 10 dB. What if the software showed an output of 90 dB SPL? Then you would assume that all is well, right? But what if it showed 90 dB, but only 80 dB was being delivered in the real ear? Now we have a problem. Unfortunately, this problem seems to exist.

Hawkins and Cook (2003), using five different manufacturers, reported that there was a poor match when the measured average REIG is compared to the REIG values shown on the fitting screen. Up to about 2000 Hz, the differences appeared to resemble what you might see for individual ear differences. For the higher frequencies, however, their research showed a distinct pattern of deviation; there was an average real-ear *reduction* of high-frequency gain of 5 to 10 dB present for all manufacturers. That is, even if an audiologist selected a validated procedure, such as the NAL-NL2, and the computer display showed an excellent match to target, it was possible—if not probable,—that the real-ear gain above 2000 Hz would fall well below this prescriptive target. Similar findings to Hawkins and Cook (2003) were obtained by Aarts and Caffee (2005). And most recently, Sanders et al. (2015) report in their article that the four manufacturers who had large deviations from targets in the real ear (e.g., greater than 10 dB in the high frequencies) all had fits to targets within 1 dB on the fitting screen.

Some of the research data we are citing on this topic is somewhat dated, but we can say anecdotally that we commonly hear clinicians say that, when they fit the hearing aids to prescriptive target in the real ear using the target displayed by the probe microphone equipment, the match on the software fitting screen is nowhere close. We do not find this surprising at all. Fortunately, if you verify using probe microphone measures, you do not care what the fitting screen shows because you have data demonstrating your exact match to validated targets. That's more or less the point we've been making for the last several pages.

Professionalism and Perceptions

Recall that in Chapter 1, we discussed how following best practices can have a long term impact regarding patient loyalty—data from MarkeTrak VIII (Kochkin, 2011a) revealed that patient loyalty increased from 57 to 84% when verification and validation were conducted. In the MarkeTrak VIII findings, probe-mic measures were just one aspect of the verification process. We do have recent data, however, which provides insight regarding the effect that conducting probe-mic measures has on patient perceptions. Amlani, Pumford, and Gessling (2016) studied three groups of 20 ($n = 60$) adult listeners with mild to moderately severe sensorineural hearing loss: experienced users, owners of hearing aids who did not use them frequently, and non-adopters of amplification who experienced hearing difficulties and were interested in a trial period. One-half of each group was fit by simply selecting the manufacturer's default NAL-NL2 setting (no probe-mic verification), the other half received probe-mic verification with appropriate adjustments to meet targets for three input levels. Both groups were allowed to rate the fitting for speech inputs, and during and after the fitting process each subject was counseled on the procedures being performed by the same experienced clinician. At the conclusion of the protocol, each listener's perception towards the service received was quantified using two measures: (1) willingness-to-pay (WTP), price anchored at $250 for professional services; and (2) a modified version of the Perceived Value Measurement (PVM), designed to assess a respondent's attitude toward professional services assessed over the five dimensions of perceived quality, perceived value, behavioral intent, emotion, and price (rating on a seven-point scale in which 1 equals very satisfied).

The authors report that all three groups showed a significant increase in WTP when probe microphone measurements were included. A similar significant finding was obtained for the PVM, which revealed that the protocol including probe-mic measures improved patient satisfaction, meanwhile reducing anxiety (i.e., emotional distress) for all three groups. For example, for the experienced user group, satisfaction improved from 4.1 to 2.2 when real-ear testing was included.

In this chapter we primarily focus on the importance of probe-mic verification for the purposes of improving audibility, speech understanding, and overall patient benefit. As the above data reveal, it is worth remembering that by conducting these measures we also are improving the perceived value and patient satisfaction in the overall fitting process. As hearing aid distribution channels continue to multiply and become more diverse, it is critical that the hearing aid fitting services proved by audiologists are indeed different from providers with limited or no training. It does not matter if the audiologist works at the neighborhood Walgreens, CVS Pharmacy, or in a high-end private practice, it is crucial that we demonstrate the added value that audiologist are trained to provide along with concomitant improvements in outcomes.

The Bottom Line

Mueller (2015) reported that recent data indicate that, when we look at the number of audiologists who simply use the manufacturer's proprietary fitting and then add a second group of audiologists who select NAL-NL2 (or NL1) in the fitting software but do not verify, we are left with the disturbingly low number of about 15 to 20% of hearing aids that actually are being fitted based on a validated prescriptive method (Mueller, 2015). Yet, we know that the patient's success with amplification will be greater when fitted to a validated prescriptive method or, at the least, when aided audibility is appropriate. There is no other way to reliably verify that this has occurred except through the use of probe microphone measures. Failure to do so is poor clinical practice, and often results in the poorer audibility, benefit, and satisfaction of our patients. Given these data, we agree it may even be a violation of the ethics of our professional organizations. We hope we have convinced you that these measures are critical for fitting hearing aids; now let's move on to the nuts and bolts of how this testing is conducted.

Probe Microphone Equipment

Probe microphone testing was conducted in the laboratory as early as the 1940s (e.g., the classic work of Wiener and Ross, reported in 1946); however, it was not until the late 1970s that a dispenser friendly system was available for testing hearing aids in the real ear. In this case, the term dispenser friendly is used somewhat loosely. The late 1970s equipment that we are referring to was first described in a paper that was presented by Earl Harford in September of 1979 at the International Ear Clinics' Symposium in Minneapolis. At this meeting, Earl reported on his clinical experiences of testing hearing aids in the real ear using a miniature (by 1979 standards) Knowles microphone. The microphone was coupled to an interfacing impedance matching system (developed by David Preves, who at the time worked at Starkey Laboratories) that could be used with existing hearing aid analyzer systems (see Harford, 1980, for review of this early work). Unlike today's probe *tube* microphone systems, this early method of clinical real-ear measurement involved putting the entire microphone (about 4 mm by 5 mm by 2 mm) in the ear canal down by the eardrum of the patient. If you think cerumen is a problem with probe microphone measurements today, you should have seen the condition of this microphone after a day's work!

Even though this early instrumentation was a bit cumbersome, we quickly learned the advantages that probe microphone measures provided in the fitting of hearing aids. We frequently ran into calibration and equalization problems, not to mention a yelp or two from the patient, but the resulting information was worth the trouble. Help soon arrived. In the early 1980s, the first computerized probe-tube microphone system, the Rastronics CCI-10 (developed in Denmark by Steen Rasmussen), entered the U.S. market (Nielsen & Rasmussen, 1984). This system had a silicone tube attached to the microphone (the transmission of sound through this tube was part of the calibration process), which eliminated the need to place the microphone itself in the ear canal. By early 1985, three or four different manufacturers had introduced this new type of computerized probe microphone equipment, and this hearing aid verification procedure became part of the standard protocol for many audiology clinics.

Due to changes in signal processing in hearing aids, it would be difficult to even do an okay job of verifying modern hearing aid gain and output using probe microphone equipment from the 1980s. This mainly relates to the fact that the majority of modern hearing aids use signal processing that provides differing amounts of gain for speech than for non-speech stimuli, as was used in early test equipment. Fortunately, there have been considerable improvements over the years in probe microphone equipment so that these systems have generally kept pace with changes in hearing aid technology. These improvements include new test signals, signal analysis, special tests for specific hearing aid features, and types of processing and portability. Today's equipment certainly has different looks, ranging from full size and portable clinical units (Figure 16–6) to the very portable system of MedRx, for which the equipment includes a probe microphone assembly and a break out box that is only slightly more than three inches long and plugs into the USB port of your computer (Figure 16–7). Regardless of the size or the complexity, all of these units have some basic components, which have not changed too much since the first Rastronics unit was released in 1982.

Test Signals

Although not equipment per se, we will start our discussion with the test signals that are available for the

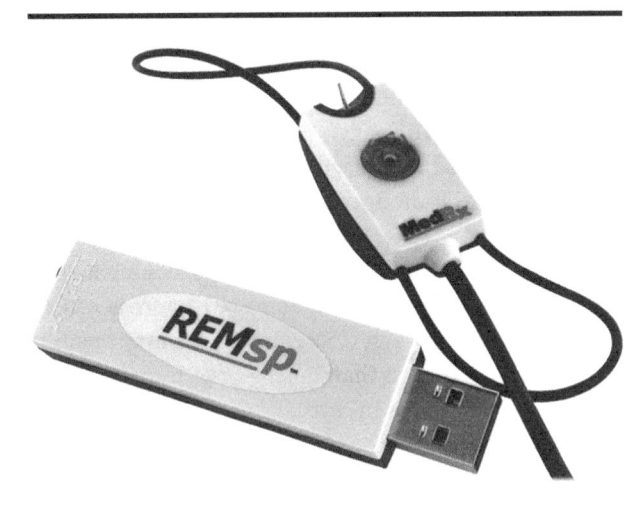

Figure 16–7. An example of a portable probe microphone setup, here showing the ear loop and the flash drive that is to be plugged into a PC. (Photo courtesy of MedRx.)

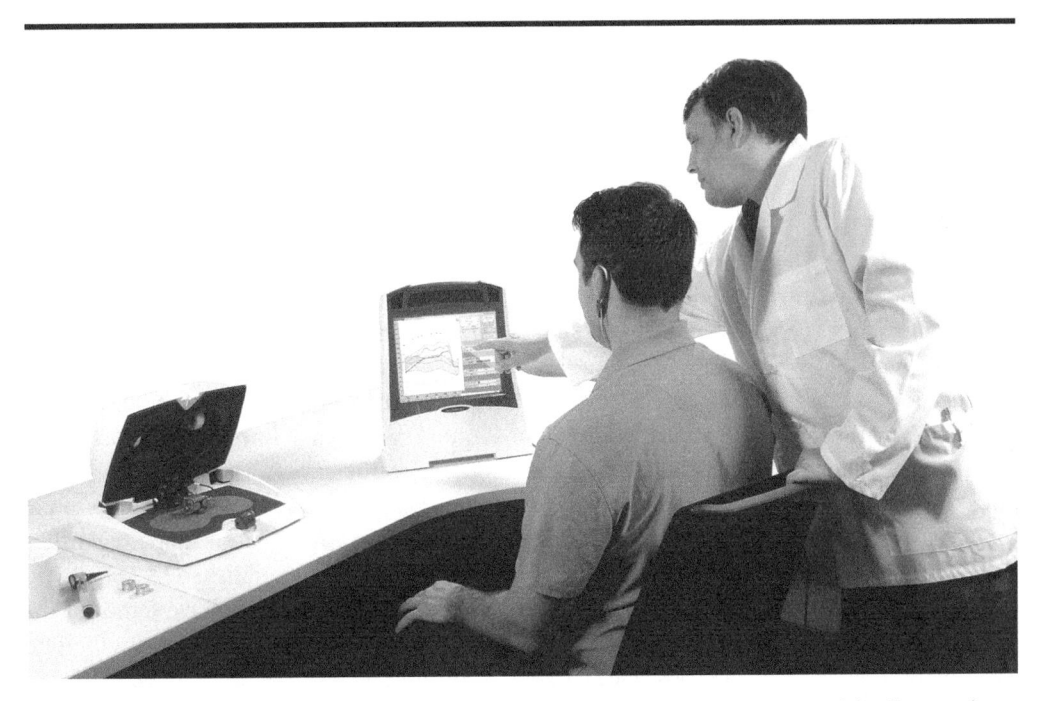

Figure 16–6. An example of a probe microphone setup. (Photo courtesy of Audioscan.)

different systems. Some of these are common among all or most manufacturers; others are unique to a particular system. Test signals can be categorized into three types:

- Signals that are intended to be used to verify validated prescriptive gain targets for speech inputs
- Signals that are intended to test the operation or provide quality control for specific features, including MPO, and
- Signals that are intended to be used for demonstration or counseling purposes.

It should be noted that there is considerable overlap among these categories, and some signals can be useful in multiple ways. Consequently, we may mention specific signals more than once as we discuss each of these three categories in turn.

Prescriptive Target Verification

As we discussed previously, the most important goal of most validated prescriptive fitting methods is to provide optimal levels of speech. It is therefore imperative that signals used for verification of prescriptive targets are categorized as speech by the specific hearing aid processing being evaluated—otherwise the concurrent processing of DNR or feedback cancellation, for example, may indicate gain and output values that are not realized in a speech-laden environment. Moreover, because it is often desirable to test the instruments in their *use settings*, these features should remain *on* during the verification process.

Simple test signals (e.g., sinusoidal, pink noise, composite noise) have one advantage over speech, however. Because they are often stable over time, the length of the test signal can be made very short, reducing testing time when multiple measures are taken. Regardless, to determine how speech is processed by modern hearing aids a test signal is needed that emulates as many of the most relevant properties of natural speech as possible. Additionally, for hearing aid verification measures to be comparable to each other, it is necessary, or at least desirable, to have standardized stimuli that can be used across clinics or with different probe microphone systems within the same clinic.

Many types of speech-like signals have been used over the years, but all share the common feature of being *speech weighted*. That is, the signal is shaped (filtered) to match that of some LTASS. Some of the simplest signals used are speech-weighted steady-state noise or a rough approximate such as pink or brown noise (pink and brown noise decrease in level at a rate of 3 dB and 6 dB per octave, respectively, when compared to white noise;

**THINGS TO REMEMBER:
THE EFFECT OF VOCAL EFFORT ON LTASS**

The characteristic pattern for average vocal effort reveals a peak around 500 Hz and a spectral slope (drop in level across frequency) of about 9 dB/octave (e.g., ANSI, 1997a; Dreschler et al., 2001; Pavlovic, 1989; Pavlovic & Studebaker, 1984). This shape, however, is affected by vocal effort. Most studies have suggested that the spectral slope is slightly steeper for soft and average vocal effort and becomes flatter as speech level increases. The frequency of the spectral peak also is higher for shouted speech than lower vocal effort levels. If you record shouted speech and play it at the same level as soft speech, one of the most striking (and perhaps surprising) features is that the shouted speech has a higher apparent pitch. Whereas some probe microphone manufacturers apply the same spectral shape regardless of testing levels, others apply the level appropriate shaping based on published LTASS. Based on reanalysis of published data, some probe microphone manufacturers have removed the distinction between soft and average vocal effort and only apply a different spectrum for loud and/or shouted vocal effort levels (see Chapter 4 for graphic representation of the effect of vocal effort on spectrum).

see Chapter 4). Slightly more complex than these simple signals is a combination of pure tones, such as the composite noise provided by Frye Electronics to simulate the speech spectrum. This test stimulus is a speech-weighted composite of multiple (79) pure-tones that are continuously presented in unison (more recently also pulsed off and on). As we will discuss, however, this test stimulus did not have other characteristics of actual speech, and has been replaced by most probe equipment manufacturers by the real thing.

By the mid-to-late 1990s, it became clear to manufacturers of probe microphone equipment that more realistic test signals were needed because of early types of digital noise reduction processing in hearing aids. This processing commonly operates by providing less gain for signals that have amplitude modulations that are either faster or slower than those associated with speech signals.

Some of the earliest modified signals included those termed DigiSpeech, Dynamic Roving Tone, Digital Speech in Noise, and Modulated Speech Noise. In general, these signals were developed by applying the overall amplitude modulations that mimic speech to speech-weighted noise, randomly interrupting composite noises or speech-weighted noises (e.g., pulsing the signal off and on a few times a second at rates similar to speech modulations), or presenting short pulses of pure tones that *hop* in a semi-random fashion over the frequency range of speech. When examined as a group, the levels of these pure tones are speech weighted.

Although some of these signals are still in use, increasingly sophisticated hearing aids are better than ever at differentiating speech from nonspeech signals. Consequently, some very sophisticated digital noise reduction schemes will classify at least some of these test signals as noise (e.g., Scollie & Seewald, 2002). Another problem arises with test signals that have tonal components. In some cases the hearing aid identifies tonal portions of the test signal as feedback, which the feedback suppression algorithm then attempts to cancel. In general, modern hearing aids typically apply compression and include adaptive characteristics that are applied based on signal analysis and classification. Consequently, they process speech much differently from non-speech signals like sine waves and unmodulated noise.

In a further step to be even more speechlike, ICRA signals (pronounced *ik-rah*) were developed (Dreschler, Verschuure, Ludvigsen, & Westermann, 2001). ICRA is an acronym for International Collegium of Rehabilitative Audiology, an international group of hearing aid researchers, and the signals were prepared by a working group dubbed Hearing Aid Clinical Test Environment Standardization (HACTES). The signals were developed by beginning with real-speech signals. This was followed by a process of filtering into three bands, reversing some segments (called Schroeder processing), recombination of the bands, and then smoothing of the spectrum was applied. This process resulted in noise signals that have the same modulation properties as the original speech in each of the three bands but are completely unintelligible and have flat spectra. Spectral shaping was then applied to this modulated noise to reflect the appropriate level and shape of a variety of materials. In total, nine different ICRA signals are available that reflect single or multiple talkers of both genders for different vocal effort levels (normal, raised, loud).

A number of probe microphone manufacturers include ICRA signals, but whereas ICRA signals share many characteristics with speech, they are not without criticism or problems. Most importantly, they lack speechlike co-modulation characteristics (e.g., fundamental frequency) and are often classified by hearing aid algorithms as *noise* not *speech*. Another important problem with the ICRA signal is that it does not allow a clinician to assess whether a product was distorted in terms of listening tasks during measurement. One of the authors of this book performed a sound quality study using the ICRA signal in an attempt to differentiate different hearing aid signal processing schemes. The outcome of this study was not published because, on the average, patients rated the sound quality of all of the signals as poor. That is, the unnatural sound quality of this signal limited its utility. In such cases its utility for verification purposes can certainly be questioned and standardized speech signals, including the ISTS, may be preferable options. Other manufactures apply the ICRA spectral shape to random noise or composite noise; however, these signals do not retain the natural amplitude modulations that are part of the ICRA signal.

Of course, the most speechlike signal is speech itself. Recordings of a single talker (or one talker at a time) shaped to the desired LTASS are now used in some probe microphone systems. Even though recordings of real-speech signals have exceptional face validity, speech within any frequency range fluctuates greatly in level

> **TECHNICAL TIP: OBTAINING THE ICRA NOISES?**
>
> The ICRA noises can be obtained on compact disc (CD) from W. Dreschler, AMC University Hospital, Amsterdam, Holland. There is a nominal fee intended solely to cover the costs of shipping. No copyright is claimed and the CD can freely be copied. The noise files can also be downloaded from several websites, such as http://www.ICRA.nu, or by entering the term ICRA noise into your favorite search engine.

and the spectrum changes as a function of phonemic content, co-articulation, and a variety of other factors present some challenges. To obtain a stable, repeatable, output measure across the wide range of gain processing available in response to the desired input spectrum is not entirely trivial. It sometimes requires compromises, such as making measurements over wider frequency ranges and the use of test signals that are longer in duration than the steady-state signals used in testing. That is, it is common for speech test stimuli to be several (10–60) seconds long in order to obtain a stable and repeatable measure. It is assumed that at least a 10-second sample of speech is needed to provide a reliable LTASS measure. As we discuss later in this chapter, longer signals may be necessary for some types of gain processing, such as compression processing with very long time constants. The average levels, as well as the output dynamic range for a single vocal effort (e.g., speech banana), of the speech signal over the entire duration of the signal can be calculated and displayed as shown in Figure 16–8.

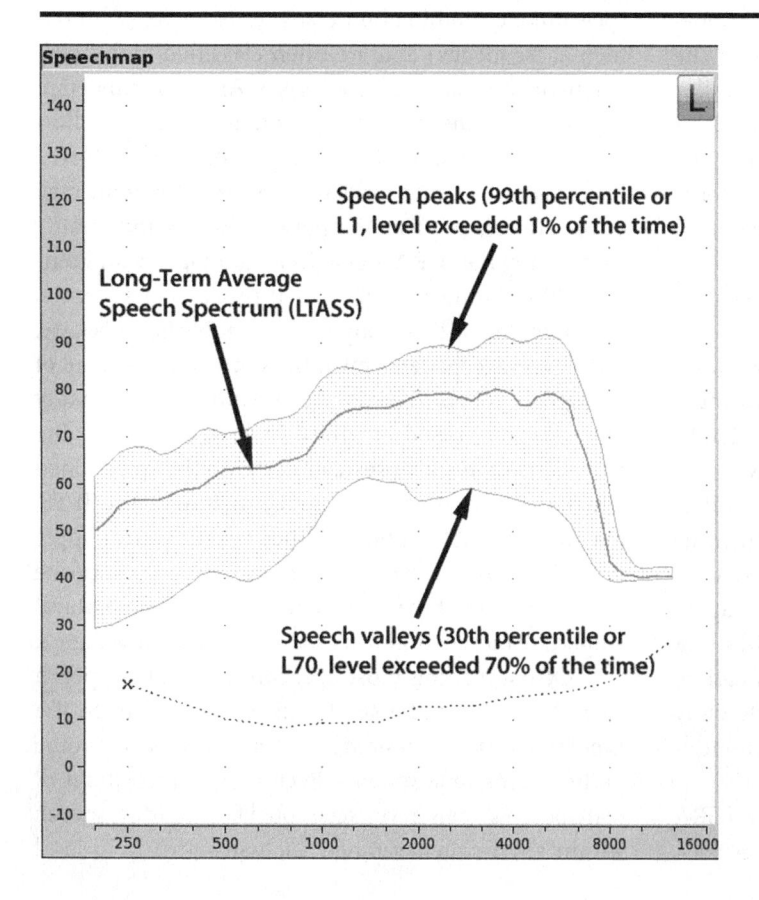

Figure 16–8. An example of the speech signal output from the Audioscan probe microphone system. The dynamic characteristics of the amplified signal are represented by the shaded area, meanwhile the average levels are shown by the solid line in the center. The shaded area is often referred to as the speech banana, whereas the average levels are referred to as the long-term average speech spectrum (LTASS).

Depending on the test equipment, speech signals may be available for male and female talkers as well as a child speech sample. These single talker samples may be shaped to multiple standard LTASSs to reflect conditions such as different vocal effort levels (casual, loud, shouted), or may remained unshaped (commonly no shaping is applied to child talkers). A specific LTASS shaping must be applied for accurate verification of validated hearing aid fitting procedures if that shape was also used in generating prescriptive output targets. Most systems will guide you regarding the preferred input signal for target verification. For some shapes, there may not be fitting targets available.

One criticism of real-speech signals, even those which are shaped, is that they represent one specific language and gender. We think this is probably fine for the purposes of verification as most validated prescriptive gain procedures derive their targets for a specific LTASS shape, one gender at a time, and derived from a single language. The work of Byrne et al. (1994) revealed that the differences among gender and different languages are not as great as we might think.

In the interest of comparing hearing aid behavior in a more generalizable way, the International Speech Test Signal (ISTS) was developed (Holube, Fredelake, Vlaming, & Kollmeier, 2010). The goal of its development was to create a reproducible, standard test stimulus that included as many of the relevant properties of speech as possible including average speech spectrum, modulation spectrum, variation of the fundamental frequency together with appropriate harmonics, and the co-modulation in different frequency bands.

TECHNICAL TIP: THE LTASS AND PRESCRIPTIVE FITTING APPROACHES

Although similar, several different speech spectra are used in clinical audiology and the fitting of hearing aids. It is of note that the two primary fitting algorithms, the National Acoustic Laboratories Nonlinear version 2 (NAL-NL2), and the Desired Sensation Level version 5.0a (DSL v5.0a) assume different speech spectra, as discussed in Chapter 14.

- NAL-NL2: The development of the NAL-NL1 and NL2 algorithms has been based on the assumed input signal represented by the one-third-octave levels of the international long term average speech spectrum (ILTASS) published by Byrne et al. in 1994.
- DSL v5.0a: The evolution of the DSL fitting scheme has focused on placement of third octave speech levels at a desired sensation level for a given hearing loss. The actual values for that speech are an average of male/female/child recordings of speech obtained 30 cm in front of the talker and recordings taken at ear level of the child. The LTASS used is based on that recommended by Cox and Moore (1988).

KEY CONCEPT: MODIFYING SIGNALS FOR TESTING FM SYSTEMS

We mention that speech signals often are shaped for use with probe microphone measures. This could be related to male versus female versus child, or to vocal effort. With some probe microphone systems, the signals are additionally shaped to be used in the fitting of FM systems (FM only). The 84 dB SPL level and appropriate spectrum may be applied for a chest microphone location or a 93 dB SPL level and appropriate spectrum for a boom microphone location.

The ISTS was created by segmenting (into 500 ms units) and then splicing back together the recordings of female speakers reading the internationally known passage, The North Wind and the Sun, in six different languages (American English, Arabic, Chinese, French, German, and Spanish). Because of splicing and segmentation, the ISTS is largely unintelligible. The final reassembled signal was then filtered to match the average female LTASS as described by Byrne et al. (1994). The resulting ISTS has been lauded for its speechlike characteristics including a realistic 20 to 30 dB dynamic range, as well as having relatively natural combinations of voiced and voiceless speech segments.

There is at least one clinical disadvantage to this stimulus: The ISTS is somewhat longer than other speech samples with the original signal at 60 seconds long. If the entire sample is used, this can make probe microphone verification more cumbersome when multiple adjustments are made followed by repeated verification. Shorter, 10- and 15-second versions commonly are being used by clinicians to move through the process more efficiently. Generally, we find that to be adequate, as long as the impact of the signal processor can be accurately measured with the shorter durations. When fitting a hearing aid with long time constants (for example, with slow attack and release times, or slow-acting noise suppression), however, a 10- or 15-second stimulus may not be sufficient to capture the characteristics of the hearing aid output when fully engaged.

In Figure 16–9, we show the unaided spectrum of the ISTS of different durations. These recordings were obtained by placing the tip of the probe tube at the regulating microphone of the probe microphone equipment, and therefore represent the input to the hearing aid. Observe, that there are only very minor differences among the three graphs. In Figure 16–10, we show the output of two hearing aids known to have different processing speeds (Panel A = slow; Panel B = fast). Observe that in the low frequencies (below 1000 Hz) there are now considerable differences as a function of the signal duration. Consequently, to obtain an accurate measure in the low frequencies, it may be necessary to use a speech test signal that has a duration of at least 15 to 20 seconds for probe measures of hearing aids with slow time constants (this is true for all speech signals, not just the ISTS). In many cases, by simply watching the screen it is apparent when the processing is still settling in. From a practical standpoint however, this will really only have a significant impact when fitting listeners with considerable low-frequency hearing loss and limited venting.

In Figure 16–11, we show the LTASS of the ISTS compared with other common spectra used in hearing aid fittings. It is clear that there is little difference in level in the 250 to 6000 Hz range across samples.

The ISTS is copyrighted and belongs to the European Hearing Instrument Manufacturers Association (EHIMA). It is free and available for download (www.ehima.com) for use in the field of hearing aid testing. For use in other fields, permission must be obtained from EHIMA.

Dynamic Range of Speech. The dynamic range for a single vocal effort—often referred to as the speech banana—is traditionally displayed by the distribution of one-third-octave band levels calculated for short time periods (120–128 ms). The level in each band that is exceeded only by 1% of the total number of samples is commonly referred to as the 99th percentile and is representative of the speech maxima. For long samples of speech, this level is about 12 to 15 dB above the LTASS. The level that is exceeded by 70% of the total number of samples is commonly referred to as the 30th percentile and is representative of the speech minima. For long

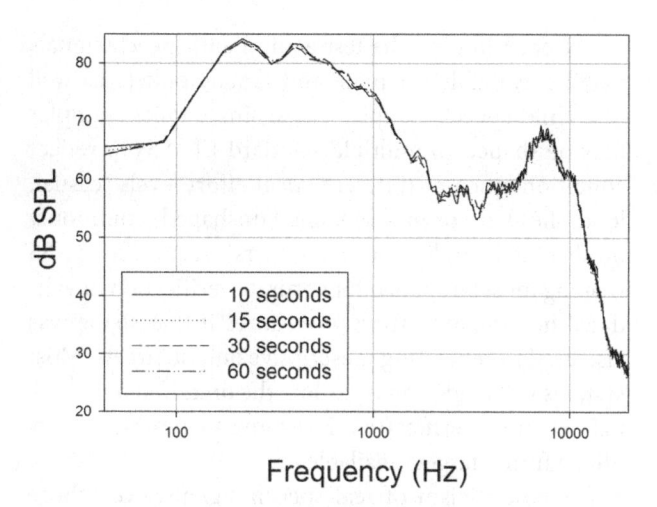

Figure 16–9. Spectra of the ISTS of different durations (10, 15, 30, and 60 seconds). These recordings were obtained by simply placing the tip of the probe tube at the regulating microphone of the probe microphone equipment, and therefore represent the input to the hearing aid.

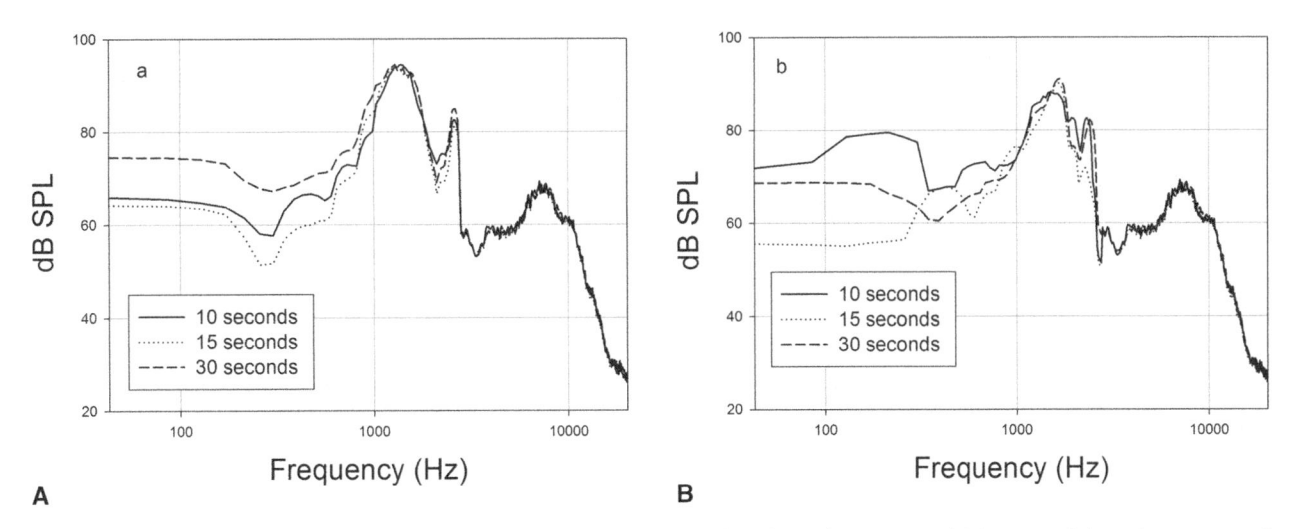

Figure 16–10. Spectra of the ISTS of different measurement durations (10, 15, and 30 seconds) at the output of two hearing aids. **A.** Hearing aid with a slow signal processor (slow attack and release times). **B.** Hearing aid with a fast signal processor. Although the spectrum into the hearing aid was identical (see Figure 16–9), the spectrum at the output varies as a result of the measurement time.

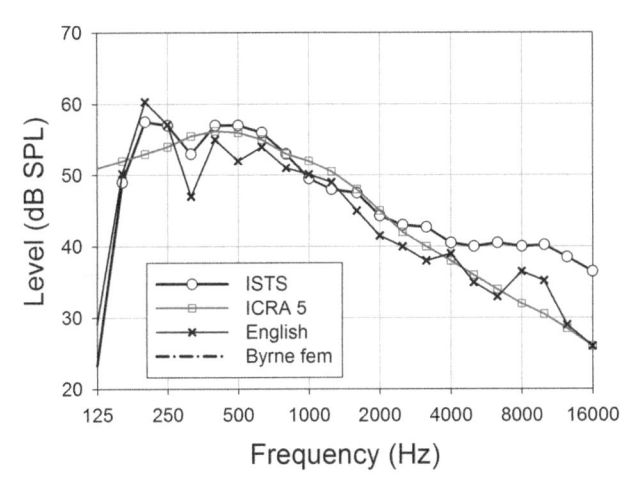

Figure 16–11. Long-term average spectrum of the ISTS (*circles*), the ICRA-5 signal (*squares*); the American-English speaker (*crosses*); and the international spectrum for female speech taken from Byrne et al. (1994) (*dashed line*), not visible because of its coincidence with the ISTS. (Reprinted with permission from Holube, Fredelake, Vlaming, and Kollmeier, 2010.) Adapted from Holube et al., 2010.

samples of speech, this level is about 15 to 18 dB below the LTASS.

Several probe microphone manufacturers not only display the approximate average (50th or 65th percentile) output or gain levels for single talker speech, ISTS and/or ICRA test signals, but also give some indication of this range (typically the percentile dependent real-ear output or gain levels for the 99th and 30th percentiles). This dynamic range information (sometimes referred to as *percentile analysis*) can be very useful in two ways: (1) by reminding us of the effect of the compression on the banana, and (2) by reminding us that even in cases when the speech information present at *average levels* fall at or slightly below a listener's thresholds, considerable speech information may still be accessible to the listener. Refer back to Figure 16–8, which shows an example of the percentile analysis used by the Audioscan Verifit®. In this example, the shaped spectrum for the male speaker (commonly called the *carrot passage*) was presented at 65-dB SPL input, with the hearing aid set to the patient's preferred listening level (after initial verification to NAL-NL2 targets). The top curve of this range is the level exceeded 1% of the time (speech peaks, typically referred to as the 99th percentile), the lower curve is the level exceeded 70% of the time (speech valleys, typically referred to as the 30th percentile). The middle curve (dark line) is the average (LTASS).

The percentile analysis developed for the ISTS is similar. As described by Holube (2015), the 30th percentile represents the soft parts of speech, the 65th percentile is similar to average speech, and the 99th percentile describes the peaks of speech. Note that both of these analyses use the 30th percentile, not the 1st percentile, as the latter one would be much more dependent on background noise in the measurement condition (and relatively impossible to measure, given the noise floor in most test environments). The difference between the 99th and the 30th percentile, then, describes the dynamic range or banana of the particular speech signal. Holube (2015) provides examples of this ISTS analysis, shown in Figure 16–12, the LTASS and the percentile analysis for the ISTS at the output of two different hearing aids. The left panel suggests a fast-acting compressor that reduces the speech range more than the slow-acting compressor in the right panel.

Percentile analysis is an excellent method to observe how the processing of the hearing aid affects the speech signal. The differences in output for slow- versus fast-acting amplitude compression, for example, easily can be observed. Unfortunately, some audiologists think of this as more or less a fitting method—that is, a replacement for using the NAL-NL2 or DSL 5.0 validated prescriptive targets. In stark contrast to what has been found during the validation of current popular prescriptive methods, some clinicians mistakenly believe that the goal of the fitting is to make all of the speech as audible as possible (e.g., the 30th percentile should be at or above the patient's threshold). Where this usually is an issue is in the higher frequencies, as most hearing losses we are fitting are downward sloping. This is certainly *not* an approach that we would recommend, and here are two reasons why:

- Each hearing aid user has a preferred loudness level. When we are shaping our frequency response, we have to decide where we obtain the best bang-for-our-buck regarding loudness. If we add considerable high frequencies, we likely will exceed the loudness limit, and the patient will turn down gain. It is not possible for them to just turn down gain for the highs, however, so this will result in less audibility for all the lower frequencies too. For most hearing losses, we would not want to sacrifice audibility at 2000 Hz for audibility at 4000 Hz.
- For downward sloping cochlear hearing losses, there is a point of *effective audibility* (see Ching, Dillon, Katsch, & Byrne, 2001, for review). Audibility beyond that point no longer has a significant impact on speech recognition, and, in fact, can make speech understanding worse.

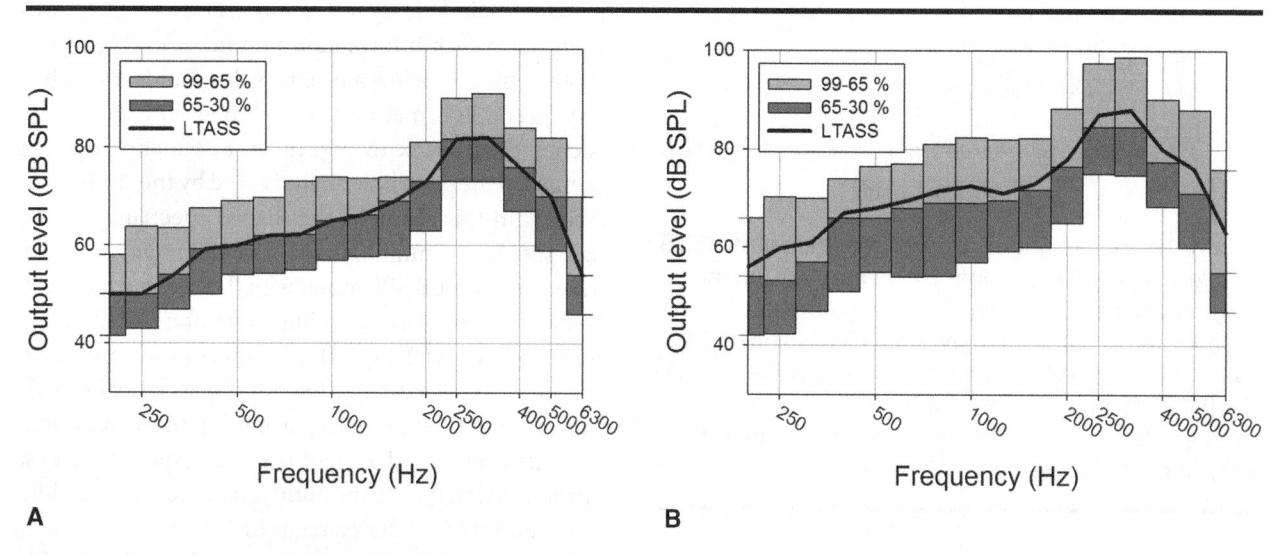

Figure 16–12. Percentile analysis of the output of two different hearing aids, with short (**A**) and long (**B**) release times. The overall gain of the instrument was not altered, only the time constants. Adapted with permission from Holube et al., 2010.

Test Signals for Evaluation of Specific Features

Several special test signals are included in probe microphone systems to test special hearing aid features. Whereas the speechlike signals described in the previous section can be useful for testing certain hearing aid features, such as the functioning of a hearing aid's feedback suppression system (e.g., additional gain before feedback or maximum gain/output before feedback) or quality control testing of the directional microphone system (e.g., front-to-back or front-to-side ratio), other special test signals often are needed to test features when the behavior for speech inputs is not of interest.

Evaluation of a hearing aid's MPO is one example of testing that often is completed with other types of signals. Specifically, warble tones, a pure-tone sweep, or bursts of pure tones (e.g., Audioscan systems implement 128 ms bursts with 128 ms gaps) are commonly used for evaluation of the MPO. These tonal signals are usually presented at either 85 or 90 dB SPL, referred to as the real-ear aided response (REAR) for these levels (REAR85 or REAR90). The maximum output of the hearing aid will be higher using a tonal input than with a broad-band signal. This 15 to 20 dB higher output when a pure tone is used rather than a complex signal provides a good worst case scenario, which is the very reason why it is used (see Chapter 17 for more details).

Since digital noise reduction processing is aimed at reducing the level of nonspeech signals, it provides another example of when signals that *are* speechlike do not work very well. Many other signals, however, are available for evaluation of noise reduction processing ranging from steady state noise (e.g., pink, white, brown), to composite noise, to recordings of specific environmental noises (vacuum cleaners, air conditioners, airplanes), to recordings of music signals. Typically these signals are available over a range of levels so the level-specific behavior of the noise reduction processing can be accurately evaluated (e.g., the strength of the noise reduction often varies as a function of the intensity of the input signal).

Probe microphone manufacturers also sometimes attempt to distinguish themselves by introducing signal types for evaluation of specific features or outcomes that are not widely adopted or are novel to a specific manufacturer. At least one probe microphone system has narrow-band noise signals that can be used for aided loudness verification, both aided and unaided. Although loudness measures were advocated for hearing aid fittings in the 1990s when fitting methods related to loudness normalization were popular, these methods are seldom used anymore (we think with good reason). That said, aided loudness verification can sometimes be useful for ensuring a patient's threshold of discomfort is not exceeded—and for the occasional patient who exhibits a very unusual loudness growth pattern necessitating changes to a standard fitting. For example, we have seen a few patients who, despite having a residual dynamic range of 50 dB, exhibited a most comfortable loudness level approximately 5 dB below their LDL. Even though some clinicians may find it useful to do aided loudness measures using probe microphone equipment, most clinicians simply use an audiometer and a loudspeaker.

Another special type of signal that we will discuss is aimed at assessing frequency-lowering technologies. At least one probe microphone manufacturer begins with a real-speech signal that has been shaped with the appropriate LTASS for verification of validated prescriptive targets. This signal is then filtered to reduce the level of the one-third octave bands above 1 kHz by 30 dB with the exception of a single high-frequency one-third octave band. Three different signals are included with a high-frequency band centered at either 4000, 5000, or 6300 Hz (Figure 16–13). These three signals may be used to determine the amount of frequency shift provided by frequency lowering technology, as well as the average sensation level of the lowered components of the speech signal after averaging over the length of the sentence. Importantly, this is not representative of audibility of the speech peaks at these frequencies. While these signals have been in common use for the past few years, there are several limitations, as pointed out in University of Western Ontario (UWO) Protocol for the Provision of Amplification (2014). They cite the following issues:

- The 1/3 octave band is narrower than the frication band of naturally produced speech sounds (e.g., /s/ or /ʃ/). This may lead to a conservative estimate of audibility.
- The 1/3 octave band is presented at the level of the LTASS at the test frequency. This presentation level is slightly lower than the

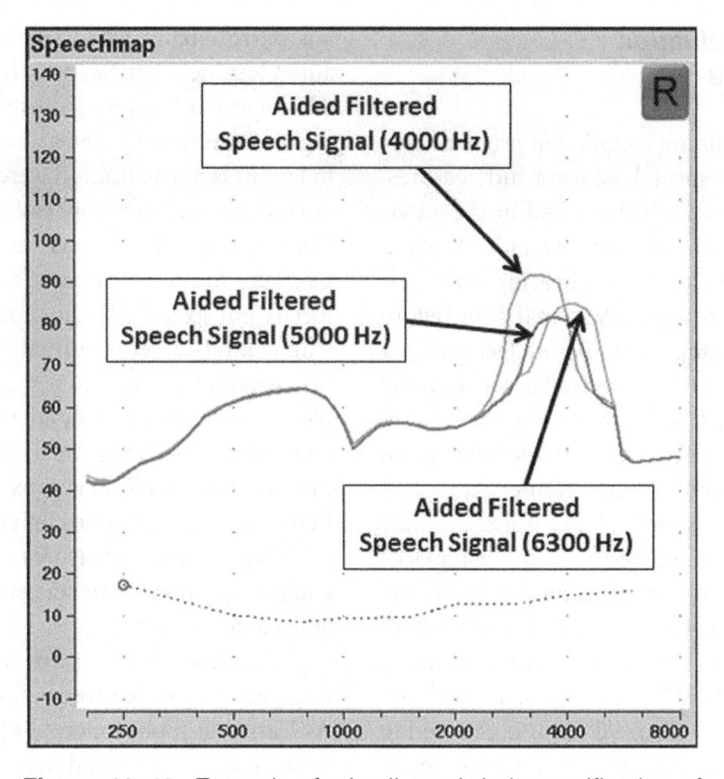

Figure 16–13. Example of stimuli used during verification of frequency-lowering technology. These signals may be used to determine the amount of frequency shift provided by frequency-lowering technology, as well as the average sensation level of the lowered components of the speech signal after averaging over the length of the sentence.

level of /s/ or /ʃ/ would be in speech that is similar to the ISTS passage.
- This test signals available only allow for evaluation to 6300 Hz, while a female /s/ is typically higher in frequency.

More recently, probe microphone manufacturers have introduced recorded Ling sounds and excised phoneme sounds for evaluation of frequency-lowering technologies. These signals can be quite helpful for evaluation of changes in speech audibility for specific sounds and overlaps and other distortions that can result when applying frequency-lowering technologies too aggressively. In some systems, industrious clinicians or researchers can even develop and upload their own stimuli for use in verification.

The /s/ and /sh/ test signals have been developed by the researchers at UWO, and have been adopted by some of the probe microphone manufacturers. The researchers state that in order to obtain calibrated /s/ and /sh/ signals with fricatives, they extracted these phonemes from the ISTS, and measuring each fricative's average spectrum. Synthetic fricatives were then generated that match the observed spectra. They report that these fricatives fall close to the peaks of speech, and represent average female production of the fricatives. It's important to point out that excised ISTS sound samples are different from the Ling /s/ and /sh/ signals—the latter were developed for threshold testing with children, not for adjustment of frequency lowering. The UWO group cites the following advantages of using the excised ISTS signals:

- The signal has been calibrated to a consistent level and frequency to improve replicability of measures. This improves test-retest reliability.

- Calibrated speech signals offer an accurate representation of the frication band. This allows the audiologist to estimate hearing aid output of the fricative.
- Measurement of the frication band of /s/ and /ʃ/ allows the audiologist to assess the spectral separation (i.e., how far apart do /s/ and /ʃ/ lie in the frequency domain), which is correlated with the listeners' ability to discriminate between these two sounds (/s/ and /ʃ/).

The measurement of the occlusion effect also involves somewhat unique signals, as we describe in more detail in Chapter 17. The most commonly used is the person's own voice—the vocalization of a vowel such as the /ee/, held constant at a determined SPL (e.g., 75–80 dB SPL) for a few seconds. Alternatively, the occlusion effect can be roughly assessed by using pure tones (e.g., 250 and 500 Hz) generated by a bone oscillator placed on the patient's head, either delivered from the probe system itself or by a portable audiometer.

Signals for Demonstration or Counseling Purposes

In addition to verification of validated prescriptive methods, it is sometimes of interest to demonstrate the amount of audibility a listener may have for specific signal types. For instance, we may want to show a patient how much more of a signal falls above his or her threshold when aided. Live voice is often used for this purpose. For example, a patient might be shown how much of his or her spouse's voice was missed with unaided hearing and how much more the patient can hear aided. We can also use this information to counsel patients that we are not making all sounds audible to them so they will still have some difficulties in some situations. A variety of other recordings that serve this demonstration purpose are also available with probe microphone equipment: male, female and child voices produced at various vocal effort levels for instance. Some systems even have speech signals that emulate a patient's own voice with regard to level and frequency shaping. Examining audibility for these speech signals *should not* be viewed as a way to fit hearing aids or as a guide for adjusting hearing aids (see associated Points to Ponder). Rather, they can provide useful information for counseling and demonstration purposes, when conducted *after* the hearing aids have been programmed correctly to match validated prescriptive targets.

We mentioned earlier the measurement of the effectiveness of the digital noise reduction through the use of a nonspeech signal. Although it is sometimes important to quantify the exact degree of reduction for different frequencies, this also can be a useful demonstration. By using the noise signals that are available with probe

---

POINTS TO PONDER: TOO MUCH AUDIBILITY

Some probe microphone systems calculate the total percentage of audibility. This is commonly referred to as percentile analysis, and it can be completed for demonstration signals as well as when completing verification of a validated prescriptive method. Somewhat similarly, other systems calculate the aided Speech Intelligibility Index (aSII) or aided Articulation Index (aAI).

We must keep in mind that audibility of *all* speech components is *not* the typical goal of hearing aid fitting. Full audibility might be achieved by very high levels of amplitude compression and/or frequency lowering. Data have clearly demonstrated, however, that too much frequency lowering or amplitude compression can actually decrease speech recognition, even when it also results in more of the speech signal being audible (e.g., Souza, Arehart, Kates, Croghan, & Gehani, 2013; Davies-Venn, Souza, Brennan, & Stecker, 2009). Although audibility is clearly important, *maximum* audibility should not be confused with *optimal* audibility. Consequently, percentile analysis and aAI must be interpreted and used with caution. Even though they both can provide important information, the more is better adage is clearly not always the case with these measures.

microphone systems, we can show patients in real-time, while they are listening, how noise levels will be reduced with noise reduction processing and how gain will be restored when speech is also presented. This also will reveal the time constants of the noise reduction (just watch the screen to see the action!), which also can be helpful for patient counseling. Real-world noise signals are available on most probe microphone equipment.

Presentation Loudspeaker

To conduct probe microphone measures, it is necessary to have a loudspeaker (or maybe even two) to present the test signals. The preferred location of this loudspeaker differs somewhat among manufacturers. All systems recommend loudspeaker placement relatively near the patient (usually within 1 meter/3 feet). Although probe microphone verification should be completed in a relatively quiet room, some noise can be tolerated. In order to obtain an accurate measure, however, the noisier the room, the closer the loudspeaker will need to be to the reference microphone as we discuss later in this chapter.

Mead Killion and Larry Revit wrote an article back in 1987 titled, "You Want Me to Put My Loudspeaker WHERE?" In this article, they examined optimal loudspeaker placement. Because head shadow can affect signal level, and patients can and do move sometimes during testing, they pointed out that the most reliable measure can be obtained by placing the loudspeaker near the ear being tested (at around a 45-degree angle), slightly elevated from the horizontal plane of the ear. For this reason, some probe microphone systems recommend this angle for testing. One problem with using this angle, however, is the loudspeaker (or patient) must be moved to a different position for each of the two ears or two separate loudspeakers must be used. A second issue is that the patient will sometimes want to turn to see the video monitor during testing. Consequently, most probe microphone systems forgo the added reliability (about 1 dB) and instead place the loudspeaker directly in front of the patient, often directly above the video monitor. That is, a 0-degree horizontal and vertical azimuth. At least one other system uses two small and separate loudspeakers that are mounted a few inches from each of the patient's ears. With this high degree of variability in procedures, it is important to consult the manual for the specific probe microphone system to ensure the recommended loudspeaker position is used.

One other difference across systems is the quality of the loudspeakers. A small, light loudspeaker is commonly used in smaller and more portable systems. Although greatly enhancing portability, such loudspeakers typically have limited output. Depending on the system, it may not be possible to test high speech input levels (greater than 70–75 dB SPL) without first adding an external loudspeaker with higher output. The addition of a higher output loudspeaker is possible with some smaller probe microphone systems but not others.

Monitor, Reference, or Regulating Microphone

Each probe microphone system has a microphone at the ear that is used to monitor the test signal. You will hear it referred to as the controlling microphone, reference microphone, regulating microphone, or monitor microphone. This microphone is intended to be near the head and the microphone of the hearing aid. As a result, the regulating microphone usually is located just under the earlobe (Figure 16–14) or on the head, just above the ear

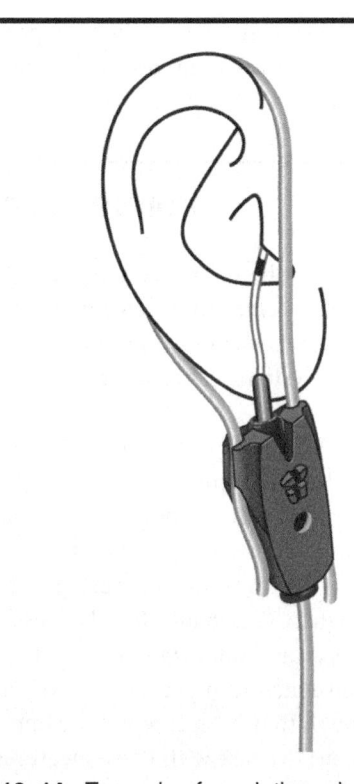

Figure 16–14. Example of regulating microphone placed just below the ear.

(Figure 16–15). ANSI S3.46-2013 refers to calibration using a reference microphone placed in this position as the modified-pressure method of equalization, although other types of calibration can be done with a reference microphone. In total, the reference microphone can be used for three different calibration applications:

- Modified-pressure method with concurrent equalization (or just concurrent equalization for short). This method measures the stimulus level during the measurement process or controls it in the equalization process. Commonly used for all fittings that do not use open coupling.
- Modified-pressure method with stored equalization (or stored equalization for short). The reference microphone is in the test position on the patient and the hearing aid is in place, but equalization is completed with the hearing aid muted. This equalization is stored and then testing begins. Commonly used for open fittings.
- Substitution method of equalization. Equalization is based on data recorded during a prior measurement of the soundfield at the position of the patient but without the patient present. (Note: This method may also be completed concurrently or based on stored data; however, it is rarely used for clinical measures).

Hawkins and Mueller (1992) reviewed the effects of different placements of the regulating microphone when concurrent equalization was used. The differences were small, especially for the frequencies below 4000 Hz. In general, although the regulating microphone position can affect the frequency response due to body baffle and reflection effects, those differences, for the most part, are accounted for by each individual system. That is, you really don't have to worry about the effects as long as you place the regulating microphone in the recommended position.

Measurement Microphone

For most probe microphone equipment, the measurement microphone is encased in the same module as the regulating microphone. This microphone is designed so that a silicone probe tube can be attached—hence the name *probe-tube microphone* or *probe microphone*. The probe tube is long enough so that the tip can reach to the patient's eardrum while attached to the microphone. Except for some of the equipment from Fonix, which uses a standard tube that results in a flat frequency response, each probe tube must be calibrated before use.

Signal Analysis

An additional factor that differs across manufacturers is the type of signal analysis used. The analyses differ both with regards to the frequency resolution and the temporal resolution. When a speech stimulus is presented, most systems use a temporal window of 120, 125, or 128 ms). Averaging of these temporal windows then occurs over the duration of the stimuli. As mentioned previously, it is common to present the output dynamic range of the speech based on the 99th and 30th percentiles. With regard to frequency resolution, some systems use partial octave analysis (commonly one-twelfth and/

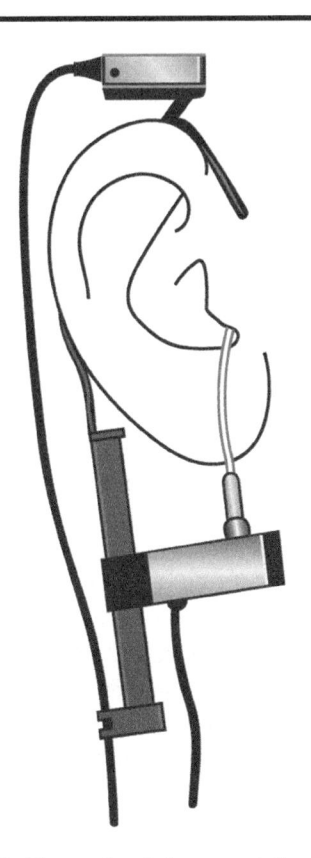

Figure 16–15. Example of the regulating microphone placed on above the ear, sometimes on a headband.

or one-third-octave), whereas others use a Fast Fourier Transform (FFT), which can have a frequency resolution as small as 87 Hz or smaller. One advantage to the greater frequency resolution is that we are able to see very narrow peaks and dips in the frequency response that may be smoothed over using a wider, partial octave analysis. Some clinicians may state a preference for the wider analysis band, however, because the representation of a response without narrow peaks will look smoother and prettier. This can be misleading because those peaks are still there. The width of the analysis window also often depends on the test signal. Specifically, whereas narrow windows are sometimes applied for pure tones and steady-state signals, nearly all systems use one-third-octave wide analysis windows when measuring the hearing aid output for a speech signal to help smooth the multiple fluctuations that occur in natural speech.

Output Display

The display of the testing can be viewed on a laptop or computer screen for computer-based systems, via an external monitor or, with some systems, a screen contained within the equipment itself. Most clinics use a traditional computer monitor for the display, although 42-inch or larger wall-mounted monitors are used in some offices. The appearance of the screen usually can be changed to be viewed as a single, full-screen, or dual (both ears), side-by-side panels. In some systems, the probe system screen can be viewed in real time on the fitting computer so a single monitor can be used for both fitting and verification. More recently, it has even become possible to view the probe microphone display via a tablet using manufacturer-specific apps. Usually a graphical display is used, but a tabular format sometimes is an option.

Monitor Headphones

Although not commonly used, many probe microphone systems have the option of plugging in headphones so that the audiologist or an interested observer can listen to the output being measured in the ear canal (or coupler during simulated real-ear measurements). Listening in can ensure that the processing is smooth and unwanted distortions are not present. This also can be helpful when troubleshooting patient complaints. It is possible to detect such things as intermittent feedback, and the occlusion effect often will be quite noticeable. One note of caution, however, if the headphones are loose fitting and the clinician turns the volume up too much, the combination can provide an additional path for feedback to occur. Consequently, we recommend tighter fitting headphones be used with higher gain open fittings.

Test Procedures and Conditions

There are several procedural considerations when conducting probe microphone measures, and most of them can influence the test results (see Hawkins and Mueller, 1992, for review). Some mistakes can lead to errors of 10 dB or more. It is reasonably easy, however, to follow some simple steps to assure good test validity and reliability.

Introduction to Common Probe Microphone Measures

In Chapter 17, we discuss the different test conditions and measures that can be conducted with the probe microphone equipment. We provide a short introduction here to assist in making sense of the different procedures we will discuss. The following is a summary of the probe microphone tests included in the ANSI Standard S-3.46-2013. We have also included the primary clinical use for each measure.

- REUR (Real-Ear Unaided Response). SPL as a function of frequency at a specified measurement point in the ear canal, for a specified soundfield with the ear canal unoccluded. *Primary clinical application: Serves as reference for the calculation of REIG.*
- REOR (Real-Ear Occluded Response). SPL as a function of frequency at a specified measurement point in the ear canal, for a specified soundfield with the hearing aid (and its acoustic coupling) in place and turned off. *Primary clinical application: Determine the tightness of the coupling in the ear canal.*

> **KEY CONCEPT: BINAURAL ANALYSIS WITH PROBE MICROPHONE MEASURES?**
>
> You might see in the promotional advertising from probe microphone manufacturers mention of *binaural analysis*. First, we believe the term should be *bilateral*, not binaural. Binaural suggests that you are measuring some combined processing of the two ears—such as what we do when we conduct soundfield binaural aided loudness discomfort measures (see Chapter 15). To assess binaural processing with a probe microphone, however, would require placing the probe tube somewhere in the low brainstem, which we believe would be an uncomfortable procedure for the audiologist, and even more so for the patient. These products do, however, allow you to hook up a probe microphone assembly to each ear and, at the same time, measure the output in each ear, although we assume that you will still need to adjust and fit each hearing aid independently. So, we are talking about *bilateral* testing. In fact, at the time of this writing, at least one probe microphone manufacturer recommended fitting each ear independently even when in the bilateral analysis mode. This is due to the fact that such measures create calibration issues related to the reference microphones that will need to be addressed and evaluated in each system before we know that simultaneous hearing aid fitting can be completed reliably—some unique calibration procedures have been developed. Even with this limitation, these systems do have a slight advantage for the clinician relative to verification of a validated prescriptive method. Rather than moving the assembly to the other ear when you finish the first, you can leave one side hooked up while testing the other. We don't see a specific measurement advantage for this type of verification unless you are using a long signal presentation, such as the 60-second version of the ISTS.
>
> We should add, however, with the availability of products that have wireless audio data transfer between hearing aids, there may be an increased interest in bilateral simultaneous measures. Specifically, simultaneous bilateral measurements allows us to quickly confirm that sound transmitted to one hearing aid is being routed to the other or that signals routed wirelessly from an external source are reaching both hearing aids.

- REAR (Real-Ear Aided Response). SPL as a function of frequency at a specified measurement point in the ear canal, for a specified soundfield, with the hearing aid (and its acoustic coupling) in place and turned on. *Primary clinical application: Verification of prescriptive targets, either as absolute values (often referred to as speech mapping), or for the calculation of the REIG.*
- REIG (Real-Ear Insertion Gain). Difference in decibels, as a function of frequency, between the REAG and the REUG, taken with the same measurement point and the same soundfield conditions. *Primary clinical application: Verification of prescriptive targets.*
- REAR85 or REAR90 (Real-Ear Aided Response for an 85 or 90 dB Input), previously referred to as Real-Ear Saturation Response (RESR). SPL as a function of frequency at a specified measurement point in the ear canal, for a specified soundfield with the hearing aid (and its acoustic coupling) in place and turned on, and with the VC adjusted to full-on (or just below feedback if full-on isn't possible). The input signal is sufficiently intense to operate the hearing aid at its maximum output level, usually 85 or 90 dB SPL as noted in the acronym. *Primary clinical application: Determine the real-ear MPO of the hearing aid.*

- RECD (Real-Ear Coupler Difference). Difference in decibels, as a function of frequency, between the SPL produced near the tympanic membrane in an occluded ear canal by a coupled sound source having a high acoustic impedance (see ANSI/ASA S1.1) and that produced in the HA-1 configuration of the 2cc coupler by the same coupled sound source. *Primary clinical application: Use with the RETSPL to convert thresholds and thresholds of discomfort from HL to ear canal SPL and to convert output from 2cc coupler to accurate estimate of real-ear SPL (typically in infants and children).*
- REDD (Real-Ear Dial Difference). Difference in decibels, as a function of frequency, between the SPL produced near the tympanic membrane by an audiometric sound source and the hearing level indicated by the audiometer driving the sound source. *Primary clinical application: Derive ear canal SPL display of audiometric and prescriptive output data for REAR verification.*

With that brief introduction, we will now review the conditions, techniques, and procedures required to obtain these measures.

Test Environment

In the early days of probe microphone testing, it was fairly common to place the equipment in an audiometric test booth, primarily because audiologists were accustomed to fitting hearing aids in the test booth, going back to the speech testing methods of the 1950s to 1960s and the popularity of functional gain measures in the 1970s. Even though it is still acceptable to conduct these measures in the test booth, most audiologists would like to free up this space for other testing, and have established fitting rooms. These fitting rooms typically work well, but there are a couple of important points to consider:

- One of the goals of the fitting is determine whether we have made soft speech audible. The best way to determine this is to present soft speech that has an input level of 50 or 55 dB SPL. It is possible, if not probable, that if the ambient noise level of your test environment exceeds this level (which easily can happen with a loud heating or air conditioning system), the resulting measures will not be valid. Hence, whereas the test area does not need to be sound isolated, the room does need to be relatively quiet. An example of how ambient noise can impact the measurement is shown in Figure 16–16. In panel A, the amplified speech—presented at 50 SPL in a quiet room—shows nearly perfect match to the intended targets (crosses). In panel B, you see the results when a low-level noise, such as that of an air conditioner, was added to the room. Observe that the output is clearly altered and the apparent dynamics of the speech signal (i.e., the banana) are compressed as well.
- A second point about the test environment is that the patient should not be seated next to any reflective surface. A common culprit is a wall mirror, which audiologists often have in the fitting room. But any wall or hard surface can generate measurement errors. Softer reflective surfaces, such as well-meaning audiologists, can be a problem too, so we need to make sure that we don't stand too close to the patient when the testing is conducted. Sound reflections from nearby surfaces can cause large measurement errors or unusual dips or bumps in the output, especially if stored equalization rather than concurrent equalization is being used (more on that later). With some equipment, standing waves from nearby walls or objects will cause speaker overdrive errors. We recommend seating the patient so that he or she is about two meters (5–6 feet) from any reflective surface.

Calibrating the Probe Tube

As we mentioned in our discussion of the measurement microphone, a key player in real-ear measures is the silicone probe tube. Before testing is started, it is necessary to place a new tube on the inlet located on the housing of the reference and measurement micro-

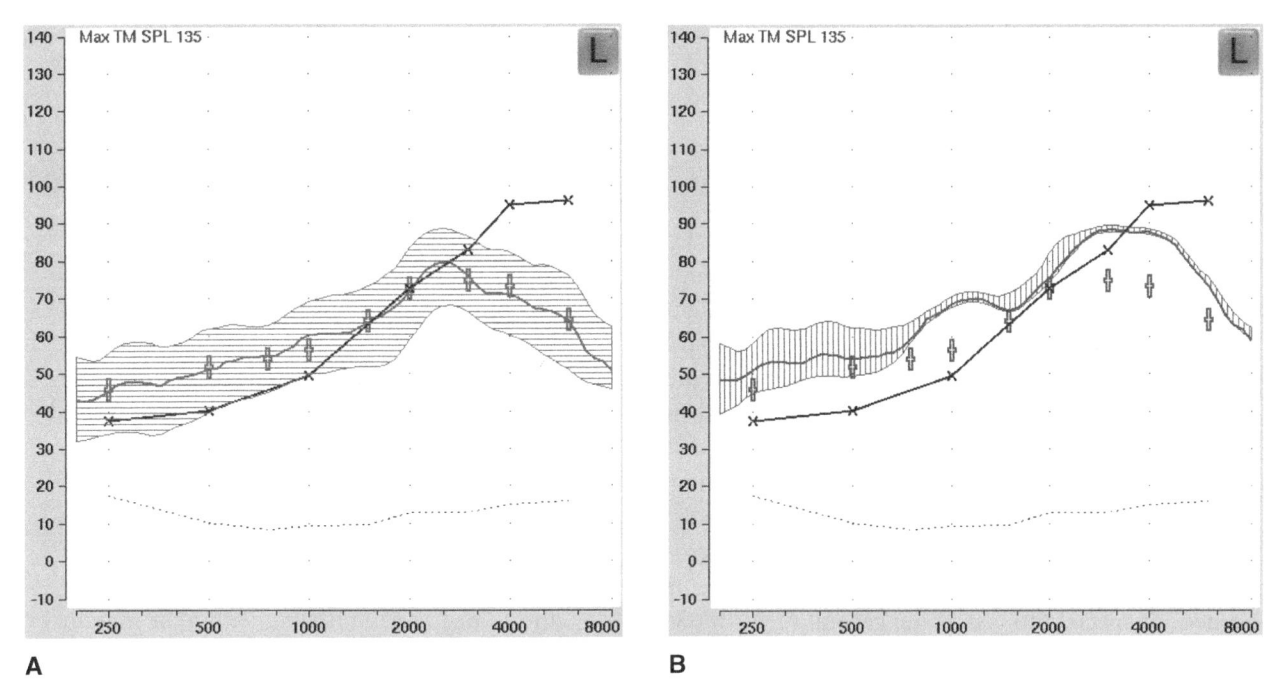

Figure 16–16. Measurement results with and without background air-conditioner noise. **A.** The *carrot passage* was presented at 50 SPL in a quiet room. **B.** The same passage was presented but with a low-level (and steady state) noise in the background.

phones. For the majority of test equipment, the tube must then be calibrated. The notion is to make the tube acoustically invisible, so that when the tip of the tube is near the ear drum, the measurement is the same as if the microphone itself were in that position. The tubes have natural resonances, and will also roll off the high frequencies, two factors which need to be corrected by the calibration process. While the tubes are machined to be all the same, there can be variances, and we therefore would always recommend doing a new calibration whenever a tube is changed. This usually is for a new patient, but if you're fighting gooey cerumen in the ear canal, which plugs the tip of the tube, it could be several times for the same patient.

The probe tubes are typically around 70 mm long with an adapter on the end. Most also have a moveable ring marker. The purpose of the marker is to assist in establishing the correct depth placement of the tube tip in the ear canal, which we will discuss in a few pages. It might be tempting to think that the probe-tube manufacturer places the marker at the correct point for testing (e.g., 30 mm from the tip for adult males). This may not be true, however, so you will want to position it appropriately before use.

To calibrate, place the tip of the tube next to the opening of the reference microphone. Most manufacturers provide a holder/dock for the tube at this location to make the process easier. Once the tube is in place, hold the microphone case with the tube attached at the approximate horizontal/vertical location of where the patient's head will be during testing. Given that it is a relative measure, the exact distance from the loudspeaker doesn't matter too much, but stay within three feet. Once everything is in place, go to the calibration mode of the system and present the calibration signal (predetermined by the manufacturer). For most equipment, you will observe on the monitor the output of the signal that has passed through the tube, which will reveal the acoustic effects we mentioned earlier. At this point you more or less have to have faith that the equipment corrected the variances observed. If you're skeptical, or simply curious, you could go to the fitting screen, present a signal that is equalized across frequencies, hold the probe apparatus in the same calibration position, and you should observe a flat output equal to the input.

Positioning the Patient

To maximize both validity and reliability, it is important to position the patient appropriately relative to the loudspeaker presenting the test signal. Although you might think this would be a simple thing to get right, we have seen the loudspeakers presenting the test signal on the floor, pointing at the patient's stomach, or from a shelf three feet above his head. We know of one clinic that placed the speakers at 90 degrees for a monaural fitting, and at a 0-degree azimuth for a patient fitted bilaterally! For specific guidance, please refer to the probe microphone systems manual (there are some adjustments needed for special fittings). Some general rules follow:

- The patient should be close to the speaker, usually not more than a meter (~3 feet), referenced to the center of the head. Many audiologists simply attach a string of the desired length to their loudspeaker, and use this for head placement calibration. Many patients do not like to sit this close to something, so repositioning of the patient may be necessary during the testing. For manufacturers that use a 45-degree angle, an even closer placement may be recommended. For example, the Fonix Company recommends a soundfield speaker placement approximately 12 inches from the patient's head at 45 degrees for the most accurate, repeatable measurements. The manufacturer goes on to say, however, that for bilateral testing . . . it may be more convenient to use a zero degree azimuth. The zero degree azimuth may be slightly less repeatable than the 45-degree azimuth, but within the margin of error for clinical use (Fonix Operator's Manual, 2013).
- The loudspeaker should also be placed at a 0-degree vertical azimuth. As we mentioned

---

KEY CONCEPT: CLOSE IS GOOD!

Some patients do not like their personal space invaded by a loudspeaker, but keeping the patient close to the test signal is a good idea. Here are three reasons why distance is important.

- When testing hearing aids with low compression kneepoints, you'll often want to use a low-level input to obtain the best estimate for gain for soft speech. This input must be above the noise floor of the test room for the equipment to operate properly. As the patient sits closer to the loudspeaker, you improve the signal-to-noise ratio, which allows for testing at lower inputs. We like to be able to test at 50 dB SPL whenever possible, certainly at 55 dB SPL.
- When testing using high inputs (75–80 dB or higher), it is possible to overdrive the loudspeaker of the system (some units will abort the run when this happens). This usually isn't a problem if the patient is seated two to three feet from the loudspeaker rather than four to six feet (remember the old half-the-distance rule).
- For loudspeakers that are directly in front of the listener, head shadow can be a problem if the loudspeaker is too close; small head movements can also generate errors. For this reason most probe microphone manufacturers that use a loudspeaker placed directly in front of the listener suggest a minimum distance, which is usually in the range of 18 to 24 inches.

earlier, this rule seems to be difficult to follow for many clinicians, as we see a lot of stomach and chest testing—probably because the equipment simply was placed on whatever table was handy. If for some reason you were to vary from the recommended 0-degree vertical azimuth, it is best to go higher than ear level rather than lower. In fact, at least one study that we mentioned earlier in this chapter revealed that the test–retest reliability (average standard deviation) was about 0.5 to 1.0 dB better for a 45-degree elevation (Killion & Revit, 1987).

Placing the patient in the correct location initially is important, but keeping him or her in place during the testing is equally important. As discussed earlier, in most cases, we do have a reference microphone active on the test ear, but even so it is important that the patient stays in the test position. To illustrate this, observe the test results shown in Figure 16–17. In this case, we used the *stored equalization* calibration technique commonly used with open-fitted hearing aids (see review in Chapter 17). Using this technique the reference microphone is used to calibrate the signal initially and then is disabled for all further testing. Consequently, it is assumed that the patient does not move! With the patient seated correctly, we initially fitted him or her to NAL-NL2 targets with the hearing aid on the right ear, and those results are shown. Without changing any setting on the hearing aid, we had the patient change position slightly in three different ways: turn head to the right, turn head to left, and lean forward. These were not exaggerated movements, but simply what we have often observed patients doing during testing—usually to look at the results on the monitor or see what the audiologist is doing. As shown in Figure 16–17, patient movements can impact the match to target by 10 dB or more. What then happens with many clinicians is that they then begin to make adjustments based on these invalid measurements, possibly moving away from what would be a perfect fit to target when testing is conducted correctly.

TECHNICAL TIP: GETTING THE LOUDSPEAKER PLACED CORRECTLY

As we've mentioned, correct placement of the loudspeaker is critical if you want valid and reliable results. Consider this: A loudspeaker placed too low could result in a measurement that is 6 to 8 dB below what is actually present at around 4000 Hz. This in turn will prompt you to increase gain for this region by 6 to 8 dB to match prescriptive targets. The patient leaves the clinic and now turns down overall gain by 8 dB because high frequencies are too shrill. This then means he doesn't have enough gain for the important frequencies of 1000 to 3000 Hz and decides that hearing aids aren't very helpful—all because he wasn't positioned correctly. Here are three relatively inexpensive items to purchase to improve the quality of your probe microphone assessments:

1. If you have probe microphone equipment with a built-in speaker, a table taller than usual for the equipment can be very useful. We've found that 36 inches works well (height of standard kitchen counter). We typically place the loudspeaker in a more desirable location if you don't have an external speaker and a wall-mount arm or floor stand.
2. A swivel chair that also has an up-down adjustment (for the unusually short or tall patient).
3. If you have a system that uses an external loudspeaker, we suggest using an adjustable wall-mount arm for your loudspeaker. This makes it easy to place loudspeaker at the desired location and even conduct the testing from the 12-inch distance and 45-degree angle location if desired. Minimally you will want a speaker stand that has an easy height adjustment.

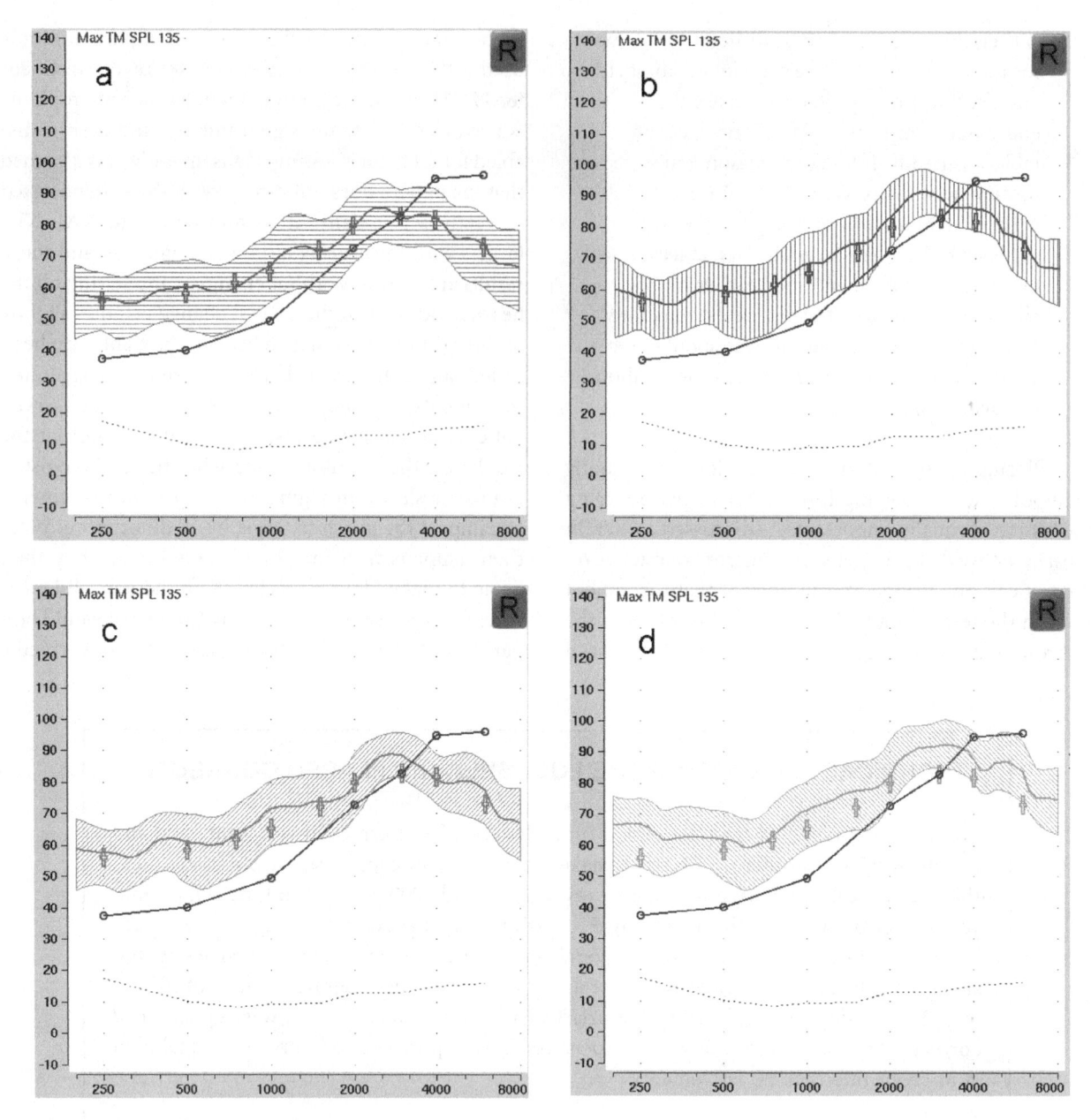

Figure 16–17. Examples of probe microphone results as a function of horizontal changes in speaker location. **A.** The patient is seated appropriated relative to the loudspeaker. We initially fitted him to NAL-NL2 targets with the hearing aid on the right ear. Without changing any setting on the hearing aid, we had the patient change position slightly in three different ways: lean forward (**B**), turn head to the right (**C**), and turn head to the left (**D**).

Placement of the Probe Tube

The probe tube has been calibrated to be *acoustically invisible*, so you can think of the tip of the tube as a miniature microphone. The general rule (for reasonably accurate measures through 6000 Hz) is that you would like to have the tip of the probe tube within 5 mm of the TM, and 3 to 5 mm beyond the medial tip of the hearing aid, eartip, or earmold. Although it is important to consider both factors, with most fittings, if you accomplish one you will also be okay with the other. Unless you have a very deep fitting, if you are within 5 mm of the TM, you probably also will be 3 to 5 mm beyond the tip of the hearing aid/earmold. The 3 to 5 mm position beyond the tip of the hearing aid relates to the fact that that in this region the sound wave is making a transition from the narrow opening from the hearing aid/fitting tip to the larger ear canal, and measures in this region may not be valid. In deep fittings, however, when only a 5 to 7 mm residual distance to the TM remains, we're okay with only 2 to 3 mm beyond the tip. An earlier study by Don Dirks and Gerald Kincaid provides perhaps the best reference for practicing clinicians (Dirks & Kincaid, 1987). As shown in Figure 16–18, the difference from the true SPL at the eardrum is most often manifested as a high-frequency error—the higher the frequency, the greater the error. As can be seen on the graph, at 1 cm (10 mm) from the eardrum, the error for 4000 Hz is only 2 dB, but increases to 4 dB for 6000 Hz, and to nearly 10 dB for 8000 Hz. Although we are not likely to get placement wrong by that much (10 mm versus 5 mm) very often, the impact on the high frequencies can easily lead to programming errors (e.g., unnecessarily increasing high-frequency gain). More recently, Vaisberg, Macpherson, and Scollie (2016), demonstrated improved test-retest reliability at the highest test frequencies with increasing probe microphone depth. These authors examined the effect of increasing insertion depth (measured from the intertragal notch) from 24 mm to 30 mm in 14 normal hearing listeners. Average test-retest differences at 8000 and 10000 Hz measured using 1/24th octave bands decreased from approximately 3 and 4 dB for the 26 and 28 mm insertion depths to approximately 2 dB for the 30 mm insertion depth. These authors concluded that a 28 mm insertion depth could provide reasonably reliable measures through 8 kHz, and potentially accurately predict levels up to 10 kHz, if one is very careful about placement of the probe tube. Unfortunately, the actual level at the eardrum was not measured in this study, so even though good reliability was demonstrated, the actual accuracy and the most accurate values that could be used to predict levels at 10 kHz could not be conclusively confirmed.

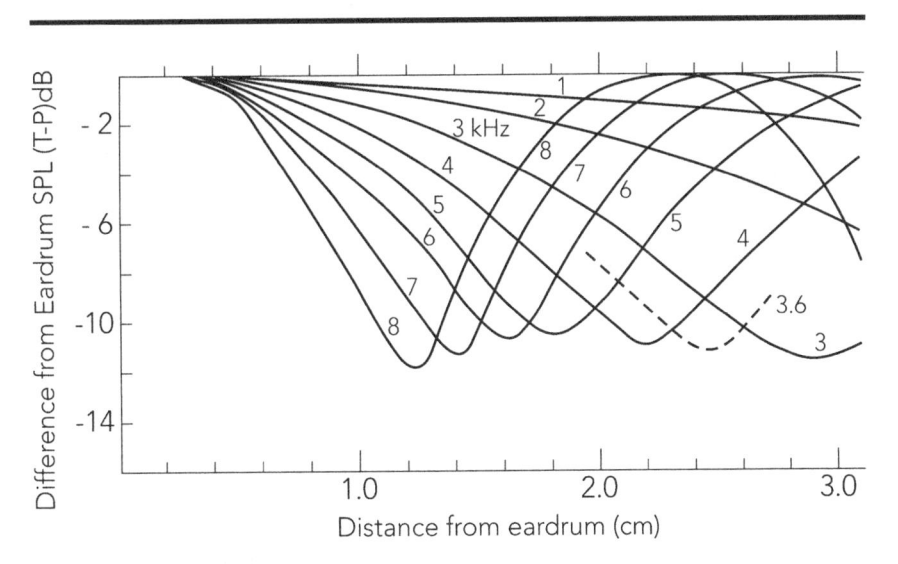

Figure 16–18. Difference between eardrum and probe-measured SPL at eight frequencies as a function of distance of the probe from the eardrum. To determine measurement error, select a distance from the eardrum (x-axis), for example 10 mm (1.0 on this cm chart), then go straight up until you reach the line of a frequency of interest (e.g., 4000 Hz), next observe the point directly to the left of this intersection on the y-axis—for this example that would be about 2–3 dB. That would be your measurement error. (Reprinted with permission from Dirks and Kincaid, 1987.)

Four commonly used procedures can help you accomplish appropriate probe placement in adults:

- Visually assisted positioning method (also referred to as the Intertragal Notch Rule or the constant insertion depth method). We know that the average ear canal is about 25 mm long and the average distance from the opening of the ear canal to the intertragal notch is 10 mm—a total of 35 mm. As discussed earlier, most probe tubes come with an adjustable sleeve that can be moved along the tube. So if we put the probe tube sleeve marker 30 mm from the tip and slide the tube down the ear canal until the marker is at the intertragal notch, we should be about 5 mm from the TM. Figure 16–19 shows the probe placed for testing, with the sleeve marker located at the intertragal notch. If the tube does not have a sleeve, use a marker pen to indicate the distance. If it is obvious that a person has a short ear canal (usually a petite female), or there is a shorter-than-average distance between the intertragal notch and the opening of the ear canal, place the marker at around 25 to 27 mm. This method is not recommended for infants and children, as the dimensions of their ears are of course smaller and quite variable. A depth of 20 to 25 mm is recommended if you do attempt to apply this method in children.
- Geometric positioning (earmold or hearing aid as a guide). This is the method that many people use when measuring the RECD in children. Position the probe tube along the inferior portion of the child's earmold or custom hearing aid, extending the tip of the tube 2 or 3 mm beyond the tip of the earmold (hearing aid), and then place the sleeve marker equal to the inferior lateral portion of the earmold (hearing aid). This should result in the marker being placed in the region of the intertragal notch. When used with adults, have the tube extend 5 mm beyond the hearing aid/earmold (Figure 16–20). A shortcoming of this approach with adults, however, is that if they have a relatively short fitting tip and a long ear canal, this approach might not get you within 5 mm of the TM, and you could be underestimating true ear canal SPL for the higher frequencies. How deeply the earmold/tip/dome fits in the canal is important for this technique.
- Acoustic positioning (standing wave notch). By observing standing waves in the ear canal, the distance between the probe-tube tip and the eardrum can be predicted fairly accurately. First, the examiner finds the position of the tube in the ear canal where a 6000 Hz warble tone is at its minimum, which will be close to 14 to 15 mm from the eardrum for most adults (refer back to Figure 16–18). The tube then can be further inserted a known distance to reach the desired point; that is, an additional insertion of 8 mm would place the

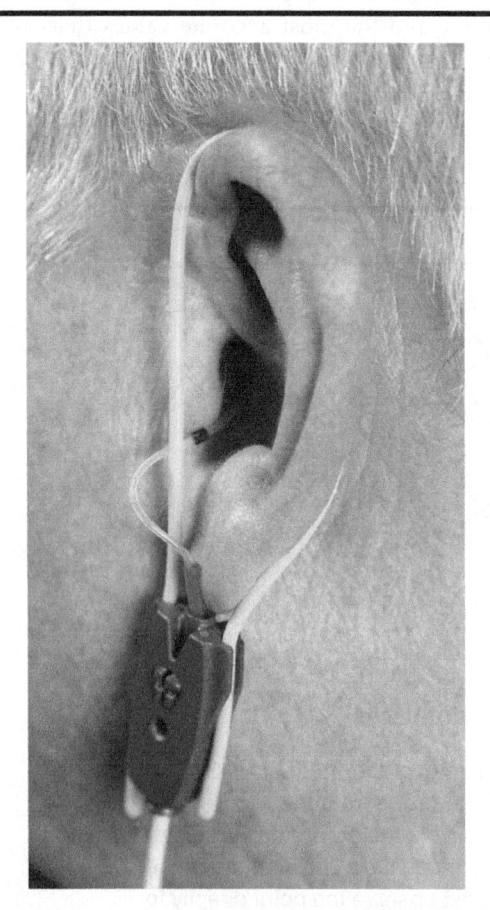

Figure 16–19. An example of the probe placed for testing with the sleeve marker located at the intertragal notch. (Photo courtesy of Audioscan.)

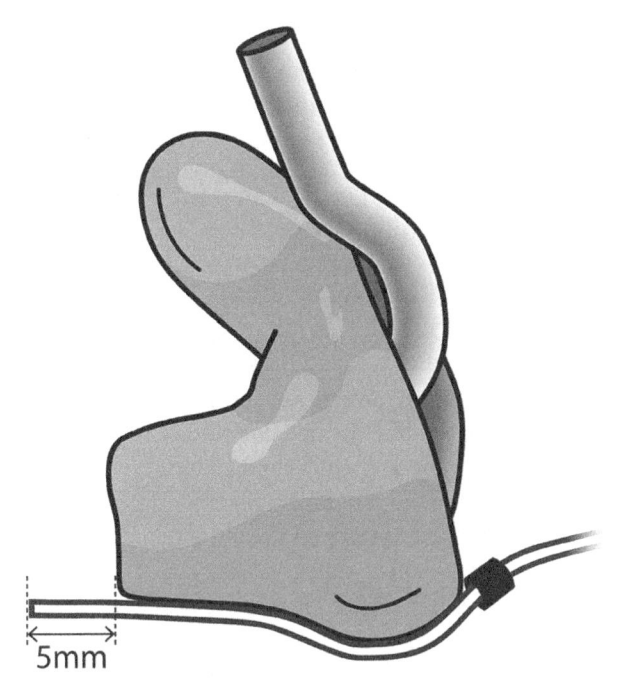

Figure 16–20. An example of lining the probe tube up to extend 5 mm beyond the hearing aid/earmold.

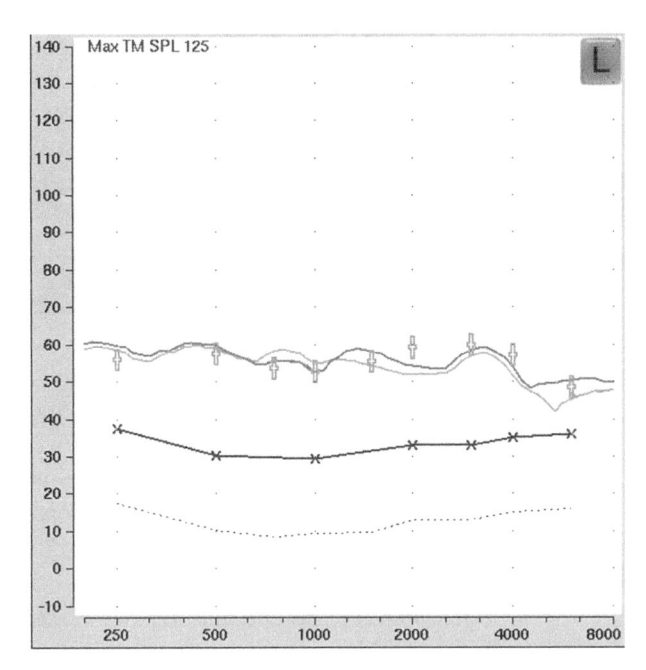

Figure 16–21. Evidence of the standing wave notch. In the first measures the probe tube was placed close to the eardrum. In the next measure the probe was moved out 3 mm. It is apparent that the notch becomes lower in frequency.

tube approximately 6 mm from the tympanic membrane. This procedure was first suggested by Sullivan in 1988, and more recently reviewed by Storey and Dillon (2001). The method also can be used in a more indirect manner: Simply monitor the output in the range above 6000 Hz to assure that no notch is present. Figure 16–21 shows how the standing wave notch can be used to ensure appropriate probe tube placement. In these measures, we started with the probe tip placed relatively close to the TM. In the subsequent measure we pulled the tube tip back 3 mm. Observe that as we pulled the tube back, the notch was present at a lower frequency. The visibility of this notch will vary from system to system, depending on the degree of smoothing of the measured output.

- Acoustically assisted positioning. Essentially a combination of the two methods above. First, the visually assisted positioning method is applied. Then, as a second step, the acoustical positioning method is applied to increase accuracy.
- Bump-and-pull. This method is used on occasion, although often not intentionally. In fact, if you haven't ever done the bump-and-pull, we are guessing that you are new to probe microphone measures or you haven't been placing the probe tube deeply enough. Using this approach, the probe tube is gently slid down the ear canal until the tip of the tube bumps the patient's TM. Don't worry, the patient will tell you when you are there. Warn the patient in advance that he or she might feel a little tickle. Once you obtain the patient's response, pull the tube back a little, and you know you are deep enough. This method is not recommended for infants and children or highly excitable patients (or for any real patient for that matter!). It actually is a very handy method, however, when you are by yourself and want to do a quick probe self-measure.

Comparisons of the first three methods in adult listeners suggest they are roughly equivalent for the average patient (Dirks, Ahlstrom, & Eisenberg, 1994). For the higher test frequencies (4000 Hz and above), however, patients with long ear canals (>25 mm) can demonstrate slightly higher (and more accurate) levels using the standing wave notch method.

We need to mention that, with all of these methods, you would first start with a good otoscopic exam, and then take another peek into the ear canal after the

---

TECHNICAL TIP: KEEPING THE TUBE IN PLACE

Probe tubes tend to be a little bouncy, and there are times when they will pop back just when you have them placed perfectly. Probe microphone manufacturers have developed gadgets that are designed to hold the probe in place. Some audiologists like them, other audiologists get rid of them. Other tricks can be used: (1) putting the tube in a small rigid *U* device; (2) slipping the probe behind the wire/cord that is holding the probe assembly in place (if an under-the-ear assembly is being used); (3) adding some lubricant to the middle of the tube (being careful not to plug the end of the tube), which helps the tube adhere to the skin of canal, stay in place, and minimize slit leaks; and (4) using retention clips to secure the probe housing cable underneath the patient's chin and across to the opposite shoulder and/or using another retention clip to hold the module and probe tube in place should the patient move.

THINGS TO REMEMBER: PROBE DEPTH AND VERIFICATION STRATEGY

As discussed in Chapter 7, there are two similar but different ways to verify your hearing aid fitting using probe microphone measures: REIG and the REAR. We bring this up now because the method selected does have some influence on probe-tube placement. Here is why. If you use the REAR for verification, you will be looking at an absolute measure of ear canal SPL. It is critical, therefore, that the probe-tube tip is deep enough so that high-frequency signals (at least through 4000–5000 Hz) are measured accurately. With the REIG, however, *if* you use a measured real-ear unaided response, then you are calculating a relative difference between two measures (the REAR minus the REUR). In this case it is not as critical that the probe tube is deep (within reason), but it is more important that the tip is the same place for both measures. For example, if the tip is somewhat shallow and a 5 dB mistake at 4000 Hz is made (output 5 dB less than it should be), and if the tube is kept in the same location, this mistake will be made for both the REUR and the REAR, and the calculated REIG will be the same as if the tube had been deep for both measures (Hawkins & Mueller, 1992). Yes indeed—two wrongs can make a right!

For a variety of good reasons that we will discuss in the next chapter, the REAR procedure is currently the more popular technique. It is easier to see if you have the wrong depth when using the REIG procedure (because of the REUR measure; we have a general idea of what the REUR should look like with a deep placement), however, and it is easier to make a mistake regarding probe depth when measuring REAR. Therefore, it is particularly critical that we really pay attention to probe depth for the REAR in order to avoid providing too much high-frequency gain (a short placement will underestimate true gain, and the prudent audiologist will compensate for this by programming more gain—that really wasn't needed)!

tube has been placed. There are times, often because of a cerumen-induced detour, the probe tube will curl and the actual depth of the tip is not as deep as you would predict from the location of the sleeve marker.

Commonly Asked Questions Regarding Probe Tube Use and Placement

The probe tube and its placement is a critical part of the test procedure. Simple mistakes easily can cause a 5 dB measurement error, which would result in a 5 dB programming error, which could affect hearing aid benefit and satisfaction. Here are our responses to some commonly asked questions about probe tubes and their use.

How do I know if the probe tube is plugged? If the tube is truly plugged, you'll know it: The output displayed will be less than the input signal. What you will see will look something like that shown in Figure 16–22. Note that the output falls below the input (average speech of 65 dB). Fortunately, the tube is usually either totally plugged or totally open—there isn't an in-between stage, which would be more difficult to detect. There are times, however, when things don't look quite right, and we wonder if this is the case. An easy way to check is to take the probe out of the ear and place it next to the regulating microphone as you would for calibration. Run a curve, and you should see a flat line (output = input). If you do, the probe is okay. If you don't, grab a new tube, calibrate, and go at it again.

Do you always need a new tube when the tube is plugged? A plugged tube usually is a throw-away situation, and if you are dealing with a patient with gooey cerumen, a persistent clinician can go through many tubes during a single test session. Cleaning the tubes does not work very well (you do not want moisture in the tube), but if your clinic is on a tight budget, there could be a solution. *If* your probe microphone system calibrates the probe tube as we talked about earlier (and most do), then you simply could snip off the tip that is plugged, recalibrate the tube, and continue to use it for testing. As we mentioned previously, this is not recommended by some probe microphone manufacturers, but it will likely work for one or two shortcuts.

Can one manufacturer's tubes be used with the equipment from a different manufacturer? We would recommend using the tubes provided by the manufacturer of the equipment you are using, but in a pinch, this probably would work as long as you are using equipment that requires calibration of the tube. If you do the calibration with the rogue tube and you see a flat line on recheck (input = output), then you may be good to go. A potential problem with this approach, however, is that the probe tube may not seal tightly to the sound outlet. As we mentioned earlier, use of a nonstandard tube may also result in a warning that the tube is not within tolerances and may not be able to be used.

Should probe tubes be thrown away after each use? Absolutely yes. Infection control is a concern in any office or clinic. We certainly hope that no one would use the same tube on different people, but we have heard of clinics that have a protocol that recommends taping the tube in the patient's chart for use on follow-up visits. Not good. This simply allows time for the growth of bacteria. The last time we checked, probe tubes were selling for less than $2.00 each. Because that they are normally used for testing hearing aids that sell for thousands of dollars, a $2 investment for infection control does not seem like an unreasonable expenditure.

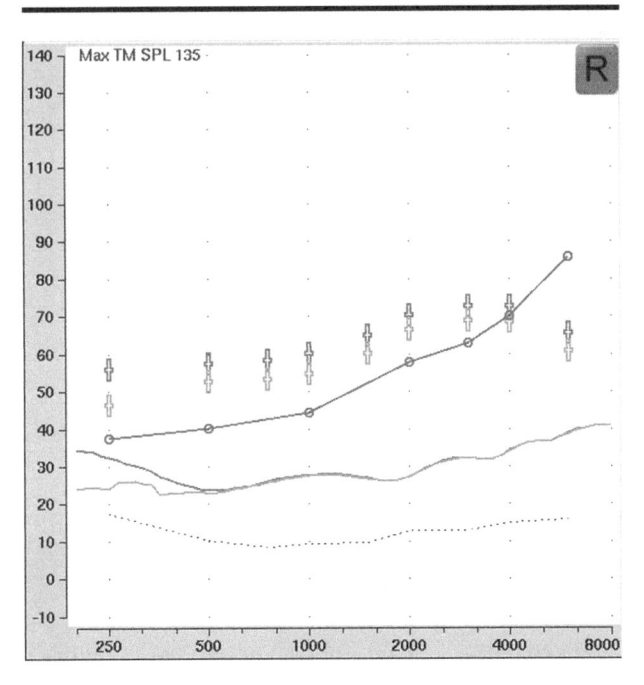

Figure 16–22. An example of the resulting plot if the probe tube is plugged. Note that the output from the probe microphone measure is below the threshold values (represented by the connected circles).

What about probe tube placement when there is cerumen in the ear? Well, the first choice of course would be to remove the cerumen, but we recognize that that is not always possible. If it is gooey, you are in for a battle. You may have to hope that your manufacturer's software will get you close, and then do your probe microphone measures on a repeat visit. We usually give it two or three tries before we give up. If it is hardened cerumen, however, your otoscopic exam will usually reveal a good path to get by it. Often, the cerumen ledge is about midway down the canal, and once you get by it the ear canal is clean. Does this cerumen in the canal change your findings? Not by much, and certainly not to the degree that you would skip the testing.

Is it okay to place the probe tube through the hearing aid vent? It sure is tempting to put it there, isn't it? If your tube is small and your vent is big, it's okay. Remember, however, that one thing being measured when we conduct probe microphone testing is the acoustic effect of venting. If the probe tube fills all or most of the vent, the resulting measurement will not represent true gain (the greatest mistake will be in the low frequencies). On the other hand, if the vent is larger than 2 mm, and you are using one of today's thin probe tubes, we doubt that placing the probe tube through the vent will influence the test results significantly.

For patients, such as children, who are followed every three months or so, is it worth ordering a probe tube vent for their earmold? Your earmold manufacturer can place a vent in the earmold for the purpose of conducting RECD and other important probe microphone measures (since probe tubes come in different diameters, it might be good to send a sample tube of what you use along with the ear impression). When you do the testing, the probe tube is threaded through this vent (it is usually difficult to do—you will need to use a good lubricant) and can be held in place with Fun-Tak® during testing. This procedure helps ensure that that the tip of the probe tube extends beyond the tip of the earmold. A second advantage is that you have only one thing to hold on to when you place the earmold in the ear. When testing is completed, the vent is plugged. Is it worth the time and effort? We know people who frequently test children who *do not* use this approach, and instead use a very thin tape to keep the probe in place on the inferior portion of the earmold when using it to measure individual RECD. If you are fairly new to pediatric evaluations, it might add some comfort to the test procedure knowing that you have a good placement of the probe-tube tip, if you can manage to get it through the vent!

For a tight fitting, is it common that the probe tube gets squashed and gives unreliable results? We have heard that this happens, but we wonder if maybe it is that the clinician just didn't have the tip of the tube past the end of the hearing aid. Or perhaps it was deep and then curled in the canal. In general, this should not be a problem. Consider that back in the 1990s, there were two studies that compared REIG to functional gain for deep, tightly fitted CICs (Mueller & Ebinger, 1997; Seewald, Cornelisse, Black, & Block, 1996). This is the type of fitting where you might expect some squash effect to occur, and if it did occur, you would expect it to show up in the higher frequencies. In both of these studies, mean REIG was equal to mean functional gain at 4000 Hz.

Quick Summary

Here is quick summary of what to remember for the test setup:

- Select a quiet room with low ambient noise and away from the hustle and bustle of the clinic/office.
- Select a sturdy office swivel chair that can be adjusted for height.
- Seat the patient approximately two meters (at least 5 to 6 feet) away from any reflective surface. Remember that you too are a reflective surface, so move back when you do actual measurements.
- Position the patient relative to the loudspeaker at the angle and within the distance recommended by the manufacturer (often directly in front at a distance of 0.5 to 1 meter—1.5 to 3 feet).
- Position the loudspeaker presenting the test signal at or slightly above the vertical azimuth of the patient's head.
- Place the microphone relatively close to the opening of the ear canal.

- The tip of the probe tube measurement microphone should be placed so that it is within 5 mm of the TM.
- Instruct the patient to sit still and look forward during the testing.
- Sit back and enjoy the science aspect of fitting hearing aids (the *art* part is yet to come).

In Closing

We have presented a rationale regarding the use of validated prescriptive approaches as a starting point for the selection of gain and output for our patients. Concurrently, we describe why probe microphone measures must be used to verify that these desired prescriptive targets are present in the patient's ear canal. Failure to complete this testing will most certainly lead to less-than-optimal fittings, and many would consider this breach of best practice evidence of unethical clinical behavior. Probe microphone verification is the only option available—there is no second choice or Plan B.

Of course, these measures must be valid and reliable. We described many considerations, techniques, and procedures to assure that accurate results are obtained, and that these real-ear findings provide meaningful information regarding the quality of the fitting. Armed with this background and procedural information, it is time to start doing some testing. We launch that in the next chapter.

17
Probe-Microphone Measures: Clinical Uses

In Chapter 16, we introduce probe microphone equipment and measures, and some of the techniques important for collecting valid and reliable information. We also briefly describe some of the most common clinical probe microphone measures. In this chapter, we discuss each one of these probe microphone measures in greater detail. Some of these measures are used in the clinic much more routinely than others, so note that the length of our discussions does not reflect how commonly each measure is currently used. For example, although still used routinely by some clinicians, certain measures (e.g., real-ear unaided gain or REUG, and real-ear insertion gain or REIG) are used far less often—if at all—when compared to others (e.g., REAR). We believe, however, there are two main reasons for providing a full discussion of each measure. First, clinical practice is ever-changing and the underlying reasons for doing things in a particular way also often change. Therefore, it is important to understand multiple ways to perform each type of measurement. Second, understanding all available measures gives us a better understanding of the measures we do use. In almost every case, there is a tradeoff in the information we have when we make a measure. For example, REAR measures allow us to view frequency-specific audibility, whereas REIG measures allow us to easily visualize frequency-specific gain. Knowing what we are gaining or giving up when we choose a particular measure can be informative. Such underlying information is important for interpreting results, even if we don't routinely complete the measures.

A Little Background

When clinical probe microphone measures were first introduced (early 1980s) the Prescription Of Gain and Output (POGO) and Libby one-third prescriptive fitting methods were at the peak of their popularity, and a revised NAL (National Acoustic Laboratories) procedure (NAL-R) was just being published. All three of these methods were verified using functional gain, but insertion gain could be substituted easily, so manufacturers included calculation of these prescriptive targets as part of the probe microphone equipment software.

Audiologists, frustrated with the tedious and unreliable functional gain procedure they had been using, soon developed a fascination with matching real-ear results to prescriptive targets on a computer monitor. To do so, it was necessary to conduct a calculation called the real-ear insertion gain (REIG), which is derived by measuring the real-ear unaided gain (REUG) and subtracting it from the real-ear aided gain (REAG). That

> **POINTS TO PONDER: AUTOMATED REAL-EAR VERIFICATION?**
>
> Currently, closed loop self-fitting hearing aids using real-ear verification are available from only a few manufacturers. We predict that, in the relatively near future, however, most hearing aids will autofit to the desired prescriptive targets after the clinician enters thresholds, appropriately places the probe tube and the reference microphone from the probe microphone system, and places the hearing aid to the ear. Several of these automated methods have already been introduced. As we describe later in this chapter, integrated probe microphone and hearing aid fitting systems that automatically fit to targets have been available for more than a decade—in some cases, as a unified system from a single manufacturer; in other cases, as a partnership between a hearing aid manufacturer and a probe microphone manufacturer with the systems interacting through Noah software or other means. Because this combination uses two existing and proven methods, we have little doubt that such systems can provide a reliable fit much more quickly than can be done by hand (a skilled clinician is still necessary to assure positioning, probe microphone placement, etc.). Why haven't they caught on yet? The big hurdle in the past was that these systems often locked the audiologists into a single probe microphone system and brand of hearing aid. It is a hurdle that can, and we think will, be overcome.
>
> More recently, hearing aids that can fit themselves without the need for probe microphone equipment have been introduced, although there are some concerns regarding their reliability and validity. So why a whole chapter on probe microphone verification if it will become automated? Two reasons: First it is important to understand basic verification so that we can troubleshoot and treat problems that may arise. More importantly, basic verification procedures are the foundation for all the advanced verification techniques we describe in more detail in the second half of this chapter. Indeed, we look forward to the automation of basic verification techniques. If a computer can help us do a part of our job more quickly and accurately, we should let it! Doing so frees up valuable clinical time for tasks that only a highly trained professional can perform, including (1) advanced verification techniques; (2) quantification of hearing aid outcomes; and (3) using pre-fitting measures, outcome measures, and patient input to individually optimize hearing aid fittings and counselling with the goal of maximizing patient outcomes.

is, REAG minus REUG equals REIG, and, of course, REAR minus REUR also equals REIG. Confused? Don't be. These are just some of the measures that are conducted clinically using probe microphone equipment. These measurements—and the acronyms used to identify them—will be much clearer by the time you reach the end of this chapter.

As you can see from the preceding paragraph, it is difficult to talk about real-ear testing without getting into the acronyms that are the vital components of probe microphone lingo. Some people cringe when they come upon acronyms, but they do provide an easy way for us to talk to each other—buying SCUBA gear or flying under the RADAR just wouldn't be the same without them.

The first ANSI standard regarding probe microphone measures was published in the late 1990s (S3.461997) and helped to define the procedures and clarify some of the already common acronyms (ANSI, 1997b). Deciding on the appropriate terminology, however, was apparently not an easy task. In 1986, Dave Preves was quoted in the *The Hearing Journal*, as stating:

> An Acoustical Society of America study group will meet this month [May 1986] to begin discussing the standardization of real-ear measurement terminology.

As you see from the 1997 date of the ANSI reference, more than ten years passed before the standard was published. Like good wine, standards take time to reach maturity. While waiting for the phantom standard to emerge, some people published papers and book chapters using the terminology that was rumored to be part of the standard and that already was being used in journal articles (e.g., Mueller, 1990; Schweitzer, Sullivan, Beck, & Cole, 1990; Mueller, 1992a). These terms were accepted and were commonly used by manufacturers, researchers, and clinicians. For the most part, the terms in the probe microphone standard were similar to what was then well-known terminology. In fact, it's now been 30 years since those acronyms were first suggested, and very little has changed in the current and revised probe microphone standard (S3.46-2013).

Term Ends in a G or an R?

As we go through the terminology, it is important to remember that, if a measure represents *SPL in the ear canal*, the term ends in an R for Response—for example, the REUR. If a measure represents *a difference value* (e.g., the input has been subtracted from the output), the term ends in a G for Gain—for example, the REUG. This difference often is confusing. Here is an example. If we were to say to audiologist Dr. Michael Valente, Hey Mike, what's your REUG at 3000 Hz? he would reply, 17 dB. (He knows this because he has measured his REUG several times.) But what if we were to ask, Hey Mike, what's your REUR at 3000 Hz? There is no way he could answer this question because he would have to know the input level that was used to measure the REUR. If the input was 50 dB SPL, then the answer would be 67 dB SPL; if the input was 60 dB, then the answer would be 77 dB, and so on. Consider also, that gain is *always* a difference value (e.g., REIG), so the REIR term, beloved and used by many in the 1990s, no longer exists (see related Technical Tip later in this chapter).

At this point, we have briefly mentioned several probe microphone test procedures. It is now time to discuss how and when to use each of these procedures in the everyday fitting of hearing aids. The definitions that we use for each term are taken from ANSI Standard S3.46-2013: Methods of Measurement of Real-Ear Performance Characteristics of Hearing Aids.

Real-Ear Unaided Response (REUR)/ Real-Ear Unaided Gain (REUG)

Definitions:

- REUR. *SPL as a function of frequency, at a specified measurement point in the ear canal, for a specified soundfield, with the ear canal unoccluded.*
- REUG. *Difference in decibels between the SPL as a function of frequency at a specified measurement point in the ear canal and the SPL at the field reference point, for a specified soundfield, with the ear canal unoccluded.*

When the REIG was commonly used for verification, the REUG was the first measure conducted in the probe microphone verification process because, at the time, the REUG was the preferred method for calculating the REIG. That is, it served as the baseline for determining gain in the ear (although it is possible, and some even say preferred, to use the average REUG, which is readily available on probe microphone equipment). If you, like most clinicians in the United States, verify performance using the REAR (e.g., speech mapping), the REUG is of little interest, and typically is not used at all in the fitting decision—more on that later in this chapter.

Figure 17–1 shows the average REUG for adults, and Table 17–1 shows values for key frequencies (from

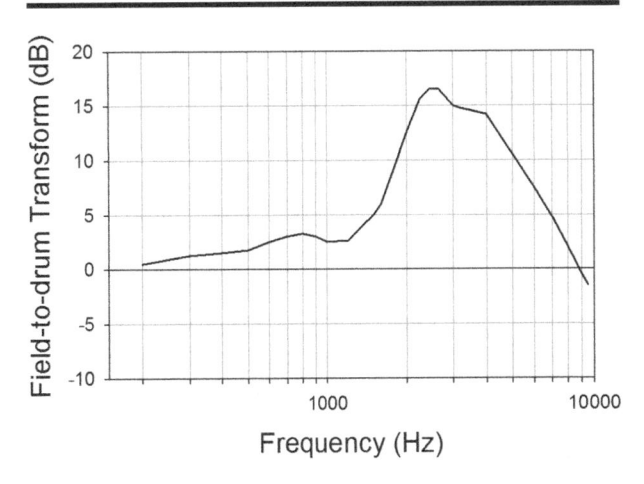

Figure 17–1. Average real-ear unaided gain (REUG), also referred to as the free field-to-eardrum transformation.

Table 17–1. Average REUG Values in Adult Listeners for Key Frequencies

	Frequency (kHz)									
	.25	.5	.75	1	1.5	2	3	4	6	8
REUG (dB)	1.0	1.8	3.0	2.6	5.1	12.0	15.4	14.3	7.3	1.8

Source: From Seewald et al. (1997).

Seewald, Cornelisse, Richert, & Block, 1997). Prior to the days of probe microphone equipment, the laboratory measure of the REUG was referred to as *free-field to eardrum transfer function*. This term is important because it reminds us that the resulting measure depends on several factors. In clinical parlance, it is sometimes simply called the *ear canal resonance*. Although the resonance of the ear canal is nearly always the primary factor, the concha and pinna can also contribute significantly. And, depending on the type of equalization system used for the input signal (e.g., modified pressure, stored, or substitution), the head, neck, and torso can also alter the measurement by a small degree.

Much of the basic research studying the acoustic effects of the external ear was conducted by E.A.G Shaw with cadavers; his 1974 article is a good summary of his work. In our Supplemental Information chapter at the end of this book (see Figure 20–9), we illustrate the average contributions of the head, torso, neck, concha, pinna flange, ear canal, and eardrum. The eardrum is included because middle ear impedance can influence this measure. The effects of the concha are also shown in Figure 20–9 and directly relate to localization.

The data from Shaw clearly show the peak of the ear canal resonance around 2500 Hz, and the peak from the concha just above 5000 Hz. The combined effect (the curve labeled T in Figure 20–9) is very similar to what we display in Figure 17–1. These values also can change based on the geography of the individual's ear. If we consider basic acoustics and resonance, we know that the peak frequency of the ear canal resonance is higher or lower depending on the size of the ear canal. People with small ear canals might have a resonance peak as high as 3500 Hz or higher. People with large ear canals often have resonance peaks as low as 2000 Hz, or even lower. Similarly, the size of the concha will have an effect. A person with a somewhat smaller ear canal (moving this peak higher) and a somewhat larger concha (moving this peak lower) might have an REUG with one single peak around 3000 to 3500 as the two acoustic components have merged.

Figure 17–2 shows the REUG variability that's commonly observed in the clinic. This figure shows the REUG of eight patients. Note that several patients have an REUG very similar to average but not all of them do. In fact, the frequency region of the peak of the response varies from near 2000 to 4000 Hz. The maximum intensity at the peak varies from about 14 to 24 dB. The teaching point here is that the actual measured REUG might not look like the expected/average REUG.

Now it is time to move on to a discussion of hearing aid fitting. If you're using the REIG for verification, the REUR (either measured or average) is always subtracted from the REAR. In general, REAR curves tend to be relatively smooth. So it is common that bumps in the REUR become dips in REIG, and that dips in the REUR become bumps in the REIG. An example of this is shown in Figure 17–3.

Figure 17–3A shows the results of a mini-BTE RIC with a stock closed dome fitted to an individual with a downward sloping hearing loss. Note that the individual's REUR is fairly average and that the resulting REIG is a good fit to the NAL-NL2 target (65 dB SPL real-speech input). Figure 17–3B shows how we fitted the same hearing aid (no changes to the programming) to a different individual with very similar hearing loss, so we entered the same audiogram to show a one-to-one comparison. The difference, however, is that the second patient doesn't have a typical REUR. This unusual REUR has a significant effect on the calculated REIG and, depending on your fitting philosophy, how the hearing aid will be programmed. This is because the REAR is very similar for both patients—many of the factors that make REURs differ are no longer in play when the input signal is fed through a BTE (microphone above the ear) and the ear canal is plugged with an earmold. Also, consider that these REUG differences are not revealed during audiometric testing, as the ear canal is plugged with an insert earphone.

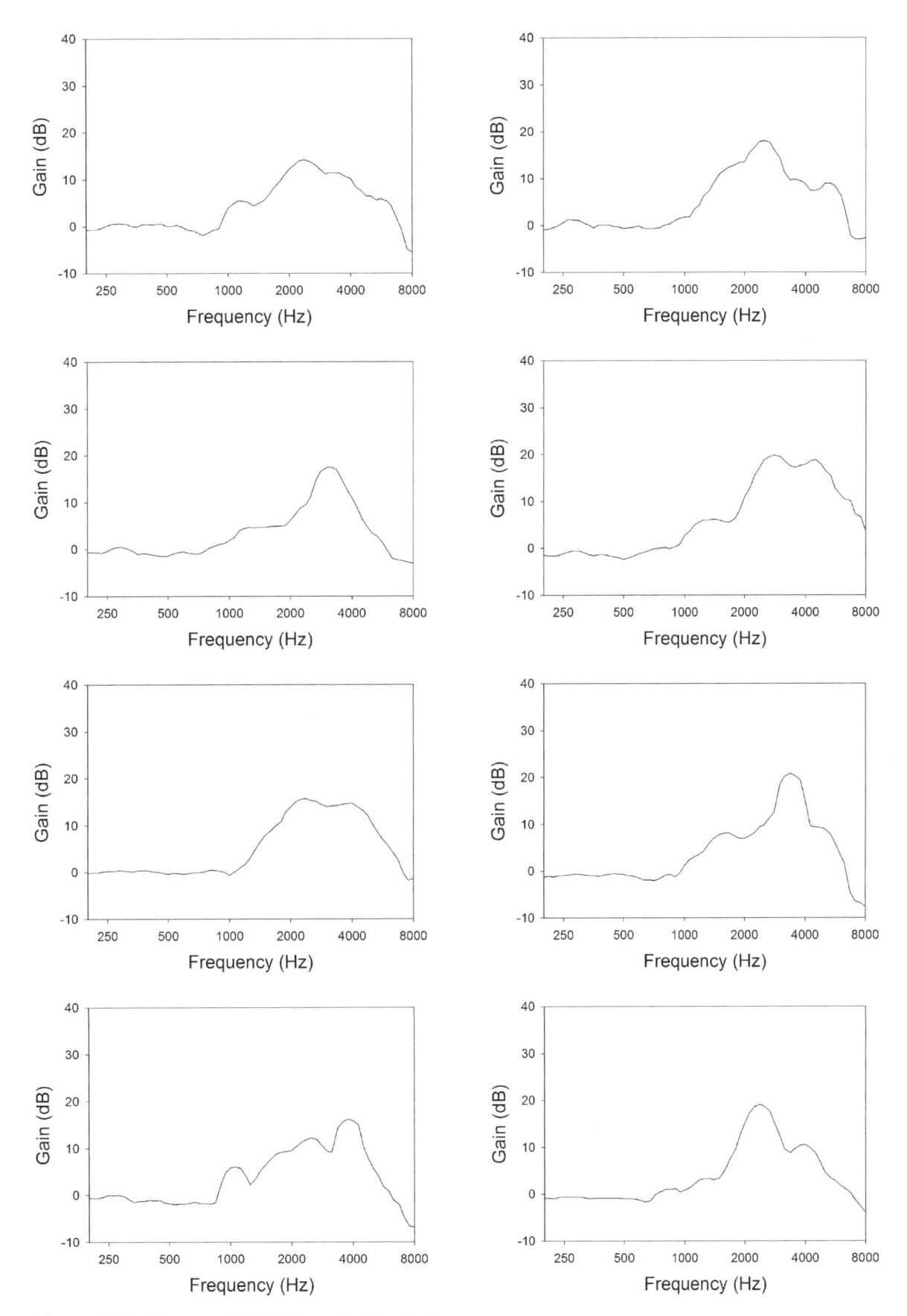

Figure 17–2. Measured REUG from eight patients.

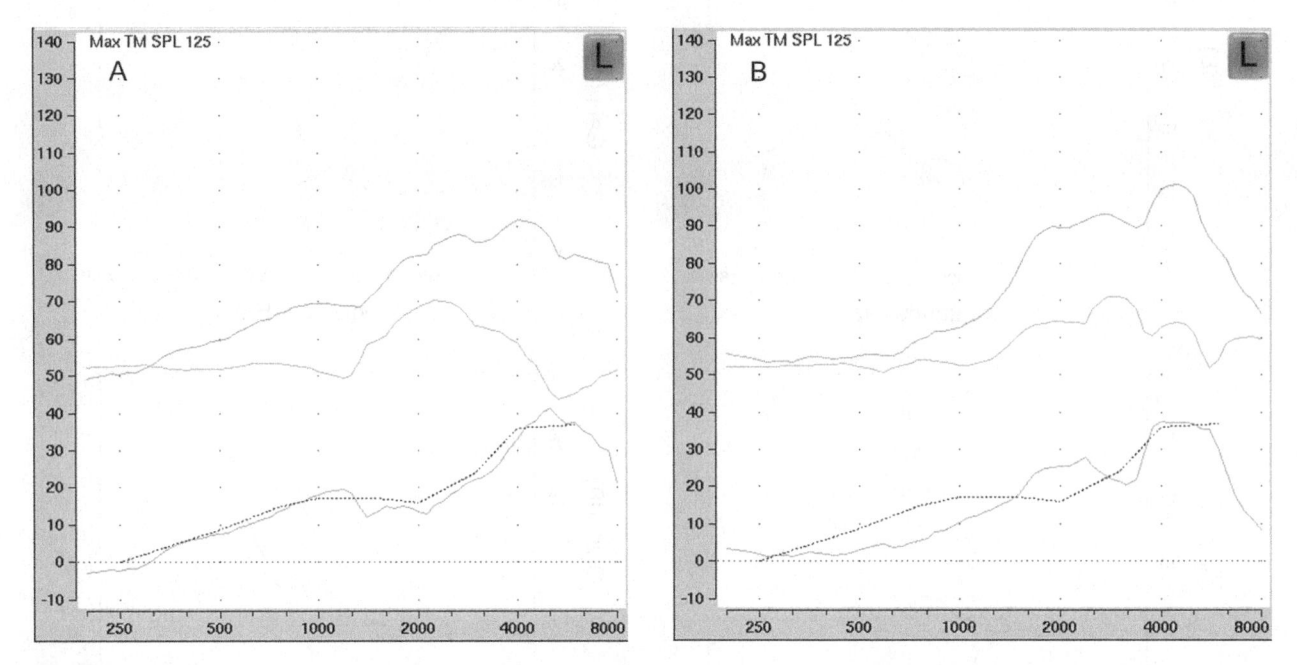

Figure 17–3. Examples of how the REUR affects the match to target. **A.** The REUR is fairly average (*middle curve*), and the resulting REIG is a good fit to the NAL-NL2 target (*bottom curve*). **B.** The same hearing aid to a different individual with an atypical REUR (*middle curve*). Note the poor fit to NAL-NL2 target (*bottom curve*).

In Figure 17–3B, the REUR of the patient is probably not a typical finding, although it occurs often enough to warrant discussion. Most probe microphone systems show an example of an average REUR or REUG, and you can compare the patient's measurement to average. In Figure 17–4, we show a measured REUR compared to average. Note that, in this case, we see with the measured REUR a distinct peak around 2500 Hz (ear canal) and a second peak around 4000 Hz (concha). This REUR is 5 dB or more greater than average at 1500 to 2500 Hz, which means that *if* you are using the REIG for verification and *if* you use the measured REUR shown here, you need to program 5 dB more gain into the instrument for this frequency range than if you use an average REUR. If this logic seems correct to you, then you are a good candidate to verify using REIG and individually measured REUR. If it seems a bit strange, you probably will be happier using average REUR or the soon to be explained REAR. The arguments for choosing to use the average REUG versus the individually measured REUG are provided in the following section and the next Points to Ponder.

Because REIG bumps and dips usually are unsightly, and the goal of the fitting is to obtain gain that is a good match to the NAL-NL2 target, if you use the REIG for verification it is common to try and make the REAG resemble the REUG more closely so that the REIG has a smoother appearance and is a closer match to the target gain curve. Given today's hearing aids with multiple channels and sophisticated programming features, doing so is usually fairly easy, although you may end up with a rather unusual looking REAR (which of course is what the patient hears).

Some prescriptive fitting methods in manufacturer's software allow you to enter the patient's REUG and, if these values are different from average, desired 2cc-coupler gain is influenced accordingly. Note we said 2cc-coupler gain—the *desired REIG* (i.e., the REIG gain targets) will remain the same because they are not affected by the REUG.

When you enter the patient's REUG, in essence, you have created a partially individualized CORFIG (see Chapter 16). Recall that the components of the CORFIG include the REUG, the RECD, and the microphone location effects (MLEs) of the hearing aid that is being fitted (in general, MLEs become larger as the microphone inlet is recessed in the concha or ear canal). You calculate the CORFIG by subtracting the RECD and the

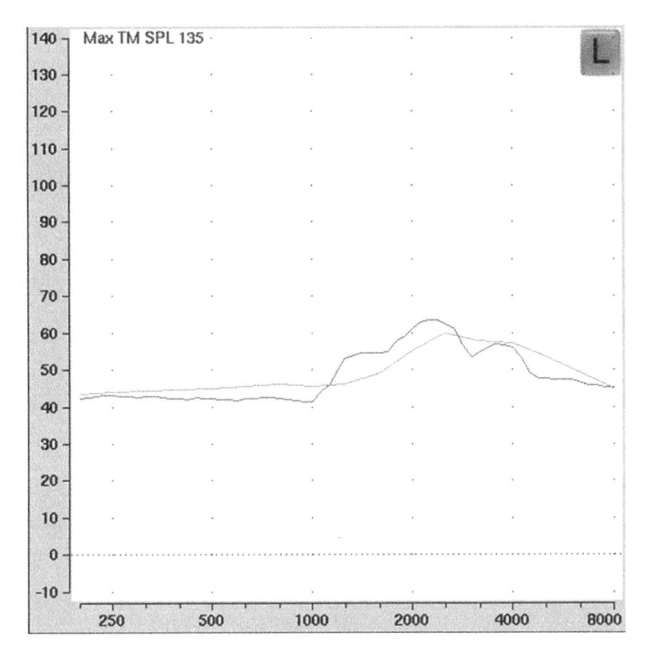

Figure 17–4. Average REUR compared to a patient's REUR. Note the higher resonance but at a lower frequency.

MLE from the REUG. Therefore, the bigger the REUG, the more positive the CORFIG. The CORFIG is added to the REIG to obtain desired 2cc-coupler gain, so the bigger the REUG, the bigger the desired 2cc coupler gain.

On the surface, correcting the CORFIG for the patient's REUG seems like a reasonable thing to do if you want to fit the REIG to a prescriptive target. Although understanding the concept is important, it is certainly not worth investing too much time entering these values into the fitting software because you can easily make these adjustments during the fitting while conducting speech mapping.

There are times when this correction for an unusual REUG can result in some rather bizarre desired 2cc-coupler values or REARs. Unusual desired values commonly occur when you have a patient with little or no hearing loss at 2000 Hz and his REUG (we say his because the patient is usually a male with a big ear canal) is 10 dB or so larger than average at 2000 Hz. By correcting for the REUG, you end up with a very unusual increase in the aided speech spectrum for a region where he may have normal or near normal hearing. Often for such cases, the use of average REUG values will provide a more desirable REAR spectrum.

POINTS TO PONDER: MEASURED OR AVERAGE REUG?

In general, we prefer using the average REUG over the measured for REIG calculation; we've mentioned examples of why the measured REUG can cause some problems. But one could, at least in theory, build a case to support the use of the measured REUG: If a person has always listened to speech through a different amplifier (his unusual REUG), it might be in his or her best interest to modify the amplified signal to match that speech spectrum. By correcting for the unusual REUG, the REAR will have a spectrum more similar to what the patient is used to. Moreover, if we do examine the individual REUG, we're more apt to apply desired prescriptive gain—again, this assumes that gain is the verification tool, not ear canal SPL at the eardrum. Consider that, if the hearing aid doesn't provide significant gain where the REUG has an unusually large peak, the ear piece is occluding and eliminates the REUG, and the patient doesn't have much hearing loss at this frequency, it is possible that the patient's audibility will be worse using the hearing aid than if the patient simply used his or her REUG.

As early as 1991, Larry Revit was writing about the pitfalls of using the measured REUG and was advocating simply using an average value. This notion was based in part on the fact that prescriptive methods are referenced to soundfield thresholds, yet we typically use earphone thresholds for target calculations. If you're interested in using average values, note that most probe microphone units offer this option, although little data exist for average REUGs for infants and children.

Some clinics rely on the REIG verification and use the measured REUG approach. To accommodate these audiologists and make their fittings more efficient, some probe microphone equipment automatically adjusts the gain of the hearing aid to compensate for an unusual REUG. That is, once you have the patient's REUG measured, it is stored in the system's fitting software. This communication between the probe microphone equipment and the manufacturer's fitting software occurs in

> **TECHNICAL TIP: THE REUG AND TM PERFS**
>
> Earlier in the chapter, we discussed how the REUG depends heavily on the size of the ear canal because the ear canal resonance is the primary factor. So what happens when a TM perforation occurs and the volume now includes a portion of the middle ear cavity? As you might likely expect, the usual resonance around 2700 Hz is gone because the ear canal volume is much greater than is typical. The concha effects, however, remain the same, and you tend to have a curve with two large peaks separated by a valley around 2500 to 3000 Hz. Although the primary clinical purpose for conducting the REUG is to obtain the values for calculating the REIG, observing the configuration of the REUG can also provide useful information regarding the status of the middle ear. Now you might say, Wouldn't you already know that there was an eardrum perforation from your otoscopic exam? Maybe. But some perforations are difficult to visualize, especially if you don't have years of experience. If you see many patients with hearing aids and routinely do probe microphone measures (including REURs), there's a pretty good chance that you'll detect a TM perforation, previously unknown to both you and the patient. If you are simply doing a REAR for verification, you may be fooled into thinking something bizarre is going on with the hearing aid. For more information on the effects of middle ear pathology on the REUG, see the review by De Jonge (1996).

the automated real-ear systems we described earlier. It's actually a pretty amazing thing to sit back and watch the match happen on the fitting screen, and this approach is a real timesaver.

Measurement of the REUG

- Calibrate or equalize the probe microphone system.
- Position the patient appropriately.
- Position the probe tube at the correct depth in the ear canal.
- Present a calibrated signal to the open ear.
- The input-level of the signal is not too critical—the REUG will remain the same across a wide range of signals. It makes sense, however, to use a signal within the range of typical hearing aid gain verification—50 to 80 dB SPL. We usually use 65 dB SPL.
- Theoretically, the type of signal doesn't matter, especially for the REUG, but the visualization of the REUR will be easier if the signal has equal level across frequency. Therefore, we recommend displaying the REUG or REUR for a test signal that is displayed as a flat frequency response in the soundfield without a hearing aid or patient present. If you use a shaped signal such as speech, considerable experience is needed to recognize the typical shape and what deviations from that shape look like if the probe microphone manufacturer does not display it on the screen.
- Observe the recorded REUG (or REUR if you are in that display mode).

Clinical Applications of the REUG

- Primary: To serve as a baseline for the calculation of the REIG; this value will be subtracted from the REAG.
- Secondary: To provide reference for REOG testing.
- Secondary: To correct 2cc-coupler data to derive an individualized 2cc-coupler fitting target.
- Secondary: To assist in determining if the tip of the probe tube is at an appropriate depth (e.g., notch effect discussed in Chapter 16).
- Secondary: To detect abnormal middle ear conditions, such as a perforation of

> **KEY CONCEPT: TEST SIGNAL FOR THE REUR**
>
> A REUR is a REUR is a REUR, and for the most part, the signal that you use does not change the effect measured. If you are interested in observing the individual characteristics of the REUR and how a given patient's REUR differs from average, however, then it is best to use a signal that has the input equalized across frequencies. When the REUG is displayed, a direct comparison to an average REUG can be made regardless of input signal shape. If you use a real-speech signal, where the spectrum is rolling off in the higher frequencies, it is difficult to visualize the average REUR reference shape, as shown in Figure 17–5. For one measure of REUR (A), we used pink noise as the input signal. Because that signal is equalized across frequencies, this patient's REUR (left curve) appears to be average (is you are used to looking at REURs). Note that the primary peak is at about 70 dB at 2500 Hz and that there is a second peak of about 60 dB at 4000 Hz. For comparison, we also measured the REUR for a real-speech signal (right panel B). Armed only with this visual, it would be difficult to say whether this patient's REUR (or REUG) is typical. There is no real discernable peak in the displayed output (because the REUG tends to provide gain where average speech rolls off, the end result is a relative flat spectrum). How close is this REUR to the REUR average? This comparison illustrates why the equalized input signal can be advantageous for this assessment.

the eardrum (unusual peaks and dips in response).

■ Secondary: With the SPL-O-Gram fitting approach, it can be used for conversion of soundfield audiometry from dB HL to dB SPL (Sinclair, Cole, & Pumford, 2001).

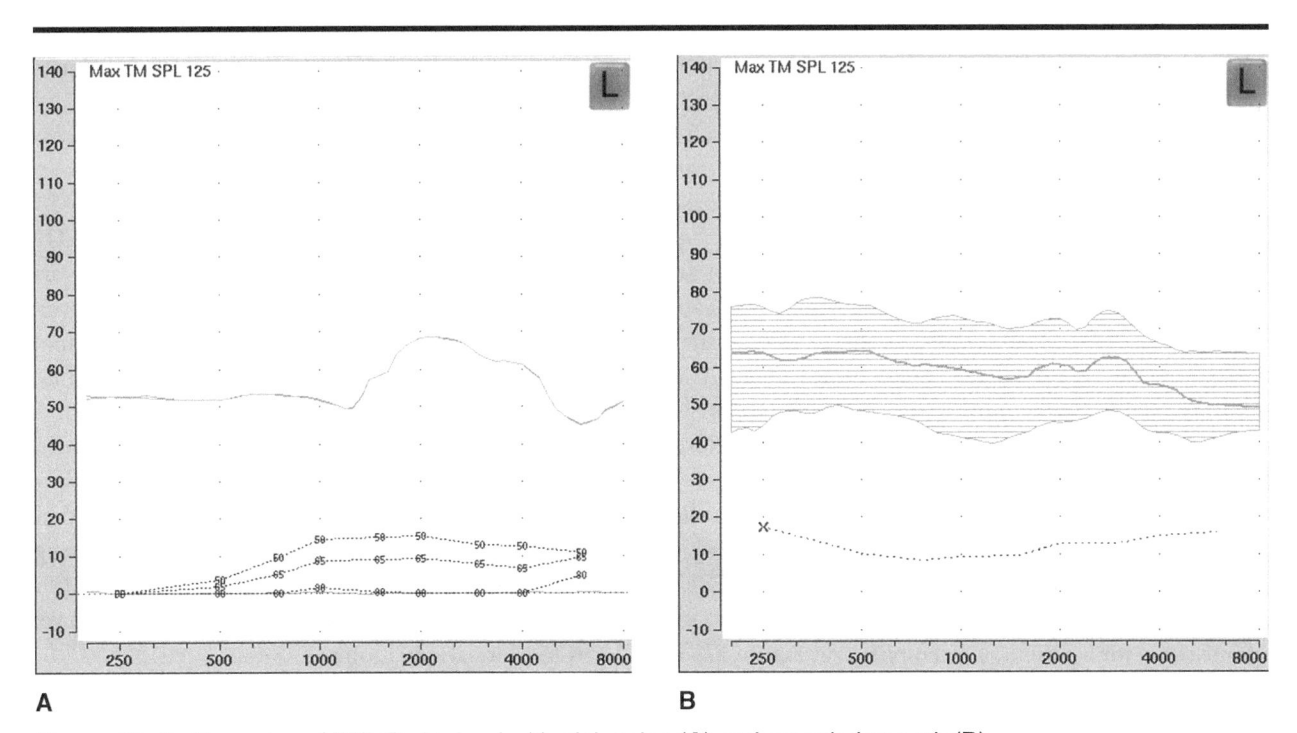

Figure 17–5. Examples of REUR obtained with pink noise (**A**) and recorded speech (**B**).

The Real-Ear Occluded Response (REOR) and Real-Ear Occluded Gain (REOG)

Definitions:

- *REOR (Real-Ear Occluded Response). SPL as a function of frequency at a specified measurement point in the ear canal, for a specified soundfield, with the hearing aid (and its acoustic coupling) in place and turned off*
- *REOG (Real-Ear Occluded Gain). Difference in decibels between the SPL as a function of frequency at a specified measurement point in the ear canal and the SPL at the field reference point, for a specified soundfield, with the hearing aid (and its acoustic coupling) in place and turned off*

The REOG is a measure of how the hearing aid or earmold has changed the REUG and the degree to which the hearing aid or earmold is serving as an earplug. Although some research has attempted to relate individual REOG values to speech understanding in background noise (e.g., Chasin, Pirzaniski, Hayes, & Mueller, 1997), the primary clinical application is to observe the sound inflow caused by an open fitting, purposeful venting, or slit-leak venting. For example, if you have a patient with normal hearing at 500 Hz and want to know whether the combined effects of slit leak and a pressure-relief vent allow 500 Hz signals to pass to the TM without attenuation, the REOG will give you this information (e.g., an REOG of 0 dB will show that sound is passing through without attenuation). You can, therefore, use repeated REOG testing to ensure that vents are sized appropriately, to monitor the acoustic effects of vent modifications, and to help predict potential feedback problems (we assume that inflow values are predictive of outflow).

With today's common use of open fittings, the REOG will quickly reveal whether the fitting is truly open, partially open, or not open at all, and the REOG or REOR is a helpful way to select the most appropriate dome or tip for a patient, as exemplified in Figure 17–6. The top curve is the patient's REUR. The curve immediately below that is the patient's REOR for an open fitting

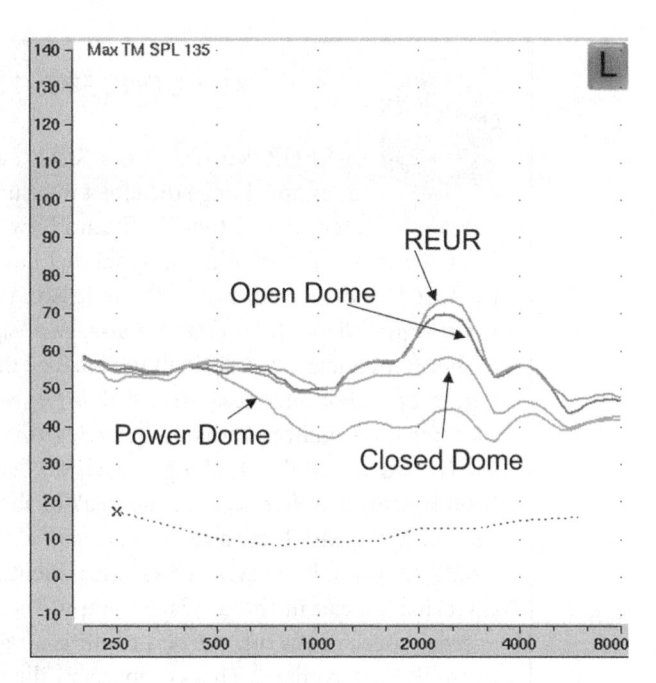

Figure 17–6. Example of REOR for different canal occlusions. The top curve is the patient's REUR. The curve immediately below that is the patient's REOR for an open-fitting tip. Note that the REOR is not identical to the REUR because the eartip changes the volume of the ear canal causing a slight shift in the resonance peak. The next lower curve is the REOR for a closed-fitting dome. The bottom curve is for a tighter fitting, a double-dome tip. Although there is no attenuation for 500 Hz and below, it's clear that 10 to 15 dB of attenuation is present in the middle to high frequencies.

tip. Note that this tip truly is open because the REOR is nearly identical to the REUR. You can see they are not completely identical, however, because the presence of the eartip changes the volume of the ear canal, causing a slight shift in the resonance peak. The next lower curve is the REOR for a closed fitting dome. For the closed dome, the ear canal resonance and concha effects are missing, but the fitting isn't tight enough to provide attenuation. That is, the output is not less than the input signal. The bottom curve is for a tighter fitting, a double-dome tip. Although there still is no attenuation for 500 Hz and below, we now see that above that level, 10 to 15 dB of attenuation is present.

In general, the REOG is determined by three factors:

- The degree that the earmold or hearing aid fills the concha, thus reducing concha effects (although this won't be a factor if the canal is completely closed, even if the concha is left open).
- The degree that the earmold or hearing aid fills the ear canal, thus altering ear canal resonance. If the canal is closed, a new resonance will be present based on the shortened length of the tube (i.e., the ear canal) and that now the tube is closed on both ends, rather than open on one end. These two factors will move the residual ear canal resonance to a point that it no longer plays a part in the amplified signal (see Chapter 9). Clinically, we often say that patients have lost their ear canal resonance, although at some higher frequency, it is still there.

POINTS TO PONDER: REOG AND INSERTION LOSS

You will read in some papers that the REOG is used to determine *insertion loss*. Over the years, the term insertion loss has been used in different ways regarding hearing aid measurement; only in one of these definitions is the REOG directly involved. In short, insertion loss is not typically defined as the REOG. Here is a brief description of the three uses of the term:

- In some cases, insertion loss has been used to describe the difference between coupler gain and real-ear (or manikin) gain (Erickson & Van Tasell, 1991). This concept is related to the CORFIG, which, as we mentioned earlier, is calculated by subtracting the RECD and the MLE from the REUR. In the case of the CORFIG, if real-ear gain for a closed earmold is compared with coupler gain, there indeed will be insertion loss in the higher frequencies for some hearing aid models, especially those with a poor microphone location, such as BTEs.
- In the early days of probe microphone measures, it was common to verify hearing aid performance via the in situ response, which we now refer to as the real-ear aided response or REAR. It was observed that the in situ response was greater than insertion gain (what we now call the real-ear insertion gain or REIG) and that difference was referred to as insertion loss. In other words: REAR minus REIG = insertion loss. The REIG is calculated by subtracting the real-ear unaided response (REUR) from the REAR; therefore, insertion loss by this definition was simply the REUG (real-ear unaided gain). What if the REUG is not totally lost when the earmold plumbing tip is placed in the ear canal, as it is with most open-canal (OC) fittings? Is it still okay to subtract the REUG and use REIG calculations? The simple answer is yes—for a review of these effects on open fittings, see Mueller and Ricketts (2006).
- The third use of the term insertion loss relates to our discussion of the REOG, which nearly always falls below the REUG and often is negative (lower than the input signal). It is tempting to subtract the REOG from the REUG and think of this as insertion loss. Because the REUG in the high frequencies is usually around 15 to 17 dB and the earplug effect of the hearing aid plumbing or the custom instrument often results in an REOG of −10 to −20 dB in the highs, the UG-OG difference can be quite large. This calculation has led some to conclude that, in a closed fitting, the amplifier must add as much as 40 dB of extra gain to compensate. Why is this logic wrong? This amount of insertion loss would apply only if the patient never turns on the hearing aid—more on this later.

- The degree that the earmold or hearing aid attenuates sound. Earmolds and custom hearing aids can act as an earplug that will attenuate sounds mostly in the higher frequencies—unless it is a very tight fit, in which case low frequencies also will be reduced. This attenuation can be 10 to 20 dB with a relatively tight fitting, and, therefore, negative REOGs are common.

Considering the three preceding factors, it is understandable that an REOG can take on many different shapes. If it is an open fitting, the REOG may look similar to the REUG. If it is a closed tight fitting, the REOG will be 20 to 30 dB less than that for an open fitting. As we mentioned earlier, although we state that the concha effects can be a REOG factor, with a closed fitting (tight fitting CIC, for example), even if the concha effects are present, they will not impact the REOG because they don't have a pathway to the measurement point at the TM.

Given that we normally are interested in openness of the fitting, the acoustic effects of venting, or modification of venting, it seems reasonable to routinely conduct an REOG whenever hearing aids are fitted. We find it particularly useful when fitting custom instruments with venting and when fitting mini-BTE instruments using noncustom eartips that are at least partially occluding—these values will help determine when the eartip needs to be more open or more closed. In these cases, little extra time is required; simply run a quick curve with the hearing aid muted before turning on the hearing aid and conduct the REAR. This will take an extra 15 seconds or so of test time.

Now that we have talked about what the REOG *does* measure, it is important to mention what it *does not* measure:

- It does not measure the occlusion effect. The occlusion effect is related to sound pressure levels in the ear canal generated by a bone-conducted signal (usually one's own voice). The REOG, unless it is reasonably similar to the REUG (e.g., a very open fitting), is a rather poor predictor of the magnitude of the occlusion effect. For one thing, some people, because of their voice quality and other characteristics, have little or no occlusion effect for their own voice regardless of how tightly the ear is plugged. In the absence of an occlusion effect, a patient's REOG could still range anywhere from 0 to −30 dB. For example, if the canal portion of a custom instrument is very shallow (allowing considerable venting), the REOG will be at or near 0 dB in the low frequencies, and there probably will not be a significant occlusion effect (especially if the patient's primary occlusion effect is below 500 Hz). Compare this to a very different fitting in which the canal of the custom instrument fits tightly and terminates in the bony margin of the ear canal (e.g., a deep-fitted CIC). This will produce an REOG of approximately −20 to 30 dB, but again, there probably will not be a significant occlusion effect (for review, see Mueller, Bright, & Northern, 1996). In further contrast, consider a shallow, tight-fitted ITC with little venting. We have seen the fitting of these instruments resulting in an REOG of −20 dB and an occlusion effect of more than +20 dB.
- The REOG does not predict required hearing aid gain, nor can it be used to assist in predicting real-ear gain. Consider these two cases: Patient A has an REOG of −10 dB, and Patient B has an REOG of −30 dB. At first glance you might say, Patient B needs more gain because he has more insertion loss. It's important to remember, however, that once the hearing aid is turned on, sound has a new pathway to reach the TM (through the hearing aid), and the negative REOG differences (the differences that exist below the 0 dB gain point) have been equalized. What have not been equalized are the effects that the insertion of the hearing aid had on the REUG, but those effects are taken care of by the way the insertion gain is calculated. Hence the REOG is not a player in gain selection except indirectly—if the REOG is similar to the REUG, we know we have a very open fitting and will have to consider the loss of gain in the low frequencies. Although initially it may seem counterintuitive, it is common that the patient who starts off with the least SPL at the TM with the hearing aid turned off will have the most SPL with the hearing aid turned on.

> **TECHNICAL TIP: USING THE REOG FOR DETECTION OF VENT-ASSOCIATED RESONANCE**
>
> One clinical application of the REOG is to detect when vent-associated resonance is present and when that resonance adversely affects the real-ear gain. Although bothersome, vent-associated resonance is a fairly rare occurrence. Nonetheless, it can be very annoying to the patient, and the problem often is misdiagnosed by the clinician. Vent-associated resonance, which is sometimes observed to be 10 dB or higher, usually is observed as increased gain in the 500 to 600 Hz region and frequently occurs when the vent diameter is 1 to 2 mm. The patient may complain that his voice sounds hollow or booming, and the clinician might implement treatment strategies for the occlusion effect, which will not solve the problem. Because vent-associated resonance is an acoustic event, not an electroacoustic event, it is present with the hearing aid turned off—the measurement procedure for the REOG.
>
> As we mentioned, vent-associated resonance usually happens with a medium-size vent, and the reason that a medium-size or larger vent normally is employed in a custom instrument (ITE or ITC) is that the patient has limited hearing loss and little hearing aid gain programmed in the low frequencies. Hence, the people for whom vent-associated resonance is the most bothersome are the very people who are the most likely to have it. If the patient has hearing loss in the low frequencies and 10 dB or so of hearing aid gain is present, then the 10 dB of vent-associated resonance gain is less noticeable (adding decibels will at most result in a 3 dB increase). It is also possible the output of the hearing aid is phase-reversed with the input, and in this case, the gain shown in the REOG might not be as great as it will be when the hearing aid is turned on (because of cancelation due to the phase interaction of the through-the-vent signal versus the through-the-hearing aid signal). So it's always good to observe both the REOG and the REAG/REIG.
>
> Figure 17–7 shows an example of vent-associated resonance for a custom instrument with a 2-mm vent. In the REIG, observe the peak just above 500 Hz, which is undesirable for this patient with normal hearing for this frequency range. Had the REOG findings not been available, the audiologist programming the hearing aid probably would have tackled this problem by turning down gain for this frequency region—which probably already was adjusted to a low level. If we look at the REOG, however, we see that the origin of much of this output—10 dB or so—is from the vent resonance and not produced by the hearing aid amplifier.

Measurement of the REOG

- Calibrate or equalize the probe microphone system.
- Position the patient appropriately.
- Position the probe tube at the correct depth in the ear canal.
- Place the earmold and/or custom instrument in the ear, but do not turn on the hearing aid.
- Present a calibrated signal, typically the same as used for the REUR.
- The input-level of the signal is not too critical; the REOG will remain the same across a wide range of signals. An input level the same as used for the REUR is typical.
- As with the REUG, the type of signal doesn't matter. In order to see effects clearly, we strongly recommend either (1) displaying REOG (this allows for easiest visualization); (2) displaying REOR in response to a test signal that is displayed as a flat frequency response in the soundfield without a hearing

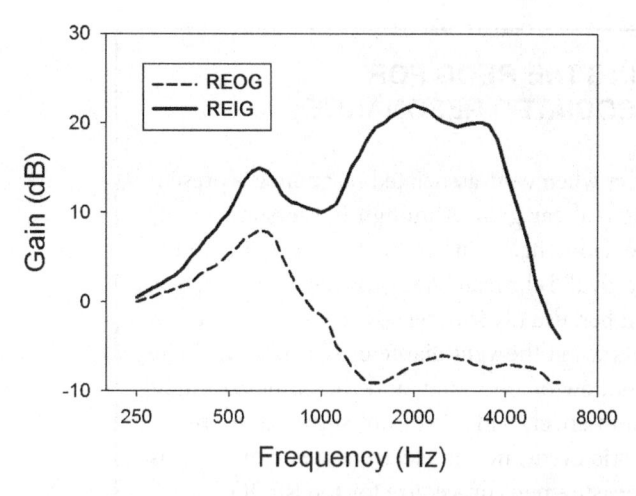

Figure 17–7. Example of vent-associated resonance for a custom instrument with a 2-mm vent. The bump near 500 Hz in both the occluded responses (hearing aid turned off) and the insertion responses (gain with hearing aid turned on) indicate the resonance characteristics.

aid or patient present, or if you are using a shaped signal such as real speech; or (3) displaying REOR and REUR on the same screen. Observe the recorded REOG (or REOR if you are in that display mode).

Clinical Application of the REOG

- Primary: To determine overall tightness of the fitting.
- Secondary: To select appropriate eartip or earmold.
- Secondary: To detect vent-associated resonance.
- Tertiary: To estimate the occlusion effect, but only if REOG closely resembles REUG.

Rear-Ear Aided Response (REAR)/ Real-Ear Aided Gain (REAG)

Definitions:

- REAR. SPL as a function of frequency at a specified measurement point in the ear canal, for a specified soundfield, with the hearing aid (and its acoustic coupling) in place and turned on.
- REAG. Difference in decibels between the SPL as a function of frequency at a specified measurement point in the ear canal and the SPL at the field reference point, for a specified soundfield, with the hearing aid (and its acoustic coupling) in place and turned on.

Of all the measures we make using probe microphone equipment, the most important—and fortunately the easiest to understand—is the REAR. As the ANSI definition states, the REAR is simply the output in the ear canal with the hearing aid in place and turned on—more or less an ear canal measure of what we have been assessing with a coupler since the 1940s. It doesn't matter if the input signal is a swept tone or real speech, or if the input level is 50 dB or 80 dB SPL, the measurement is still referred to as the REAR. Today, when audiologists use an input of real speech or some speech-like signal, there is a tendency to refer to the process as speech mapping. Indeed one manufacturer trademarked the term SpeechMap™ to describe its' speech based REAR measure. We agree that these terms do sound a bit cooler than REAR, but they really just describe a REAR or a series of REARs.

As we discuss later in the chapter, there are a variety of uses for the REAR regarding the assessment of hearing aid special features and the collection of general information on ear canal-aided output. For the moment, however, we will limit our discussion to the two primary uses: verification of prescriptive targets using the REAR values themselves and verification of prescriptive targets using the REIG, which is calculated using REAR values. Currently, the most popular way to verify a validated prescriptive hearing aid fitting procedure using a probe microphone is the REAR. It is certainly our preferred method because of several advantages we discuss in the remainder of this section.

Using the REAR to verify the fitting is quite logical, as everything is referenced to ear canal SPL, and we can easily visualize the portion of the speech signal that is audible for individual patients in their own ear. The SPL-O-Gram format means that louder outputs indeed fall *above* softer outputs. The common upward sloping audiogram takes some getting used to because it seems upside down compared to the traditional HL audiogram, but it's well worth the effort.

> ### POINTS TO PONDER: REIG VERSUS REAR—A LITTLE HISTORY
>
> When clinically friendly probe microphone equipment was introduced in the early 1980s, there was some discussion about whether the preferred verification measure was the REAR (then referred to as the *in situ response*) or the calculated insertion gain, soon to be called the REIR, now the REIG. The Madsen equipment, for example, originated in Europe and defaulted to the in situ setting. Audiologists by far, however, favored the REIG for several reasons:
>
> - All the popular prescriptive methods had gain targets.
> - REIG is essentially the same as functional gain, which was a common verification procedure at the time,
> - It's just simply a lot easier to talk about fitting hearing aids using gain terminology.
>
> So insertion gain became the preferred method of prescriptive target verification for the next 20 years or so. The exception for some audiologists was for pediatric fittings in which the DSL prescription was used as this fitting method did not have REIG targets (see Chapter 14).
>
> In the early 2000s, two factors converged that started to move audiologists toward using the REAR rather than the REIG for target verification. First, the NAL-NL1 had just been introduced and, unlike previous versions of this fitting algorithm, REAR prescriptive targets were now available. A second contributing factor was that the equipment company Audioscan introduced the Verifit®. It had a calibrated real-speech signal that could be used with the NAL-NL1 targets, which had been converted to ear canal SPL for the NAL-NL1 LTASS and were displayed on the fitting screen. Other probe microphone manufacturers soon followed with similar ear canal SPL fitting methods, and verification using the REAR rapidly grew in popularity. In their 2010 survey, Mueller and Picou asked dispensers who routinely use probe microphone measures what their primary method of prescriptive target verification was: 78% said the REAR and only 22% said the REIG. We suspect that even fewer audiologists are using the REIG today.
>
> That said, using the REAR as the verification approach does have two possible limitations. First, as we discuss in Chapter 16, with the REAR it is not as obvious when the probe tube is not deep enough as it is with the REUR measure. Second, since REAR targets are for a response instead of gain, it is sometimes unclear how much gain there is or how much should be present. As we discuss later in this chapter, this uncertainty can create specific issues in the low frequencies for open fittings.

Shown in Figure 17–8 is a typical fitting screen using the REAR for verification. The example here is for a real-speech 65 dB SPL input—the complete verification process would also include a soft and loud input signal (e.g., 55 and 75 dB SPL). The HL audiometric thresholds and the patient's LDLs have been converted to ear canal SPL using the REDD. This conversion is done automatically by the probe microphone equipment. Some equipment will use the patient's own RECD for this conversion, if it is entered, to provide a more accurate reflection of the patient's true threshold in dB SPL and for calculation of prescriptive targets. This calculation, however, also depends on the transducer used for the hearing assessment. In this example, we are looking at the NAL-NL2 fitting targets represented by the crosses. The shaded area represents the amplitude range of the amplified signal (30th to 99th percentiles), with the LTASS the dark line near the middle. The goal, accomplished very nicely here, is to make the LTASS equal to the prescriptive targets. The amplitude range of

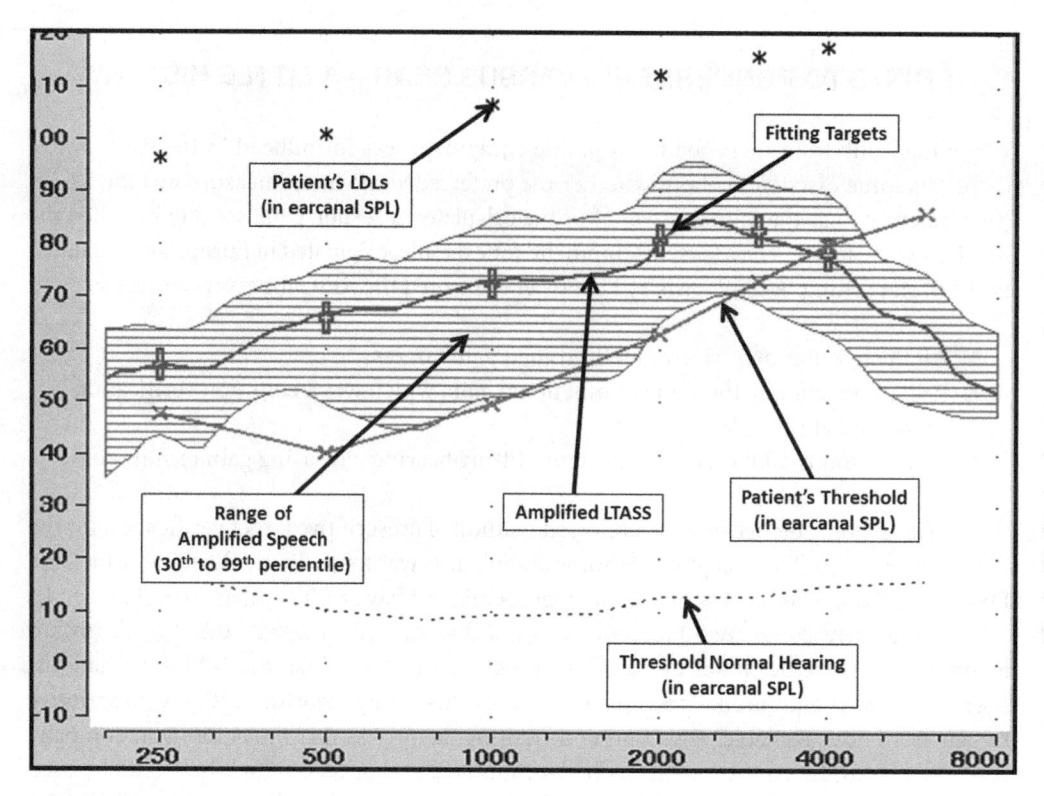

Figure 17–8. Example of fitting screen. Thresholds are converted from dB HL to dB SPL in the ear canal. Prescriptive targets are shown as crosses; the patient's LDLs are shown as asterisks. The amplified speech (65 dB SPL input) is shown both as the average LTASS and as the range (30th to 99th percentile). (Courtesy of Audioscan.)

the amplified speech signal also provides some insights regarding compression; note that the range is smaller for the higher frequencies where compression is the greatest.

Here are a couple of important points to consider when using the REAR to verify prescriptive targets:

- First, as we discuss in Chapter 16, the placement of the probe tip is very important. Because the measure is the absolute ear canal SPL, and poor probe-tip placement (shallow rather than deep) tends to mostly influence high frequencies, a less-than-ideal placement can significantly alter the recorded values. This in turn could prompt the audiologist to change the overall fitting. Figure 17–9 shows an example of this. Observe that the top curve is a nearly perfect match to the REAR targets for the patient with a moderate hearing loss. This measure was taken with the probe tip at the preferred location—within 5 mm of the patient's TM. Notice that the lower curve on the chart falls 5 to 10 dB below the targets in the higher frequencies. This output was obtained with the tube about 8 mm to 10 mm from the TM, a common mistake if one isn't careful. But what if the audiologist conducting this testing assumed the shallow placement was correct? This would probably lead to increasing gain up to 10 dB in the highs to match target. Now the patient leaves the clinic with excessive gain in the highs, which will no doubt prompt him or her to turn down overall gain, and we now have less audibility throughout the rest of the speech range—not a good outcome.

- A second consideration is to ensure that the input signal used corresponds to the targets on the fitting screen. That is, the fitting targets must be calculated using the LTASS being used for testing, which is why it is important

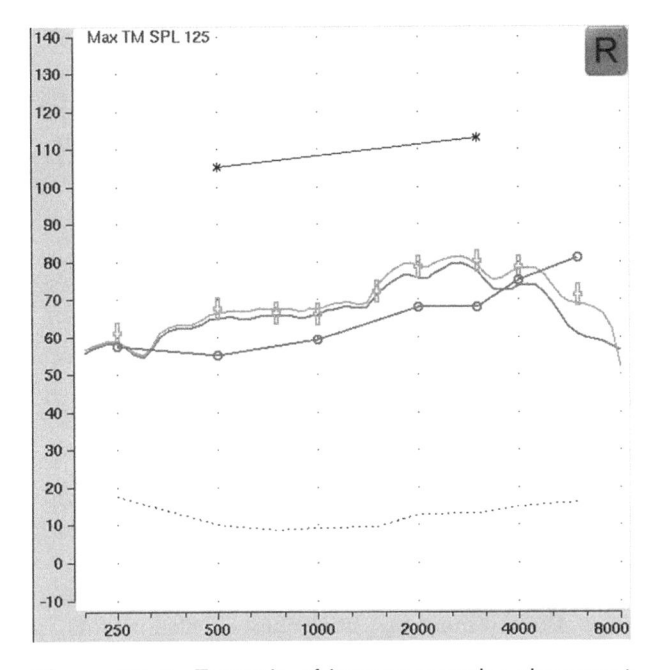

Figure 17–9. Example of how poor probe placement can lead to poor overall fitting. The top curve is a nearly perfect match to the REAR targets for the patient with a moderate hearing loss; the measure was taken with the probe tip at the preferred location—within 5 mm of the patient's TM. The lower curve falls below the targets in the higher frequencies; the measure was obtained with the tube about 8 to 10 mm from the TM.

to use a calibrated signal. This is why the on-screen targets will change with some probe microphone equipment if the input signal is changed. Alternatively, you may not see any fitting targets at all (which is certainly better than providing incorrect ones).

Test Protocols for REAR Verification of Prescriptive Targets

When using the REAR for verification, there are a couple of things to consider related to the level of the input signals: what levels to use and in what order to use them. First, we'll talk about the best input levels to use. As we have said many times, we want to obtain measures for soft, average, and loud speech. Soft speech is considered to be 50 to 55 dB SPL, average is 60 to 65 dB SPL, and loud is 75 to 80 dB SPL. So we could select inputs with a 30 dB range (a 50-65-80 dB SPL) or only a 20 dB range (a 55-65-75 dB SPL). Both of these two options are popular, and some clinics use a combination of the two. Although the 50-65-80 dB SPL gives us a larger range of measures, there are some limitations with this approach. In some offices, ambient noise makes it difficult to test at 50 dB SPL, and the loudspeaker of some probe microphone

---

TECHNICAL TIP: SPECIAL FEATURES ON OR OFF?

Hearing aids have several special features that, depending on the type of test signal, interact with the REAR measure. The most notable one is *digital noise reduction* because, if you are using an input signal that the hearing aid classifies as noise, the signal will be reduced, and the subsequent output will not represent the gain that the patient will have when listening to speech. This was a big problem when digital noise reduction was introduced, as most input signals used at that time indeed were classified as noise by the hearing aids. This led to the cry that you can't do probe microphone testing with digital hearing aids, which pleased more people than it should have (see Mueller, 2001). Fortunately, this issue was solved in the short term by using only short bursts of noise. It was permanently solved shortly thereafter when almost all probe microphone systems provided a real-speech or speech-like signal (see Chapter 16 for a review of these test signals). Now that we have these speech signals, we certainly recommend conducting verification with features such as directional technology and noise reduction activated. Given that they will be activated for the patient's everyday use, we want to determine how the hearing aid will function for the use condition—it is likely that there will be no effect, but if there is, we want to know about it. One possible exception to the "everything activated" philosophy is frequency lowering. We discuss evaluation of frequency lowering later in this chapter.

equipment tends to overdrive for the 80 dB SPL speech signal. For these reasons, we tend to prefer the 55-65-75 dB SPL approach. Because most of the products today have WDRC with kneepoints of 50 dB SPL or lower, we have found that, if the output for the 55 dB SPL input is okay, the output for the 50 dB SPL input is probably okay, too. And if the output for the 75 dB SPL input is okay, the output for the 80 dB SPL input is probably close enough.

After you decide which three input levels to use, the next decision involves the ordering of the verification levels. The goal is to obtain a target match for all three levels as efficiently as possible. The main thing that leads to inefficiency occurs when the programming for one input messes up the output for another input that you already programmed. In such a case, you have to go back and forth trying to obtain the best match or compromise. We can't think of a good reason for starting with loud, so let's eliminate that choice. A case can be made, however, for starting with either soft or average.

- Starting with soft: Many products have a kneepoint about the same level of soft speech (e.g., 50 dB SPL around 500 Hz); therefore, compression will have a minimal effect on the soft speech level. Therefore, we can start by adjusting overall gain (may be labeled gain for soft or gain for 50 dB input or something similar in fitting software) until we reach our desired targets. Using this approach, the next input presented will be loud. At this point, we no longer change gain but now alter the kneepoints/ ratios for the WDRC until a match is obtained (this is typically labeled gain for loud, gain for 80 dB input, or something similar in the fitting software). This second adjustment should have little or no effect on the gain for soft already programmed. If the WDRC system uses constant compression ratios (e.g., is relatively linear as opposed to curvilinear), then the output for the 65 dB input should be fairly close to prescriptive target, as it falls midway between the 55 and 75 dB SPL inputs. If not close enough, changes in gain for 65 dB SPL must be made, and gain for the 75 dB input should be rechecked.

- Starting with average: Although starting with the soft input may be the best choice for some hearing aid brands and models, there are two good reasons to start with average for other brands and models. First, depending on the patient's hearing loss and the compression system of the hearing aids being fitted, it may not be possible to obtain a precise fit for all three inputs. Typically, the hearing aid will simply not allow enough compression to meet all three targets, and you end up underfitting the soft targets and overfitting the loud targets no matter what you do. This limitation commonly occurs with slow release times in

---

POINTS TO PONDER: CHOOSING THE BEST PRESCRIPTIVE PROCEDURE IN THE SOFTWARE

We have noticed that, for some manufacturers, the prescriptive method you need to select to obtain a match to the correct compression parameters may have a different name than the method to which you are fitting. It might seem strange that you get a better match to the compression parameters you need for an NAL-NL2 fit when you select the manufacturer's proprietary fitting method or one that is labeled NAL-NL1, but we have seen both happen. In particular, compression release times may vary substantially from one software-fitting algorithm to another (and are not adjustable within a given algorithm). Consequently, it may be worth experimenting a bit with your favorite manufacturer's software to see if one of its built-in prescriptive methods leads to a close match to the compression parameters being prescribed by your chosen prescriptive method. If you find one, you can apply the average input first procedure we described and save a little time in the long run.

combination with speech test stimuli. In some of these hearing aids, adjusting gain for loud does indeed affect gain for soft. In such a case, we argue that it is best to start with average inputs. If you are only able to match targets for one input level it is likely best to match gain for average input levels, and then adjust MPO settings to make sure that loud sounds do not exceed discomfort levels. That is, if you use a hearing aid for which you effectively cannot increase the compression ratio after the initial fitting, all you can do is program average correctly and then measure soft and loud to see how far off they are.

The second and better reason to start with average is for the case in which your manufacturer typically gets the compression right when you enter the thresholds into the fitting software and select the correct prescriptive method. In this case, you adjust overall gain to obtain a good fit to average targets and then simply verify that your match to soft and loud are correct. In some cases, you can do this with no additional adjustments for soft and loud inputs—now that is time-efficient!

Using the REAR for Overall Assessment of Audibility

As we mentioned, probe microphone equipment converts audiometric thresholds and LDLs to the SPLO-Gram format (using average or measured REDD corrections), as illustrated in Figure 17–8. In the absence of prescriptive targets, this approach does provide a general window of acceptability for the fitting. It is fairly intuitive that, if the goal of the fitting is to make soft sounds audible, then the REAR for the soft speech inputs must be above the threshold curve. And, if we want to ensure that loud inputs are not too loud, the REAR for high inputs (swept tones) must be below the top LDL curve. This method lacks the preciseness of a validated prescriptive fitting; however, Mueller and Picou (2010) report that about one-third of audiologists who routinely use probe microphone measures, use this general approach rather than match specific targets. It does at least provide some basic evidence regarding audibility of speech and certainly is better than not conducting probe microphone measures at all, but there are some important limitations. For example, making soft speech audible is, of course, important, but what percent of the 30 dB range of soft speech should be above the patient's threshold? 100%? 50%? Is 25% good enough? And, in a downward sloping hearing loss, when do you concede that the hearing loss is so great that it may not be possible, or perhaps even desirable, to make soft speech audible? 70 dB? 80 dB? 90 dB? And how should the required percent of speech that needs to be audible change as a function of hearing loss? The goal of fitting a hearing aid is rarely to make all of speech audible. Patients reject such fittings as far too loud. By the time you try to sort all of this out and make all of the necessary decisions, you might as well be using a prescriptive method that already has researched these very factors, such as the NAL-NL2 or DSL v5, which is what we recommend in the first place.

Measurement of the REAR (Assuming a 3-mm Effective Vent Size or Smaller)

- If necessary, calibrate the probe tube (not all systems require this step).
- Position the patient appropriately.
- Position the probe tube at the correct depth in the ear canal.
- After muting, place the earmold and/or custom instrument in the ear with hearing aid programmed to desired starting point (e.g., manufacturer's implementation of a validated fitting method for the patient's hearing loss).
- If necessary, calibrate/level the loudspeaker using the reference microphone (not all systems require this step).
- Activate the hearing aid with all special features on (unmute), with the possible exception of frequency lowering, depending on fitting goals.
- Present a calibrated real-speech or speechlike signal; use an input level consistent with fitting protocol (see previous discussion).
- Observe the recorded REAR; if fitting to prescriptive targets, make programming changes to obtain the desired output.

Clinical Application of the REAR

- Primary: To obtain output match to desired prescriptive fitting targets
- Primary: To obtain general information regarding aided audibility
- Secondary: To calculate REIG (see next section)
- Secondary: To assess special features (e.g., directional, noise reduction, frequency lowering, etc.)
- Secondary: To assess assistive listening technology

Real-Ear Insertion Gain (REIG)

Definition:

- REI. *Difference in decibels, as a function of frequency, between the REAG and the REUG, and taken with the same measurement point and the same soundfield conditions.*

As we have already discussed, the clinical application of the REIG is to verify prescriptive fitting targets. The REIG is not a measurement per se but, rather, a calculation based on two other measures that we've already discussed: the REUR subtracted from the REAR, or the REUG subtracted from the REAG. Consider that when we discussed using the REAR for verification in the preceding section, we were looking at placing the amplified speech signal at a desired SPL in the ear canal. With the REIG, we're looking at the *gain* that is needed to accomplish the same task. When we assess the gain the patient has with the hearing aid, we have to consider the gain that he or she first had with the open ear—which takes us back to the REUR.

Although the REUG is more or less ignored when we verify with the REAR, when comparing REIG findings to prescriptive targets, the patient's REUG can have a huge influence (assuming a measured REUG is used). When we first started conducting probe microphone testing in the mid-1980s, the hearing aid technology at the time had little insertion gain above 3000 Hz. Audiology students often would ask, "How can I obtain more insertion gain at 4000 Hz?" The answer was always the same: "Find a patient who has an REUG of 0 dB at 4000 Hz!" A bit absurd, yes, but the point is that you can nearly always predict the goodness of the REIG as soon as you've measured the REUG. For example, let's say that Patient A and Patient B both have an identical 50 dB hearing loss at 3000 Hz, and we're conducting probe microphone testing using a 55 dB input. We'd like to see about 30 dB of insertion gain for this soft input signal. Patient A has a REUG of 10 dB at 3000 Hz, and Patient B's REUG is 25 dB for this frequency. What might very

---

TECHNICAL TIP: THE REIR DIDN'T MAKE THE CUT

In the early days of probe microphone testing when insertion gain was measured, it was referred to as the real-ear insertion response (REIR). If we talked about gain at a specific frequency, we referred to it as real-ear insertion gain (REIG). As pointed out in the standard (correctly, of course), insertion gain is gain, and therefore cannot be a response. It's always an REIG. This was a good change because calling it a response tended to get one thinking that it indeed was a response rather than a difference curve. When looking at the REIR (now the REIG), audiologists would often say, "I need to get rid of that 'bump' right there," when in fact it really wasn't a bump in the frequency response but only an area where gain was greater, which easily could have been caused by a dip in the unaided response (REUG), and so had nothing to do with what might be a very smooth REAR. The bottom line is that, even though most probe microphone measures do have an acronym containing an R at the end, REIG is always REIG. Don't be surprised, however, to see the acronym REIR used in literature prior to the release of the 1997 standard.

likely happen is that on our first measure following the manufacturer's first fit, our REIG for Patient A is exactly what we want, so we deem it a good fitting; whereas for Patient B, we are 15 dB below our fitting target, so we deem it a bad fitting. Yet, the REAR for the two fittings might be exactly the same. So was one really a good fit and the other a bad fit if speech were placed at the same ear canal SPL for both patients?

It's these types of questions that generate interesting lunchtime discussions among audiologists fitting hearing aids, especially if one favors REAR speech mapping and another favors the REIG approach. The earlier example had two patients with quite different REUGs, and indeed if your patient has an unusual REUG, you will end up with a considerably different fitting when the REIG is used rather than the REAR for a target match. But in general, for average REUGs, you would expect the match-to-target results to be similar.

Figure 17–10A shows a patient fitted to NAL-NL2 prescriptive gain for a 65 dB input using the REIG as verification. In Figure 17–10B, the REAR that resulted for the target REIG fitting is displayed in the speech mapping mode. Observe that when the insertion gain targets were matched for the average input signal, the REAR targets were also matched for the same signal.

Real Speech and REIG Calculations

Some probe microphone equipment limits the type of input signal that can be selected when insertion gain calculations are conducted compared to those available when speech mapping is selected. That is, the signal for the REIG measures does not include a speech type signal. This can be a problem because some special features, such as digital noise reduction, will now interact with the REIG measurement. It is possible, however, to conduct measures for REIG calculation using your favorite speech signal. Shown in Figure 17–11 are the REUR and the REARs obtained using the ISTS 65-dB SPL input. The REIG targets are not displayed on this fitting screen but could be referenced easily on the REIG screen. This particular equipment does not automatically calculate the difference between these two curves, but that, too, could be obtained easily with the on-screen curser (in Figure 17–11, the curser is set to 2000 Hz, for

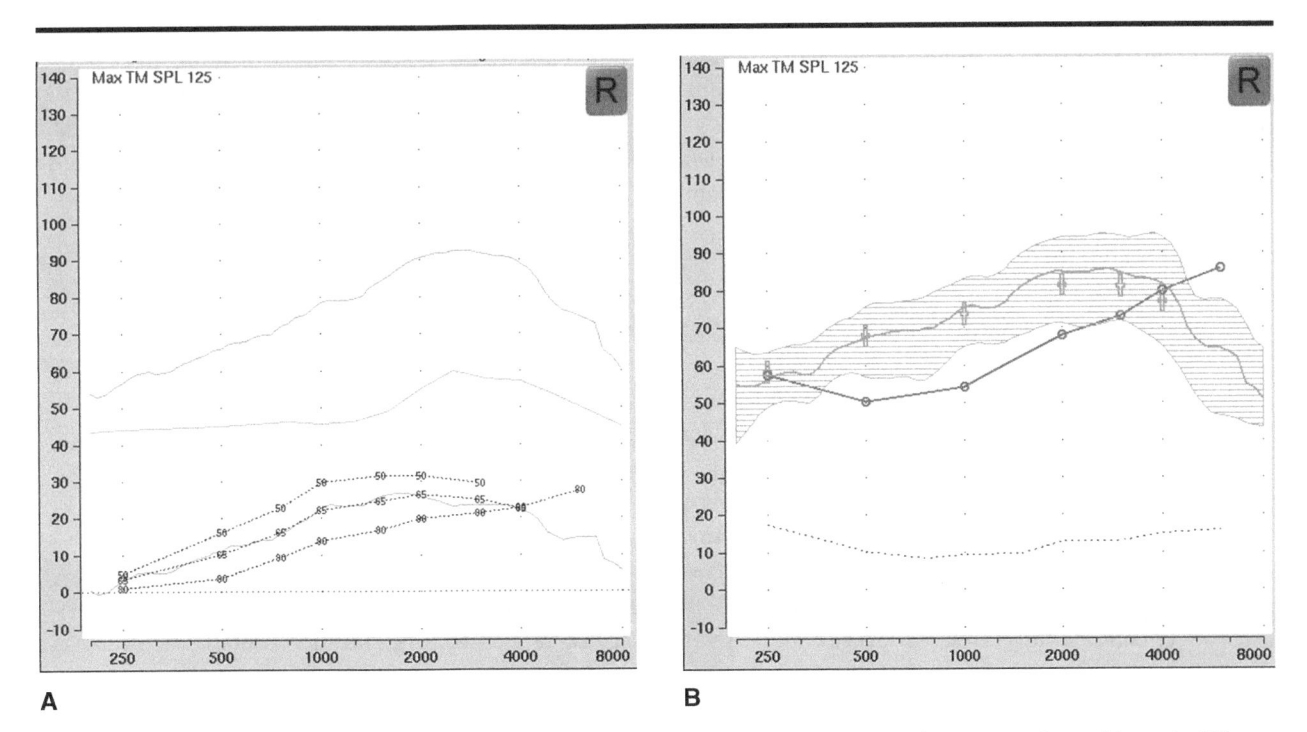

Figure 17–10. Example of matching insertion gain targets (**A**) and resultant match to output-based targets (**B**).

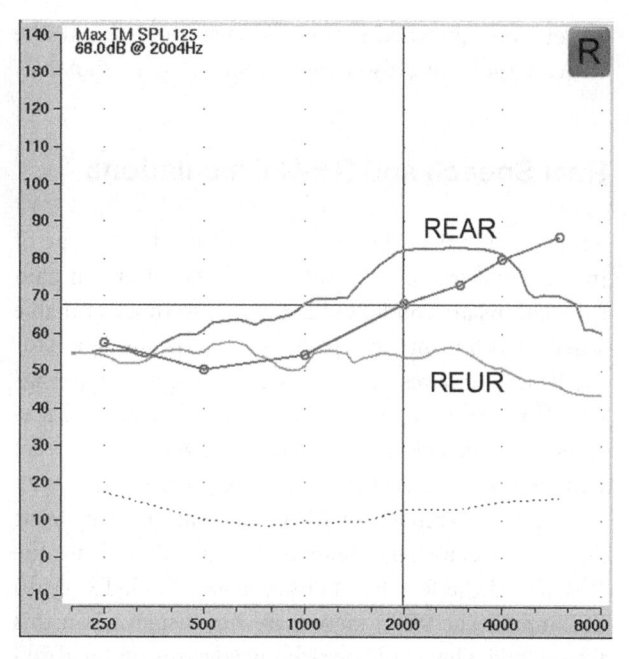

Figure 17–11. Example of REUR and REAR obtained with ISTS stimulus. Cursor at 2000 Hz shows difference between those two curves or insertion gain at 2000 Hz of nearly 30 dB.

TECHNICAL TIP: PLACEMENT OF PROBE TUBE FOR REIG MEASURES

As we discuss in detail in Chapter 16 and in the previous REAR section, placement of the tip of the probe tube in the ear canal is critical. When in doubt, deep is usually the best approach, particularly when attempting to accurately match prescriptive gain targets at 4000 Hz and above. There is some forgiveness, however, when REIG values are used for verification. If you use a measured REUG, then it also is important that the probe-tube tip is the same place for both the REUR and REAR measures—but it doesn't really have to be deep (within reason). That is, if your probe is a little too shallow for the REUR, and is also a little too shallow for the REAR, the resulting REIG will be as accurate as if a deep placement had been used for both fittings—one of the few times that two wrongs make a right! See Mueller (1992) for research findings on this topic.

---

example). So real-speech signals and REIG measures are not mutually exclusive using any probe microphone equipment. It is just that a little more effort is sometimes required to obtain the REIG calculations.

As with the REAR, the REIG can be used to verify several different hearing aid features. It's probably easier to conduct these measures using only the REAR, but if the REIG is used for verification, then it may be easier to continue to use this same reference when observing the effects of digital noise reduction, adaptive feedback, and other dynamic hearing aid signal processing.

POINTS TO PONDER: HOW CLOSE IS CLOSE ENOUGH?

It is unfortunate that prescriptive targets usually are displayed as a single value because they really represent a range for an acceptable fitting. The single target value, often displayed for the dispenser and patient to see, encourages some people to try to attain a level of preciseness that may not be necessary. As we discussed in Chapter 14, background research with the development of the NAL-NL2 revealed that +/−3 dB of target (a 6 dB window) is satisfactory for the preferred listening level of about 60% of patients. Each office or clinic must establish its own rules for what is close enough, but given the lack of preciseness in threshold measurement (5 dB steps), the common use of average correction factors, and the variability of applying average prescriptive targets to individual listeners, a +/−3 to 5 dB deviation from REIG or REAR targets certainly seems acceptable. At least one manufacturer does provide a vertical bar rather than a single point representing an acceptable range for the fitting target.

Reliability of the Measures

When probe microphone measures were first introduced, there was some concern regarding the reliability of these measures and how this reliability might vary from machine to machine. All research findings on this topic, however, were encouraging. Mueller and Sweetow (1987) found that REIGs measured on three different systems were very similar, and Hawkins and colleagues (1991) provided test–retest data, showing results that certainly are adequate for clinical work. As shown in Table 17–2, they found that the 95% confidence intervals (CIs) were 2 to 3 dB at 3000 Hz and below and 4 to 5 dB at 4000 and 5000 Hz. As expected, the mean test–retest differences for the REAR/REIG were a little higher (because now we have the variable of hearing aid or earmold insertion), but these values were still respectable with CIs of 2 to 3 dB below 1000 Hz, 3 dB in the 1000 to 2000 Hz region, and 4 to 6 dB at 3000 Hz and above. Similar findings were reported by Valente et al. (1990), and we certainly would expect findings as good or better with today's equipment.

Calculation of the REIG Assuming a 3-mm Effective Vent Size or Smaller)

- If necessary, calibrate the probe tube (not all systems require this step).
- Position the patient appropriately.
- Position the probe tube at the correct depth in the ear canal.
- If necessary calibrate/level the loudspeaker using the reference microphone (not all systems require this step).
- Measure the REUR and store (or use the average REUR in your probe microphone system).
- After muting, place the eartip or earmold and/or custom instrument in the ear, with hearing aid programmed to desired starting point (e.g., manufacturer's implementation of a validated fitting method for the patient's hearing loss).
- Activate the hearing aid with all special features on (unmute), with the possible

Table 17–2. Mean Signed Test-Retest Differences, SDs and 95% CIs for the REUR, REAR, REIG Measures

	Frequency (kHz)								
	.25	.5	.75	1	1.5	2	3	4	5
REUR									
Mean	0.3	0.3	0.4	0.0	−0.2	0.0	0.1	0.4	2.0
SD	0.7	1.3	1.8	1.0	1.1	1.4	1.6	2.7	1.9
95% CI	1.4	2.6	3.6	2.0	2.2	2.8	3.2	5.4	3.8
REAR									
Mean	−1.3	−0.6	−0.6	−0.4	−0.2	−0.2	−0.3	−0.4	−0.2
SD	*	*	*	1.6	1.4	1.7	2.0	2.7	3.0
95% CI	*	*	*	3.2	2.8	3.4	4.0	5.4	6.0
REIG									
Mean	1.4	0.9	−0.9	−0.4	0.1	0.1	−0.3	−0.8	−0.6
SD	*	*	*	1.7	1.5	1.6	2.0	2.2	2.5
95% CI	*	*	*	3.4	3.0	3.2	4.0	4.4	5.0

Note. *Values not reported due to variable leakage around earmold resulting in inflated test–retest variability.
Source: From Hawkins et al. (1991).

exception of frequency lowering, depending on fitting goals.
- Present a calibrated real-speech or speech-like signal; use an input level consistent with fitting protocol (see previous REAR discussion).
- Observe the calculated REIG; if fitting to prescriptive targets, make programming changes to obtain the desired output.

Clinical Application of the REIG

- Primary: To obtain gain match to desired prescriptive fitting targets.
- Secondary: To assess special features (e.g., directional, noise reduction, etc.).
- Secondary: To estimate aided thresholds (see example later in this chapter).

Real-Ear Aided Response for an 85 dB or 90 dB Input (REAR85 or REAR90)

Definition:

- SPL as a function of frequency, at a specified measurement point in the ear canal, for a specified soundfield, with the hearing aid (and its acoustic coupling) in place and turned on, with the VC adjusted to full-on (or just below feedback if full-on isn't possible). The input signal is sufficiently intense to operate the hearing aid at its maximum output level. Usually 85 dB or 90 dB SPL as noted in the acronym. Previously referred to as Real-Ear Saturation Response (RESR).

This measure became part of the ANSI standard after the latest revision, but the use of the RESR term (and the measurement) dates back to the early days of probe microphone testing. As the definition states, this test is conducted with the volume control (VC) full-on (or just below feedback) using an 85 or 90 dB SPL input signal. You can think of it as conducting the 2cc coupler OSPL90 measure in the real ear, although this is only partially true, as the measurement is taken with the hearing aid's maximum output adjusted for the patient, which often will not be the maximum. In other words, we want to create a worse case measure in the clinic to ensure that there isn't excessive aided loudness in the real world. If the patient's hearing aid does not have a VC, then the programmed use-gain is the level used for conducting the measure. The clinical application of conducting this measure is twofold: to ensure that the hearing aid's maximum output does not exceed the patient's comfort levels and to ensure that the maximum output does not exceed safe levels.

The general use of the REAR85 or REAR90 in clinical practice is to verify that the MPO that was set based on the unaided LDL measures is appropriate. Refer back to Figure 17–8 and you see that the patient's LDLs have been converted to ear canal SPL and are displayed on the fitting screen. We can think of these as the REAR85/90 targets—targets in the sense that we don't want to exceed these levels. If our unaided LDLs (in HL) during the initial audiometric evaluation were conducted carefully, and we then used these values (converted to 2cc coupler using the RETSPL) to program the hearing aid's MPO, there should not be any surprises. In fact, it is common that the REAR85/90 values are well below the upper level, simply because the output is being limited by the WDRC, rather than the AGCo or some other type of output limiting. But, if there are peaks in the output, these can be handled by using the channel-specific output limiting controls in the software.

A concern that has been associated with this measure since it was first introduced is the potentially high levels of sound that can be present in the ear canal while conducting this procedure. In a worst-case scenario, a linear power hearing aid with a coupler output of 135 to 140 dB SPL could be driven to its maximum if the VC is set to max and the input is a pure tone. If the residual ear canal volume is small (e.g., deep earmold, small ear canal), the output in the ear canal could be 150 dB SPL or higher. This raises the concern of acoustic trauma during the test procedure. We assume that a prudent dispenser will ensure that levels of 150 dB are never delivered to a patient; however, it could happen. Probe microphone equipment does have safeguards for this, as you can set the maximum output measured by the system to a specific value (e.g., 120 dB SPL), and it will shut down the input signal when this output is reached.

If you do choose to conduct REAR85 measurements, it is important to remember that the input signal can influence the results significantly—the spectrum level of the output at a particular frequency using a broadband signal will be lower than the total rms output, as illustrated in Figure 17–12. Observe the difference between the output for swept tone and the speech signal, both presented using an input of 85 dB. The question then becomes, do you want to set the maximum output of the hearing aid for the most common signals the patient hears (broadband signals like speech) or do you want to set the maximum output of the hearing aid for the occasional narrowband signals the patient hears? A conservative approach is to adjust the maximum output of the hearing aid using pure-tone inputs, as many signals that the user experiences do have a narrowband spectra and will drive the hearing aid output close to this level (see Stelmachowicz, 1991).

Measurement of the REAR85/90

- If necessary, calibrate the probe tube (not all systems require this step).
- Position the patient appropriately.
- Position the probe tube at the correct depth in the ear canal.
- After muting, place the eartip or earmold and/or custom instrument in the ear, with hearing aid programmed to desired starting point (e.g., manufacturer's implementation of a validated fitting method for the patient's hearing loss).
- If necessary, calibrate/level the loudspeaker using the reference microphone (not all systems require this step).
- Activate the hearing aid with all special features on (unmute), with the exception of frequency lowering. Frequency lowering must be deactivated in order to measure an accurate REAR85/90 in response to tonal signals.
- If patient has a VC, adjust to full-on or just below feedback. If patient does not have a VC, conduct testing at use-gain settings.
- Present a calibrated swept pure tone (or tone pips) of either 85 dB or 90 dB SPL.
- Observe the recorded real-ear MPO; make programming changes to obtain the desired output.

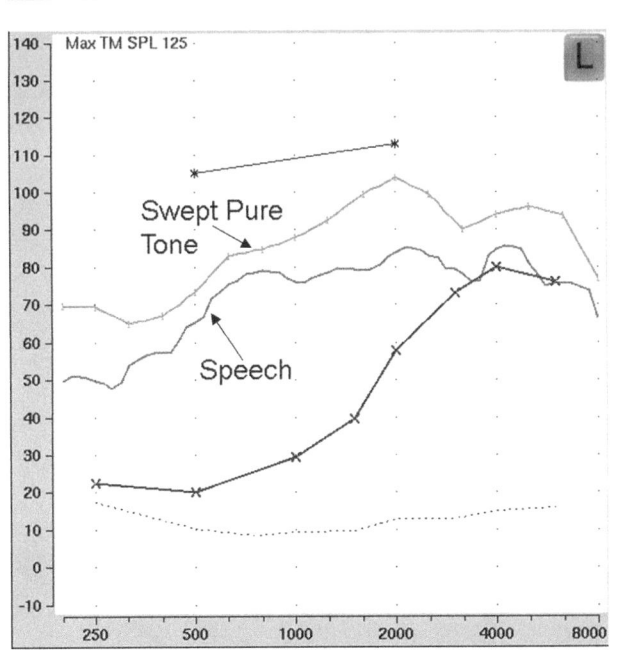

Figure 17–12. Example of the output of a hearing aid for both a speech signal and a pure-tone sweep of the same input level.

TECHNICAL TIP: SETTING THE VC FOR THE REAR85/90 MEASURE

As mentioned in the definition for the REAR85/90 measure, the hearing aids should be set to full-on if possible. Although we like to follow rules laid out in standards, there may be times when this one can be broken. The primary purpose of doing this testing is to ensure that the MPO of the hearing aid will not exceed the patient's LDLs. We understand that, if the patient is using a hearing aid with a VC, it is certainly possible that he or she may be listening to something soft with the VC turned up when a sudden loud sound might occur. But what if the patient doesn't have a VC, as is the case for approximately 25% of fittings? Does it make sense to turn the hearing aid to full-on gain for this testing when we know that the patient will never have the gain at this level in the real world? We don't think so. We propose doing the testing at the patient's use-gain setting.

Clinical Application of the REAR85/90

- Primary: To ensure that MPO doesn't exceed patient's LDLs.
- Primary: To ensure that MPO is safe.
- Secondary: To ensure that MPO is not unreasonably low, unnecessarily restricting headroom.

Real-Ear Coupler Difference (RECD)

Definition:

- RECD. *Difference in decibels, as a function of frequency, between the SPL produced near the tympanic membrane in an occluded ear canal by a coupled sound source having a high acoustic impedance (see ANSI/ASA S1.1) and that produced in the HA-1 configuration of the 2 cm3 earphone coupler by the same coupled sound source.*

The RECD is a new addition to the ANSI probe microphone standard, and as you can see by the caveats in our associated Technical Tip, there is considerable concern about the measure being conducted correctly. Although this procedure was not in the standard until recently, the RECD has been a common measurement conducted with children since the late 1980s (e.g., see Feigin, Kopun, Stelmachowicz, & Gorga, 1989). If you fit hearing aids to infants and children and do not own probe microphone equipment, the ability to conduct this procedure alone justifies its purchase. If we know a child's RECD, we have information that will assist us in selecting the appropriate hearing aid output and in predicting the output in the child's ear (OSPL90 + RECD = Predicted Real-Ear MPO, or 2cc coupler + RECD + MLE = Predicted RealEar Output). Moreover, on the day of the fitting, the majority of the patient-specific hearing aid adjustments can be made in the 2cc coupler, reducing the time and cooperation required from the child. Matching hearing aid gain to validated prescriptive targets in a coupler by applying average or individually measured RECDs can also be useful with some adult patients. We have all seen difficult-to-test patients

---

TECHNICAL TIP: THREE RECD CAVEATS

The current ANSI standard for real-ear measurements (ANSI S3.46-2013) has three caveats to the measurement of the RECD:

- Caveat 1. The HA-1 configuration of the 2cc earphone coupler is described in ANSI/ASA S3.7 and excludes any coupling tubing.
- Caveat 2. If the coupled sound source is the same for both the ear canal and the coupler SPL measurements, and if the magnitude of its acoustic impedance is significantly higher than the magnitudes of the acoustic impedances of the ear canal and of the 2cc coupler, the RECD will be a measure of the magnitude of the acoustic impedance of the ear canal relative to that of the 2cc coupler, independent of the coupled sound source. Otherwise, the SPL difference between the ear and the coupler is dependent on the coupled sound source utilized in its measurement.
- Caveat 3. Because the HA-2 configuration of the 2cc coupler described in ANSI/ASA S3.22 contains 25 mm of 2 mm inside diameter (i.d.) tubing plus 18 mm of 3 mm i.d. tubing, which in most cases will be different from that in the individual earmold or eartip used for the ear canal measurement, its use for the coupler portion of RECD measurements will result in a different coupled sound source for the two measurements. The resulting RECD will not be a measure of the magnitude of the acoustic impedance of the ear canal relative to that of the 2cc coupler. For this reason, its use in the determination of RECD is strongly discouraged.

who are unable to sit quietly motionless for enough time to adjust the hearing aid to REAR targets. A short RECD measure greatly lessens this time and will typically result in an accurate fitting. In some cases, we are even unable to measure RECDs. Fitting the hearing aid in a coupler with an age-specific average RECD value in these cases

> **THINGS TO REMEMBER: THE ANSI STANDARD RECD AND PAST CLINICAL PRACTICE**
>
> In the past, the two different uses for the RECD (application for hearing aid fitting, adjustment of threshold for calculation of accurate prescriptive targets) were somewhat in conflict. Specifically, because the primary application was hearing aid fittings in children, the hearing aid was being fitted with a specific plumbing (tubing and venting) in a BTE earmold. Conversely, thresholds were measured with insert earphones in the absence of this plumbing. A common recommendation of the time was to assess the RECD using the child's earmold and, to be most accurate, consider remeasuring thresholds through the individual's earmold as well. Furthermore, many probe microphone systems measured and referenced the RECD to the HA-2 coupler. The advantage of this method was that it allowed the clinician to fit the hearing aid in the coupler before the child arrived (for closed earmolds/ eartips). As pointed out in the notes from ANSIS3.46-2013, however, this was problematic since the plumbing assumed in a HA-2 coupler (a stepped bore horn) rarely reflects what the patient is actually fitted with, and impedance issues also were a factor. In order to address these issues, the new standard recommends measurement using an insert transducer that is calibrated relative to the HA-1 coupler, a considerably different measurement than the RECD calibrated in a HA-2 coupler (Figure 17–13). In other words, the plumbing effects are removed from the RECD, and it reflects only the acoustic differences between the ear and a 2cc coupler. Consequently, the same RECD can now be applied when correcting individual thresholds for target calculation as when fitting a hearing aid in the coupler. The plumbing is then accounted for when the hearing aid is programmed by attaching the hearing aid with all plumbing (e.g., the earmold and tubing) to a HA-1 coupler. Overall, we agree this standard should improve consistency and accuracy across clinical fittings that apply the RECD; however, some equipment requires that we have the earmold in hand when programming the hearing aid. Consequently, introduction of the new standard had a considerable impact on clinical practice in some clinics, particularly those that were fitting hearing aids using a HA-2 coupler before obtaining the earmold.
>
> In order to circumvent this issue, at least one probe microphone manufacturer allows for fittings to validated prescriptive targets in a HA-2 coupler using an HA-1 referenced RECD. This fitting is accomplished using a HA-2 to earmold simulator correction factor that is applied by the probe microphone manufacturer. This procedure has the advantage of not requiring the patient's earmold prior to fitting to targets, as well as being a very repeatable measure (ensuring that the hearing aid earmold is oriented correctly in a HA-1 coupler and well-sealed with putty takes considerable care). When fitting with this procedure, the match to target on the HA-2 coupler will be very similar to that obtained in a HA-1 coupler using standard tubing and an unvented earmold (and consequently in the ear of the patient using REAR procedures). Of course, the accuracy of using this HA-2 based fitting procedure will be lessened when the earmold tubing is shorter or longer than assumed by the correction factor and when there is any venting introduced.

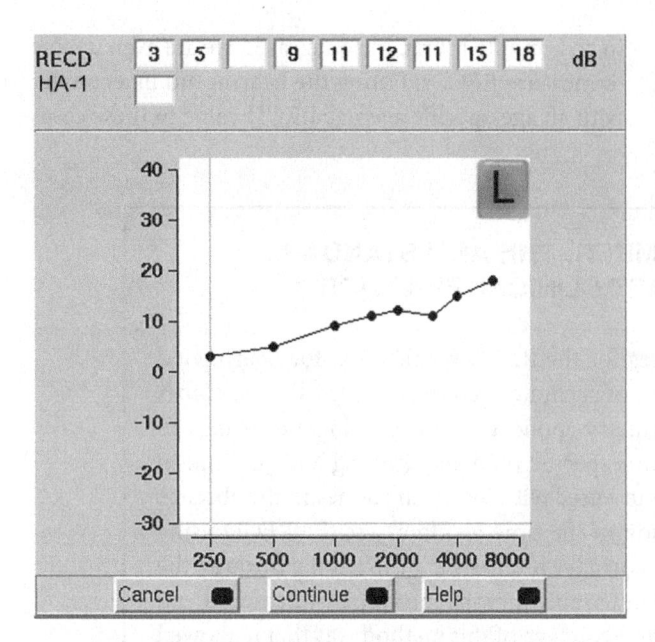

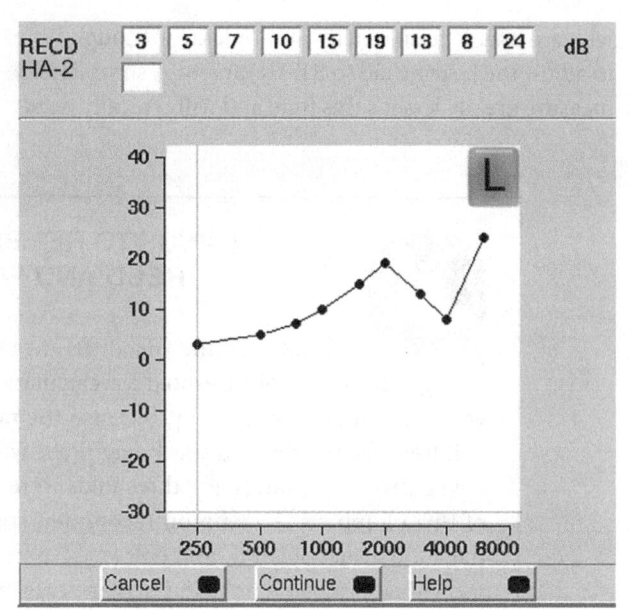

Figure 17–13. The average, age-specific RECD values relative to calibration in HA-1 (**A**) and HA-2 (**B**) couplers. Note the differences in the numerical values at the top.

will typically result in a fitting that is considerably closer to the desired real-ear targets than simply applying a manufacturer's first fit.

The RECD also can be used with adults to refine the fitting. As we describe in Chapter 5, one study reported that adult RECD standard deviations are 3.1 dB for 1000 Hz, 3.5 dB for 2000 Hz, and 5.4 dB for 4000 Hz (Saunders & Morgan, 2003). Hence entering the patient's RECDs rather than using average values will add preciseness to the threshold measures and, in turn, increase the accuracy of the calculated prescriptive targets.

In 1994, Moodie, Seewald, and Sinclair described an RECD procedure that utilized insert earphones, a HA-2 coupler, and the child's own earmold. Even with the recent standard, we expect this method is still commonly used in some clinic protocols. Specifically, the procedure they described is as follows:

- Conduct appropriate calibration and configure the software of the probe microphone equipment for RECD measurements (this procedure will vary depending on manufacturer of the probe microphone equipment).
- Connect the insert earphone to the loudspeaker output terminal of the probe microphone equipment using a matching phone plug.
- Thread the probe tube through the calibrator adapter plug so that the tip of the tube extends no more than 3 mm above the surface of the plug.
- Place the calibrator adapter plug into the microphone port of the HA-2 2cc coupler.
- Connect the probe tube to the probe microphone.
- Connect the insert earphone tip to the tubing of the HA-2 2cc coupler.
- Deliver a speech-weighted signal of 50 dB SPL, and record the coupler output. Save this as the "unaided measure" (REUR).
- Remove the probe microphone apparatus from the coupler and place the tube in the patient's ear with the probe tip at the appropriate depth.
- Place the patient's earmold in patient's ear.
- Attach the insert earphone tip to the tubing of the earmold (the length of the earmold tubing should be appropriate for BTE hearing aid use).

- Deliver a speech-weighted signal of 50 dB SPL, and record the real-ear output. Save this as the "aided measure" (REAR).

- Either automatically or through software command, the probe microphone equipment will calculate an REIG, which in this case

---

KEY CONCEPT: FACTORS COMPLICATING THE RECD MEASUREMENT

We now have a standard describing an RECD procedure, but as we just noted, there have been several variations of how these measures were conducted over the years. These differences complicated the precise description of the measurement, hence the need for the standard. A description of some of the complicating factors follows including two that still apply.

These factors no longer apply:

- If the measurement was conducted using the patient's own hearing aid (which is one approach that had been suggested), MLEs become part of the RECD (assuming the testing is conducted in the sound field; if direct audio input is used, then the MLE is not included). If a given prescriptive fitting approach (such as DSLv5 or NAL-NL2) or a manufacturer's software already includes average MLEs and they allow you to enter the patient's RECD, then it's possible that the MLE would be added twice. Recall that the CORFIG is calculated by the formula: REUG − RECD + MLE, which assumes that the MLE is not part of the RECD.
- The MLEs for a hearing aid tested by using a moderate input level are not the same as the MLEs when the hearing aid is in saturation. One of the uses of the RECD is to predict the output of the hearing aid when it's in saturation, yet the hearing aid REAR measurement often is conducted using a 60 dB input.
- If the patient was fitted with a WDRC instrument, then it is necessary to consider the effects of WDRC on the MLE. That is, if a 60 dB signal at 4000 Hz becomes a 70 dB input because of an MLE of 10 dB (CIC fitting), the increase in output will not be proportional if the input signal is compressed (e.g., if the compression ratio is 2:1, the MLE will now yield only a 5 dB change in output).
- If a HA-1 coupler is used, then the RECD will be different than if a HA-2 coupler is used.

These factors still apply:

- If an insert earphone is used, the output impedance effects need to be the same as for the patient's hearing aid. If a foam plug is used, the placement depth in the ear canal should approximate the depth of the patient's hearing aid or earmold.
- Even when depth is controlled, the RECD using a foam tip will be somewhat different from the RECD using the patient's earmold.
    When applied to open fittings, the RECD is really only useful to correct threshold values for calculation of prescriptive targets. As we describe later in this chapter, it is not possible to complete an open fitting accurately using typical simulated gain (RECD) techniques.

is not an REIG but an RECD. What will be displayed is the coupler output subtracted from the real-ear output for all test frequencies.
- Positive values are added to the OSPL90 to predict the RESR and subtracted from ear canal SPL targets to determine appropriate 2cc-coupler output. By also adding the MLE to the RECD, values can be used to predict real-ear SPL for other inputs of interest.

This procedure has been used successfully for several years and has been found to be a highly accurate predictor of real-ear output. Using this approach, Seewald, Moodie, Sinclair, and Scollie (1999) compared the predicted REAG and RESR to the respective measured values for 14 children fitted with BTE hearing aids (head diffraction and MLE effects were included for the REAG prediction). Their results showed a 95% confidence interval of +/−2.3 dB for the REAG and an average error range of 4.4 dB for the RESR. These findings illustrate that, if appropriate probe microphone measures are employed with infants and children, the certainty of the hearing aid fitting is probably greater than the certainty of their audiometric thresholds.

Measurement of the RECD

The approach described by Moodie et al. (1994) really needs only minor modifications that mainly relate to calibration details to be in line with the current ANSI standard. Our modified version of these instructions follows:

- Connect an insert earphone or RECD transducer to the probe microphone equipment.
- Configure the software of the probe microphone equipment for RECD measurements and conduct appropriate calibration of the transducer referenced to a HA-1 coupler (this procedure will vary depending on manufacturer of the probe microphone equipment).
  - One method is to attach the transducer via foam insert eartip to the HA-1 coupler. Another is to attach the transducer to the individual's earmold with all venting blocked and putty the earmold to the HA-1 coupler. A broadband speech-weighted or pink noise signal is typically used for calibration.

Note: At least one probe microphone manufacturer currently calibrates the transducer in a HA-2 coupler (without an insert eartip or earmold), and then applies a correction so that the measure is referenced to a HA-1 coupler. We assume that this procedure is applied to improve reliability compared to attaching a transducer to a HA-1 coupler. Some systems also use a 0.4cc coupler and connector adaptor to allow the transducer to be easily coupled to the coupler, and then automatically provide an equivalent HA-1 referenced RECD for compatibility with other equipment and fitting software.

- Place the probe tube in the patient's ear with the probe tip at the appropriate depth.
- Remove the transducer from the HA-1 coupler (with earmold or foam insert attached) and insert it in the patient's ear.
- Deliver the same signal used in calibrating the transducer in the HA-1 coupler through the loudspeaker and measure the output in the ear. The difference between the coupler and real-ear values is the individual's RECD. These values are typically calculated automatically by the probe microphone system.

Clinical Application of the RECD

- Primary: To predict hearing aid output in the ear canal when 2cc coupler values are known.
- Primary: To determine desired OSPL90 and coupler output settings.
- Primary: To apply when programming the hearing aid in the coupler to equivalent real-ear targets.
- Secondary: To individualize REDD corrections so as to provide a better estimate of hearing thresholds for calculation of real-ear prescriptive targets.

> **TECHNICAL TIP: APPLICATION OF RECD FOR REAL-EAR EQUIVALENT VERIFICATION**
>
> When considering young children or other difficult-to-fit patients, one important use of the RECD is the simulated REAR. Once you measure an individual's RECD, a fitting procedure that accurately reflects verification in the real ear can be completed using the following steps:
>
> - Configure your probe microphone software for a simulated REAR, enter the patient's thresholds and LDLs, and identify the validated prescriptive fitting method you plan to use.
> - Measure or enter the patient's RECD.
> - If a BTE instrument is being fitted, attach the patient's earmold or eartip with the tubing length size appropriate for the patient and all plumbing configured as it will be for the patient. Attach the earmold or ear shell (in the case of a custom hearing aid) to a HA-1 coupler using putty. As noted earlier in this chapter, at least one probe microphone system will allow you to use a BTE and a HA-2 coupler and will automatically apply anHA-2 to earmold simulator correction factor.
> - Adjust hearing aid gain in the coupler to match prescriptive targets. Typically, this will use methods that are very similar to REAR verification procedures.
>
> Although this procedure typically yields fittings that are equivalent to those measured in the real ear, there is one considerable limitation related to venting. Specifically, larger vents must be wholly or partially plugged to avoid uncontrollable feedback that occurs because of the reflective surfaces within the hearing aid test box. Therefore, it is not possible to use this procedure with open fittings—in addition to the feedback issue, it is also very difficult to accurately simulate an open fitting using a coupler, although a standard open coupler is currently under development.

Real-Ear Dial Difference (REDD)

Definition:

- *REDD. Difference in decibels as a function of frequency between the SPL produced near the tympanic membrane by an audiometric sound source and the hearing level indicated by the audiometer driving the sound source.*

Note: The REDD can be used to convert hearing level (HL) behavioral measures obtained with an audiometer to ear canal SPL for comparison to the measured real-ear quantities described in the standard. The REDD is specific to the audiometer and sound source used in its measurement.

A final probe microphone term that you may not be too familiar with is the REDD, a term has been in use since 1995 (Mueller, 1995). The REDD is another calculation that was just added to the current ANSI standard. The primary purpose of the REDD is to allow you to plot SPL-o-Grams—the REDD is added to the HL thresholds (and LDLs, if available) to obtain a plot of these values in ear canal SPL. Most of today's probe microphone equipment will do this calculation and plotting for you using average or measured REDD values. Consider that the REDD is really a combination of two other correction factors: the RETSPL, which takes us from the audiometer to the 2cc coupler (see associated Key Concept); and the RECD, which then takes us from the 2cc coupler to the real ear—RECD + RETSPL = REDD. For example, the average RECD for an adult

> **KEY CONCEPT: REMEMBER THE RETSPL**
>
> We've talked about the RETSPL before, but because it is a component of the REDD, we'll do a quick review. These correction factors allow us to convert HL values to 2cc coupler SPL as discussed in our Supplemental Information Chapter at the end of this text. This correction factor isn't directly related to probe microphone measures, but it certainly relates to hearing aid selection and verification. Most clinics today have their audiometer calibrated by a local Special Instruments Dealer (SID) that is probably a member of NASED (National Association of Special Equipment Dealers). Today's audiometers nearly always can be calibrated within 0.3 to 0.5 dB of the ANSI standard values, so you should be able to assume that the values listed in ANSI S3.6-1996 are reliable RETSPLs for you to use (in this maze of acronyms, it is important to remember that audiometers have RETSPLs, people don't). In addition to REDD calculations, a common clinical application of RETSPLs is to convert LDL values to 2cc-coupler values when considering the appropriate maximum output of a hearing aid.

at 3000 Hz is around 9 dB, and the RETSPL for insert earphones is 3 dB (we'll assume that the audiometer is appropriately calibrated). So we would expect the average REDD at 3000 Hz for insert earphones to be around 12 dB (9 + 3 = 12). RETSPLs are somewhat different for insert versus supra-aural earphones, and the REDDs will then be slightly different also.

It is not too difficult to measure individual REDDs, but very few people do it. For one thing, it does require that your audiometer and probe equipment are located fairly close to each other. If you'd like to try it, see the step-by-step procedure outlined by Mueller (2001). If your equipment is not in close enough proximity, another easy way to obtain individualized REDDs is to measure the individual's RECD and add the RETSPL.

Clinical Applications of the REDD

- Primary: To convert HL hearing thresholds to ear canal SPL.
- Secondary: To convert HL LDLs to ear canal SPL.

If you're somewhat new to hearing aids, all these terms and correction factors can be a little confusing. When do you add what to what to get . . . whatever? Several years ago, Larry Revit put together a chart to simplify things, and called it the "circle of decibels" (Revit, 1997). We think it's still helpful today, and have included it here in Figure 17–14.

Now that we have reviewed all the specific probe microphone measures, it is time to talk in a bit more detail about how you can use this ear canal information in your everyday fitting of hearing aids. As we have said before, the use of this testing is limited only by your imagination, but to help you out a little, in the following section we provide examples of several uses for probe microphone testing in your daily practice.

Verification of Prescriptive Targets Using the REAR (including Speech Mapping)

We begin this section with the most common probe microphone measure conducted by audiologists—verification of prescriptive targets using speech mapping. We use the term verification, but this has the unstated implication that a fair amount of adjustment is also required before the final verification of our fit to prescriptive targets. It is very unlikely that the manufacturer's software-derived setting will be an acceptable match for even one input level, and certainly not all three (see Saunders, Stoody, Weber, & Mueller, 2015; and our discussion in Chapter 16). The process, of course, begins with selecting a validated fitting algorithm (e.g., NAL-

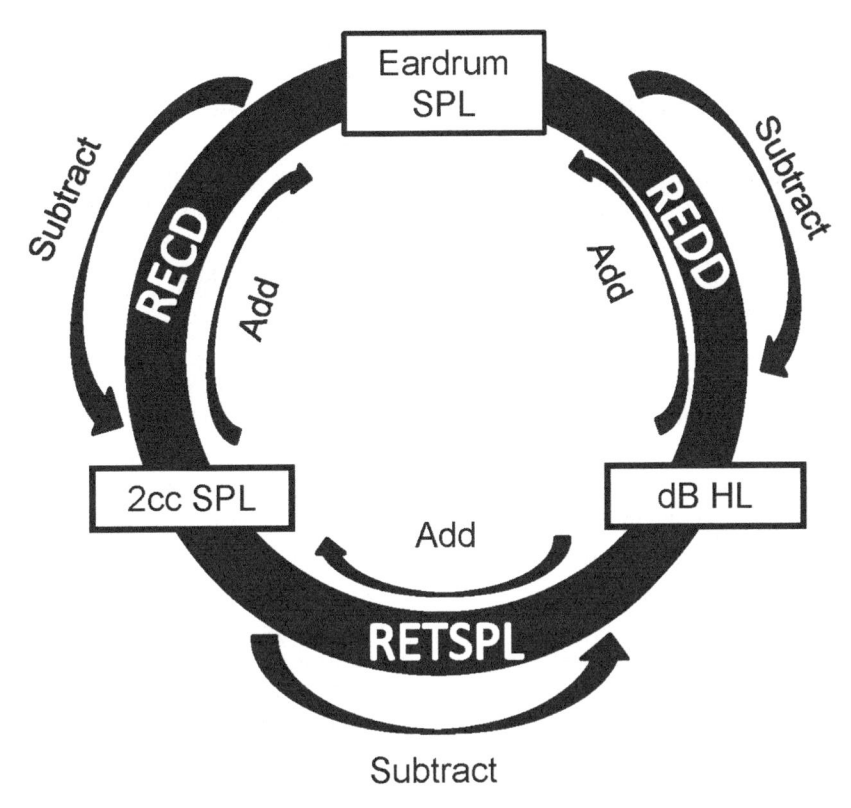

Figure 17–14. The circle of decibels showing the formulation of correction factors from dB hearing level (HL) 2cc-coupler and eardrum SPL measures. (Adapted from Revit, 1997.)

NL2 or DSL v5) and ensuring that these real-ear targets are available with your probe microphone equipment (which should not be a problem unless your equipment is quite dated). The task then becomes measurement-tweaking-measurement-tweaking until you obtain a close match to the desired output. We talked a lot about this procedure in the first part of this chapter and gave a general protocol when we introduced the REAR, so let's go directly to the application of the REAR to fitting and verification.

Test Protocol

- Enter patient's audiogram and measured LDLs. If conductive loss is present, enter bone conduction thresholds (conductive losses impact calculated targets). LDLs will affect targets for the DSL, not the NAL.
- Select your choice of validated prescriptive method in the probe microphone fitting software, and also select appropriate variables that could influence target calculation (e.g., adult versus child, gender, experience, transducer type, unilateral versus bilateral fitting—not all choices are available with all manufacturers or all fitting methods).
- Program hearing aid to desired fitting algorithm using manufacturer's software control process (again, select appropriate patient and fitting factors).
- Select appropriate speech or speech-like signal (e.g., shaped real speech, ISTS).
- If necessary, calibrate the probe tube (not all systems require this step).
- Position the patient appropriately.
- Position the probe tube at the correct depth in the ear canal.

- After muting, place the earmold and/or custom instrument in the ear with hearing aid programmed to desired starting point (e.g., manufacturer's implementation of a validated fitting method for the patient's hearing loss).
- If necessary, calibrate/level the loudspeaker using the reference microphone (not all systems require this step).
- Unmute the instrument and begin testing, using the first input level in your personal protocol (see discussion of test order earlier in this chapter). Adjust frequency-specific gain to achieve a reasonable match to target.
- Continue until a match is obtained for all three input levels. We suggest a final check of all levels to ensure that programming for one did not significantly influence another.

Sample Findings

Figure 17–15 is an illustration of REAR verification using the ISTS input at three levels: 55, 65, and 75 dB SPL. Although it might be interesting to see the entire amplitude range of the amplified signal (e.g., the banana) when plotting all three curves together, doing so becomes a bit too much information, so only the LTASS is shown here. This patient has a fairly typical hearing loss, although he or she does have a rather substantial drop at 4000 Hz (to 80 dB HL, which might not be obvious on this type of plot). We have done a pretty good job of matching targets. We are just a little shy of desired gain at 4000 Hz for soft, but the output for the other inputs, even at 4000 Hz, look good. At first glance, you might be questioning whether we have enough audibility at 4000 Hz—we address that in an associated Key Concept. Or you might also question whether frequency lowering should be activated above 3000 Hz. That is probably a patient-specific decision, but could be considered in this case. Notice that in the 1500 to 3000 Hz range, the LTASS output range is now about 10 dB for the inputs that differed by 20 dB (55–75 dB), suggesting a compression of the speech signal of about 2:1. We suspect that this hearing aid has a fairly short release time because otherwise you probably wouldn't see this degree of compression (e.g., even though the fitting software may say 2:1, effective compression may be only 1.3:1 or so for real speech for WDRC with slower release times). If you use the protocol of fitting to soft inputs first and if the compression has a slow release, it may not be possible to match the prescriptive targets for the 75 dB input, even with WDRC set to max (which usually is 3:1 or 4:1).

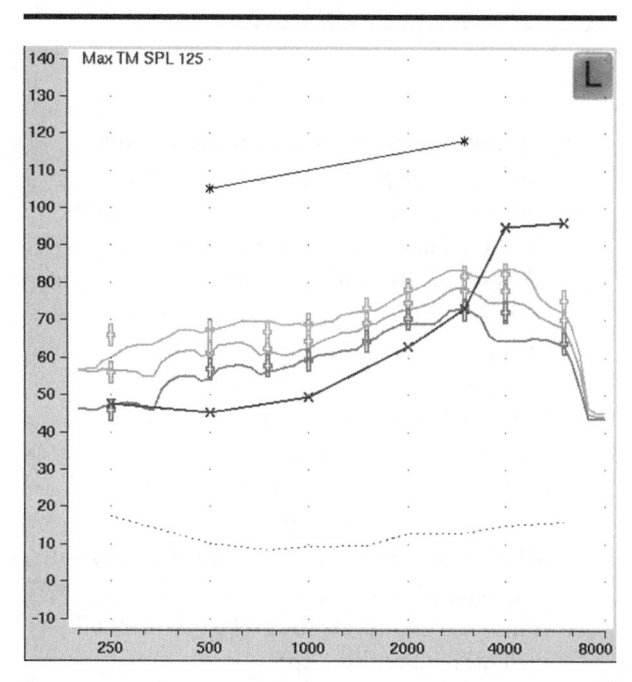

Figure 17–15. Example of REAR measures obtained with ISTS stimulus, shown for three input levels (55, 65, 75 dB inputs).

Fitting Tips

- We recommend conducting speech mapping with all special features activated. The exception to this is frequency lowering, which should be turned off unless the specific purpose is to measure the lowered signals (see the Frequency Lowering section later in this chapter).
- We mention in the preceding section that the fit to target can be influenced by the release times of the WDRC. We know that at least one manufacturer uses fast release times if you select NAL-NL2 in the fitting software, and long release times if you select its proprietary fitting. If your goal is to fit to the NAL-NL2 targets and you can get there from different

TECHNICAL TIP: WHAT IS THAT "MYSTERY DIP"?

When attempting to match the REAR to prescriptive target, there are times when you might see a notch in the response around 1000 to 1500 Hz of 5 dB or so, or even greater. It is there even when programmed gain is the same for the entire frequency region. It's sometimes difficult to fix. An example in is shown in Figure 17–16 from a recent patient. It is tempting to think that it's some kind of anti-resonance in the ear canal, which could be related to the location of the tip of the probe tube or the eartip itself. That is possible, but we know that, in at least some cases, the dip remains even when we have changed probe placement and eartips. Another possibility in an open fit is that there is approximately zero real-ear gain from the hearing aid and the amplified signal mixes with the direct signal coming in around the eartip, which might be out of phase, thus causing a cancellation. If this is it, the dip should go away when you either increase or decrease gain significantly in the region of the dip. If not, there is also some possibility that it is not a dip at all! How could that be? Look again at Figure 17–16 and let's assume we turn the hearing aid off and measure the REOR for the open fit. In some cases you will see you precisely match the REAR of all frequencies below the notch (in this case 1000 Hz). In this case what you are seeing as a dip is simply the effect of the REOR below 1000 Hz (sound entering the ear without gain) and the REAR above 1000 Hz (sound entering the ear with hearing aid gain applied). In other words, it is not really a dip at all, it is simply that the hearing aid is not providing gain—nothing needs to be fixed in this case. Our best guess, when the dip does not occur because of one of these explanations, it is related to the filters of the hearing aid and there is some type of interaction happening at the filter crossover frequency region. You might see that it occurs at slightly different regions for different manufacturers. It's annoying, but if it is not fixable by adding extra gain to this region, it is often narrow enough that it is not noticeable by the patient.

Figure 17–16. The REAR measured for a 65 and 75 dB SPL ISTS input. Note the "mystery dip" in the frequency response around 1000 Hz.

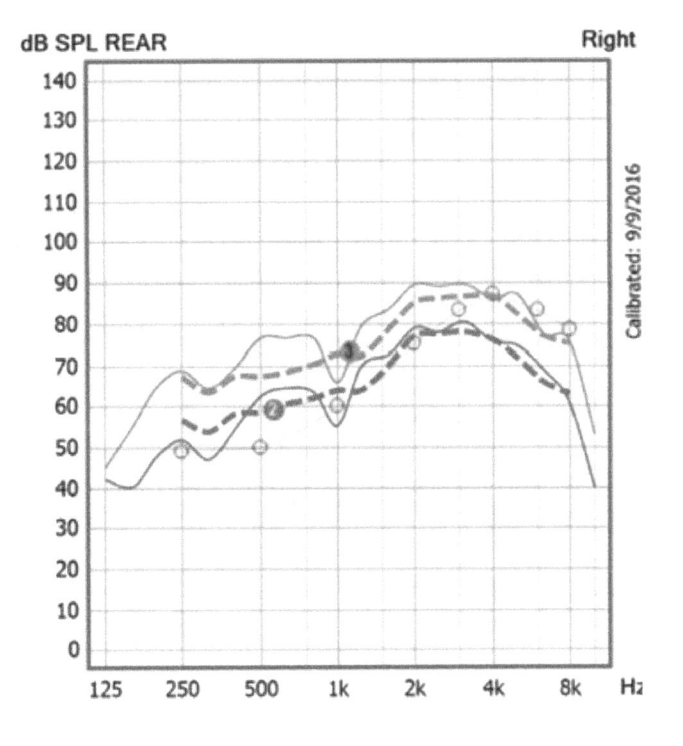

starting points, we advise starting off with the manufacturer's NAL algorithm rather than their proprietary default setting.

Verification of Prescriptive Targets Using Insertion Gain (REIG)

As we have discussed, even though the majority of audiologists (at least in the United States) use the REAR for verification, some audiologists still prefer to stick with an old friend: insertion gain. Because this is just a different approach to accomplish the same thing, much of what we have said about REAR verification also applies. As shown earlier in Figure 17–10, for a given hearing aid programmed to specific gain and output levels, you expect to see the same good or poor match to prescriptive targets with either approach. The exception is a patient with an unusual REUG. If in this case the measured REUG is used, rather than using the average REUG for calculation of the REIG, then the match to target will vary from the REAR match, roughly by the difference between average and measured REUG.

> ### KEY CONCEPT: HOW MUCH GAIN IS "ENOUGH GAIN" IN THE HIGH FREQUENCIES?
>
> We all agree that audibility is a good thing, but there are times when making things too audible can have a negative effect. We talked about this back in Chapter 16, but it's important enough to bring up again here. Observe that the patient in Figure 17–15 has a hearing loss that drops significantly at 4000 Hz (80 dB HL, about 95 dB in ear canal SPL). Also observe that the target for the LTASS for the NAL-NL2 fitting is below his threshold at the frequency, even for the 75 dB input signal. This bothers some audiologists, and they will be tempted to make speech in that area as audible as possible—maybe to the limits of the hearing aid if feedback is not an issue. As you can see by the targets, the developers of the NAL-NL2 obviously don't think this is a wise move, and we agree with them. Here are three reasons why:
>
> - First, it is important not only to consider the LTASS but also to view the entire range of amplified speech. Because the peaks of the speech signal fall about 12 to 15 dB above the LTASS, it may indeed be the case that some speech information is audible.
> - All patients have a preferred level of loudness. Adding more highs will add to that overall loudness level, and if the overall fitting was appropriate prior to adding the highs, speech will now be too loud. This result will prompt the patient to turn down overall gain, reducing audibility for the 1500 to 3000 Hz range, where audibility is more important than 4000 Hz. The key is to use the total signal loudness as effectively as possible by providing the greatest audibility for the most important speech frequencies.
> - There is a point, referred to as *effective audibility*, where increased audibility doesn't lead to an increased understanding of speech. The NAL-NL2 targets have attempted to account for this issue in the algorithm.
>
> The preceding points are particularly true for downward sloping configurations, but apply to some degree for all types of hearing loss. Our comments, however, are based on fittings for adults with acquired hearing loss—the fitting philosophy might be quite different for infants and children.

Test Protocol

- Enter patient's audiogram and measured LDLs. If conductive loss is present, enter bone conduction thresholds (conductive losses impact calculated targets). LDLs will impact targets for DSL, not the NAL.
- Select your choice of validated prescriptive method in the probe microphone fitting software, and also select appropriate variables that could influence target calculation (e.g., adult versus child, gender, experience, and unilateral versus bilateral fitting—not all choices are available with all manufacturers or all fitting methods).
- Program hearing aid to desired fitting algorithm using the manufacturer's software control process (again, select appropriate patient and fitting factors).
- Select appropriate speech or speech-like signal (e.g., shaped speech, ISTS). *Note*: Not all equipment will allow for automatic REIG calculation using speech signals. If you are forced to use a noise-type signal, check to see if it has amplitude modulations similar to speech (e.g., ICRA noise). If not, the signal might activate DNR if it is not disabled, which will give you an invalid REIG for speech.
- If necessary, calibrate the probe tube (not all systems require this step).
- Position the patient appropriately.
- Place the probe tube in the ear at an appropriate depth and conduct the REUR, or enter average REUR (our recommendation). *Note*: The input level for the REUR doesn't matter; it will be subsequently adjusted to correspond to the REAR levels selected.
- After muting, place the earmold and/or custom instrument in the ear with hearing aid programmed to desired starting point (e.g., manufacturer's implementation of a validated fitting method for the patient's hearing loss).
- If necessary, calibrate/level the loudspeaker using the reference microphone (not all systems require this step).
- Unmute the instrument and begin testing, using the first input level in your personal protocol (see discussion of test order earlier in this chapter). Adjust frequency-specific gain to achieve a reasonable match to target.
- Continue until a match is obtained for all three input levels. We suggest a final check of all levels to ensure that programming for one did not significantly influence another.

Sample Findings

Figure 17–17 shows the findings for REIG verification for a patient with a downward sloping hearing loss (same patient as shown for REAR verification in Figure 17–15), fitted to NAL-NL2. The REIGs are shown on the lower portion of the display, and above are the REARs for the three levels tested. Also shown is the *average* REUR, which was used for this calculation. This particular equipment displayed REIG targets only for 50, 65, and 80 dB SPL, so that is what was used for this testing.

Overall, we consider this a good fitting—a very nice match for both the 50 dB and 65 dB SPL inputs. It does appear that we could use about 8 to 10 dB more gain in the 3000 Hz region for the 80 dB SPL input. We are not too bothered by this, but if we were, the first

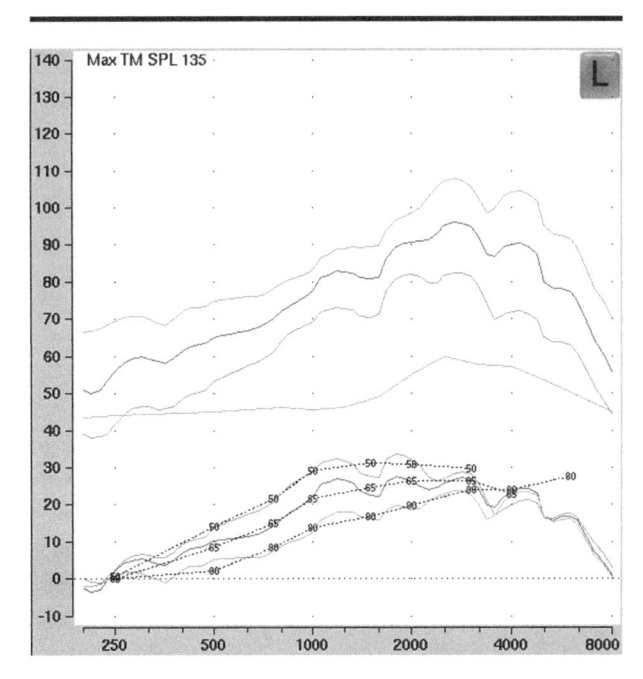

Figure 17–17. Example of REIG measures obtained with ISTS stimulus, shown for three input levels (50, 65, 80 dB inputs).

TECHNICAL TIP: USING REIGS TO CONSTRUCT AIDED AUDIOGRAM

Those of you in clinical practice know that every now and then you will be asked to provide an aided audiogram. In some cases, this is to facilitate counseling for parents and teachers. In other cases, it may be because of a government form left over from the 1950s, or constructed by someone who thinks that this is something that we routinely do. Given that research has shown that insertion gain is the same as functional gain, and functional gain does indeed provide an aided audiogram, it seems reasonably okay to us to use the REIG findings (for soft inputs) to construct an estimated aided audiogram. That is, you simply take the REIG findings and improve the earphone thresholds by that amount (e.g., if earphone thresholds are 60 dB at 2000 Hz and the REIG for soft inputs are 35 dB, then the predicted aided threshold will be 25 dB). Yes, there are some concerns with expansion and compression, but these same issues will exist when the patient uses the hearing aids in the real world. At least one manufacturer of probe microphone equipment has simplified this process for you—it automatically adjusts the earphone thresholds by the REIG and provides the data on a handy audiogram. Figure 17–18 shows an example of this for the right and left ears.

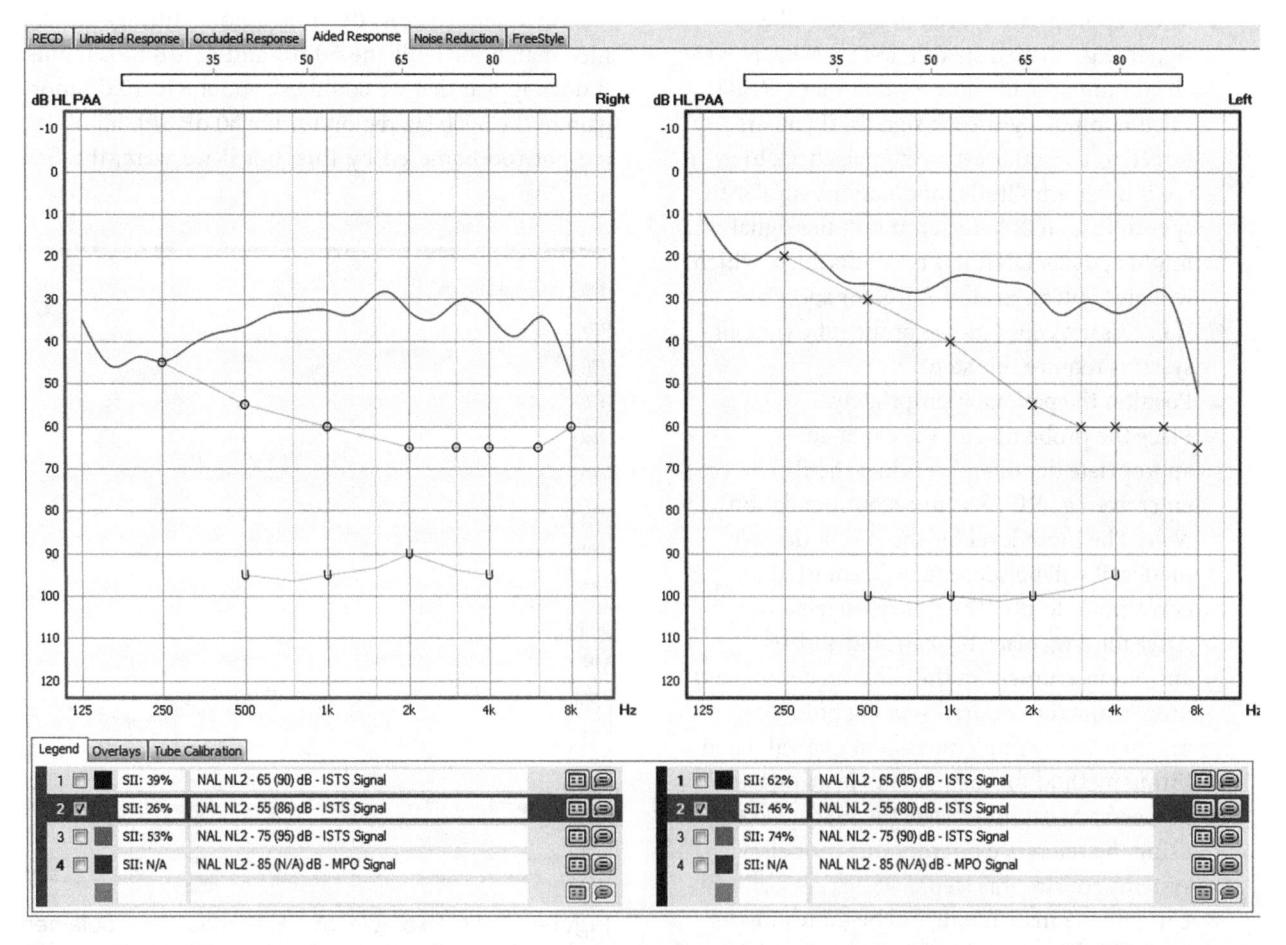

Figure 17–18. Example of one manufacturer's use of correcting the earphone thresholds using the REIG to obtain predicted aided thresholds on the same graphic, which can be used in counseling and in cases in which an aided audiogram is requested.

thing to check out is whether we've reached the MPO kneepoints, which would then be what is limiting gain. We wouldn't expect WDRC to create a gain pattern like this, and we know from our 50 dB SPL input findings that adequate gain has been programmed, so a low MPO setting is likely the case. Raising the MPO in this frequency range might allow us to obtain the desired gain. But the MPO is where it is because we set it there based on the patient's LDLs. So we need to make sure we don't create a new problem while trying to solve this one, which is why we'd probably just accept this fitting. If you're wondering why targets are not present for 4000 Hz, it is because the NAL-NL1 (changed in NAL-NL2) imposes a rule that once the hearing loss reaches a certain level (80 dB in this example) for some configurations, targets are not calculated.

Fitting Tips

- The targets provided in Figure 17–17 are unique to this equipment, which is why we used the 50-65-80 dB SPL inputs. Although these inputs are fine, we typically use the same 55-65-75 dB SPL inputs for REIG calculation as we do for speech mapping for reasons we discussed earlier.
- The display shown here illustrates one of the things we don't like about using the REIG for verification. Observe that, at 3000 Hz, we have about 25 dB of gain for soft inputs. But did we make soft sounds audible? How do we know?

Open Ear Canal Fittings

Open fittings are very common, with some clinics fitting more than 50% of their patients with this earmold configuration. For the most part, probe microphone verification is the same whether the fitting is open or closed, but there is one significant difference: the on-ear calibration process for the input signal. As we discuss in Chapter 16, there is a reference microphone at the ear for all probe systems. Traditionally, we've used a concurrent modified-pressure method of equalization: The reference microphone continually monitors the input signal during presentation. With open fittings, however, there can be issues using this approach. Amplified sound leaking out of the ear canal can lead to erroneous measurements at the reference position, which will then lead to an erroneous signal from the loudspeaker and a subsequent mistake in the observed real-ear output (less output than actually present). For this reason, we use a stored modified-pressure equalization approach when we assess open fittings (see Chapter 16 for a complete explanation).

If we fail to switch to the stored equalization mode and conduct testing using the concurrent equalization method, several factors will impact the degree of the measurement error:

- Gain/output of hearing aid. The greater the gain, the greater the mistake.
- Feedback reduction algorithm. The better the feedback reduction system, the greater the potential size of the mistake, as you are able to keep increasing gain without feedback.
- Location of reference microphone. The closer the reference microphone is to the ear canal opening, the more likely we are to have a measurement error.
- Openness of the fit. The more open the fitting, the more sound leaks out, and the more likely we are to have a measurement error.
- Residual ear canal resonance of the patient. The measurement error usually occurs at the point of ear canal resonance; the mistake will be greater if the patient has a large resonance and the ear is left mostly open.

Test Protocol

- Change equalization method from modified pressure to stored equalization (*Note:* On most systems, this simply requires selecting "open" or a similar descriptor of the hearing aid style.)
- Enter patient's audiogram and measured LDLs. If conductive loss is present, enter bone conduction thresholds (conductive losses impact calculated targets). LDLs will affect targets for DSL, not NAL.
- Select your choice of validated prescriptive method in probe microphone fitting software and also select appropriate variables that could

influence target calculation (e.g., adult versus child, gender, experience, and unilateral versus bilateral fitting—not all choices are available with all manufacturers or all fitting methods).
- Program hearing aid to desired fitting algorithm using manufacturer's software control process (again, select appropriate patient and fitting factors).
- Place the probe tube in the ear at an appropriate depth, mute the hearing aid, and fit it to the patient's ear.
- Conduct stored-equalization, free-field calibration, then unmute the hearing aid. (*Note:* Probe microphone system manufacturers refer to this process using several different terms, including open calibration, equalization, and leveling.) Some manufacturers do not require this step to be completed before measurement, however, it should always be completed to ensure an accurate REAR.
- From this point forward, all speech mapping testing is the same as for the traditional modified-pressure approach, *except* the patient must keep his or her head in the calibration position and cannot move it during test signal presentation.
- If the patient moves, it is important to mute the hearing aid, repeat the equalization procedure, unmute the hearing aid, and continue. Failure to complete this step can lead to fitting errors as great as 10 dB or more.

Sample Findings

To illustrate the potential mistake that can be made in real-ear output, we conducted speech mapping for an open fitting using both types of equalization. In Figure 17–19A, observe the bottom LTASS output curve tracing, which is a close match to NAL-NL2 targets, although it falls slightly below in the 3000 Hz region. This output was recorded using the concurrent equalization approach. The LTASS that is slightly higher at 3000 Hz was recorded using stored equalization—this is the correct output. In this case, you would think you were about 3 to 4 dB below target at 3000 Hz, when in fact you're 3 to

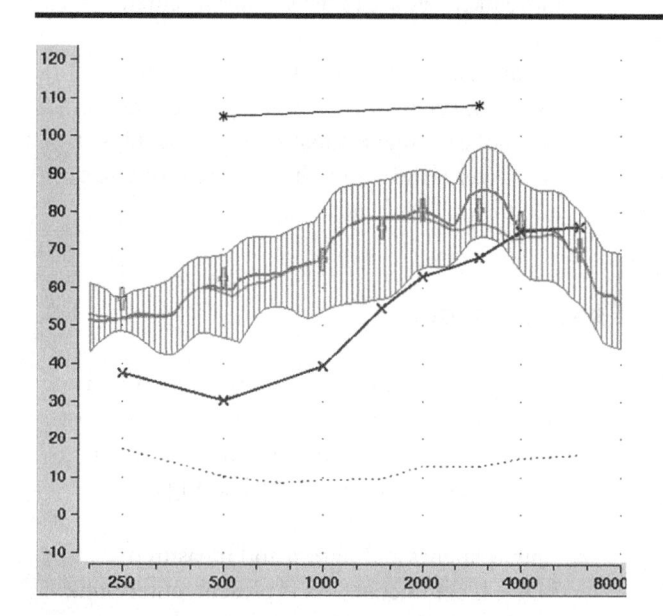

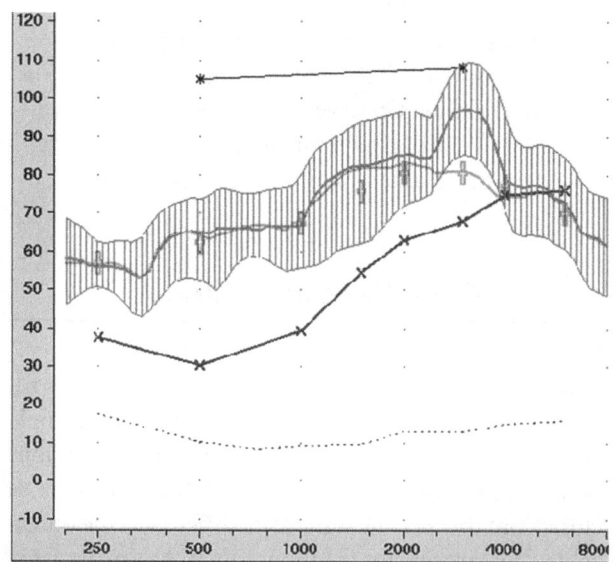

Figure 17–19. Repeat testing for an open fitting for the same patient using both modified pressure and stored equalization at-ear calibration procedures. **A.** Note that the output for the two measurement procedures is essentially the same except for a 5 dB or so increase around 3000 Hz for stored equalization (this is the true ear canal output). **B.** Gain has now been increased in the 3000 Hz region, and the output for the stored equalization is now nearly 20 dB greater (this is the true output) than what was obtained using the modified-pressure approach.

4 dB *above* target at this frequency. Not a huge problem, but significant nonetheless—a net difference of 6 to 8 dB.

Let's assume, however, that the audiologist doing this fitting failed to use the stored equalization approach, and wasn't happy with falling 3 to 4 dB below target at 3000 Hz, so the audiologist raises gain at this frequency until the target is reached. After this change we repeat our testing using the concurrent equalization approach—see the bottom LTASS output curve in Figure 17–19B. Observe that, indeed, there is now a perfect match to target at 3000 Hz. But what *real output* is being delivered to the ear? That is shown in the upper LTASS, obtained using the stored equalization procedure. What had been a measurement mistake of around 6 dB is now nearly a 20 dB error. Why? Because as the audiologist turned up gain, leakage increased (essentially at a 1:1 rate), and the fitting error increased accordingly. Imagine that an audiologist is using the wrong equalization process in a real fitting (and it *does* happen), the patient is saying, "That is really harsh sounding," and the audiologist is thinking, "I'm right at targets; I don't understand why this patient has a problem with that."

Fitting Tips

- Probe microphone manufacturers have made it very easy to access the stored equalization mode. There may be a software setting for "open" or something similar.
- Remember, when using the stored equalization approach, the patient must keep his or her head in the same position as when the equalization is conducted, and not move it during the testing (usually not a problem with adults).
- The measurement error is usually present only when the fitting is considerably open and gain is at least 18 to 20 dB or so, but given the simplicity of using stored equalization, we see no reason not to simply use it routinely whenever an open or even partially open fitting is assessed. In fact, there is also no harm in using it with closed fittings as long as the patient's head and body movements aren't an issue.

POINTS TO PONDER: ONE LIMITATION OF REAR FOR OPEN FITTINGS

As we have indicated a few times, we prefer to use REAR over REIG verification procedures for a number of good reasons. Sometimes a REAR limitation is related to not having an obvious picture of hearing aid gain. When completing an open fitting, we sometimes see a good match to targets at 500 Hz and below, and at 2000 Hz and above, but no matter how much we increase mid-frequency gain, we just can't reach targets (Figure 17–20A). Sometimes, this problem is evident as a relatively narrow notch around 1500 Hz, which results from a phase cancellation interaction between the amplified and direct signal pathways. This notch artifact is not easily remedied but is often narrow enough that it does not affect sound quality (see Mueller and Ricketts, 2006). A different problem is represented in Figure 17–20A, where we can visualize an under-fitting over a relatively wide range of middle frequencies. Given that this is an open fitting and that more amplification is needed in the low frequencies to overcome gain lost to venting, it may seem strange that we're having trouble with the middle (not low) frequency gain—that is, until we consider REIG instead (Figure 17–20B). In this figure, we can easily visualize that the hearing aid just isn't capable of much gain below 2000 Hz. The patient had normal-hearing thresholds at 500 Hz and lower, however, so we were able to match REAR targets because no gain was required (i.e., what we are observing is the delivered speech input passing directly to the tip of the probe tube). Knowing that more amplification was generally needed may lead to the use of a more powerful receiver. Although we would eventually come to this conclusion clinically without the REIG, it's an example of how not having a simple picture of gain can lead to a misinterpretation. Of course, we can glean this same information from the REAR if we also measure the REUR on the same screen.

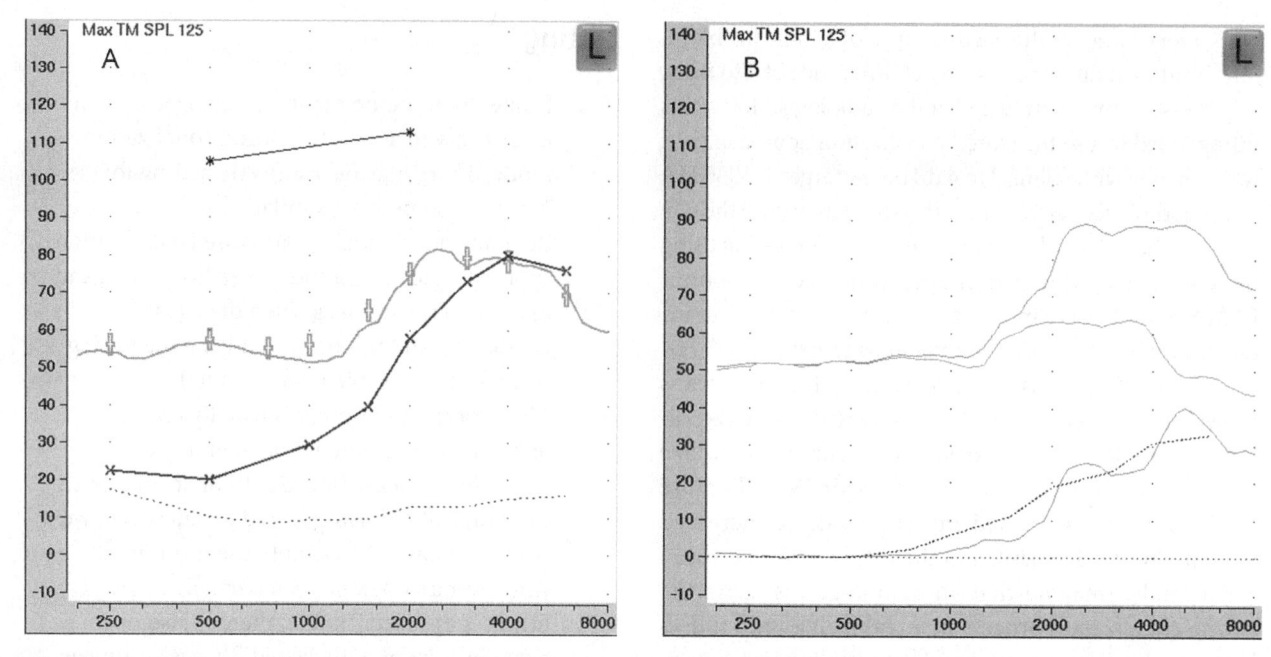

Figure 17–20. A. Example of good match to targets at 500 Hz and below and at 2000 Hz and above with REAR. **B.** When we consider REIG instead, it is clear the hearing aid wasn't capable of much gain below 2000 Hz.

Verification of MPO

As we discuss earlier in this chapter, getting the maximum output right is an important aspect of fitting hearing aids. You certainly don't want the output too high, but you don't want it too low either, as that reduces headroom, and possibly decreases the quality of speech and, especially, music. Verification to ensure that the aided output is correct is a three-pronged process: aided loudness ratings using speech material, aided loudness measures using obnoxious noises, and real-ear measures of the hearing aid's MPO—the topic of focus here. As you saw earlier in the chapter, the new probe microphone standard refers to this as REAR85 or REAR90; previously it was referred to as the real-ear saturation response (or RESR, although not in the standard). For simplicity, we simply use the REAR85 for our discussion and sample findings here.

Some audiologists have expressed concern that driving the hearing aid to an output this high is risky business because of the potential for loudness discomfort, acoustic trauma, or even inducing tinnitus. We do not consider this procedure to be a significant risk for the following reasons:

- You already have the hearing aid programmed to a level below the patient's LDL, so discomfort caused by loudness will not be an issue (this assumes you conducted frequency-specific LDLs and adjusted to MPO accordingly).
- The signal is very brief.
- The hearing aid likely will be driven to this level in the real world so, if a problem exists, it is best to fix it now.
- The level will be no louder than what the patient will experience when feedback occurs.

Test Protocol

- This procedure is completed using the REAR approach described earlier in this chapter. It is completed on the individual patient after verification of a validated prescriptive method.

- Adjust the overall gain of the instrument to just below feedback or to max user gain if no feedback is present. If the patient does not have control of gain with either a VC or remote device, conduct testing at the programmed use gain.
- Even if you use REIG for verification, go to the REAR screen. The measured LDLs should be displayed and referenced to ear canal SPL.
- Provide the patient with the Cox loudness anchors chart (see Chapter 5).
- Deliver a frequency-swept tone at 85 dB SPL; observe the output relative to LDL targets, and have the patient rate the signal on the loudness chart (the objective and subjective findings should agree).
- If the output is either too high or too low, make appropriate changes and retest until REAR85 output falls to desired levels. (*Note*: The patient can also note exact frequency ranges where fine-tuning of the response may be required.)

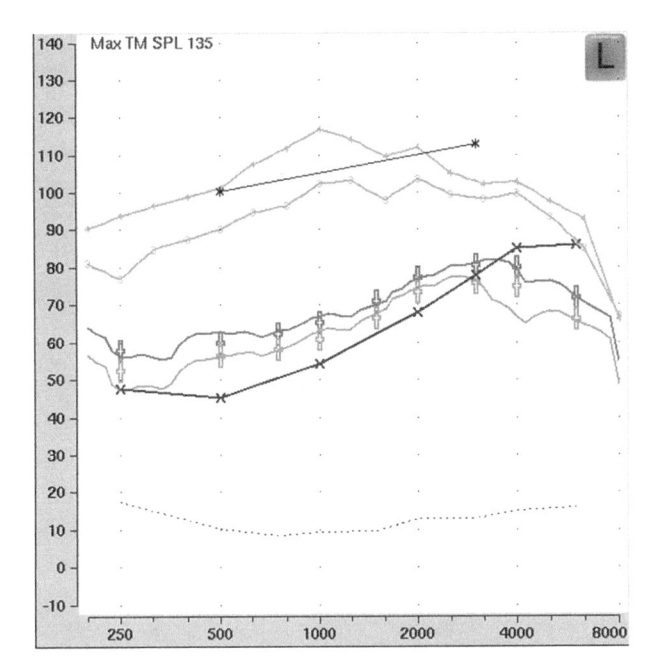

Figure 17–21. Example of maximum output set too high. The measured LDLs are represented by the horizontal line going from 100 dB at 500 Hz to 110 dB at 3000 Hz. The top curve was the initial REAR85 measure. After adjustment, the maximum output falls below the LDLs.

Sample Findings

Figure 17–21 shows the test results for the REAR85. The measured LDLs are represented by the horizontal line going from 100 dB at 500 Hz to 110 dB at 3000 Hz. In this instance, the audiologist did not go into the software and set the MPO kneepoints to correspond with the LDLs but used the manufacturer's default settings instead. The initial REAR85 measure is shown in the top curve, which peaks around 1000 Hz. It exceeds the patient's LDL by 10 dB. To no surprise, the patient also rated this as uncomfortably loud (some patients will actually point to screen to show where it was uncomfortably loud—it was quite obvious in this case). The lower REAR85 curve shows the final setting that was achieved after some adjustments of the MPO (lowering AGCo kneepoints in the corresponding channels). Note the advantage of multichannel AGCo, as we were able to lower the mid-frequencies by almost 20 dB, while only changing the MPO by 5 to 10 dB for other frequencies. In the not-too-distant past, with a single channel AGCo, we had to lower all frequencies by the same amount just to achieve the desired outcome where the peak existed.

Figure 17–22 provides an example in which the REAR85 is too low (at least by our standards). Note that the MPO of this instrument is limiting the output at a point that is 10 dB or more below the patient LDLs (except at the very high frequencies). What you can't tell from this chart is that we already raised the MPO setting by 5 dB and the REAR85 didn't change. What does this tell us? That output is being limited by the WDRC, and this is why we also included the speech map results for the 75 dB SPL input for you to view. Observe that we are pretty much on target for loud speech. So, if we make the WDRC less aggressive to raise the MPO and increase headroom, we will have too much gain for 75 dB SPL (unless the hearing aid had a second or third AGCi kneepoint at 75 dB SPL, which it does not). The solution? We would probably try a compromise and involve the patient in helping us decide whether loud speech is becoming too loud as we increase the MPO by making the WDRC less aggressive. A point to remember: Do not assume that the MPO setting in the software is necessarily controlling the MPO.

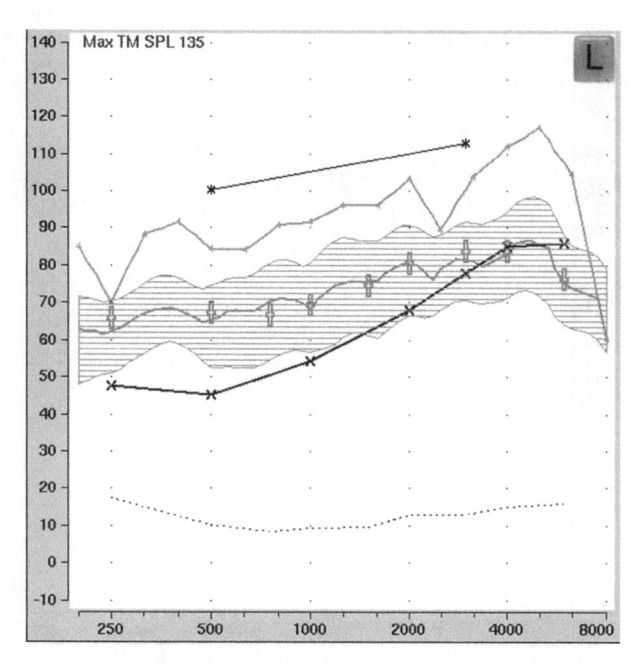

Figure 17–22. Example of maximum output set too low. The measured LDLs are represented by the horizontal line going from 100 dB at 500 Hz to 110 dB at 3000 Hz. The maximum output curve falls below the LDLs. The 30th to 99th percentiles of the amplified speech signal (ISTS) for a 75 dB input is shown below the MPO output.

Fitting Tips

- It is useful to explain to the patient why we are conducting this test: We want to create a loudness situation that is as bad as you will ever encounter in the real world, so if there is a problem, we can fix it now.
- Even after appropriate instructions, what sometimes happens is that when the first REAR85 run is conducted, even when the output falls below the patient's LDLs, the patient will indicate that the signal was uncomfortably loud on the loudness chart. We suggest repeating the testing once or maybe even twice to see if this is a constant rating before you start changing the MPO. Sometimes the initial run startles the patient a bit, and he or she reacts to this sound, rather than process whether the output is truly uncomfortable.
- It is tempting to think that, when fitting a relatively mild gain mini-BTE instrument with an open fitting, MPO issues will never be a problem. This is not true, however, as it is very possible that with some hearing aids the MPO will be higher with an open fitting than with a closed fitting (Mueller, 2014a). This is because the open-ear resonance (REUG) often is maintained, which boosts the ear canal hearing aid output by that amount (with a closed mold this resonance is no longer a factor).
- Another concern with open fittings, the ones that are truly open, is that the maximum output that you see on the fitting screen might not represent the MPO of the hearing aid but rather the signal going directly to the TM. This can be even more of a problem for higher level test signals (e.g., REAR90). We know of audiologists who have worked diligently to lower the MPO in the software only to discover later that no hearing aid adjustment changed the output. If a person has a large REUG—note from Figure 17–2 that a 20 dB peak is not that uncommon—then an ear canal SPL of 105 dB or so certainly is possible, which could exceed the person's LDLs if they were somewhat lower than average.
- We have often recommended conducting an obnoxious noise test as part of the MPO verification. We find it helpful to conduct ear canal SPL measures while we're doing this testing because it helps to determine if there is a peak and what channel of MPO might need to be reduced. This real-ear testing is conducted in the live speech or spectral analysis mode of probe microphone systems (see Figure 17–23 for an example). This is the output for rattling marbles in a glass jar, indeed an obnoxious noise, written about by Robyn Cox (2009). In this case, the noise was rated as uncomfortably loud by the patient, so we will lower the MPO. By observing the real-ear output, we clearly see that the peak is around 2000 Hz, and we'll lower the MPO for this region. If these data were not available, we would have to guess about what MPO channel was causing the problem or perhaps unnecessarily lower MPO across all frequencies. Granted, the patient may never

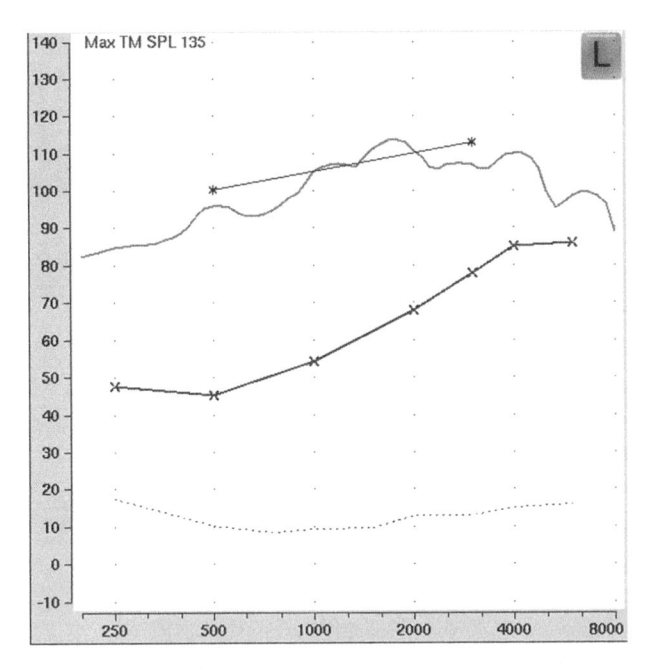

Figure 17–23. Example of REAR obtained by shaking a jar full of marbles. Note that the output of the hearing aid exceeds the LDL values in the mid-frequencies.

hear rattling marbles in a glass jar again, but there are other intense environmental sounds that can create the same real-ear aided output.

Directional Microphone Technology

Many different special features can and should be assessed with probe microphone measures, and directional microphone technology is among the most commonly examined ones. As we reviewed previously, several 2cc-coupler test box systems allow for the measurement of directionality, so you might ask, "Why do the testing in the real ear rather than the coupler?" A reasonable question. First, it isn't really an either/or thing. We recommend conducting the coupler measures when the hearing aid arrives for quality control purposes, as explained in Chapter 13. But even if the hearing aid passes this testing, as most will, there are still several reasons to also consider testing in the real ear:

- The selection of the directional setting may influence gain (e.g., output, particularly in the low frequencies, might not be the same for directional compared to omnidirectional).
- The positioning of the hearing aid on the ear will influence directivity.
- The tightness of the fitting (magnitude of venting) will influence directivity, particularly in the lower frequencies.
- The process of doing the testing and having the patient present to view the results provides an opportunity to counsel the patient about the use and potential benefit of directional technology.

When this testing is conducted, it is important to remember that the purpose is to determine whether the hearing aid is functioning appropriately and to help with counseling, not to compare one product to another. Different products have different polar patterns, and real-ear measures from a single specific azimuth do not reliably predict the overall directional effectiveness when a typical diffuse noise is present (e.g., Ricketts, 2000). As we describe in Chapters 13 and detail later in this section, compression can also affect the clinically measured directivity, but not actually affecting the patient's directional benefit.

Here is how you might use directional probe microphone measures clinically. Let's say that you usually fit one of two models of directional instruments, either a Sonotone or a Radioear. After testing four or five different models of the Sonotone, which default to a cardioid directional pattern, you find that the typical real-ear front-to-back difference (REAR at 180° subtracted from the REAR at 0°) for the 1000 to 4000 Hz range is around 12 dB with typical compression settings. The Radioear defaults to a supercardioid pattern, and the typical front-to-back difference for this product is 6 dB with typical compression settings. This gives you some clinical norms to work with. Now, if you're testing a patient with his or her new directional Sonotones and you see only a 5 dB front-to-back difference, you know something is wrong.

Test Protocol

- This procedure is completed by following the verification of prescriptive targets using either the REAR or REIG approach.

- Program the hearing aid to the "fixed directional" setting.
- Disable digital noise reduction if you want to use a noise test signal. (*Note*: If the attack time on the DNR is slow enough, you might be able to use noise and take the measure quickly before DNR begins to reduce gain.)
- With the patient sitting in the usual test position (0° degree horizontal and vertical azimuth), conduct REAR measure using

> **KEY CONCEPT: COMPRESSION AND DIRECTIONALITY MEASURES**
>
> When conducting probe microphone measures with directional technology, it is quite probable that the input levels will exceed the kneepoint of the instrument's multichannel WDRC. Because of this, the directional effect assessed in the clinic will be less than that observed by the patient in the real world. The reason for this was explained by Mueller (2001), and we will summarize it here. We all know that when WDRC is employed greater gain is applied as the signal becomes softer. So consider this example: Your patient's WDRC hearing aid (2:1 compression ratio) is programmed to apply 20 dB of gain for a 70 dB input. The patient is in a room where there is a 70 dB input originating from in front of him or her (the other person speaking), and there is also 70 dB originating from behind the patient (party noise). With an omnidirectional setting, in theory, the amplified SNR will be 0 dB. But you wisely fit the patient with a directional instrument, and we'll say that it reduces the input from the back by 12 dB. You might think that the front-to-back ratio (FBR) will be +12 dB (70 + 20 = 90; 58 + 20 = 78; 90 − 78 = 12 dB); this would be true for linear processing. Remember, however, that as the input goes down, gain goes up for a WDRC instrument. Therefore, with a 2:1 compression ratio, the 58 dB input will receive 6 dB more gain than the original 70 dB input; hence, the gain will be 26 dB, not 20 dB. In other words, the WDRC is adding back in one-half of the gain that the directional microphone so diligently took away, and the measured FBR will be only 6 dB. This doesn't sound like a good thing.
>
> This effect, however, is present only when the different test signals from different azimuths occur in isolation with no other sounds present—an unlikely event in the real world and a situation in which directional amplification isn't needed. In all real-world situations of interest, the signals from the front and back are occurring at the same time; therefore, the same hearing aid gain is applied to both after directional processing. Based on this reality, it is perhaps not surprising that Ricketts, Lindley, and Henry (2001) clearly showed that, for real-world use, directionally processing coupled with WDRC will be just as effective as when it is used with a linear fitting.
>
> As we describe in Chapter 13, it is possible to obtain a fairly accurate estimate of true FBR in the test box using a method that produces and analyzes two signals simultaneously from the front and back location. A speech signal can also be introduced during testing so that DNR processing doesn't also affect the results. This type of testing is also available with some probe systems for real-ear evaluation. When this method is used, the FBR is the same for both the WDRC and linear settings of the hearing aid. The bottom line of this Key Concept is that the probe microphone assessment of directionality isn't to predict the degree of directionality in the real world but to determine whether the instrument is working as expected and to help with counseling patients.

standard real speech (e.g., ISTS), a shaped speech signal, or a speech-shaped noise at an input of 75 dB SPL.
- Swing the patient around 180 degrees (carefully; preferably he or she is in a swivel chair) and conduct a second REAR at the same input level from the back.
- By comparing these two outputs on the fitting screen, you will have a good estimate of the directional function—that is, are the results about what you would expect for that instrument?

Rather than eyeball the differences in the REAR curves, you might want to have the probe microphone equipment plot the frequency-specific front-to-back difference. If so, then try out the following test protocol:

- Program the hearing aid to the "fixed directional" setting.
- Set your probe microphone equipment for REIG calculations. We hope you can do these measures using real speech. If not, disable DNR in the hearing aid if you want to use a noise test signal. (*Note:* If the attack time on the DNR is slow enough, you might be able to use noise and take the measure quickly before DNR begins to reduce gain.)
- Turn your patient around 180 degrees so that you conduct the first measure with the loudspeaker of the probe system located behind the patient using a 75 dB input signal. Tell your probe system that this run is the REUR.
- Turn the patient back so that he or she is in the normal test position and conduct a second measure. Tell your probe system that this run is the REAR.
- Because the probe system thinks you are doing an REIG, it will automatically subtract the first run from the second. What is then presented on the monitor is the frequency-specific front-to-back ratio (FBR) of the directional hearing aid.

Sample Findings

Figure 17–24 shows front-to-back directional testing for a mini-BTE RIC product. Figure 17–24A is for a standard eartip (moderate tightness), and Figure 17–24B is for a more open fitting; the hearing aid is programmed the same for both measures. First, we consider this a product with good directivity, and it likely is programmed with very little compression. With the partially closed eartip (A), note that we have a front-to-back difference of 25 dB or so for much of the

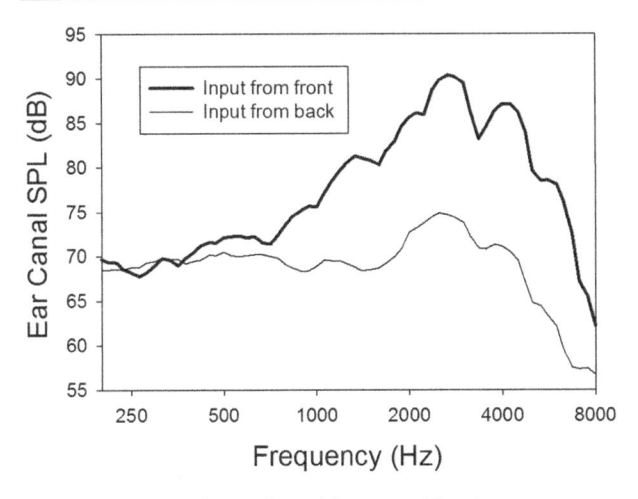

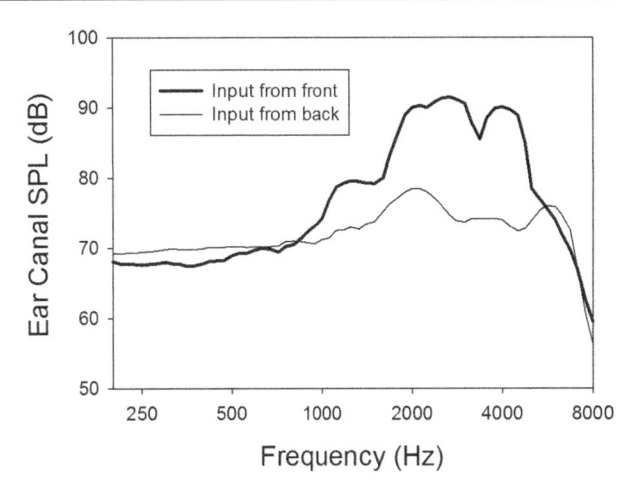

Figure 17–24. Examples of front and back curves measured for mini-BTE product. **A.** Results for a standard eartip (moderate tightness). **B.** Results for a more open fitting. The hearing aid is programmed the same for both measures.

frequency range. Directivity begins to disappear around 500 Hz because we have leakage from the eartip, and we do not have much gain programmed for this lower frequency range. Notice that, when we move to an open fitting (B), directivity for the higher frequencies stays about the same, but from around 1500 Hz and moving downward, directivity is reduced because of increased leakage from the open fitting and the direct path of the input signal to the tympanic membrane.

Results are not always as impressive as shown in Figure 17–24. We conducted the same testing for a mini-BTE RIC, fitted with an open eartip, from a different manufacturer. Those findings are shown in Figure 17–25. Except for a 10 dB effect around 4000 Hz, this product is functioning like an omnidirectional product, although set to "directional." The difference between this hearing aid and its mini-BTE competitor shown in Figure 17–24B is quite significant, certainly significant enough to be noticed by a patient in some listening environments—an obvious reason why this type of testing is important.

Fitting Tips

- The primary cause of poor directional function is dirt and debris in the inlet ports of the microphones. Therefore, it is as important to evaluate directional processing on repeat visits as on the day of the fitting. It is necessary, however, also to have a measurement on the day of fitting or during the initial electroacoustic evaluation to provide a baseline.
- It is very common to fit mini-BTEs that are designed to be cosmetically appealing and to fit comfortably behind the ear. Those two factors may work in opposition to good directional processing. When doing real-ear directional testing with these instruments, you will find that the directionality can vary significantly relative to how they are positioned on the ear. It is hard to say how you should base your final decision, but we can say that the best directionality often will not be the position that is the most comfortable or the prettiest. Because we certainly can't have a hearing aid that is uncomfortable, this matter may turn into a counseling issue regarding the limitations of benefit.
- We recommend conducting your probe microphone assessment of directionality with the hearing aid programmed to "fixed directional." If you are curious (and who isn't, really), however, you can easily determine the trigger for directionality for a given product by setting directional processing to "automatic," and then testing at input levels of increasing intensity starting at 50 to 55 dB or so. When you first see a separation between the 0-degree and 180-degree signals, you know you've exceeded the activation point.
- Related to the preceding Fitting Tip, when you have directionality set to "automatic directional," it is then controlled by the signal classification system. The hearing aid will not switch to directional unless certain parameters are met, which include an intensity of a certain level (variable among manufacturers, but probably around 60 to 70 dB SPL) and detection of some type of background noise. Hence, whenever conducting directional testing with the instrument in the automatic setting, be sure that you are using a fairly intense input (70 dB SPL or so should work)

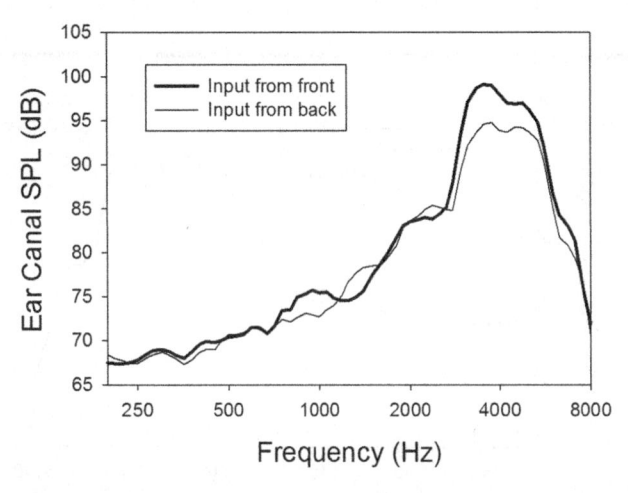

Figure 17–25. Examples of front and back curves measured for mini-BTE product with an open eartip. Except for the separation in tracings at 4000 Hz, the hearing aid, in the directional setting, is functioning as an omnidirectional instrument.

and a signal that *will not* be classified as speech in quiet.
- Because you will be using a nonspeech signal, it is probable that noise reduction will be activated. Hence, unless your goal is to observe the combined effects of directionality and noise reduction, we suggest that you disable noise reduction when the directional effects are assessed.

Digital Noise Reduction

As we discuss in Chapter 11, most of today's hearing aids have two or more different types of noise reduction, working simultaneously and independently in each channel. The most common of these is modulation-based, which reduces gain in a channel when the dominant signal is identified as steady-state noise. Other types include fast-acting spectral subtraction or *Wiener filtering*, designed to clean the signal by subtracting noise in gaps between words or syllables. As with modulation-based noise reduction, this filtering method also reduces steady-state noise in the absence of speech (ambient room noise, for example). In addition, some hearing aids also have a fast-acting, impulse noise reduction algorithm that reduces the amplitude peaks of impulse noises (e.g., the clinking of dishes in a busy restaurant). Whereas the latter two are very fast-acting, modulation-based noise reduction may have a relatively slow onset and/or offset (even up to several seconds), which does vary among manufacturers. Manufacturers' software typically allows for changing the magnitude of the noise reduction for a given patient (e.g., min to medium to max), although, among different manufacturers and among different products from the same manufacturer, the range from min to max may vary from as low as 5 to 6 dB to as much as 12 to 20+ dB.

In the previous section, we talked about how, with directional technology, the positioning on the ear can have a very significant effect, and the processing easily can be affected by other issues regarding the sound reaching the two microphones (e.g., dirt and debris in microphone inlet ports). These are not concerns with DNR. If you know how a given manufacturer's product XYZ worked for Mary, you can pretty much be assured it will work the same way for Bob—except that the tightness of the fitting will have an effect (see the following sample findings). If you are unfamiliar with a product, it is helpful to evaluate the DNR at least once to better understand the workings, but is it really worthwhile to conduct real-ear DNR measures with all patients? Maybe not, but there are a couple of reasons why you might want to consider it with some patients:

- As we mentioned, the tightness of the fitting will affect DNR significantly in the low frequencies to the extent that there may be no effect at all. This will help determine situations when increasing DNR will not solve a patient's complaint about a given noise.
- Ever had a patient ask why hearing aids are so expensive? Conducting this testing with the patient watching the screen can be quite impressive and leads to many counseling opportunities. Moreover, both you and the patient will be able to observe the time constants of the effect firsthand.
- For some manufacturers, the amount of gain reduction for noise inputs increases with increasing signal levels. In such cases, a demonstration of this effect to a patient can help manage expectations relative to function in his or her everyday environments.

Test Protocol

- This procedure is completed after the verification of prescriptive targets using either the REAR or REIG approach has been completed.
- Although for most testing we want to use real speech, in this case, select a signal that is truly noise. This could be speech noise, white or pink noise, or different noises that might be available on your probe microphone equipment for this purpose (e.g., air conditioner, bus, vacuum cleaner).
- Conduct a REAR with the DNR turned off using a 75 dB input to establish a baseline.
- Program hearing aid to the DNR planned for the patient's everyday use and conduct REAR—leave noise on for 10 seconds or so to ensure maximum reduction has occurred.

(*Note*: For a few models, maximum reduction may take up to 20 to 30 seconds!) Observe difference from baseline REAR and note time required to reach maximum reduction. (*Note*: Rather than requiring a baseline, some systems require only a single measure that compares the level very soon after the presentation begins to the level after the signal has been presented for a period of time.)
- Check DNR effects for different programs if DNR is programmed differently, or check the effect of different settings of DNR for future reference.

Sample Findings

Shown in Figure 17–26 are the effects of DNR set to four different strengths. Observe that the change in REAR shows a change in output across all frequencies above 500 Hz. Figure 17–27 illustrates the DNR effects for an individual using a hearing aid with an open fitting. Note that the effects in the high frequencies are rather large—about 15 dB when set to maximum. But, because the ear canal is open and little gain is present, the low-frequency effects are minimal, even at the maximum DNR setting.

Fitting Tips

- Some products have DNR that increases with increasing intensity—that is, the effect may be only 5 dB for a 60 dB input but 10 dB for an 80 dB input. Although we suggest routinely using a 75 dB input, it may be useful to check softer inputs for different products on occasion just to gain information regarding how different algorithms work.
- To observe the release time of the DNR, you can try talking while the noise is present (raise your voice well above the noise). You should observe the release of the DNR on the screen (the time for this to happen will vary among instruments, but it usually is quite fast—one second or less).

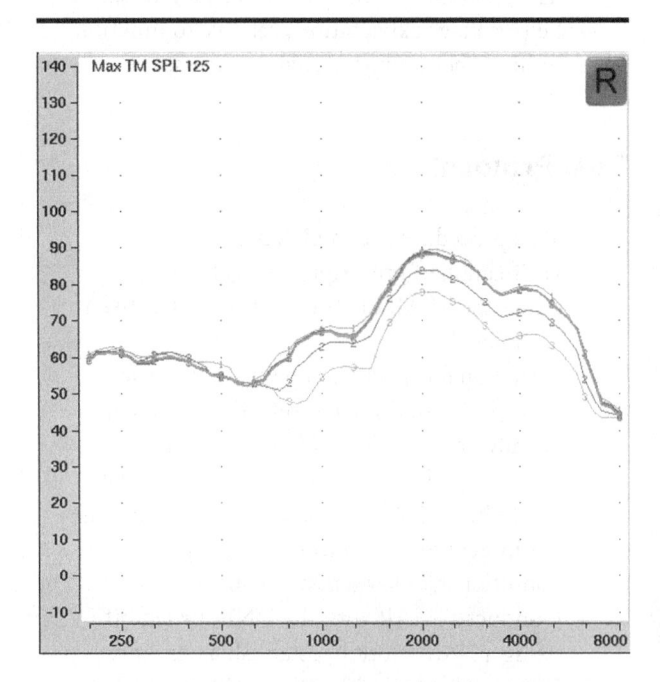

Figure 17–26. Example of DNR testing for different levels of DNR. The top output is DNR set to off. Note that at each of the DNR settings, there is a small change in output across the entire frequency range.

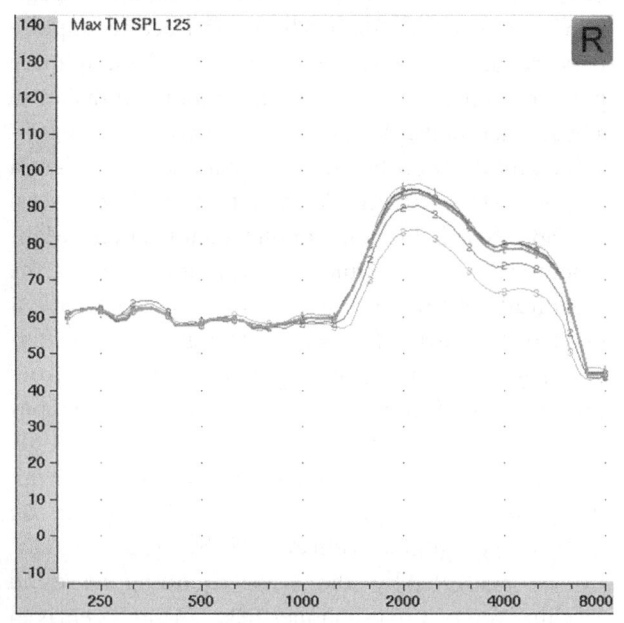

Figure 17–27. Example of DNR testing with an open-fit hearing aid. The top output is the reference DNR-off condition. Note that at each of the DNR settings, there is little change in the lower frequencies.

- DNR should have no effect when the patient is listening to speech. To confirm this, you may want to check products by simply conducting a REAR using real speech with the DNR turned on versus off at a relatively high input level (e.g., 75 dB SPL).

Frequency Lowering

With downward sloping hearing loss, there are times when the loss in the high frequencies reaches a level of severity at which it is not realistic to make speech audible with conventional amplification. For these patients, we sometimes simply choose to roll off gain to help prevent feedback. A second option is to use frequency lowering to make speech in this area audible, albeit at a different frequency. As we discussed in detail in Chapter 12, frequency lowering can be accomplished using a variety of different techniques.

Regardless of the approach used to lower the frequencies, the fitting application remains the same—move high-frequency speech (and environmental sounds) from a frequency range where they are inaudible to a frequency range where they are audible (or reinforce a particular frequency range by boosting the energy present in a lower frequency region). As we show in our sample findings, it is fairly easy, using probe microphone measures, to determine whether the algorithm has been activated, as you will observe frequencies missing from the usual aided speech spectrum when speech mapping is conducted and/or you will see an increase in energy in a lower frequency region. Determining whether the high-frequency sounds have been made audible at a lower frequency, however, is a more difficult task because the lowered signal will blend in with the amplified signals that originate at this frequency.

In Chapter 13 we detailed several test stimuli that have been developed specifically for evaluation of frequency lowering in the hearing aid test box including the Ling 6-Sound Test and /s/ and /sh/ sounds excised from the ISTS. In some cases the level of these sounds represents the actual peak level we would expect in running speech. One system has filtered the standard speech passage so that only higher segments of speech are present (options include speech segments centered at 3150, 4000, 5000, or 6300 Hz), which then allows for observation of each signal when it is lowered. Many of these same test signals are also available when completing probe microphone measurements. In the absence of recorded speech, live voice presentation of the /s/ and /sh/ sounds will provide a rough idea of the effects of the lowering. We recommend using a calibrated speech signal whenever possible, however, if you are interested in not only the amount of frequency lowering but also the audibility of the lowered signal in the individual patient (See review of frequency-lowering verification procedures by Scollie et al, 2016.)

Test Protocol

- This procedure usually is completed after the routine verification of prescriptive targets has been conducted using either the REAR or REIG approach.
- Conduct speech mapping for 65 dB input for reference; display the full amplitude spectrum of the amplified signal.
- If your system has an excised /s/ stimulus, present it at 65 dB SPL. If the stimulus does not fall above the patient's threshold, frequency lowering may be warranted to improve audibility and should be activated. (*Note:* Deactivate noise reduction for all testing using excised /s/ and /sh/ stimuli.)
- Activate frequency lowering and present the speech signal; observe change in speech spectrum showing that frequency lowering indeed has been activated.
- Deliver one or more high-frequency signals to observe the placement and level of the lowered signal.
- If the signal does not appear to be audible, adjustment may be needed regarding either the target location frequency or the gain at the lowered region, or both. For example, if your system has the excised /s/, fine tune until the signal falls just above threshold using the weakest frequency-lowering setting possible. In some cases, the signal may still be audible even though it does not appear to be so—more on that later in this chapter.
- Optional: Play a slightly lower frequency stimulus (e.g., /sh/) that is band-limited

around 5000 Hz and make sure there is frequency separation. If the output from the two signals overlap too much, the listener may have difficulty perceiving them as two different speech sounds.

- After activating noise reduction, have the listener listen to ensure that he or she can distinguish between /s/ and /sh/.

Sample Findings

It is initially of interest to observe whether the frequency compression has indeed been activated, but our real interest is its effect on the test signal. Figure 17–28A (from Mueller, Alexander, & Scollie, 2013) shows the output for a 65 dB SPL speech input with frequency lowering deactivated and with two nonlinear frequency compression settings: one starting at 2000 Hz with a 2.2:1 frequency compression ratio, and another starting at 1500 Hz with a 3.2:1 frequency compression ratio, for the same hearing aid programming. No gain adjustments were made as the settings were changed. As shown, the output for the frequency compressed regions (between the start frequency and response rolloff) is essentially the same as it is without frequency lowering, which suggests that the lowered signals are being treated as though they originated at their new frequencies. It is also possible to observe the presence of frequency lowering by viewing the REAR85. Illustrated in Figure 17–28B is the real-ear MPO of this same hearing aid for the same two different frequency compression settings. As we noted previously, REAR85 and REAR90 measurements using swept pure tones are invalid when frequency lowering is activated. In fact, it is not unusual to see a REAR85 for a swept pure tone that appears to be lower than the REAR observed in response to a 65 dB SPL-shaped real-speech signal! This artifact occurs because, during signal acquisition, a filter is used by many probe microphone systems that surround the test frequency and sweeps along with it. Because the output frequency is not the same as the input frequency after frequency compression, this filter does not correspond to the test frequency and the REAR is artificially lowered. This really does not affect operation of the hearing aid in the real world. It just means we need to disable

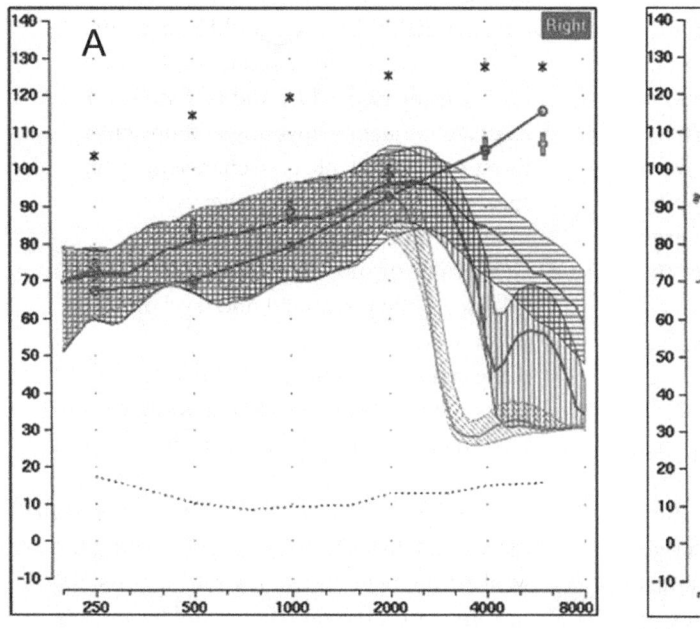

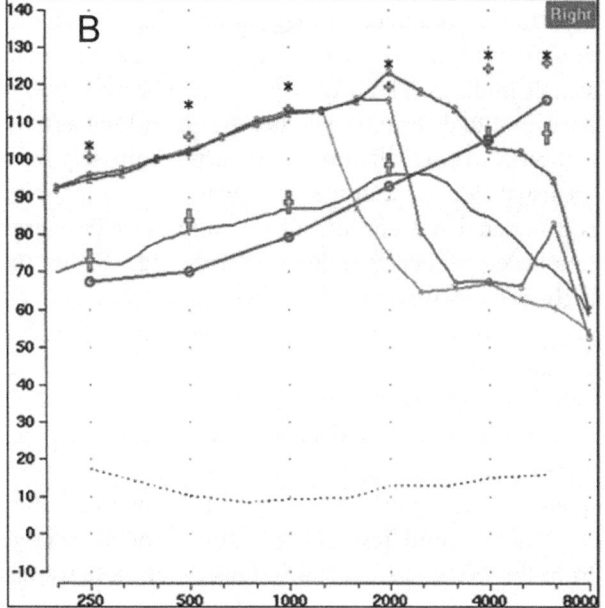

Figure 17–28. A. The output for a 65 dB SPL speech input with frequency lowering deactivated, and with two nonlinear frequency compression settings: one starting at 2000 Hz with a 2.2:1 frequency compression ratio, and another starting at 1500 Hz with a 3.2:1. **B.** The real-ear MPO of this same hearing aid for the same two different frequency compression settings. (Adapted from Mueller et al., 2013.)

frequency lowering in order to measure REAR85 and REAR90 accurately.

In Figure 17–29, we show the findings for a patient whose hearing loss drops to 80 to 90 dB at 4000 to 6000 Hz; in this case we decided to apply frequency lowering for these frequencies. We used the equipment's calibrated and filtered speech with high frequency energy preserved around 4000 Hz and 6300 Hz and the hearing aid manufacturer's default setting for the testing. In Figure 17–29A, you see the output for these two signals following activation of frequency lowering in the default mode. The 6300 Hz signal is now around 4000 Hz, and the 4000 Hz signal is now around 3000 Hz. From this figure, it might appear that the signals are clearly *inaudible*. Actually, they probably are not *totally* inaudible, however. Previously, we described how speech peaks could be audible even when the LTASS is below the threshold and the signal appears to be inaudible. The same issue is present here. Specifically, because the LTASS averages over time (and energy is not present at all frequencies all of the time) and speech segments vary in level, the speech peaks are not captured by this average. Instead, the speech peaks fall approximately 10 to 15 dB above the filtered LTASS shown in this figure. Applying this information, only the very peak of the high-frequency signal energy centered at 4000 Hz is likely audible, and the entire signal centered at 6300 Hz falls below threshold. Because it is not possible to see directly the peak energy using this test signal, we encourage you to assume the peak is 12 to 15 dB above the line you see and also test with actual excised /s/ and /sh/ signals (from the ISTS) to get a better picture of the true audibility provided. As mentioned, this example is the hearing aids manufacturer's default setting, with programming set to the manufacturer's proprietary algorithm. We show you this to point out that many manufacturers take a very conservative approach to frequency lowering, and you will find that their default settings often do not accomplish the desired goal. (Of course, if you did not conduct this type of probe microphone testing, how would you know?)

In Figure 17–29B, you see these same two signals after adjustments are made. Observe that we changed the target destination to the 2000 to 2700 Hz range and increased gain slightly to obtain increased signal audibility. These two test signals roughly represent the

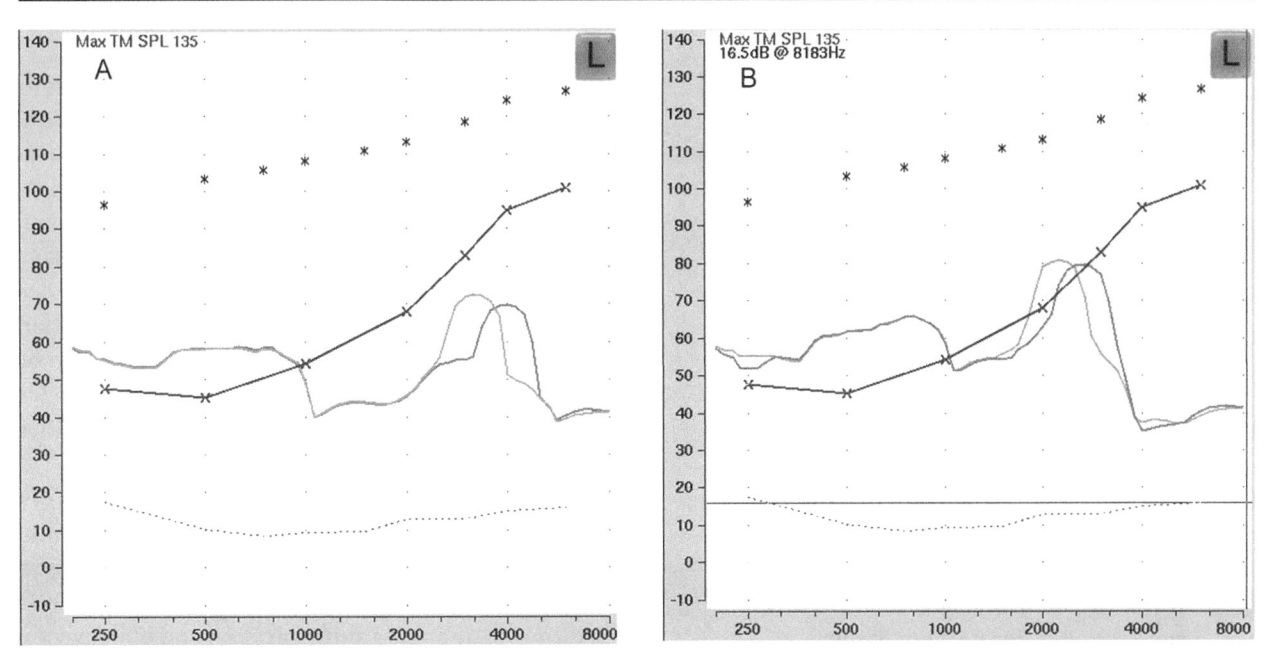

Figure 17–29. A. Shows the output of this manufacturer's high-frequency speech bands, centered at 4000 Hz and 6300 Hz for the manufacturer's proprietary fitting and default frequency-lowering settings. **B.** Shows the same patient after adjustments have been made to gain and the frequency compression parameters. The 6300 Hz signal is now around 3000 Hz, and the 4000 Hz signal is lowered to the 2000 Hz region.

frequency of /sh/ and /s/, and we do want to maintain separation of the signals after lowering, as shown here. We, of course, involve the perceptions of the patient during this testing to confirm that the signals are audible, but not to the extent of distorting the overall speech signal. In this case, we were probably too aggressive, in that the LTASS falls above threshold, even for speech energy centered at 6300 Hz. This excessive aggressiveness was confirmed by patient complaints of that sounds were too hissy. When we reduced the frequency so that the band-limited 6300 Hz test signal fell a couple of dB below the patient's threshold, peak energy was still 8 to10 dB above threshold, which led to a patient who was satisfied with the sound quality. Even though we eventually got it right, the use of the excised /sh/ and /s/ test signals during our initial fitting would have made actual audibility more clearly evident and saved us some time, reinforcing the utility of using the two types of test signals in tandem. This benefit is even more clearly evident with patient's for which it is difficult to get reliable feedback (e.g. young children).

Fitting Tips

- It is important to remember that the gain applied to the lowered signal is the same as a signal originating at the frequency. Therefore, as we demonstrated in Figure 17–29, if the hearing aid was not programmed appropriately originally (e.g., due to use of the manufacturer's proprietary fitting), then it is unlikely the lowered signals will be optimally audible.
- Related to the preceding fitting tip, when attempting to make the lowered signals audible, it is tempting to keep increasing gain for the lowered region. We cannot forget, however, that this is also affecting signals originating at the target frequency, and you may end up with a fitting that has strayed far from the NAL-NL2 targets. A compromise often is necessary.
- If your probe system does not have specific speech sounds for use with frequency-lowering testing, you can download a Ling 6-Sound Test app that is compatible with iPhone, iPad, and iPod Touch—optimized for iPhone 5. This app allows for delivery of the sounds at a consistent SPL. Ling 6 test signals and /sh/ and /s/ signals excised from the ISTS are also available as .wav files which can be used for digital delivery using tablets, computers, or other devices from the DSL website at the University of Western Ontario (http://www.dslio.com/?page_id=166).
- Not all frequency lowering technologies are fitted the same way. We encourage you to also consider individual manufacturer's recommendations related to application of frequency lowering, especially when supporting data are also provided.

Assessment of Feedback Suppression

For some hearing aid features, such as compression, there may be considerable similarities across at least some manufacturers in how the features work as well as the expected outcome. For others, such as DNR, there are some differences across manufacturers in how the feature operates and how it affects the patient's listening experience. As discussed in Chapter 12, one feature with considerable published differences across manufacturers is digital feedback suppression (DFS).

Over the past decade or so, DFS has significantly affected how we select and fit hearing aids. Without feedback suppression, open fittings are restricted to listeners with no greater than mild-to-moderate high-frequency hearing loss. Therefore, the current popularity of mini-BTE hearing aids when used with open and other non-custom eartips has often been attributed in large part to effective DFS technology. The differences in how well the DFS technology works, however, greatly influence the hearing loss configurations and the degree of high-frequency hearing loss that can be fitted appropriately.

We assume that you will be completing probe microphone measures on each patient, so determining the effectiveness of DFS on every individual patient is not necessary (or even particularly informative). In addition to the large differences in the effectiveness of this technology across manufacturers, however, the effectiveness often changes with each new generation of hearing aids. These differences include how much gain is available before feedback, as well as any audible artifact that is introduced by the feedback suppression system—sometimes referred to as *entrainment*. The speed with which a feedback suppression system can adjust to eliminate feedback generated by the introduction of a cell phone or other new surface is also of interest. In addition, considerable differences (approximately +/− 10 dB) occur across individuals in the maximum stable gain before feedback within the same product. Although we can't do a lot to control for individual differences across patients, having a general idea of the effectiveness of a DFS technology is tremendously useful for both selection of an appropriate hearing aid and effective counseling. Consider a patient who has normal hearing in the low frequencies, sloping to a moderately severe hearing loss in the highs. This patient is an excellent candidate for an open fitting because hearing thresholds are normal through 1000 Hz. With some models of mini-BTE hearing aids, you will not be able to reach high-frequency NAL-NL2 targets without significantly decreasing the amount of venting. With other products, we can match targets with a non-custom open eartip but only with audible artifacts. With still other products, we easily can match targets with a non-custom open eartip without entrainment. If you do not previously evaluate the hearing aids with your probe microphone tests, how do you know which is which? So, whereas you don't need to do this testing with each patient, information that is highly useful clinically can be gained from testing each product.

Test Protocol

- This procedure can be completed by using either a REAR or REIG approach. Select a speech or speechlike test signal (e.g., shaped speech, ISTS).
- Select a patient for testing. It might be useful to have access to the same individual multiple times for assessment of multiple new instruments as they are introduced over time. The magnitude of hearing loss does not matter that much as long as the individual is willing to listen to feedback for a short period of time; even a coworker with normal hearing will work.
- Change the equalization method from concurrent to stored equalization. (*Note*: On most systems this simply requires selecting "open" or other similar descriptor as the hearing aid style.) Select an average patient's audiogram and LDLs that reflect a good candidacy for open fitting (e.g., normal hearing in the low frequencies sloping to moderate hearing loss in the high frequencies).
- Select the verified prescriptive method in the probe microphone fitting software that you use for a typical patient and usual fitting factors.
- Program the hearing aids to the desired fitting algorithm using the manufacturer's software control process (select the same patient and fitting factors entered into the probe microphone software).
- Place the probe tube in the ear at an appropriate depth and measure the REUR.
- Fit the hearing aid to the patient's ear with a fully open, non-custom eartip.
  - Activate feedback suppression and calibrate the feedback suppression system if recommended by the manufacturer.
  - If there is more than one DFS setting, consider repeating this entire protocol for all available DFS settings.
- Mute the hearing aid and conduct stored-equalization, free-field calibration.
- Unmute the instrument and begin testing and making gain adjustments using a 55 dB input level. A lower signal level is used because compression processing will provide increased gain with decreased input, increasing the likelihood of feedback.
- Adjust frequency-specific gain to achieve a reasonable match to target. It may be the case that you are unable to match the gain targets because of feedback or gain limiting resulting from the hearing aid's feedback calibration routine, or because you reach the gain limits of the hearing aid. If so, either (1) attempt to match the same gain shape as the targets, or (2) consider using better thresholds for the hearing loss that you enter into the probe microphone system.
- Once you match the shape, increase overall gain across all frequencies until (1) you or the

patient hear feedback, (2) you reach the hearing aid gain limits, or (3) you reach the gain limit imposed by the feedback calibration routine.

- If you reach audible feedback, decrease and increase overall gain slightly—talk, whistle, and have the patient open and close her mouth until you determine the gain setting that is just below the presence of feedback for typical listening conditions.
- Remeasure the REAR to display the maximum REAR before feedback. If you are interested, compare these values to the REUR; this difference is the maximum real-ear gain before feedback.
- Turn gain down a couple of dB, and if available, plug monitor headphones into your probe microphone system in order to listen in to the sounds in the patient's ear. Have the patient sit quietly while you talk, whistle, and make other sounds. Listen for any artifacts or problems with the sound quality.
- If the maximum additional gain before feedback is of interest for quick comparisons to other products and manufacturers, repeat the maximum REAR procedure with the feedback suppression system disabled. In this way, you can calculate the difference between DFS-on and DFS-off REARs.
- Repeating the sound quality procedure we just described with DFS disabled is also useful as a benchmark for comparing possible degradation in sound quality related to DFS processing.
- It may also be informative to increase the thresholds entered into the probe microphone software until the prescriptive targets are similar to the maximum REAR you measured. This procedure provides an indication of the maximum hearing loss you're able to fit before feedback.

Sample Findings

We selected a new hearing aid from Bob's-Pretty-Good Hearing Aids to test its new DFS processing. This is a mini-BTE instrument, and we fitted it to a patient's ear using a pediatric open eartip. This manufacturer recommends completing the DFS calibration routine in its software, so we did. Two separate DFS settings, normal and turbo, were available; we tested turbo first. A sloping hearing loss (normal in the low frequencies sloping to 65 dB HL thresholds in the high frequencies) was entered into the probe microphone system and we adjusted gain to match NAL-NL2 targets. Gain was then increased. Rather than reaching feedback, we stopped seeing gain increases in the high frequencies after increasing overall gain a few steps. This gain limit, the maximum REAR before feedback, is shown in the upper curve in Figure 17–30. Given that this curve falls 5 to 10 dB above our original targets, we estimated we could successfully match targets even for a patient with high-frequency hearing thresholds of 70 to 75 dB, or perhaps greater at some frequencies. We then lowered gain, disabled the DFS, and searched for feedback. We found it quickly! In fact, we had to lower gain a few clicks to reach the stable REAR with DFS deactivated, resulting in the lower curve in Figure 17–30. By comparing these two curves, we can see that approximately 20 dB of additional high-frequency gain was available before feedback after activating the DFS system—clearly, this is a DFS system that works, and works well! We then

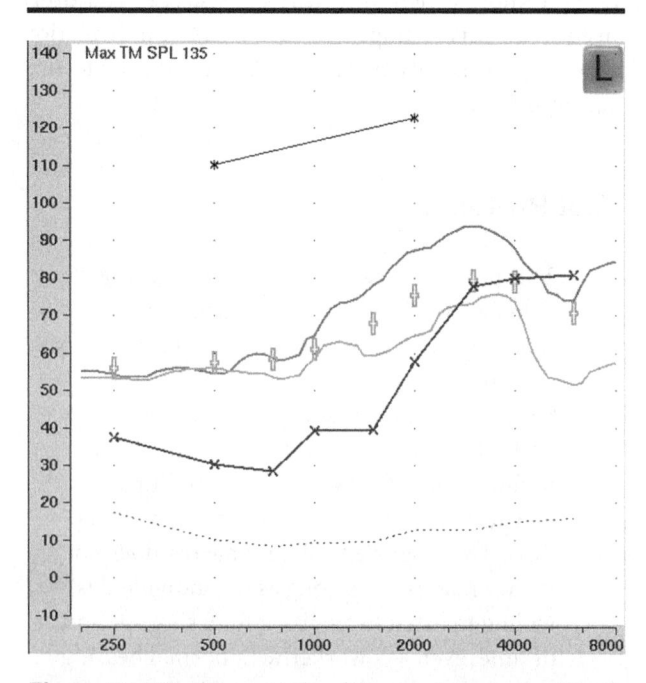

Figure 17–30. An example of the maximum ouput available before feedback with the feedback cancellation turned on (*upper curve*) and off (*lower curve*).

turned gain down two clicks (about 2 dB in this instrument) and plugged headphones into the probe microphone system. Right away we heard a soft but audible roughness that sounded a bit like a distant motorboat. We then repeated the entire procedure on the normal setting, which resulted in a decrease in maximum REAR of about 4 dB and the elimination of roughness in the sound quality. From this information, we know we can fit a wide range of high-frequency hearing loss with this product. We further know that we probably want to activate the turbo setting only if we cannot reach targets with the normal feedback reduction setting. Finally, we know that if the patient has a range of normal hearing, counseling may be necessary for acceptance of the turbo setting, or there may be a tradeoff involving decreasing venting and using the normal setting to achieve desired target gain.

Fitting Tips

- It is often useful to examine not only the limits of high-frequency gain and REAR corresponding to the DFS function but also the gain in the middle and low frequencies. A lower power receiver can greatly limit low-frequency gain in open fittings. Therefore, consider using a power receiver to really test the maximum limits of additional gain before feedback in a product.
- Plugging in headphones to the probe microphone system to search for audible artifacts will add another potential path for feedback. Therefore, consider not plugging the headphones in until you reach this testing phase. Furthermore, it may be necessary to limit headphone gain and/or reduce hearing aid gain to ensure there is no feedback during the sound quality assessment.

CROS Fittings

When a patient has an unaidable ear, head shadow can reduce speech recognition in specific listening situations (speech from the bad side). One way to improve performance is to place a microphone on the ear that is unaidable (usually housed in a hearing aid), which wirelessly transfers signals from this side to a hearing aid on the good ear. This is referred to as a Contralateral Routing of Offside Signal fitting or *CROS fitting*. If the better hearing ear has a hearing loss, then a microphone is activated for this side, too, and the fitting is termed a *bi*lateral CROS or *BiCROS*.

Fitting the on-side hearing aid when a BiCROS is employed is no different from fitting any other unilateral hearing aid. Fitting the signal from the off-side microphone, however, requires some adaptation to the usual probe microphone test approach, particularly when the patient has normal hearing in the better ear, which often is the case. When normal hearing is present, the goal of the fitting is simply to eliminate the head shadow effect. So, we want to place the signal originating from the side of the bad ear into the good ear but apply 0 dB insertion gain (no gain but no loss). In other words, the REAR should equal the REUR; therefore, the REUR is our fitting target. For BiCROS fittings, the REAR targets for the better ear are also the targets for the signal directed to the poorer ear. Some probe systems have a dedicated method for conducting CROS/BiCROS fittings on their systems using two probe modules.

Test Protocol

- Initially, position the patient as you do for conventional probe microphone testing. Properly position the probe tube in the better ear.
- Use stored equalization to calibrate the system (as you do for an open fitting).
- Measure the REUR using a standard real-speech signal (e.g., shaped speech or ISTS). This now becomes the fitting target. For a BiCROS fitting, you can skip measuring the REUR and instead simply use the targets for the better ear.
- Fit the CROS system to both ears and, with it muted, measure the REOR to confirm that it is similar to the REUR. Remember the goal is that there is an open fitting on the good ear and the eartip does not serve as an earplug. Unmute the system. For a BiCROS system, begin by fitting the better ear to targets using the standard REAR fitting we described previously.

- Swivel patient in chair so that the loudspeaker is directly facing the bad ear (i.e., 90° or 270°). The patient's head should be the same distance from the loudspeaker. In the case of a CROS, conduct the REAR using a speech signal at 65 dB SPL (the probe tube remains in the good ear). Adjust programming until the aided output matches the previously measured REUR. In a true CROS fitting, this typically involves increasing gain only in the high frequencies. In the case of a BiCROS, adjust programming until the aided output matches the better ear's REAR targets.

Sample Findings

Shown in Figure 17–31 are the findings for a CROS fitting for a patient with an unaidable left ear and essentially normal hearing for the good (right) ear (thresholds around 15 dB HL). For conducting the fitting, with the hearing aid turned off, we first obtained the REUR for the right ear (with the patient at 0° azimuth). We then positioned him so that the loudspeaker was directly facing his left ear (270° azimuth relative to the patient).

For counseling purposes, we conducted a REOR measurement (hearing aid turned off) to illustrate the head shadow effect—this is shown in Figure 17–31A. The upper response is the patient's REUR, and the lower response is the signal presented from the off-side. This finding is fairly typical if the fitting is truly open, showing a 10 to 12-dB head-shadow effect for the higher frequencies. We then turned the off-side microphone on and conducted a REAR. As shown in Figure 17–31B, we programmed the hearing aid to mirror the REUR, falling just a few dB higher for most frequencies.

Fitting Tips

- Hearing aids generally do not provide much amplification for frequencies above 5 to 6 kHz. Consequently, for a true CROS fitting some patients will prefer a fitting that is a few dB higher than the REUR, similar to what we provided in the example above.
- There has been some work with fittings termed *transcranial CROS,* which is when a power instrument is placed in the unaidable ear, and the desired signal is transferred to the good ear

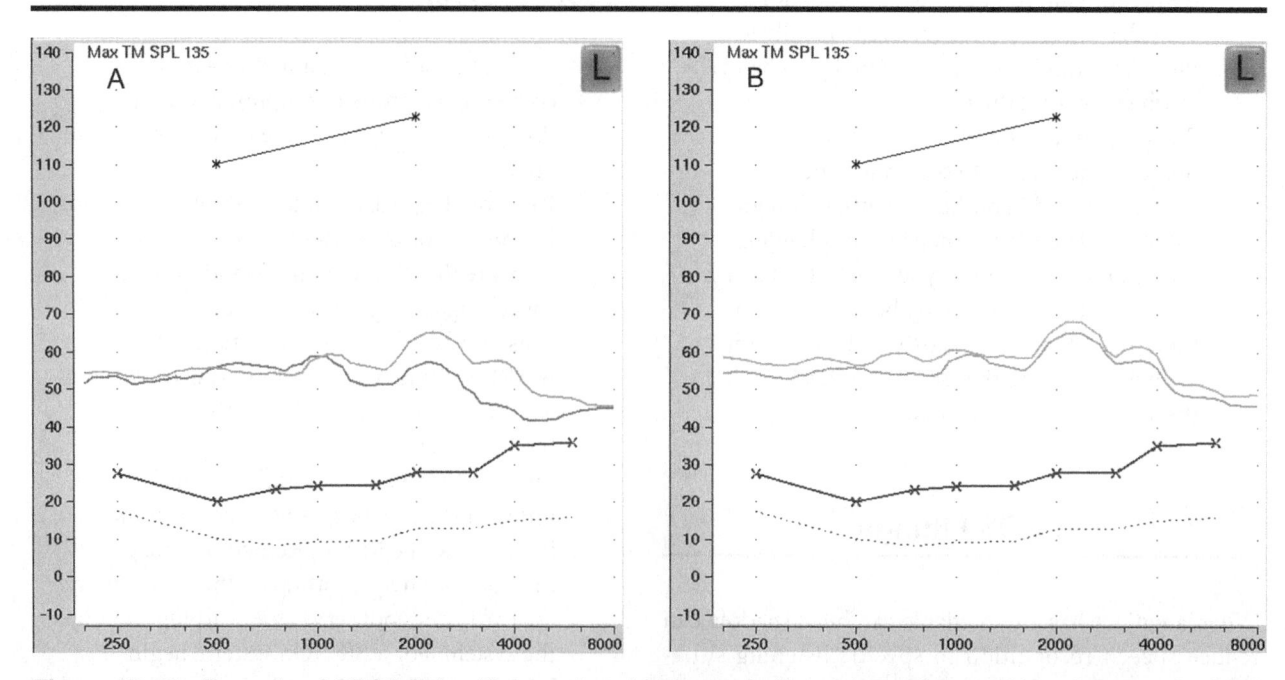

Figure 17–31. Example of CROS fitting. The hearing aid is turned off and the patient positioned so that the loudspeaker is directly facing his good/left ear (270° azimuth relative to the patient). **A.** The head shadow is present. **B.** After the hearing aid is turned on, the head shadow is gone, indicating the functionality of the CROS.

via bone conduction vibrations generated in the ear canal. If you want to try this interesting fitting approach, you'll find your probe microphone measures will come in handy to determine specific crossover levels for the fitting (Valente, Potts, Valente, & Goebel, 1995).

Telephone and Streaming Devices

Wireless streaming from telephones, personal music systems, wireless microphones, television, and a variety of other devices has gained considerable traction in the past few years as a convenient way to bring aided signals to a patient's ears and, in some cases, provide considerable benefits when compared to traditional routing methods (e.g., Picou & Ricketts, 2011, 2013). As we describe in Chapter 13 with respect to electroacoustic evaluation, fitting wireless streaming is typically completed in the test box by matching the frequency response from the streaming signal to the hearing aid's frequency response after fitting to a validated prescriptive target using the techniques we described earlier in this chapter. There are at least two reasons we may want to complete probe microphone measures for demonstration and counseling purposes, however. First, we may want to demonstrate wireless streaming from a telephone while completing probe microphone measures to allow the patient to visualize the audibility of the streamed signal using speech mapping techniques. Both electromagnetic handsets and bilateral measurements available from some probe microphone systems can be useful to demonstrate specific conditions, such as streaming telephone signals from one ear to the other and streaming all types of signals to both ears. Having the patient call a telephone number with a standard message like the weather number can also be useful for this demonstration.

Another, more important reason to complete probe microphone assessment relates to the bandwidth of streamed signals. Modern hearing aids differ considerably in audible bandwidth, with the high-frequency limit ranging from as low as 3 to 4 kHz to as high as perhaps 8 to 10 kHz. The effect that these audible high frequencies have on sound quality depends on the listener. That is, extended high-frequency audibility could be either negative or positive (Ricketts et al., 2008), so it is useful to know how high into the high frequencies audibility extend here. Venting can contribute to an even greater extent to a reduction in the sound quality of wireless streamed signals, particularly music. Specifically, a large vent as is typical in open-fit hearing aids can preclude delivery of the low-frequency energy from a streamed source and result in music that sounds tinny and unacceptable. This problem is not observed for sounds in the listener's environment because the low frequencies reach the listeners' ears through the vent. Therefore, this potential problem is unique to wireless streaming.

Test Protocol

- This protocol should occur after the hearing aid is already fitted to a validated prescriptive target using the REAR or REIG techniques previously described, so we are assuming that you have already entered the patient's audiogram and measured LDLs, placed the probe tube and hearing aid, and calibrated the probe system appropriately.
- Set equipment to spectral analysis mode, which may be the same as "live speech mapping" for some equipment.
- Activate wireless streaming in the hearing aid from a smartphone or personal music player. Some audiologists we know keep a Bluetooth-capable wireless music player on hand for this specific testing purpose—this can be a great use for that old smartphone you replaced last year.
- Select and play music of the patient's choosing.
- View the audible bandwidth and discuss the sound quality in consultation with the patient.

Sample Findings

Our patient came to us as a typical open fitting and had normal hearing at 750 Hz and below. He indicated no real difficulties on the telephone but was interested in streaming music, text to speech, and other signals from his smartphone. We activated his music program and streaming and had him play one of his favorite songs. The resulting REAR is marked Open in Figure 17–32. The patient indicated that it sounded tinny and very shrill. Just to see the difference, we tried replacing the open eartip with closed tips. The patient indicated that things sounded much better but were still shrill and that the high pitches sounded like mechanical noise. We

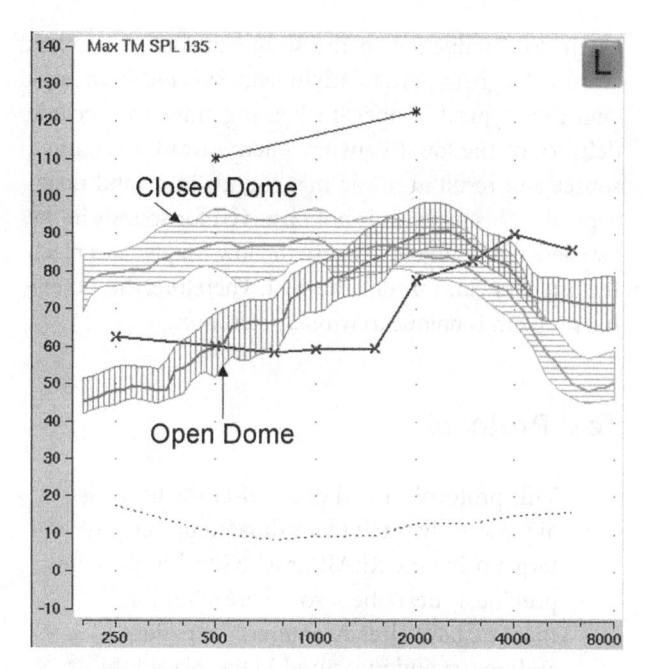

Figure 17–32. Example of verification of a wireless accessory. The two curves represent the output measured for the same music signal with an open eartip (Open) and a closed eartip (Closed). In both cases, the REAR was matched to the patient's NAL-NL2 targets through 4000 Hz, but gain was reduced in the higher frequencies for the closed fitting per the patient's request.

then reprogrammed the hearing aid master program so that there was again a match to NAL-NL2 targets with his new closed domes. Based on this complaint of shrillness, we then turned down gain above 5000 Hz in his music program until the patient indicated he was happy with the sound quality. The resulting output is labeled Closed in Figure 17–32. As you can see, even though the same low-frequency REAR targets were matched for the open and closed fittings, the open fitting resulted in a reduction in the low frequencies for the streamed signal of about 30 dB—no wonder it sounded tinny!

But have we just created other problems? Somewhat surprisingly, the patient indicated he liked the sound of the hearing aids in general with the closed domes and felt satisfied with the sound of his own voice. A quick measure of the occlusion effect with the closed fitting (as we describe in the next section) indicated it was much greater than with the open tip, but not terribly high (about 12 dB). After trying the closed domes for a couple of weeks, the patient indicated he was very satisfied overall with how the hearing aids worked—so this fitting worked out pretty well. We would not have been surprised, however, if he had returned and asked for some middle ground, with a little more venting.

Fitting Tips

- For some patients, it may be necessary to select a more closed eartip to obtain desirable sound quality from streamed media. If so, it will be necessary to refit the hearing aid to targets and ensure that the sound quality for external sounds and the patient's own voice are still acceptable. Finding the right balance in this trading relationship for patients can take a bit of effort. With some patients who prefer a completely open hearing aid fitting, the best solution will be to remove the hearing aids and listen to music through headphones or insert earphones.
- When you are attempting to maximize sound quality for extended high frequencies, probe microphone testing may be less useful because standing wave issues make accurate assessment of the higher frequencies challenging without getting very close to the TM. In these cases, it's also sometimes best to rely on patient feedback and/or audibility assessment in the coupler using simulated REAR and average RECDs. Some newer probe microphone systems use a variety of techniques to provide a visual representation of hearing aid output through 10 kHz or even higher.

Assessing the Hearing Aid Occlusion Effect

When the ear is occluded with a hearing aid or earmold, low-frequency sounds generated in the ear canal when the patient talks can no longer escape. This annoying effect is referred to as the *occlusion effect,* and it may increase the level of sounds below approximately 500 to 750 Hz by up to 20 to 30 dB in the occluded ear canal when compared to the level in the open ear canal. The occlusion effect causes the person wearing the hearing aid to report that his or her own voice sounds hollow or booming or that he or she is talking in a barrel (see

Chapter 8). Not all patients will have a significant occlusion effect for their own voice when their ear canals are occluded, but when they do you can often solve this problem with an open fitting. This situation still continues to be an issue for many patients, nonetheless, to the extent that they may not use their hearing aids (in Chapters 8 and 18 we provide additional information on the cause and treatment of the occlusion effect).

The patient can provide us with a subjective report of this problem, although in these reports we do need to differentiate between the occlusion effect and low-frequency gain of the hearing aids. Also, 10 dB of occlusion effect may be terribly bothersome for one patient and not even noticed by another. Hence, for detecting the occlusion effect and for monitoring the magnitude during the treatment of the problem, it's very handy to have objective real-ear data of the effect. This isn't something we'd suggest measuring for all patients, only those who have the common complaints associated with the occlusion effect.

Test Protocol

- Set equipment to spectral analysis or live monitoring mode. This may be termed "live speech mapping" in some equipment. Other equipment may have special software for assessing the occlusion effect.
- Place the probe tube in the ear at an appropriate depth.
- Without the hearing aid in place, have patient vocalize /ee/ at 75 dBA and hold for five to eight seconds. Some equipment will have a monitoring microphone to show the SPL of the vocalization. If not, an inexpensive sound level meter or smartphone app can be used. (*Note:* Some probe microphone equipment will monitor the level at the probe microphone, not the reference microphone—this level cannot be used for this purpose.) Some older patients may have difficulty holding this level. If so, 70 dBA will also work.
- Place earmold/hearing aid in ear but don't turn on.
- Again have patient vocalize /ee/. This vocalization needs to be at the same input level as the open-ear measure on the smartphone app.
- Compare the two outputs. The degree that the occluded output is greater than the open-ear output is the occlusion effect.

Sample Findings

Figure 17–33 shows the before (A) and after (B) testing for a woman with a moderately severe hearing loss who was treated following her complaint of the occlusion effect. She originally was fitted with a double-dome tip for her RIC hearing aid. In Figure 17–33A, you see the open ear (*bottom curve*) and occluded (*top curve*) for her vocalization of the /ee/ with the double-dome tip in place. These findings clearly explain why she was bothered, since the occlusion effect was about 25 dB at 500 Hz and below. Not all occlusion effects peak in the low frequencies, but when they do, there is a good chance the problem can be helped with venting. Some probemic equipment will measure the total occlusion effect, which can be misleading. We believe it is important to know the magnitude at which the effect is at its maximum, and therefore favor the approach shown here.

Her double-dome molds were replaced with tips that didn't fit as tightly. With the new tips, she reported a big improvement and stated that the hollowness was mostly all gone. This is shown nicely in Figure 17–33B. The curve just above the open-ear output is what we're seeing for the new eartip. Note that essentially all the low-frequency effects are gone, and all that remains is 10 dB or so of occlusion from 500 to 1500 Hz, where this degree of venting doesn't have a substantial effect. Following these occlusion measures, we then programmed the hearing for the new eartip. Fortunately, we were still able to obtain desired gain without feedback issues. This is not always the case and sometimes a compromise between occlusion and desired gain must be made.

Fitting Tips

- If open fittings are truly open (e.g., the REOG is very similar to the REUG), the occlusion effect will nearly always be no more than a few dB—see research by MacKenzie (2006) comparing eartips/earmolds of different sizes and tightness.
- Annoyance from occlusion is rated slightly higher for a bilateral fitting than a unilateral

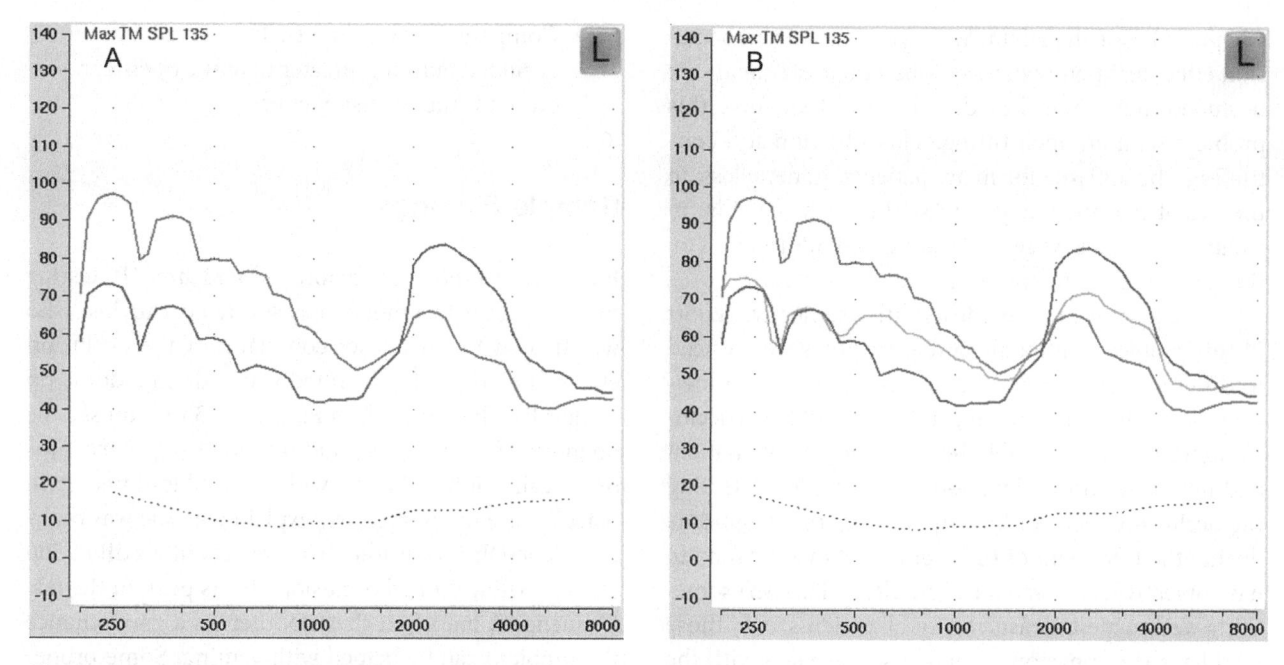

Figure 17–33. Example of occlusion effect. **A.** The open ear (*bottom curve*) and occluded (*top curve*) response for her vocalization of the /ee/ with the double-dome tip in. **B.** Replacing the double-tip domes with standard domes reduced occlusion, as shown by the middle curve.

one (Jespersen, Groth, Kiessling, Brenner, & Jensen, 2006). Some patients report using only one of their two hearing aids for this reason.

- We are not aware of convincing data to support this, but our general notion is that, if you can reduce the occlusion effect to no more than 8 to 10 dB, it will no longer be bothersome for most patients.
- For patients who simply cannot sustain an /ee/ vocalization, it is possible to conduct these measures using bone-conducted signals from an audiometer (for review, see Stender & Appleby, 2009).

In Closing

For those of us who use probe microphone measures routinely, it is difficult to imagine how hearing aids could be fitted without this testing. Certainly, using either the REAR or the REIG is essential for verification of prescriptive targets and determining appropriate audibility of the amplified signals—there is no alternative choice. Along with being the most important clinical measure, as we have described in this chapter, this procedure is also helpful in assessing and adjusting several hearing aid features and in troubleshooting post-fitting problems. Moreover, conducting these measures can be fascinating and educational, and sharing the results with the patient is a very effective counseling procedure. Clearly, the routine use of probe microphone assessment and making reasoned decisions based on the findings, in combination with other important information is one of the most important components in the overall fitting of hearing aids. Without this information we are forced to make choices based on guesses or clinical intuition instead of data. This is certainly not something we want to do if we are truly interested in providing evidence-based services.

18
Hearing Aid Orientation and Troubleshooting

In the preceding chapters, we have discussed the importance of determining that hearing aids meet certain quality-control standards, fit comfortably in or on the ear, and meet some criteria for optimal gain and output as experienced by the individual and as verified with probe microphone measures.

Now that we have completed discussion of the initial phases of fitting and verification, in this chapter we discuss the importance of the orientation stage and the follow-up during the first few weeks after the fitting. Although many fittings go perfectly from day one, on other occasions, issues arise that need attention. We discuss those issues and offer suggestions for solving them, or at the least, offer a reasonable compromise (not all problems can be completely solved).

As we have mentioned before, the overall procedure for fitting a hearing aid is a systematic process requiring a blend of art and science. The first phase of the fitting process involves a lot of science. You need to know how special features work and which ones are best for which patients, how to weigh the potential tradeoffs when considering the benefits and limitations of all specific technologies, the ins and outs of prescriptive fitting procedures, how to check the hearing aid in the coupler, and then how to verify that you are at a reasonable starting point for gain/output through the application of probe microphone measures.

The second phase of the fitting process, which is where we are in this chapter, requires you to be an effective listener, teacher, communicator, and troubleshooter. You will need to go through the many details of use, care, and maintenance in a methodical fashion. This guidance often needs to be repeated and it will likely be most beneficial when provided in both verbal and written formats. The post-fitting process requires a lot of thinking, attention to detail, and sometimes problem solving.

First Things First

Whether the patient is a new hearing aid user or a long-term, experienced user, it is important to complete the following steps. Each new purchase requires unique understanding and effort on the part of the patient, and it is incumbent upon us to ensure that the patient is well-informed before leaving our office. We summarize some easy-to-follow steps in the following Things to Remember.

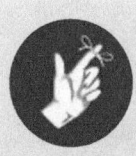

THINGS TO REMEMBER: OVERVIEW OF HEARING AID ORIENTATION

Step 0 (before you start). Put on their hearing aids so they can hear.

Step 1. Provide paperwork.

1. Warranty forms
2. Insurance options
3. Invoice and instructional brochure

Step 2. Discuss parts of the hearing aid and their functions (brief summary for experienced users).

1. Describe function of various parts of the hearing aid.
2. Have a hearing aid just like theirs in front of them.
3. Show the controls to the patient (volume, remote, toggle buttons, switches), if applicable, and how they function.
4. If applicable, briefly demonstrate additional hardware (e.g., wireless streamers, remote microphones).

Step 3. Batteries (very brief summary for experienced users). For individuals using rechargeable batteries, much of this is not necessary—use instructions provided by the manufacturer for patients using rechargeable batteries in their hearing aids.

1. Write down the type of battery their hearing aid uses.
2. Give battery life estimates, in days or weeks.
3. Inform them how and where to obtain batteries (many audiologists suggest their patients return to them for their batteries—a nice way to stay connected with patients. Knowledge of alternate battery sources can also be helpful for your patients, as is having a complete picture of the large variations in pricing.)
4. Demonstrate proper insertion and have the patients do it several times.
5. Mention buildup of debris in battery compartment and how to clean it.
6. Reinforce that there is no reason to buy a large supply of batteries at one time.
7. Mention battery testers (may be more critical for parents of hearing-impaired children).
8. Emphasize removing battery from the contacts (by opening the battery door) when not using hearing aid, as drainage may continue.
9. Describe warning signs of weakening battery (e.g., beeping hearing aid).
10. Provide patient with Battery Ingestion Hotline information: (202) 625–3333
    a. Remind him or her to keep batteries out of reach of children.
    b. Remind him or her *not* to store batteries in proximity to pills.

Step 4. Discuss the earmold, eartip, or custom hearing aid case (very brief summary for experienced users).

1. Describe the three main functions: to anchor, to direct sound into ear, and to help prevent feedback.
2. For new users, point out parts and, on an artificial ear, show where they fit into the ear.

3. Demonstrate insertion on the artificial ear using an earmold made for that ear. Be patient; consider age and motor difficulties. Modify mold or case, if necessary, for comfort and/or ease of insertion.
4. Discuss feedback. Let the patient know why it occurs, when to expect it, and what it indicates (e.g., warning of improper insertion).
5. Discuss care of earmold/eartip.
   a. If the patient is fitting with a traditional BTE, reinforce that earmolds must be removed from BTE for washing; that they can be washed with warm water and soap, not alcohol; and that all water must be allowed to evaporate before reconnecting to the hearing aid.
   b. Show how to re-attach tubing to the ear hook in the proper orientation.
   c. If the patient has good dexterity, demonstrate proper use of the cleaning brush and wax loop.
   d. If the patient has good dexterity, demonstrate proper removal and replacement of non-custom eartips (RIC and RITA devices) and thin tubing (RITA devices).
   e. If the patient has good dexterity, demonstrate how to clean the thin tubing of the RITA device with the cleaning wire.
6. Emphasize that if soreness occurs, the patient should return and have the hearing aid, earmold, or eartip modified.

Step 5. Maintenance instructions should include the following:

1. Avoid temperature extremes.
2. Avoid moisture when possible (high humidity, rain, perspiration). If these are likely, recommend (and offer) Dri-Aid Kit options.
3. Do not use hair spray or hair dryers around the hearing aids.
4. Do not take the hearing aid apart.
5. Keep hearing aid away from children and pets (discuss how dogs and cats can be drawn to feedback—and even the smell of the owner's earwax!).

During the first few weeks that patients use new hearing aids, many of them are still learning how to insert the battery correctly, how to remove and replace the earmold or eartip, and even how to insert the device properly and comfortably. During this time (and thereafter), a number of things can go wrong: The hearing aid might stop working or start whistling, the amplified sound might be weak or distorted, and so on. We don't cover all of these symptoms and potential outcomes in detail with the patient, but sometimes it is useful to give him or her a worksheet that helps them troubleshoot during the adjustment period. Table 18–1 provides that information.

Because there are many things to review, considerable time and effort are associated with the orientation of a hearing aid. This orientation can be laborious, but it is critically important. Remember that the manufacturer of the hearing aids must provide an instructional booklet for the purchaser's use. Often, those booklets provide excellent schematics of the very topics we talk about in our orientation sessions (e.g., telephone orientation, battery insertion, and so on).

To help focus and segment the process, we have organized the orientation phase of the fitting appointment into three general areas that need to be addressed:

1. Explain use of hearing aid.
   - Instruct patient on how to insert and remove the devices (a mirror is very useful here). Have the patient attempt to do so with you in your office. Show the patient how to hold the hearing aids during the insertion process

Table 18–1. Sample Table for New Hearing Aid Users Describing Potential Problems and Solutions

Symptom	Cause	Possible Remedy
Hearing instrument has no sound.	Hearing instrument is turned off.	Check to ensure that the hearing instrument is turned on.
	Battery is upside down.	Be sure the battery is in the correct orientation (plus, +, side up for custom instruments).
	Battery is depleted or dead.	Replace the battery.
	Microphone protector is plugged.	Consult your audiologist.
	Hearing instruments, earmolds, slim tubes, and/or domes are blocked with earwax.	Clean ear molds and/or domes. Use cleaning wire to dislodge earwax in slim tubes. Use wax loop to remove wax from the sound outlet. Consult your audiologist.
	Hearing instrument is damaged or defective.	Consult your audiologist.
Hearing instrument isn't loud enough.	The volume is set too low.	Turn up the volume. Consult your audiologist for models without a manual volume control or if problem persists.
	Battery is depleted or dead.	Replace the battery.
	Hearing instruments, earmolds, slim tubes, and/or domes are not inserted properly.	Remove and reinsert carefully.
	Hearing instruments, earmolds, slim tubes, and/or domes are blocked with earwax.	Clean earmolds and/or domes. Use cleaning wire to dislodge earwax in slim tubes. Use wax loop to remove wax from the sound outlet. Consult your audiologist.
	Microphone protector is plugged.	Consult your audiologist.
	Your hearing has changed.	Consult your audiologist.
Hearing instruments are whistling.	Noise or whistling when a hand and/or clothing are near ear.	Move hand and/or clothing away from ear.
	Hearing instruments, earmolds, slim tubes, and/or domes are not inserted properly.	Remove and reinsert carefully.
	Hearing instruments, earmolds, slim tubes, and/or domes are blocked with earwax.	Clean earmolds and/or domes. Use cleaning wire to dislodge earwax in slim tubes. Use wax loop to remove wax from the sound outlet. Consult your audiologist.
	Hearing instruments, earmolds, and/or slim tubes are fitting poorly.	Consult your audiologist.
	Battery is depleted or dead.	Replace the battery.
	Microphone protector is plugged.	Consult your audiologist.
Sound is distorted or unclear.	Battery is depleted or dead.	Replace the battery.
	Hearing instruments, earmolds, and/or slim tubes are fitting poorly.	Consult your audiologist.
	Hearing instrument is damaged or defective.	Consult your audiologist.
Performance is inconsistent.	Battery is depleted or dead.	Replace the battery.
	Battery contact is dirty.	Consult your audiologist.

Table 18–1. *continued*

Symptom	Cause	Possible Remedy
Hear beeps.	Battery is depleted or dead.	Replace the battery.
Earmolds, slim tubes, and/or domes are falling out of ear.	Hearing instruments, earmolds, slim tubes, and/or domes are not inserted properly.	Remove and reinsert carefully.
	Hearing instruments, earmolds, and/or slim tubes are fitting poorly.	Consult your audiologist.
The sound is weak on the telephone.	Hearing instrument requires adjustment.	Consult your audiologist.
	Telephone is not positioned properly.	Move telephone receiver around ear for clearer signal.

Source: Adapted from Unitron, Inc.

(do this training over something "soft," as the hearing aids *will be* dropped). Instruct the patient on adjusting the volume control, the remote switch, and any additional switches on his or her hearing aid.

- Demonstrate to patient how to use the telephone with their new hearing aids. It is important to create a real-world situation—for example, have him or her answer a ringing telephone. If the hearing aids have wireless streaming, ensure that the patient knows how to operate this feature. If he or she uses a telecoil (t-coil) or acoustic telephone program, show the patient appropriate activation procedures (e.g., pushing a switch, using a magnet for an auto-coil or auto-phone program) and how to orientate the telephone: (1) near the hearing aid case for a t-coil; (2) near the microphone for an acoustic telephone program; and (3) directly over the opening of the ear canal for open-fitted mini-BTEs in patients with good low-frequency hearing. The figures from the instruction booklet will be helpful for this instruction.
- Instruct patient on care and maintenance. Patients need to be shown how to clean their hearing aids. This involves showing them how cerumen is removed from the end of the hearing aid. Cerumen impaction in the receiver and/or tubing is one of the leading causes of hearing aid failure. If listeners with sufficient dexterity are instructed on how to remove wax from the sound outlet tubing using a wax loop or a cleaning wire in the thin tube of a RITA instrument, they may not need to visit your office as often.
- Educate patient about moisture. This can be problematic, especially for patients living in regions with high humidity. A variety of drying solutions for hearing aids are available, ranging from inexpensive solutions using silica gel crystals to active drying systems. Those systems that use silica gel can typically be reconditioned several times by baking the silica gel insert in an oven or a microwave oven. Remind your patients, however, that only the insert, not the whole system, should be baked! Part of care and maintenance is also instructing patients on how to change the battery and how to store the instruments when they are not being worn.

2. Establish realistic expectations.
   - When fitting new hearing aid users, we suggest that you place them on a wearing schedule. A wearing schedule allows patients to gradually adjust to the new sounds they will hear. As a rule of thumb, new hearing aid users might benefit from first wearing their hearing aids in a relaxed and quiet situation for a few days before wearing them in more

demanding situations like restaurants. New users generally need about a week to begin full-time use. The main point is that they need to go from relatively easy to more difficult listening situations. You may also want to encourage some patients, particularly those who are relatively inactive or who have a "set it and forget it" attitude, to wear their hearing aids as much as possible. In such cases, however, it is important to counsel them to ease into wearing the hearing aid more each day if the "jump-all-in" strategy is not working for them.
- We know that new users often tend to be bothered by louder noises when they start using their hearing aids, even if you programmed gain for loud sounds correctly. It is important to encourage them to attempt to adjust to these sounds over time because their annoyance level will reduce (assuming that their hearing aids were programmed correctly initially).
- We know that many new users expect the hearing aids to provide improved speech understanding in all listening environments—including extreme background noise. During this initial orientation, we recommend that you remind them that there are certain situations in which improvement will be limited. This is also a good time to suggest that there may be additional solutions. For example, you can work with Hearing Assistive Technologies (HATs) if they are dissatisfied with their ability to understand speech in noisy situations. This is a time when self-assessment scales like the COSI can be very helpful (see Chapters 7 and 19).

3. Offer reassurance.
   - In Chapter 3, we discuss the potential negative emotions surrounding hearing loss and the use of hearing aids. Many of these emotions are still present on the day of the fitting. It is important to be patient and to offer support for each individual, especially during the initial foray with hearing aids.
   - If a patient expresses a negative emotional feeling, it is important that we acknowledge this feeling as valid and provide the appropriate empathetic response.

Using a Checklist

Before sending patients home with new hearing aids, it is helpful to review a simple checklist with them. Doing so ensures that you have covered all the main points that often cause confusion or unnecessary stress for patients. Here are some data about informational counseling provided by Margolis (2004a):

- Only about 50% of the information provided by health care providers is retained. Depending on conditions, 40 to 80% of the information may be forgotten immediately.
- Of the information that patients do recall, they remember about half *incorrectly*. So half is forgotten immediately and half of what is remembered is wrong; that only leaves 25% of correct information retained. If you remove 50% of the facts you told the patient about his or her hearing loss and hearing aids, and then distort half the remaining information, the result will be a highly misunderstood message.
- Research has found that after counseling, patients and the health care provider agreed on problems that required follow-up only 45% of the time.

These data about informational counseling certainly point out the importance of sending information home with the patient. A hearing aid checklist is a good starting point. Table 18–2 provides a sample of what can be included in the checklist.

Short-Term Follow-Up Procedures

One procedure that we recommend to help ensure that your patients are adjusting to their new hearing aids is to call them a day or two after the initial fitting. This small gesture is an excellent way to uncover any problems; it could be something as simple as having trouble insert-

Table 18–2. Sample Checklist for Use During Patient Orientation

	Verified prescriptive match of gain/output target using probe-microphone measures
	Ensured that loud sounds were not uncomfortable loud
	Ensured that patient found the quality of the programmed gain and output "acceptable"
	Ensured no acoustic feedback in typical use conditions
	Ensured hearing aids fit properly (not too loose or too tight)
	Instructed patient on insertion and removal of hearing aids; patient now able to put hearing aids in and take them out
	Demonstrated how to use hearing aids with telephones
	Instructed patient on proper use of volume control and/or remote control
	Counseled patient on initial use of the hearing aids and realistic expectations
	Instructed patient on care, cleaning, proper storage, and batteries
	Provided phone number to call with questions or problems

ing the hearing aids into their ears. At the same time, it sends a positive message to each patient by showing that your service doesn't end the moment the patient walks out the door. During this call, it is useful to ask patients questions about how many hours a day they are using the hearing aids, what listening situations they are using them in, and what problems they are having.

Some audiologists say that they simply are too busy to provide these follow-up services to all their patients. If so, we suggest triaging the patients and selecting the ones who might be "at risk" for successful adaptation to hearing aid use based on the results of your pre-fitting testing (see Chapters 5, 6, and 7). For example, you may want to earmark the patients who have a large ANL, unusually low LDLs, a poor score on the QuickSIN, high expectations on the ECHO, unrealistic expectations on the COSI, or other factors, and target them for additional attention during the first week or two after the fitting.

Troubleshooting Common Problems

During the first few weeks of using a hearing aid, it is common for your patients to encounter some problems. Most can be solved through a phone call, text, or e-mail. Others require a patient visit. Some are easy to fix, some require careful thinking, and others simply may not be solvable—a compromise may be necessary. We call this section "troubleshooting" because we first have to define the problem and the cause before initiating treatment. Diagnose the situation incorrectly and apply the wrong treatment, and the patient who walked in with one problem may walk out with two (yes, this can happen). And yes, sometimes even the correct treatment will create a new problem (e.g., solving an earmold comfort problem may result in acoustic feedback). In the following sections, we discuss some of the problems you are likely to see.

The Occlusion Effect

As we review in detail in Chapter 8, the occlusion effect is best described as an echo, "boomy" (as in an overabundance of low-frequency energy), or hollow sensation occurring when the patient is speaking or chewing. Older patients may describe it as sounding as though they are "talking in a barrel" (young people don't talk in barrels as much). This sensation can be highly annoying, and it is more likely to be annoying for patients having better than 30 to 40 dB HL thresholds in the low frequencies. Addressing the possibility of the occlusion effect is part of the verification process, and it is relatively easy to measure with your probe microphone equipment at the time of the fitting. Nevertheless, there will always be situations in which a patient was not bothered by the occlusion effect initially but, after using the hearing aids for a while, finds it distracting. Some patients report using only one hearing aid rather than two to minimize the annoyance, which of course is not the preferred solution. Hopefully, this issue can be resolved during follow-up visits.

The most common way to fix the occlusion effect problem is through venting. When a vent of 2 mm or more is created, sound energy can readily escape. The larger you make the vent, the more likely you are to solve the occlusion problem. If you are using the manufacturer's eartips or domes for the fitting, the same general application applies: Switch to a more open or looser fitting style—more on this later.

In many cases today, the patient is fitted with a mini-BTE and an open or relatively open mold, often a non-custom dome. These couplings don't have a vent per se, but their "openness" (using the most open dome) commonly results in the venting equivalent of a large traditional vent. In some cases, however, what is labeled an "open" fitting tip may be occluding for someone with a small ear canal. Probe microphone measures of the REOG will quickly determine whether the ear canal is open or not. If the fitting is not open, probe microphone measures of the occlusion effect described in Chapter 17 will tell us precisely how much occlusion is present.

The general treatment process for the post-fitting complaint of occlusion goes something like the following:

- Determine that indeed the patient is reporting the occlusion effect, and not a general dissatisfaction related to too much low-frequency amplification:
  - For fittings not expected to be open, measure the magnitude of the occlusion effect using probe microphone techniques.
  - If the occlusion effect is less than 5 dB or so, the complaint may be related to low-frequency gain, not the occlusion effect. Many patients do not find the occlusion effect to be particularly bothersome until it reaches 8 to 10 dB.
- For fittings using an open eartip, determine whether the fitting is open through the use of REOG measures or by measuring the occlusion effect. If the REOG shows the fitting is open (or nearly open) or that the occlusion effect is near zero, reconsider whether the complaint is truly the occlusion effect.
- If the fitting is not open, use increased venting or a different fitting tip to allow for a more open ear canal (again, you can monitor this with REOG measures).
- If the fitting was made more open, before the patient leaves the clinic ensure that two key conditions hold:
  - You have not created a feedback problem.
  - The increased venting did not remove necessary low-frequency information needed for speech understanding (i.e., you still have adequately matched your desired low-frequency gain targets).

Illustrative Case Study

To illustrate how we might handle occlusion effect problems in the clinic, we have a case study of a 55-year-old woman with a unilateral hearing loss (sudden onset at age 52) who was fitted with a mini-BTE RIC instrument using a double-dome eartip (reasonably tight fitting). She had a relatively flat hearing loss (40 dB in the lows, sloping slightly to 65 to 70 dB in the highs). The degree of hearing loss in the lows is what prompted the audiologist to select a relatively tight-fitting dome. The patient returned to the clinic after one week of using her hearing aid, reporting that the hollowness of her own voice was very annoying to the point that she was not using the hearing aid. Here is the step-by-step procedure an audiologist might use to address this patient's issue:

- Step 1. We ask the patient to read a passage that contains vowels that trigger the occlusion effect with the hearing aid on and also turned off. We suggest the following passage (see related Technical Tip): *"Through three cheese trees three free fleas flew."* If the problem is truly an occlusion effect, it should be present not only with the hearing aid on but also with the hearing aid turned off.

- Step 2. For this patient, we want to see whether using a dome that is not as tight fitting can solve the problem—without creating a new one. Our probe microphone equipment will provide the data to ensure that we are approaching things correctly. We first measure the REOG for the dome she is using and for a second dome that does not fit as tightly. We also measure her REUG just to have a reference regarding the degree of openness. These results are shown in Figure 18–1A. Observe that, indeed, the REOG for the replacement dome (Dome B) is more similar to the REUG than the original dome (Dome A), suggesting that the fit is more open. So we know we're going in the right direction.
- Step 3. The REOG, of course, is not a direct measure of the occlusion effect, so our next step is to assess the occlusion effect directly. In the clinic, we may skip Step 2 and jump straight to Step 3 to save time, if we planned to measure the occlusion effect all along.

Figure 18–1B shows the occlusion effect for the open ear (for reference), the original tighter fitting dome (Dome A), and the new dome (Dome B), which is more open. Notice that with the original dome, this patient had more than 20-dB occlusion effect with a peak around 250 Hz. With the new dome, we reduced this occlusion effect by approximately 15 dB. The patient also reports a very noticeable improvement.

- Step 4. Now that we have successfully reduced the occlusion effect, we must determine what effect this looser fitting dome has on the hearing aid output. We expect some reduction in the low frequencies because the increased venting caused the reduction in the occlusion effect. Figure 18–2 shows the speech mapping results (65-dB input; NAL-NL2 targets) for the hearing aid fitted to NL2 with the original dome (Dome A) and the results we have now with the new dome (Dome B). Note that there is a ~10 dB reduction in output for the new dome from 750 to 3000 Hz (and above 4000 Hz), and we also are no longer at target in those frequency ranges. This needs to be

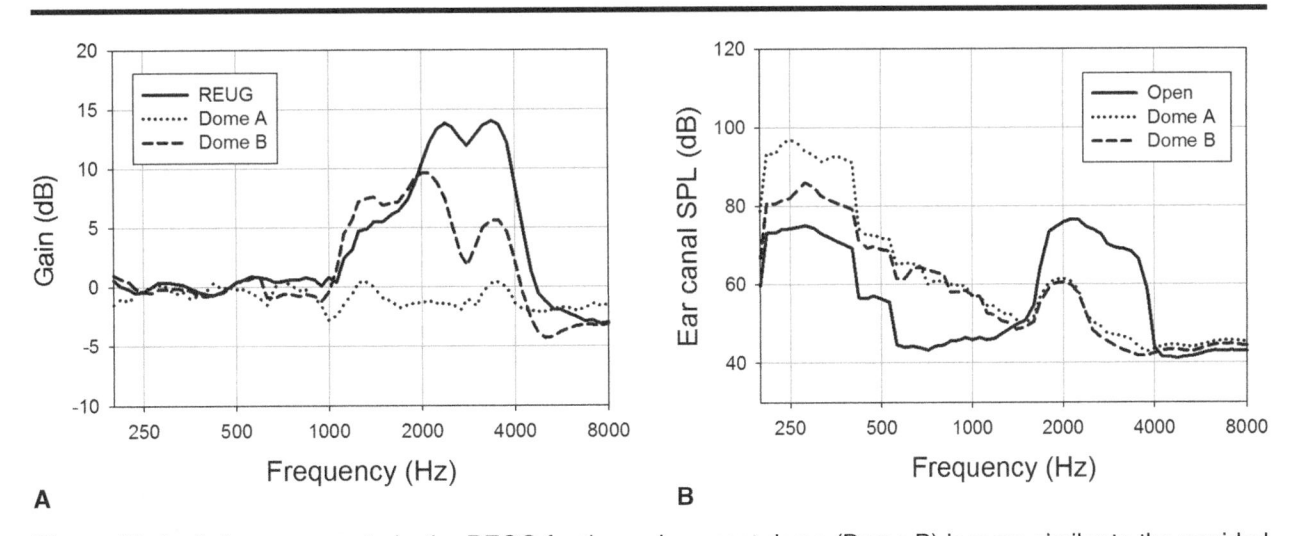

Figure 18–1. A. In our case study, the REOG for the replacement dome (Dome B) is more similar to the unaided curve (REUG) than the original dome (Dome A), suggesting that the fit is more open. **B.** In our case study, the occlusion effect for the open ear (for reference), the original tighter fitting dome (Dome A) and the new dome (Dome B), which is more open, are shown. Notice that with the original dome, our patient had over 20 dB occlusion effect, with a peak around 250 Hz. With the new dome, we reduced this occlusion effect by approximately 15 dB.

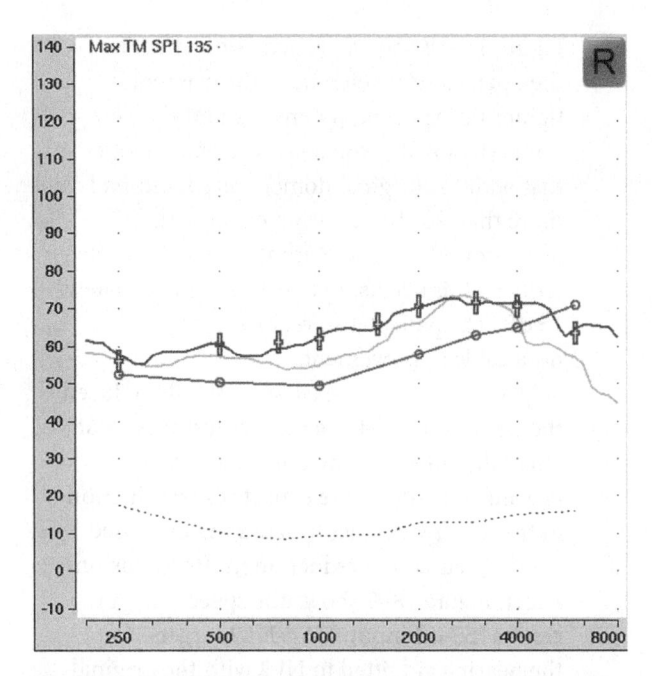

Figure 18–2. Screenshot of speech mapping results (65-dB input; NAL-NL2 targets) for the hearing aid fitted in our case study. Target values are shown as open crosses, original dome (Dome A) output is shown as the darker line, and the new dome (Dome B) output is shown in the lighter line. Eliminating the occlusion effect resulted in a 10 dB drop from the targets (750 to 300 Hz), which must now be corrected.

fixed, so we adjust gain in the hearing aid to rematch prescriptive target values using our probe microphone equipment.
- Step 5. After the hearing aid is reprogrammed, we ensure that this "more open" fitting does not create a feedback issue.

What Doesn't Work Very Well

It is important to talk about treatments that do not reduce the occlusion effect, so let's briefly review what we stated back in Chapter 8. Recall that the effect is produced by a signal traveling along the mandible to the ear canal, *not* a signal traveling through the hearing aid. So it is only logical that changing the programming of the hearing aid (reducing low frequencies, for example) will *not* reduce the occlusion effect. In fact, this approach could have a negative effect if a person needs the low-frequency amplification in order to understand soft speech. If you have a follow-up patient with the complaint of the occlusion effect, and if turning down low-frequency gain made the occlusion effect go away, then the problem probably wasn't the occlusion effect in the first place—it probably was too much gain for the low frequencies, which is a different problem.

Some have suggested that you *add* low-frequency gain to fix the occlusion effect. The rationale is that the gain of the hearing aid will sound more natural than that produced by the occlusion effect (and this may be true because the occlusion effect is different for different vowels). The extra-low frequencies from the occlusion will still be there, but the effect might be masked. The added low frequencies from the hearing aid might work against understanding speech in background noise, however, so again, this isn't the preferred solution.

Acoustic Feedback

Audible acoustic feedback occurs as a result of sound leaking around or through the earmold or ear shell, going back to the microphone inlet at a level in excess of unity gain, and then getting fed back through the hearing aid. The resulting whistling or screeching sound is not only annoying to the user and others, it also contributes to poor sound quality for the user. Also, this feedback often prompts the user to use less gain (turn the hearing aid gain down), which then, of course, reduces the overall benefit of the hearing aid. In some cases, if the hearing aids are known to generate feedback during routine use, the patient will simply stop using them. Feedback problems, therefore, need to be treated effectively.

Most hearing aids have the potential to feed back under certain conditions from time to time. It is important to determine whether the patient's concern is related to conditions known to cause feedback (e.g., when a hand is cupped over the hearing aid that is on the ear, or when the hearing aid is being inserted or removed) or if feedback is occurring during routine use. Feedback is always present but typically does not result in oscillation leading to audible feedback unless the sound level leaking out of the ear exceeds the unamplified sound in the environment at the microphone inlet. Therefore, feedback is most likely to occur when the input is low because the amplitude compression used in hearing aids results in the most gain for the lowest level inputs,

> ### TECHNICAL TIP: OCCLUSION EFFECT OR NOT?
>
> When patients say that their voice sounds "hollow" or "booming," we usually assume it is the occlusion effect, but the complaint could be related to too much low-frequency gain. A quick test is to have the patient read a passage with the hearing aid turned on, and then again with it off. If the hollow sound goes away with the hearing aid turned off, it's *not* the occlusion effect. As we mentioned earlier, we suggest a sentence using words with vowels that trigger the occlusion effect such as, *"Through three cheese trees three free fleas flew."*

and these higher levels of amplification result in more sound leaking out of the ear. As we review in Chapter 10, with a hearing aid with a very low (20 dB SPL) compression threshold and a high (3.2:1) compression ratio, gain might be only 20 to 25 dB for average speech-level inputs, but might reach 40 dB or more for the lowest input levels.

Today's feedback reduction algorithms have significantly reduced the occurrence of feedback-related post-fitting problems. But, even when the audiologist carefully ensures that no problem with acoustic feedback existed on the day of the fitting, some patients will return with feedback issues, and some troubleshooting may be necessary. Here are some reasons why feedback that did not exist initially may be present following the fitting:

- The patient quickly adjusted to amplification and is now using more gain than he or she considered acceptable on the day of the fitting. That is, the patient is turning up the volume.
- A common use condition, such as listening on the telephone, was not tested on the day of the fitting.
- At the time of the fitting, the patient was never in a room as quiet as one he or she experiences at home (e.g., quiet living room). If ambient noise is decreased, the gain of the hearing aid increases, which, in some cases, is just enough to cause feedback.
- The audiologist activated an "automatic gain increase" algorithm, which increased the output gradually over time.
- The patient is not putting the earmold or eartip or hearing aid (in the case of a custom fitting) in the ear canal appropriately. The placement usually is not deep enough, which is particularly common with custom earmolds and hearing aids, and the instrument can easily work out of the ears of some users. For RIC instruments, the incorrect length of the receiver wire linkage also can cause problems. Patients using non-custom eartips may also experience this problem or may be inserting the eartip too far or at an angle so that the sound outlet is near an ear canal wall, thus reflecting sound out of the ear.
- There is a defect with the earmold plumbing or a crack in tubing, loose tubing, and so on. This is most likely after a significant wearing period (i.e., six months or longer). Some designs of receiver-in-the-aid (RITA) instruments seem particularly vulnerable to this problem because the linkage between the thin tubing and hearing aid body breaks down with use, resulting in leakage.
- The thin wire or tubing becomes stiffer with age, increasing the likelihood of mechanical coupling and resulting in mechanical feedback. Designs of RIC instruments appear to be particularly vulnerable to this problem.
- Excessive cerumen develops in the ear canal, which reflects enough sound to cause feedback.

Treating Feedback Problems on Post-Fitting Visits

When a patient returns with a feedback problem, the first step is to be sure that this indeed is a problem that has a negative impact on routine hearing aid use, and is not an isolated occurrence (e.g., "When I'm standing near a wall and then lean my head against the wall,

I get a whistle"). Once it has been established that it is a real problem, we suggest first examining the easy-to-fix possible causes, such as excessive cerumen in the ear canal, a problem with the tubing or earmold, or poor placement of the earmold or hearing aid by the patient. Another easy fix for RIC and RITA instruments is to bend the wire or tubing to ensure that the sound outlet is directed away from the ear canal wall. Sometimes this bending is made easier and more permanent by applying a little heat (e.g., some clinicians use a hair dryer on RITA or standard BTE tubing). When these factors are eliminated, the following treatments can be considered:

- Extend the depth of the ear canal portion of the earmold (or custom hearing aid). This usually reduces the leakage. It means another patient visit, however, as this is not a "while you wait" fix.
- Fit an earmold with less leakage, which could be as simple as using a different fitting tip or dome or changing a select-a-vent. With the popularity of today's open fittings, many times this means abandoning the use of the non-custom tips or domes and ordering a custom earmold for the patient. This treatment, of course, is working counter to our previous treatment recommended for the occlusion effect, as you will probably have a fitting that is more closed.
- Increase the aggressiveness of the digital feedback suppression algorithm (DFS). Some manufacturers include multiple settings. The most aggressive settings may generate additional artifact on their own, however, so it is important to ensure that this fix does not create a new problem by decreasing sound quality or introducing annoying audible artifacts.
- Activate digital frequency compression (if available). Although not an optimal solution, as it may result in reduced sound quality for some listeners if activated too aggressively, many of these methods (those that do not maintain the original high-frequency amplification), may allow a little more gain before feedback with the same venting configuration. See Chapter 11 regarding the pros and cons of activating frequency compression.
- Reduce gain in the area of the feedback. Throughout this book, we repeatedly stress the importance of audibility; there are times when a slight tradeoff or compromise might be necessary. That is, if reducing gain by 5 dB at a peak around 4000 Hz means that the patient can now turn up overall gain by 5 dB, the net effect for speech understanding probably will be positive. Moreover, in some cases, feedback is occurring at a frequency where the chances of audibility for average speech are slim anyway (i.e., the high-frequency speech inputs plus the hearing aid gain at these frequencies do not exceed the patient's thresholds). Remember, as quantified by SII and AI procedures, the higher frequencies (above 4500 Hz) do not carry a lot of important speech information. Therefore, it is often best to try reducing gain in the highest frequency band first and then work your way down. Furthermore, if feedback primarily occurs in quiet environments, reducing gain only for soft inputs (often the outcome is to reduce gain and increase the compression threshold) can sometimes eliminate feedback problems without compromising gain for average and loud speech inputs. Many hearing aids have a "feedback manager" algorithm that finds the feedback location and automatically reduces gain (Figure 18–3). Generally, we find these strategies to be a little overaggressive and we prefer reducing the gain ourselves—probe microphone testing should reveal the frequency at which feedback is occurring. Or, you can compare the findings of the open loop gain measure to the real-ear output.

Sounds Are Too Loud

The first two common problems reviewed in this chapter mainly deal with mechanical solutions requiring the clinician to make a physical change in the earmold or shell to solve them. We now turn our attention to some other common problems that may require programming adjustments.

In Chapter 5, we discuss how the LDLs are measured during pre-fitting testing, and in Chapters 15 and 17,

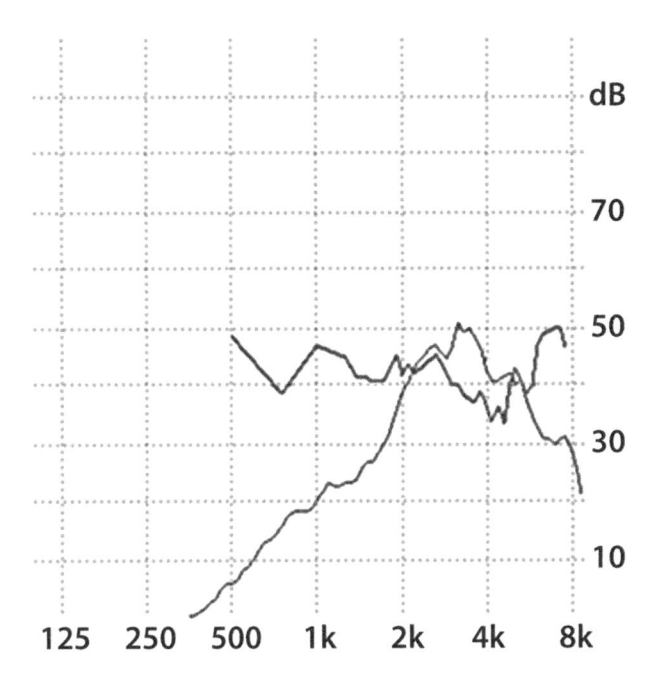

Figure 18–3. Example of open-loop gain measured for an open-fit hearing aid in which feedback was a problem. The frequencies at which feedback will occur (or is occurring) are where the bottom curve and upper curve are similar—in this case, about 2500 to 5000 Hz.

we discussed how loudness is verified at the time the hearing aid is fitted. Consider that we first adjust the MPO based on the patient's frequency-specific LDLs (by adjusting channel-specific AGCo), we program WDRC using a validated prescriptive method, we conduct probe microphone measures to verify both gain and output, and then we conduct aided behavioral loudness measures to account for other summation and signal-specific factors. All these tests are conducted (or at least should be conducted) before the patient leaves the clinic with the hearing aids. You might ask, "After all that, how could there be problems with loudness perceptions?" Trust us, it still happens.

Later in this chapter, we discuss the issue of adaptation for loudness, but for now let's assume that the perceptions reported by the patient a few weeks after the initial fitting are not going to change. On the post-fitting visit, a comment from the patient may be something like this: "I really hear a lot of things I've never heard before, and I do think I'm doing better understanding speech, but things are a little too loud." So your first task in solv-

ing this problem is to determine what these "things" are and what are the bothersome intensity level and frequency range. Some patients mean that they now hear their own footsteps when they are walking on carpet (yes, people really do complain of this!). Other patients might be referring to the crowd noise at their grandson's basketball game. Two very different loudness issues with different treatment strategies (*if* your strategy is to change hearing aid programming). In general, we want to know if the "too loud" is related to soft-level sounds, average sounds, or loud sounds.

For starters, let's consider a problem with loud inputs. One might first assume that the MPO was not set correctly. First it is important to determine whether the sounds reported are truly uncomfortable (#7 on the Cox Contour Anchor List—see Chapter 5) or if the sounds are just louder than what the patient is accustomed to but are really still okay (#6 on the Cox Contour Anchor List). If, after repeating the aided loudness testing we discuss in Chapter 15, loud environmental sounds are rated #6, then your treatment might be nothing more than counseling; the patient simply needs to know that the world is louder than what he or she remembers.

If, however, a patient is complaining about loud sounds being too loud and the loudness ratings are indeed #7, you have three choices regarding how to fix the problem (see related Technical Tip). But first, you need to determine the frequency range of the signals the patient is complaining about. If they are broadband, the adjustments will be over the full range of frequencies. In some cases, however (e.g., emergency sirens, dogs yapping, the bass drum at a club), a general frequency range (typically higher or lower) can be identified. In such cases, you may try making adjustments to the gain, compression, or MPO controls only in the target frequency range—if frequency-specific controls are available (some AGCo circuits are single-channel).

Loudness issues regarding soft and average inputs are a little more difficult to deal with. If a patient states certain sounds, when amplified, are uncomfortable, this is something that needs to be dealt with promptly. LDLs do not generally increase with hearing aid use, and the problem is not going to go away. Loudness perceptions for soft and average inputs, however, sometimes change over the course of getting used to amplification. Let's consider a new hearing aid user, fitted to NAL-NL2, who returns and says that both soft and average sounds are too loud. We really don't know if he or she just needs

> ## TECHNICAL TIP: FIXING THE "LOUD SOUNDS ARE TOO LOUD" PROBLEM
>
> As we've discussed, a common problem reported by patients at follow-up visits is that loud sounds are too loud. Once you establish that these loud sounds truly are too loud (#7 on Cox Loudness Chart), you can fix the problems in three different ways:
>
> - The preferred method is to lower the hearing aid MPO. Do this in 2 dB increments while presenting a loud signal to the patient until the patient gives you a #6 rating. In some instances, even when the MPO is at its lowest setting, the patient still states that loud sounds are #7 (uncomfortable). Before going any further and potentially messing up the entire fitting, turn the hearing aid off and present the same signal. In some cases, if it is an open fitting and the patient has unusually low LDLs, the direct sound to the tympanic membrane (TM) is causing the discomfort. Obviously, in these cases, changing the hearing aid setting will not make things better.
> - Assuming the preceding situation is not the case, another method to lower the output for high inputs is to increase (make larger) the WDRC ratio (e.g., go from 2:1 to 3:1). With most hearing-aid-fitting software, this problem can be addressed by adjusting the control called "gain for loud sounds." Doing so generally increases the compression ratio over some range of input levels (depending on the specific implementation and the number of compression kneepoints within each channel). Unfortunately, this may (depending on the specific manufacturer's design) also lower the output for average speech, and now average speech might be lower than desired levels (typically this will initially be the match-to-target gain for average input levels), something you'll need to verify again.
> - Finally, lowering overall gain, of course, decreases the output for loud sounds. This is the least desirable option because it might place average speech below the patient's preferred listening level, and could very well make soft speech inaudible. If the patient has a way of lowering the volume of his or her hearing aids, this is probably what the patient is already doing. Hopefully this solution can be avoided.

a few more weeks to adjust to amplification or if the patient's preferred listening levels are low—perhaps a standard deviation or so below the NAL-NL2 average. Because preferred listening levels represent an *average*, several patients will fall into this category. Do we simply reduce gain and make this person happy, knowing that we likely will also be reducing speech recognition? Or do we make no program changes and use the "don't worry, you'll get used to it" counseling adage? This approach could easily backfire and result in rejection of hearing aids during this important early adjustment period. Remember that, even though speech recognition benefit typically decreases with decreasing gain, an in-the-drawer hearing aid provides no benefit at all! Tough decisions.

Continued Problems Understanding Speech in Noise

Many, if not most, patients purchase hearing aids because of problems associated with understanding

> **POINTS TO PONDER: LOUDNESS—
> THE CLINIC VERSUS THE REAL WORLD**
>
> We typically do considerable testing to be sure that the loudness of the hearing aids is set appropriately before the patient leaves the office; this includes testing pre-fitting LDLs and aided loudness measures for speech and environmental sounds. So it is puzzling that patients sometimes return to the office saying that loud sounds are too loud (although this certainly occurs much more often if pre-fitting LDLs are *not* obtained). Why, after this testing, do patients still occasionally have loudness issues? We have a couple of theories why this might happen. First, the clinic is a rather sterile environment for the patient to make decisions. They may give "expected" responses. Additionally, we ask them to make a quick decision about a task that they may not completely understand. (It's like when you try on a pair of shoes in a store, think they are okay, and purchase them; then after walking around your house with them on, you decide they really didn't fit correctly.) The patient's real-world experiences may be different enough from what was experienced in the clinic to alter his or her perceptions of aided loudness. Maybe you didn't present obnoxious noises (which commonly are more annoying and rated louder)?
>
> A related factor is that in a relaxed listening situation, the patient has some time to evaluate independently all the different factors that were packed into a 15-minute segment in the clinic. Audibility of speech? Understanding of speech? Speech quality? Background noise? Given the expense involved in purchasing a pair of hearing aids, it is reasonable for the patient now to want each one of these factors—along with loudness perceptions—optimized.

> **TECHNICAL TIP: DON'T FORGET YOUR PAL!**
>
> As we discussed previously, when a patient returns with loudness issues, it's a good idea to repeat the aided loudness scaling using the Cox Contour Anchors used during the verification process. But other tools are also helpful. As we discuss in Chapter 19, the PAL is an outcome measure specifically designed to assess the patient's judgments in the real world. Before making programming changes, take a look at the PAL findings from the patient's aided experiences. If the patient reports loudness impressions that are similar to those of normal-hearing individuals, then the treatment might simply be counseling rather than tweaking of the programming. The aided aversiveness or AV subscale of the APHAB may also provide useful information related to loud inputs. It is probable that the aided AV scores will be worse than at pre-fitting, so it is best to compare your patient's findings with those of successful hearing aid users, rather than with his or her pre-fitting score.

speech in the presence of background noise. Understandably, this is then one of the first things that the patient evaluates following the purchase of hearing aids. When the aided performance does not meet the patient's expectations, he or she is back in your office hoping you can make things better. This is probably the most common troubleshooting problem you will encounter, and it is likely to be the most challenging. There are many underlying components to the problem and there may not be a simple solution.

Here are a few things to consider:

- What were the patient's pre-fitting scores on the ECHO or other expectations profile? Were expectations for speech understanding reasonable?
- What goals did the patient have regarding speech understanding as identified by the COSI or other tools? Are those goals currently being met? Have the patient's expectations changed after using the hearing aids?
- Was the patient's pre-fitting speech recognition in noise ability measured by the QuickSIN, WIN, or some other measure? If scores were poor relative to the normative data, is the patient now expecting to understand speech in very adverse SNRs? (For example, a patient with an unaided QuickSIN SNR Loss of +12 dB, even when fitted with the best technology, will not do well in a busy restaurant where the SNR may be approaching 0 dB.)
- Conversely, if speech understanding in noise was better than average or at least average, and current listening situations are typical, question whether the hearing aids are programmed correctly.
- Are the hearing aids programmed to validated targets, or did the patient request (and receive) large reductions in gain, thus limiting the potential for benefit?
- Does the patient have a VC? If so, is it being used appropriately)? Check the data logging. Data logging can also reveal the possibility of other common problems, such as a patient who has been wearing an instrument with a dead battery or who is not switching programs appropriately (e.g., t-coil for everyday use or nonuse of manual programs for noisy and other specific listening environments). Data logging might also reveal that the patient rarely is in background noise and, therefore, the problem is not as great as expressed.
- Is it possible a special feature is working against speech understanding? For example, some feedback reduction algorithms, when implemented, alter the frequency response. Frequency lowering, if too aggressive, can affect speech understanding negatively. Noise reduction, if too aggressive, can limit speech understanding at the beginning of utterances. Even though directional microphones can improve speech recognition when facing a talker, they can be detrimental when attempting to understand a talker who is behind the hearing aid wearer.

This is only a partial list of what needs to be considered. At some point, it's going to boil down to the question: "Do I need to change the programmed features, gain, or output of the hearing aids?" If the answer is "yes," then what do you do? In general, we think (and the data strongly support the contention) that more audibility is good for speech understanding. If the patient initially was fitted below typical target-gain levels, then increasing gain, particularly in the higher frequencies (1500 to 3000 Hz), will usually improve speech recognition. But what if the patient already is fitted to prescribed target levels? Is it still okay to increase gain? Maybe, but more often than not this may lead to patient complaints related to the hearing aid being too loud; there also are times when too much gain reduces speech understanding. In difficult cases, additional speech testing can be of assistance (see Chapter 15).

Of course, the starting point for resolving the speech-perception-in-noise problems is ensuring that the patient has realistic expectations and that optimum performance is yet to be reached. If gain is appropriate based on prescriptive targets, expectations are reasonable, and speech recognition in noise remains at unsatisfactory levels, the most effective solution involves improving SNR through hearing assistive technology (HAT) solutions. Although not always accepted well by patients for reasons related to cosmetics and convenience, remote microphones, including "spouse microphones," FM systems, and handheld beamformers (enhanced directionality), can lead to tremendous improvements in speech recognition in noisy environments, particularly when a single talker is the target. A well-motivated patient will often consider one of these options if he or she continues to struggle with understanding speech in noisy environments. Furthermore, advances in spouse mics—including reduced cost, automatic activation, improved cosmetics, and the implementation of multiple microphones with automatic switching between them—are expected to increase

> **THINGS TO REMEMBER: REMOTE MICROPHONES AND SNR IMPROVEMENT**
>
> We mention the advantages of using remote microphones as a solution to understanding speech in background noise problems. For some listening situations, the improvement in SNR is very dramatic, and often the user of this technology will understand speech better in that situation than someone with normal hearing. This was demonstrated by Thibodeau (2014), who compared the performance of adults with moderate-to-severe bilateral hearing impairment using remote microphone technology to a group of young adults with normal hearing. Sentence recognition in quiet and in noise and subjective ratings were obtained in three conditions of wireless signal processing. The results showed that performance by the hearing-impaired listeners, when using the remote microphone technology, was up to 62 percentage points better than people with normal hearing in the same high-noise condition!

acceptance of this technology. Other HAT technologies like TV listeners can also be useful for specific listening situations. The bottom line is that it is important that we do not forget about technology solutions beyond the hearing aid that are extremely effective in addressing patient complaints related to speech understanding in noise.

Problems Understanding on the Telephone

For many patients, understanding speech using the telephone is as important as general conversations. As we discuss in Chapter 14, providing the patient with a telephone solution and then confirming that this solution is working for the patient are parts of the overall fitting process. This solution could involve the telecoil of the hearing aid, simply pressing the phone to the ear (with an open-fitted hearing aid), using the hearing aid as an amplifier (acoustic telephone), using a speakerphone, or using some type of wireless streaming solution. In addition, these solutions are activated in a variety of different manners, including a button or a remote control, proximity to a magnet (auto-coil and auto-phone), and a user switch or toggle on the hearing aid.

With all of these possibilities, a number of trade-offs, confusions, and complications can arise. One of the most common confusions for patients relates to remembering how to use the technology best. Particularly for new hearing aid users, but also for patients who are using a new telephone technology, reinstruction at a subsequent office visit may be necessary. Commonly, reinstruction includes how to activate the technology (e.g., which button to push, where to place and how to use the activating magnet, what to do if it is not activating automatically) and use of any intermediary streaming devices. In the following sections, we describe a few other common problems that are encountered after the patient leaves the office.

Phone Placement

One common issue that may require instruction or reinstruction is placement of the phone for optimal reception. Figure 18–4 shows examples of signal-to-noise ratios for two patients, one who was more successful at telephone placement (Good Location) and one who was less successful at telephone placement (Poor Location) relative to the t-coil. That difference in SNR could be the difference in acceptable conversations on the phone and failure to converse on the phone.

Although it is common practice to train a hearing aid user to angle the telephone correctly to use a t-coil most effectively or to place the telephone outlet near the hearing aid microphone (but not so near as to engender feedback) when using an acoustic phone program, special considerations sometimes arise when using the popular mini-BTE styles with relatively open, or fully open, fittings. The patients fitted with such devices typically

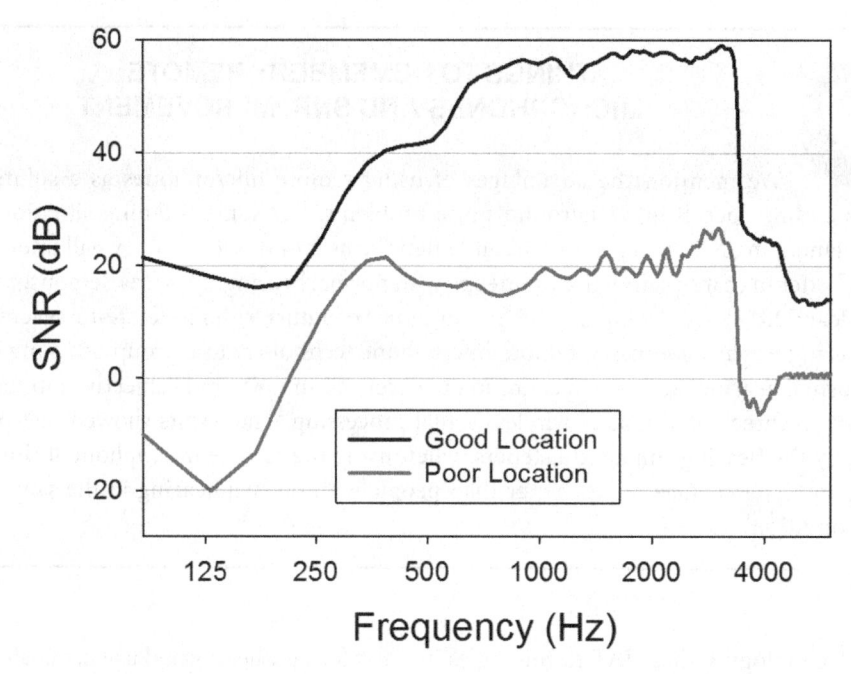

Figure 18–4. Example of signal-to-noise ratios for two patients, one who was more successful at telephone placement (Good Location) and one who was less successful at telephone placement (Poor Location) relative to the t-coil. (Adapted from Picou & Ricketts, 2013, with permission.)

have low-frequency hearing thresholds near normal and may report little or no difficulty on the telephone. Consequently, they may or may not be instructed on telephone use during the fitting appointment. Conversely, if these listeners are past users of other hearing aid-based telephone solutions, they may have been (for example) instructed on how to hold the telephone to optimize use of an acoustic telephone program. If these hearing aid wearers are fitted with wireless telephone streaming technologies, they will no longer have to worry about where the phone is as it will likely work just as well if it remains in a purse or pocket. Open-fit hearing aid wearers may complain about the sound quality of wirelessly streamed signals, however, because of the lack of low-frequency transmission (lost through venting) and limited subsequent bandwidth (see Chapter 17).

So what is the best configuration for users of open-fit mini-BTE hearing aids with low-frequency hearing thresholds that are near normal? We find that most patients are happiest when bypassing the hearing aid altogether. That is, they are simply instructed to press the phone to their ear. In fact, research suggests this solution will lead to the best SNR and, therefore, the best speech recognition in noise for this population and type of fitting (Picou & Ricketts, 2011). Furthermore, this solution is expected to provide the best sound quality because it retains low-frequency energy that is lost through the vent when routed through the hearing aid.

Using the Acoustic Telephone Program in Background Noise

As the degree of hearing loss increases, particularly in the low frequencies, it is likely the amount of venting will decrease and consequently more amplified low-frequency sound bandwidth will be maintained. As discussed in Chapter 8, one phone solution for such hearing aid wearers is an acoustic telephone program. Such programs are being used increasingly because modern feedback-suppression algorithms can limit feedback as long as not too much gain is required. That said, these algorithms often do not provide the SNR benefits associated with a t-coil or more modern wireless streaming technologies. In fact, as shown in Figure 18–5, research

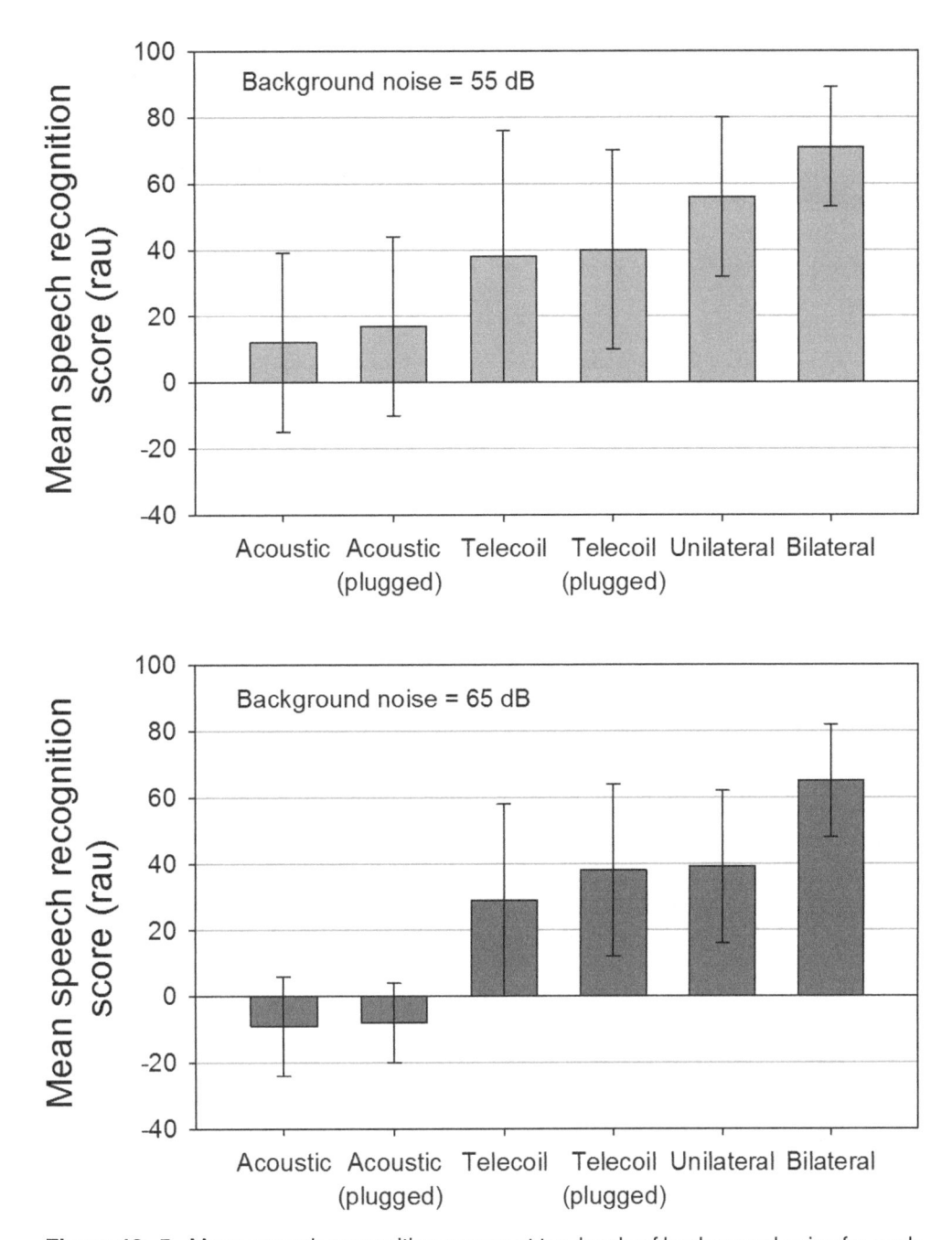

Figure 18–5. Mean speech recognition scores at two levels of background noise for each of six telephone coupling options: acoustic, acoustic with the opposite ear plugged, telecoil, telecoil with the opposite ear plugged, unilateral streaming, and bilateral streaming. (Adapted from Picou & Ricketts, 2013, with permission.)

suggests an acoustic telephone program is not useful at all in noisy environments for listeners with more severe hearing loss (Picou & Ricketts, 2013). Therefore, we need to explore other options for patients who are dissatisfied with the performance of an acoustic phone program in noisy environments, such as the following:

- **Phone placement.** Counsel patients to place the phone directly over the ear if low-frequency hearing is near normal (as described earlier).
- **Phone equipment choices.** Use an amplified telephone or speaker phone.
- **Signal choices.** Switch the patient to t-coil or other wireless streaming technologies for telephone use.

This same research suggests it is important to make sure the listener can accurately hold the telephone in the correct position to optimize reception from the t-coil. Although the SNR delivered to the patient's ear for t-coil or any wireless streaming strategy should be approximately equivalent, assuming optimal orientation (Figure 18–6), variations in exactly how the patient holds the telephone can greatly affect the SNR of the t-coil signal delivered in noisy rooms. This may be difficult for some listeners; therefore, a wireless streaming solution that is relatively insensitive to the specific angle and position of the telephone (as long as it is near enough) may be preferable.

Maintaining Balance Between Phone Use and Environmental Monitoring

The most advanced telephone-listening strategies allow a wide range of configuration options that vary greatly in their effects on listening. The most important changes are related to signal routing and environmental microphones, specifically: (1) Signals from the telephone can be routed to one or both ears, and (2) One or both hearing aid microphones can be activated for environmental monitoring, sometimes with varying strength. So what is the best setting? It really depends on the hearing aid wearer's listening needs and his or her ability to communicate in a noisy environment. It is sometimes difficult to determine the answer prior to the fitting. Does the patient often listen on the phone in very noisy environments and have considerable trouble understanding in background noise? If so, the existing data clearly demonstrate that the best outcomes occur when the telephone signal is routed to both ears and the environmental microphones are disabled (Picou & Ricketts, 2011, 2013). If we apply this configuration, particularly with limited venting, however, monitoring the outside

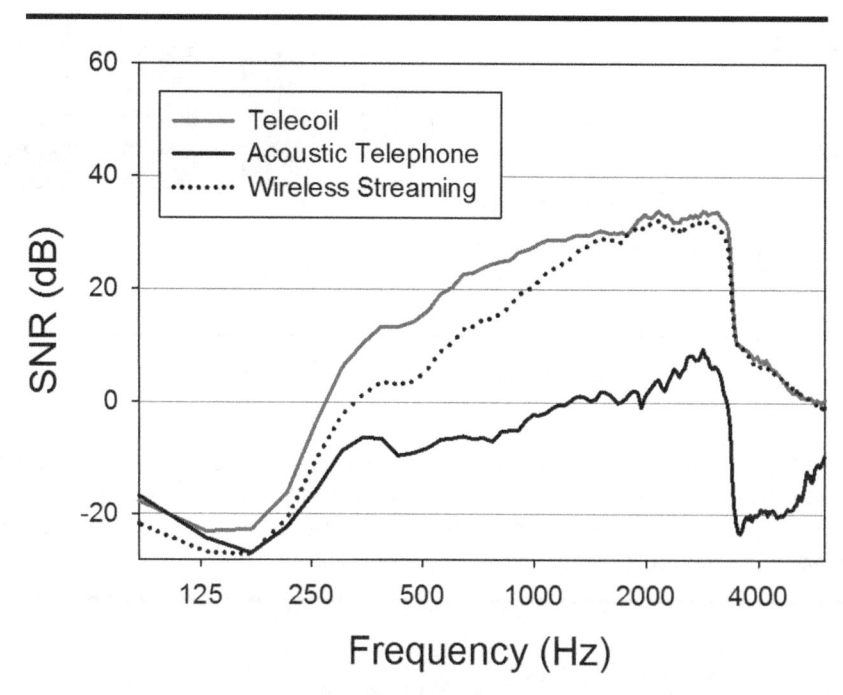

Figure 18–6. Example of the signal-to-noise ratio advantage for patients across three different coupling options with optimal positioning of the hearing aid. (Adapted from Picou & Ricketts, 2013, with permission.)

> **POINTS TO PONDER: PLUG THE OTHER EAR WHEN LISTENING ON THE PHONE IN NOISE?**
>
> Most of us have tried plugging our other ear when listening on the phone in noise to try to hear the phone signal better. Does it really help us understand the person talking on the phone? To examine the effectiveness of such strategies, Picou and Ricketts (2011) tested a variety of configurations for the contralateral ear to be used in conjunction with unilateral wireless telephone streaming. These configurations included (1) leaving the hearing aid in and turned on, (2) taking the hearing aid out, and (3) plugging the ear. Somewhat surprisingly, they found no differences at all among these strategies for speech recognition in noise. We really don't know why people continue to plug their ear given these findings, but there must be an advantage. We speculate that it may help with concentrating on the telephone signal, or perhaps even help to reduce informational masking from other talkers in the environment. Regardless, it does not appear to be as effective as we hoped!

environment may be difficult. Consequently, many patients may prefer to activate the hearing aid microphones on one or both sides and/or route the telephone signal to just one ear, even though doing so makes it more difficult to communicate in noise on the phone. So it is useful to quantify how much difficulty the individual patient has in real-world noisy environments on the phone and the importance of monitoring external sounds while listening on the phone. Sometimes this is a balancing act requiring a little trial and error. For some patients, routing the signal bilaterally and then activating the environmental microphone of one of the hearing aids can provide a good starting place.

Taking Time to Adjust

So far, we have reviewed a few factors that may need some attention in the first few weeks following the hearing aid fitting. We want to address one more issue that is not troubleshooting per se but, to some extent, is related to possible troubleshooting issues. "Don't worry, you'll get used to it after a while" is a counseling phrase used by nearly everyone who has ever fitted hearing aids. In the phrase "get used to it," the "it" could mean hearing aid noise, ambient noise, environmental sounds, unwanted high-frequency gain, too much gain for loud sounds, listening at higher levels in general, or a number of other things. The assumption behind this counseling statement is that the hearing aids have been programmed correctly, and that the patient will experience some degree of acceptance over time to the bothersome acoustic signal(s). After a few weeks of hearing aid use, this fitting and counseling technique usually results in one of four outcomes:

- The patient adapts to whatever it was that was bothersome. All is well.
- The patient is still bothered by the annoying acoustic feature(s) (maybe a little less than initially), but the benefits of using hearing aids outweigh the nuisance, so he or she is a fairly happy full-time hearing aid user.
- The patient is still bothered by the annoying acoustic feature(s), so much so that he or she reserves use of his or her hearing aid for isolated listening situations and is a fairly unhappy part-time hearing aid user.
- The patient is still bothered by the annoying acoustic feature(s) and either has returned the hearing aids or keeps them in his or her possession but never uses them.

It is obvious that the third and fourth choices are undesirable for the audiologist and, most importantly, for the patient. So what should we do to prevent this from happening?

As we discuss in Chapter 14, in most cases we start the fitting process by programming the hearing aids to a validated prescriptive fitting strategy. Substantial research has indicated that these strategies (e.g., NAL-NL2 or DSL V5) provide an appropriate fit for *average* patients, given their specific audiometric characteristics. An appropriate fit refers to maximizing speech intelligibility, obtaining acceptable speech quality, restoring normal loudness perceptions, or some combination of these and other factors. It is difficult to know, however, at the time of the fitting whether the real-world environments will result in the right level of loudness for new hearing aid users. As we mention in Chapter 16, most manufacturers believe that for the new user, prescriptive fittings such as the NAL-NL2 may not be appropriate for Day 1, but rather are more appropriate as a *final* fit after some period of adjusting to the louder levels. The question then becomes: are these validated prescriptive fitting targets a reasonable *starting* point for the average patient? Should there be a difference between first fit and final fit? And if so, can we assume that some sort of auditory adaptation is going to take place? Manufacturers have provided options for clinicians that allow for reduced gain/output based on previous hearing aid experience. As we discuss in Chapter 11, there also are algorithms that increase gain automatically over the first few weeks of hearing aid use.

Terminology

Both manufacturers and audiologists have used several terms to describe what happens (or at least usually happens) when perceptual judgments change after the fitting of hearing aids. Here is a review of some of the commonly used terms:

- Acclimatization. Adapting to a new environment (in this case, auditory) or, as defined by Darwin, the process of inuring to a new climate or the state of being so inured. We posit that acclimatization can occur when an auditory system is exposed to novel stimulation, as is the case with cochlear implant users. There is an assumption or implication of some "brain rewiring" occurring to allow for the change in perception.
- Adaptation. The process of adapting to something such as environmental conditions (in this case, auditory); the responsive adjustment of a sense organ. This is a reasonable term (suggested as a replacement for acclimatization in 1995 by Palmer), as it has long been used in reference to the eye. In the world of auditory physiology, however, that term carries a specific meaning related to a reduction in neural firings following repeated stimulation.
- Adjustment. Making or becoming suitable; adjusting or accommodating to circumstances. This term also describes the process quite well as long as we mean adjustment to the hearing aid rather than adjustments *made* to the hearing aid.

So, we have several terms that can be used to describe the patient's experience of growing accustomed to sounds processed through hearing aids. For the most part, we believe the new user faces a period of adjustment to the device *and* to the sounds that are now available.

Clinical Relevance

An adjustment period *is* something to think about following the fitting of hearing aids because of the wide range of acoustic changes to which the patient must adjust. These changes range from low-level ambient noise to louder-than-usual soft sounds to the newly acquired audibility of high-frequency speech signals. The underlying mechanisms may not be the same for all of these conditions during the adjustment period, but we need to be cognizant of the need for concern.

Soft Input Levels

For the past few decades, hearing aids typically have been fitted with compression kneepoints of 40 to 50 dB SPL or lower. As we discussed previously (see Chapter 10), the lower the kneepoint, the more gain we provide for low-level sounds. This, of course, is good for the audibility of soft speech, but often patients are not happy with the increased loudness of soft environmental sounds. When counseling patients about this issue, it is sometimes useful to say something like the following: "You have to hear what you don't want to hear to know what you don't want to hear."

> **KEY CONCEPT: ACCLIMATIZATION OR JUST PLAIN ADJUSTMENT?**
>
> The notion of auditory acclimatization has been used relating to hearing aids since at least the 1930s. At that time, it was believed that, through continued training that required people to listen to sounds above their LDLs, we could expand their dynamic range. In 1993, however, the term "acclimatization" became much more popular in clinical parlance when Stuart Gatehouse published an article showing that, when individuals were fitted with increased high-frequency gain, word recognition improved significantly following the use of hearing aids but only after several weeks of hearing aid use. He termed this *perceptual acclimatization*. These data were quickly adapted for counseling purposes by almost everyone selling hearing aids, as it was a pseudo-scientific way to explain to people why they didn't understand as well as they thought they should in the first few weeks following the fitting of their hearing aids. A consensus conference was held in Copenhagen, Denmark, in 1995, at which the following statement was formulated by the 15 international researchers in participation: "Auditory acclimatization is a systematic change in auditory performance with time, linked to a change in the acoustic information available to the listener. It involves an improvement in performance that cannot be attributed to task, procedural, or training effects" (Arlinger et al., 1996, p. 87S). The effect has been documented to be in the range of 0% to 10% change in speech perception ability across a wide range of speech materials and presentation conditions. This magnitude of change is unlikely to be observed in a clinical setting but may be recorded across larger group data.
>
> We share the opinion of many authors that new users of amplification often require some time to adjust—and even report improvement in listening ability—but we attribute that to factors such as increased confidence or familiarity with their hearing aids. As we discuss later in this chapter, most recent data suggest there is no evidence of acclimatization in the form of improved speech recognition with modern hearing aids. Today the term is often misused to mean "adjustment to" a hearing aid and its processing or features. In concert with the intended definition, acclimatization is rarely observed in a clinical setting. This is due to (1) insensitivity of our speech tests to show real differences of 2 to 5%, and (2) the reality that individuals with mild to moderately severe hearing loss who use hearing aids don't actually have "novel" stimulation to which they can adjust. That is, as per the consensus group, acclimatization can occur when the auditory system must recode novel stimulation. That recoding (rewiring) process takes an extended period of time. Cochlear implant patients are often shown to have changes in speech perception ability over an extended period of time because the patient is better able to code the novel stimulation of the electrical impulses—this is a good example of acclimatization. Most hearing aid users are provided with increased audibility, not novel stimulation. One might argue that the increased audibility provides for novel stimulation, but that is the case only for the more severely impaired hearing aid recipients. The term has also been used to describe adjustment to newfound loudness, audibility of soft sounds, and so on. We posit that what is really happening here is better labeled "adjustment" because it is unlikely that any brain rewiring is happening for the majority of our hearing aid patients.

In our counseling, we often use the example of a person who lives by a railroad track and after several months, no longer hears the trains. A good story, but does this really happen with hearing aids? Mueller and Powers (2001) reported on a study in which new hearing aid users and experienced users were fitted with new hearing aids with gain for soft inputs programmed according to DSL 4.1 or NAL-NL1 fitting targets. All subjects were given the PAL on the day of the fitting and at one, four, and eight weeks after the fitting. Within one week of using a hearing aid, PAL scores for those subjects experienced with using hearing aids, the four items related to soft sounds fell within the expected range (Figure 18–7). In contrast, even after four weeks of hearing aid use, the new hearing aid users still showed average PAL scores for soft sounds that were two loudness categories above the desired levels (e.g., they rated soft sounds at the level that individuals with normal-hearing rated average-level sounds). After eight weeks of hearing aid use, however, these new users were showing PAL results close to the desired loudness range. These results suggest that the average patient does adjust to the greater gain for soft sounds, although the length of time to do so may be longer than desired by either the audiologist or the patient, and therefore adjustments over time may be desirable.

Loud Input Levels

Can the patient adapt to loud sounds, and, if so, do we want to fit people intentionally with too much output to see whether we can push their LDLs to a higher level? Over the years, some research has shown that it might be possible to raise an individual's LDL with repeated tolerance training, although it is possible that these changes were simply reflecting a practice effect for the LDL test procedure (see Byrne & Dirks, 1996). Even if this were true, it is not practical to fit individuals with output that exceeds their LDL because excessive output is one of the leading causes for rejection of hearing aids and, at the very least, will prompt the patient to turn down gain. Research has shown that when hearing aids are initially programmed so that the maximum output corresponds to the patient's LDL, the unaided LDL does not appear to increase significantly after the prolonged use of hearing aids (Bentler & Cooley, 2001).

With that said, there is an interesting caveat regarding LDLs and unilateral fittings based on research reported by Hamilton and Munro (2010), which was a follow-up study of Munro and Trotter (2006). Hamilton and Munro studied adults with symmetrical high-frequency hearing impairment: 48 listeners with unilateral experience, 13 listeners with bilateral experience, and a control group of 47 listeners with no hearing aid experience. They found that the group using only one hearing aid showed a statistically significant inter-

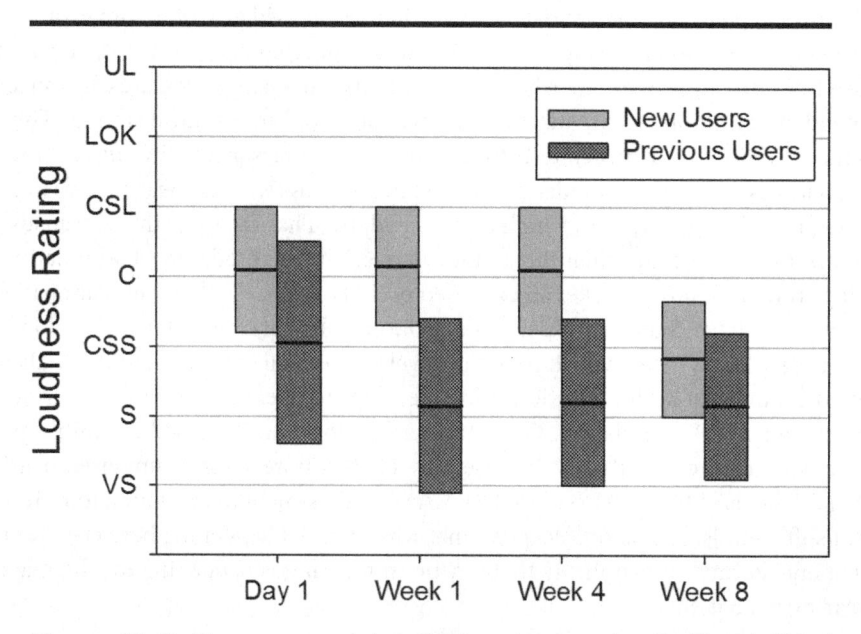

Figure 18–7. Mean scores (+/−1 S.D.) scores on the Profile of Aided Loudness (PAL) test for the four test items related to soft sounds over the eight-week post-fitting period for new and experienced hearing aid users. (Adapted from Mueller & Powers, 2001, with permission.)

aural asymmetry of 3 to 5 dB, with the trend of higher LDLs in the fitted ear and lower LDLs in the non-fitted ear. When matched for hearing loss, however, the LDLs for the bilateral aided group were symmetrical and similar to the control group. Hence, it appears, as has been found in other research, that the use of hearing aids does not alter LDLs, but that the use of a single hearing aid may have some effect, which the authors attribute to a central gain mechanism.

Change in Speech Understanding

When new hearing aid users return to the clinic and express disappointment in their ability to understand speech with their new hearing aids, it is tempting to tell them that this will likely get better as they adjust to amplification. This counseling ploy appears to be based more on wishful thinking than evidenced-based research. As noted earlier in this chapter, several studies have failed to show increased hearing aid benefit over time following hearing aid use (for reviews, see Turner & Bentler, 1998; Bentler, Holte, & Turner, 1999); some earlier studies that did show significant effects were either related to design flaws or specific to the design, and not generalizable to the typical clinical patient.

A study by Dawes, Munro, Kalluri & Edwards (2014) addressed several of the earlier design flaws and found no evidence for acclimatization in their study. Because some earlier investigations suggested that the effect might be present only for high-level stimulation, investigators of the more recent study tested speech recognition in noise for 65 and 75 dB presentation levels, for 16 unilateral and 16 bilateral hearing aid users at one-week and 12-week post-fittings. A control group of experienced hearing aid users ($n = 17$) was tested over the same time span. The researchers found no evidence of auditory acclimatization—in terms of improvement in aided speech recognition—above the approximately 4% improvement that was shown in the unaided ear and the control group, which was attributable to a training effect.

So, telling a new hearing aid user that his or her speech understanding will probably improve over time is not prudent counseling. Of course, if the patient adapts to amplification to the extent that he or she begins using more gain, audibility will be enhanced, and improvement in speech understanding may follow. But that is a different issue than what we are discussing here.

Trainable Hearing Aids and Automatic Gain Increase Algorithms

In response to patient complaints, some audiologists believe it is better to fit new users below the levels prescribed by validated prescriptive gain methods and to increase gain slowly over time to allow the patient time to adjust to these new, higher levels. Other audiologists simply fit to targets and counsel the patient that he or she will get used to it. For those in the first camp, fitting hearing aids in years past required one or more follow-up fitting visits at which time gain was increased. More recently hearing aid processing has been introduced that systematically increases gain on a fixed schedule from a lower level to the desired target levels defined by the audiologist. These automatic algorithms provide a way to increase gain slowly over a period of time (typically weeks or months) without further intervention by the audiologist.

Another type of gain adjustment is achieved with trainable hearing aids. In trainable hearing aids, the gain adapts to new levels over a predefined period of time based on patient adjustments to the volume level. Depending on the manufacturer and/or product, automatic gain managers, trainable algorithms, or both may be available. When both types of processing are implemented, the most common recommendation is to implement automatic gain increase first immediately following fitting for a limited period of time (e.g., two weeks to two months). After this period, the trainable algorithm is implemented for a limited period of time (two weeks to a few months). Regardless, the audiologist typically can adjust the timing of the gain adjustments. Refer to Chapter 11 for a complete description of these algorithms, the pros and cons, and fitting tips on how they can be applied on the day of the fitting and revised on post-fitting visits.

In Closing

In closing, from the moment your patient is first fitted with new hearing aids and onward for the next several months, it is important to provide information, training, and follow-up opportunities in order to get it right—or *more* right. For the new patient, the process may be overwhelming; for the experienced patient, there are many new things to learn about the newer technology and its options.

As we move on to the next chapter of this book on outcome measures, it is important that we point out what we *did not* discuss directly in this chapter on orientation and counseling: group and individualized auditory rehabilitation. Rehabilitative audiology is, of course, a critical part of the overall hearing aid fitting process. The fact that we did not dedicate chapters to this topic is not because we believe it is unimportant, but just the opposite—the topic is too complex and multifaceted to cover adequately in a book on hearing aids and hearing aid fitting. There are many other excellent books devoted to rehabilitative audiology.

Today, several types of hearing aid delivery models are available, ranging from over-the-counter sales to internet sales to big-box stores to experienced audiologists in offices and clinics. What is the differentiation? In many cases, the strengths of the dispensing audiologist shine through in follow-up visits when minor problems are correctly identified and fixed, and in the provision of appropriate counseling. The audiologist is the hearing health-care provider most trained to *serve* these individuals by choosing the most appropriate hearing aid and features, at a price they can accept, with a candid discussion of realistic expectations. But in this phase of the rehab process, it is most important that we *listen* to the concerns and equip ourselves with the tools to respond to whatever questions or problems arise.

19

Validation: Self-Report Outcomes

Earlier in this book we discuss pre-fitting testing tools to help in the decision-making stages of audiologic management. Specifically, in Chapter 7 we overview self-assessment scales to complement the objective findings. We encourage the use of some type of formal questionnaire to be completed by patients that relates to their hearing difficulty and communication needs to help us determine the best strategies for the management of the indicated hearing loss. Many of these same pre-fitting tools are used as outcome measures in the validation stage. The results of these outcome measures are useful in and of themselves and, when compared to pre-fitting test results, they allow us to determine the benefit afforded by the intervention. We begin this chapter by defining validation and considering the various domains that outcome measures can encompass.

An outcome measure allows us to quantify the effect of the management or treatment scheme. In Chapters 13, 15, 16, and 17 we discussed the various verification stages of hearing aid provision. The *outcomes* discussed in those chapters focus on determining whether the hearing aid met quality control standards (as per ANSI S3.22), fit comfortably in the ear, approximated some predetermined target for gain and output, and did not cause loudness discomfort for high-level stimuli. Those outcomes are part of the verification stage. As we discuss in some detail in Chapter 6, some outcomes can be classified as either verification or validation. In this chapter, we discuss measures that are most assuredly *validation* outcomes. They are useful for answering the following important clinical questions:

- How did the intervention impact the individual?
- Did the management improve the communication abilities of the individual?
- Did our intervention improve the person's overall lifestyle?
- And most important clinically, did we meet our intervention goals that were identified during the hearing needs assessment?

The Need for Outcome Measures

You might ask: Why do we need self-report measures of real-world outcomes? Why not stick with probe microphone measures and speech perception scores as *indicators* of success? We can think of at least three reasons. First, for largely economic reasons, health care is becoming more consumer-driven. In this evolving system, the consumer decides what treatment is selected and when it is complete. The major index of quality of service is self-reported outcome and satisfaction. Consumer-driven health care places an added emphasis on the patient's point of view. Therefore, it is critical to measure the real-world benefit and satisfaction of hearing aid use. Because today's patients are, on average, more savvy and better informed than our grandparents, they want to know how much benefit they are receiving in everyday listening situations. Using a self-report of hearing aid outcome allows us to measure and report to patients how they are doing compared to an average. Second, self-report measures of outcome are gaining importance, due, in part, to the fact that many real-world experiences simply cannot be measured effectively in laboratory conditions. The traditional hearing aid outcome measures (e.g., speech recognition in quiet and in noise) do not capture the true experiences of hearing aid use in everyday listening situations. Consider hearing aids with automatic and adaptive directional technology. The effectiveness of features such as these depends heavily on the lifestyle and listening environments of the individual patient. In order to quantify the true impact of hearing loss and its associated treatment on activity limitations, lifestyles, and so on, self-report measures need to be used. Third, even when laboratory conditions are used to simulate real-world listening situations, they do not always resemble the patient's impression of the actual real-life situation. Assessing speech perception in noise with a defensible signal-to-noise ratio (SNR) is rarely perceived by patients as bearing any resemblance to their own experiences. Self-report outcome measures give us a scientifically defensible way to measure the real-life success of the hearing aid fitting.

Evidence-based practice (EBP) is taking foothold in audiology (see Chapter 1). An evidence-based practice paradigm requires that clinicians demonstrate that their hearing aid fittings are providing benefit in real-world conditions. For this reason, self-reports of outcome are becoming the new "gold standard" for measuring and reporting success. The norms tell you how your patient compares to other patients of similar demographics. The critical difference values allow the clinician to make a statement of true difference in scores, as with the speech recognition testing discussed earlier in Chapter 6.

Finally, if you choose *not* to use outcome measures, it is likely that your patients will find other ways to report their satisfaction or lack of satisfaction. There are several internet sites devoted to rating doctors and other health care providers, and we suspect that these will become even more commonly used in upcoming years. Increasingly, hospitals and clinics are sending out provider satisfaction surveys following a clinic visit. And although this is not a direct rating of satisfaction with amplification, Kochkin (2010) has identified this factor as an important component of satisfaction with hearing aids. Many prospective patients will likely view these ratings before making an appointment—just as your patients now use TripAdvisor or Yelp to decide where

---

KEY CONCEPT: DOMAINS OF OUTCOMES

There are many dimensions or domains of outcomes for our consideration. We could argue that any of the following are appropriate outcomes to address clinically, so as you can see, we have a large and diverse collection of domains to choose from:

- Listening effort
- Use time
- Quality of life
- Naturalness of sound
- Sound quality (especially for music)
- Annoyance for loud environmental sounds
- Sound awareness (especially for soft environmental sounds)
- Social interaction
- Satisfaction with device
- Reduced burden for the significant other(s)
- Speech understanding

to have dinner. It makes good sense, therefore, to obtain these ratings yourself so that, if there are problems, you can take care of them before they are made public.

Types of Validation Measures

A number of methods are available for validating that the intervention strategy was a successful one. Perceptual measures of sound quality and/or speech perception are often attempted after the individual has had sufficient time to adjust to the intervention. Reports from significant other persons (SOPs) can be useful in understanding success. The most common approach, however, is through the use of self-report measures, thus allowing the hearing aid wearer an opportunity to provide information relative to the real-world effectiveness of the current management scheme. It cannot be ignored that the clinician is often faced with a limited timeframe in which to obtain the measurements of success after some period of hearing aid use. Let's look at the options available to us, and determine which tests provide the most information relative to our amplification choices.

One could argue that *speech testing* falls better under the *verification* stage of the hearing aid fitting. That argument is a good one. If verification implies determining whether all of our fitting goals (audibility, comfort, and so on) were met, then it might be more logical to consider speech testing (often a measure of audibility) as a step in that stage. Estimations of the speech perception ability—based on weighted audibility provided with AI or SII calculations—provide evidence of audibility during the verification stage (as we discuss in Chapter 6). In fact, there are many speech tests to choose from, and the notion is that we select a specific test to answer a specific question we might have about the patients: How much are they bothered by background noise while wearing their new hearing aids? How well do they understand speech in background noise with directional microphone technology? It is often the case in a clinical setting that a speech test is used to compare two ears, two hearing aids, or the *acclimatization* effect of new hearing aids. But wait! Is that a validation outcome? We argue that such a test fits better in the verification stage: Did the hearing aid intervention provide enough audibility to allow for improved communication?

Some clinicians (and manufacturers) use *return rate* as a validation of successful fittings. If the hearing aids don't get returned, they must be fit successfully. Right? Wrong. Although true data are difficult to secure for this concern, various MarkeTrak surveys have suggested that as many as 6 to 10% of all purchased hearing aids end up in a dresser drawer somewhere and are neither worn nor returned!

A related proposed measure of successful hearing aid fittings is "use time." Historically, hearing aid *use* time has been employed as a measure of "successful" amplification (e.g., Brooks, 1979, 1981; Haggard, Foster, & Iredale, 1981). The most common measure of use time is the user's self-report of how many hours a day the hearing aid is in operation (or turned on). One of the dilemmas facing clinicians and researchers is whether these data can be accepted as accurate. Using an early data logging algorithm, Taubman, Palmer, Durrant, and Pratt (1999) found that subjects both underestimate and overestimate hearing aid use time compared to actual recorded use time (even when aware that the time is being monitored electronically) in a manner that cannot be accounted for by phenomena such as social acceptability or impression-management. In another investigation of preferred amplification processing options, using the same early data logging algorithm, blatant discrepancies were apparent when the subjects were *not* aware of the electronic monitoring (Bentler & Nelson, 1997). Data from Walker et al. (2013) found that parents tend to overreport daily hearing aid use by approximately two hours per day. A more recent focus has been on consideration of the fact that all hearing aid users don't need to use their devices 12 to 14 hours a day. Laplante-Lévesque, Jensen, Dawes, and Nielsen (2013) argue that *optimal* hearing aid use could be less than the clinician might anticipate and still meet the patient's needs. That is, if some patients really only "need" their hearing aids for four hours/day, then if they use them four hours/day this would be considered a successful fitting.

As we discuss in Chapter 12, hearing aid technology is now available in which a data log can be maintained for a variety of *use* parameters including total hours of use; average daily use; number of hours or percent of time spent in different environments; number of times the hearing aid is turned off, on, up, or down; and so on. Looking through available logged information can be useful in a variety of ways. Besides conveying a sense of management concern for patients during their adjustment phase, the logged information can often validate the patients' complaints relative to difficulties encountered during their adjustment phase. Or, on the other hand, these data may identify potential problems not mentioned by the patient.

Self-Report Measures

The tool currently most favored for validation of fitting efforts is the self-report inventory. Self-report inventories are used primarily for two purposes: as assessment for rehabilitative planning and as assessment for rehabilitative (including hearing aid) effectiveness. In this chapter, we discuss those tools most useful for assessing the effectiveness of the intervention. But first, let's remember that patients have always provided clinicians with real-world assessments of outcomes from their hearing aids, and frequently these reports are used for counseling and hearing aid adjustments. Until quite recently, most real-world assessments of outcome involved informal discussions between the patient and the professional. Although quite useful, such informal assessments can be susceptible to a number of errors, including those that follow:

- Increased bias of patients to provide an answer the clinician is looking for
- Failure to ask the most important or salient questions
- Use of questions that are either unreliable or invalid (or both)
- Failure to record problems (or failure to act on problems and simply commenting on the patient encounter in the patient report)

In the past 20 years, a number of well-designed and validated self-assessment inventories have been introduced. The goal now is to make these inventories part of the protocol for routine hearing aid fitting. Information gleaned from the inventories can also be used to alter the individual management strategy as well as to evaluate practices and personnel (see related Things to Remember).

In 2005, Robyn Cox described some of the fundamental characteristics that we should consider when selecting a self-assessment inventory. The following section is adapted from her article. Cox (2005b) suggests that the audiologist should consider four practical elements: clinical burden, patient burden, scoring, and utility. These are factors that impact the everyday use and success of the inventory. We briefly describe each factor here:

- Clinician burden. This relates to the challenges for the audiologist in learning how to administer, score, and interpret the test. Does learning about the test require a one-day instructional course or a five-minute YouTube tutorial? Obviously, the test cannot be used if there is not time to learn how to use it correctly. Moreover, if it is known as a difficult test, this may prompt clinicians to avoid it before even trying it.
- Patient burden. This refers to the difficulty encountered by the patient in reading, understanding, and completing the items of the questionnaire. The reading level and cognitive level of both items and instructions should be considered. Consider that what is suitable for one clinic population may not work in another. This is important when deciding if a scale can be mailed to the patient in advance or if it needs to be completed knee-to-knee with the patient in the clinic. Also, some scales are designed specifically for computer or internet administration. Although convenient for the audiologist, this approach may be an unreasonable burden for some patients. A paper-and-pencil option may be necessary.
- Scoring. Busy clinical audiologists are looking for a questionnaire that is convenient, quick, objective, and easy to score. Automated scoring usually is preferred but is not always available. Most of us have little trouble scoring the Hearing Handicap Inventory for Elderly (HHIE) by hand, but for the Abbreviated Profile of Hearing Aid Benefit (APHAB) . . . without automation, the scoring process involves more math and time than we want to invest. Computerized scoring can be accomplished through direct keyboard entry by the patient (e.g., using an iPad in your waiting room), although usually the audiologist keys in answers from

> **THINGS TO REMEMBER: OTHER USES FOR OUTCOME MEASURES (BEYOND INDIVIDUAL PATIENT MANAGEMENT)**
>
> 1. Comparison of different dispensing sites or personnel: If you are the manager of a clinic that has several different offices, you might want to compare the patient-reported outcomes as a form of quality control.
> 2. Comparison of different fitting procedures across groups of patients: If you always fit your hearing aids to the NAL-NL2 targets with careful verification and adjustment using probe microphone measures, and another audiologist defers to the manufacturer's first-fit setting, will both groups of patients have the same benefit and satisfaction with hearing aids in the real world?
> 3. Comparison of circuitry across groups of patients: As new circuitry and features become available, it is important to know in your own setting whether "new means better," especially when the newer circuitry adds several hundred dollars to the cost of the hearing aids. If your patients were fitted with that feature, would they observe/report improved speech understanding in noise in their everyday use situations?
> 4. Counseling effectiveness across groups of patients: Does extra effort result in improved real-world satisfaction and benefit with hearing aids? That is, if you have changes in counseling techniques or time commitments, do the outcomes change for your patients?
> 5. Documentation of service effectiveness: You know you do a good job, but do you have data to prove it? Are your patients more satisfied than the average person fitted with hearing aids? For example, how often do their IOI-HA scores exceed national norms? How often are their COSI goals obtained?
> 6. Research has shown that patients are significantly more satisfied with their hearing aids when they have been given a formalized outcome measure asking them if they are satisfied with their hearing aids. That's right, you can improve patient outcomes simply by measuring them!

a completed paper-and-pencil measure. As reviewed by Cox (2005b), computer-based scoring has at least three advantages: (1) the scores are obtained quickly and accurately; (2) comparison with norms, previous sessions, and so on can be accomplished readily; and (3) a database of patient records can be built up without additional effort or time. We might add that this report also then easily can become part of the patient's electronic records.

- Utility. This characteristic relates to the extent to which the data from the scale can be readily applied for treatment, planning, or counseling. Dillon and So (2000), for example, report that clinicians are more apt to take the time to use outcome measures if they see some immediate use of the findings. A scale with good utility is the Client Oriented Scale of Improvement (COSI), as the patient response relates directly to a listening condition identified by the patient.

In her article, Cox (2005b) also identifies four technical elements that we should consider when evaluating different self-assessment inventories: norms, reliability, validity, and sensitivity.

- Norms. The availability of published normative data is very helpful to the audiologist for patient counseling. Patients typically are very interested in hearing how they are performing compared to others with similar hearing loss, people their age with normal hearing, or even young normal-hearing listeners. Norms are also very useful in determining when a fitting change is needed, compared to when the patient is

> **TECHNICAL TIP: WHAT DOES "PSYCHOMETRICALLY SOUND" MEAN ANYWAY?**
>
> Several times throughout this chapter, we state the importance of choosing a tool with psychometric strength. Entire books are written on development of questionnaires and surveys, and we won't try to summarize those here. Instead, we want to encourage the use of outcome measures that provide information such as normative data (for several populations), critical difference values (so the clinician can compare scores over different administrations), and written instructions (so the clinician uses the tool in the manner intended by the developers and results are reliable). Other important psychometric information such as appropriate eigenvalues, Cronbach's alphas, and factor-loading can be assumed, if the test development has undergone the rigor of peer review.

simply performing as expected (e.g., based on the norms, we expect the AV score of the APHAB to become worse following the fitting of hearing aids).

- Reliability. This relates to the consistency of responses for a given inventory across different tests and different testers. This is critical for the audiologist because, before changes to the fitting or specific counseling are conducted, it is important to know to what extent the patient's responses would vary simply by chance, if the test were administered on another day or by another person. Critical differences have been calculated for several inventories and can be used in the same manner as when conducting speech-in-noise testing (see Chapter 6). That is, if the patient is tested at two different intervals or two different fittings are employed, the findings from the inventories can be compared to determine whether the differences in scores reflect a true change in the patient's opinion.
- Validity. We consider an outcome measure valid if it truthfully measures what it purports to measure. Benefit? Satisfaction? Quality of Life? In this regard, the inventory should produce scores that have a predictable relationship with other validated outcome measures that are purporting to measure the same domain. For example, we expect the benefit rating on the COSI for understanding in background noise to be similar to the background noise (BN) subscale of the APHAB. As we discussed earlier, determining how many hours/day a given patient uses his hearing aids may not be a valid measure of benefit or satisfaction because "use" generally differs from benefit.
- Sensitivity. A final technical issue is the sensitivity of the questionnaire. That is, will it detect performance or changes in performance that are of interest to the audiologist? A bilateral versus a unilateral fitting? New technology versus the patient's old hearing aids? Premier hearing aids versus a pair of personal sound amplification products (PSAPs)? The difference between noise reduction "on" versus "off"? It is very possible that a scale may effectively differentiate aided versus unaided but will not be very good at pulling out more subtle amplification differences. A short scale probably will not be able to detect small differences on an individual basis.

We can look at various outcome measures and assign grades based on the eight different factors identified by Cox (2005b). Obviously, the scores will have to be weighted for a given setting: "quick to administer and score" is more important for some clinics than others. An example of how this might be conducted was presented by Cox (2005b). She included the (unbiased we assume) grading of her own outcome measure, the APHAB. In Figure 19–1, you can see Cox's scoring of three outcome measures: the APHAB, the HHIE, and the International Outcome Inventory of Hearing Aids (IOI-HA). It is obvious that all inventories are not created equal!

Report Card for APHAB Questionnaire				
Features	Poor	Fair	Good	Very Good
Burden	X (pt.)	X (clin.)		
Scoring				X
Utility			X	
Norms				X
CDs				X
Problem Sensing			X	
Device Sensing		X		

Report Card for IOI-HA Questionnaire				
Features	Poor	Fair	Good	Very Good
Burden				XX
Scoring				X
Utility	X			
Norms				X
CDs	X			
Problem Sensing			?	
Device Sensing		?		

Report Card for HHIE Questionnaire				
Features	Poor	Fair	Good	Very Good
Burden				XX
Scoring			X	
Utility		X		
Norms		X		
CDs	X			
Problem Sensing				X
Device Sensing	X			

Figure 19–1. Report cards based on the eight different factors identified by Cox, 2005b. *APHAB* = Abbreviated Profile of Hearing Aid Benefit; *IOI-HA* = International Outcomes Inventory for Hearing Aids; *HHIE* = Hearing Handicap Inventory for the Elderly; *CDs* = critical differences.

POINTS TO PONDER: SENSITIVITY OF THE OUTCOME MEASURE?

As we discuss in this section, many outcome measures may not have the sensitivity to detect small differences in hearing aid performance that are of interest to the audiologist. We see an example of this in research conducted by Ricketts, Henry, and Gnewikow (2003) that related to the benefit of directional microphone technology in the real world. The authors used the Profile of Hearing Aid Benefit (PHAB) self-assessment inventory and added two new subscales that were developed to specifically address situations in which directional hearing aids may provide different degrees of benefit than do omnidirectional hearing aids. When the results of the new subscales were examined, the expected benefit of directional technology was present, but it was not present for the PHAB. If only the PHAB had been used, the conclusions of the research would have been somewhat different. On the other hand, the new subscales had not undergone the reliability scrutiny of the more established PHAB.

> **KEY CONCEPT: LOOKING FOR THE TRUTH!**
>
> New hearing aid technology continues to emerge and, as would be expected, manufacturers promote the potential benefit of this technology to their customers (e.g., audiologists). Historically, "proof" that the technology was better often was based on efficacy testing in an anechoic chamber or audiometric test booth, sometimes under rather contrived conditions. In recent years, clinical studies have more frequently included a real-world effectiveness component to the clinical study: Participants use the new technology in the real world and then complete a self-assessment inventory regarding the benefit. As you might expect, some technologies show benefit in the laboratory but not in the real world. How do we explain this?
>
> - Opinion #1: Audiologists who truly believe in the technology might say that if you see a significant advantage in behavioral testing, albeit under rather ideal conditions, this still shows that the benefit is there. They might add that it is likely the real-world outcome measure that was used simply was not sensitive enough to detect the benefit. Perhaps special real-world inventories are needed when specific features are studied.
> - Opinion #2: Skeptical dispensing audiologists might say that they really don't care how the hearing aid performs in the laboratory; they want to know how it works for their patients in the real world. They might then add that, if this special feature or algorithm really did provide significant benefit, then that benefit would be significant enough that the patient would notice and that, therefore, it would show up on the standardized scales we already have, and no special scale is needed. So where is the truth? Probably somewhere in between!

> **POINTS TO PONDER: WHEN TO ADMINISTER THE SELF-REPORT INVENTORIES?**
>
> The question of exactly when to administer a self-report of outcome plagues many clinicians. If the self-report is completed too soon, patients may not have had enough time to become familiar with the fundamental daily care and maintenance of the devices such as cleaning and insertion into, or removal from, the ears (e.g., Vestergaard, 2006). Additionally, the re-introduction of the audibility of an array of soft sounds might still be a little overwhelming. As a result, their satisfaction, benefit, or overall success may not be optimized. On the other hand, if a clinician waits too long to conduct self-report measures, the entire fitting process may be unnecessarily prolonged, needed changes might not be detected, and/or the patient may no longer appreciate the benefits that were originally obvious. Robyn Cox has studied this question of optimal timing and concludes: "Outcomes are best after three weeks of use and then go down, on average, across all domains."

Reasons to Use Post-Fitting Self-Assessment Scales

To get started, we first list a few areas where self-assessment tests might be helpful for the overall process of fitting hearing aids. Our examples include names of specific tests. You will be familiar with many of these tests as they were discussed in Chapter 7. Here are four good reasons (we think) for using standardized scales as part of the fitting and validation process:

- Assist in determining the success of the hearing aid fitting by comparing the patient's score to normative data. Example: A patient has a very mild hearing loss; normal hearing through 2000 Hz, dropping down to a 40 dB loss in the 3000 to 6000 Hz range. His unaided APHAB scores showed significant handicap and considerable communication problems. Following the fitting of new hearing aids and a reasonable adjustment period, the patient's aided APHAB scores suggest fewer communication problems. In fact, the patient's aided APHAB reveals that he is performing at the 40th percentile of people with normal hearing.
- Assist in determining if pre-fitting goals are met or if additional intervention is needed. Example: The patient identified "easier to understand my daughter on the phone" as a pre-fitting goal on the COSI. After three weeks of wearing the hearing aids, the patient indicates continued difficulty and no benefit in this area. Additional hearing assistive technologies including amplified telephones, wireless streaming, and speakerphone solutions are explored.
- Assist in determining if pre-fitting goals are met or if additional counseling is needed. Example: On the GHABP, the patient established the goal of wearing his or her new hearing aids in more listening environments. Because the inventory can be used to monitor progress, it becomes apparent after three months of use that the patient is not using the hearing aids as he or she had hoped. More counseling regarding the difficulties encountered as well as ways to achieve more successful use of the hearing aids could be key to future success.
- Assist in determining need for post-fitting adjustment. Example: The patient's results for the aversiveness scale of the APHAB revealed that the patient has a low tolerance for loud sounds with his or her new hearing aids. This was not the case on the pre-fitting assessment with the APHAB. This information might suggest adjusting the hearing aid MPO settings again, but might also represent a newfound perception of loudness that will be only appreciated after a few weeks of adjustment to the hearing aids.

In this chapter, we review several different self-assessment scales that can be used in the validation process. We recognize that it is unlikely you will use *all* of them for a given patient, but you may find a couple of favorites for routine use and save the others for special cases. As we discuss in Chapter 7, audiologists often comment that it would be nice to use several scales, but they just don't have the time. This may be true, but there are some ways to facilitate administration. Many of these scales can be mailed to the patient and completed at home before the clinic visit. Other scales could be completed in the waiting room, with assistance from support personnel if needed. As the average patient becomes more computer-savvy, you may be able to use modern technology to facilitate administration and scoring—using a tablet or smartphone, the patient simply completes a couple of scales and then hands them to you when you begin the initial pre-fitting counseling.

Most of the earlier outcome inventories were more general assessments of success, whereas current tools focus on specific domains of benefit or success and are typically developed to be used as open-ended (or user-specified) or closed-ended tools, or both. Open-ended self-report measures allow patients to nominate and target their own areas of expected improvement with amplification. The assumed advantage of an open-ended scale is that it can be tailored to the true communication needs of the individual patient. That is, if you and your patient work together carefully, the items selected will represent true, difficult listening situations for that patient, rather than arbitrary listening situations collected from average patients. One disadvantage with this type of inventory is that it is difficult to compare your patient's performance to a large pool of other hearing aid users because the specific listening situations they nominate might be quite unique.

> **TECHNICAL TIP: CHOOSING THE ASSESSMENT TOOL**
>
> Assessment tools are primarily used for two purposes: as assessment for rehabilitative planning and as assessment for rehabilitative (including hearing aids) effectiveness. As we discuss later in this chapter, effectiveness can be measured in terms of residual activity limitation (disability reduction), participation restriction (handicap reduction), areas of communication difficulty, other areas of concern (e.g., service, fit, use time), or general satisfaction. Different inventories have been developed for these purposes, depending upon the goals of the authors. Most inventories were developed for the general adult population, although some are specifically for older adults (e.g., the Communication Scale for Older Adults by Kaplan, Bally, Brandt, Busacco, & Pray, 1997), prelingually deafened adult (e.g., Communication Self-Assessment Scale Inventory for Deaf Adults by Kaplan, Bally, & Brandt, 1995), or for nursing home residents (Nursing Home Hearing Handicap Index by Schow & Nerbonne, 1976, 1977). Other inventories are designed to be administered to staff or to significant others. For clinicians to be able to choose the appropriate existing outcome measure for their clinical purposes, a table on the companion website provides some information about length, internal structure, and stated purpose of each. Other important psychometric data can be found by referring to the original articles, as referenced.

We selected eight of our favorite self-assessment inventories that can be used in the validation stage, and we describe each inventory in detail in the following pages. Because each inventory provides somewhat different information, each one is uniquely useful in specific situations. Here is a brief summary (with details to follow):

- Abbreviated Profile of Hearing Aid Benefit (APHAB). Provides "percent of problems" the patient has for three different listening conditions involving speech understanding (in quiet, in background noise, and in reverberation) and problems related to annoyance of environmental sounds (aversiveness scale). These values can be obtained as a pre-fitting or unaided measure, as an aided measure, or—by looking at the aided to unaided difference score—as a benefit measure.
- Glasgow Hearing Aid Benefit Profile (GHABP). Accesses a number of different components of disability and benefit via a mixture of pre-specified and subject-specified listening circumstances of relevance to the hearing-impaired client.
- Satisfaction with Amplification in Daily Life (SADL). Designed to evaluate the patient's satisfaction with a new or current hearing aid, or to assess differences between previous and new hearing aids.
- Device Oriented Subjective Outcome (DOSO). Designed to measure hearing aid outcomes focusing on the device itself in a manner that is relatively independent of wearer's personality.
- International Outcome Inventory for Hearing Aids (IOI-HA). Covers a minimal set of seven core outcome items that are sufficiently general to apply to many different types of investigations carried out in different countries in the world.
- Client Oriented Scale of Improvement (COSI). Measures early and final abilities for specific communication situations important to the patient; used as a pre-test to define goals and to plan management and quantify expectations, and as a post-test to assess the success of the management in meeting the patient's goals.
- Profile of Aided Loudness (PAL). Assesses the patient's loudness perceptions and satisfaction with these perceptions for 12 different everyday environmental sounds.
- Speech, Spatial, and Qualities of Hearing Scale (SSQ). Assesses hearing disability (participation restriction) across the domains of speech, spatial hearing, and sound quality.

Abbreviated Profile of Hearing Aid Benefit (APHAB)

The APHAB was developed by Robyn Cox and her colleagues at the University of Memphis. Cox (1997) offers four potential clinical uses of the APHAB that span the whole pre-fitting to follow-up process:

- Predict success from unaided scores
- Compare results with different hearing aids
- Evaluate fittings in an absolute sense
- Measure benefit from a fitting

In this chapter, we focus on the last three uses of the tool.

Background

The origins of the APHAB are from other, more extensive, self-assessment scales that were also developed at the University of Memphis: the PHAP and the PHAB (see Chapter 7 for complete review). As a review, the APHAB comprises 24 items that are scored in four subscales (six questions each). The subscales are as follows:

- Ease of Communication (EC). The strain of communicating under relatively favorable conditions. *When I am in a small office, interviewing, or answering questions, I have difficulty following the conversation.*
- Reverberation (RV). Communication in reverberant rooms such as classrooms. *It is hard for me to understand what is being said at lectures or church services.*
- Background Noise (BN). Communication in settings with high background noise levels. *I have trouble understanding others when an air conditioner or fan is on.*
- Aversiveness (AV). The unpleasantness of environmental sounds. *The sound of a fire engine siren close by is so loud that I need to cover my ears.*

Administration and Scoring

The APHAB can be administered as a paper-and-pencil test or by using a computer software version (e.g., the APHAB is included in the Questionnaire Module of the Noah software). The 24 items of the APHAB are scored on a seven-point scale. See Chapter 7 for review of administration and scoring, which is the same whether the scale is used as a pre-fitting test or an outcome measure.

Clinical Application

Cox (1997) developed the APHAB for a number of uses, as we have discussed. Unaided and/or aided difficulty can be compared to published norms, which is a powerful counseling tool. Perhaps the most common use is in calculating benefit with amplification. To do this, we must first have the unaided baseline for comparison, which one hopes was obtained during the pre-fitting testing discussed earlier.

When using the APHAB results for counseling, it is helpful to examine the scores for each one of the four subscales. The following are the results for Mr. Smith, a 68-year-old golfing buddy of Mr. Jones, whom we met back in Chapter 7. He also has a mild-to-moderate downward sloping hearing loss—dropping to 80 dB in the 3000 to 4000 Hz area. He does a lot of volunteer work at the local VA hospital, which involves considerable communication with others, sometimes in background noise. Here are his average *unaided* APHAB percent of problems for each subscale:

- EC: 34%
- RV: 58%
- BN: 67%
- AV: 20%

Following three months of hearing aid use, the APHAB was administered again (recall from Chapter 7 that looking at previous answers is okay). Here are his current percent of problems for each subscale in the aided condition:

- EC: 14%
- RV: 19%
- BN: 35%
- AV: 53%

We can consider these scores by themselves or compare them to the unaided scores, which allows us to consider the benefit afforded by the new hearing aids. In her original development of this tool, Cox and Alexander (1995) established norms for patients wearing hearing of that era, linear analog hearing aids. In 2010, those norms were re-examined with users of both linear hearing aids and wide-dynamic range compression (WDRC). Except for the aversiveness subscale (AV), there was little change in the norms. That is, newer hearing aids resulted in less aversiveness than the earlier technologies, no doubt because of the increased use of both input and output compression. The current 2010 norms, according to the developers, "reflect the real-world effectiveness of WDRC-capable hearing aids with current technology and fitting practices" and can be found in Table 19–1 for global (the average of EC, RV, and BN) scores as well as for each of the four subtests independently.

Table 19–1. Normative Data for WDRC-Capable Hearing Aids with Current Technology and Fitting Practices Shown for Global Score (GS) and Each Subscale for the APHAB

Percentile	Subscale				
	EC	RV	BN	AV	GS
Unaided					
95	99	99	99	70	99
80	83	87	89	35	86
65	75	81	81	21	79
50	63	71	75	14	70
35	56	65	67	9	63
20	46	58	58	3	54
5	26	47	41	1	38
Aided					
95	86	79	82	82	82
80	39	57	58	64	51
65	29	46	49	53	41
50	23	37	40	38	33
35	17	29	32	23	16
20	12	21	22	14	18
5	5	12	14	2	10
Benefit					
95	76	70	56	16	67
80	52	52	47	0	50
65	46	41	39	–8	42
50	38	34	33	–13	35
35	29	27	23	–25	26
20	19	16	12	–41	16
5	10	–3	–1	–61	–5

Note. The table shows data for the four subscales of Ease of Communication (EC), Reverberation (RV), Background Noise (BN), and Aversiveness (AV). Data Are Given for Each Response Mode: Unaided, Aided, and Benefit.

Source: From Johnson et al. (2010).

For our own Mr. Smith, aided and benefit scores are plotted onto the visual representation of those norms in Figures 19–2, 19–3, and 19–4. It is apparent that he doesn't have a lot of problems in quiet environments (EC subscale) or with aversive sounds (AV subscale). His real area of concern is background noise (BN subscale) and, even for that subscale, his problems are only at the 50th percentile. Looking at the difference between the scores, we can consider the benefit provided by these hearing aids. The benefit scores for each subscale are as follows:

- EC: 20%
- RV: 32%
- BN: 37%
- AV: −23%

It becomes obvious that our Mr. Smith is obtaining a good deal of benefit with his hearing aids in reverberant environments (RV subscale) and for aversive sounds (AV subscale) where his benefit scores put him well above the 50th percentile. His benefit for easy-listening environments (EC subscale) shows only 30th percentile, but recall he had few problems to overcome there—benefit scores always are low when the initial problems are few! His benefit in the background noise realm (BN subscale) places him around the 25th percentile, which might be the focus of further rehabilitative efforts.

A final way to evaluate the APHAB scores of this patient, which can be very useful for counseling, is to compare his aided percent of problems to those of people in his age range who have normal hearing. Note that, when aided, he is roughly at the 50th percentile for listening in quiet and in reverberation (Figure 19–5). Those are excellent findings and should be passed along to the patient. Even in background noise, where we mentioned we may still have some work to do, he is at the 80th percentile—in other words, he is outperforming (according to his perceptions) 20% of people with normal hearing. That kind of news gives patients a good perspective of their performance and is what many new

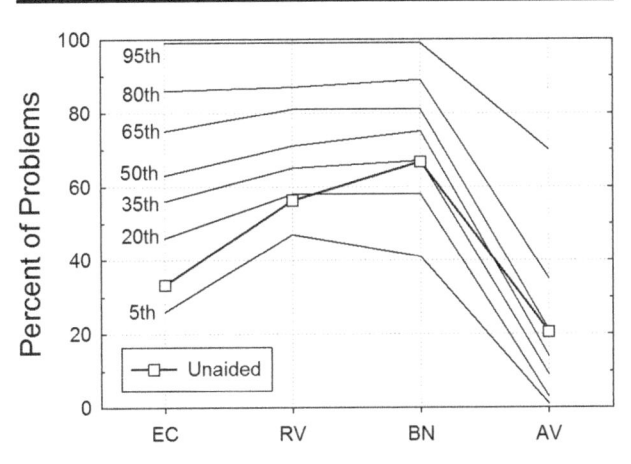

Figure 19–2. Comparison of patient's unaided APHAB scores to unaided norms as provided by Johnson et al., 2010.

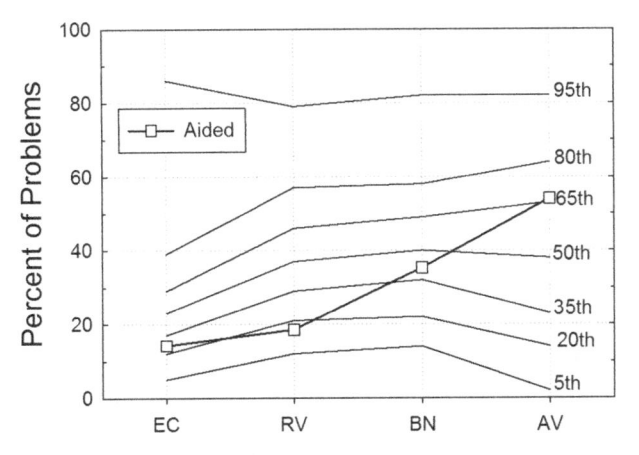

Figure 19–3. Comparison of patient's aided APHAB scores to aided norms as provided by Johnson et al., 2010.

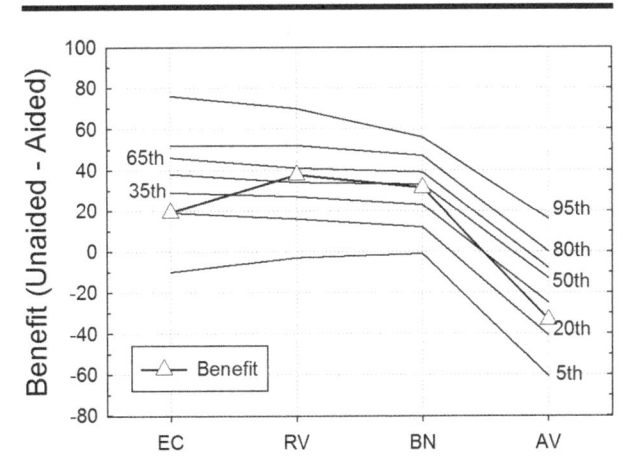

Figure 19–4. Comparison of this patient's benefit, as determined by the APHAB, to the benefit norms as provided by Johnson et al., 2010.

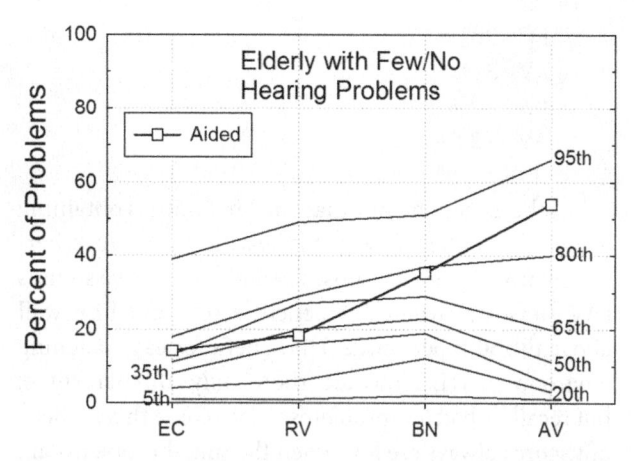

Figure 19–5. Comparison of patient's aided scores to the unaided norms for "Elderly with few/no hearing problems" from Cox (1997). This information may be useful in counseling the patient.

Table 19–2. 90% and 95% Critical Differences (in %) for APHAB Subscales Shown for Unaided, Aided, and Benefit Scores

	Subscale			
	EC	RV	BN	AV
Unaided				
90% CD	22	24	23	17
95% CD	26	28	27	21
Aided				
90% CD	22	18	22	31
95% CD	26	22	27	36
Benefit				
90% CD	26	28	27	31
95% CD	31	33	33	37

patients need to hear to continue using their hearing aids even in difficult, noisy situations.

Looking at Differences

We believe that the use of critical difference values is essential for understanding the impact of our efforts in the successful management of hearing loss. Let's consider Mr. Smith again. Perhaps on his first visit to our clinic, he chose *not* to pursue hearing aids. When he returned for his annual evaluation, we re-administered the APHAB in its unaided form. He showed changes across all subscales of 20%; that is, he was reporting 20% more problems hearing in quiet (EC), reverberation (RV), and background noise (BN). Our first inclination is to assume that Mr. Smith has gotten much worse over the year. That is where the critical difference values come into play! Table 19–2 shows critical difference values for the unaided, aided, and benefit scores across all subscales. Values are given for 90% and 95% confidence intervals. This is how we can read them: *If we want to be 90% confident that the difference we see in scores from last year is a real difference, there must be a change of " x" in that subscale.* For BN, that difference needs to be 23 points. If we are interested in being more statistically secure in our management, we might rather use the 95% CDs: *If we want to be 95% confident that the difference we see in BN scores from last year is a real difference, there must be a change of 27 points in that subscale.* The same use can be made of aided scores and benefit scores across different hearing aids. The eyeball is no longer the meter! We can use some statistical confidence in our counseling, our management, and even our report for reimbursement. Relative to Mr. Smith, his 20% increase in problems, as measured for each of the subscales, doesn't reach statistical significance; that is, the 20% difference that we recorded is not a real difference in his recorded communication problems, with 90 or 95% confidence levels considered.

The same decision can be made using the CDs for aided performance or benefit. If our patient were to try two different hearing aids as a part of our evaluation, we could compare either the aided scores or the benefit score using the CDs for those conditions. Rather than compare each subscale independently, as we did before, we might want to look at a global assessment of the unaided versus the aided scores. To do so, we examine the differences for the three listening categories collectively; if a trend is present, the differences do not need to be as large as if we compared each subscale independently. Cox (1997) reports that if EC, RV, *and* BN are all superior by at least five points, you can be fairly certain that this is a true difference. She goes on to state that if the difference between scores is at least 10 points

> **TECHNICAL TIP: USING ANSWERS TO INDIVIDUAL QUESTIONS**
>
> One feature of the APHAB and other measures of its type is that each subscale asks about a range of specific environments within a category of environments. For example, the following two items are from the BN subscale:
>
> 1. When I am in a crowded grocery store, talking with the cashier, I can follow the conversation.
> 19. I can communicate with others when we are in a crowd.
>
> This structure has the advantage of capturing hearing aid benefit across a wide range of listening situations. One limitation of this structure, however, is that the interaction between specific hearing aid technologies and specific environments is sometimes concealed. For example, a directional hearing aid will provide benefit (relative to omnidirectional) if the patient is facing the talker of interest, but will be detrimental if the talker is behind, even though both situations represent "listening in background noise." Consequently, although general measures such as the APHAB may do a good job of capturing whether there is overall benefit when weighing the advantages and limitations across all situations, the specific benefits and limitations are not apparent from simply examining the subscale scores. Consequently, it is sometimes useful to look over answers to individual questions for the purposes of counseling and hearing aid adjustment. For example, if a patient demonstrates hearing aid benefit on one subscale, but problems are evident for a specific listening situation, counseling by focusing on improving communication strategies in that specific situation may be useful.

for all three subscales, the likelihood of this occurring by chance is only about 2%. Going back to our previous example, where the differences were 20% for each subscale but were not individually significant, based on the global performance (EC, RV, *and* BN) we can quite confidently say that the two sets of scores are different.

Glasgow Hearing Aid Benefit Profile (GHABP)

Many self-assessment inventories deal with a single outcome, such as benefit or satisfaction; other outcome measures examine several different dimensions. The GHABP was developed by Stuart Gatehouse (2000) and was designed to assess, across six dimensions, the efficacy and effectiveness of rehabilitation intervention on reducing disabilities and handicap for hearing-impaired individuals in order to demonstrate the value of hearing aids and related services to the National Health Service in the United Kingdom.

Background

In developing the GHABP, Gatehouse and colleagues stated that it could be argued that traditional disability and benefit measures that can be completed in clinically acceptable time frames can (1) ignore important components or dimensions of disability and benefit, (2) rely on data not relevant to individual clients, and (3) result in insufficient discriminatory power for the targeting of management or the assessment of intervention. They sought to overcome these limitations in the GHABP.

The following is a brief overview of this outcome measure:

- Consists of four fixed listening situations and four listener-specified situations;

- Assesses six dimensions: initial disability, handicap, satisfaction, reported hearing aid use, residual disability, and reported benefit;
- Designed to be used clinically to gather multidimensional information in a short amount of time;
- Is sensitive enough to differentiate between the benefit of two different hearing aids;
- Exists in paper-and-pencil version as well as a computer version.

The GHABP is not limited to a fixed number of questions that may or may not apply to, or are infrequently encountered by, a hearing aid user. Instead, there are four preset listening conditions and up to four hearing aid user-set listening conditions. The preset conditions cover listening to the television with others, having a one-on-one conversation in quiet, having a group conversation, and having a conversation in a busy location. These preset situations serve as an example to the hearing aid user who may cite using the telephone or hearing the speaker during religious services as user-specified areas where hearing is very important (Gatehouse, 1999a, 2000).

Each of the situations is evaluated on whether or not the hearing aid user experiences the condition; from there, six dimensions are assessed. The six dimensions considered include initial disability, handicap, reported hearing aid use, reported benefit, residual disability, and satisfaction (Gatehouse, 1999a, 2000). For questions 5 through 8, the patient nominates up to four more situations that are important and answers the questions related to the six dimensions in the same manner.

The first two dimensions measure hearing ability without amplification and the degree of difficulty caused by the hearing loss in that situation. These two dimensions may be evaluated before interventions to influence the course of intervention and guide the counseling process (Gatehouse, 2000).

The other four dimensions are used to gauge how an individual is faring after rehabilitation using amplification. Typically, hearing aid outcome measures ask the patient to report daily hearing aid use, but the GHABP asks subjects to report how much of the time they use amplification during each situation. Although knowing the total number of hours a patient wears the hearing aids is useful, it is not as informative as knowing how much he or she uses them in conditions where he or she needs help (Gatehouse, 2000). If a patient is not wearing his or her hearing aids much in a certain situation but is still having a great deal of difficulty, it may indicate that further counseling or setting adjustments are warranted.

The next dimension, benefit, asks the users to rate how well they can hear with their hearing aids versus unaided. Directly asking the patient about the benefit (deficit) from hearing aid use is more sensitive than subtracting pre- from post-fitting data. The residual disability dimension focuses on the areas where the hearing aid user is still experiencing some difficulty and may need further intervention. The satisfaction dimension is meant to cover the other factors that are not directly related to hearing ability such as comfort and self-image (Gatehouse, 2000).

The GHABP has been shown to have good validity and high internal reliability (Gatehouse, 1999a).

Administration and Scoring

The GHABP is meant to be administered through interview by the clinician. It is not meant to be handed to the patients to be filled out by themselves. The scale is densely worded and may be difficult for older patients to read or follow. Regarding the user-specified situations, the developers suggest that we ask the patients to be as specific as possible about conditions where hearing is of great importance to them rather than what situations cause their disability. It is also important not to suggest specific circumstances (e.g., listening on the telephone) to patients, but rather ask them what tasks they do and what environments they are in on a regular basis. Those important environments may or may not cause disability. Also, if a certain listening situation is important but covered broadly by another section, the developer encourages the exploration of the specific situation in the user-specified section (Gatehouse, 2000). For each condition specified, patients respond whether they encounter the situation and then respond to the six dimensions. Each dimension has five possible answers (1 through 5), or actually six if you consider Not Applicable (NA) as one possible answer. The others are as follows:

1. No difficulty
2. Only slight difficulty

3. Moderate difficulty
4. Great difficulty
5. Cannot manage at all

The score of each scale can vary between 0 and 100. Once the questionnaire is completed, the scores for each column are averaged. Sections where the answer was "Not Applicable" are omitted from the average.

For example, following are the responses from our Mr. Jones across the eight questions on the inventory (recall that four are predetermined, and four are nominated by the patient):

- Initial Disability: 4, 1, NA, 3, 3, 4, 3, NA— Average = 3
- Handicap: 3, NA, NA, 4, 5, 5, 3, NA— Average = 4
- Use: 4, NA, NA, 2, 5, 2, 4, NA—Average = 3.4
- Benefit: 3, NA, NA, 3, 3, 2, 3, NA— Average = 2.8
- Residual Disability: 2, NA, NA, 3, 2, 4, 2, NA—Average = 2.6
- Satisfaction: 3, NA, NA, 2, 3, 2, 3, NA— Average = 2.6

The average score is scaled to a number between 0 and 100 instead of 1 and 5. To do this, subtract 1 from the average score and then multiply it by 25. After this is completed, the scores are initial disability, 50; handicap, 75; use, 60; benefit, 45; residual disability, 40; and satisfaction, 40. If the GHABP software is used, the score is calculated automatically, which is the approach we recommend.

Scores can be looked at individually or compared to the norms of hearing aid users with similar characteristics (Gatehouse, 2000). To illustrate this, examples of normative data combined from two clinics in the United Kingdom are plotted for unaided, aided, and the general population in Figure 19-6. Our patient had an initial disability score of 50, placing him just above the 60th percentile for unaided individuals. His residual disability (aided) score of 40 places him at the 80th percentile for this normative group. The developer encourages each clinical facility to generate reference data that is specific to the circumstances of its clinic population (Gatehouse, 1997).

Another interesting analysis by the developers was consideration of how improvement in audibility

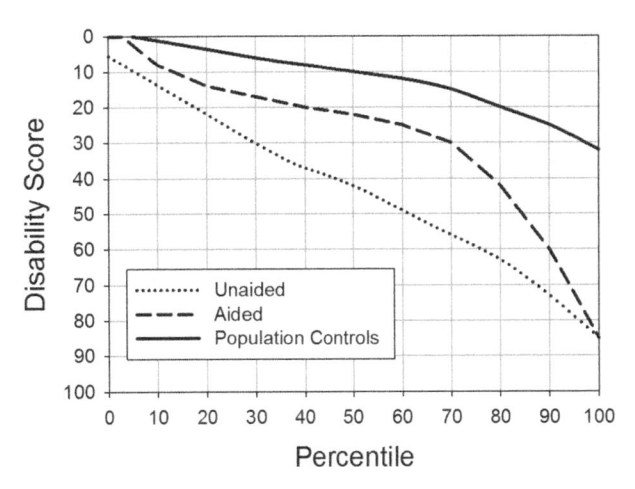

Figure 19-6. Percentile distribution of the disability scores from the GHABP for unaided and aided conditions and for the aggregated population controls. This graph shows which percentile patients with and without hearing aids, as well as normal-hearing people, fall into in terms of disability. Because these norms were established within two hospital settings in England, they are not intended as norms for other populations; rather, the developers suggest generating norms in each clinical setting of use. (Adapted from Gatehouse, 1997.)

relates to each of these domains: use, benefit, satisfaction, and handicap. They determined that reported use and reported benefit are predictable from increased SII or audibility.

Clinical Application

The GHABP may be used in different ways. Before intervention, the patient may fill out the initial disability and handicap scales and then complete the form after intervention. Or, the GHABP may be used to evaluate the effectiveness once intervention is complete (Gatehouse, 2000). Comparing the user's scores to the appropriate norms lets the user know if he or she is doing better, worse, or about the same as the typical hearing aid user. The GHABP may also be used to evaluate a goal of rehabilitation. For example, if the goal is to have the patient wear his or her hearing aids in more situations, the GHABP can be used to monitor the progress. When the patient responds that he or she wears the hearing aids "all of the time" in all circumstances where the hearing aids are needed, then that goal can be considered met.

A disadvantage of the GHAPB is that it is subject to recall bias. The hearing aid users must remember how much difficulty they were experiencing prior to hearing aid fitting. Various electronic and paper versions of the GHABP have been posted by the Medical Research Council: Institute of Hearing Research. Although these documents are freely available, the web address to which they are posted sometimes moves. Therefore, we encourage interested readers to simply search for "Glasgow Hearing Aid Benefit Profile" to obtain a copy.

Satisfaction With Amplification in Daily Life (SADL)

When the SADL was developed, many outcome measures were focused on hearing aid benefit. Although benefit is closely related to the performance of the hearing aid, it does not encompass other factors that affect the satisfaction of the hearing aid user, such as services or cost. The SADL, therefore, was developed to find a hearing aid user's overall satisfaction score, as well as break the score down into specific problem areas (Cox & Alexander, 1999).

Background

The SADL is an indirect measure of satisfaction and was developed by Cox and Alexander (1999). The items are very similar to those of the Expected Consequences of Hearing Aid Ownership or ECHO (Cox & Alexander, 2000), which was described in Chapter 7. A summary of the scale is as follows:

- The scale consists of 15 items.
- The scale has four subscales: positive effect, service and cost, negative features, and personal image.
- All items are rated on a 7-category scale: not at all, a little, somewhat, medium, considerably, greatly, tremendously.
- The scale takes less than about 10 minutes to complete.

The current clinical setting requires that outcome measures be easy to administer and time-efficient. The SADL items are written at a seventh-grade reading level; it takes less than 10 minutes to complete. It is an indirect measure because it does not directly ask the hearing aid users to rate their satisfaction but quantifies it through questions regarding different dimensions of hearing aid satisfaction (Cox & Alexander, 1999).

Each of the four subscales of the SADL covers a different aspect of satisfaction and was decided upon by interviewing many hearing aid users with at least one year of experience. According to the interviews of those hearing aid users, the domains of satisfaction are cosmetics and self-image, comfort and ease of use, sound quality/acoustics, cost, benefit, and service. Further exploration showed that comfort and ease of use didn't significantly contribute to user satisfaction. Although it is unclear why comfort and ease of use were not significant factors, we speculate that it is unlikely that a hearing aid wearer will purchase and keep a hearing aid that is either uncomfortable or too difficult to use. If so, these may still be important factors to hearing aid wearers; they just don't show up as significant when listeners who wear a particular set of hearing aids are evaluated.

We find a Global Satisfaction score by combining the four SADL subscale scores detailed below (Cox & Alexander, 1999):

1. Positive Effect. This scale has twice as many (six) items as any of the other scales and contributes more to the variance in satisfaction than any other subscale. Questions in this subscale cover acoustic benefit, sound quality, and psychological aspects of satisfaction. Positive Effect Example Question #6: "Do you think your hearing aid(s) is worth the trouble?"
2. Service and Cost. Hearing aid users assert that the cost of the instruments and the services they receive from clinicians greatly influence their satisfaction. Service & Cost Example Question #14: "Does the cost of your hearing aid(s) seem reasonable to you?"
3. Negative Features. Each of the items in this scale focus on different specific problem areas in hearing aid use, such as the telephone, feedback, and unwanted background noise. Satisfaction scores in this subscale may take longer than others to become stable (McLeod, Upfold, & Broadbent, 2001). Negative Features Example Question #7: "Are you frus-

trated when your hearing aid(s) picks up sounds that keep you from hearing what you want to hear?"
4. Personal Image. This subscale centers around the stigma associated with hearing aid use as well as the hearing aid user's self-image. Although this is important to hearing aid users, it is not as influential on satisfaction as communication benefit or services received. Personal Image Example Question #4: "How content are you with the appearance of your hearing aid(s)?"

As with any outcome measure, the SADL has some limitations. For hearing aid users who receive their instruments through the VA or through a third-party payer, cost may not be an issue, so item 14 should be omitted (Cox & Alexander, 1999). The scale contains four items that are scored in reverse, and this might lead to misinterpretation of the responses on the part of the patients, which would result in invalid global, negative features, and personal image scores (Hosford-Dunn & Halpern, 2000). Although more time-consuming, it may be worthwhile to administer this and other outcome measures with "reversed items" orally to patients that might have difficulty with written comprehension.

Research has shown that the SADL has good test–retest reliability for the Global score (Cox & Alexander, 1999), good construct and cross validity (Cox & Alexander, 2001), and good content, factorial, and statistical validity for private practice patients (Hosford-Dunn & Halpern, 2000).

Since the SADL questionnaire does not actually mention the word "satisfaction," Cox and Alexander (2001) compared the Global score of 196 respondents with the single-item satisfaction question: "How satisfied are you with your hearing aids?" Subjects answered the question on a scale from 1 (very dissatisfied) to 5 (very satisfied). Results showed that a Global score of 4.1 on the SADL corresponded to an answer of "dissatisfied" on the single-item scale. Therefore, patients who report scores of 4.0 and lower can be interpreted as dissatisfied with their hearing aids (Cox & Alexander, 2001).

Hosford-Dunn and Halpern (2001) looked at the effects of individual variables on the SADL Global and subscale scores. Subjects ($n = 282$) in this study were English-speaking adults who had been fit with hearing aids between 1996 and 1997 and had worn their hearing aids for at least one year. The variables examined included age, style of hearing aid, duration of hearing aid use, daily use, degree of hearing loss, processing technology, and cost of hearing aids. They found small but significant relationships between many of the variables and SADL scores. Their results showed that adults over 59 years old had more negative global and positive effect scores than their younger counterparts. Even though the older adults tended to have more hearing loss, the authors found that adults who had more hearing loss and used the hearing aids for longer periods each day had higher positive effect scores. Those adults with greater amounts of hearing loss and a longer duration of hearing aid use reported lower (poorer) negative feature scores. The authors attribute this to the effect issues with feedback that accompany greater amounts of gain (Hosford-Dunn & Halpern, 2001).

In the same study, results showed that patients with smaller hearing instruments (ITCs and CICs) reported less dissatisfaction in the negative features subscale and higher satisfaction in the personal image subscale than those with larger instruments (traditional BTEs and ITEs). The authors reported that the patients with smaller instruments tended to be younger with less hearing loss who therefore had less hearing difficulty. The study also found a small positive relationship between higher-priced hearing instruments and patients with higher Personal Image scores. When the authors looked at the different types of processing in the hearing aids (analog vs. digital), they found no difference in SADL scores (Hosford-Dunn & Halpern, 2001). This study and the SADL norms were conducted before the surge in popularity of mini-BTE open-fit hearing aids and the feedback management systems that made them possible. Those two factors might affect current SADL scores.

To assess the stability in SADL scores over time, researchers in Australia gave the questionnaire to a specific group of patients (McLeod et al., 2001). All of the patients in the study were more than 60 years old at the time of their fitting, retired, and were fit with the same hearing aid by the same two audiologists. The patients were divided into two groups determined by the time interval between their fittings and filling out the questionnaire. One group, referred to as the 2-week group, consisted of 45 participants who were given the scale at the two-week follow-up to their hearing aid fitting. The other group, referred to as the 12-month group, consisted of 75 participants who had been fitted between 12 and 24 months earlier and were mailed the questionnaire. When the scores of each group were compared, global and all subscales were lower for the 12-month group than for the 2-week group. The only subscale that was not significantly different between the two timeframes was the personal image subscale, and the subscale with the largest difference was negative features.

Results from this study suggest that some aspects (personal appearance, communication improvement) are stable over time but not others (background noise interference, feedback) and take time to become apparent in outcome measures. Therefore, the authors argue, two weeks post fitting is likely too soon to assess satisfaction in hearing aid patients. As we discussed earlier in this chapter, there may be no one ideal time to conduct such a measure. On one hand, we want the outcome results early so that we can nip any problems that might exist in the bud—and to be practical, this needs to happen during the 30-day return policy. Yet, we know that it may be 60 days or more before many patients are able to effectively rate the performance of their hearing aids.

Administration and Scoring

For each of the 15 items of the SADL, the patient has the choice of seven answers:

- Not At All
- A Little
- Somewhat
- Medium
- Considerably
- Greatly
- Tremendously

The patient reads each scale item and then answers the questions with one of the preceding choices. The scale can be scored manually or by a computer program. For most of the items, an answer of "Not At All," which indicates low satisfaction, receives one point and "Tremendously," which indicates high satisfaction, receives seven points. There are four items (2, 4, 7, and 13) where scoring is reversed, and an answer of "Not At All" indicates high satisfaction and receives seven points, whereas "Tremendously" indicates low satisfaction and receives only one point (Cox & Alexander, 1999).

The global satisfaction score is computed by averaging the score of all of the items. Satisfaction scores for each of the subscales are found by averaging the scores of each of the subscale items. If a patient skips some of the items, the subscale scores are only valid if two-thirds of the questions are answered. The global score can be computed only when each subscale has a valid score (Cox & Alexander, 1999).

The norms for interpreting the scores are listed in Table 19–3. These norms were first reported in Cox and Alexander (1999) and were validated in Cox and Alex-

---

TECHNICAL TIP: SADL VERSUS MARKETRAK?

Humes et al. (2002) compared the SADL scale to the MarkeTrak IV survey (Kochkin, 1994a, 1994b, 1996, 1997, 1998) to see whether the two questionnaires led to similar conclusions. The MarkeTrak IV satisfaction survey is direct in that it asks hearing aid users how satisfied they are with certain aspects of hearing aid use. Although both surveys look at hearing aid user-satisfaction, the SADL consists of 15 items, whereas the MarkeTrak surveys contain about 40 items. In the Humes (2002) study, 43 elderly hearing aid users were fit with the same style of WDRC ITC hearing aids. One month after they were fit, the subjects filled out the two questionnaires. The global scores for each of the surveys had moderately strong positive correlation ($r = .75$), which was statistically significant. The correlation scores of the subscales were lower, but were still statistically significant (0.42 to 0.62). This study suggests that the same information can be gathered with the much shorter and more clinically convenient SADL as with the longer, more detailed MarkeTrak-IV satisfaction survey (Humes et al., 2002). The MarkeTrak satisfaction survey, however, does address many specific issues that are not directly mentioned on the SADL, which may be of interest to some audiologists.

Table 19–3. Normative Data for the SADL

Score	Mean	SD	80th	20th	Application
Global*	4.9	1.0	5.9	4.2	3rd Party Pay
Global	4.9	0.8	5.6	4.3	Private Pay
Service & Cost*	5.4	1.2	6.5	4.5	3rd Party Pay
Service & Cost	4.7	1.2	5.7	4.0	Private Pay
Positive Effect	4.9	1.3	6.1	3.8	All Patients
Negative Features	3.6	1.4	5.0	2.3	All Patients
Personal Image	5.6	1.1	6.7	5.0	All Patients

*"Reasonable Cost" is omitted.

Source: Adapted from Cox and Alexander (1999) with permission.

ander (2001). Scores obtained from patients that are lower than the norms can be interpreted as dissatisfaction in the areas with the poor scores.

Clinical Application

There are three main applications of the SADL in the clinical setting. The scale can be used to compare a hearing aid user's satisfaction to normative data and to compare the scores from the same hearing aid user under two different conditions—such as choosing between two hearing aids during the fitting process—and the subscale scores can be used to find the reasons why a patient's global satisfaction score is low (Cox & Alexander, 1999).

Sometimes it is useful for a hearing aid user to see how his or her scores compare to a typical group of peers; for example, to see whether they are more or less satisfied than others with the outcome of their fitting, or if others have similar issues with their hearing aids (Cox & Alexander, 1999). There are several ways to do so. Our 77-year-old patient has decided it is time for a new set of hearing aids. After several months of use, he is asked to fill out the SADL inventory. It is apparent from Figure 19–7 that he is at or above the 50th percentile for the global score and two of the four subscales (positive effect and personal image). He is still below the 50th percentile for service and cost and negative features.

We can plot our patient's outcomes in a slightly different manner. In Figure 19–8, the 90th and 10th percentiles for satisfaction are shown as line functions. The same information can be gleaned, but here is an interesting note: In the pre-fitting phase of our hearing aid work, we obtained ECHO scores as we described in Chapter 7. It is apparent from the comparison of Figures 19–8 and 19–9 that our patient's expectations were in relatively good alignment with his self-reported satisfaction. Even the personal image subscale seems logical when you consider that our patient was not all that concerned (low expectations) about that domain, yet his satisfaction was above the 90th percentile for the published norms.

To compare a hearing aid user's satisfaction under different conditions, we must once again consider critical difference (CD) scores. As we have discussed, the CD score is a statistically based way to see whether the difference in scores is a result of chance or is truly a significant change in satisfaction. Critical difference scores for the SADL are given for 90% and 95% confidence intervals in Table 19–4.

Our 77-year-old patient is struggling with his new set of hearing aids. He has worn hearing aids bilaterally for the past ten years. His SADL scores with his previous hearing aids are shown in Table 19–5. Looking at the global score, it appears that he is more satisfied with his previous hearing aids, but the difference between the two scores is 0.5 and does not meet the CD score of 0.9 (for 90% confidence), so we cannot be confident that the difference is a real one. When we look at the negative features score, there is a significant difference of 2.3, which meets the 95% CD interval, indicating that his old

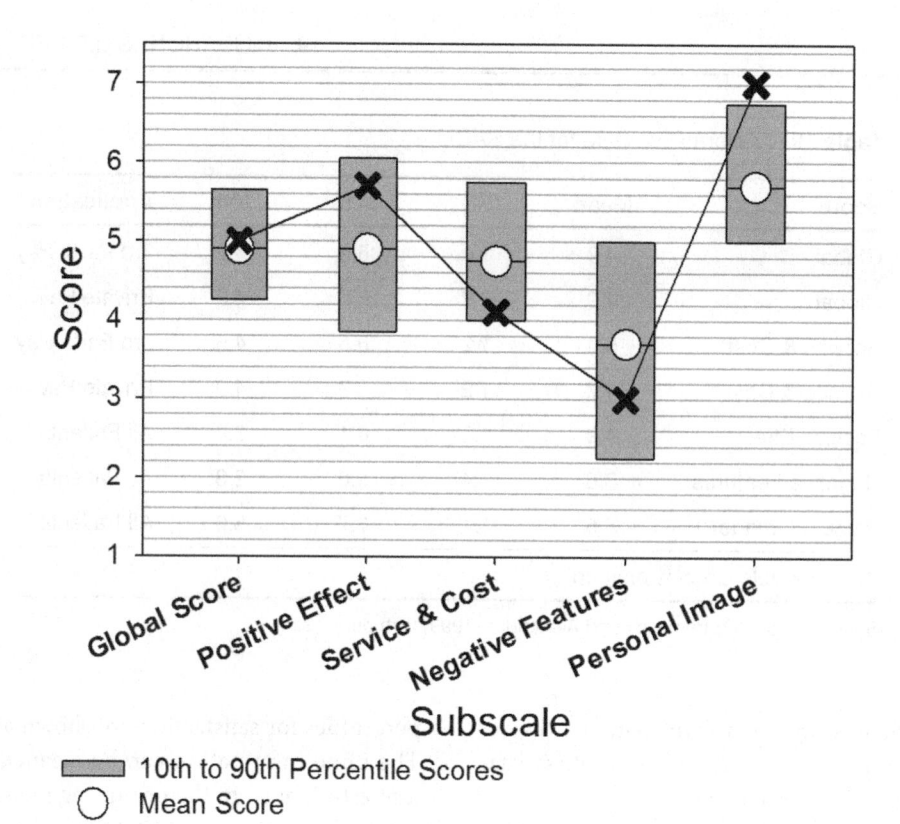

Figure 19–7. SADL normative data for hearing aid users who were not VA-connected; that is, patients paid for hearing aids. Scores for a 77-year-old patient shown by "X" marks.

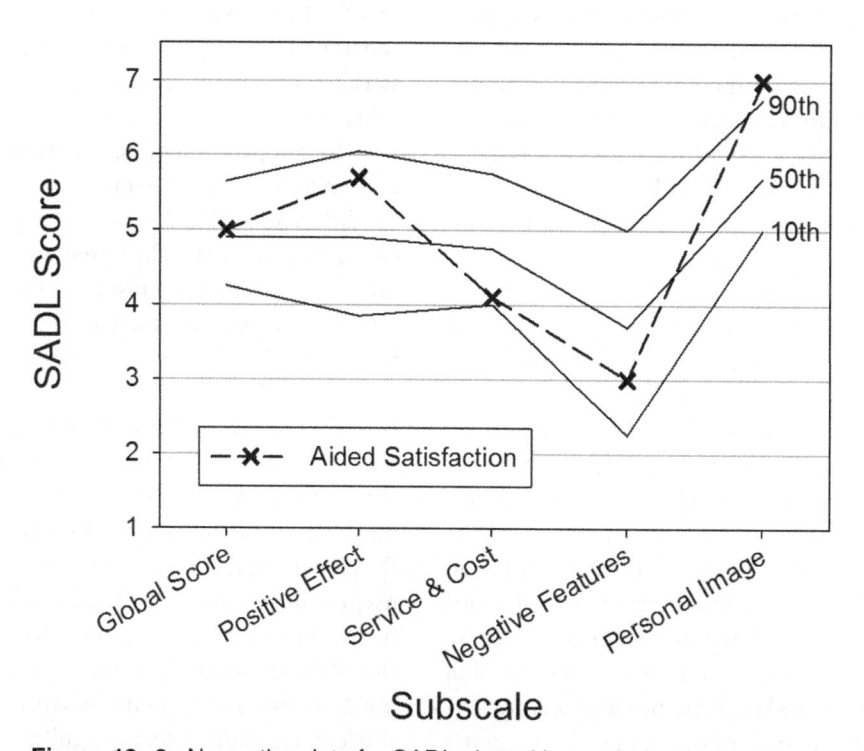

Figure 19–8. Normative data for SADL plotted in another manner.

756

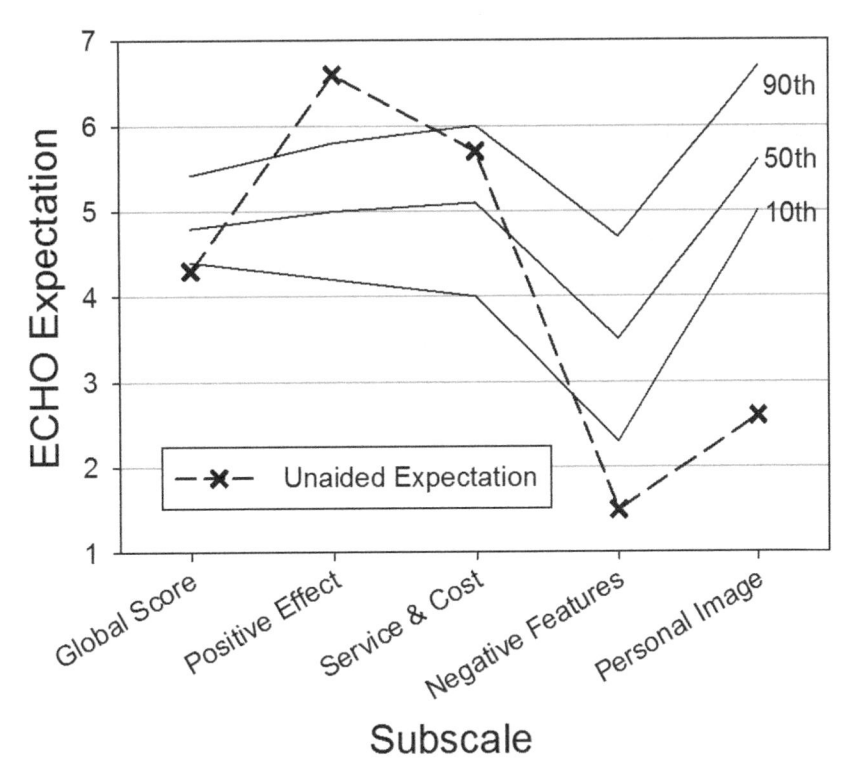

Figure 19–9. Example expectation scores.

Table 19–4. Critical Difference (CD) Values for SADL Global Score and Subscales at 90% and 95% Confidence

Score	90% CD	95% CD
Global	0.9	1.0
Positive Effect	1.3	1.6
Service & Cost	1.3	1.6
Negative Features	2.0	2.3
Personal Image	1.6	2.0

Source: Adapted from Cox and Alexander (1999) with permission.

Table 19–5. Two Sets of SADL Scores from a 77-Year-Old Patient

	Global	Positive Effect	Service & Cost	Negative Features	Personal Image
Previous HA	5.1	4.6	4.7	6	6
Current HA	4.6	3.8	4.7	3.7	6

Note. The differences in scores (global and across subscales) can be compared to the CDs to determine whether there are real differences.

> **POINTS TO PONDER: ARE OLDER NORMS STILL VALID?**
>
> As we have mentioned, the norms for some of the scales we are using were collected 15 or more years ago. Are these norms still valid today? After all, hearing aid technology has changed. Do these changes impact overall benefit and satisfaction? One way to at least obtain a general impression of the impact of technology is to compare MarkeTrak surveys taken over the years. The methodology for these serial surveys was very similar and, of course, the number of participants was much higher than that observed for other surveys of this type (e.g., n = over 2000 for most categories). Figure 19–10 shows a comparison of overall satisfaction for the MarkeTrak survey taken in 1997 and the survey taken in 2008 (Kochkin, 2010). Data are shown both for all users and for only the new users (one year or less of hearing aid use). There seems to be good news, in that overall satisfaction increased—54 to 74% for all users. Observe, however, that dissatisfaction rates and the percent of in-the-drawer hearing aids did not change substantially. Note also that there are significantly fewer neutral ratings for the 2008 survey. We suspect this is because the Likert scale used in 2008 was a seven-point scale, whereas it was only a five-point scale in 1997. The categories "Somewhat Satisfied" and "Somewhat Dissatisfied" were added. It's possible that part of the satisfaction increase for 2008 was because of the "Somewhat Satisfied" patients, who might not have given a "Satisfied" rating had they used the five-point scale from the 1997 survey. We see a similar trend if we look at specific items related to satisfaction. For example, for whistling/feedback, satisfaction increased from 43 to 69%, but dissatisfaction only improved slightly (24 to 18%). So are the norms from 10 to 15 years ago still okay to use? We would say "probably yes" because overall, at least for satisfaction ratings, it appears that there is a trend for better performance, but significant changes aren't apparent. But we will add the caveat that the 2008 MarkeTrak data are *now* somewhat dated. And of course, we also need to consider the findings of MarkeTrak9 (Abrams et al., 2014), although a different sampling method was used.

hearing aid resulted in more satisfaction relative to the negative features associated with hearing aid use! From there we can look back at his answers to the items in that subscale in order to reprogram his hearing aids or to counsel him regarding the new devices.

In this case, comparing the negative features subscale score to the norms may also be beneficial. The mean score for a typical hearing aid user on this scale is 3.6, which is very close to the score of 3.7 with our patient's current aid. His score of 6 on the same scale for his previous hearing aids is well above one standard deviation (80th percentile).

Obtaining the SADL/A

An electronic PDF version of the questionnaire, scoring instructions, and norms can be downloaded at the University of Memphis Hearing Aid Research Lab's website. Here are the links to the Questionnaire, the Scoring Document, and the Norms Template, respectively:

http://www.memphis.edu/ausp/harl/downloads/SADL15.pdf

http://www.memphis.edu/ausp/harl/downloads/SADLScoring.pdf

http://www.memphis.edu/ausp/harl/downloads/SADLPlot.pdf

You can download the scoring software for $30 at the following website: http://www.memphis.edu/ausp/auspsoft/purchase.htm

The SADL has also been translated into Danish, Spanish, Brazilian-Portuguese, German, Mandarin, Cantonese, Swedish, and Odia and can be downloaded from this website: http://www.memphis.edu/csd/harl/sadl.htm

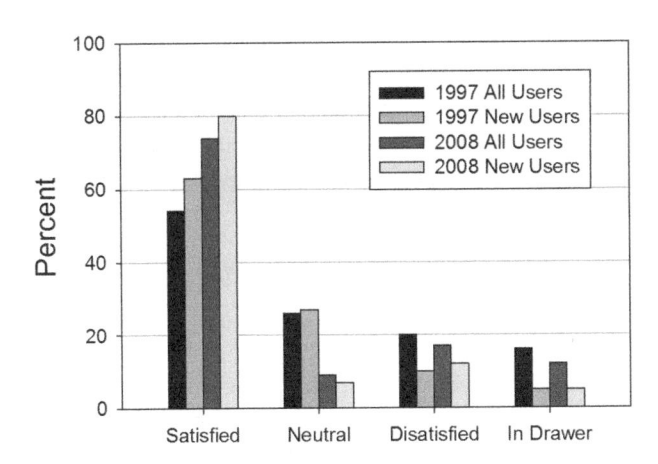

Figure 19–10. Comparison of overall satisfaction for the MarkeTrak survey taken in 1997 and the most recent survey, taken in 2008. (Adapted from Kochkin, 2010.)

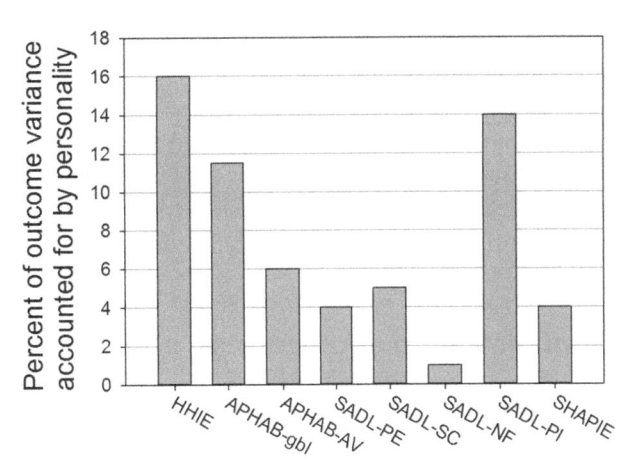

Figure 19–11. Study of the extent to which various outcome measures are related to personality. *HHIE* = Hearing Handicap Inventory for the Elderly (Ventry & Weinstein, 1982), *SHAPIE* = Shortened Hearing Performance Inventory of the Elderly (Dillon, 1994), *APHAB* = Abbreviated Profile of Hearing Aid Benefit (Cox & Alexander, 1995), *SADL* = Satisfaction with Amplification in Daily Life (Cox & Alexander, 1999). (Adapted from Cox et al., 2014, with permission.)

Device Oriented Subjective Outcome (DOSO)

The Device Oriented Subjective Outcome (DOSO) was developed, as the name implies, to measure the benefit of the device, and to be less sensitive to the personality of the hearing aid wearer (Cox, Alexander, & Xu, 2009).

Background

In their 2007 study, Cox, Alexander, and Gray found that many questions on self-report questionnaires were more closely related to the hearing aid users' personalities than to their audiometric hearing loss. The DOSO attempts to separate outcomes with the device from the influence of personality (Cox, Alexander, & Xu, 2009). Figure 19–11 depicts the extent to which outcome data from several popular questionnaires can be attributed to personality (Cox et al., 2007), showing substantial differences among the different scales, or subscales. For example, the handicap measured with the HHIE (Ventry & Weinstein, 1982), the disability measured by the APHAB (Cox & Alexander, 1995), and the satisfaction measured by the SADL (Cox & Alexander, 1999), were more strongly associated with personality than the other outcome measures tested. That certainly creates confusion in trying to determine the outcomes of our intervention strategies!

Cox et al. (2009) suggest that regardless of the outcome domain (handicap, benefit, satisfaction, etc.), self-reported hearing aid outcomes fall into two broad categories: device-oriented and wearer-oriented. The authors conclude that wearer-oriented outcomes are associated with user personality, but device-oriented outcomes are not (or very little). The potential problem here is that, if the outcome measure depends partly on the personality of the patient, then these measures may not be very sensitive to differences between hearing aids, and are not optimal for evaluating new technology or comparing processing strategies. This led to the development of the DOSO, which, as the name indicates, is device-oriented and not wearer-oriented.

Some general background regarding the DOSO includes the following:

- The scale has three different forms, two equivalent short forms—DOSO(a) and DOSO(b)—and one long form (DOSO).
- The number of items on the forms is 28 (short forms) and 40 (long form).

- The measure has six subscales: speech cues, listening effort, pleasantness, quietness, convenience, and use.
- All items (other than those for the use subscale) are rated on a seven-category scale: Not At All, A Little, Somewhat, Medium, Considerably, Greatly, and Tremendously.

Administration and Scoring

For each of the items in the speech cues, listening effort, pleasantness, quietness, and convenience subscales of the DOSO, the patient has the choice of seven answers with seven different point values: Not At All (1), A Little (2), Somewhat (3), Medium (4), Considerably (5), Greatly (6), and Tremendously (7). The subscales address "how good is your hearing aid" across five factors: speech cues, listening effort, quietness, pleasantness, and convenience. Sample questions from the general categories are shown for each subscale in Table 19–6.

The Hearing Aid Research Lab (HARL) at the University of Memphis provides guidelines for test administration at its website (http://www.harlmemphis.org). The patient reads each scale item and then answers the questions with one of the choices listed. The scale can be scored manually or by a computer program. Each answer is given a numerical value from 1 to 7, with higher numbers associated with better outcomes. For the three items of the use subscale, answers are given values from 1 to 5. Again, higher values indicate a better outcome. For the two questions regarding use in terms of hours per day and days per week, an answer with the shortest amount of time receives 1 point, and the greatest amount of time receives 5 points. For the question regarding use in situations where improvement in hearing is needed, an answer of "Always" receives 5 points, whereas an answer of "Never" receives only 1 point. As the use time decreases, so does the value associated with the answer.

Once the answers are converted to numerical data, responses for each subscale are averaged to calculate the score of the subscale. It is not uncommon for a patient to skip some of the items, but subscale scores are valid only if two-thirds of the questions are answered. Table 19–7 shows the number of completed items required for a valid score for each form.

Table 19–7. Number of Completed Items Required per Form for a Valid DOSO Score

	Number of Items	
Subscale	Forms A and B	Long Form
Speech Cues	5	10
Listening Effort	4	7
Pleasantness	3	3
Quietness	4	4
Convenience	3	3
Use	2	2

Table 19–6. Content of Six Subscales of the DOSO With Sample Item From Each

	How Good Are the Hearing Aids for . . .
Speech Cues	Recognizing different voices?
Listening Effort	Distinguishing between male and female voices?
Quietness	Keeping loud sounds from being uncomfortable?
Pleasantness	Keeping the volume at a pleasing level?
Convenience	Being easy to put in and out of your ears?
Use	How many days a week do you usually wear your hearing aids?

Source: Adapted from Cox (2009).

Figure 19–12 and Table 19–8 show a norms template for interpreting the subscale scores. The norms were reported in Cox, Alexander, and Xu (2009). Scores obtained from patients that are lower than the norms can be interpreted as dissatisfaction in those areas.

Clinical Application

In the clinical setting, the DOSO is useful for measuring differences between devices or technologies. Questions in the DOSO are worded to minimize the effect of

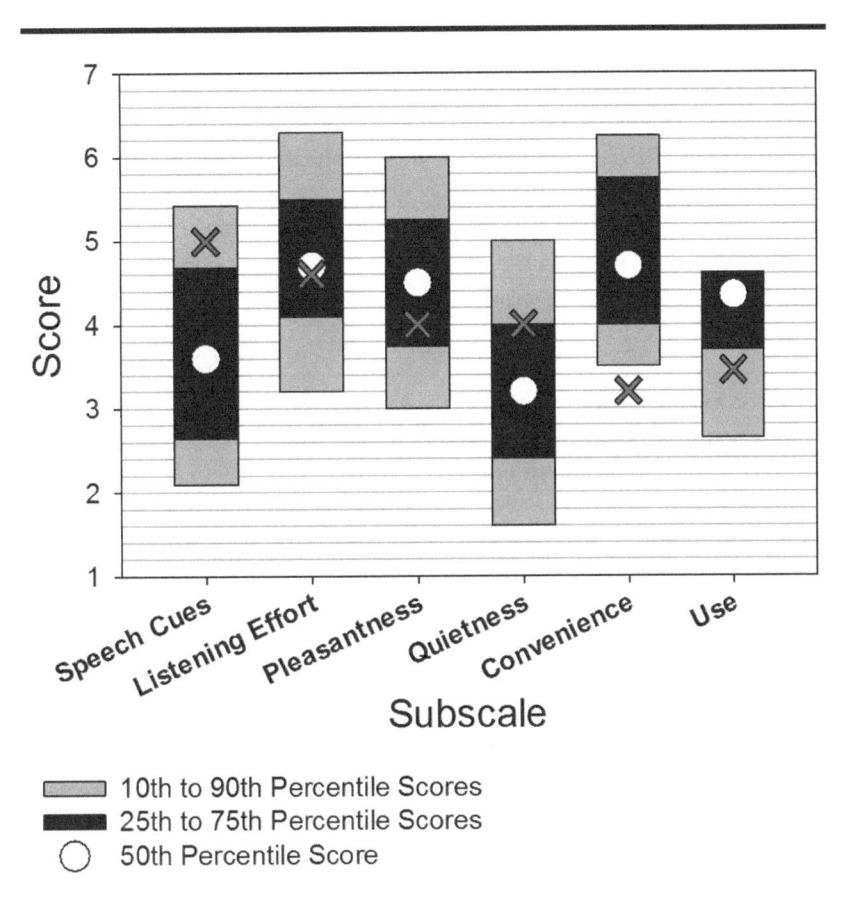

Figure 19–12. Normative data for the DOSO. No critical differences (CDs) have been established for this tool, but the norms can support counseling and management decision. Sample patient scores shows by "X." (From Cox, 2014.)

Table 19–8. A Norms Template for Interpreting the DOSO Subscale Scores

Subscale	Percentile Score						
	5	10	25	50	75	90	95
Speech Cues	1.9	2.1	2.7	3.6	4.7	5.4	5.8
Listening Effort	2.7	3.2	4.1	4.8	5.5	6.3	6.5
Pleasantness	2.5	3.0	3.8	4.5	5.3	6.0	6.4
Quietness	1.4	1.6	2.4	3.2	4.0	5.0	5.8
Convenience	3.3	3.5	4.0	4.8	5.8	6.3	6.5
Use	2.3	2.7	3.7	4.3	4.7	4.7	4.7

personality and to point toward the hearing instrument (Cox, Alexander, & Xu, 2009). Therefore, if a patient cannot decide between two different pairs of hearing aids or between two different programs on the same pair of hearing aids, the DOSO can be administered to compare the technologies. When clear differences in hearing aids or technologies are apparent, this outcome measure can aid in the decision-making process.

Recall that Forms DOSO(a) and DOSO(b) each consist of 28 items. The difference between them relates to the items in the speech cues and listening effort subscales. They are equivalent forms, however, and you can use them for repeated administrations to produce scores for all six subscales. The long form DOSO comprises all 40 items and produces scores for all six subscales. Interim norms have been developed using the DOSO (long form), but they are also applicable to the DOSO(a) and DOSO(b) short forms (Cox, Alexander, & Xu, 2014). These were obtained from 179 clinic and private practice patients who participated in the development of the questionnaire.

As an example of the usefulness of this tool, let us consider a patient who has been relatively vocal, in a negative way, during his or her care in your clinic. The obvious concern in obtaining outcomes of our management efforts is ascertaining how much of his vocalized concerns are related to *the patient*, and not to the success or failure of your management strategy. Upon completion of the DOSO(b), results show that he or she is well below the norms on the convenience subscale. With that new information, you can address possible difficulties that the patient may not have expressed relative to insertion and removal of the battery and/or the hearing aids, any dexterity concerns—for either side—and other non-hearing factors that seem to impact his or her overall satisfaction with the new hearing aids.

Obtaining the DOSO

An electronic PDF version of the questionnaires, scoring instructions, and norms can be downloaded at the University of Memphis Hearing Aid Research Lab's website. Here are the links to the Questionnaire, the Scoring Document, and the Norms Template, respectively:

http://www.harlmemphis.org//index.php?cID=148

http://www.harlmemphis.org/files/6213/5041/6232/manual_scoring_instructions.pdf

http://www.harlmemphis.org/files/4213/5041/6231/doso_template.pdf

You can find the link to the scoring software at http://www.memphis.edu/csd/auspsoft/purchase.htm. The DOSO has also been translated into Mandarin and can be downloaded from this website: http://www.harlmemphis.org//index.php?cID=148

The International Outcome Inventory for Hearing Aids (IOI-HA)

The IOI-HA is a short inventory used to quantify the effectiveness of hearing aid treatment and to facilitate cooperation between researchers/clinicians in var-

---

KEY CONCEPT: IS THE DOSO FREE OF PERSONALITY INFLUENCE?

As we have stated, one of the goals in developing the DOSO was to have an outcome measure that was Device-oriented, and not significantly influenced by the wearer's personality. So were they successful in attaining this goal? Cox and colleagues (1997) reported on preliminary data related to this question and, based on those findings, the answer is "sort of." These authors compared the association between scores on the DOSO for the six different subscales and the Positive and Negative Affect Schedule (PANAS) personality test. The data suggest that four of the subscales are independent of personality, but the listening effort and convenience subscales are somewhat associated with personality.

ied settings (Cox & Alexander, 2002). This inventory is unique in that it addresses several domains related to hearing aid use and is the outcome measure that is available in the greatest number of different languages, allowing for hearing aid outcome comparisons around the world.

Background

The IOI-HA is a product of a workshop entitled, "Measuring Outcomes in Audiological Rehabilitation Using Hearing Aids," held in 2000 in Eriksholm, Denmark. The IOI-HA is a result of the expressed need for a "universal" outcome measure. Even when outcome measures address the same topics and are written in the same language, the differences in the data are such that they often cannot be directly compared. In the field of audiology, the sample sizes in many studies are relatively small, and outcome measures are not particularly sensitive. In order to reach statistical significance and draw conclusions from data, it is beneficial for researchers to pool their data to evaluate different treatment options (Cox et al., 2000; Cox & Alexander, 2002). Despite the research goal central to the development of the IOI-HA, it can also be useful for clinical comparisons across groups based on differences in clinical setting, treatment option, or specific clinician. Alternatively, it can be used as a very quick way to evaluate patient outcomes to reinforce the positive impact of our clinical services.

The IOI-HA consists of seven items that focus on different domains of hearing aid outcomes. The domains that are assessed are benefit, daily use, satisfaction, impact on significant others, residual activity limitation, residual participation restriction, and quality of life. Because the inventory is short, it is intended to be a supplement to the outcome measures used in a given study with minimal added resources and is general enough that it can apply to many different research questions. These factors allow data from similar studies across cultures and countries to be assembled to strengthen statistical power (Cox & Alexander, 2002; Cox, Alexander, & Beyer, 2003).

The IOI-HA items were originally written in easy-to-understand English and have been translated into 22 different languages. So that psychometric properties can be established, only one official version has been translated per language (Cox & Alexander, 2002). Currently, the inventory is available in Arabic, Chinese, Danish, Dutch, English, Finnish, French, German, Greek, Hebrew, Italian, Japanese, Korean, Mandarin, Malay, Norwegian, Polish, Brazilian Portuguese, Russian, Serbian, Sinhalese, Slovenian, Spanish, and Welsh. There are two other versions of the outcome measure. Noble (2002) adapted the inventory to obtain the view of significant others (International Outcome Inventory for Hearing Aids—Significant Other; IOI-HA-SO) and to assess other amplification intervention such as television devices or amplified telephones (International Outcome Inventory for Alternative Interventions; IOI-AI). Cox, Alexander, and Beyer (2003) established norms for the IOI-HA. An eighth item was added to the inventory: "How much hearing loss do you have when you are not wearing your hearing aids?" This item was intended to identify how much perceived difficulty the participants had. The authors chose a subject population that was, at the time, widely representative of the typical hearing aid user. The subjects ($n = 154$) all wore bilateral,

---

**THINGS TO REMEMBER:
KEY POINTS REGARDING THE IOI-HA**

- Seven items/domains: benefit, daily use, satisfaction, impact on significant others, residual activity limitation, residual participation restriction, and quality of life.
- Appropriate for adult hearing aid users with mild to severe hearing losses.
- Intended for new hearing aid users but can be used for all hearing aid users.
- Proposed to be used in addition to specific outcome measures utilized in research studies so that data can be compared across countries and cultures.
- Assesses the quality-of-treatment intervention (Cox et al., 2000), so it is useful for comparing outcomes across clinicians or clinical sites.

programmable analog, compression ITE instruments and obtained them from a private practice. All subjects had purchased their hearing aids six to 12 months prior to filling out the inventory.

Results from their study revealed that the IOI-HA was affected by subjective hearing difficulty without amplification. Analysis indicated that participants with more subjective hearing difficulty without amplification had significantly different scores on four of the inventory items than those with less difficulty. Participants with more subjective hearing difficulty were shown to use their hearing aids longer on a daily basis, were more satisfied with their hearing aids, had more improvement in their quality of life, and felt that they were more of an inconvenience to others because of their hearing losses than those with less subjective hearing difficulty. Therefore, there are separate norms for those with mild-to moderate subjective hearing difficulty and those with moderate-to-severe subjective hearing difficulty. The norms for the IOI-HA are summarized in Figure 19–13 and Table 19–9 (Cox, Alexander, & Beyer, 2003).

More than any other variable, the daily use item was affected by other factors. Specifically, participants who used two hearing aids all of the time, paid full price for their aids, and had prior hearing aid experience reported wearing their hearing aids significantly longer than other participants. Therefore, clinicians may want to pay particular attention to that item as an indication that the hearing aids may not be set optimally (Cox, Alexander, & Beyer, 2003).

Administration and Scoring

Each of the IOI-HA items has five answers that range from the worst outcome on the left to the best outcome on the right. Answer choices are equidistant in meaning in English. The inventory is meant to be given in paper-and-pencil form. It is very self-explanatory, and there are no formal instructions (Cox & Alexander, 2002).

To score the outcome, each answer is given a number value 1 (worst) through 5 (best). For this measure,

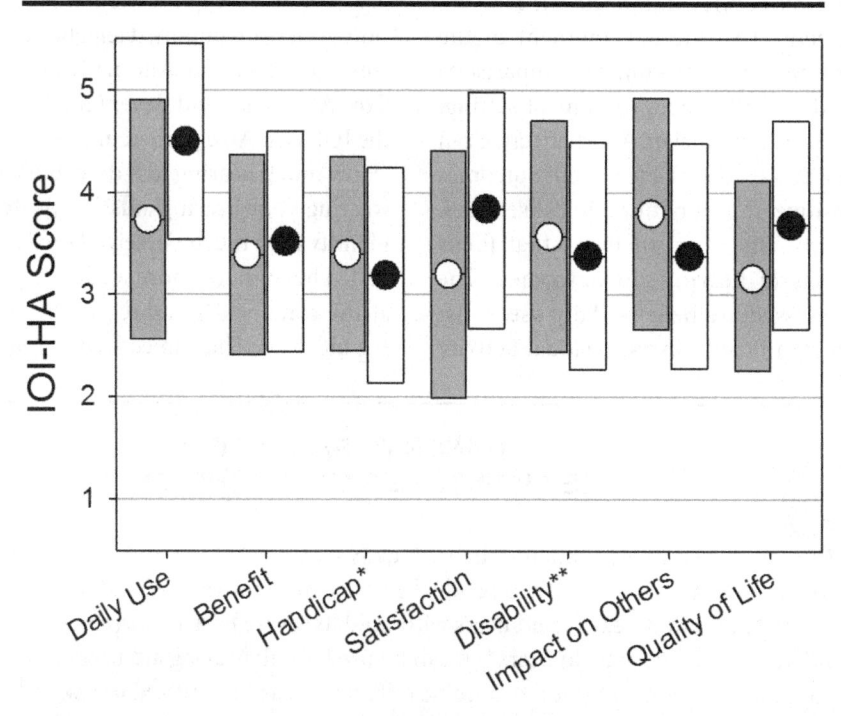

Figure 19–13. Graphic comparison of the norms for hearing aid users with mild-to-moderate hearing loss (*open bars*) and moderate-to-severe hearing loss (*filled bars*). (From Cox et al., 2003.)

a higher score is indicative of a better outcome (Cox & Alexander, 2002). For example, item 4 asks, "Considering everything, do you think your present hearing aids are worth the trouble?" The choices are

- Not at all worth it (1 point)
- Slightly worth it (2 points)
- Moderately worth it (3 points)
- Quite a lot worth it (4 points)
- Very much worth it (5 points)

Referring to the norm templates in Figures 19–14 and 19–15 and reproduced from Cox et al. (2003), if a patient answered the preceding question as "slightly

Table 19-9. IOI-HA Normative Data for Persons with Mild-to-Moderate Loss and Moderate-to-Severe Loss

Item	Mild to Moderate		Moderate to Severe	
	Mean	SD	Mean	SD
Daily Use	3.73	1.17	4.50	0.96
Benefit	3.39	0.98	3.52	1.08
Residual Activity Limitation	3.40	0.95	3.19	1.05
Satisfaction	3.20	1.21	3.84	1.17
Residual Participation Restriction	3.57	1.13	3.38	1.11
Impact on Others	3.79	1.13	3.38	1.10
Quality of Life	3.19	0.93	3.68	1.02

Source: From Cox et al. (2003).

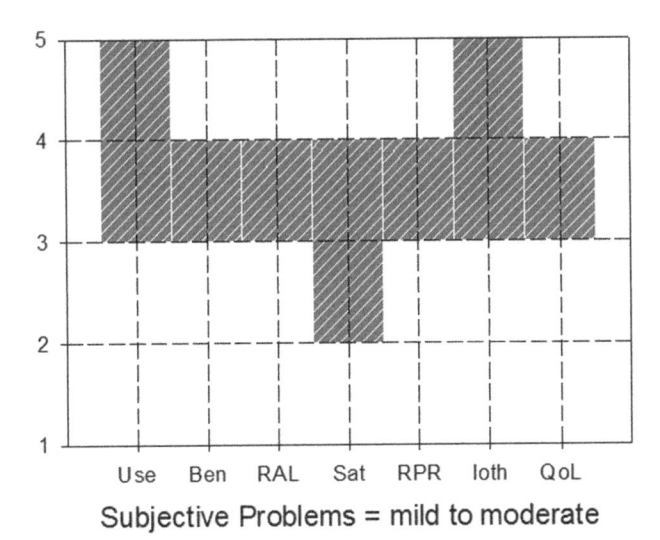

Figure 19–14. Normative data for the IOI-HA for persons with mild-to-moderate degrees of hearing loss. The shaded boxes indicate acceptable outcomes for each of the subscales. (From Cox et al., 2003.)

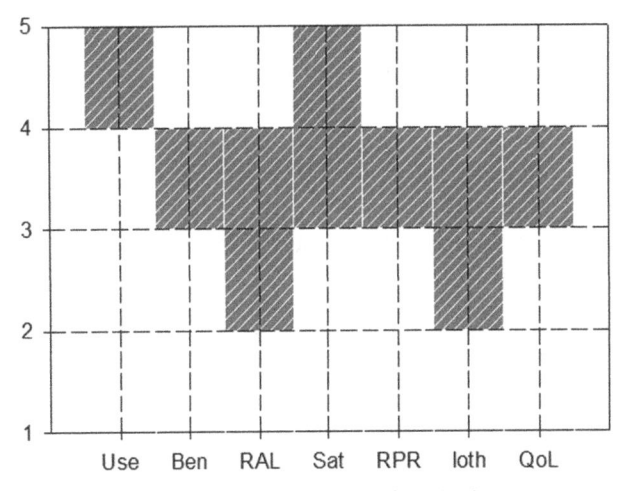

Figure 19–15. Normative data for the IOI-HA for persons with moderate-to-severe degrees of hearing loss. The shaded boxes indicate acceptable outcomes for each of the subscales. (From Cox et al., 2003.)

worth it," whether it fell within the norms depends on how much difficulty he or she perceived when not wearing his or her hearing aids. If the patient responded as having mild difficulty, then the response is within the norms, whereas a response of moderately-severe hearing difficulty indicates dissatisfaction. In general, if a patient reports a score of three or lower, it is indicative of a poor treatment outcome.

Clinical Application

The IOI-HA was originally intended to be a supplemental research outcome, but it may also be used as a stand-alone measure of hearing aid treatment.

Depending on the personality of the patients, they might or might not let the clinician know when they are having issues with their instruments. The IOI-HA is a quick way to get a general overview of how the patients feel about their hearing aid settings and how they are doing with them. For example, you might consider having every patient in your clinic fill out the IOI-HA each time they came into the office for follow-up visits while they are waiting for their appointments. By looking over the survey before seeing patients, you can focus your questions on their specific problem areas.

Take, for example, item #3, "Think again about the situation where you most wanted to hear better. When you use your present hearing aids, how much difficulty do you still have in that situation?" Patients often write out the reasons why they chose a certain answer in addition to answering the question. They might write: "I still have trouble hearing the TV" or "I cannot understand my grandchildren as well as I would like to." The survey can help clinicians go straight to their patients' issues and spend more time on counseling after adjusting the hearing aid settings. Remember the point we made at the beginning of this chapter—simply giving your patients an outcome measure and asking about satisfaction can actually improve satisfaction. This particular scale requires very little time to administer and score.

Obtaining the IOI-HA/A

A PDF version of the scale in English and for all translations can be downloaded from the following source: Link to Questionnaire/Norms:

http://www.memphis.edu/ausp/harl/downloads/IOIfiles/EnglishNormsVersion.pdf

Client Oriented Scale of Improvement (COSI)

The COSI is one of the most frequently used self-assessment tools utilized in the pre-fitting stage of auditory habilitation, and also is probably the most commonly used post-fitting outcome measure. In fact, as a pre-test and post-test, this tool has both efficiency and specificity (to the individual). One issue related to most all standardized self-assessment scales is that the items must be relevant for the hearing aid user. This is the main strength of the COSI (see Chapter 7 for review).

Background

The COSI concept was first introduced in an article by Harvey Dillon and colleagues in 1997. In short, the COSI allows patients to design their own questionnaire. This tool is an open-ended scale in which patients target up to five listening situations for improvement with amplification. It was normed on 1770 adults in Australia who had hearing loss. The goal of the COSI is for the patient to target up to five specific listening situations and to report the degree of benefit obtained compared to that expected for the population in similar listening situations. Many hearing aid manufacturers now include the COSI in their fitting software.

Dillon, James, and Ginis (1997) recommend the COSI for routine clinical use for five reasons:

- It fits into a well-conducted clinical interview in a nonintrusive manner by finding out what problems the patient is having, how much these problems are alleviated by the hearing aid fitting and counseling, and how well the patient is now doing in situations that are important to him or her.
- It is useful to the audiologist for formulating a treatment plan and determining whether additional action needs to be taken. Likewise, the patients view the measure as being relevant and as providing individual attention.

> **TECHNICAL TIP: CATEGORIZING COSI SITUATIONS**
>
> If the COSI is used as an outcome measure and the information is quantified and analyzed according to each listening situation, then the listening category for each situation also should be recorded. At the bottom of the COSI form are 16 different general listening situations that can be used for this purpose. The item number is then placed in the category column on the form for each situation. If you don't expect to conduct a group analysis of the data or if the COSI will be used only to measure expectations, then this categorization probably is not necessary.

- The correlation between the COSI improvement measure and other longer scales assessing improvement with hearing aids is reasonable.
- The test–retest reliability is reasonable, especially when considering the test contains only three to five items.
- Clinicians rate the COSI method as useful and convenient for them to use.

Administration and Scoring

One example of the COSI tool is shown in Figure 19–16. This one was provided by the National Acoustic Laboratories, but it should be evident that the clinician can start out with a blank sheet. The process begins by having the patient identify up to five specific listening situations in which he or she would like to hear better. Some patients will happily list six or seven; other patients struggle to come up with three. We encourage having at least three whenever possible.

As we reviewed in Chapter 7, it is important to make each item as specific as possible: "hearing in background noise" is not specific enough. After some questioning, this item might be narrowed to "hearing my friends while playing in the pool league in the Ryder bar". Once one situation is identified, you then move on and establish other situations. After all situations are identified, it is then helpful to go back and review and rank all situations. Simply place a "1" for most important, "2" for second most important, and so on in the box to the left of the item. Often, the item that the patient mentions first is something that just happened recently but is not the most important.

We suggest that what we just described be conducted on the day of the fitting or even on the day that the hearing aids are ordered. It is also possible to measure the patient's expectations for these nominated items at that time (see Chapter 7). Regardless whether expectations were initially assessed, when the patient returns for his or her post-fitting visit, the previously completed COSI form is then brought out for the patient's ratings. It is common that the patient doesn't remember all of the exact items he or she selected (and may have new items based on recent listening experiences). Mormer and Palmer (2001) report that after three weeks of hearing aid use, 96% nominated two items the same, but no patient who originally nominated four items nominated the same four items on the return visit. Although this lack of consistency can slow down the process a little, because the COSI is such a flexible instrument, item selection can be dealt with quite easily. It is easy to cross out listening tasks that are no longer meaningful, add new ones, or simply have the patient rate only the situations that are consistently on the list.

Notice that with the COSI (see Figure 19–16), benefit can be assessed in two different ways: degree of change (improvement provided by the hearing aids) and final hearing ability with hearing aids (an absolute measure of communication ability). It is typical to see a similar pattern for these two different ratings, but sometimes a difference is noted. For example, a patient with a fairly severe hearing loss who works in a demanding listening situation might rate his degree of change as "Much Better" but have only a final hearing ability of 50%. We suggest having the patient rate both categories because doing so may bring up key issues that need to be addressed.

NAL CLIENT ORIENTED SCALE OF IMPROVEMENT

Name: Kirby Mueller **Category:** New X Return

Audiologist:

Date: 1. Needs Established
2. Outcome Assessed

Final Ability (with hearing aid) — Person can hear: 10% 25% 50% 75% 95%

SPECIFIC NEEDS

Indicate Order of Significance

#	Specific Need	Worse	No Difference	Slightly Better	Better	Much Better	CATEGORY	Hardly Ever	Occasionally	Half the Time	Most of Time	Almost Always
#5	Hearing friends while shooting pool in Ryder Bar.			X						X		
#4	Understanding numbers called during Bingo.					X						X
#2	Understanding wife when she is in another room.			X						X		
#3	Not have to turn the TV up so loud.					X						X
#1	Understanding soft voices of grandchildren when they visit.					X					X	

Figure 19–16. Completed COSI form showing the four items initially nominated by the patient including the ratings of the importance of these items from 1 to 4 and the expectations of how much benefit would be obtained, all of which is gathered at the pre-fitting appointment. The final ability scoring was done three months after the fitting of the hearing aids and represents the amount of time the patient is successful in those listening situations.

TECHNICAL TIP: WEIGHTINGS FOR THE DIFFERENT NOMINATED ITEMS?

As mentioned, after the patient nominates three to five items for the COSI worksheet, we suggest rank-ordering the items regarding their importance. This is helpful for counseling when the patient rates the improvement following hearing aid use. Interestingly, however, Dillon et al. (1997) report that, when comparing the COSI scores to other measures of benefit and satisfaction, weighting the improvement scores by the priority assigned by the patient neither increased nor decreased the COSI's correlation with other measures. So, although they are useful for counseling, there is no reason to use the patient's priorities when deriving a summary improvement score.

Clinical Applications

A pool-playing grandfather is back in our office after using his hearing aids for three weeks. The first thing he said when he walked in the door was "these things are great"—that's the news we want to hear, but we still move forward and sit down with him to complete the COSI. We don't show him the sheet he completed earlier regarding his expectations—we'll bring that out later. His completed COSI is shown in Figure 19-16. The good news—he reports doing "much better" in three of the five categories. He notes some improvement with hearing his wife from a different room, but we are falling below his expectations for this category (see Figure 19-16). It may be that given his degree of hearing loss, and the difficulty of this listening situation, this might be as good as it gets. We already have soft sounds programmed to NAL-NL2 fitting targets, but we could try increasing them a few dB. Overall, we would consider this a successful fitting, and indeed we met or exceeded expectations for most of the nominated categories. Moreover, the use of the COSI in this manner facilitates post-fitting counseling.

Obtaining the COSI

The form for the COSI can be downloaded from:

http://www.nal.gov.au/pdf/COSI-Questionnaire.pdf

Profile of Aided Loudness (PAL)

At this point, we have discussed outcome measures that in one way or another relate to the patient's ability to understand speech and communicate effectively. We know, however, that it is also important to the patient that the world sounds "normal"—things that are supposed to be soft, sound soft; and things that are supposed to be loud, indeed are loud (but not too loud). Like other tests that we have discussed here, the PAL also can be used as a pre-fitting tool, as we discuss in Chapter 7. Although it is important to know how potential hearing aid users rate many of their everyday/environmental sounds before the hearing aid fitting, it is particularly critical to understand what the hearing aids are doing to the loudness perception of those sounds. In other words, you can use the PAL as both a pre-fitting tool and a post-fitting tool. First, let's revisit the development of this outcome measure.

Background

The PAL was introduced by Mueller and Palmer in 1998, with administration and scoring details provided the following year (Palmer, Mueller, & Moriarty, 1999). Additional data for test interpretation (loudness rating distributions for test items for normal-hearing individuals) were provided in 2000 by Palmer and Mueller. This tool was designed as an outcome measure to determine whether the fitting goal of maintaining a normal loudness perception has been accomplished.

The selection of the 12 items on the final version of the PAL began with a list of 95 sounds that new hearing aid users had reported hearing during their first few weeks of hearing aid use. Normal-hearing subjects between the ages of 20 and 65 rated the loudness of each sound based on the seven-point loudness scale of the Cox Contour Test (see Chapter 5). Importantly, this was not a laboratory measure; rather, each subject rated the loudness as he or she remembered hearing it. The 95 items were reduced to the current 12 items using the following criteria:

- Items were consistently rated the same. Items that did not have a test–retest 0.7 or greater Pearson correlation coefficient and had a two-tailed p value of > 0.05 were not included.
- Items were rated the same across age groups. Items that did not have the same ratings across age groups were eliminated.
- Items had clustered loudness ratings. Items that did not have ratings clustered around three loudness categories were eliminated.
- Items met desired ratings. The loudness ratings for the final items needed to cluster around targets of either #2 (soft), #4 (average), or #6 (loud), with an equal number of items for each category.
- Items experienced by majority of hearing aid users. A small subset was administered to hearing aid users, and the final 12 items were based on acceptable test–retest and that the

item was experienced by most hearing aid users.

The 12 items of the PAL include four items relating to soft sounds (target is a #2 rating), four items for average (target is a #4 rating), and four items for loud (target is a #6 rating). Because of the rigid criteria used for item selection, it is possible that your patient may not have experience with some of the items (e.g., a religious leader during a sermon, which is one of the items).

In addition to the loudness categories, there also are satisfaction ratings for each item ranging from #5 (best) to #1 (worse). There aren't norms per se for satisfaction, although when it is used as an outcome measure, any satisfaction rating below a #3 (Okay) needs to be discussed. The highest satisfaction rating of #5 is not necessarily good (for the patient). For example, a patient could rate "Your Own Breathing" as a #0 (Do not hear—desired rating is #2) on the loudness scale, yet rate this as #5 (Just right) for satisfaction. Our clinic patient of the day rated our practice question, the "Hum of the Refrigerator," as a #3 (Comfortable, but slightly soft) on the loudness scale, and this was rated as #5 (Just right) for satisfaction. Refer to Figure 19–17.

Administration and Scoring

The PAL is a paper-and-pencil administered scale and can be conducted in the waiting room during the follow-up clinic visit or it can be mailed to the patient following the fitting. Some audiologists administer it knee-to-knee by reading the questions to the patient. The 12 items from the three different loudness categories are randomized on the form (i.e., the four items with a normative rating of #2 do not follow each other). The instructions are as follows:

Please rate the following items by both the level of loudness of the sound and by the appropriateness of that loudness level. For example, you might rate a particular sound a "Very Soft" (#1). If Very Soft is

Sample Item: The hum of a car's turn signal:

Loudness Rating

0. Do Not Hear
1. Very Soft
2. Soft
3. Comfortable, But Slightly Soft
4. Comfortable
5. Comfortable, But Slightly Loud
6. Loud, But Okay
7. Uncomfortably Loud

Satisfaction Rating

5. Just Right
4. Pretty Good
3. Okay
2. Not Too Good
1. Not Good At All

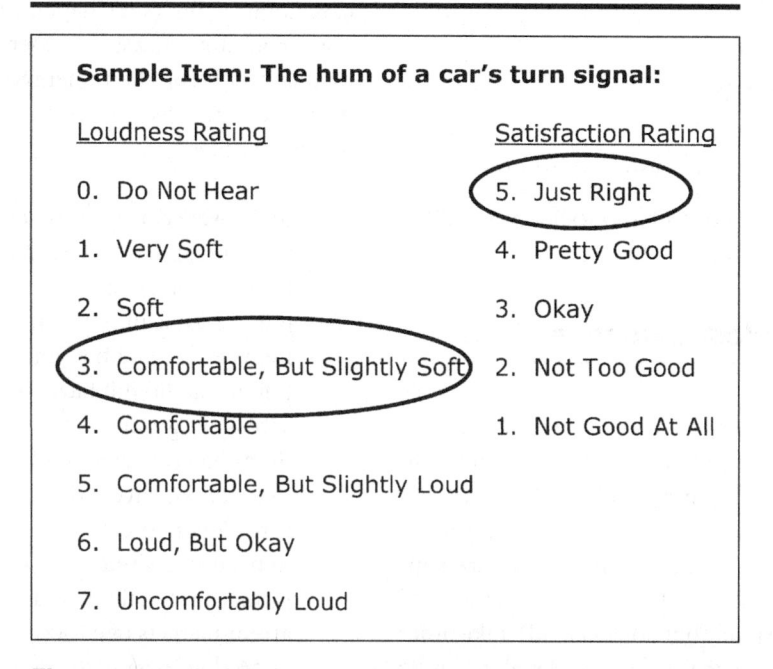

Figure 19–17. In this example, the patient rated the loudness level of the refrigerator hum while wearing his new hearing aids as "Comfortable, But Slightly Soft," and rated his loudness satisfaction for this sound as "Just Right." This satisfaction rating indicates that the patient believes that it is appropriate for that typical environmental noise to sound "Comfortable, But Slightly Soft."

your preferred level for this sound, then you would rate your loudness satisfaction as "Just Right." If on the other hand, you think the sound should be louder than "Very Soft," then your loudness satisfaction rating might be #2: "Not Too Good" or even #1: "Not Good At All." The Loudness Satisfaction rating is not related to how pleasing the sound is to you, but rather, the appropriateness of the loudness.

It is also important to inform the patient that it is okay to skip an item if it is not something they recall hearing and, therefore, don't have a loudness perception for it. Once the patient completes the inventory, scoring is quite straightforward. Using the PAL scoresheet (Figures 19–18 and 19-19), enter the patient's loudness and satisfaction ratings for each of the 12 items and then calculate an average of the responses. *Note*: If your patient does not respond to one of the items, don't enter "0"; instead, leave the item blank on the form and average across the number of scores entered for each level (soft, average, loud).

The example shown in Figures 19–18 and 19–19 show the PAL ratings for a patient with a mild-to-moderate downward sloping hearing loss. Observe that this patient is rating soft sounds somewhat above norms (3.0), but the satisfaction rating is quite good (3.25). The loudness ratings for average are also slightly above norms, typical of first-time wearers of hearing aids (4.5–4.0 is target rating); again, satisfaction is good. Ratings for loud sounds and satisfaction with those loud sound levels are okay. Still, the conscientious clinician might want to look at the dog-barking rating. Is it possible that some impulsive noise-reduction scheme might be in order? Or are the AGCo kneepoints set too high for this frequency range?

Clinical Applications

The PAL ratings can be used to make decisions about overall gain, compression kneepoints, and ratios and/or output limiting, in order to bring the patient into better alignment with normal-hearing perception of these everyday sounds. Many times no adjustment is needed—it's a matter of counseling the patient regarding what is normal.

The results also allow patients to offer their own judgment as to the satisfaction they perceive with the loudness of the environmental sounds now that the hearing aids have provided amplification. In Figure 19–18, our patient's scores are shown alongside the normative data. Even if his or her ratings don't align perfectly with the norms, if the patient is happy with the loudness, that information is valuable to the clinician. You can use the same PAL at a longer term follow-up as well to ensure that initial perceptions—and satisfaction with those perceptions—have not changed. Usually, you can counsel patients regarding how they differ from people with normal hearing.

Four Possible PAL Outcomes

When looking at PAL findings, you need to consider two factors: Does the patient have aided loudness perceptions that are similar to individuals with normal hearing, and is the patient satisfied with the aided loudness perceptions that you have provided with amplification? There are four possible outcomes:

1. Loudness perceptions good, satisfaction good. This is an easy one. Pat yourself on the back and enjoy a long relationship with a happy patient.

TECHNICAL TIP: THE PAL AND THE APHAB

The reason to conduct a battery of tests is to collect new information with each measure. There may be some overlap across the measures, however. If you conduct both the PAL and the APHAB, for example, we expect to see agreement between the PAL ratings for the four "Loud, but OK" questions and the APHAB subscale score for aversiveness. If the results from these scales indicate the patient has a low tolerance for louder sounds, you might take a look at your pre-test LDL and ANL findings (see Chapters 5 and 6). With the same patient, same ears, and same brains used for all testing, things should (and usually do) fit into a predictable pattern.

Normative data for PAL

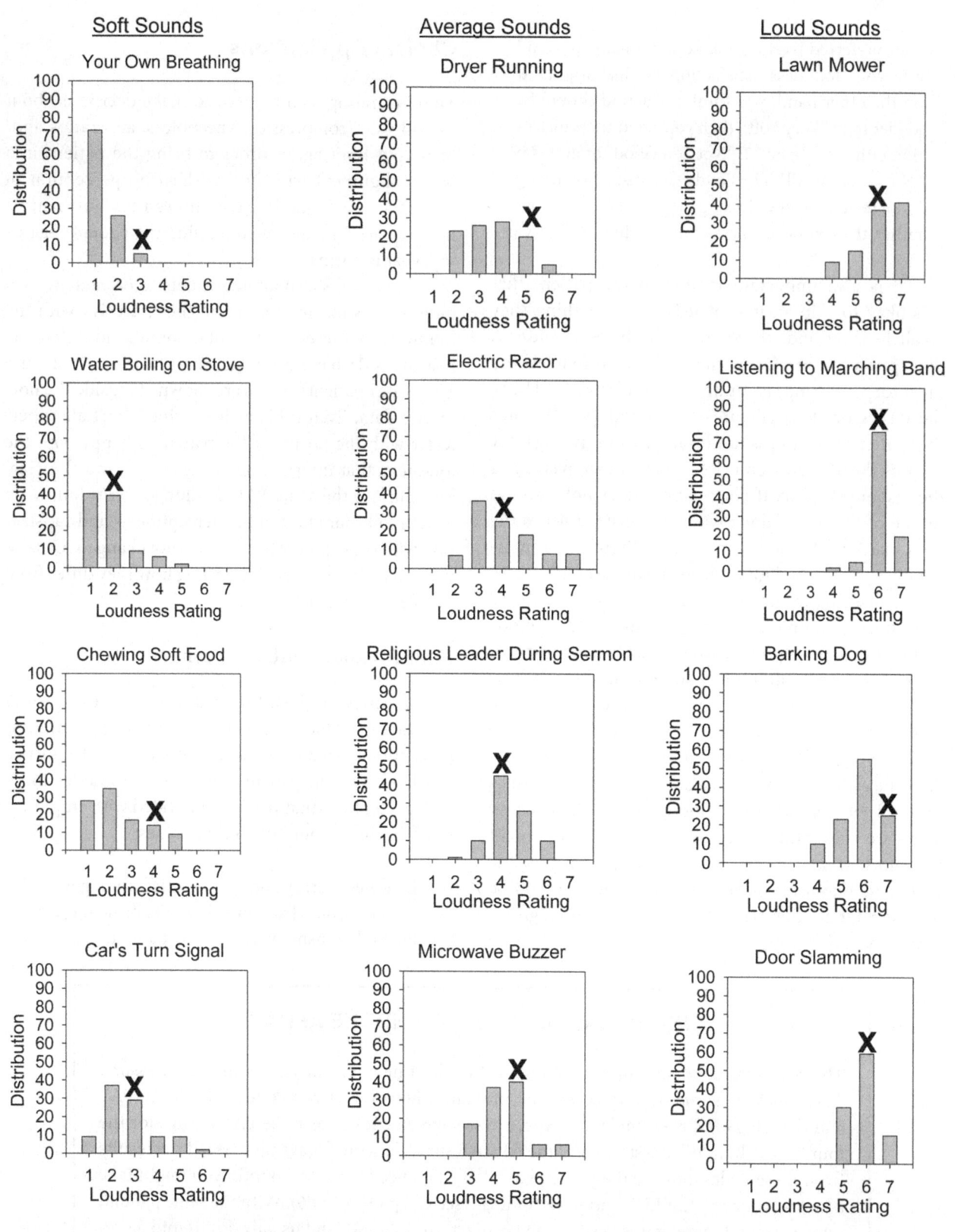

Figure 19–18. Patient's loudness perceptions while wearing her newly fitted hearing aids is shown for the 12 different PAL items that are plotted ("X" markings) on the normative distribution scale for each item.

PATIENT SUMMARY
Profile of Aided Loudness (PAL)
Aided Performance

Soft sounds	Q3	Q4	Q5	Q8	Category average
Loudness	3	2	4	3	3 (target = 2)
Satisfaction	3	5	2	3	3.25

Average sounds	Q1	Q6	Q7	Q12	Category average
Loudness	5	4	4	5	4.5 (target = 4)
Satisfaction	3	3	5	3	3.5

Loud sounds	Q2	Q9	Q10	Q11	Category average
Loudness	6	6	7	6	6.25 (target = 6)
Satisfaction	3	3	2	4	3

Figure 19–19. Score sheet for compiling and averaging PAL loudness ratings, and the patient's satisfaction with those loudness perceptions.

2. Loudness perceptions good, satisfaction not-so-good. This is not an uncommon finding. As we have mentioned, many patients, especially new ones, find that, initially, the world is much louder than they remember. Everything from the sound of their shoes on carpet to the crackling of newspaper to a pan moving across a stove burner—these sounds, some of them previously inaudible because of the hearing loss, are judged as being "too loud." As we discuss in Chapter 18, over the first month of hearing aid use we often see a change in PAL scores for soft inputs; once the patient adjusts to hearing all these sounds, their significance will be reduced, which likely will lead to them being viewed as more satisfactory. In this case, we explain to the patients that they simply are perceiving these sounds the same way normal-hearing individuals perceive them, and that with continued use of their hearing aid(s), they will be likely to find the hearing aid(s) satisfactory. Grabbing your mouse and making changes is not always the best course of action.

3. Loudness perceptions not-so-good, satisfaction good. To develop a treatment plan for this outcome, we first need to determine whether the poor loudness ratings are because things are being perceived as too soft or too loud. If the findings are "too soft" (maybe similar to unaided), our first guess is that we did not provide adequate gain—a typical finding when a manufacturer's proprietary fitting is used. It is predictable that the patient is satisfied because the amplified signal is not substantially different from unaided. Happy patients are good, but we will still repeat our verification procedures to ensure that we are delivering an appropriate amount of gain, and increase gain if necessary. It is pretty unusual to have a PAL outcome where the loudness perceptions are too high and the patient is satisfied, but it could happen. This is probably most common for

previous users, usually with a more severe hearing loss, who have become accustomed to placing the world toward the top end of their dynamic range. For this PAL outcome, we probably wouldn't make any gain or output changes.

4. Loudness perceptions not-so-good, satisfaction not-so-good. This is a tough one. You first might think it's time to start over, but in fact this is the typical finding when fitting someone who hasn't heard soft sounds for many years and for whom you have now provided good audibility for soft sounds. It is common for these patients to rate soft sounds a #4—the rating that should be given for average-level inputs. And these patients typically are not satisfied with this renewed audibility. For this PAL outcome, we check to make sure our fitting is at or near our desired fitting targets and, if so, then see if we can convince the patient to continue using the hearing aids a few weeks longer. At that time, we will repeat the PAL, and hopefully both the loudness perceptions and the satisfaction ratings will be moving in the right direction. At times, of course, this PAL outcome does mean that reprogramming the hearing aid is necessary, and you more or less start over. Perhaps the most common example is when the MPO is programmed too high, resulting in items that should be rated #6 being rated as #7. Like most things in fitting hearing aids, however, there is not is not a cookbook solution to any of these PAL outcomes. Deductive reasoning and common sense usually are required, and experience helps!

Obtaining the PAL

The PAL is not copyrighted. We suggest you use the forms available in the introductory articles we cited earlier. There is no computerized version or scoring system for this scale.

Speech Spatial Qualities of Hearing Scale (SSQ)

The Speech Spatial Qualities of Hearing Scale (version 5.6) was designed to assess many different hearing disabilities across several domains. The goal of the questionnaire is to answer two questions: (1) "What is disabling about hearing impairment?" and (2) "How do these disabilities determine experience of the handicap?" (Gatehouse & Noble, 2004).

Background

Here is a brief overview of the SSQ:

- The original scale is made up of 49 items.
- The scale has three subscales: speech hearing (14 items), spatial hearing (17 items), and qualities of hearing (18 items).
- All items are rated on a 0 to 10 scale, with 0 representing the greatest disability and 10 representing greatest ability.
- There are six versions of the SSQ (SSQ, SSQ-B, SSQ-C, SSQ12, SSQ5, and SSQ15).

The original SSQ is not a short survey. It includes 49 items. The items are further divided into three different scales: hearing speech, spatial hearing, and other qualities. An example of an item in each subscale is shown in Figure 19–20. The hearing speech scale items cover listening to speech in a variety of environments. The spatial hearing subscale items cover detection of the direction and movement of sound. The qualities of hearing subscale cover the other aspects and features of hearing that do not fall into the first two categories. This subscale includes items such as naturalness and clarity of speech/music, segregation of sounds, and ease of listening (Gatehouse & Noble, 2004).

When the developers of this scale, Stuart Gatehouse and Bill Noble, were collecting normative data, they noticed that one-third of the study participants had asymmetrical hearing thresholds between their right and left ears (Gatehouse & Noble, 2004; Noble & Gatehouse, 2004). They found a significant difference in spatial disability, especially in direction, movement, and distance, for the asymmetrical group. These participants had a difference between the two ears > 10 dB when the thresholds at 500, 1000, 2000, and 4000 Hz were averaged and compared. From this finding, they concluded that the SSQ is sensitive to the differences between unilateral and bilateral hearing aid fittings.

To assess the ability of the SSQ to measure the benefit differences between unilateral and bilateral hearing

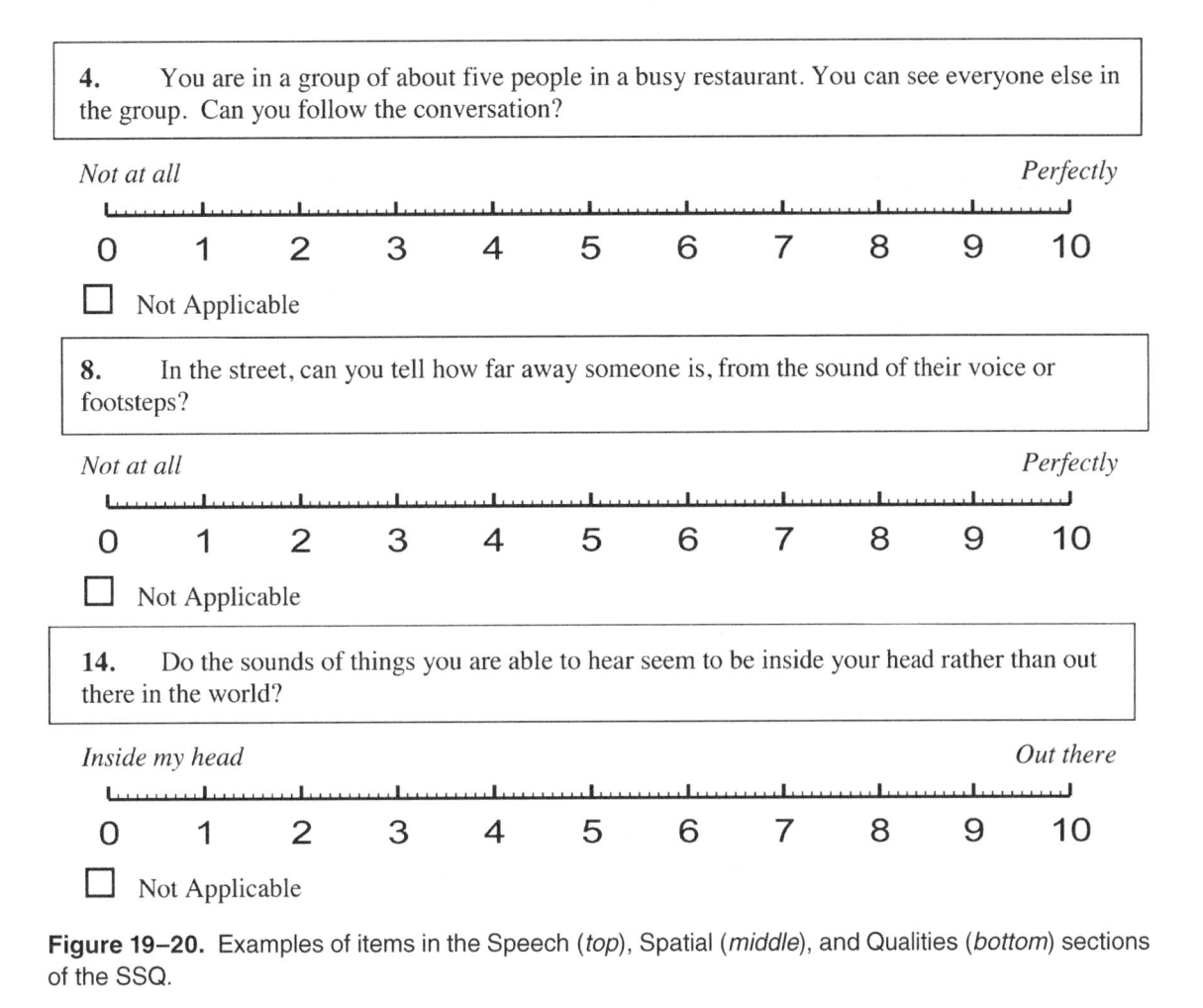

4. You are in a group of about five people in a busy restaurant. You can see everyone else in the group. Can you follow the conversation?

Not at all   *Perfectly*

0   1   2   3   4   5   6   7   8   9   10

☐ Not Applicable

8. In the street, can you tell how far away someone is, from the sound of their voice or footsteps?

Not at all   *Perfectly*

0   1   2   3   4   5   6   7   8   9   10

☐ Not Applicable

14. Do the sounds of things you are able to hear seem to be inside your head rather than out there in the world?

Inside my head   *Out there*

0   1   2   3   4   5   6   7   8   9   10

☐ Not Applicable

Figure 19–20. Examples of items in the Speech (*top*), Spatial (*middle*), and Qualities (*bottom*) sections of the SSQ.

aid fittings, Noble and Gatehouse (2004) compared the results from matched unaided, unilaterally aided, and bilaterally aided participants. Results of the study showed some clear differences for participants with moderate-to-severe hearing losses when fit with one versus two hearing aids. For traditional listening conditions (one-on-one and group conversations with and without noise), benefit was observed for one hearing aid over no aids, but the results showed no significant benefit increase when a second hearing aid was added. But in situations where the participants had to switch the focus of their attention between conversational partners or when attending to more than one stimulus, the participants showed the most benefit with two hearing aids. In the spatial hearing domain, unilateral participants perceived benefit for discriminating the direction of the source of sound with no added benefit with a second aid, and bilaterally aided participants had further benefit in judging distance and movement. The results for the other qualities scale showed an increase in benefit for naturalness, clarity, recognizability, and segregation of sounds with one hearing aid. Further benefit was noted for ease of listening with the addition of a second hearing aid.

Singh and Pichora-Fuller (2010) analyzed the test–retest reliability for interview and self-report methods of administration of the SSQ. Four groups of 40 older adult participants completed the SSQ twice at an interval of about a half year. The SSQ was administered using an interview method, and/or it was self-administered and then returned by mail. Although the method of administering the test did not systematically affect scores on the SSQ, the highest test–retest correlation ($r = 0.83$) was observed using the interview method at both test times, making it the better choice for the purpose of demonstrating the effectiveness of interventions.

Administration and Scoring

For each of the 49 items of the SSQ, patients rate their ability on a 0 to 10 scale, as shown in Figure 19–21. A reported ability of "0" on the scale represents "complete inability," the total absence of the quality described in the item or the need for great effort, depending on the item. A reported ability of "10" represents "complete ability," the "complete presence of a quality," or absence of the need for effort in that listening condition (Gatehouse & Noble, 2004). Therefore, a higher score indicates less disability.

The patient fills out the inventory, either using pencil-and-paper or a computer, and the scores are tallied for each subscale. The mean and standard deviation for interpreting patient scores by scale are available for each of the subscales. In addition, the means and standard deviations for each question provide the clinician with some insight into the residual disability (activity restriction) after hearing aid use. These charts can be found at the MRC website (https://www.ihr.mrc.ac.uk/pages/products/ssq).

Other Versions of the SSQ

In many clinical settings, the time it takes to complete the original SSQ hinders its usefulness. Assessing a difference between two hearing aid conditions by administering the original 49-item SSQ twice at two different points in time is problematic on several levels including time demands and possible ceiling effects. To address these problems, Eriksholm established a cooperation between William Noble (University of New England, Australia) and Michael Akeroyd (MRC Institute of Hearing Research, Glasgow, Scotland). As a result of this collaboration, there are two additional versions of the test: SSQ-B (B for Benefit) and SSQ-C (C for Comparative) in addition to three shortened versions: SSQ5, a screening version consisting of five questions (Demeester et al., 2012); SSQ12, another version consisting of 12 questions (Noble, Jensen, Naylor, Bhullar, & Akeroyd, 2013); and SSQ15, for epidemiological settings (Kiessling, Grugel, Meister, & Meis, 2011).

The basic idea behind the development of the SSQ-B and SSQ-C was to reuse all the items appearing in the original SSQ, but instead of rating ability or experience on an absolute scale (as in the SSQ), the differential versions use a relative scale to compare the perceived ability or experience in a present condition with that in a previous condition. The SSQ-B compares aided and unaided conditions, and the SSQ-C compares two aided conditions. For research purposes, the recommended approach is to apply the original SSQ at the end of the first test period. This provides an absolute assessment of condition, and familiarizes the respondent with the SSQ items. The SSQ-C is then applied at the end of the second test period to assess the difference between conditions A and B. Instead of rating their ability on a 0 to 10 scale as in the original, the respondents rate it on a −5 to +5 scale. A response of −5 always corresponds to a much poorer ability or worse performance than with the previous hearing aid, a response of 0 corresponds to no noticeable change, and a rating of +5 corresponds to a much better ability or much better performance with the new hearing aid over the previous hearing instrument. Various electronic and paper versions of the SSQ have been posted by the Medical Research Council: Institute of Hearing Research. Although these documents are freely available, the web address to which they are posted sometimes moves. Therefore, we encourage interested readers to simply search for "SSQ quality" to obtain a copy.

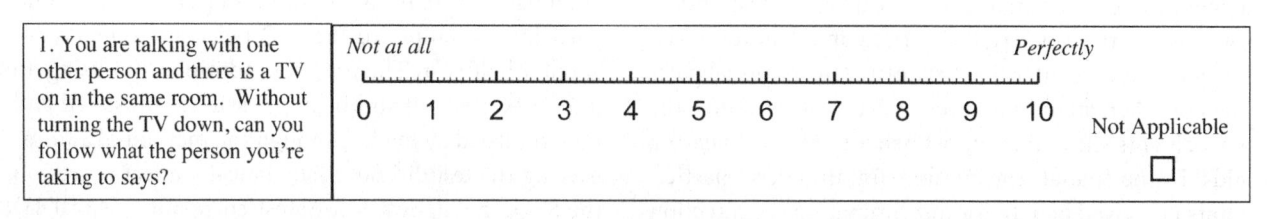

1. You are talking with one other person and there is a TV on in the same room. Without turning the TV down, can you follow what the person you're taking to says?	Not at all　　　　　　　　　　　　　　　　　　　　　　　　Perfectly 0　　1　　2　　3　　4　　5　　6　　7　　8　　9　　10	Not Applicable ☐

Figure 19–21. Example of a test item and the "ruler" used to rate ability as used by the SSQ.

> ## TECHNICAL TIP: THE SHORTENED VERSIONS
>
> As we mention, there are shortened versions of the SSQ. The 12 items of the SSQ12 reported in an abbreviated form include the following:
>
> 1. Talking with one person with TV on
> 2. Talking with one person and follow TV
> 3. Following one conversation when many people talking
> 4. Having conversation with five people in noise with vision
> 5. Following conversation without missing start of new talker
> 6. Locating dog barking
> 7. Judging distance of vehicle
> 8. Identifying whether a vehicle is approaching or receding
> 9. Listening when sounds appearing jumbled
> 10. Identifying instruments in music
> 11. Judging clarity of everyday sounds
> 12. Needing to concentrate when listening
>
> For the five items of the SSQ5, original full version items were chosen. Per the developers, the average score of these items should be used as an outcome for "general degree of disability," which correlates very well with the average of all SSQ-items. The five items are:
>
> - Can you have a conversation with someone when another person is speaking whose voice is the same pitch as the person you're speaking to?
> - You are sitting in between two people. One of them starts to speak. Can you tell right away whether it is the person on your left or your right without having to look?
> - Can you tell how far away a bus or a truck is based on its sound?
> - Do everyday sounds that you can hear easily seem clear to you (not blurred)?
> - Do you have to concentrate very much when listening to someone or something?

> ## TECHNICAL TIP: INTERESTED IN REAL-WORLD LOCALIZATION?
>
> We mention that a portion of the SSQ is the Spatial Hearing Scale. If your interest is real-world localization, you may want to use the Disabilities and Handicaps Associated with Localization, DHAL (Noble, Byrne, & LePage, 1994), which uses questions very similar to the SSQ. This questionnaire has a total of 25 items, consisting of 14 questions regarding difficulties in everyday sound localization (localization disabilities) and 11 questions related to limitations and disadvantages caused by these disabilities (localization handicap). Normative data for this scale also are available (see Ruscetta, Palmer, Durant, Grayhack, & Ryan, 2005).

The SSQ12 was narrowed down based on ten subscales determined by Gatehouse and Akeroyd, using a factor analysis of the 49 original items (Akeroyd, Guy, Harrison, & Fuller, 2014). When average performance on the SSQ12 was compared to the original, they were shown to generate very close results (Noble et al., 2013).

The SSQ12 was determined to be more sensitive to differences in hearing status. This can be seen in Figure 19–22 as the steeper slope of the SSQ12 scores when compared to the original. Given that the developers purposefully included more items asking about challenging contexts than easier ones, no items about listening to speech in quiet are included in the scale. The authors assert that, although the full-length SSQ is better, the SSQ12 can give clinicians and researchers a clear picture of an individual's pre-intervention hearing disability and handicap (Noble et al., 2013).

In a study by Demeester et al. (2012), the researchers further narrowed the original SSQ to five items by cluster analyses and binary logistic regression analyses. Their aim was to find the SSQ items with the highest probability of predicting hearing disability. Because the original SSQ can be time-consuming to administer, the SSQ5 can be used to gain a first impression of an individual's hearing ability. The authors stress that this shortened group of questions cannot replace behavioral measures but that it is better able for assessing hearing disability than simply asking: "Do you have a hearing loss?"

This tool has been translated into Danish, French, German, Polish, Afrikaans, Spanish, Turkish, and Italian.

Clinical Application

In the clinical setting, the SSQ can be used to evaluate how well a patient is doing with his or her hearing aid(s) in a variety of situations. Subsequently, the results can be used as a counseling tool or as a guide on how to further fine-tune the instruments.

Because the SSQ has been shown to be sensitive to unilateral versus bilateral fitting differences, it can also be used to facilitate that decision as well. If a clinic patient is struggling to decide whether to keep a second

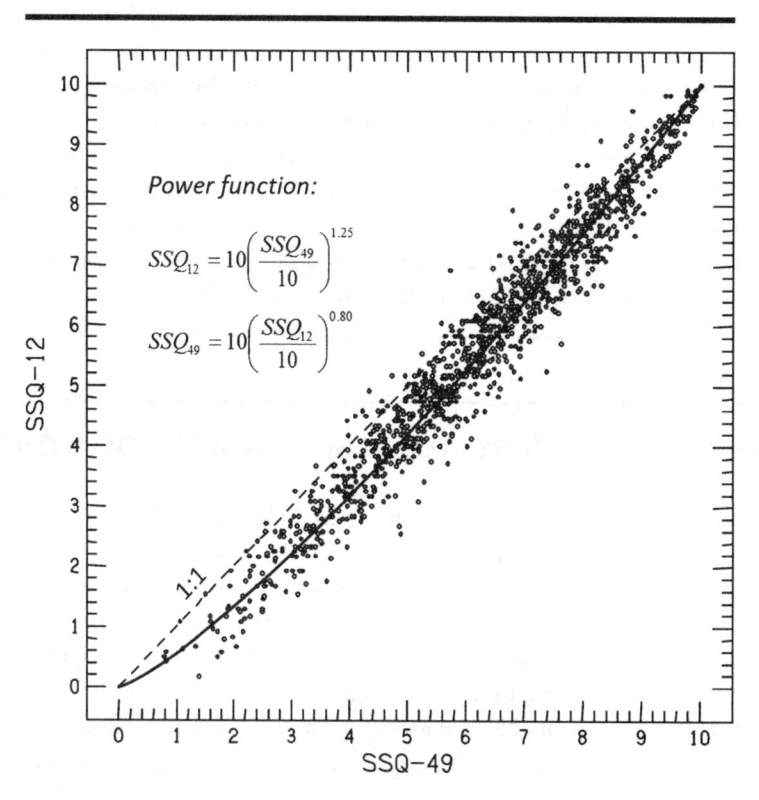

Power function:

$$SSQ_{12} = 10\left(\frac{SSQ_{49}}{10}\right)^{1.25}$$

$$SSQ_{49} = 10\left(\frac{SSQ_{12}}{10}\right)^{0.80}$$

Figure 19–22. SSQ12. (Reprinted with permission from Informa Healthcare. Noble, et al., 2013). *International Journal of Audiology*, *52*(6), 409–412.)

hearing aid, this tool may be used to assess whether benefit is gained from using a second aid (Noble & Gatehouse, 2006).

Let's consider Tommy Toms, a 70-year-old male on a limited income with symmetrical, mild-to-moderate sensorineural hearing loss and two newly fit hearing aids. He is nearing the end of his adjustment period and is struggling to decide whether to keep both aids or simply use one. Up until this point, he has worn both hearing aids most of the time. His audiologist has him fill out the SSQ based on using two hearing aids and based on his experiences without hearing aids. She then lengthens his trial period and sends him out with the instructions to use just the right one for two weeks. When he returns to the audiologist, he again fills out the SSQ. The audiologist then sends him out with instructions to use only the left aid. He then returns to the clinic and fills out the SSQ for the left aid. The comparison of the results allows the audiologist to help Tommy make the decision about keeping the second hearing aid.

What About Quality of Life?

We mentioned that outcomes cross many domains including quality of life. For many years, studies have linked hearing loss to many negative outcomes. Any of these outcomes can impact the patient's quality of life:

- Irritability, negativism, and anger
- Fatigue, tension, stress, and depression
- Avoidance or withdrawal from social situations
- Social rejection and loneliness
- Reduced alertness and increased risk to personal safety
- Impaired memory and ability to learn new tasks
- Reduced job performance and earning power
- Diminished psychological and overall health

Many researchers have studied the impact of hearing aid use on quality of life (QoL). In fact, the American Academy of Audiology (AAA) Task Force on the Health-Related Quality of Life Benefits of Amplification in Adults conducted a systematic review of all of the published evidence and concluded that hearing aids improve adults' QoL by reducing the psychological, social, and emotional effects of hearing loss. The report suggests that when the outcome measure is generic—for example, Medical Outcomes Study short form, or MOS SF-36 (Ware & Sherbourne, 1992)—it is hard to show the impact. On the other hand, if the outcome measure is disease-specific—for example, the Auditory Disability Preference Index-Visual Analog Scale, or ADPI-VAS (Joore, Potjewijd, Timmerman, & Anteunis, 2002)—the impact is significantly positive.

Sergei Kochkin has taken another approach to understanding how hearing aids can impact QoL in his series of MarkeTrak surveys. By sending surveys to 1500 people who own hearing aids, he found that nine in ten users of hearing aids say use of hearing aids improves their quality of life (MarkeTrak VII at http://www.betterhearing.org). The study also showed that the hearing aid users' feelings and confidence in self and relationships at work improved because of their hearing aid use. Results from MarketTrak9 were similar, with 40% reporting that hearing aids improved their quality of life occasionally, and 48% reporting that the improvement was regular (Abrams & Kihm, 2015).

In another review of a large number of surveys, the findings also show that the use of hearing aids causes significant improvement in the quality of life in many ways (Shield, 2006).

- Hearing aids improve overall quality of life for most users.
- Hearing aid users enjoy better overall health than nonusers.
- Hearing aid users are perceived by their families to have better cognitive functioning than nonusers and to be less introverted.
- The most beneficial effects of hearing aids are found in the users' social lives—taking part in group activities and family relationships.
- Hearing-impaired people with hearing aids have greater self-confidence, stronger self-image, and better communicative functioning, resulting in overall higher self-esteem than those without aids.
- Hearing aids help reduce deterioration in psychological functioning as a result of hearing impairment.

- Hearing aids can reverse social, emotional, and communication dysfunctions caused by hearing impairment.
- Hearing aid users are more likely than nonusers to engage in activities involving other people.
- Hearing aids improve most aspects of emotional life, and hearing aid users have greater warmth and less negativity in personal relationships than nonusers.

Finally, when we think of quality of life, we cannot ignore interrelated factors involving cognitive function, social isolation, and early dementia—and whether hearing aid use affects these factors. Although we are not aware of a direct cause and effect, there is compelling research that suggests a potential link between untreated hearing loss and higher incidence of cognitive decline. Work in this area is still limited so no firm conclusions can be drawn at this point, but it is certainly an area to watch!

In Closing

We have reviewed a number of different self-assessment scales, all of which measure somewhat different aspects regarding the success of the hearing aid intervention. We have reviewed some of our favorites, but we should mention that there are even more tools available for use to determine the success—across many domains—of a hearing aid fitting. For example, the Hearing Handicap Inventory for Elderly/Adults (HHIE/A) was discussed in Chapter 7, as an option for assessing handicap—specifically, as related to the emotional and social aspects of having a hearing loss. This tool has been around for more than 30 years and can be administered in either the long (25 items) or short (10 items) form. The Hearing Aid Performance Inventory (HAPI) developed by researchers from Walter Reed Army Medical Center 30 years ago is still used as a measure of benefit. The HAPI uses 64 items based on 12 bipolar communication features (e.g., visual cues present/absent). The goal of the HAPI is to assess the effectiveness of amplification on a variety of everyday listening situation. The HAPI has been normed on 128 hearing aids users, 119 of whom were men. Another tool that remains in use today is the Hearing Aid Users Questionnaire (HAUQ), an 11-item questionnaire designed to assess hearing aid use, benefit, and satisfaction (Dillon, Birtles, & Lovegrove, 1999). The HAUQ uses a four-point score for each of the 11 questions. The goal of the HAUQ is to measure problems that may affect a person's ability to use and benefit from hearing aids. It has been normed on 4,421 adults with hearing loss.

We recognize that it is not feasible or even necessary to conduct all of our suggestions for a single patient. Instead, the clinician is urged to develop a battery that works the best for individual settings, or different batteries for different patients. Unfortunately, surveys such as MarkeTrak VIII (Kochkin, 2010) reveal that most individuals fitted with hearing aids are never given any outcome measure, even though the same studies show that patient satisfaction increases when outcome measures are used.

And how many scales really are enough? In part that depends on what we want to measure, how well we want to do it, and how much time we are willing to invest. The most important take-home point from this chapter is that successful use of hearing aids is a multidimensional construct. Depending upon the outcome domain of interest, different tools exist for consideration. In this era of evidence-based practice and accountability, it is important that we document—using psychometrically strong instruments—the impact of our efforts. People are watching!

20

Supplemental Information: Corrections, Conversions, and Calculations

Audiologists deal in acronyms, correction factors, conversions, and calculations more than many disciplines. The activities might apply to field measurements, audiometric diagnostic testing, or conversions necessary when hearing aids are fitted; going from HL—to 2cc—to ear canal SPL is not always an easy process. Fortunately, much of the work of the corrections and calculations is now done within the hearing aid fitting and probe microphone system software. Nonetheless, it is important to understand the origins as well as the applications of many of these corrections, conversions, and calculations. Here are a few conversions that you will want to store in memory or keep handy in your office.

Testing Related to Hearing Aid Selection

When programming the patient's hearing aids, it all starts with your prescriptive algorithm. This algorithm, of course, is based on the hearing thresholds (and maybe also the loudness discomfort levels [LDLs]) that were obtained during the routine audiometric evaluation. Incorrect thresholds will result in incorrectly programmed gain, which could result in diminished benefit and/or satisfaction with the hearing aids. Consider, for example, a test booth that has a high ambient noise level. This probably would cause elevated thresholds in the low frequencies, which in turn would result in programming more gain than needed for the frequency range. Or consider the errors that might be present when an audiologist conducts testing with supra-aural earphones using an audiometer calibrated for insert earphones. In this section, we'll address some of the corrections and conversions that are used to ensure that our test booth measures are valid and reliable.

Ambient Noise Levels

Even before the hearing testing begins, we need to consider the background noise in our test area. If the ambient noise levels in the testing area are excessive, the hearing thresholds will be inaccurate. As with many measurements, there is an ANSI Standard for permissible noise levels (ANSI S3.1-2010). One can see on the charts to follow that we use the term MPANLs, which represents Maximum Permissible Ambient Noise Levels. Audiologists are responsible for ensuring that their test areas are adequately quiet in order to ensure accuracy of thresholds. That is really the first step in the process of optimal fitting of hearing aids. Table 20–1 shows the minimum octave and one-third octave levels for unoccluded ear testing, which is conducted in the sound field to determine the softest sound that can be heard across the frequencies. This type of testing is most commonly completed with young children who, for one reason or another, cannot be fitted with or will not tolerate earphones. In these cases, soundfield thresholds may be used initially to determine programming parameters, and then also used for a cross-check verification, in conjunction with the probe microphone/real-ear-to-coupler difference (RECD) calculations.

For most of our air-conduction hearing testing, the patient is of course wearing earphones on both ears. These earphones provide some additional attenuation (more for insert phones than supra-aural), and therefore, the permissible room levels are somewhat higher. Tables 20–2 and 20–3 show the minimum octave and one-third octave noise level that is acceptable for testing when the ears are covered. By comparing the data from Table 20–1 and Table 20–2 we can see the attenuation effects of the earphones; for insert phones this difference is 40 dB or more for some frequencies. These tables also illustrate the well-recognized advantage of using insert earphones rather than supra-aural. For example, if you are not testing a frequency lower than 500 Hz (see 500–8000 Hz range in Table 20–2); there is a 29 dB advantage when using inserts at 500 Hz (21 versus 50 dB SPL permissible noise).

Hearing Threshold Measurement

As we are sure you have observed throughout this book, our decision-making relative to hearing aid fitting is affected by the patient's audiometric thresholds. That is, our patients come to us with a complaint of not hearing well, and in best-practice style, we check the hearing levels to confirm that report. Thresholds obtained using standardized equipment are recorded in dB HL or decibels re: Hearing Level. Those hearing levels (ANSI S.3.6, 2010) are related to the threshold of audibility that we all studied in our beginning course work. Recall that the "thresholds of audibility" or "minimum audibility curve" defines the softest sound, as a function of frequency, that an average human can hear. Exactly what those values are depends on a number of factors related to the measurement technique: ears can be tested separately or at the same time, testing can be accomplished under earphones

Table 20–1. Minimum Octave and One-Third Octave Levels for Unoccluded Ear Testing

Center Frequency	Octave Band			One-Third Octave Band		
	125–8000 Hz	250–8000 Hz	500–8000 Hz	125–8000 Hz	250–8000 Hz	500–8000 Hz
125	29.0	35.0	44.0	24.0	30.0	39.0
250	21.0	21.0	30.0	16.0	16.0	25.0
500	16.0	16.0	16.0	11.0	11.0	11.0
800	–	–	–	10.0	10.0	10.0
1000	13.0	13.0	13.0	8.0	8.0	8.0
1600	–	–	–	9.0	9.0	9.0
2000	14.0	14.0	14.0	9.0	9.0	9.0
3150	–	–	–	8.0	8.0	8.0
4000	11.0	11.0	11.0	6.0	6.0	6.0
6300	–	–	–	8.0	8.0	8.0
8000	14.0	14.0	14.0	9.0	9.0	9.0

Note. Table shows maximum permissible ambient noise levels (MPANLs) with ears not covered for supra-aural earphones and for insert earphones for three test frequency ranges (in dB re: 20 µPa to nearest 0.5 dB).

Table 20-2. One-Third-Octave Band (OB) Maximum Permissible Ambient Noise Levels (MPANLs) for Insert Earphones for Three Test Frequency Ranges

One-third OB Intervals	Supra-Aural Earphone			Insert Earphone		
	125–8000 Hz	250–8000 Hz	500–8000 Hz	125–8000 Hz	250–8000 Hz	500–8000 Hz
125	30.0	34.0	44.0	54.0	62.0	73.0
250	20.0	20.0	30.0	48.0	48.0	59.0
500	16.0	16.0	16.0	45.0	45.0	45.0
800	19.0	19.0	19.0	44.0	44.0	44.0
1000	21.0	21.0	21.0	42.0	42.0	42.0
1600	25.0	25.0	25.0	43.0	43.0	43.0
2000	29.0	29.0	29.0	44.0	44.0	44.0
3150	33.0	33.0	33.0	46.0	46.0	46.0
4000	32.0	32.0	32.0	45.0	45.0	45.0
6300	32.0	32.0	32.0	48.0	48.0	48.0
8000	32.0	32.0	32.0	51.0	51.0	51.0

Note. Ears covered for supra-aural earphones and for insert earphones (re: 20 µPa to nearest 0.5 dB).

Table 20-3. Octave Band (OB) Maximum Permissible Ambient Noise Levels (MPANLs) for Three Test Frequency Ranges.

OB Intervals	Supra-Aural Earphone			Insert Earphone		
	125–8000 Hz	250–8000 Hz	500–8000 Hz	125–8000 Hz	250–8000 Hz	500–8000 Hz
125	35.0	39.0	49.0	59.0	67.0	78.0
250	25.0	25.0	35.0	53.0	53.0	64.0
500	21.0	21.0	21.0	50.0	50.0	50.0
1000	26.0	26.0	26.0	47.0	47.0	47.0
2000	34.0	34.0	34.0	49.0	49.0	49.0
4000	37.0	37.0	37.0	50.0	50.0	50.0
8000	37.0	37.0	37.0	56.0	56.0	56.0

Note. Ears covered for supra-aural earphones and for insert earphones (re: 20 µPa to nearest 0.5 dB).

or in a "field," the type of earphone that is used and so on. As shown in Figure 20–1, the threshold of audibility, expressed in SPL, is clearly not a straight line. Lower and higher frequency sounds require more sound pressure to be heard than the middle frequency sounds. The audiogram, then, is a graphic representation of the threshold of audibility across frequencies for an individual relative to the standard threshold of audibility (the lowest level at each frequency an individual with normal hearing can hear), defined as the 0 dB HL reference.

The 0 dB HL reference has changed over the years as new data have been collected. The most significant changes occurred in the 1950 to 1970 time frame (see related Key Concept).

As we mentioned earlier, to go from the hearing thresholds expressed in dB SPL, which differ by 20 dB

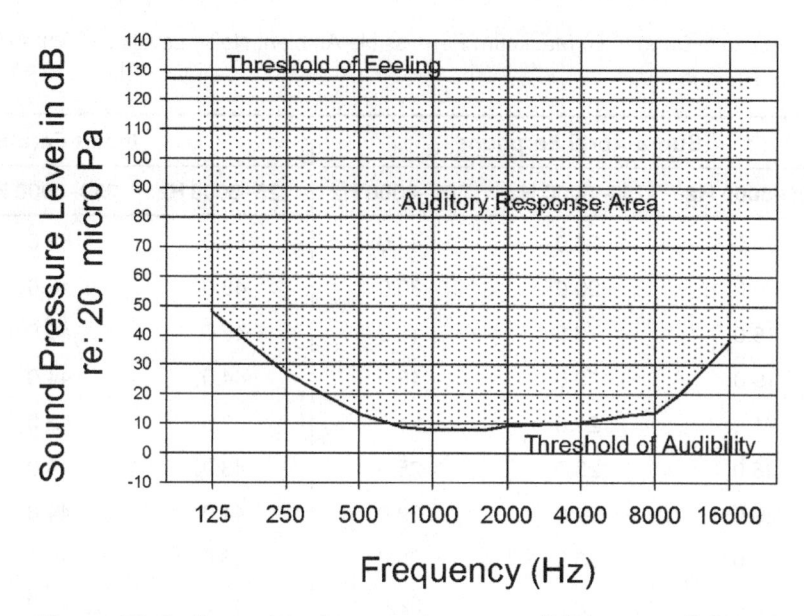

Figure 20–1. Illustration of average human audibility range. (Adapted from Stach, 1998.)

KEY CONCEPT: CHANGES TO THE 0 DB HL REFERENCE OVER THE YEARS

- American Standards Association (ASA): In 1951, the ASA used the data from a large study by Beasley (1938) to establish audiometric standards, which were then used by all clinics.
- British Standard: Because of conflicting research data (e.g., the work of Sivian and White, 1933), the British adopted a different audiometic standard about the same time as the ASA standard was introduced. There was a significant difference between the two standards—between 10 and 15 dB for the 250 to 2000 Hz range.
- International Organization for Standardization (ISO): The ISO reviewed the two different standards, and in 1964 adopted a standard that was very similar to the British. This new standard was endorsed by the American Speech and Hearing Association and began to be used in some U.S. clinics. During this period, there was considerable clinical confusion. Because the ISO had a lower reference for audiometric zero, if a patient previously had been tested using ASA, it would now appear that his or her hearing thresholds had dropped by 10 dB when the ISO standard was used. During testing, it was necessary to use paper-and-pencil correctional factors, as audiometers had been calibrated to ASA 1951.
- American National Standards Institute (ANSI; formerly ASA): In 1969 the ANSI adopted the ISO standards. Although there have been minor changes regarding measurement procedures since this time, the zero reference levels are basically the same today as they were then.

or so between 250 and 1000 Hz, to making the reference "0 dB HL" for all frequencies, requires correction factors that differ from frequency to frequency. These corrections, however, vary depending on whether the testing was conducted under earphones or in the sound field.

MAP Versus MAF

When testing hearing, the lowest level sounds that a human ear can (typically) hear are referred to as minimal audible pressure (MAP) when the values are obtained using an earphone, and minimum audible field (MAF) when the values are obtained in a sound field. The difference between the MAP and MAF curves is assumed to be about 15 dB in the mid to high frequencies, a value which relates directly to the free-field-to eardrum transformation (e.g., head diffraction, pinna effects, and ear canal resonance). In the clinic, these effects are clearly reflected in our measures of real-ear unaided gain (REUG). The two terms are not necessarily synonymous. The REUG, as discussed in Chapter 6, typically only incorporates pinna effects and ear canal resonance due to the calibration used in the measurement—a modified-pressure approach. If the substitution method (not common in the clinic) is used for the REUG assessment, then a true free-field transformation will be obtained. The factors contributing to the free-field-to-eardrum transformation combine to make MAF thresholds lower (better) than MAP thresholds. If binaural MAFs are used in the comparison, there are other effects that come into play. For example, we usually observe 2 to 3 dB binaural summation for threshold measures. Additionally, in the field, the response will always be from the better ear; whereas the research subjects used in the development of correction factors had "normal hearing," there still may have been a slight asymmetry between ears.

The MAP values shown in Table 20–4 are from Killion (1978). They are derived from MAF values from ISO R226 (1961). As we point out in this section there are clear differences between dB HL and dB SPL; however, the specific magnitude of these differences are greatly dependent on where and how they are measured. In other words, precise calibration is a key factor. In part due to these calibration issues, the threshold of audibility curve is applied indirectly in the fitting of hearing aids, as we describe in the following section.

Earphones and RETSPLs

For many hearing aid applications, it would be easier if hearing thresholds were simply measured and recorded in dB SPL, but as we have discussed, it was decided long ago that the audiogram be turned upside down, and we express everything relative to audiometric zero (0 dB HL). For purposes of calibration, therefore, both during hearing testing and during real-ear verification, we need to know the frequency specific differences between dB SPL and dB HL; specifically, the *dB SPL* in a coupler for a specific transducer that corresponds precisely to *0 dB HL* in the same coupler. These corrections are referred to as reference equivalent threshold sound pressure

---

POINTS TO PONDER: MISSING 6 DB?

As we pointed out, we would expect that there would be a sizable difference between MAP and MAF in the higher frequencies due to the external ear advantages present only in the MAF condition. But interestingly, in some studies it was found that, even when MAP and MAF were referenced to ear canal SPL, there still was a discrepancy of about 6 dB. In audiology circles, this became known as "the missing 6 dB."

This unexplained difference led to an article by Killion in 1978 entitled, "Revised Estimates of Minimum Audible Pressure: Where Is the Missing 6 dB?" and another a few years later by Rudmose (1982), "The Case of the Missing 6 dB." If all this has concerned you at some time in your career, we are pleased to report that most of the missing 6 dB has been found. And relevant to this chapter, these dB were found because the very correction factors that we are discussing here were applied appropriately.

Table 20–4. Derivation of Minimum Audible Pressure at the Eardrum from Minimum Audible Field Data

Frequency (Hz)	MAF (ISO R226 corrected)[a]	P_D/P_{FF} at $0°$[b]	MAP (binaural)	MAP (monaural)
100	33	–	33	35
150	24	–	24	26
200	18.5	0.5	19	21
300	12	1.3	13.3	15.3
400	8	1.6	9.6	11.6
500	6	1.7	7.7	9.7
700	4.7	2.8	7.5	9.5
1000	4.2	2.6	6.8	8.8
1500	3	5	8	10
2000	1	12	13	15
2500	–1.2	16.8	15.6	17.6
3000	–2.9	15.4	12.5	14.5
3500	–3.9	14.8	10.9	12.9
4000	–3.9	14.2	10.3	12.3
4500	–3	12.8	9.8	11.8
5000	–1	10.7	9.6	11.6
6000	4.6	7.4	12	14
7000	10.9	4.3	15.2	17.2
8000	15.3	1.8	17.1	19.1
9000	17	–0.7	16.3	18.3
10000	16.4	–1.6	14.8	16.8

Note. Data expressed in decibels.

[a]A constant 2 dB was added to the ISO values to convert binaural to monaural thresholds. [b]P_D/P_{FF} is the ratio of eardrum pressure to free-field pressure as given by Shaw, 1974.

THINGS TO REMEMBER: USES OF RETSPLS RELATED TO THE FITTING OF HEARING AIDS

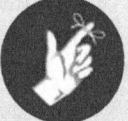

The RETSPL might be a new term for you and you may wonder how you will use it in your clinical practice. Here are the four most common uses:

1. Calibration of the audiometer, first and foremost;
2. Transformation of LDLs or thresholds of discomfort to 2cc values for the purpose of setting the MPO of the hearing aid;
3. Display of simulated real-ear gain and output curves in hearing aid fitting software;
4. Calculation (in conjunction with the RECD) of ear canal SPL thresholds and LDLs for display in probe microphone equipment.

levels (RETSPLs; pronounced *Rhet spulls*) and can be found in the ANSI standard that regulates the calibration of audiometers (ANSI 3.6, 1989).

As shown in Tables 20–5 and 20–6, there are RETSPLs for each kind of earphone that we use in our hearing testing, both for pure tones as well as for speech. From a clinical standpoint, it is important to note the RETSPL differences between standard aural (TDH-50) and standard insert (EAR-3A) earphones. This reminds us that you can't arbitrarily unplug one type of earphone

Table 20–5. Reference Equivalent Threshold Sound Pressure Levels (RETSPLs) for Supra-Aural and Insert Earphones

Frequency Hz	Supra-Aural Earphone		Insert Earphone	
	TDH 39	TDH 49/50	HA-2 with rigid tube	HA-1[a]
	NBS 9A	NBS 9A		
125	45.0	47.5	26.0	26.5
160			22.0	22.0
200			18.0	19.5
250	25.5	26.5	14.0	14.5
315			12.0	15.0
400			9.0	10.5
500	11.5	13.5	5.5	6.0
630			4.0	4.5
750	8.0	8.5	2.0	2.0
800			1.5	1.5
1000	7.0	7.5	0.0	0.0
1250			2.0	1.0
1500	6.5	7.5	2.0	0.0
1600			2.0	1.5
2000	9.0	11.0	3.0	2.5
2500			5.0	4.5
3000	10.0	9.5	3.5	2.5
3150			4.0	2.5
4000	9.5	10.5	5.5	0.0
5000			5.0	1.5
6000	15.5	13.5	2.0	−2.5
6300			2.0	−2.0
8000	13.0	13.0	0.0	−3.5
Speech	19.5	20.0	12.5	12.5

Note. [a]Values are valid when the end of the foam eartip or other eartip is inserted to a depth of 12 to 15 mm from the entrance to the ear canal. Values are based on a foam eartip having the length of 12 mm. (re: 20 µPa.)

Source: ANSI 3.6-1989 (R2010).

Table 20–6. Reference Equivalent Threshold Sound Pressure Levels (RETSPLs) for Speech Materials

Earphone Type	Reference Level for 1000 Hz dB SPL	Correction in dB	Computed Reference Level for Speech in dB SPL
WE 705-A	6.5+	12.5	= 19.0
TDH-39, TDH-39p	7.0+	12.5	= 19.5
TDH-49, TDH-49p	7.5+	12.5	= 20.0
TDH-50, TDH-50p	7.5+	12.5	= 20.0
TELEX 1470-A	6.5+	12.5	= 19.5

Note. (dB re: 20 µPa)
Source: From ANSI 3.6-1989 (R2010).

and plug in another. Instead, the audiometer calibration must be changed for the specific earphone type. Some audiometers simplify this process by having separate connections for different earphone types.

Most of the above uses of the RETSPL occur in the background (calculations are made automatically by the fitting software), and are more or less transparent to the audiologist. The exception is the use of the RETSPL to adjust the hearing aid's maximum power output (MPO). This is something that we recommend for each hearing aid patient. To make this calculation we simply add the RETSPL to the frequency-specific LDL that we mea-

---

TECHNICAL TIP: FACTORS THAT INFLUENCE HEARING THRESHOLD MEASURES

Our focus in this chapter is the acoustic corrections and conversions that relate to hearing aid fittings, but there are also psychophysical factors that can influence measurement of hearing thresholds. It's reasonable to ask—if a patient has his or her hearing threshold tested in Clinic A, and then goes down the street and is tested again in Clinic B—what factors would affect the probability that the results would be the same, from both a correctness and reliability standpoint. The following eight acoustic or psychophysical factors are adapted from Yost and Killion, 1997:

1. Accuracy of the calibration of the sound source, which is typically performed with the listener absent;
2. Effects of the individual listener's ear (and the head in the case of soundfield testing) on the stimulus delivered to the listener's eardrum;
3. Accuracy of the zero reference SPL used for the calibration of the sound source;
4. Level of background noise entering the listener's ear canal;
5. Listener's willingness and ability to cooperate in the threshold assessment task;
6. Method of stimulus presentation (e.g., pulsed versus continuous tone);
7. Other psychophysical factors (e.g., ascending versus descending approach); and,
8. Number of responses averaged to obtain a single threshold estimate.

sured in dB HL. This gives us the LDL in dB SPL referenced to a 2cc coupler. We now can talk the language of the fitting software, which also uses this same reference. We can then set the MPO value to the corrected LDL target value for all frequencies of interest. If the math is correct, then we would expect that the REAR85 will fall at or below the LDL targets when we complete probe microphone verification. We provide a step-by-step procedure for this, with illustrative cases in Chapter 4 of *Modern Hearing Aids: Pre-Fitting Testing and Selection Considerations*.

A Little Basic Acoustics

Many of the corrections we use with hearing aids require some understanding of acoustics. Consequently, we review a few important basic principles in this section.

Pressure Versus Power

Although this is not a textbook on acoustics, terms such as *power* and *pressure* may be confusing when assessing hearing levels or hearing aids. Power is the capacity to do work expressed in watts. In the case of acoustics, absolute sound power is the rate at which sound energy is transferred through a medium. Because we are usually interested in the sound power applied to a particular area, we translate sound power into sound intensity by defining the sound power in watts for a given area.

The normal human ear is sensitive to a wide range of intensities. The threshold of pain or feeling in a listener with normal hearing has an intensity that is 1,000,000,000,000,000,000 times greater than that of the lowest level sound they can barely perceive at threshold. Because this very large range makes it unwieldy to deal with absolute units of intensity, convention has led to presenting relative intensity in terms of 10 times the log of ratios between a given sound intensity and a standard reference. The standard reference we use for sound intensity is 10^{-12} watts/m^2, which corresponds to the relative sound intensity of 0 dB intensity level. Most often, however, we measure sound using a sound level meter. This device is actually set up to measure force per are, rather than intensity per area. Our standard reference for force is 20 µP which corresponds to a 0 dB SPL. Conveniently 20 µP of sound pressure is equivalent to 10 to 12 watts/m^2 of sound intensity so measuring the dB SPL of a source with a sound level meter also gives us the intensity level. Consequently, as a convention we typically describe the sound level in dB SPL.

"Adding" dB

Combining (or adding) dB is another concept that comes in handy in our audiology work. In most situations, it is power that is being combined rather than pressure. Consequently, to combine dB we convert from dB SPL to relative sound intensity using the formula dB SPL = 10 log $x/10^{-12}$ watts/m^2 and solving for x. We can then combine the intensities and then convert back into dB SPL by applying the formula in reverse (e.g., dB SPL = 10 × antilog $x/10^{-12}$ watts/m^2) and solving for dB SPL. Some quick math will show us that if we combine two sources of the exact same level, doubling the intensity increases the total level by 3 dB (3 dB = 10 × antilog 2/1). Consequently, if you have two sounds that differ in intensity, you will always be adding less than 3 dB to the higher level. Fortunately there are online calculators that will also do this math for us (e.g., https://www.noisemeters.com/apps/db-calculator.asp). If you want to avoid the math, using Table 20–7 is a convenient shortcut. Find the difference (in dB SPL) between the two sounds. Add the corresponding increment to the larger original dB value—and voilà!

When combining two sources the chart in Table 20–7 works just fine. When you have more than two sources, however, particularly when there are multiple levels that do not differ by exactly 3 dB, you have to resort to the formulas presented earlier. For example, we were recently conducting soundfield testing of hearing aid directional processing using eight loud speakers positioned around the patient at 45-degree intervals. The primary signal was delivered from the loudspeaker at 0 degrees, with noise presented from the other seven loudspeakers. The noise from each loudspeaker was carefully calibrated to be 60 dB SPL, but what we needed to know was the noise at the middle of the room: the sum of all seven. If we apply the math we see the answer is roughly 68.5 dB SPL, which was roughly what we measured. One simple trick to use if you are trying to estimate is to remember

Table 20–7. Simplified Table for Combining dB(s)

Difference in dB (between original sounds)	Increment in dB (add to larger original sound)
0	3.0
1	2.6
2	2.2
3	1.8
4	1.4
5	1.2
6	1.0
7	0.8
8	0.6
9	0.5
10	0.4
11	0.35
12	0.3
13	0.25
14	0.2
15	0.15
16	0.1

Note. Determine the difference (in dB SPL) between two sounds and add the increment to the larger original dB value.

that doubling intensity increases things by 3 dB. What if our example above only had four equal sources of 60 dB SPL? We could combine them as follows:

$$60 + 60 + 60 + 60 = 63 + 63 = 66 \text{ dB SPL}$$

If we do have sources that are equal, we can also easily modify the formula presented above to get our answer with fewer steps: dB SPL combined = dB SPL of a single source + 10 log (number of sources). For our example 68.45 dB SPL = 60 + 10 log 7.

Weighting dB

Speaking of loudness versus level, it sometimes makes sense to filter broadband sounds so that the frequency-

---

POINTS TO PONDER: ADDING POWER VERSUS PRESSURE

As is apparent from Table 20–7, when you add two different sound sources of the same level together, you get a 3 dB increase. A common and very reasonable question often asked by students is: Why don't we see a 6 dB increase, as we are adding sound *pressure*? The reality is that when we combine two sound sources of the exact same level we are typically doubling power, not pressure. Sound intensity is in fact proportional to pressure squared, so if we take our intensity formula and substitute pressure squared for intensity we have dB SPL = 10 log P^2/reference P^2. We apply a little algebra and the formula becomes dB SPL = 20 log P/reference P. Doing this math is allowable because the reference sound intensity (10^{-12} watts/m2) is equivalent to the reference for sound pressure (20 µPa) and both represent 0 dB SPL. By repeating the exercise we completed above for intensity, we can see that doubling pressure results in a 6 dB increase in level instead of a 3 dB. For most purposes the addition of two sound sources will result in a doubling of intensity, however, not a doubling of pressure. For pressure to double we must have two identical pure tones that are exactly in phase with each other. Other than combining two identical pure tones using computer software, this is a pretty rare occurrence, so generally we just need to remember we are usually combining intensities (power) not pressure (force).

In the lay press you will often see the use of "times factor," rather than specific dB level to express the change in the intensity of a sound. It sounds more dramatic to say that today's music is played 100 times louder than music in the 1950s rather than to say that today's music is played 20 dB higher in level. Our psychoacoustics background reminds us this is acoustics and not loudness; we would express loudness in sones or phons. For completeness, we have included Table 20–8 for various ratios—including doubling—and the resulting increase in dB SPL for both intensities and pressure.

> **POINTS TO PONDER: WHAT'S A PHON?**
>
> If it has been a while since you have taken a hearing science class you may not remember *phons* and *sones*. To establish a phon contour a listener matches the loudness of various pure tones to the level of a 1000-Hz tone presented at a specified level. Therefore, the 40-phon contour is the frequency-specific level for which the loudness is equal to a 1000-Hz pure tone presented at 40 dB SPL. The shape of this contour is roughly similar in shape to the MAP and MAF curves. That is, the lowest and highest frequencies need to be presented at a much higher level than the middle frequencies to result in the same loudness. As the level goes up (e.g., 90 dB SPL phon contour), the function flattens significantly!

Table 20–8. Ratios in Decibels of Power and Pressure

Ratio	Power (dB)	Pressure (dB)
1	0	0
2	3.0	6.0
3	4.8	9.5
5	7.0	14.0
7	8.5	16.9
9	9.5	19.1
10	10.0	20.0
11	10.4	20.8
13	11.1	22.2
17	12.3	24.6
19	12.8	25.6
20	13.0	26.0
30	14.8	29.6
40	16.0	32.0
50	17.0	34.0
60	17.8	35.6
70	18.4	36.9
80	19.0	38.0
90	19.5	39.0
100	20.0	40.0
1000	30.0	60.0
10000	40.0	80.0
100000	50.0	100.0
1000000	60.0	120.0
10000000	70.0	140.0

specific levels more accurately reflect human loudness perception. By far the most common technique is to apply a filter that approximately reflects the 40-phon loudness contour. We call application of this filter shape "A-weighting." This is contrasted with "Z-weighting" (for zero weighting—formerly called linear weighting), which in fact means you do not apply any filter at all.

In Table 20–9, corrections are provided to convert linear octave-band levels into A-weighted octave-band levels. That is, this reflects the shape of the filter being applied. For example, if the 125-Hz octave band is 60 dB, we would correct it to its dBA-weighted value by subtracting 16.1 dB for a dBA value of 43.9.

Table 20–9. Corrections (dBA Weightings) to Convert Linear Octave-Band Levels into A-weighted Octave-Band Levels

Octave-Band Center Frequency (Hz)	dBA Weighting
31.5	−39.4
63	−26.2
125	−16.1
250	−8.6
500	−3.2
1000	0
2000	+1.2
4000	+1.1
8000	−1.1

> **KEY CONCEPT: SO MANY BANDWIDTHS**
>
> If you happen to lose the table (see Table 20–9), or if you want to know the bandwidth for any other partial octave, or if you are just a lover of math, you can calculate the upper and lower cutoff frequency for any partial octave if you know its center frequency. The formulas are:
>
> $$\text{Lower frequency cutoff (FL)} = \text{antilog}(\{\log F_c\} - 0.3/2n)$$
>
> $$\text{Upper frequency cutoff (Fu)} = \text{antilog}(\{\log F_c\} + 0.3/2n)$$
>
> Where F_c is the center frequency and n is the denominator of the partial octave (e.g., 1 for full octaves, 12 for 1/12 octaves). The bandwidth is the difference between FL and Fu.

Octaves and One-Third Octaves

We indicated that a sound level for the same stimulus is sometimes reported without filtering (Z-weighted, which is also sometimes referred to as the total sound power or TP) and sometimes reported with filtering (A-weighted). This can be confusing because we are reporting what appear to be two different sound levels for exactly the same stimulus. What we have to remember though is that we are always specifying sound level within specific frequency constraints: that is, the sound level after applying some type of frequency-specific filtering. In fact, it is often useful to describe the level of a sound over a very small range of frequencies. For example, we might want to know the sound level within an octave or partial octave, or even the spectral level (roughly level per Hz). Knowing actual bandwidths, both one-third octave and octave, is helpful for both calibration and interpretation of audiometric results. The center frequencies and band limits for octave and one-third octaves are shown in Table 20–9.

The Noise Signal

For testing hearing aids, both in a coupler and for measuring speech perception, various noise types are used. The most commonly used noise is babble noise, often time-matched to the spectrum of the test signal. Other common noises include *white* noise and *pink* noise. The terms "pink" and "white" come from optics. The visual color pink has greater spectral power density at the longer optical wavelengths (lower frequencies, near the red end of the visible spectrum) than at the shorter optical wavelengths (higher frequencies, near the violet end of the visible spectrum). Some engineers also talk about "brown noise," which is similar to pink noise except that the spectral power density decreases even more rapidly with increasing frequency (6 dB per octave). Rather than coming from optics—brown noise (also called Brownian noise or red noise) is named after botanist Robert Brown who discovered Brownian motion.

White noise, also referred to as random noise, has equal intensity and random phase at all frequencies. Pink noise, on the other hand, has equal intensity for each one-third octave band. As shown in Figure 20–2, pink noise has a high-frequency rolloff of 3 dB when plotted in spec-

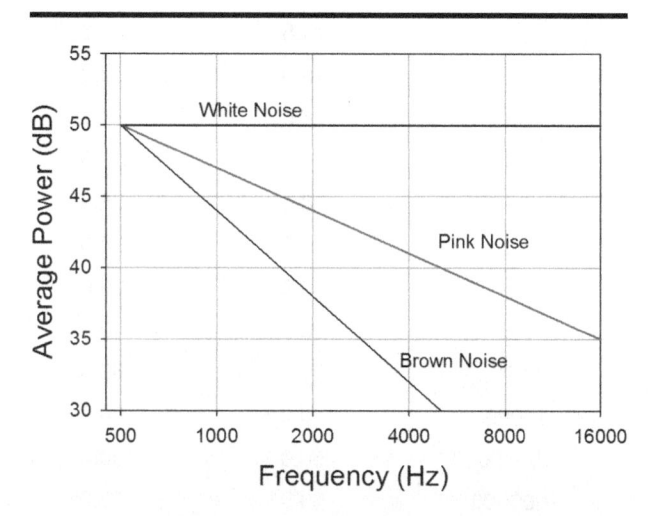

Figure 20–2. The amplitude spectra of all three noises: white, pink, and brown shown in spectrum level (one Hz wide). (Adapted from Yost, 2007.)

> **TECHNICAL TIP: SPECTRA OF THE TEST NOISES (PINK AND WHITE)**
>
> Different manufacturers of hearing aid test equipment (probe microphone systems and test boxes) use pink and/or white noise as test stimuli. The appearance on the screen is not always consistent with the expectation of shape. The differences in appearance are related to the filtering bank used (see related Points to Ponder). For example, as noted, white noise has a uniform spectrum level. If you measure white noise using a fractional octave filter, as is done with several of the probe microphone systems, you will obtain a level that rises at 3 dB per octave. For example, the equation for a one-third octave band is L = 10*log [fm*(2^1/6–2^1/6)] + S where L is the SPL in the one-third octave band centered at fm and S is the spectrum level. For the band at 1 kHz, L = 23.6 + S and for the band at 2 kHz, L = 26.6 + S. So, if you measure pink noise (which falls at 3 dB per octave) with a fractional octave filter (which measures white noise rising at 3 dB per octave), you obtain a flat line—as you do in the Audioscan Verifit® (following the calibration of the probe tube). In fact, the definition of pink noise from ANSI S1.1 states: "Noise for which the spectrum density varies as the inverse of frequency" (p. 5).

trum level/density values (one Hz wide bands). For example, the level at 500 Hz is 3 dB less than the level at 250 Hz; the level at 4000 Hz is 3 dB less than the level at 2000 Hz.

Understanding Figure 20–3 requires a relative understanding of the difference between spectrum level (power in a single-frequency band) and band level—or total power (TP) in a given bandwidth (BW). Sometimes TP of a given BW is referred to as overall level (OAL). One can move between these values with the following formula:

$$TP = 10 (\log BW) + \text{Spectrum Level}$$

From Figure 20–3 we can see that the Spectrum Level is equal to 50 dB and the BW is equal to 1000 Hz. Using the formula, TP = 10 (3) + (50) or 80 dB.

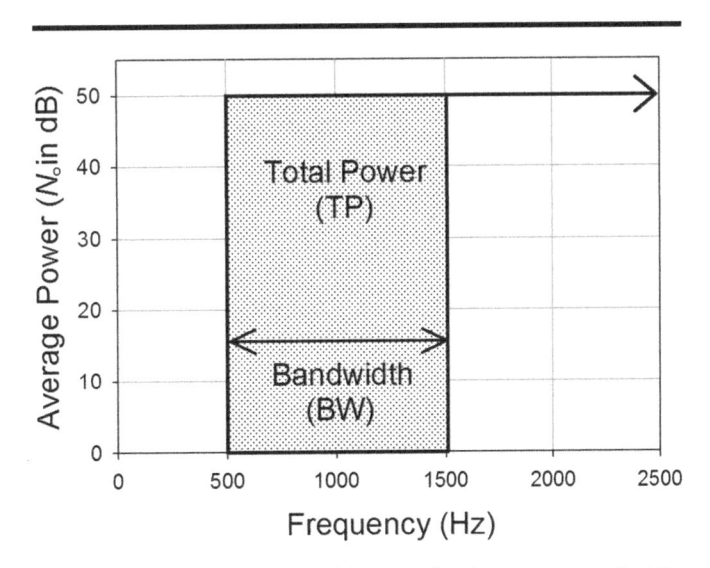

Figure 20–3. Schematic of the amplitude spectrum of white noise. The total power (TP) of white noise is equal to the summed power of all the sinusoids in the noise bandwidth.

> ### POINTS TO PONDER: WHICH LEVEL IS CORRECT?
>
> When doing probe microphone testing, we may measure the real-ear unaided response (REUR) and it may be displayed as the real-ear unaided gain (REUG): the REUR with the input signal subtracted. Although it is easy to recognize the expected shape of the average REUG and individual patient deviations from that shape, it is sometimes more difficult to recognize what an average REUR should look like because it is affected by the spectral shape of the signal you use for testing. You decide you want to measure REUR in several patients' ears so you know the shape for a 70 dB SPL pink noise input signal. You first measure the average level in the patient's ear using a Frye Fonix® 8000 probe microphone system. You are surprised at the results of this measure because you notice that the level on the screen is less than 70 dB SPL (Figure 20–4). To double check you decide to make the same measure using an Audioscan Verifit®. You see the levels are higher, and the shape is different in that the level drops off much less in the high frequencies than it did for the Fonix®. What is happening? Is your test equipment malfunctioning?
>
> Actually, these results are correct and as expected. The differences are due to how the sound is measured in the systems. The Fonix® analyzes sound level using an FFT with a spectral resolution of around 87 Hz. In other words, the level displayed is the 87 Hz wideband level. We see levels much lower than 65 dB SPL because we would need to add all of these individual bands together in order to get the TP level of the signal. In contrast, the Verifit® uses 1/12th octave-band analysis. This has two effects: first 1/12th octave bands are wider than 87 Hz, particularly in the highest frequencies so the levels displayed will be higher; second, partial octave analysis results in increasing bandwidth with increasing frequency (Table 20–10). Because more frequencies (larger bandwidths) are summed together as frequency increases, the effect is a relative frequency shape that increases with increasing frequency when compared to an analysis for which the analysis bandwidth is constant regardless of frequency.

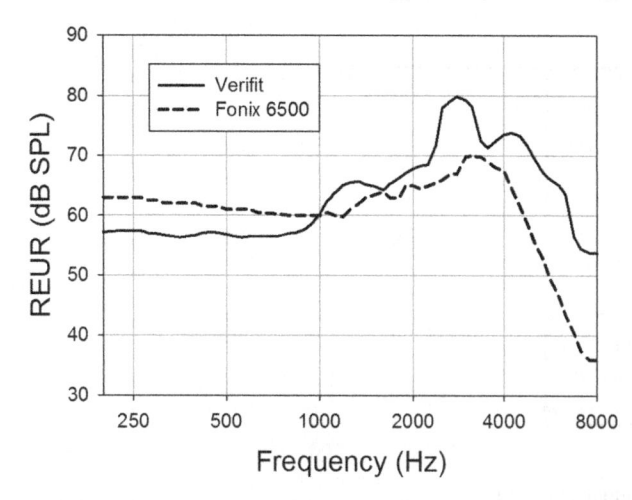

Figure 20–4. Example of the real-ear unaided response (REUR) obtained from two different real-ear systems but with the same input level.

Now back to Figure 20–2: The average power of pink noise drops off by 3 dB per octave. If we were to replot this figure using one-third octave or octave-levels as our y-axis rather than spectrum level, we would see a very different picture. Plotted in one-third octave (bandwidth) levels, pink noise looks flat, white noise looks as though it is rising (by 3 dB per octave), and brown noise only drops 3 dB per octave. Using the formula above, the student of audiology can prove this!

The Speech Signal

Understanding the speech signal and how it is used in hearing aid fitting is useful basic knowledge for all audiologists. Since the primary reason for obtaining hearing

Table 20–10. Center Frequencies and Band Limits for Octave and One-Third Octave Bands

Octave		One-Third Octave	
Center Frequency (Hz)	Band Range (Hz)	Center Frequency (Hz)	Band Range (Hz)
16	11–22	16	14.1–17.8
		20	17.8–22.4
		25	22.4–28.2
31.5	22–44	31.5	28.2–35.5
		40	35.5–44.7
		50	44.7–56.2
63	44–88	63	56.2–70.8
		80	70.8–89.1
		100	89.1–112
125	88–177	125	112–141
		160	141–178
		200	178–224
250	177–355	250	224–282
		315	282–355
		400	355–447
500	355–710	500	447–562
		630	562–708
		800	708–891
1000	710–1420	1000	891–1122
		1250	1122–1413
		1600	1413–1778
2000	1420–2840	2000	1778–2239
		2500	2239–2818
		3150	2818–3548
4000	2840–5680	4000	3548–4467
		5000	4467–5623
		6300	5623–7079
8000	5680–11360	8000	7079–8913
		10000	8913–11220
		12500	11220–14130
16000	11360–22720	16000	14130–17780
		20000	17780–22390

aids is to hear speech better, it is important to understand the details of that signal. Consequently, we review some of the details related to quantifying the speech signal here. Let's begin by describing the actual levels of the long-term average speech spectrum (LTASS). Some-*body's* LTASS is used in the generation of targets for hearing aid fittings; but we are getting ahead of ourselves. In Table 20–11, the published one-third octave levels of speech are shown from a variety of sources, including the NAL and DSL prescriptive formulas. In most cases

Table 20–11. Comparison of One-Third Octave Levels of Speech (in dB SPL) from Four Commonly Used Sources in Prescriptive Fittings

Frequency (Hz)	NAL	DSL	Cox & Moore	International
100	–	39.1	–	54.4
125	–	39.9	–	57.7
160	–	46.3	–	56.8
200	63.0	59.6	–	60.2
250	62.0	62.8	60.0	63.3
315	60.0	60.1	57.0	59.0
400	62.0	61.6	61.0	62.1
500	61.0	64.3	62.0	62.1
630	58.0	63.1	59.0	60.5
800	55.0	60.1	56.5	56.8
1000	50.0	56.4	55.0	53.7
1250	51.0	53.7	54.5	53.0
1600	51.0	52.1	52.0	52.0
2000	49.0	51.0	49.0	48.7
2500	48.0	48.8	48.0	48.1
3150	47.0	45.0	46.5	46.8
4000	48.0	42.3	46.0	45.6
5000	45.0	41.5	44.0	44.5
6300	46.0	42.1	45.5	44.3
8000	0.0	40.9	0.0	43.7
10000	0.0	38.0	0.0	43.4
Overall	70.0	70.9	70.0	70

they are obtained in the same manner: a microphone 30 cm from the talker's mouth, using travelogue type reading material, spoken at an average vocal effort. Occasionally, the LTASS is defined more specifically, as in the case of the DSL fitting formula. In generating that LTASS for use with the DSL formula, the originators (Seewald, Zelisko, Ramji, & Jamieson, 1991) were most interested in providing audibility for children. As a result they considered two factors: (1) the relationship between the hearing aid microphone and the source of the speech, and (2) the self-monitoring children do of their own voices. That is, most other LTASS values are taken with the talkers speaking into the microphone at 30 cm away in order to obtain a clear signal. These levels are typically then corrected—based on the decrease in level with increasing distance—to reflect the level that would be produced with the same vocal effort but measured at a distance of one meter. In this case, the DSL developers also recorded the speech using a microphone placed at the ear of the child. Their final LTASS is composed of averaged male/female/child recordings of the speech obtained directly in front (30 cm) of the talkers averaged with recordings taken at the ear level of the child. It is apparent that they are similar but not identical across sources.

For comparison, Table 20–12 shows the spectrum level (1 Hz wide) of speech from the ANSI S3.5 standard and critical band center frequencies. Shown in Table 20–13 are spectral, one-third and octave-wide levels of speech for the more commonly used octave frequencies from 250 to 4000 Hz. As a final comparison, from the early work of Pearsons, Bennett, and Fidell (1977), the most often cited source of speech levels, are shown in Figure 20–5 and Table 20–13.

A few words of clarification: The ANSI standard (S3.5-1997) on Methods for Calculating the Speech Intelligibility Index defines the *standard* speech spectrum as "spectrum level of speech measured one meter directly in front of the talker's lips, in a free field, for a specified vocal effort, in quiet, averaged across a large group of adult male and female talkers" (ANSI, 1997a, p. 6). The ANSI standard (S3.42 or IEC 60118-15) on Methods for Characterizing Signal Processing in Hearing Aids with a Speech-like Signal considered average speech to have an OAL of 65 dB: "The nominal overall sound pressure level is defined over the band from

Table 20–12. Standard Speech Spectrum Level for Stated Vocal Effort

Critical Band		Standard Speech Spectrum Level for Stated Vocal Effort, Db			
Center Frequency (Hz)	Band Limits (HZ)	Normal	Raised	Loud	Shouted
350	300–400	34.14	38.62	43.68	47.14
450	400–510	34.58	39.84	44.08	48.46
570	510–630	33.17	39.44	45.34	50.17
700	630–770	30.64	37.99	45.22	51.68
840	770–920	27.59	35.85	43.60	51.43
1000	920–1080	25.01	33.86	42.16	51.31
1170	1080–1270	23.52	32.56	41.07	49.40
1370	1270–1480	22.28	30.91	39.68	49.03
1600	1480–1720	20.15	28.58	37.70	47.65
1850	1720–2000	18.29	26.37	35.62	45.47
2150	2000–2320	16.37	24.34	33.17	43.13
2500	2320–2700	13.80	22.35	30.98	40.80
2900	2700–3150	12.21	21.04	29.01	39.15
3400	3150–3700	11.09	19.56	27.71	37.30
4000	3700–4400	9.33	16.78	25.41	34.41
4800	4400–5300	5.84	12.14	19.20	29.01
5800	5300–6400	3.47	9.04	15.37	25.17
Overall SPL, dB		62.35	68.34	74.85	82.30

Note. In that standard, the overall levels for the four vocal efforts is provided: average (62.35), raised (68.34), loud (74.85), and shouted (82.30).

Source: Adapted from ANSI (1997a) (3.5-1997 R2012).

Table 20–13. Example of LTASS Level Shown for Various Vocal Efforts Using Spectral, One-Third Octave, and Octave Measurement Bandwidths

		Soft	Normal	Raised	Loud	Shouted
250	S. Level	–	34.75	38.98	41.55	42.50
	One-Third Octave	48.00	52.38	56.61	59.18	60.13
	Octave	–	57.25	61.48	64.05	65.00
500	S. Level	–	34.27	40.15	44.85	49.24
	One-Third Octave	50.00	54.88	60.76	65.46	69.85
	Octave	–	59.77	65.65	70.35	74.74
1000	S. Level	–	25.01	33.86	42.16	51.31
	One-Third Octave	42.00	48.65	57.50	65.80	74.95
	Octave	–	53.52	62.37	70.67	79.82
2000	S. Level	–	17.32	25.32	34.39	44.32
	One-Third Octave	40.00	43.96	51.96	61.03	70.96
	Octave	–	48.84	56.84	65.91	75.84
3000	S. Level	–	11.55	20.15	28.21	38.13
	One-Third Octave	33.00	40.18	48.78	56.84	66.76
	Octave	–	–	–	–	–
4000	S. Level	–	9.33	16.78	25.41	34.41
	One-Third Octave	32.50	38.96	46.41	55.04	64.04
	Octave	–	43.86	51.31	59.94	68.94

Source: Adapted from Pearsons, Bennett, and Fidell, 1977.

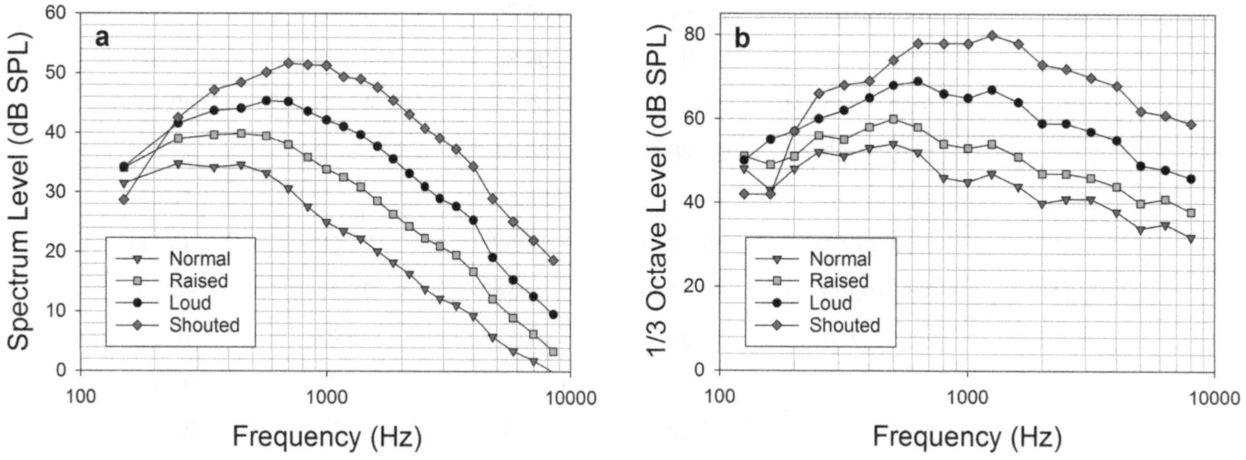

Figure 20–5. The speech spectra for various vocal efforts in both spectrum level (**A**) and one-third octave band level (**B**). (From Pearsons, Bennett, and Fidell, 1977.)

200 Hz to 5 kHz. This level is 65 dB which is considered to be the level of normal conversational speech at 1 m distance (p. 14)." So when someone refers to the *average* level of speech, they could be referring to the Pearsons et al. data or one of the ANSI standards (with differing definitions) (Table 20–14). It has also been suggested

Table 20–14. Mean Sound Pressure Levels in One-Third-Octave Bands for Speech at Five Vocal Efforts by Three Groups of Talkers

Frequency (kHz)	.125	.160	.200	.250	.315	.400	.500	.630	.800	1.0	1.25	1.6	2.0	2.5	3.15	4.0	5.0	6.3	8.0
Females																			
Casual	26	36	47	44	39	45	45	44	39	36	36	36	35	31	30	30	30	32	33
Normal	26	37	48	47	42	49	50	48	46	42	43	42	38	36	38	40	36	36	34
Raised	25	35	48	53	49	53	57	55	54	52	53	52	47	45	45	45	42	40	39
Loud	20	34	45	55	55	55	59	62	62	61	62	62	57	54	53	53	49	47	45
Shouted	20	30	40	50	55	61	64	68	70	72	74	74	70	67	67	64	60	57	55
Males																			
Casual	44	42	46	46	44	47	48	45	38	37	39	39	35	33	33	35	34	33	32
Normal	48	43	48	52	51	53	54	52	46	45	47	44	40	41	41	38	34	35	32
Raised	51	49	51	56	55	58	60	58	54	53	54	51	47	47	46	44	40	41	38
Loud	50	55	57	60	62	65	68	69	66	65	67	64	59	59	57	55	49	48	46
Shouted	42	42	57	66	68	69	74	78	78	78	80	78	73	72	70	68	62	61	59
Children																			
Casual	23	25	42	47	39	43	49	48	43	39	37	38	38	33	33	33	33	33	33
Normal	24	29	42	51	47	47	53	52	49	44	43	43	41	38	39	40	38	36	37
Raised	25	30	41	51	54	53	55	58	57	54	54	54	50	46	47	48	45	43	43
Loud	24	29	41	51	54	58	60	60	63	61	62	63	60	54	54	54	52	49	48
Shouted	24	45	43	49	53	61	66	66	67	72	72	72	71	65	66	66	63	57	54

Source: Tabular data from Pearsons et al. (1977).

> ### THINGS TO REMEMBER: WHAT IS THE "CORRECT" OVERALL LEVEL FOR THE LTASS?
>
> Most of the prescriptive methods used a 70 dB overall level (OAL) for their LTASS because most earlier hearing aids (at the time of development) would never have met target without serious feedback or loudness discomfort issues had they used 60 dB; that is, the gain to be prescribed would need to be 10 dB higher. ANSI S3.42 (IEC 60118-15) considers 65 dB to be the OAL for normal conversational speech at one meter, but most studies have found the OAL at one meter to be around 60 dB. Cox, Matesich, and Moore (1988) found 61 dB OAL for males and 59 dB OAL for females, whereas Pearsons et al. (1977) found 58 dB OAL for males and 55 dB OAL for females. The use of 65 dB in ANSI S3.42 was largely a compromise between being correct (closer to 60 dB) and being able to obtain an adequate signal-to-noise ratio for measurements at higher frequencies.
>
> Bottom line: People have chosen to use OALs that are not typical of normal speech at one meter for various practical reasons.

that the 70 dB SPL used in hearing aid prescriptions better represents the input to a hearing aid microphone for a hearing aid user. Do we tend to speak up when we see someone wearing hearing aids?

Speech in the Verification Stage

There are various ways speech stimuli and the spectrum of speech can be used in the verification process. In its simplest version, clinical application of the AI (SII) by counting-the-dots of importance-weighted audibility helps us counsel the patient when explaining the concept of audibility, the effects on hearing handicap, and potential benefits of amplification. It is possible to use calculated insertion gain to alter the audiogram to predict aided thresholds, which will provide a new aided AI. Some probe microphone equipment does this calculation automatically. We provide three different clinical AI options for use: (1) Killion and Mueller, (2) Humes, and (3) Pavlovic (Figures 20–6, 20–7, and 20–8). Notice they each assume a different speech spectrum (e.g., the shape of the "speech banana") because each assumed a different speech signal to start with!

For those clinicians who are interested in the more general AI, the formula is thus:

$$AI/SII = \sum_{i=1} I_i \, A_i$$

Where n is the number of bands, I_i is the function that characterizes the importance of the ith frequency band to speech intelligibility (band importance function [BIF]), A_i represents the proportion (a value between 0.0 and 1.0) of the speech dynamic range in the ith frequency band that contributes to speech intelligibility.

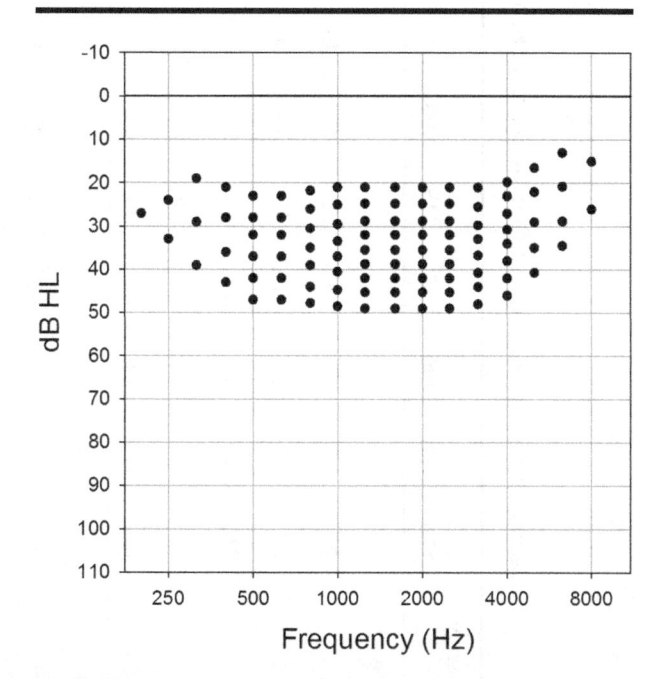

Figure 20–6. An example of a count-the-dot audiogram. (From Killion and Mueller, 2010.)

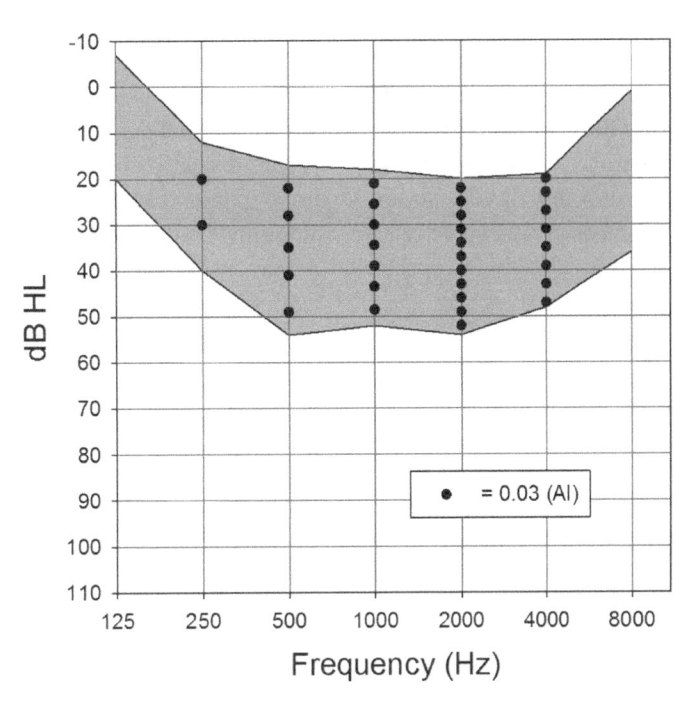

Figure 20–7. An example of count-the-dot audiogram. (From Humes, 1991.)

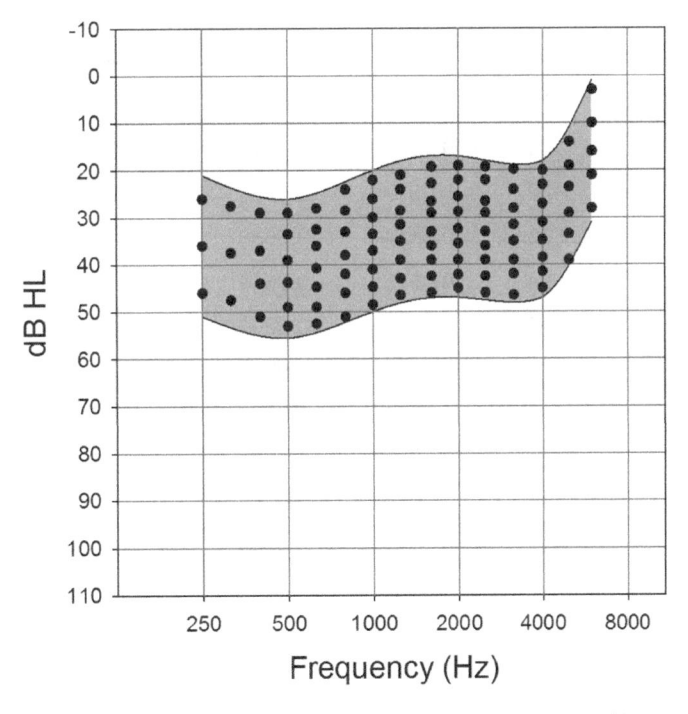

Figure 20–8. An example of count-the-dot audiogram. (From Pavlovic, 1991, as rendered by Conrad Lundeen, 1996.)

One correction factor of interest when considering hearing aid fittings is the *band importance function* (BIF) for different speech materials. As BIFs refer to the weighting applied to the frequency bands, the analogy would be the density of the dots on the count-the-dot audiograms. The relative density (shape of the BIF) is affected most by the amount of context provided by the speech material. For example, for nonsense syllables (e.g., /ba/, /da/, and /ga/) the frequency regions around 2000 and 3000 Hz are the most important to hear because you need to hear each phoneme to be able to distinguish it from others. Increasing the amount of context (e.g., moving from nonsense syllable to running speech) shifts more importance to the lower frequencies. This is because context and our knowledge of running speech allow us to fill-in missing information associated with lower level, high-frequency phonemes. How might this affect clinical practice? Consider a very young child who has not yet acquired speech and language and therefore has limited use of context. When developing a prescriptive hearing aid fitting method, one might assume a nonsense syllable BIF to ensure greater audibility of high-frequency phonemes. Conversely, for a postlingually hearing-impaired adult with an acquired hearing loss, one might assume less importance in the higher frequencies and therefore place less emphasis on ensuring that high-frequency phonemes are as audible as possible. To highlight just how different these functions can be we provide the published BIFs for a number of clinically used speech materials in Tables 20–15, 20–16, 20–17, and 20–18.

Table 20–15. One-Third Octave Band Importance Functions for Various Speech Tests

Band Number	Midland Frequency, Hz	NNS[a]	CID-22[b]	NU6[c]	DRT[d]	Short Passages[e]	SPIN[f]
1	160	0.0000	0.0365	0.0168	0.0000	0.0114	0.0000
2	200	0.0000	0.0279	0.0130	0.0240	0.0153	0.0255
3	250	0.0153	0.0405	0.0211	0.0330	0.0179	0.0256
4	315	0.0284	0.0500	0.0344	0.0390	0.0558	0.0360
5	400	0.0363	0.0530	0.0517	0.0571	0.0898	0.0362
6	500	0.0422	0.0518	0.0737	0.0691	0.0944	0.0514
7	630	0.0509	0.0514	0.0658	0.0781	0.0709	0.0616
8	800	0.0584	0.0575	0.0644	0.0751	0.0660	0.0770
9	1000	0.0667	0.0717	0.0664	0.0781	0.0628	0.0718
10	1250	0.0774	0.0873	0.0802	0.0811	0.0672	0.0718
11	1600	0.0893	0.0902	0.0987	0.0961	0.0747	0.1075
12	2000	0.1104	0.0938	0.1171	0.0901	0.0755	0.0921
13	2500	0.1120	0.0928	0.0932	0.0781	0.0820	0.1026
14	3150	0.0981	0.0678	0.0783	0.0691	0.0808	0.0922
15	4000	0.0867	0.0498	0.0562	0.0480	0.0483	0.0719
16	5000	0.0728	0.0312	0.0337	0.0330	0.0453	0.0461
17	6300	0.0551	0.0215	0.0177	0.0270	0.0274	0.0306
18	8000	0.0000	0.0253	0.0176	0.0240	0.0145	0.0000

Note. [a]NNS various nonsense syllable tests where most of the English phonemes occur equally often. [b]CID-W22 (PB-words). [c]NU6 monosyllables. [d]DRT (diagnostic rhyme test). [e]short passages of easy reading material. [f]SPIN mono-syllables.
Source: ANSI (1997a) (3.5-1997 R2012).

Table 20–16. Octave Band Importance Functions for Various Speech Tests

Band Number	Midland Frequency, Hz	NNS[a]	CID-22[b]	NU6[c]	DRT[d]	Short Passages[e]	SPIN[f]
1	250	0.0437	0.1549	0.0853	0.0960	0.1004	0.0871
2	500	0.1294	0.1562	0.1912	0.2043	0.2551	0.1493
3	1000	0.2025	0.2165	0.2110	0.2343	0.1960	0.2206
4	2000	0.3117	0.2768	0.3090	0.2643	0.2322	0.3022
5	4000	0.2576	0.1488	0.1682	0.1501	0.1744	0.2102
6	8000	0.0551	0.0468	0.0353	0.0510	0.0419	0.0306

Note. [a]NNS various nonsense syllable tests where most of the English phonemes occur equally often. [b]CID-W22 (PB-words). [c]NU6 monosyllables. [d]DRT (diagnostic rhyme test). [e]short passages of easy reading material. [f]SPIN monosyllables.
Source: ANSI (1997a) (3.5-1997 R2012).

Table 20–17. Band Importance Functions for SPIN Sentences and W-22 Phonetically Balanced Words

Band	High Predictability SPIN	Low Predictability SPIN	High and Low Predictability SPIN Pooled	W-22
1	0.0216	0.0441	0.0315	0.0326
2	0.0354	0.0151	0.0265	−0.0156
3	0.0423	0.0732	0.0558	0.0184
4	0.0560	0.0240	0.0420	0.0752
5	0.0344	0.0404	0.0370	0.0681
6	0.0757	0.0391	0.0597	0.0724
7	0.0718	0.0618	0.0674	0.0525
8	0.0560	0.0681	0.0613	0.0993
9	0.0521	0.0290	0.0420	0.0468
10	0.0905	0.1349	0.1099	0.1149
11	0.0560	0.0214	0.0409	0.1191
12	0.0472	0.0378	0.0431	0.0383
13	0.0551	0.0681	0.0608	0.0241
14	0.0679	0.0870	0.0763	0.1106
15	0.0570	0.0744	0.0646	0.0213
16	0.0619	0.0391	0.0519	−0.0057
17	0.0492	0.0542	0.0514	0.0482
18	0.0315	−0.0063	0.0149	0.0128
19	−0.0148	0.0177	−0.0006	−0.0071
20	0.0266	0.0542	0.0387	0.0270
21	0.0266	0.0227	0.0249	0.0468

Source: Healy, Yoho, and Apoux (2013).

Table 20–18. Band Importance Functions for Connected Speech Test (CST)

Critical Band		One-Third Octave Band		Octave Band	
Band	Importance	Band	Importance	Band	Importance
1	0.0654	1	0.0131	1	0.0928
2	0.0603	2	0.0168	2	0.186
3	0.0707	3	0.0255	3	0.1599
4	0.0556	4	0.0374	4	0.2984
5	0.0404	5	0.0637	5	0.1788
6	0.0299	6	0.0694	6	0.0842
7	0.0307	7	0.0529		
8	0.0494	8	0.0374		
9	0.0571	9	0.0441		
10	0.0677	10	0.0784		
11	0.0671	11	0.1035		
12	0.0644	12	0.1023		
13	0.0611	13	0.0926		
14	0.0529	14	0.0738		
15	0.049	15	0.0596		
16	0.0448	16	0.0454		
17	0.0376	17	0.0365		
18	0.0322	18	0.0477		
19	0.026				
20	0.0231				
21	0.0146				

Source: Sherbecoe and Studebaker (2002).

Pressure Transformations of Head and Body Including Head Shadow

Back in our basic acoustics' studies, we learned how our head, body, and ear canal affect sound traveling in space towards us. It is also important for us to understand these effects when considering hearing aid decision making and fitting. Perhaps the most familiar representation of these transformations is the graphic display in Figure 20–9, which has been reproduced in many audiology textbooks. What is clear from this figure is the cumulative effect of head, neck, and torso, and the parts of the external ear (concha, pinna flange, and ear canal). The "T" for total of those pressure transforms is very similar to what we have come to know as the free-field-to-eardrum transformation or the real-ear-unaided gain response (REUG) (see Chapter 6 for more detailed description).

These concepts are important for understanding how head and body transformations affect the fitting of hearing aids. The most obvious effect is on the total "T." In some nonoccluding fittings, such as those using the popular open non-custom eartips, the free gain associated with the REUG is still in place with only small alterations. In contrast, the total T is often completely eliminated by most custom hearing aids, custom earmolds, and occluding non-custom domes.

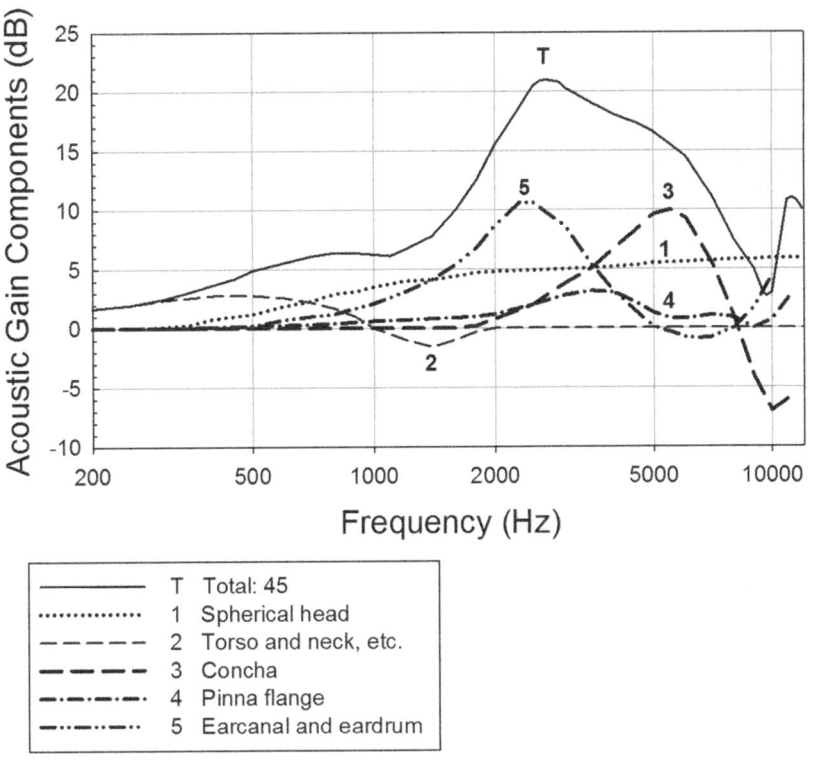

Figure 20–9. The average pressure gain contributed by the different components of the outer ear in a man with stimulus in the horizontal plane at 45-degree azimuth. (From Shaw, 1974. Reprinted, with permission, from Springer Science and Business Media.)

Also of clinical interest is how that total pressure sum changes as a function of the angle (or azimuth) of the sound source. Although there is some head diffraction that provides a boost to the input signal, the change in level as a function of angle is primarily due to head shadow. A *head shadow* or acoustic shadow refers to the region of reduced amplitude of a sound because it is obstructed by the head. The obstruction caused by the head can account for a significant attenuation (reduced amplitude) of overall intensity, particularly in the higher frequencies. The effects of head shadow are an essential element of sound localization. Specifically, the relative amplitude, timbre, and phase of a sound heard by the two ears are analyzed by the brain to facilitate in localization. Figure 20–10 shows the effect of head shadow.

The effects of head shadow must be considered relative to placement of the patient in front of a loudspeaker for testing or probe microphone testing. It also is useful when counseling patients relative to how they may be able to increase loudness just by angling their heads. Figure 20–11 shows the average pressure gain of the external ear for different orientations of the sound source (or the head, for that matter) in the horizontal plane ipsilateral to the ear. Understanding these transformations is essential to understanding how patients can use their unaided ears for localization and targeting of the important components of conversation in a degraded environment.

Field to Eardrum Transformation

In this era of probe microphone measurements, the clinician is typically knowledgeable about the REUG. In the past, however, researchers relied on calculations based on acoustic measurements taken with larger microphones and less well-calibrated acoustic manikins instead of having access to live REUG measures. Roughly equivalent to the REUG, the *free* field-to-eardrum transformation of Shaw (1974) and Shaw and

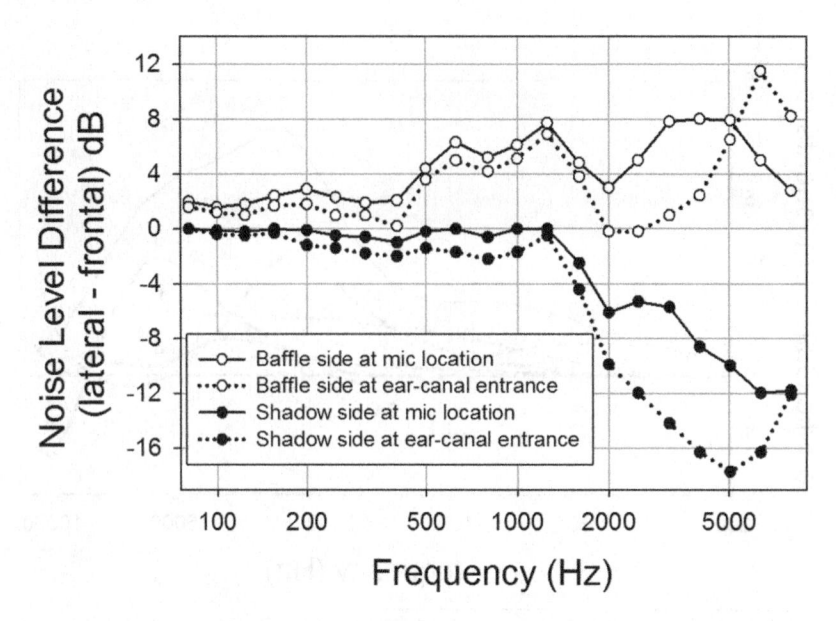

Figure 20–10. Average level differences between the noise from the front and from a lateral position, measured in one-third octave bands, as a function of frequency, measured for eight subjects. Closed symbols pertain to the shadow side of the head and open symbols to the baffle side. Level differences at the ear canal entrance are connected by dashed lines at the hearing aid and at the hearing aid microphone location with solid lines. (Adapted from Festen and Plomp, 1986.)

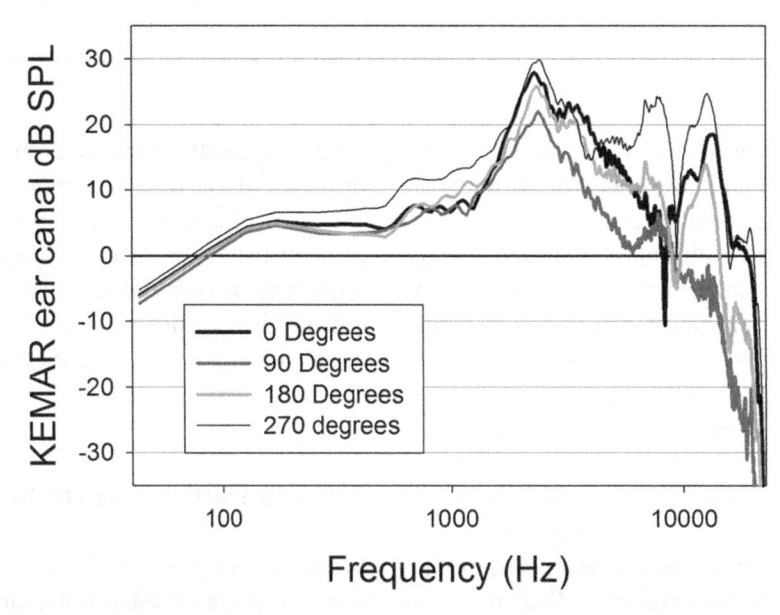

Figure 20–11. The average head-related transfer function (HRTF) in the horizontal plane for the ipsilateral ear. These values represent the average pressure gain as a function of angle.

Table 20–19. Average Real-Ear-Unaided Gain (REUG) Values for Various Loudspeaker Azimuths and Field Reference Points

Frequency	250	500	750	1000	1500	2000	3000	4000	6000	8000
0° Center of Head*	1	2	3	3	5	12	16	14	8	2
45° Over the Ear†	2	3	3	3	6	13	14	13	8	4
Diffuse, Center of Head‡	1	2	3	4	7	11	16	13	9	9

Note. Values rounded to nearest dB; some values interpolated.
*Data from Bentler and Pavlovic (1989). †Data from Frye Electronics, Inc., Tigard, OR. ‡Data from Killion et al. (1987).

Vaillancourt (1985) is shown in Table 20–19. The values were derived from averaging a pool of data from 12 studies (total of 100 subjects). The *diffuse* field-to-eardrum transformation data are from Bentler and Pavlovic (1992). Their derived values came from averaging data from Kuhn (1979), Shaw (1980), and Killion, Berger, and Nuss (1987). These are also estimates of average REUG; however, as evident from differences in their titles, the data were collected in a diffuse field (sound of random phase arriving from all angles and elevations) rather than in free field (anechoic). Kuhn obtained his values using six different artificial pinnae on an anthropomorphic manikin. A microphone in an acoustic coupler, mounted in the manikin, simulated the average impedance of a normal eardrum. Shaw obtained his values on a geometric model ear; seven pinnae replicas terminated in the same eardrum simulator. Killion et al. obtained their data from 16 subjects (eight male and eight female), using a 1-mm outside diameter silicone rubber tube placed within a couple of mm of the eardrum. All derivations are shown in Table 20–19. Note that through the frequencies of 6000 Hz there is no more than a 2 dB difference among the measures.

Transformations From the Field to Various Microphone Locations

The field to microphone transformation is referred to as the microphone location effect (MLE). Table 20–20 shows MLEs for both free-field and diffuse-field measures taken from Bentler and Pavlovic (1989, 1992). The data are useful in that they provide a good indication of the expected change in frequency response that occurs from simply changing the position of the hearing aid microphone through changing the hearing aid style. By examining the change in level as a function of sound source location, one can also gain some understanding of real-world signal-to-noise ratio effects based on MLE. For example, the pinna shadow that reduces sound levels from behind for the completely-in-the-canal (CIC) microphone location is not there for the BTE microphone location. Another real-world example is when a listener faces a talker and has noise behind him or her; in that case, the SNR is poorer for a BTE than an ITE.

Behind-the-Ear (BTE)

For free field values, the BTE MLE transforms from Bentler and Pavlovic (1989) were derived by averaging data from Madaffari (1974) and Kuhn and Burnett (1977). Using a KEMAR, Madaffari calculated the difference between the SPL in a free field (KEMAR absent) and the SPL at the entrance to the BTE microphone placed on the KEMAR at the same location. Kuhn and Burnett took pressure measurements at 348 positions around the KEMAR's head. A microphone probe was mounted on x-y-z coordinates, with the x-axis corresponding to 4 mm increments from the front to the back of the head (with 0 mm representing the notch of the pinna to the head); the y-axis corresponding to 2, 4, and 7 mm away from the head surface along the ear canal axis; and the z-axis corresponding to 0, 5 and 10 mm above the pinna notch. For the BTE MLE, the coordinates were chosen to best approximate that microphone location (x = 0 mm, y = 4 mm, z = 5 mm).

For diffuse field values, the BTE MLE transforms were derived by Bentler and Pavlovic (1989) by averaging data from Kuhn (1979) and Killion et al. (1987). Kuhn obtained his data by averaging measurements

Table 20–20. Nominal Values for Transformations from Free-field (A–D) and Diffuse-field (E–H) to Eardrum and Various Microphone Locations Shown at One-Third Octave Center Frequencies from 160 to 8000 Hz

Frequency One-Third Octave Center	A	B	C	D	E	F	G	H
200	0.5	0.5	0.3	0.0	0.4	1.5	0.3	0.5
250	1.0	0.5	0.5	0.3	0.5	0.5	0.5	0.4
315	1.4	0.8	0.8	0.3	1.0	0.5	0.8	0.7
400	1.5	1.1	1.0	0.7	1.3	0.8	1.2	1.1
500	1.8	1.2	1.8	0.0	1.7	0.9	1.3	1.6
630	2.4	1.1	2.0	0.1	2.2	1.4	1.3	1.6
800	3.1	0.9	2.0	0.4	2.9	1.5	1.3	1.9
1000	2.6	0.3	1.5	1.2	3.8	1.7	1.8	2.3
1250	3.0	0.6	0.3	–1.6	5.3	2.5	2.1	2.7
1600	6.1	2.5	–0.3	–1.9	7.2	2.7	2.4	3.3
2000	12.0	4.1	3.8	2.1	10.2	2.6	2.7	4.1
2500	16.8	3.5	5.0	4.8	14.9	2.8	3.4	5.0
3150	15.0	2.8	3.3	3.5	14.4	2.9	3.9	5.9
4000	14.3	3.7	4.3	6.4	12.9	2.7	5.4	7.9
5000	10.7	–1.2	4.3	6.6	10.8	2.8	5.5	8.9
6300	6.4	1.6	–0.4	–1.8	8.7	2.8	4.9	8.3
8000	1.8	3.3	1.0	–1.9	8.5	2.9	6.1	5.6

Note. A = free-field to eardrum; B = free-field to BTE mic location; C = free-field to ITE mic location; D = free-field to ITC mic location; E = diffuse-field to eardrum; F = diffuse-field to BTE mic location; G = diffuse-field to ITE mic location; H = diffuse-field to ITC mic location.

Source: Bentler and Pavlovic (1989); Bentler and Pavlovic (1992).

(described above for free-field-to-eardrum transformations) taken on the same anthropomorphic manikin's head and two adult subjects. Killion et al. measured the increase in SPL over diffuse field SLP using a BTE hearing aid mounted on the KEMAR.

In-the-Ear (ITE)

For free-field values, the ITE MLE transforms were obtained from Madiffari (1974). Similar to the methodology used for the BTE value, Madaffari determined the difference between the SPL in a free field with the KEMAR absent and the SPL at the entrance (the center of the filled concha) of an ITE hearing aid microphone placed on the KEMAR at that same point in the free field.

For diffuse-field values, Killion et al. (1987) measured the increase in SPL over diffuse field SPL using an ITE hearing aid mounted on the KEMAR. The investigators originally provided separate values for a full-shell ITE, a low-profile ITE, and an "average" ITE. Only the average ITE transformation values are shown in Table 20–20.

In-the-Canal (ITC)

Values for the *free*-field MLEs are actually free-field to blocked-canal transfer functions and were derived by averaging data obtained from Wiener and Ross (1946) and Shaw (1975). Weiner and Ross used human ear canals plugged with "suitable insert tips," although the material and insertion details were not provided.

Values for the diffuse-field MLE transforms were obtained by averaging data from Kuhn and Guernsey (1983) and Killion et al. (1987). Kuhn and Guernsey took measurements using the KEMAR and six different pinnae. The measurements were obtained using a 1.25 mm diameter probe placed at the center of the concha and a coupler microphone at the eardrum position. Data from Killion et al. (1987) were obtained using two sizes of ITC hearing aids, and the results were averaged.

Completely in the Canal (CIC)

As expected, the largest MLEs are present for the CIC hearing aid, assuming that the microphone inlet is now located at the opening of, or slightly within, the ear canal. This difference in location allows for some resonating of the sound—or enhancement of the level—due to the pinna and concha (Figure 20–12). Seewald, Cornelisse, Richert, and Block. (1997) measured CIC MLEs for 24 adult ears at 0 degrees and 45 degrees azimuth. To obtain these measures, "dummy" CICs were fabricated for each individual which included the CIC microphone and receiver but no amplifier. The electrical output of the microphone was hardwired directly to a dual-channel signal analyzer, which allowed for these SPL measures to be compared to the SPL of the undisturbed sound field. In Figure 20–13 the impact of the azimuth on the measured MLE can be seen.

Real-Ear-Coupler Differences (RECD)

Often in hearing aid fittings, the RECD is measured—or estimated—to improve the intended audibility goals and/or to predict real-ear output. When estimated, there are several data sets that are used by manufacturers in their fitting software. In adult patients, RECD values are typically added to the OSPL90 coupler response to

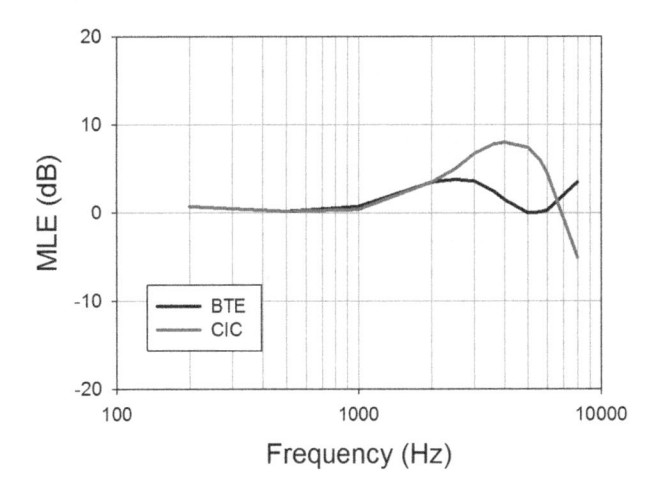

Figure 20–12. Example of the difference between the microphone location effect (MLE) between a behind-the-ear (BTE) and a completely-in-the-canal (CIC) hearing aid. See text for explanation due to microphone placement relative to the head. (Adapted from Chasin, 1997, with permission.)

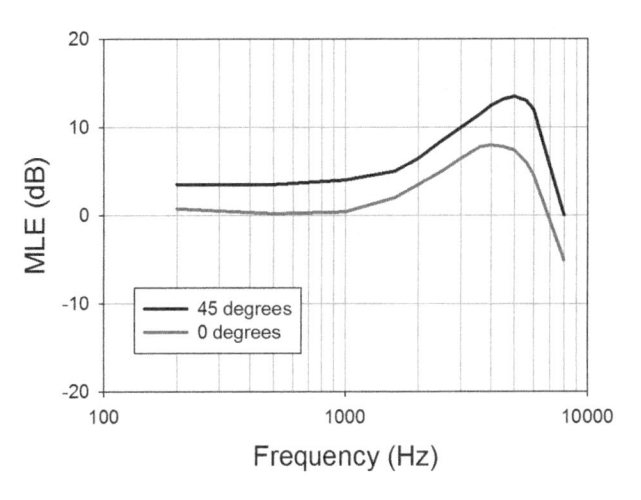

Figure 20–13. Example of the difference in the microphone location effect (MLE) for a completely-in-the-canal (CIC) hearing aid when the sound source varies from 0 to 45 degrees relative to the front. See text for explanation. (Adapted from Chasin, 1997, with permission.)

obtain estimated real-ear MPO values. Another use for RECD values is their application to threshold measures to reflect more accurately thresholds as they would be measured using the actual hearing aid coupling system. Regardless of use, however, most authors suggest measurement of RECD in individual patients rather than the use of normative data in order to be as accurate as possible.

The earliest—and most famous—RECD data were from Sachs and Burkhard (1972), who determined the eardrum pressure developed by insert receivers on 11 ears. The values are shown in Figure 20–14 and Table 20–21. In Table 20–22, we show more recent RECD data sets. In an attempt to improve existing normative data through the use of a greater number of infant ears, a collaborative study between the University of Western Ontario and Boys Town National Research Hospital completed RECD measurements on 392 children aged one month to 16 years (Bagatto, Scollie, Seewald, Moody, and Hoover, 2002). These measures were completed using either acoustic immittance eartips (141 ears) or personal earmolds (251 ears). A re-analysis of these data was used to generate age-specific RECD normative data for infants up to 36 months of age (Baggatto et al., 2005). These newer RECD values have been implemented into the several prescriptive gain calculations used by probe microphone systems at the time of this writing. The latest probe microphone standard has redefined the RECD to remove all "plumbing" factors from this measure and the RECD is now defined in reference to a HA-1 coupler in place of the old reference defined in a HA-2 coupler. This change enhances the measure's reliability and repeatability across equipment; however, it did require some corrections to the correction factors implemented in probe microphone systems. To help simplify this transition some probe microphone manufacturers provide built-in correction factors so that the average RECD may still be applied to a hearing aid measurement made in a HA-2.

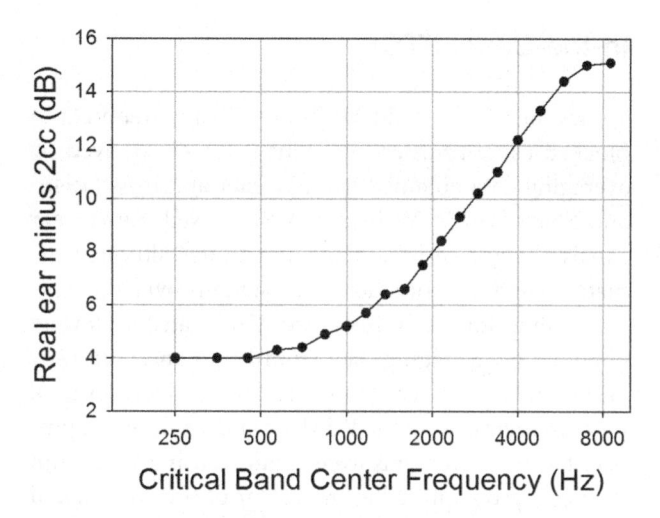

Figure 20–14. Real-ear-to-coupler differences (RECD). (From Sachs and Burkhard, 1972.)

The Transform for Estimating Real-Ear Output (TEREO)

The RECD is the appropriate transform for predicting real-ear MPO from the OSPL90 obtained in the 2cc coupler. In this instance, the MLE of the instrument is no longer a factor. We will explain. Consider that a CIC instrument may have an MLE of 10 dB or more in the higher frequencies: considerably more than a BTE. This is because the deep microphone placement allows for the impact of the collection and resonance properties of the concha. As the input signal becomes higher, the output reaches the MPO of the hearing aid, and that 10 dB boost no longer matters—all that matters is the

---

TECHNICAL TIP: RECDS AND THE INFLUENCE OF TRANSDUCER

As we've mentioned, there are four things that will impact the RECD: the acoustic impedance of the sound source, the coupling system, the coupler that is used, and the characteristic of the patient's real ear. We know that the acoustic impedance likely will be different for an insert earphone and a given hearing instrument. One might question, therefore, should the RECD be measured using the patient's own hearing aid as the transducer? In one study (Munro & Toal, 2005), the authors found significant differences between the RECDs obtained with two different hearing aids, when compared to coupler measures. With one of the hearing aids, the differences were as large as 6 dB (HA-1 coupler) and 11 dB (HA-2 coupler).

Table 20–21. Tabular Data for the Real-Ear-to-Coupler Differences (RECD)

	250	500	1000	2000	3000	4000	6000
RECD	4	4.2	5.2	8.0	10.3	12.2	14.5

Note. Values were obtained by reading them directly from Figure 3–13 graph.
Source: Sachs and Burkhard (1972).

Table 20–22. Estimated Real-Ear to 2cc Coupler-Difference (RECD) Transformations as a Function of Age and Audiometric Frequency*

HA-1 Coupler	Frequency (Hz)								
	250	500	750	1000	1500	2000	3000	4000	6000
0–12 months	5.4	9.8	10.0	13.0	14.4	14.5	18.5	21.6	22.4
13–24 months	7.3	10.2	9.9	12.6	13.7	14.2	16.1	18.5	15.5
25–48 months	4.0	8.5	8.7	11.8	13.2	13.2	15.5	16.2	15.4
49–60 months	2.8	8.0	8.5	9.8	11.9	12.7	14.0	15.0	14.8
>60 months	2.2	4.6	4.3	6.3	7.7	8.8	11.2	13.1	13.7
HA-2 Coupler	250	500	750	1000	1500	2000	3000	4000	6000
0–12 months	5.5	9.7	9.6	11.9	11.6	10.5	16.2	19.4	17.8
13–24 months	7.4	10.1	9.5	11.5	10.9	10.2	13.8	16.3	10.9
25–48 months	4.1	8.4	8.3	10.7	10.4	9.2	13.2	14.0	10.8
49–60 months	2.9	7.9	8.1	8.7	9.1	8.7	11.7	12.8	10.2
>60 months	2.3	4.5	3.9	5.2	4.9	4.8	8.9	10.9	9.1

Note. *Values for individuals >60 months were derived by Seewald, Ramji, Sinclair, Moodie, and Jamieson (1993) at the University of Western Ontario. Values for individuals <60 months were derived by applying age group data reported by Feigin, Kopun, Stelmachowicz, and Gorga (1989) to the values of Seewald et al. HA-2 coupler values were derived by applying an HA-1 to HA-2 coupler transformation (Seewald et al, 1993) to the HA-1 coupler values.

Source: "Amplification for Infants and Children With Hearing Loss," by F. H. Bess, P. A. Chase, J. S. Gravel, A. Hedley-Williams, R. C. Seewald, P. G. Stelmachowicz, A. M. Tharp, *American Journal of Audiology*, 5(1), p. 66,. Copyright 1996. Reprinted with permission from the *American Journal of Audiology*.

volume difference between the patient's ear canal and the 2cc coupler.

When we make transformations for the REAR, however, the MLE *does* matter, as now we are looking at much lower inputs and the hearing aid has not reached its MPO. This correction factor has been termed the *TEREO* (Seewald et al., 1997). Therefore, the TEREO = RECD + MLE. If you want to go from the 2cc-coupler values to the real-ear equivalent, you *add* the TEREO; to obtain the coupler equivalent when you have ear canal SPL values, you subtract the TEREO. Of course it is not necessary to consider the TERO for RECDs measured through real hearing aids as described earlier because this measure includes both the RECD and MLE in the single measurement.

Coupler Response for Flat Insertion Gain (CORFIG)

As we just discussed, the TEREO is a step beyond the RECD, as it includes the MLE. If we want to do a transform from the 2cc coupler that provides insertion gain (not just real-ear output), it is necessary to include the REUG. Killion and Monser (1980) introduced the term *CORFIG* to describe the coupler response for flat insertion gain. The formula used to derive these values is:

$$\text{CORFIG} = \text{REUG} - \text{RECD} - \text{MLE}$$

In this formula REUG refers to the real-ear unaided gain (discussed in Chapters 6 and 7), RECD refers to the real-ear coupler difference, and MLE refers to the microphone location effect.

Of course CORFIG values depend upon the coupler used (ear simulator versus 2cc) and on the location of the microphone sound entrance about the head (refer to the previous section, Transformations from the Field to Various Microphone Locations). The original CORFIG values were derived using available transformations including (1) the correction from the free field SPL to the hearing aid microphone entrance (from Madaffari, 1974), (2) the correction from a 2cc coupler to the eardrum or ear simulator (Sachs & Burkhard, 1972), and (3) the free-field-to-eardrum transformation (from Shaw, 1974). Table 20–23 shows the COR-

> **POINTS TO PONDER: A CLINICAL APPLICATION FOR CORFIG**
>
> Assume you have a mini-BTE hearing aid that is programmed to produce 35 dB of gain at 3000 Hz in the 2cc coupler. What gain will this be in the average real ear? What the patient will *lose* is the REUG—we'll say that is 15 dB at 3000 Hz. What the patient will *gain* is the MLE (2 dB for this hearing aid model at 3000 Hz) and the RECD (we'll say 8 dB for 3000 Hz). If we now plug these numbers into the CORIFG formula we have: 15 − 2 − 8 = 5 dB. That is, the patient lost 5 dB more than he gained, so we would predict that the insertion gain would be 5 dB less in the real ear, around 30 dB rather than 35, than it was in the coupler. Now, if he had been fitted with a CIC with a 10 dB MLE, and the fit had been deeper making his RECD 10 dB, we would predict that the insertion gain would be 5 dB greater than coupler gain: 40 dB rather than 35 dB.

Table 20–23. Average CORFIG Values for 0 Degrees, 45 Degrees, and Diffuse Incidences of the Sound Source

Frequency	250	500	750	1000	1500	2000	3000	4000	6000	8000
0° BTE*:	−4	−4	−3	−3	−3	0	3	−2	−8	−16
45° BTE[†]:	−1	0	−1	−2	−1	4	4	3	−1	−8
Diffuse BTE[‡]:	−3	−3	−3	−3	−2	1	3	−2	−8	−13
0° ITE*:	−4	−4	−4	−4	−1	0	2	−2	−8	−14
45° ITE[†]:	−1	−1	−2	−2	−2	2	3	−2	−6	−10
Diffuse ITE[‡]:	−3	−3	−3	−3	−2	1	2	−4	−10	−15
0° ITC*:	−3	−2	−2	−4	−1	2	1	−4	−10	−11
45° ITC[†]:	−2	−1	−2	−3	−2	1	1	−7	−9	−13
Diffuse ITC[‡]:	−3	−3	−3	−3	−2	1	0	−8	−1	−15
CIC[‡§]:	−6	−6	−7	−7	−7	−5	−7	−16	−22	−24

Note. The values in the table are rounded to the nearest dB; some values are interpolated. To convert from 2cc coupler-gain to predicted REIG, the values are subtracted from 2cc gain.

*Source: Bentler and Pavlovic (1989) (free-field reference). [†]Source: Killion and Revit (1993) (over-the-ear reference). [‡]Source: Killion et al (1987) (center-of-head reference). [§]The diffuse-field CIC values apply for all sound-source angles because the direction-dependent variables cancel in both the CORFIG calculation and the REIG measurement.

Source: Revit (2000).

FIG values previously published by Bentler and Pavlovic (1989) for 0-degree azimuth. These values were derived in this manner for BTE, ITE, and ITC hearing aids. In the table, data are shown from Killion et al. (1987) and Killion and Revit (1993) for 45-degree azimuth and diffuse fields. Other derivations were obtained using a Zwislocki coupler mounted on a KEMAR (Burnett, 1985; Cole, 1975; Hawkins & Schum, 1984; Knowles & Burkhard, 1975; Longwell & Johnson, 1980) or with probe microphone measures on *real* people (Hawkins & Mueller, 1992) have been published. For comparison, we show the Hawkins and Mueller (1992) *real* people values (Table 20–24). What should be obvious here is that no correction factor is likely to be *correct* for the potential hearing aid user sitting in front of you. In fact, there is general consensus that the usefulness of CORFIG corrections has been diminished with the availability of real-ear *output* targets!

POINTS TO PONDER: CORFIGS AND OPEN-CANAL FITTINGS

When open-canal (OC) fittings became routine more than 10 years ago, there was some discussion regarding how this might affect CORFIGs. In the CORFIG calculation, we had treated the REUG as if it was no longer present when the hearing aid (earmold) is in place. With an OC fitting, however, it's very possible that most of the REUG will remain. It seemed unfair to subtract something that is still there. The traditional CORFIG formula also uses average RECDs. But what if the canal is open? How does this impact the RECD? We certainly would not expect the RECD to be as large as if a closed earmold were fitted. This issue was indirectly studied by Mueller and Ricketts (2006) when they compared REIGs for hearing aids fitted with both an open and closed earmold. They found that, indeed, the open earmold provided an increase of gain of 5 to 10 dB around the area of the peak of the REAR (2500–3000 Hz; associated with the peak in the patient's REUR). There was considerable patient variability, however, because of the size of the ear canals (small ear canals would increase gain for the closed fitting more than the open) and the size of the REUG (large REUGs would benefit the open fitting more than the closed). So does the CORFIG formula need to change for OC fittings? Yes, but it would be very difficult to predict, as ear canals vary considerably and not all open fittings are open. We are not sure how the manufacturers accomplish this in their simulated gain curves in the fitting software. We assume an average (KEMAR) ear canal with a completely open fit is used. Under these assumptions there is a peak increase of about 8 dB around 2700 Hz.

Table 20–24. Average CORFIG Values Measured on Patients

Hearing Aid Type	Frequency						
	250	500	1000	2000	3000	4000	6000
BTE	−3	−2	−2	−7	−10	−10	0
ITE	0	0	0	−2	−6	0	3
ITC	0	0	0	−2	−3	3	7

Note. To convert from 2cc coupler-gain to predicted REIG, the values are added to 2cc gain.
Source: Hawkins and Mueller (1992).

> **TECHNICAL TIP: USE OF CORFIGS IN PRESCRIPTIVE METHODS**
>
> The two prescriptive formulas in common use at the time of this writing, NAL-NL2 and the DSL v.5, have incorporated REUG, MLE, and RECD values of their own derivation into their fitting software. Those values are discussed in more detail in Chapter 4. The developers of the DSL software have not provided CORFIG values, in that their prescription is based on output, not gain. Although NAL does provide a table of CORFIG values for consideration by the interested clinician, those developers point out that even though the CORFIG can be thought of as the combination of MLE, RECD, and REUG, the problem with combing those values is related to the common use of amplitude compression in our processing schemes (Table 20–25). Consider that the MLE occurs prior to the compressor, and the RECD and REUG occur subsequent to the compressor. Consequently, the NAL fitting software uses each of these corrections separately.

Table 20–25. Common Hearing Aid Transformations

Predicted REAR85	= OSPL90	+	RECD
Predicted REAR	= 2cc-coupler gain	+	TEREO (RECD + MLE)
Predicted REIG	= 2cc-coupler gain	−	CORFIG (REUG − RECD − MLE)

Corrections for Setting Maximum Output

There has been much said about the importance of testing and applying output limitation values that are specific to the patient's needs. Whether the LDLs or thresholds of discomfort (TDs) are obtained pre-fitting or in the verification stage, these frequency-specific values can be used to set the MPO of the hearing aid. This is accomplished by adding the RETSPL for a given frequency (see Table 20–5) to the HL LDL, and then using this value to adjust the AGCo kneepoint.

There are situations, however, when frequency-specific LDLs cannot be obtained for a patient and it is necessary to predict the LDL from the hearing threshold. Although this is better than not considering LDLs at all, it is certainly risky as there is considerable variability among people with the same hearing loss. As a reminder of this variability, Figure 20–15 shows the results from 732 ears. There was no age or gender effect in the analysis of these data.

Another early effort to quantify both most comfortable listening levels (MCLs) and uncomfortable listening levels (UCL) was attempted by David Pascoe at the Central Institute of the Deaf. His values can be

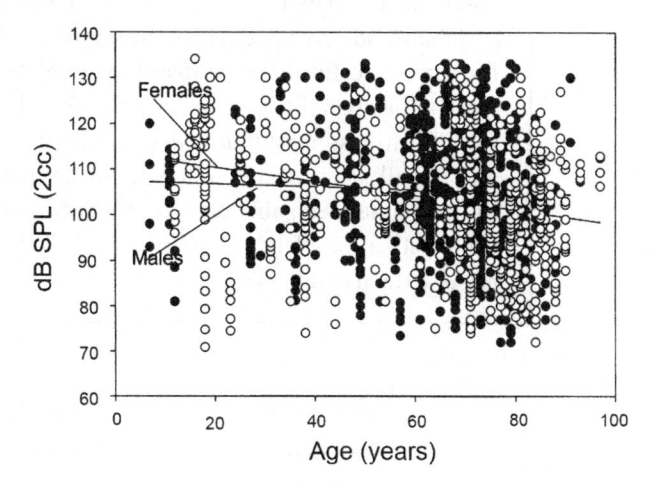

Figure 20–15. The variability of loudness discomfort levels (LDLs) is seen in this graph from Bentler and Cooley's 2000 study (2001). The filled circles represent males; the open circles represent females; all LDLs are plotted in 2cc values. There was no significant gender or age effect in this data set of 732 ears.

read from the familiar graph in Figure 20–16, and are shown as a function of hearing level. Because many audiologists do not adjust the MPO of the patient's hear-

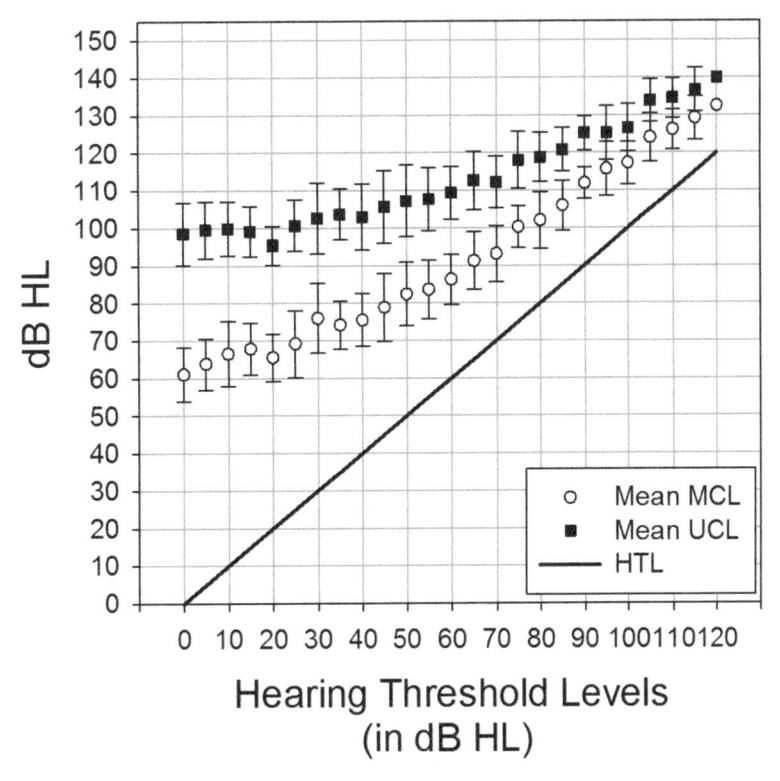

Figure 20–16. Average most comfortable levels (MCL) and uncomfortable levels (UCL) as a function of four frequency average thresholds (500, 1000, 2000, 4000 Hz). Error bars represent one standard deviation. Note the MCL and UCL are also displayed in hearing level (HL). (Adapted from Pascoe, 1988.)

ing aids based on LDL data, default settings for MPO are included in the fitting software. It is customary for manufacturers to use data like Pascoe's for this purpose.

Prescriptive formulas use UCL, LDL, or equivalent data for establishing maximum output targets as well. The NAL prescription estimates the appropriate settings using the function shown in Figure 20–17; the actual values applied within the software are shown in

---

POINTS TO PONDER: COMPARISON OF AVERAGE LDLS

By far, the two sets of LDL data shown here from Bentler and Cooley (2001) and Pascoe (1988) are the largest samples available. When comparing the two charts, keep in mind that the y-axis of the Pascoe chart is in HL, and the Bentler-Cooley chart is in 2cc coupler. If we subtract average RETSPLs to convert the Bentler-Cooley chart to HL, we can see that the Pascoe LDLs in the 40 to 60 dB hearing loss range are almost 10 dB higher. Certainly it is enough of a difference to influence the success of a hearing aid fitting. Why the difference? It could be related to the loudness anchor charts that were used for data collection. The Bentler-Cooley chart had three loudness categories above the midpoint (e.g., MCL), whereas the Pascoe chart had four. Whatever the reason, the manufacturer's default settings will be different depending on whose set of data is used.

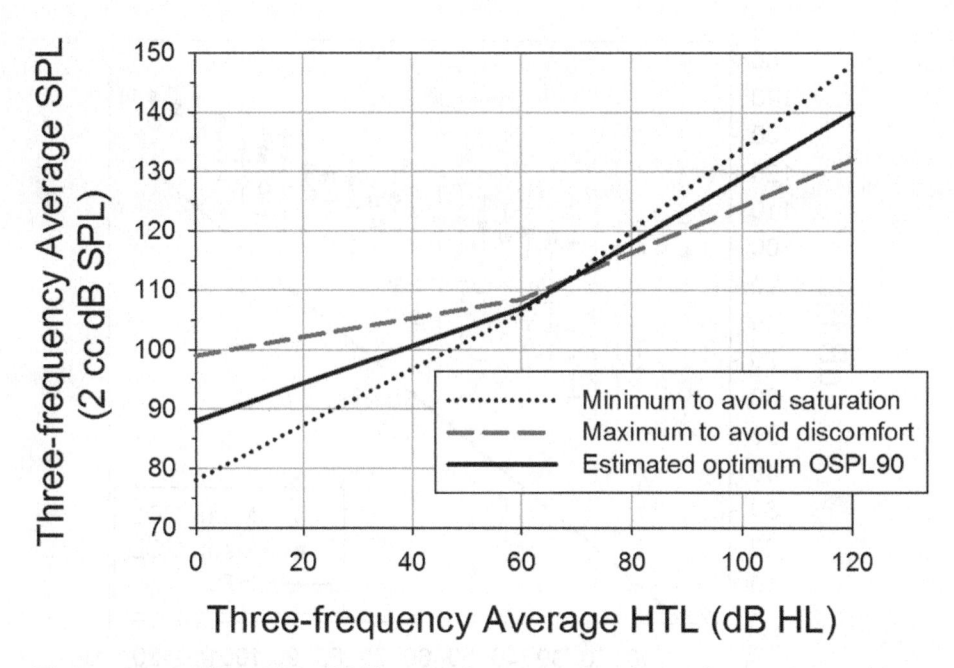

Figure 20–17. The NAL OSPL selection procedure, based on values midway between the estimated OSPL90 need to avoid discomfort and the estimated OSPL90 need to avoid saturation. (Adapted from Dillon, 2012, with permission.)

Table 20–26. The DSL prescription derives its targets for maximum output data from Pascoe's earlier work but with one additional correction: MPO is set to be one standard deviation lower than Pascoe suggested (Table 20–27).

In Closing

It may be true that an audiologist could have a successful hearing aid dispensing practice without thinking about many of the corrections and transformations we describe here; however, it wouldn't be as much fun. More importantly, understanding these corrections can help inform us when we are surprised by changes we see when using different measurement or fitting equipment. In the world of selecting and fitting hearing aids, we often need to transfer our thoughts from HL to SPL, from HL to ear canal SPL, from coupler SPL to real-ear SPL, from coupler SPL to real-world SPL, and on and on. True, many of these corrections are made for us behind the scenes by audiometers, fitting software, and probe microphone equipment, but not always. Sometimes an unexpected test result can be easily explained by the use or *mis*use of one of these transformations. When that time comes, we hope that the information provided here will be helpful.

Table 20–26. Actual Values (see Figure 20–16) of Uncomfortable Loudness Level for Frequencies (500, 1000, 2000, 4000) as a Function of Hearing Level (HL)

	500 Hz			1000 Hz			2000 Hz			4000 Hz		
HL	HL	Mean	SD	N	Mean	SD	N	Mean	SD	N	Mean	SD
0	95.4	9.9	14	101.7	6.8	6	–	–	–	–	–	–
5	97.7	8.7	22	101.3	6.4	12	–	–	–	–	–	–
10	99.1	7.3	39	100.3	6.9	15	110.0	–	1	90.0	–	1
15	97.5	6.8	57	99.1	6.5	32	100.0	–	1	100.0	–	1
20	95.0	7.8	45	100.0	7.1	26	95.0	2.9	2	91.7	2.9	3
25	100.4	8.9	40	102.4	8.5	40	100.0	9.6	5	100.0	0	2
30	102.5	8.4	54	100.8	8.1	40	100.5	9.1	11	106.7	12.6	3
35	97.9	8.7	57	103.3	7.4	51	103.3	7.3	24	110.0	–	1
40	100.2	9.7	45	102.1	9.5	63	104.6	9.0	52	105.0	7.1	15
45	106.6	9.5	35	104.2	8.9	63	105.6	8.9	63	106.3	11.4	19
50	105.3	9.8	33	108.2	9.2	47	107.7	9.1	84	107.8	10.2	34
55	106.7	8.5	27	108.4	7.8	44	107.6	8.3	82	107.8	8.9	66
60	108.2	6.1	17	108.3	6.5	26	110.6	7.1	78	110.3	8.4	67
65	108.3	7.5	6	112.9	6.8	22	115.2	8.0	30	113.9	9.3	58
70	103.8	4.8	4	114.3	6.7	7	115.5	8.4	22	115.4	7.7	61
75	116.3	6.4	8	122.5	10.6	2	116.9	7.2	24	116.6	5.7	57
80	115.0	5.8	4	120.0	10.0	3	119.7	4.6	16	120.5	6.0	33
85	125.0	–	1*	117.5	4.2	6	120.7	6.7	7	120.2	6.5	22
90	130.0	–	1	127.5	3.5	2	120.0	–	1	123.3	5.6	26
100	–	–	–	–	–	–	–	–	–	126.6	6.3	16
105	–	–	–	–	–	–	135.0	7.1	2	132.5	4.2	6
110	–	–	–	135.0	–	1	136.7	2.9	3	131.7	7.6	3
115	–	–	–	–	–	–	–	–	–	136.7	5.8	3
120	–	–	–	–	–	–	–	–	–	140.0	–	1

Note. *All values greater than 120 dB HL are extrapolated.
Source: Adapted from Pascoe (1988).

Table 20–27. OSPL Values as Prescribed in the Current NAL-NL2 Fitting Software

3FA loss (dB HL)	3FA OSPL90
0	89
5	90
10	92
15	93
20	95
25	96
30	98
35	99
40	101
45	102
50	104
55	105
60	107
65	109
70	112
75	115
80	118
85	120
90	123
95	126
100	128
105	131
110	134
115	136

References

Aarts, N. L., & Caffee, C. S. (2005). Manufacturer predicted and measured REAR values in adult hearing aid fitting: Accuracy and clinical usefulness. *International Journal of Audiology*, *44*(5), 293–301.

Aazh, H., & Moore, B. C. (2007a). Dead regions in the cochlea at 4 kHz in elderly adults: Relation to absolute threshold, steepness of audiogram, and pure-tone average. *Journal of the American Academy of Audiology*, *18*(2), 97–106.

Aazh, H., & Moore, B. C. (2007b). The value of routine real-ear measurement of the gain of digital hearing aids. *Journal of the American Academy of Audiology*, *18*(8), 653–664.

Aazh, H., Moore, B. C., & Prasher, D. (2012). The accuracy of matching target insertion gains with open-fit hearing aids. *American Journal of Audiology*, *21*(2), 175.

Abrams, H. B., Chisolm, T. H., McManus, M., & McArdle, R. (2012). Initial-fit approach versus verified prescription: Comparing self-perceived hearing aid benefit. *Journal of the American Academy of Audiology*, *23*(10), 768–778.

Abrams, H. B., & Doyle, P. J. (2000). Functioning, disability, and quality of life in the adult with hearing impairment. In *Rehabilitation research and development service merit review*. Washington, DC: Department of Veterans Affairs.

Abrams, H. B., Hnath-Chisolm, T., Guerreiro, S. M., & Ritterman, S. I. (1992). The effects of intervention strategy on self-perception of hearing handicap. *Ear and Hearing*, *13*(5), 371–377.

Abrams, H., & Kihm, J. (2015). An Introduction to MarkeTrak IX—A new baseline for the hearing aid market. *Hearing Review Online*. Retrieved from http://www.hearingreview.com/2015/05/introduction-marketrak-ix-new-baseline-hearing-aid-market/

Academy of Doctors of Audiology. (2012). *HIPAA*. Retrieved from http://www.audiologist.org/practice-management/federal-regulations/hipaa.html

Agnew, J. (1998). The causes and effects of distortion and internal noise in hearing Aids. *Trends in Amplification*, *3*(3), 82–118.

Agnew, J., & Thornton, J. M. (2000). Just noticeable and objectionable group delays in digital hearing aids. *Journal of the American Academy of Audiology*, *11*(6), 330–336.

Akeroyd, M. A., Guy, F. H., Harrison, D. L., & Suller, S. L. (2014). A factor analysis of the speech, spatial and qualities of hearing questionnaire (SSQ). *International Journal of Audiology*, *53*(2), 101–114.

Akeroyd, M. A., & Whitmer, W. M. (2015). A meta-analysis of the effects of hearing impairment and hearing aids on directional hearing. *Journal of the Acoustical Society of America*, *137*(4), 2229–2229.

Alexander, J. M. (2013a). Individual variability in recognition of frequency-lowered speech. *Seminars in Hearing*, *34*(2), 86–109.

Alexander, J. M. (2013b). 20Q: The highs and lows of frequency lowering amplification. *Audiology Online*, Article #11772. Retrieved from http://www.audiologyonline.com/articles/20q-highs-and-lows-frequency-11772

Alexander, J. M. (2014). How to use probe microphone measures with frequency-lowering hearing aids. *Audiology Practices*, *6*(4), 8–13.

Alexander, J. M. (2015). *Enhancing perception of frequency-lowered speech*. Patent No. US 9,173,041 B2. Washington, DC: U.S. Patent and Trademark Office.

Alexander, J. M. (2016a). Nonlinear frequency compression: Influence of start frequency and input bandwidth on consonant and vowel recognition. *Journal of the Acoustical Society of America*, *139*(2), 938–957.

Alexander, J. M. (2016b). Hearing aid delay and current drain in modern digital devices. *Canadian Audiologist*, *3*(4). Retrieved from http://canadianaudiologist.ca/hearing-aid-delay-feature/

Alexander, J. M. (2016c). 20Q: Frequency lowering ten years later—New technology innovations. *Audiology Online*, Article #18040. Retrieved from http://www

.audiologyonline.com/articles/20q-frequency-lowering-ten-years-18040

Allen, J. B., Hall, J. L., & Jeng, P. S. (1990). Loudness growth in 1/2-octave bands (LGOB)—A procedure for the assessment of loudness. *Journal of the Acoustical Society of America*, 88(2), 745–753.

Alpiner, J. G., Hansen, E. M., & Kaufman, K. J. (2000). Transition: Rehabilitative audiology into the new millennium. In J. G. Alpiner & P. A. McCarthy (Eds.), *Rehabilitative audiology: Children and adults*. Baltimore, MD: Lippincott Williams & Wilkins.

Alpiner, J. G., Kaufman, K. J., & Hanavan, P. C. (1993). Overview of rehabilitative audiology. In J. G. Alpiner & P. A. McCarthy (Eds.), *Rehabilitative audiology: Children and adults* (pp. 3–16). Baltimore, MD: Lippincott Williams & Wilkins.

American Academy of Audiology. (2003). *Ethical practice guidelines on financial incentives from hearing instrument manufacturers*. Retrieved from http://www.audiology.org/resources/documentlibrary/Documents/financialinfinancia.pdf

American Academy of Audiology. (2004). *Scope of practice*. Retrieved from http://www.audiology.org/resources/documentlibrary/Pages/ScopeofPractice.aspx

American Academy of Audiology. (2006). *Guideline for audiologic management of the adult patient*. Retrieved from http://www.audiology.org/resources/documentlibrary/documents/haguidelines.pdf

American Academy of Audiology. (2006). Guidelines for the audiological management of adult hearing impairment. *Audiology Today*, 18(5), 32–36.

American Speech-Language-Hearing Association. (1967). Proceedings of 1966 Conference on Hearing Aid Evaluation (ASHA Reports, 1967), 2, 1–7.

American Speech-Language-Hearing Association. (1984). Definitions of and competencies for aural rehabilitation. *ASHA*, 26, 37–41.

American Speech-Language Hearing Association. (1997). *Guidelines for audiologic screening*. Retrieved from http://www.asha.org/docs/html/GL1997-00199.html

American Speech-Language Hearing Association. (1998). Guidelines for hearing aid fitting for adults. *American Journal of Audiology*, 7, 5–13.

American Speech-Language-Hearing Association. (2001). *Knowledge and skills required for the practice of audiologic/aural rehabilitation* [Knowledge and skills]. Retrieved from http://www.asha.org/policy

American Speech-Language-Hearing Association. (2004). *Evidence-based practice in communication disorders: An introduction* [Technical report]. Retrieved from http://www.asha.org/members/deskref-journals/deskref/default

American Speech-Language-Hearing Association. (2006). *Preferred practice patterns for the profession of audiology* [Preferred practice patterns]. Retrieved from http://www.asha.org/ policy

Amlani, A. M. (2001). Efficacy of directional microphone hearing aids: A meta-analytic perspective. *Journal of the American Academy of Audiology*, 12(4), 202–214.

Amlani, A. M., Pumford, J., & Gessling, E. (2016). Improving patient perception of clinical services through real-ear measurements. *Hearing Review*, 23(12), 12.

Angelo, K., Alexander, J. M., Christiansen, T. U., Simonsen, C. S., & Jespersgaard, C. F. C. (2015). *Oticon frequency lowering: Access to high-frequency speech sounds with Speech Rescue technology*. Smørum, Denmark: Oticon. Retrieved from http://www.oticon.com/~/media/Oticon%20US/main/Download%20Center/White%20Papers/43698%20Speech%20Rescue%20White%20Paper%202015.pdf

ANSI. (1960). *American National Standard: Acoustical terminology* (ANSI S1.1-1960 R2013). New York, NY: American National Standards Institute.

ANSI. (1979). *American National Standard for an occluded ear simulator* (ANSI S3.25-1979 R2009). New York, NY: American National Standards Institute.

ANSI. (1985). *Specification for a manikin for simulated in-situ airborne acoustic measurements* (ANSI S3.36-1985 R2006). New York, NY: American National Standards Institute.

ANSI. (1989). *ANSI specifications for audiometers* (ANSI S3.6-1989 R2010). New York, NY: American National Standards Institute.

ANSI. (1991). *Maximum permissible ambient noise levels for audiometric test rooms* (ANSI S3.1-1991 R2013). New York, NY: American National Standards Institute.

ANSI. (1992). *Testing hearing aids with a broadband noise signal* (ANSI S3.42-1992 R2007). New York, NY: American National Standards Institute.

ANSI. (1994). *Acoustical terminology* (ANSI S1.1-1994). New York, NY: American National Standards Institute.

ANSI. (1995). *ANSI method for coupler calibration of earphones* (ANSI S3.7 R2008). New York, NY: American National Standards Institute.

ANSI. (1997). *The calculation of the speech intelligibility index* (ANSI S3.5-1997). New York, NY: American National Standards Institute.

ANSI. (1997a). *Methods for the calculation of the speech intelligibility index* (ANSI S3.5-1997 R2012). New York, NY: American National Standards Institute.

ANSI. (1997b). *Methods of measurement of real-ear characteristics of hearing instruments* (ANSI S3.46-1997). New York, NY: American National Standards Institute.

ANSI. (2003). *Specification of hearing aid characteristics* (ANSI S3.22-2003). New York, NY: American National Standards Institute.

ANSI. (2004). *American National Standard method of measurement of performance characteristics of hearing aids under simulated real-ear working conditions* (ANSI S3.35-2004). New York, NY: American National Standards Institute.

ANSI. (2004). *Specification for audiometers* (S3.6-2004). New York, NY: American National Standards Institute.

ANSI. (2006). *American National Standard for methods of measurement of compatibility between wireless communication devices and hearing aids* (ANSI PC63.19-2006). New York, NY: American National Standards Institute.

ANSI. (2008). Accredited Standards Committee (ASC) Operating Procedures. New York, NY: American National Standards Institute.

ANSI. (2009). *Specifications of hearing aid characteristics* (ANSI S3.22-2009). New York, NY: American National Standards Institute.

ANSI. (2011). *American National Standard methods of measurement of compatibility between wireless communications devices and hearing aids* (IEEE/ANSI C63.19-2011). New York, NY: American National Standards Institute.

ANSI. (2012). *Testing hearing aids—Part 2: Methods for characterizing signal processing in hearing aids with a speech-like signal (a nationally adopted international standard)* (ANSI/ASA/IEC S3.42-2012/Part 2/ IEC 60118-15:2012). New York, NY: American National Standards Institute.

ANSI. (2013). *Methods of measurement of real-ear characteristics of hearing instruments* (ANSI S3.46-R2013). New York, NY: American National Standards Institute.

ANSI. (2014). *Specification of hearing aid characteristics* (ANSI S3.22-2014). New York, NY: American National Standards Institute.

Arehart, K. H., Kates, J. M., & Anderson, M. C. (2010). Effects of noise, nonlinear processing, and linear filtering on perceived speech quality. *Ear and Hearing, 31*(3), 420–436.

Arlinger, S., Gatehouse, S., Bentler, R. A., Byrne, D., Cox, R. M., Dirks, D. D., . . . Willott, J. F. (1996). Report of the Eriksholm workshop on auditory deprivation and acclimatization. *Ear and Hearing, 17*(3 Suppl.), 87S–98S.

Arthur, D. (2002). The Vibrant Soundbridge. *Trends in Amplification, 8*(2), 67–72.

ASA. (1951). *Audiometers for general diagnostic purposes (Standard Z 24.5–1951)*. New York, NY: American Standards Association.

Aspell, E., Picou, E. M., & Ricketts, T. A. (2014). Directional benefit is present with audio-visual stimuli: Limiting ceiling effects. *Journal of the American Academy of Audiology, 35*(3), 339–352.

Auriemmo, J., Kuk, F., & Stenger, P. (2008). Criteria for evaluating the performance of linear frequency transposition in children. *Hearing Journal, 61*(4), 50–52.

Auriemmo, J., Kuk, F., Lau, C., et al. (2009). Effect of linear frequency transposition on speech recognition and production of school-age children. *Journal of the American Academy of Audiology, 20*(5), 289–305.

Bachorowski, J., & Owren, M. (1999). Acoustic correlates of talker sex and individual talker identity are present in a short vowel segment produced in running speech. *Journal of the Acoustical Society of America, 106*(2), 1054–1063.

Baer, T., Moore, B. C. J., & Kluk, K. (2002). Effects of low-pass filtering on the intelligibility of speech in noise for people with and without dead regions at high frequencies. *Journal of the Acoustical Society of America, 112*(3), 1133–1144.

Bagatto, M., Moodie, S., Scollie, S., Seewald, R., Moodie, S., Pumford, J., & Liu, K. P. R. (2005). Clinical protocols for hearing instrument fitting in the desired sensation level method. *Trends in Amplification, 9*(4), 199–226.

Bagatto, M. P., Scollie, S. D., Seewald, R. C., Moodie, K. S., & Hoover, B. M. (2002). Real-ear-to-coupler difference predictions as a function of age for two coupling procedures. *Journal of the American Academy of Audiology, 13*(8), 407–415.

Baguley, D. (2003). Hyperacusis. *Journal of the Royal Society of Medicine, 96*(12), 582–585.

Balfour, P. B., & Hawkins, D. B. (1992). A comparison of sound quality judgments for monaural and binaural hearing aid processed stimuli. *Ear and Hearing, 13*(5), 331–339.

Banerjee, S. (2016, May). In support of Lyric3: Study shows good speech clarity, natural sound & acceptance. *Field Study News* (Phonak AG, Stäfa, Switzerland).

Bankaitis, A. U., & Fredrickson, J. M. (2002). Otologics middle ear transducer (MET) implantable hearing device: Rationale, technology, and design strategies. *Trends in Amplification, 6*(2), 53–60.

Barcroft, J., Sommers, M. S., Tye-Murray, N., Mauze, E., Schroy, C., & Spehar, B. (2011). Tailoring auditory training to patient needs with single and multiple talkers: Transfer-appropriate gains on a four-choice discrimination test. *International Journal of Audiology, 50*(11), 802–808.

Bauer, B., Rosenheck, A., & Abbagnaro, L. (1967). External ear replica for acoustical testing. *Journal of the Acoustical Society of America, 42*(1), 204–207.

Beasley, W. C. (1938). *National health survey (1935–1936), preliminary reports. Hearing Study Series Bulletin*, 1–7. Washington, DC: U. S. Public Health Service.

Bench, J., Kowal, Å., & Bamford, J. (1979). The BKB (Bamford-Kowal-Bench) sentence lists for partially-hearing children. *British Journal of Audiology, 13*(3), 108–112.

Bentler, R. A. (2000). List equivalency and test-retest reliability of the speech in noise test. *American Journal of Audiology, 9*(2), 84–100.

Bentler R. A. (2004). *Advanced hearing aid features: Do they work?* Paper presented at the convention of the American Speech-Language-Hearing Association, Washington, DC.

Bentler, R. A. (2005). Effectiveness of directional microphones and noise reduction schemes in hearing aids: A systematic review of the evidence. *Journal of the American Academy of Audiology, 16*(7), 473–484.

Bentler, R.A. (2006). Effectiveness of directional microphones and noise reduction schemes in hearing aids: A systematic review of the evidence. *Journal of the American Academy of Audiology, 16*(7), 473–484.

Bentler, R. A., & Cooley, L. J. (2001). An examination of several characteristics that affect the prediction of OSPL90 in hearing aids. *Ear and Hearing, 22*(1), 58–64.

Bentler, R. A., & Duve, M. R. (2000). Comparison of hearing aids over the 20th century. *Ear and Hearing, 21*(6), 625–639.

Bentler, R. A., Egge, J. L., Tubbs, J. L., Dittberner, A. B., & Flamme, G. (2004). Quantification of directional benefit across different polar response patterns. *Journal of the American Academy of Audiology, 15*(9), 649–659.

Bentler, R. A., Holte, L., & Turner, C. (1999). An update on the acclimatization issue. *Hearing Journal, 52*(11), 44–49.

Bentler, R. A., & Nelson, J. (1997). Assessing the effect of varying release time in a 2-channel AGC hearing aid. *American Journal of Audiology: A Journal of Clinical Practice, 6*(1), 43–51.

Bentler, R. A., & Nelson, J. A. (2001). Effect of spectral shaping on loudness discomfort. *Journal of the American Academy of Audiology, 12*(9), 462–470.

Bentler, R. A., Niebuhr, D. P., Getta, J. P., & Anderson, C. V. (1993a). Longitudinal study of hearing aid effectiveness. I: Objective measures. *Journal of Speech, Language, and Hearing Research, 36*(4), 808–819.

Bentler, R. A., Niebuhr, D. P., Getta, J. P., & Anderson, C. V. (1993b). Longitudinal study of hearing aid effectiveness. II: Subjective measures. *Journal of Speech, Language, and Hearing Research, 36*(4), 820–831.

Bentler, R. A., Niebuhr, D. P., Johnson, T. A., & Flamme, G. A. (2003). Impact of digital labeling on outcome measures. *Ear and Hearing, 24*(3), 215–224.

Bentler, R. A., & Pavlovic, C. V. (1989). Transfer functions and correction factors used in hearing aid evaluation and research. *Ear and Hearing, 10*(1), 58–63.

Bentler, R. A., & Pavlovic, C. V. (1992). Addendum to "Transfer functions and correction factors used in hearing aid evaluation and research." *Ear and Hearing, 13*(4), 284–286.

Bentler, R., Walker, E., McCreery, R., Arenas, R. M., & Roush, P. (2014). Nonlinear frequency compression in hearing aids: Impact on speech and language development. *Ear and Hearing, 35*(4), e143–e152.

Bentler, R. A., Wu, Y. H., & Jeon, J. (2006). Effectiveness of directional technology in open-canal hearing instruments. *Hearing Journal, 59*(11), 40–42.

Bentler, R. A., Wu, Y. H., Kettel, J., Hurtig, R. (2008). Digital noise reduction: Outcomes from laboratory and field studies. *International Journal of Audiology, 47*(8), 447–460.

Beranek, L. L. (1954). *McGraw-Hill electrical and engineering series: Acoustics.* New York, NY: McGraw-Hill.

Berger, K. W. (1974). *The hearing aid: Its operation and development.* Livonia, MI: National Hearing Aid Society.

Berger, K. W. (1976a). Genealogy of the words of audiology and audiologist. *Journal of the American Audiological Society, 2*(2), 38–44.

Berger, K. W. (1976b). Prescription of hearing aids: A rationale. *Journal of the American Audiology Society, 2*(3), 71–78.

Berger, K. W., Hagberg, E., & Rane, R. (1984). *Prescription of hearing aids: Rationale, procedures and results.* Kent, OH: Herald Press.

Bergman, M. (2002). On the origins of audiology: American wartime military audiology [Monograph]. *Audiology Today, 1*, 1–28.

Bernarding, C., Strauss, D. J., Hannemann, R., Seidler, H., & Corona-Strauss F. I. (2014). Objective assessment of listening effort in the oscillatory EEG: Comparison of different hearing aid configurations. *Conference Proceedings: Annual International Conference of the IEEE Engineering in Medicine and Biology Society*, 2653–2656.

Bess, F. (1983). Clinical assessment of speech recognition. In D. Konkle & W. Rintelmann (Eds.), *Principles of speech audiometry* (pp. 127–201). Baltimore, MD: University Park Press.

Better Hearing Institute. (n.d.). *Prevalence of hearing loss.* Retrieved from http://betterhearing.org/hearing_loss/prevalence_of_hearing_loss/index.cfm

Beyer, C. M., & Northern, J. L. (2000). Audiologic rehabilitation support programs: A network model. *Seminars in Hearing, 21*(3), 257–265.

Beynon, G. J., Thornton, F. L., & Poole, C. (1997). A randomized, controlled trial of the efficacy of a communication course for first time hearing aid users. *British Journal of Audiology, 31*(5), 345–351.

Bilger, R. C. (1984). *Manual for the clinical use of the revised SPIN test*. Champaign, IL: University of Illinois Press.

Bilger, R. C., Neutzel, J. M., Rabinowitz, W. M., & Rzeczkowski, C. (1984). Standardization of a test of speech perception in noise. *Journal of Speech and Hearing Research, 27*(1), 32–48.

Bird, J., & Cohen-Cole, S. A. (1990). The three-function model of the medical interview. In *Methods in teaching consultation-liaison psychiatry* (Vol. 20, pp. 65–88). Basel, Switzerland: Karger.

Bistafa, S. R., & Bradley, J. S. (2000). Reverberation time and maximum background-noise level for classrooms from a comparative study of speech intelligibility metrics. *Journal of the Acoustical Society of America, 107*(2), 861–875.

Blamey, P. J., & Martin, L. F. (2009). Loudness and satisfaction ratings for hearing aid users. *Journal of the American Academy of Audiology, 20*(4), 272–282.

Blue, V. J. (1979). NAEL—An important part of the team. *Hearing Instruments, 30*, 16.

Blumsack, J. T., Bower, C. R., & Ross, M. E. (2007). Comparison of speechreading training regimens. *Perceptual and Motor Skills, 105*(3 Pt. 1), 988–996.

Boike, K. T., & Souza, P. E. (2000). Effect of compression ratio on speech recognition and speech-quality ratings with wide dynamic range compression amplification. *Journal of Speech, Language, and Hearing Research, 43*(2), 456–468.

Boothroyd, A. (2004). Hearing aid accessories for adults: The remote FM microphone. *Ear and Hearing, 25*(1), 22–23.

Boothroyd, A. (2007). Adult aural rehabilitation: What is it and does it work? *Trends in Amplification, 11*(2), 63–71.

Borg, G. (1990). Psychophysical scaling with applications in physical work and the perception of exertion. *Scandinavian Journal of Work, Environment & Health*, 55–58.

Boymans, M., & Dreschler, W. A. (2000) Field trials using a digital hearing aid with active noise reduction and dual-microphone directionality. *Audiology, 39*(5), 260–268.

Bradley, J. S., Reich, R. D., & Norcross, S. G. (1999). On the combined effects of signal-to-noise ratio and room acoustics on speech intelligibility. *Journal of the Acoustical Society of America, 106*(4), 1820–1828.

Bradley, M. M., Greenwald, M. K., Petry, M., & Lang, P. J. (1992). Remembering pictures: Pleasure and arousal in memory. *Journal of Experimental Psychology: Learning, Memory and Cognition, 18*(2), 379–390.

Bratt, G. W., Rosenfeld, M. A. L., Poek, B. F., Kang, J., Williams, D. W., & Larson, V. (2002). Coupler and real-ear measurement of hearing aid gain and output in the NIDCD/VA hearing aid clinical trial. *Ear and Hearing, 23*(4), 308–324.

Bregman, A. S. (1990). *Auditory scene analysis: The perceptual organization of sound*. Cambridge, MA: MIT Press.

Brennan, M., & McCreery, R. (2014). SHARP updates enable audibility estimates with nonlinear frequency compression. *Hearing Journal, 67*(3), 14–18.

Brickley, G. J., Cleaver, V. C. G., & Bailey, S. (1996). An evaluation of a group follow-up scheme for new NHS hearing aid users. *British Journal of Audiology, 30*(5), 307–312.

Brooks, D. N. (1979). Counseling and its effects on hearing aid use. *Scandinavian Audiology, 8*(2), 101–107.

Brooks, D. N. (1981). Use of hearing aids by National Health Service patients. *British Journal of Audiology, 15*(2), 79–86.

Brown, A. D., Rodriguez, F. A., Portnuff, C. D. F., Goupell, M. J., & Tollin, D. J. (2016). Time-varying distortions of binaural information by bilateral hearing aids. *Trends in Hearing, 20*, 2331216516668303.

Brungart, D., McKenna, E., & Sherlock, L. (2015). *Evaluation of extended-wear hearing aid technology for operational military use*. Bethesda, MD: The Henry M. Jackson Foundation for the Advancement of Military Medicine.

Büchler, M. C. (2002). *Algorithms for sound classification in hearing instruments*. Dissertation submitted to Swiss Federal Institute of Technology Zurich, Diss. ETH #14498 (pp. 1–136).

Burk, M. H., & Humes, L. E. (2007). Effects of training on speech recognition performance in noise using lexically hard words. *Journal of Speech, Language, and Hearing Research, 50*(1), 25–40.

Burk, M. H., & Humes, L. E. (2008). Effects of long-term training on aided speech-recognition performance in noise in older adults. *Journal of Speech, Language, and Hearing Research, 51*(3), 759–771.

Burnett, E. (1985). NBS hearing aid test procedures. In *Handbook of hearing aid measurement*. Washington, DC: Government Printing Office.

Burney, P. (1972). A survey of hearing aid evaluation procedures. *ASHA, 14*(9), 439–444.

Burton, P., Smaka, C., & Powers, T. A. (2006). Digital noise reduction: Yes, there is research supporting its effectiveness. *Hearing Review, 13*(3), 82.

Byrne, D. (1982). Theoretical approaches for hearing aid selection. In G. A. Studebaker & F. H. Bess (Eds.), *The Vanderbilt hearing-aid report: State of the art—research needs* (pp. 175–179). Upper Darby, PA: Monographs in Contemporary Audiology.

Byrne, D. (1996). Hearing aid selection for the 1990s: Where to? *Journal of the American Academy of Audiology, 7*(6), 377–395.

Byrne, D., Christen, R., & Dillon, H. (1981). Effects of peaks in hearing aid frequency response curves on comfortable listening levels of normal hearing subjects. *Australian Journal of Audiology, 3*(2), 42–46.

Byrne, D., & Cotton, S. (1988). Evaluation of the National Acoustic Laboratories' new hearing aid selection procedure. *Journal of Speech and Hearing Research, 31*(2), 178–186.

Byrne, D., & Dirks, D. (1996). Effects of acclimatization and deprivation on non-speech auditory abilities. *Ear and Hearing, 17*(3 Suppl), 29S–37S.

Byrne, D., & Dillon, H. (1986). The National Acoustic Laboratories' new procedure for selecting the gain and frequency response of a hearing aid. *Ear and Hearing, 7*(4), 257–265.

Byrne, D., Dillon, H., Tran, K., Arlinger, S., Wilbraham, K., Cox, R., . . . Ludvigsen, C. (1994). An international comparison of long-term average speech spectra. *Journal of the Acoustical Society of America, 96*(4), 2108–2120.

Byrne, D., Parkinson, A., & Newall, P. (1990). Hearing aid gain and frequency response requirements for the severely/profoundly hearing impaired. *Ear and Hearing, 11*(1), 40–49.

Byrne, D., & Tonisson, W. (1976). Selecting the gain of hearing aids for persons with sensorineural hearing impairments. *Scandinavian Audiology, 5*(2), 51–59.

Carhart, R. (1946a). Selection of hearing aids. *Archives of Otolaryngology-Head and Neck Surgery, 44*(1), 1–18.

Carhart, R. (1946b). Tests for the selection of hearing aids. *Laryngoscope, 56*(12), 780–794.

Carhart, R. (1946c). Volume control adjustment in hearing aid selection. *Laryngoscope, 56*(9), 510–526.

Carhart, R. (1947). Auditory training. In H. Davis. (Ed.), *Hearing and deafness: A guide for laymen* (pp. 276–299). New York, NY: Murray Hill Books.

Carhart, R., & Tillman, T. W. (1970). Interaction of competing speech signals with hearing losses. *Archives of Otolaryngology-Head and Neck Surgery, 91*(3), 273–279.

Carlson, E. V., & Killion M. C. (1974). Subminiature directional microphones. *Journal of the Audio Engineering Society, 22*(4), 237–243.

Carney, E., & Schlauch, R. S. (2007). Critical difference table for word recognition testing derived using computer simulation. *Journal of Speech, Language, and Hearing Research, 50*(5), 1203–1209.

Carson, A. J. (2005). "What brings you here today?" The role of self-assessment in help-seeking for age-related hearing loss. *Journal of Aging Studies, 19*(2), 185–200.

Castle, W. E. (1967). *A conference on hearing aid evaluation procedures* (ASHA Reports Number 2). Washington, DC: The American Speech and Hearing Association.

Causey, G. D., Hood, L. J., Hermanson, C. L., & Bowling, L. S. (1984). The Maryland CNC test: Normative studies. *International Journal of Audiology, 23*(6), 552–568.

Cavanaugh, W., Farrell, W., Hirtle, P., & Waters, B. (1962). Speech privacy in buildings. *Journal of the Acoustical Society of America, 34*(4), 475–483.

Chalupper, J. (2007). *What is the relationship between acclimatization, learning hearing systems, and auditory training?* Presented at the 52nd International Congress of Hearing Aid Acousticians, Nuremberg, Germany.

Chalupper, J. (2008). *Audiological rehabilitation is more than amplification.* Retrieved from https://media.sivantos.com/siemens-website/media/2014/07/2008_05_eARena.pdf

Chalupper, J., & Powers, T. A. (2007). New algorithm is designed to take the annoyance out of transient noise. *Hearing Journal, 60*(7), 42–44.

Chalupper, J., Wu, Y. H., & Weber, J. (2011). New algorithm automatically adjusts directional system for special situations. *Hearing Journal, 64*(1), 26–33.

Chasin, M. (Ed.). (1997). *CIC handbook.* San Diego, CA: Singular.

Chasin, M. (2002). Bone anchored middle ear implants. *Trends in Amplification, 6*(2), 33–38.

Chasin, M., Pirzaniski, C., Hayes, D., & Mueller, H. G. (1997). Real-ear occluded gain as a clinical predictor. *Hearing Review, 4*(4), 22–26.

Ching, T. Y., Dillon, H., & Byrne, D. (1998). Speech recognition of hearing-impaired listeners: Predications from audibility and the limited role of high-frequency amplification. *Journal of the Acoustical Society of America, 103*(2), 1128–1140.

Ching, T. Y., Dillon, H., Katsch, R., & Byrne, D. (2001). Maximizing effective audibility in hearing aid fitting. *Ear and Hearing, 22*(3), 212–224.

Ching, T. Y. C., O'Brien, A., Dillon, H., Chalupper, J., Hartley, L., Hartley, D., . . . Hain, J. (2009). Directional effects on infants and young children in real life: Implications for amplification. *Journal of Speech, Language, and Hearing Research, 52*(5), 1241–1254.

Chisolm, T., Abrams, H., & McArdle, R. (2004). Short- and long-term outcomes of adult audiologic rehabilitation. *Ear and Hearing, 25*(5), 464–477.

Chisolm, T., & Arnold, M. (2012). Evidence about the effectiveness of aural rehabilitation programs for adults. In L. Wong & L. Hickson (Eds.), *Evidence-based practice in audiology: Evaluating interventions for children and adults with hearing impairment* (pp. 237–266). San Diego, CA: Plural.

Chmiel, R., & Jerger, J. (1996). Hearing aid use, central auditory disorder, and hearing handicap in elderly persons. *Journal of the American Academy of Audiology, 7*(3), 190–202.

Churchill, E., & Truett, B. (1957). *Metrical relations among dimensions of the head and face.* Aero Medical Lab, Wright Air Development Center, WADC Tech Report (pp. 56–62).

Cienkowski, K. M., & Speaks, C. (2000). Subjective vs. objective intelligibility of sentences in listeners with hearing loss. *Journal of Speech, Language, and Hearing Research, 43*(5), 1205–1210.

Ciorba, A., Bianchini, C., Pelucchi, S., & Pastore, A. (2012). The impact of hearing loss on the quality of life of elderly adults. *Clinical Intervention Aging, 7,* 159–163.

Clark, J. G., & English, K. M. (2003). *Counseling in audiologic practice: Helping patients and families adjust to hearing loss.* Boston, MA: Pearson Education.

Clarke, C. M. (2000). Lexical neighborhood properties of the original and revised speech perception in noise (SPIN) tests. *Research on spoken language processing* (Progress Report No. 24), 305–320.

Cole, W. (1975). Hearing aid gain–A functional approach. *Hearing Instruments, 26*(10), 22–24.

Convery, E., Keidser, G., & Dillon, H. (2005). A review and analysis: Does amplification experience have an effect on preferred gain over time? *Australian and New Zealand Journal of Audiology, 27*(1), 18.

Conway, F., & Siegelman, J. (2005). *Dark hero of the information age: In search of Norbert Wiener, the father of cybernetics.* New York, NY: Basic Books.

Cooper, J. C., & Cutts, B. P. (1971). Speech discrimination in noise. *Journal of Speech and Hearing Research, 14*(2), 332–337.

Cord, M.T., Surr, R. K., Walden, B.E., & Olsen, L. (2002) Performance of directional microphone hearing aids in everyday life. *Journal of the American Academy of Audiology, 13*(6), 295–307.

Cord, M. T., Walden, B. E., & Atack, R. M. (1992). *Speech recognition in noise test (SPRINT) for H-3 profiles.* Unpublished report, Audiology and Speech Center, Walter Reed Army Medical Center, Washington, DC.

Cornelisse, L. E., Seewald, R. C., & Jamieson, D. G. (1994). Fitting wide-dynamic-range compression hearing aids: The DSL [i/o] approach. *Hearing Journal, 47,* 23–23.

Cornelisse, L. E., Seewald, R. C., & Jamieson, D. G. (1995). The input/output formula: A theoretical approach to the fitting of personal amplification devices. *Journal of the Acoustical Society of America, 97*(3), 1854–1864.

Costa, P. T., & McCrae, R. R. (1992). *NEO-PI-R Professional Manual.* Odessa, FL: Psychological Assessment Resources.

Coverstone, J. (2012). Fee-for-service in an audiology practice. *AudiologyOnline,* Article 776.

Cox, R. M. (1979). Acoustic aspects of hearing aid ear canal coupling systems. In *Monograph in contemporary audiology.* Minneapolis, MN: Maico Hearing Instruments.

Cox, R. M. (1982). Combined effects of earmold vents and suboscillatory feedback on hearing aid frequency response. *Ear and Hearing, 3*(1), 12–17.

Cox, R. M. (1983). Using ULCL measures to find frequency/gain and SSPL90. *Hearing Instruments, 34*(7), 17–21, 39.

Cox, R. M. (1985). A structured approach to hearing aid selection. *Ear and Hearing, 6*(6), 226–239.

Cox, R. M. (1988). The MSUv3 hearing instrument prescription procedure. *Hearing Instruments, 39*(1), 6–10.

Cox, R. M. (1995). Using loudness data for hearing aid selection: The IHAFF approach. *Hearing Journal, 48*(2), 10, 39–44.

Cox, R. M. (1997). Administration and application of the APHAB. *Hearing Journal, 50*(4), 32–48.

Cox, R. M. (2004). Waiting for evidence based practice for your hearing aid fittings? It's here. *Hearing Journal, 57*(8), 10–17.

Cox, R. M. (2005a). Evidence-based practice in provision of amplification. *Journal of the American Academy of Audiology, 16*(7), 419–438.

Cox, R. M. (2005b). Choosing a self-report measure for hearing aid fitting outcomes. *Seminars in Hearing, 26*(3), 149–156.

Cox, R. M. (2009). Verification and what to do until your probe-mic system arrives: The second of two parts. *Hearing Journal, 62*(10), 10–14.

Cox, R. M., & Alexander, G. C. (1983). Acoustic versus electronic modifications of hearing aid low-frequency output. *Ear and Hearing, 4*(4), 190–196.

Cox, R. M., & Alexander, G. C. (1995). The abbreviated profile of hearing aid benefit. *Ear and Hearing, 16*(2), 176–186.

Cox, R. M., & Alexander, G. C. (1999). Measuring satisfaction with amplification in daily life: The SADL scale. *Ear and Hearing, 20*(4), 306–320.

Cox, R. M., & Alexander, G. C. (2000). Expectations about hearing aids and their relationship to fitting outcome. *Journal of the American Academy of Audiology, 11*(7), 368–382.

Cox, R. M., & Alexander, G. C. (2001). Validation of the SADL questionnaire. *Ear and Hearing, 22*(2), 151–160.

Cox, R. M., & Alexander, G. C. (2002). The International Inventory for Hearing Aids (IOI-HA): Psychometric properties of the English version. *International Journal of Audiology, 41*(1), 30–35.

Cox, R. M., Alexander, G. C., & Beyer C. M. (2003). Norms for the international outcome inventory for hearing aids. *Journal of the American Academy of Audiology, 14*(8), 407–417.

Cox, R. M., Alexander, G. C., & Gilmore, C. (1987). Development of the connected speech test (CST). *Ear and Hearing, 8*(5s), 119s–126s.

Cox, R. M., Alexander, G. C., Gilmore, C., & Pusakulich, K. M. (1988). Use of the connected speech test (CST) with hearing-impaired listeners. *Ear and Hearing, 9*(4), 198–207.

Cox, R. M., Alexander, G. C., & Gray, G. A. (1999). Personality and the subjective assessment of hearing aids. *Journal of the American Academy of Audiology, 10*(1), 1–13.

Cox, R. M., Alexander, G. C., & Gray, G. A. (2003). Audiometric correlates of the unaided APHAB. *Journal of the American Academy of Audiology, 14*(7), 361–371.

Cox, R. M., Alexander, G. C., & Gray, G. A. (2007). Personality, hearing problems, and amplification characteristics: Contributions to self-report hearing aid outcomes. *Ear and Hearing, 28*(2), 141–162.

Cox, R. M., Alexander, G. C., & Rivera, I. M. (1991). Comparison of objective and subjective measures of speech intelligibility in elderly hearing-impaired listeners. *Journal of Speech and Hearing Research, 34*(4), 904–915.

Cox, R. M., Alexander, G. C., Taylor, I. M, & Gray, G. A. (1997). The contour test of loudness perception. *Ear and Hearing, 18*(5), 388–400.

Cox, R. M., Alexander, G. C., & Xu, J. (2009). *Development of the Device Oriented Subjective Outcome Scale (DOSO)*. Annual meeting of the American Auditory Society. Retrieved from http://www.memphis.edu/ausp/harl/pupblications.htm#posters

Cox, R. M., Alexander, G. C., & Xu, J. (2014). Development of the Device-Oriented Subjective Outcome (DOSO) Scale. *Journal of the American Academy of Audiology, 25*(8), 727–736.

Cox, R. M., & Gilmore, C. (1986). Damping the hearing aid frequency response: Effects on speech clarity and preferred listening level. *Journal of Speech and Hearing Research, 29*(3), 357–365.

Cox, R. M., & Gilmore, C. (1990). Development of the profile of hearing aid performance (PHAP). *Journal of Speech, Language, and Hearing Research, 33*(2), 343–357.

Cox, R. M., Gilmore, C., & Alexander, G. C. (1991). Comparison of two questionnaires for patient-assessed hearing aid benefit. *Journal of the American Academy of Audiology, 2*(3), 134–145.

Cox, R. M., Goff, C. M., Martin, S. E., & McLoud, L. L. (1994, April). *The contour test: Normative data.* Presented at the American Academy of Audiology Convention, Richmond, VA.

Cox, R. M., Hyde, M., Gatehouse, S., Noble, W., Dillon, H., Bentler, R., . . . Wilkerson, D. (2000). Optimal outcome measures, research priorities, and international cooperation. *Ear and Hearing, 21*(4), 106S–115S.

Cox, R. M., Johnson, J. A., & Alexander, G. C. (2012). Implications of high-frequency cochlear dead regions for fitting hearing aids to adults with mild to moderately severe hearing loss. *Ear and Hearing, 33*(5), 573–587.

Cox, R. M., Johnson, J. A., & Xu, J. (2014). Impact of advanced hearing aid technology on speech understanding for older listeners with mild to moderate, adult-onset, sensorineural hearing loss. *Gerontology, 60*(6), 557–568.

Cox R. M., Johnson J. A., Xu J. (2016). Impact of hearing aid technology on outcomes in daily life I: The patients' perspective. *Ear and Hearing, 37*(4), e224–237.

Cox, R. M., Matesich, J. S., & Moore, J. N. (1988). Distribution of short-term rms levels in conversational speech. *Journal of the Acoustical Society of America, 84*(3), 1100–1104.

Cox, R. M., & McDaniel, D. M. (1989). Development of the speech intelligibility rating (SIR) test for hearing aid comparisons. *Journal of Speech, Language, and Hearing Research, 32*(2), 347–352.

Cox, R. M., & Moore, J. N. (1988). Composite speech spectrum for hearing aid gain prescriptions. *Journal of Speech and Hearing Research, 31*(1), 102–107.

Cox, R. M., Schwartz, K. S., Noe, C. M., & Alexander, G. C. (2011). Preference for one or two hearing aids among adult patients. *Ear and Hearing, 32*(2), 181–197.

Cox, R. M., Taylor, I. M., Gray, G. A., & Brainerd, L. E. (1994, April). *The contour test: Applications to hearing aid selection and fitting.* Presented at American Academy of Audiology Meeting, Richmond, VA.

Craik, F. I. M., & Lockhart, R. S. (1972). Levels of processing: A framework for memory research. *Journal of Verbal Learning and Verbal Behavior, 11*(3), 671–684.

Crandell, C., & Smaldino, J. (2000). Classroom acoustics and amplification. In M. Valente, R. Roeser, & H. Hosford-Dunn (Eds.), *Audiology: Treatment* (Vol. 2). New York, NY: Thieme Medical.

Czaja, S. J., Sharit, J., Lee, C. C., Nair, S. N., Hernández, M. A., Arana, N., & Fu, S. H. (2013). Factors influencing use of an e-health website in a community sample of older adults. *Journal of the American Medical Informatics Association, 20*(2), 277–284.

Darkner, S., Larsen, R., & Paulsen, R. (2007). Analysis of deformation of the human ear and canal caused by mandibular movement. In N. Ayache, S. Ourselin, & A. Maeder (Eds.), *MICCAI 2007, Part II.* (LNCS, Vol. 4792, pp. 801–808). Heidelberg, Germany: Springer-Verlag.

Davies-Venn, E., Souza, P., Brennan, M., & Stecker, G. C. (2009). Effects of audibility and multichannel wide dynamic range compression on consonant recognition for listeners with severe hearing loss. *Ear and Hearing, 30*(5), 494.

Davis, H., Hudgins, C. V., Marquis, R. J., Nichols, R. H., Peterson, G. E., Ross, D. A., & Stevens, S. S. (1946). The selection of hearing aids. *Laryngoscope, 56*(3), 85–115, 135–163.

Davis, H., & Silverman, S. R. (1960). *Hearing and deafness.* New York, NY: Holt Reinhart and Winston.

Davis, L. A., & Davidson, S. A. (1996). Preference for and performance with damped and undamped hearing aids by listeners with sensorineural hearing loss. *Journal of Speech and Hearing Research, 39*(3), 483–93.

Davis, S. (1988). *Topics in syllable geometry.* New York, NY: Garland Science.

Dawes, P., Hopkins, R., & Munro, K. J. (2013). Placebo effects in hearing-aid trials are reliable. *International Journal of Audiology, 52*(7), 472–477.

Dawes, P., Munro, K. J., Kalluri, S., & Edwards, B. (2014). Acclimatization to hearing aids. *Ear and Hearing, 35*(2), 203–212.

De Ceulaer, G., Bestel, J., Mülder, H. E., Goldbeck, F., de Varebeke, S. P. J., & Govaerts, P. J. (2016). Speech understanding in noise with the Roger Pen, Naida CI Q70 processor, and integrated Roger 17 receiver in a multi-talker network. *European Archives of Oto-Rhino-Laryngology, 273*(5), 1107–1114.

Degertekin, L., Jeelani, K., Qureshi, S., Hasler, P., Bicen, B., Cui, W., Su, Q. T., & Miles, R. N. (2008). Miniature diffraction-based optical MEMS microphones with integrated optoelectronics. *Journal of the Acoustical Society of America, 123*(5), 3229.

Demeester, K., Topsakal, V., Hendrickx, J. J., Fransen, E., van Laer, L., Van Camp, G., . . . Van Wieringen, A. (2012). Hearing disability measured by the Speech, Spatial, and Qualities of Hearing Scale in clinically normal-hearing and hearing-impaired middle-aged persons, and disability screening by means of a reduced SSQ (the SSQ5). *Ear and Hearing, 33*(5), 615–616.

De Jonge, R. (1996). Real-ear measures: Individual and measurement error. In M. Valente (Ed.), *Hearing aids: Standards, options, and limitations* (pp. 72–125). New York, NY: Thieme Medical.

Del Dot, J., Hickson, L. M., & O'Connell, B. (1992). Speech perception in noise with BiCROS hearing aids. *Scandinavian Audiology, 21*(4), 261–264.

Deming, W. E. (1986). *Out of the crisis.* Cambridge, MA: MIT Center for Advanced Engineering Study.

Demorest, M., Wark, D., & Erdman, S. (2011). Development of the screening test for hearing problems. *American Journal of Audiology, 20*(2), 100–110.

Desjardins, J. L., & Doherty, K. A. (2014). The effect of hearing aid noise reduction on listening effort in hearing-impaired adults. *Ear and Hearing, 35*(6), 600–610.

Dickinson, W. W. (2010). Verification of Baha fitting for single-sided deafness: How, what, where and why do we measure? *Seminars in Hearing, 31*(4), 350–365.

Dietrich, V., Nieschalk, M., Stoll, W., Rajan, R., & Pantev, C. (2001). Cortical reorganization in patients with high frequency cochlear hearing loss. *Hearing Research, 158*(1), 95–101.

DiGiovanni, J. J., Davlin, E. A., & Nagaraj, N. K. (2011). Effects of transient noise reduction algorithms on speech intelligibility and ratings of hearing aid users. *American Journal of Audiology, 20*(2), 140–150.

DiGiovanni, J. & Pratt, R. (2010). Verification of in situ thresholds and integrated real-ear measurements. *Journal of the American Academy of Audiology, 21*(10), 663–670.

Dillon, H. (1982a). A quantitative examination of the sources of speech discrimination test score variability. *Ear and Hearing, 3*(2), 51–58.

Dillon, H. (1982b). The sources of speech discrimination test score variability: A reply to Thornton and Raffin. *Ear and Hearing, 3*(6), 340–341.

Dillon, H. (1985). Earmolds and high frequency response modification. *Hearing Instruments, 36*(12), 8–12.

Dillon, H. (1991). Allowing for real ear venting effects when selecting the coupler gain for hearing aids. *Ear and Hearing, 12*(6), 406–416.

Dillon, H. (1994). Shortened hearing aid performance inventory for the elderly (SHAPIE): A statistical approach. *Australian Journal of Audiology, 16*(1), 37–48.

Dillon, H. (1999). NAL-NL1: A new procedure for fitting nonlinear hearing aids. *Hearing Journal, 52*(4), 10–12.

Dillon, H. (2001). *Hearing aids.* Turramurra, Australia: Boomerang Press.

Dillon, H. (2001, December). The research of Denis Byrne at NAL: Implications for clinicians today. *Audiology Online*, Article #1200. Retrieved from http://www.audiologyonline.com/articles/research-denis-byrne-at-nal-1200

Dillon, H. (2012). *Hearing aids* (2nd ed.). New York, NY: Thieme Medical.

Dillon, H., Birtles, G., & Lovegrove, R. (1999). Measuring the outcomes of a national rehabilitation program: Normative data for the Client Oriented Scale of Improvement (COSI) and the Hearing Aid User's Questionnaire (HAUQ). *Journal of the American Academy of Audiology, 10*(2), 67–79.

Dillon, H., James, A., & Ginis, J. (1997). Client oriented scale of improvement (COSI) and its relationship to several other measures of benefit and satisfaction provided by hearing aids. *Journal of the American Academy of Audiology, 8*(1), 27–43.

Dillon, H., Koritschoner, E., Battaglia, J., Lovegrove, R., Ginis, J., Mavrias, G., . . . Macaskill, F. (1991). Rehabilitation effectiveness I: Assessing the needs of clients entering a national hearing rehabilitation program. *Australian Journal of Audiology, 13*(2), 55–65.

Dillon, H., Roe, I., & Katch, R. (1999, January). *Wind noise in hearing aids: Mechanisms and measurements.* National Acoustics Labs Australia: Report to Danavox, Phonak, Oticon and Widex.

Dillon, H., & So, M. (2000). Incentives and obstacles to the routine use of outcomes measures by clinicians. *Ear and Hearing, 21*(4), 2S–6S.

Dillon, H., & Storey, L. (1998). The national acoustics laboratories' procedure for selecting the saturation sound pressure level of hearing aids: Theoretical derivation. *Ear and Hearing, 19*(4), 255–266.

Dirks, D. D., Ahlstrom, J. B., & Eisenberg, L. S. (1994). Effects of probe insertion depth on real-ear measurements. *Otolaryngology-Head and Neck Surgery, 110*(1), 64–74.

Dirks, D. D., Kamm, C. A., Dubno, J. R., & Velde, T. M. (1981). Speech recognition performance at loudness discomfort level. *Scandinavian Audiology, 10*(4), 239–246.

Dirks, D. D., & Kincaid, G. E. (1987). Basic acoustic considerations of ear canal: Probe measurements. *Ear and Hearing, 8*(5), 68s.

Dirks, D. D., Morgan, D. E., & Dubno, J. R. (1982). A procedure for quantifying the effects of noise on speech recognition. *Journal of Speech and Hearing Disorders, 47*(2), 114–123.

Donaldson, G. S., Chisolm, T. H., Blasco, G. P., Shinnick, L. J., Ketter, K. J., & Krause, J. C. (2009). BKB-SIN and ANL predict perceived communication ability in cochlear implant users. *Ear and Hearing, 30*(4), 401.

Dorman, M. F., & Loizou, P. C. (1996). Relative spectral change and formant transitions as cues to labial and alveolar place of articulation. *Journal of the Acoustical Society of America, 100*(6), 3825–3830.

Drennan, W. R., Gatehouse, S., Howell, P., Van Tasell, D., & Lund, S. (2005). Localization and speech-identification ability of hearing-impaired listeners using phase-preserving amplification. *Ear and Hearing, 26*(5), 461–472.

Dreschler, W. A., & van der Hulst, R. J. A. M. (1987). High-frequency audiometry using headphones. *Audiology in Practice, 4*(3), 1–3.

Dreschler, W. A., Verschuure, H., Ludvigsen, C., & Westermann, S. (2001). ICRA Noises: Artificial Noise Signals with Speech-like Spectral and Temporal Properties for Hearing Instrument Assessment: Ruidos ICRA: Señates de ruido artificial con espectro similar al habla y propiedades temporales para pruebas de instrumentos auditivos. *Audiology, 40*(3), 148–157.

Dreyfuss, H. (1966). *The measure of man: Human factors in design.* (2nd ed.). New York, NY: Whitney Library of Design.

Dubno, J. R., Lee, F. S., Klein, A. J., Matthews, L. J., & Lam, C. F. (1995). Confidence limits for maximum word-recognition scores. *Journal of Speech, Language, and Hearing Research, 38*(2), 490–502.

Dubno, J. R., Lee, F. S., Matthews, L. J., & Mills, J. H. (1997). Age-related and gender-related changes in speech recognition. *Journal of Speech, Language, and Hearing Research, 40*(2), 444–452.

Duncan, K. R., & Aarts, N. L. (2006). A comparison of the HINT and quick SIN tests. *Journal of Speech Language Pathology and Audiology, 30*(2), 86–94.

Egan, M. D. (1988). *Architectural acoustics.* New York, NY: McGraw-Hill.

Egolf, D. P., Howell, H. C., Weaver, K. A., & Barker, D. S. (1985). The hearing aid feedback path: Mathematical simulations and experimental verification. *Journal of the Acoustical Society of America, 78*(5), 1578–1587.

Eisenberg, J. (2001). What does the evidence mean? Can the law and medicine be reconciled? *Journal of Health Politics, Policy and Law, 26*(2), 369–381.

Eisenberg, L. S., Dirks, D. D., Takayanagi, S., & Martinez, A. S. (1998). Subjective judgments of clarity and intelligibility for filtered stimuli with equivalent speech intelligibility index predictions. *Journal of Speech, Language, and Hearing Research, 41*(2), 327–339.

Eisenthal, S., & Lazare, A. (1977). Evaluation of the initial interview in a walk-in clinic: The clinician's perspective on a negotiated approach. *Journal of Nervous and Mental Disease, 164*(1), 30–35.

Elert, G. (1998–2017). *Electricity & magnetism*, The physics hypertextbook: A work in progress. Retrieved from http://physics.info/

Elliott, L. L. (1979). Performance of children aged 9 to 17 years on a test of speech intelligibility in noise using sentence material with controlled word predictability. *Journal of the Acoustical Society of America, 66*(3), 651–653.

Ellis, R., & Munro, K. (2013). Does cognitive function predict frequency compressed speech recognition in listeners with normal hearing and normal cognition? *International Journal of Audiology, 52*(1), 14–22.

Ellis, R. J., & Munro, K. J. (2014). Benefit from, and acclimatization to, frequency compression hearing aids in experienced adult hearing-aid users. *International Journal of Audiology, 54*(1), 3–47.

Erber, N. P., & Witt, L. H. (1977). Effects of stimulus intensity on speech perception by deaf children. *Journal of Speech and Hearing Disorders, 42*(2), 271–277.

Erdman, S. A. (2009). Audiologic counseling: A biopsychosocial approach. In J. J. Montano & J. B. Spitzer (Eds.),

Adult audiologic rehabilitation: Advanced practices (pp. 171–215). San Diego, CA: Plural.

Erdman, S. A., & Demorest, M. E. (1998). Adjustment to hearing impairment II: Audiological and demographic correlates. *Journal of Speech, Language, and Hearing Research, 41*(1), 123–136.

Erickson, F. N., & Van Tasell, D. J. (1991). Maximum real-ear gain of in-the-ear hearing aids. *Journal of Speech, Language, and Hearing Research, 34*(2), 351–359.

Etymotic Research. (2005). BKB-SIN: Speech-in-Noise Test (Version 1.03) [Computer software CD]. Elk Grove Village, IL: Etymotic Research.

Etymotic Research. (2006). QuickSIN: Speech-in-Noise Test (Version 1.3) [Computer software CD]. Elk Grove Village, IL: Etymotic Research.

Eysenck, M. W., & Eysenck, M. C. (1979). Memory scanning, introversion-extraversion, and levels of processing. *Journal of Research on Personality, 13*(3), 305–315.

Fabry, D. A., & Van Tasell, D. J. (1990). Evaluation of an articulation-index based model for predicting the effects of adaptive frequency response hearing aids. *Journal of Speech, Language, and Hearing Research, 33*(4), 676–689.

Fallon, M., Trehub, S. E., & Schneider, B. A. (2000). Children's perception of speech in multitalker babble. *Journal of the Acoustical Society of America, 108*(6), 3023–3029.

Federal Trade Commission, Office of the Federal Register, National Archives and Records Service, General Services Administration. (1975). Hearing aid industry: Proposed trade regulation rules. *Federal Register,* 26650.

Feigin, J. A., Kopun, J. G., Stelmachowicz, P. G., & Gorga, M. P. (1989). Probe-tube microphone measures of ear-canal sound pressure levels in infants and children. *Ear and Hearing, 10*(4), 254–258.

Festen, J. M., & Plomp, R. (1986). Speech-reception threshold in noise with one and two hearing aids. *Journal of the Acoustical Society of America, 79*(2), 465–471.

Fifer, R. C., Jerger, J. F., Berlin, C. I., Tobey, E. A., & Campbell, J. C. (1983). Development of a dichotic sentence identification test for hearing impaired adults. *Ear and Hearing, 4*(6), 300–305.

Flamme, G. A., Mudipalli, V. R., Reynolds, S. J., Kelly, K. M., Stromquist, A. M., Zwerling, C., . . . Merchant, J. A. (2005). Prevalence of hearing impairment in a rural midwestern cohort: Estimates from the Keokuk county rural health study, 1994–1998. *Ear and Hearing, 26*(3), 350–360.

Fletcher, H., & Galt, R. H. (1950). The perception of speech and its relation to telephony. *Journal of the Acoustical Society of America, 22*(2), 89–151.

Folkeard, P., Littmann V., & Scollie S. (2017). Using a De-reverberation Program to Improve Speech Intelligibility and Reduce Perceived Listening Effort. *Hearing Review, 24*(4), 32–33.

Fonix (2013). *Operator's manual.* Retrieved from http://www.frye.com/wp/wp-content/uploads/2013b/manuals/8000v2.41.pdf

Food and Drug Administration. (1999). *Summary of safety and effectiveness* [Bilateral fitting], (K984162-[June 28, 1999]). Retrieved from http://www.accessdata.fda.gov/cdrh_docs/pdf/k984162.pdf

Food and Drug Administration. (2013, November 7). *Regulatory requirements for hearing aid devices and personal sound amplification products—Draft guidance for industry and Food and Drug Administration staff.* Retrieved from http://www.fda.gov/medicaldevices/deviceregulationandguidance/guidancedocuments/ucm373461.htm

Fortune, T. W., & Preves, D. (1994). Effects of CIC, ITC, and ITE microphone placement on the amplification of wind noise. *Hearing Journal, 47*(9), 23–27.

Frankel, R., & Stein, T. (1999). Getting the most out of the clinical encounter: The four habits model. *Journal of Medical Practice Management, 16*(4), 184–191.

Frankel, R. M., & Stein, T. (1999). Getting the most out of the clinical encounter: The four habits model. *Permanente Journal, 3*(3), 79–83.

Franks, J. R. (1982). Judgments of hearing aid processed music. *Ear and Hearing, 3*(1), 18–23.

Fraser, S., Gagné, J. P., Alepins, M., & Dubois, P. (2010). Evaluating the effort expended to understand speech in noise using a dual-task paradigm: The effects of providing visual speech cues. *Journal of Speech, Language, and Hearing Research, 53*(1), 18–33.

Freed, D. J., & Soli, S. D. (2006). An objective procedure for evaluation of adaptive antifeedback algorithms in hearing aids. *Ear and Hearing, 27*(4), 382–398.

French, N. R., & Steinberg, J. C. (1947). Factors governing the intelligibility of speech sounds. *Journal of the Acoustical Society of America, 19*(1), 90–119.

Freudenthal, H. (1992). Norbert Werner. In C. C. Gillispie (Ed.), *Dictionary of scientific biography* (Vol. 20, pp. 131–148). New York, NY: Scribner.

Freyaldenhoven, M. C., Nabelek, A. K., Burchfield, S. B., & Thelin, J. W. (2005). Acceptable noise level (ANL) as a measure of directional benefit. *Journal of the American Academy of Audiology, 16*(4), 228–236.

Freyaldenhoven, M. C. (2007). Acceptable noise level (ANL): Research and current application. *Audiology Online,* Article #956. Retrieved from http://www.audiologyonline.com/articles/acceptable-noise-level-anl-research-956

Freyaldenhoven, M. C., Nabelek, A. K., & Tampas, J. W. (2008). Relationship between acceptable noise level and the abbreviated profile of hearing aid benefit. *Journal of Speech, Language, and Hearing Research, 51*(1), 136–146.

Freyman, R. L., Helfer, K. S., McCall, D. D., & Clifton, R. K. (1999). The role of perceived spatial separation in the unmasking of speech. *Journal of the Acoustical Society of America, 106*(6), 3578–3588.

Froehlich, M., Freels, K., & Powers, T. A. (2015, May). Speech recognition benefit obtained from binaural beamforming hearing aids: Comparison to omnidirectional and individuals with normal hearing. *Audiology Online*, Article #14338. Retrieved from http://www.audiologyonline.com/articles/speech-recognition-benefit-obtained-from-14338

Froehlich, M., & Powers T. A. (2015). Improving speech recognition in noise using binaural beamforming in ITC and CIC hearing aids. *Hearing Review, 22*(12), 22.

Gabriellson, A. (1979). Dimension analyses of perceived sound quality of sound reproducing systems. *Scandinavian Journal of Psychology, 20*(1), 159–169.

Gabrielsson, A., Schenkman, B. N., & Hagerman, B. (1988). The effects of different frequency responses on sound quality judgments and speech intelligibility. *Journal of Speech and Hearing Research, 31*(2), 166.

Gagné, J. P. (2000). What is treatment evaluation research? What is its relationship to the goals of audiological rehabilitation? Who are the stakeholders of this type of research? *Ear and Hearing, 21*(4 Suppl.), 60S–73S.

Gagné, J. P., Dinon, D., & Parsons, J. (1991). An evaluation of CASTA: Computer-Aided Speechreading Training Program. *Journal of Speech, Language, and Hearing Research, 34*(1), 213–221.

Gagné, J. P., Southall, K., & Jennings, M. B. (2009). The psychological effects of social stigma: Applications to people with acquired hearing loss. In J. Montano & J. B. Spitzer (Eds.), *Advanced practice in adult audiologic rehabilitation: International perspective* (pp. 63–92). New York, NY: Plural.

Galster, J. A., Valentine, S., Dundas, J. A., & Fitz, K. (2011). *Spectral IQ: Audibility improving access to high-frequency sounds*. Eden Prairie, MN: Starkey. Retrieved from http://www.spectraliq.com/pdfs/spectral-iq-wht-paper.pdf

Gardner, W., & Martin, K. (1994). *MIT Media Lab Machine Listening Group*. Cambridge, MA: The MIT Media Laboratory.

Garstecki, D. C., & Erler, S. F. (1998). Hearing loss, control, and demographic factors influencing hearing aid use among older adults. *Journal of Speech, Language, and Hearing Research, 41*(3), 527–537.

Garstecki, D. C., & Erler, S. F. (1999). Older adult performance on the communication profile for the hearing impaired gender difference. *Journal of Speech, Language, and Hearing Research, 42*(4), 785–796.

Gatehouse, S. (1992). The time course and magnitude of perceptual acclimatization to frequency responses: Evidence from monaural fitting of hearing aids. *Journal of the Acoustical Society of America, 92*(3), 1258–1268.

Gatehouse, S. (1994). Components and determinants of hearing aid benefit. *Ear and Hearing, 15*(1), 30–49.

Gatehouse, S. (1997, April). *The Glasgow hearing aid benefit profile: A client-centered scale for the assessment of auditory disability, handicap, and hearing aid benefit*. Poster session presented at the Annual Conference of the American Academy of Audiology, Fort Lauderdale, FL.

Gatehouse, S. (1999a). Glasgow Hearing Aid Benefit Profile: Derivation and validation of a client-centered outcome measure for hearing aid services. *Journal of American Academy of Audiology, 10*(2), 80–103.

Gatehouse, S. (1999b). A self-report outcome measure for the evaluation of hearing aid fittings and services. *Health Bulletin, 57*(6), 424–436.

Gatehouse, S. (2000). The Glasgow Hearing Aid Benefit Profile: What it measures and how to use it. *Hearing Journal, 53*(3), 10–12.

Gatehouse, S., & Akeroyd, M. A. (2006). Two-eared listening in dynamic situations. *International Journal of Audiology, 45*(Suppl. 1), S120–S124.

Gatehouse, S., Naylor, G., & Elberling, C. (2006). Linear and nonlinear hearing aid fittings—1. Patterns of benefit. *International Journal of Audiology, 45*(3), 130–152.

Gatehouse, S., & Noble, W. (2004). The speech, spatial and qualities of hearing scale (SSQ). *International Journal of Audiology, 43*(2), 85–99.

Gates, G. A., Murphy, M., Rees, T. S., & Fraher, A. (2003). Screening for handicapping hearing loss in the elderly. *Journal of Family Practice, 52*(1), 56–62.

Gebert, A., & Saltykov, O. (2013). A conical 0.4 cc coupler. Presentation to ANSI S3 Working Group 48, April 3, Anaheim, CA.

Gelfand, S. A. (1979). Usage of CROS hearing aids by unilaterally deaf patients. *Archives of Otolaryngology-Head and Neck Surgery, 105*(6), 328–332.

Gelnett, D., Sumida, A., Nilsson, M., & Soli, S. D. (1995). *Development of the hearing in noise test for children (HINT-C)*. Paper presented at the annual meeting of the American Academy of Audiology, Dallas, TX.

Gil, D., & Iorio, M. C. M. (2010). Formal auditory training in adult hearing aid users. *Clinics, 65*(2), 165–174.

Gillispie, C. C., Holmes, F. L., Koertge, N. & Gale, T. (2008). *Complete dictionary of scientific biography* (pp. 342–347). Detroit, MI: Scribner.

Giolas, T. G., Owens, E., Lamb, S. H., & Schubert, E. D. (1979). Hearing performance inventory. *Journal of Speech and Hearing Disorders, 44*(2), 169–195.

Glasberg, B. R., & Moore, B. C. J. (1990). Derivation of auditory filter shapes from notched-noise data. *Hearing Research, 47*(1–2), 103–138.

Glaser, R., & Traynor, R. (2013). *Strategic practice management: A patient-centric approach* (2nd ed.). San Diego, CA: Plural.

Glista, D., Hawkins, M., & Scollie, S. (2016). An update on modified verification approaches for frequency lowering devices. *Audiology Online*, Article #16932. Retrieved from http://www.audiologyonline.com/articles/update-on-modified-verification-approaches-16932

Glista, D., & Scollie, S. (2009). Modified verification approaches for frequency lowering devices. *Audiology Online*, Article #871. Retrieved from http://www.audiologyonline.com/articles/modified-verification-approaches-for-frequency-871

Glista, D., Scollie, S., & Sulkers, J. (2012). Perceptual acclimatization post nonlinear frequency compression hearing aid fitting in older children. *Journal of Speech, Language, and Hearing Research, 55*(6), 1765–1787.

Gnewikow, D., Ricketts, T., Bratt, G., & Mutchler, L. (2009). Real-world benefit from directional microphone hearing aids. *Journal of Rehabilitation Research and Development, 46*(5), 603–618.

Graf, R. F. (1999). *Modern dictionary of electronics* (7th ed.). Boston, MA: Newnes Books.

Grande, D., Frosch, D., Perkins, A., Barbara, E., & Kahn, B. (2009). Effect of exposure to small pharmaceutical promotional items on treatment preferences. *Archives of Internal Medicine, 169*(9), 887–893.

Grant, L., Bow, C., Paatsch, L., & Blamey, P. (2002, December). *Comparison of production of /s/ and /z/ between children using cochlear implants and children using hearing aids*. Poster session presented at the Ninth Australian International Conference on Speech Science and Technology, Melbourne, Australia.

Grayson, A. W., & Liang, B. (2000). Interview with Bryan Liang, M.D., Ph.D., J.D. and Arthur W. Grayson professor of law and medicine, Southern Illinois University schools of law and medicine. *Audiology Online*, Article #1822. Retrieved from http://www.audiology-online.com/interviews/interview-with-bryan-liang-m-1822

Green, D. S. (1969). Non-occluding earmolds with CROS and IROS hearing aids. *Archives of Otolaryngology-Head and Neck Surgery, 89*(3), 512–522.

Groen, J. J. (1969). Social hearing handicap: Its measurement by speech audiometry in noise. *International Journal of Audiology, 8*(1), 82–83.

Guenette, L. A. (2006). How to administer the dichotic digit test. *Hearing Journal, 59*(2), 50.

Gustafson, S., Ricketts, T. A., & Tharpe, A. M. (2017). Hearing technology use and management in school-age children: Reports from data logs, parents, and teachers. *Journal of the American Academy of Audiology*. Advance online publication. doi:10.3766/jaaa.16042

Guthrie, L. A., & Mackersie, C. L. (2009). A comparison of presentation levels to maximize word recognition scores. *Journal of the American Academy of Audiology, 20*(6), 381–390.

Haggard, M. P., Foster, J. R., & Iredale, F. E. (1981). Use and benefit of postaural hearing aids in sensorineural hearing loss. *Scandinavian Audiology, 10*(1), 45–52.

Hall, J. W. (2013). 20Q: Treating patients with hyperacusis and other forms of decreased sound tolerance. *Audiology Online*, Article #11679. Retrieved from http://www.audiologyonline.com/articles/20q-what-can-done-for-11679

Hallgren, M., Larsby, B., Lyxell, B., & Arlinger, S. (2005). Speech understanding in quiet and noise, with and without hearing aids. *International Journal of Audiology, 44*(10), 153–171.

Halpin, C. (2002). The tuning curve in clinical audiology. *American Journal of Audiology, 11*(2), 56–64.

Hamilton, A. M., & Munro, K. J. (2010). Uncomfortable loudness levels in experienced unilateral and bilateral hearing aid users: Evidence of adaptive plasticity following asymmetrical sensory input. *International Journal of Audiology, 49*(9), 667–671.

Hanks, W. D., & Johnson, G. D. (1998). HINT list equivalency using older listeners. *Journal of Speech, Language, and Hearing Research, 41*(6), 1335–1340.

Harbour, R., & Miller, J. (2001). A new system for grading recommendations in evidence based guidelines. *BMJ: British Medical Journal, 323*(7308), 334.

Harford, E. R. (1980). The use of a miniature microphone in the ear canal for the verification of hearing aid performance. *Ear and Hearing, 1*(6), 329–337.

Harford, E. R. (2000). Professional education in audiology. In H. Hosford-Dunn, R. Roeser, & M. Valente (Eds.), *Audiology practice management* (pp. 17–40). New York, NY: Thieme Medical.

Harford, E., & Barry, J. (1965). A rehabilitative approach to the problem of unilateral hearing impairment: The contralateral routing of signals (CROS). *Journal of the Speech Language Hearing Association, 30*(3), 121–138.

Harford, E., & Dodds, E. (1966). The clinical application of CROS. *Archives of Otolaryngology-Head and Neck Surgery, 83*(5), 455–464.

Harlmemphis.org. (2012). *Manual scoring instructions*. Retrieved from http://www.harlmemphis.org/files/6213/5041/6232/manual_scoring_instructions.pdf

Harnack Knebel, S. B., & Bentler, R. A. (1998). Comparison of two digital hearing aids. *Ear and Hearing, 19*(4), 280–287.

Hawkins, D. B. (2005). Effectiveness of counseling-based adult group aural-rehabilitation programs: A systematic review of the evidence. *Journal of the American Academy of Audiology, 16*(7), 485–493.

Hawkins, D. B., Beck, L. B., Bratt, G. W., Fabry, D. A., Mueller, H. G., & Stelmachowicz, P. G. (1991). Vanderbilt/VA hearing aid conference 1990 consensus statement. Recommended components of a hearing aid selection procedure for adults. *Journal of the American Speech-Language Hearing Association, 33*(4), 37–38.

Hawkins, D. B., & Cook, J. A. (2003). Hearing aid software predictive gain values: How accurate are they? *Hearing Journal, 56*(7), 26–28.

Hawkins, D. B., Hamill, T., & Kukula, J. (2006). Ethical issues in hearing. *Audiology Today, 18*(4), 22–29.

Hawkins, D. B., Hamill, T., Van Vliet, D., & Freeman, B. (2002). Potential conflicts of interest as viewed by the audiologist and the hearing-impaired consumer. *Audiology Today, 14*(5), 27–33.

Hawkins, D. B., Montgomery, A. A., Prosek, R. A., & Walden, B. E. (1987). Examination of two issues concerning functional gain measurements. *Journal of Speech and Hearing Disorders, 52*(1), 56–63.

Hawkins, D. B., & Mueller, H. G. (1992). Procedural considerations in probe-microphone measurements. In H. G. Mueller, D. Hawkins, & J. Northern (Eds.), *Probe microphone measurements: Hearing aid selection and assessment* (pp. 67–91). San Diego, CA: Singular.

Hawkins, D. B., & Schum, D. J. (1984). Relationships among various measures of hearing aid gain. *Journal of Speech and Hearing Disorders, 49*(1), 94–97.

Hawkins, D. B., Walden, B. E., Montgomery, A., & Prosek, R. A. (1987). Description and validation of the LDL procedure designed to select SSPL90. *Ear and Hearing, 8*(3), 162–169.

Haynes, B. (1999). Can it work? Does it work? Is it worth it?: The testing of healthcare intervention is evolving. *British Medical Journal, 319*(7211), 652–653.

Healy, E. W., Yoho, S. E., & Apoux, F. (2013). Band importance for sentences and words reexamined. *Journal of the Acoustical Society of America, 133*(1), 463–473.

Hearing Industries Association. (1984). *Market survey: A summary of findings and business implications for the U.S. hearing aid industry*. Washington, DC: Author.

Hellman, R. P., & Meiselman, C. H. (1990). Loudness relations for individuals and groups in normal and impaired hearing. *Journal of the Acoustical Society of America, 88*(6), 2596–2606.

Hellman, R. P., & Meiselman, C. H. (1993). Rate of loudness growth for pure tones in normal and impaired hearing. *Journal of the Acoustical Society of America, 93*(2), 966–975.

Henry, P., & Ricketts, T. (2003). The effects of changes in head angle on auditory and visual input for omnidirectional and directional microphone hearing aids. *American Journal of Audiology, 12*(1), 41–51.

Henshaw, H., Clark, D. P., Kang, S., & Ferguson, M. A. (2012). Computer skills and internet use in adults aged 50–74 years: Influence of hearing difficulties. *Journal of Medical Internet Research, 14*, e113.

Henshaw, H., & Ferguson, M. A. (2013). Efficacy of individual computer-based auditory training for people with hearing loss: A systematic review of the evidence. *PloS ONE, 8*(5), e62836.

Herbig, R., Barthel, R., & Branda, E. (2014). A history of e2e wireless technology. *Hearing Review, 21*(2), 34–37.

Hétu, R. (1996). The stigma attached to hearing impairment. *Scandinavian Audiology, 25*(Suppl. 43), 12–24.

Hétu, R., Jones, L., & Getty, L. (1993). The impact of acquired hearing impairment on intimate relationships: Implications for rehabilitation. *International Journal of Audiology, 32*(6), 363–380.

Hétu, R., Riverin, L., Lalande, N., Getty, L., & St-Cyr, C. (1988). Qualitative analysis of the handicap associated with occupational hearing loss. *British Journal of Audiology, 22*(4), 251–264.

Hicks, C. B., & Tharpe, A. M. (2002). Listening effort and fatigue in school-age children with and without hearing loss. *Journal of Speech, Language, and Hearing Research, 45*(3), 573–584.

Hickson, L., Worrall, L., & Scarinci, N. (2007). A randomized controlled trial evaluating the active communication education program for older people with hearing impairment. *Ear and Hearing, 28*(2), 212–230.

Hill, C. R., & Thompson, B. (2004). Computing and interpreting effect sizes. In J. C. Smart (Ed.), *Higher education: Handbook of theory and research* (Vol. 19). Dordrecht, Netherlands: Springer.

Hill, S. L. III, Marcus, A., Digges, E. N., Gillman, N., & Silverstein, H. (2006). Assessment of patient satisfaction with various configurations of digital CROS and BiCROS hearing aids. *Ear, Nose, and Throat Journal, 85*(7), 427–430, 442.

Hillenbrand, J., & Nearey, T. (1999). Identification of resynthesized /hVd/ utterances: Effects of formant contour. *Journal of the Acoustical Society of America, 105*(6), 3509–3523.

Hirsh, I. (1952). Intelligibility of speech. In *The measurement of hearing*. New York, NY: McGraw-Hill.

Hol, M. K. S., Bosman, A. J., Snik, A. F. M., Mylanus, E. A. M., & Cremers, C. W. R. J. (2004). Bone-anchored hearing aid in unilateral inner ear deafness: A study of 20 patients. *Audiology and Neurotology*, 9(5), 274–281.

Holder, J. T., Picou, E. M., Gruenwald, J. M., & Ricketts, T. A. (2016). Do modern hearing aids meet ANSI standards? *Journal of the American Academy of Audiology*, 27(8), 619–627.

Holube, I. (2015). 20Q: Getting to know the ISTS. *Audiology Online*, Article #13295. Retrieved from http://www.audiologyonline.com/articles/20q-getting-to-know-ists-13295

Holube, I., Fredelake, S., Vlaming, M., & Kollmeier, B. (2010). Development and analysis of an international speech test signal (ISTS). *International Journal of Audiology*, 49(12), 891–903.

Hopkins, K., Khanom, M., Dickinson, A. M., & Munro, K. J. (2014). Benefit from non-linear frequency compression hearing aids in a clinical setting: The effects of duration of experience and severity of high-frequency hearing loss. *International Journal of Audiology*, 53(4), 219–228.

Hornsby, B. W. (2013). The effects of hearing aid use on listening effort and mental fatigue associated with sustained speech processing demands. *Ear and Hearing*, 34(5), 523–534.

Hornsby, B. W., & Dundas, J. A. (2009). Factors affecting outcomes on the TEN (SPL) test in adults with hearing loss. *Journal of the American Academy of Audiology*, 20(4), 251–263.

Hornsby, B. W., Johnson, E. E., & Picou, E. (2011). Effects of degree and configuration of hearing loss on the contribution of high- and low-frequency speech information to bilateral speech understanding. *Ear and Hearing*, 32(5), 543–555.

Hornsby B. W., & Mueller, H. G. (2008). User preference and reliability of bilateral hearing aid gain adjustments. *Journal of the American Academy of Audiology*, 19(2), 158–170.

Hornsby, B. W., & Mueller, H. G. (2013). Monosyllabic word testing: Five simple steps to improve accuracy and efficiency. *Audiology Online*, Article #11978. Retrieved from http://www.audiologyonline.com

Hornsby, B. W., & Ricketts, T. A. (2003). The effects of hearing loss on the contribution of high- and low-frequency speech information to speech understanding. *Journal of the Acoustical Society of America*, 113(3), 1706–1717.

Hornsby, B. W., & Ricketts, T. A. (2006). The effects of hearing loss on the contribution of high- and low-frequency speech information to speech understanding. II. Sloping hearing loss. *Journal of the Acoustical Society of America*, 119(3), 1752–1763.

Hornsby, B. W., & Ricketts, T. A. (2007). Effects of noise source configuration on directional benefit using symmetric and asymmetric directional hearing aid fittings. *Ear and Hearing*, 28(2), 177–186.

Hornsby, B. W., Ricketts, T. A., & Johnson, E. E. (2006). The effects of speech and speechlike maskers on unaided and aided speech recognition in persons with hearing loss. *Journal of the American Academy of Audiology*, 17(6), 432–447.

Hosford-Dunn, H., & Halpern, J. (2000). Clinical application of the Satisfaction in Daily Life scale in private practice I: Statistical, content, and factorial validity. *Journal of the American Academy of Audiology*, 11(10), 523–539.

Hosford-Dunn, H., & Halpern, J. (2001). Clinical application of the Satisfaction in Daily Life scale in private practice II: Predictive validity of fitting variables. *Journal of the American Academy of Audiology*, 12(1), 15–36.

Hougaard, S., Ruf, S., Egger, C., & Abrams, H. (2016). Hearing aids improve hearing—and a lot more. *Hearing Review*, 23(6), 14–17.

Houtgast, T. (1981). The effect of noise on speech intelligibility in classrooms. *Applied Acoustics*, 14(1), 15–25.

Houtgast, T., & Steeneken, H. J. M. (1971). Evaluation of speech transmission channels by using artificial signals. *Acustica*, 25(6), 355–367.

Houtgast, T., & Steeneken, H. J. M. (1973). The modulation transfer function in room acoustic as a predictor of speech intelligibility. *Acustica*, 28(1), 66–73.

Houtgast, T., & Steeneken, H. J. M. (1985). A review of the MTF concept in room acoustics and its use for estimating speech intelligibility in auditoria. *Journal of the Acoustical Society of America*, 77(3), 1069–1077.

Houtgast, T., Steeneken, H. J. M., & Plomp, R. (1980). Predicting speech intelligibility in rooms from the modulation transfer function: I. General room acoustics. *Acustica*, 46(1), 60–72.

Hua, H., Karlsson, J., Widén, S., Möller, C., & Lyxell, B. (2013). Quality of life, effort and disturbance perceived in noise: A comparison between employees with aided hearing impairment and normal hearing. *International Journal of Audiology*, 52(9), 642–649.

Hull, R. H. (2013). Breaking news: Going beyond the basics in aural rehabilitation. *Hearing Journal*, 66(1), 14–15.

Humes, L. E. (1991). Understanding the speech-understanding problems of the hearing impaired. *Journal of the American Academy of Audiology*, 2(2), 59–69.

Humes, L. E. (2002). Factors underlying the speech-recognition performance of elderly hearing-aid wearers. *Journal of the Acoustical Society of America*, 112(3), 1112–1132.

Humes, L. E. (2003). Modeling and predicting hearing aid outcome. *Trends in Amplification, 7*(2), 41–75.

Humes, L. E., Dirks, D. D., Bell, T. S., Ahlstrom, C., & Kincaid, G. E. (1986). Application of the articulation index and the speech transmission index to the recognition of speech by normal-hearing and hearing-impaired listeners. *Journal of Speech and Hearing Research, 29*(4), 447–462.

Humes, L. E., Halling, D., & Coughlin, M. (1996). Reliability and stability of various hearing aid outcome measures in a group of elderly hearing aid wearers. *Journal of Speech and Hearing Research, 39*(5), 921–935.

Humes, L. E., & Krull, V. (2012). Evidence about the effectiveness of hearing aids in adults. In L. Wong & L. Hickson (Eds.), *Evidence-based practice in audiology: Evaluating interventions for children and adults with hearing impairment* (pp. 61–92). San Diego, CA: Plural.

Humes, L. E., Rogers, S. E., Quigley, T. M., Main, A. K., Kinney, D. L., & Herring, C. (2017). The effects of service-delivery model and purchase price on hearing-aid outcomes in older adults: A randomized double-blind placebo-controlled clinical trial. *American Journal of Audiology, 26*(1), 53–79.

Humes, L. E., Wilson, D. L., Humes, L., Barlow, N. N., Garner, C. B., & Amos, N. (2002). A comparison of two measures of hearing aid satisfaction in a group of elderly hearing aid wearers. *Ear and Hearing, 23*(5), 422–427.

Hurley, R. M. (1999). Onset of auditory deprivation. *Journal of the American Academy of Audiology, 10*(10), 529–534.

Hurley, R. M., & Sells, J. P. (2003). An abbreviated word recognition protocol based on item difficulty. *Ear and Hearing, 24*(2), 111–118.

Hutcherson, R. W., Dirks, D. D., & Morgan, D. E. (1979). Evaluation of the speech perception in noise (SPIN) test. *Otolaryngology-Head and Neck Surgery, 87*(2), 239–245.

IEEE. (1969). *IEEE recommended practice for speech quality measurements* (IEEE Report No. 297). Appendix C. Boulder, CO: Global Engineering Documents.

Inglis, A. H., Gray, C. H. C., & Jenkins, R. T. (1932, April). A voice and ear for telephone measurements. *Bell System Technical Journal, 11*(2), 293.

Ingvalson, E. M., Lee, B., Fiebig, P., & Wong, P. C. (2013). The effects of short-term computerized speech-in-noise training on postlingually deafened adult cochlear implant recipients. *Journal of Speech, Language, and Hearing Research, 56*(1), 81–88.

International Society of Audiology. (2005). *Good practice guidance for adult hearing aid fittings and services*. Isa-audiology.org. Retrieved from http://www.isa-audiology.org/members/pdf/gpg-adaf.pdf

ISO. (1961). *Normal equal-loudness contours for pure tones and normal threshold of hearing under free-field listening conditions, R226-1961*. Geneva, Switzerland: International Organization for Standardization.

Jacobson, G. P., Newman, C. W., Fabry, D. A., & Sandridge, S. A. (2001). Development of the three-clinic hearing aid selection profile (HASP). *Journal of the American Academy of Audiology, 12*(3), 128–141.

Jacobson, G. P., Newman, C. W., Sandridge, S. A., & McCaslin, D. L. (2002). Using the hearing aid selection profile to identify factors in hearing aid returns. *Hearing Journal, 55*(3), 30–33.

Jadad, A. R., Moore, R. A., Carroll, D., Jenkinson, C., Reynolds, D. J. M., Gavaghan, D. J., & McQuay, H. J. (1996). Assessing the quality of reports of randomized clinical trials: Is blinding necessary? *Controlled Clinical Trials, 17*(1), 1–12.

Jensen, J., & Pedersen, M. S. (2015, April). Analysis of beamformer directed single-channel noise reduction system for hearing aid applications. In *Acoustics, Speech and Signal Processing (ICASSP), 2015 IEEE International Conference on* (pp. 5728–5732). IEEE.

Jenstad, L. M., Pumford, J., Seewald, R. C., & Cornelisse, L. E. (2000). Comparison of linear gain and wide dynamic range compression hearing aid circuits II: Aided loudness measures. *Ear and Hearing, 21*(1), 32–44.

Jenstad, L. M., Van Tasell, D., & Ewert, C. (2003). Hearing aid troubleshooting base on patients' descriptions. *Journal of the American Academy of Audiology, 14*(7), 347–360.

Jerger, J. (Ed.). (1969). *Modern developments in audiology*. New York, NY: Academic.

Jerger, J. F. (2006). Informational masking. *Journal of the American Academy of Audiology, 17*(6), 1.

Jerger, J. F. (2009). *Audiology in the USA*. San Diego, CA: Plural.

Jerger, J., Chmiel, R., Allen, J., & Wilson, A. (1994). Effects of age and gender on dichotic sentence identification. *Ear and Hearing, 15*(4), 274–286.

Jerger, J., Stach, B., Johnson, K., Loiselle, L., & Jerger, S. (1990). Patterns of abnormality in dichotic listening. In J. Jensen (Ed.), *Presbyacusis and other age related aspects*. Copenhagen, Denmark: Stougaard Jensen.

Jespersen, C. T., Groth, J., Kiessling, J., Brenner, B., & Jensen, O. D. (2006). The occlusion effect in unilateral versus bilateral hearing aids. *Journal of the American Academy of Audiology, 17*(10), 763–773.

Jirsa, R.E., & Norris, T. W. (1982). Effects of intermodulation distortion on speech intelligibility. *Ear and Hearing, 3*(5), 251–256.

Johnson, E. E. (2012). Comparing the latest NAL and DSL prescriptive targets. *Audiology Online*. Retrieved from http://www.audiologyonline.com/articles/20q-same-or-different-comparing-769?report=reader

Johnson, E. E., & Dillon, H. (2011). A comparison of gain for adults from generic hearing aid prescriptive methods: Impacts on predicted loudness, frequency bandwidth, and speech intelligibility. *Journal of the American Academy of Audiology, 22*(7), 441–459.

Johnson, E. E., Mueller, H. G., & Ricketts, T. A. (2009). Statistically derived factors of varied importance to audiologists when making a hearing aid brand decision. *Journal of the American Academy of Audiology, 20*(1), 40–48.

Johnson, E. E., Ricketts, T. A., & Hornsby, B. W. Y. (2007). Effects of digital feedback reduction algorithms in modern digital hearing aids on sound quality. *Journal of the American Academy of Audiology, 18*(5), 404–416.

Johnson, J. (2014). Lyric 24/7 hearing: Could it help those with tinnitus? *ENT and Audiology News, 23*(5), 84–86.

Johnson, J. A., & Cox, R. M. (2009, March). *QuickSin™ HFE and LP lists: Learning effect, equivalence and sensitivity.* Paper presented at the annual meeting of the American Auditory Society, Scottsdale, AZ.

Johnson, J. A., Cox, R. M., & Alexander, G. C. (2010). Development of APHAB norms for WDRC hearing aids and comparisons with original norms. *Ear and Hearing, 31*(1), 47–55.

Johnson, J. A., Xu, J., & Cox, R. M. (2017). Impact of hearing aid technology on outcomes in daily life III: Localization. *Ear and Hearing.* Retrieved from https://insights.ovid.com/crossref?an=00003446-900000000-99057

Jones, C., Feilner, M. (2014). What do we know about the fitting and daily life usage of hearing instruments in pediatrics? In J. Northern (Ed.), *A sound foundation through early amplification: 6th International Conference Proceeding* (pp. 97–104). Stafa, Switzerland: Phonak AG.

Jongman, A., Wayland, R., & Wong, S. (2000). Acoustic characteristics of English fricatives. *Journal of the Acoustical Society of America, 108*(3), 1252–1263.

Jonkman, J. (2015). *Wideband RECD on Verifit2.* Dorchester, Ontario: Audioscan.

Joore, M. A., Potjewijd, J., Timmerman, A. A., & Anteunis, L. J. C. (2002). Response shift in the measurement of quality of life in hearing impaired adults after hearing aid fitting. *Quality of Life Research, 11*(4), 299–307.

Kahneman, D. (1973). *Attention and effort.* Englewood Cliffs, NJ: Prentice-Hall.

Kahneman, D. (2011). *Thinking, fast and slow.* New York, NY: Farrar, Straus and Giroux.

Kalikow, D. N., Stevens, K. N., & Elliott, L. L. (1977). Development of a test of speech intelligibility in noise using sentence materials with controlled word predictability. *Journal of the Acoustical Society of America, 61*(5), 1337–1351.

Kamm, C. A., Dirks, D. D., & Mickey, M. R. (1978). Effects of sensorineural hearing loss on loudness discomfort level and most comfortable loudness. *Journal of Speech and Hearing Research, 21*(4), 668–681.

Kamm, C. A., Morgan, D. E., & Dirks, D. D. (1983). Accuracy of adaptive procedure estimates of PF-max level. *Journal of Speech and Hearing Disorders, 48*(2), 202–209.

Kaplan, H., Bally, S., Brandt, F., Busacco, D., & Pray, J. (1997). Communication scale for older adults (CSOA). *Journal of the American Academy of Audiology, 8*(3), 203–217.

Kaplan, H., Bally, S. J., & Brandt, F. (1995). Revised communication self-assessment scale inventory for deaf adults (CSDA). *Journal of the American Academy of Audiology, 6*(4), 311–329.

Kaplan, H., & Hesse, J. (2000). National and state policies effecting hearing aids and assistive listening devices. In M. Valente, H. Hosford-Dunn, & R. J. Roeser (Eds.), *Audiology treatment* (pp. 307–322). New York, NY: Thieme Medical.

Karlsen, B. L., Flynn, M. C., & Eneroth, K. (2006, August). *The benefit of high-frequency bandwidth for hearing-impaired people under speech in noise conditions.* Paper presented at the 2006 International Hearing Aid Research Conference (IHCON), Lake Tahoe, CA.

Kates, J. M. (1999). Constrained adaptation for feedback cancellation in hearing aids. *Journal of the Acoustical Society of America, 106*(2), 1010–1019.

Kates, J. M. (2008). *Digital hearing aids.* San Diego, CA: Plural.

Keidser, G., & Alamudi, K. (2013). Real-life efficacy and reliability of training a hearing aid. *Ear and Hearing, 34*(5), 619–629.

Keidser, G., Brew, C., & Peck, A. (2003). Proprietary fitting algorithms compared with one another and with generic formulas. *Hearing Journal, 56*(3), 28–32.

Keidser, G., & Dillon, H. (2006). What's new in prescriptive fittings Down Under? In C. V. Palmer & R. Seewald (Eds.), *Hearing care for adults 2006* (pp. 133–142). Stafa, Switzerland: Phonak AG.

Keidser, G., & Dillon, H. (2012). Siemens expert series: NAL-NL2—Principles, background data, and comparison to other procedures. *Audiology Online.* Retrieved from http://www.audiologyonline.com/articles/siemens-expert-series-nal-nl2-11355

Keidser, G., Dillon, H., & Convery, E. (2008). The effect of the base line response on self-adjustments of hearing aid gain. *Journal of the Acoustical Society of America, 124*(3), 1668–1681.

Keidser, G., Dillon, H., Dyrlund, O., Carter, L., & Hartley, D. (2007). Preferred low- and high-frequency compression ratios among hearing aids. *Journal of the American Academy of Audiology, 18*(1), 17–33.

Keidser, G., O'Brien, A., Latzel, M., & Convery, E. (2007). Evaluation of a noise-reduction algorithm that targets non-speech transient sounds. *Hearing Journal, 60*(2), 29–39.

Keidser, G., Rohrseitz, K., Dillon, H., Hamacher, V., Carter, L., Rass, U., & Convery, E. (2006). The effect of multichannel wide dynamic range compression, noise reduction, and the directional microphone on horizontal localization performance in hearing aid wearers. *International Journal of Audiology, 45*(10), 563–579.

Keidser, G., Yeend, I., O'Brien, A., & Hartley, L. (2011). Using in-situ audiometry more effectively: How low-frequency can affect prescribed gain and prescription. *Hearing Review, 18*(3), 12–16.

KEMAR, T. (2006). Where in the world is KEMAR? *Hearing Journal, 59*(4), 10–16.

Kent, R. D., & Read, C. (2002). *Acoustic analysis of speech* (2nd ed.). Canada: Thomson Learning.

Kiessling, J., Brenner, B., Thunberg Jespersen, C., Groth, J., & Jensen, O. D. (2005). Occlusion effect of earmolds with different venting systems. *Journal of the American Academy of Audiology, 16*(4), 237–249.

Kiessling, J., Grugel, L., Meister, H., & Meis, M. (2011). German translations of questionnaires, SADL, ECHO and SSQ and their evaluation. *Zeitschrift fur Audiologie, 50*(1), 6–16.

Killion, M. C. (1978). Revised estimate of minimum audible pressure: Where is the "missing 6 dB"? *Journal of the Acoustical Society of America, 63*(5), 1501–1508.

Killion, M. C. (1979). *Design and evaluation of high-fidelity hearing aids* (Unpublished doctoral dissertation). Northwestern University, Evanston, IL.

Killion, M. C. (1980). Problems in the application of broadband hearing aid earphones. In G. A. Studebaker & I. Hochberg (Eds.), *Acoustic factors affecting hearing aid performance*. Baltimore, MD: University Park Press.

Killion, M. C. (1981). Earmold options for wideband hearing aids. *Journal of Speech and Hearing Disorders, 46*(1), 10–20.

Killion, M. C. (1988). Earmold design: Theory and practice. In J. Jensen (Ed.), *Hearing aid fitting: Theoretical and practical views* (pp. 155–174). Copenhagen, Denmark: Stougaard Jensen.

Killion, M. C. (1993). Transducers and acoustic couplings. In G. A. Studebaker & I. Hochberg (Eds.), *Acoustical factors affecting hearing aid performance* (2nd ed., pp. 31–50). Boston, MA: Allyn & Bacon.

Killion, M. C. (1994). *Fig6.exe software: Hearing aid fitting targets for 40, 65 & 95 dB SPL inputs (version 1.01D)*. Elk Grove Village, IL: Etymotic Research.

Killion, M. C. (1997). SNR loss: I can hear what people say, but I can't understand them. *Hearing Review, 4*(12), 8–14.

Killion, M. C. (2003). Earmold acoustics. *Seminars in Hearing, 24*(4), 299–312.

Killion, M. C., Berger, E. H., & Nuss, R. A. (1987). Diffuse field response of the ear. *Journal of the Acoustical Society of America, 81*(S1), S75–S75.

Killion, M. & Carlson, E. (1970). A wide-band miniature microphone. *Journal of the Audio Engineering Society, 18*(6), 631–635.

Killion, M. C., & Monser, E. L. (1980). CORFIG: Coupler response for flat insertion gain. In G. A. Studebaker & I. Hochlberg (Eds.), *Acoustical factors affecting hearing aid performance* (pp. 149–168). Boston, MA: Allyn & Bacon.

Killion, M. C., & Mueller, H. G. (2010). Twenty years later: A new count-the-dots method. *Hearing Journal, 63*(1), 10–17.

Killion, M. C., Mueller, H. G., Pavlovic, C. V., & Humes, L. E. (1993). A is for audibility. *Hearing Journal, 46*(4), 29.

Killion, M. C., & Niquette, P. A. (2000). What can the pure-tone audiogram tell us about a patient's SNR loss? *Hearing Journal, 53*(3), 46–53.

Killion, M. C., Niquette, P. A., Gudmundsen, G. I., Revit, L. J., & Banerjee, S. (2004). Development of a quick speech-in-noise test for measuring signal-to-noise ratio loss in normal-hearing and hearing-impaired listeners. *Journal of the Acoustical Society of America, 116*(4), 2395–2405.

Killion, M. C., & Revit, L. J. (1987). Insertion gain repeatability versus loudspeaker location: You want me to put my loudspeaker WHERE? *Ear and Hearing, 8*(5), 74s.

Killion, M. C., Schulien, R., Christensen, L., Fabry, D., Revit, L., Niquette, P., Chung, K. (1998). Real world performance of an ITE directional microphone. *Hearing Journal, 51*(4), 24–26, 30, 32–36, 38.

Killion, M. C., & Villchur, E. (1993). Kessler was right partly: But SIN test shows some aids improve hearing in noise. *Hearing Journal, 46*(9), 31–35.

Killion, M. C., Wilber, L., & Gudmundsen, G. I. (1988). Zwislocki was right. *Hearing Instruments, 39*(1), 14–18.

Kim, J. S., & Bryan, M. F. (2011). The effects of asymmetric directional microphone fittings on acceptance of background noise. *International Journal of Audiology, 50*(5), 290–296.

Kimlinger, C., McCreery, R., & Lewis, D. (2015). High-frequency audibility: The effects of audiometric configuration, stimulus type, and device. *Journal of the American Academy of Audiology, 26*(2), 128–137.

Kimura, D. (1961a). Cerebral dominance and the perception of verbal stimuli. *Canadian Journal of Psychology, 15*(3), 166–171.

Kimura, D. (1961b). Some effects of temporal lobe damage on auditory perception. *Canadian Journal of Psychology, 15*(3), 156–165.

Klein, W., Plomp, R., & Pols, L. C. W. (1970). Vowel spectra, vowel spaces, and vowel identification. *Journal of the Acoustical Society of America, 48*(4B), 999–1009.

Knowles, H., & Burkhard, M. (1975). Hearing aids on KEMAR. *Hearing Instruments, 26*(1), 19–21.

Koch, D. B, Nilsson, M. J., & Soli, S. D. (2004). Using the HINT test on compact disk. House Ear Institute—Qsound. Licensed by Starkey Laboratories.

Kochkin, S. (1990). One more time . . . What did the 1984 HIA market survey say? *Hearing Instruments, 42*(11), 11–13.

Kochkin, S. (1991). MarkeTrak II: More MDs give hearing tests, yet hearing aid sales remain flat. *Hearing Journal, 44*(2), 24–35.

Kochkin, S. (1994a). MarkeTrak IV: Impact on purchase intent of cosmetics, stigma, and style of hearing instrument. *Hearing Journal, 47*(9), 1–7.

Kochkin, S. (1994b). MarkeTrak IV: Will CICs attract a new type of customer—And what about price? *Hearing Journal, 47*(11), 49–54.

Kochkin, S. (1995). Customer satisfaction and benefit with CIC hearing aids. *Hearing Review, 2*(4), 16–26.

Kochkin, S. (1996). MarkeTrak IV: 10-year trends in the hearing aid market—Has anything changed? *Hearing Journal, 49*(1), 1–6.

Kochkin, S. (1997). MarkeTrak IV: What is the viable market for hearing aids? *Hearing Journal, 50*(1), 31–38.

Kochkin, S. (1998). MarkeTrak IV: Correlates of hearing aid purchase intent. *Hearing Journal, 51*(1), 30–38.

Kochkin, S. (2001). MarkeTrack VI: The VA and direct mail sales spark growth in hearing-aid market. *Hearing Review, 8*(12), 16–24, 63–65.

Kochkin, S. (2002). MarkeTrak VI: 10-year customer satisfaction trends in U.S. hearing instrument market. *Hearing Review, 9*(10), 14–25, 46.

Kochkin, S. (2007). MarkeTrak VII: Obstacles to adult non-user adoption of hearing aids. *Hearing Journal, 60*(4), 27–43.

Kochkin S. (2009). MarkeTrak VIII: 25-year trends in the hearing health market. *Hearing Review, 16*(10), 12–31.

Kochkin, S. (2010). MarkeTrak VIII: Consumer satisfaction with hearing aids is slowly increasing. *Hearing Journal, 63*(1), 19–32.

Kochkin, S. (2011a). MarkeTrak VIII: Reducing patient visits through verification & validation. *Hearing Review, 18*(6), 10–12.

Kochkin, S. (2011b). Mini-BTEs tap new market, users more satisfied. *Hearing Journal, 24*(3), 17–24.

Kochkin, S. (2012). 20Q: More highlights from MarkeTrak. *Audiology Online*, Retrieved from http://www.audiologyonline.com/articles/more-highlights-from-marketrak-6830

Kochkin, S. (2014). A comparison of consumer satisfaction, subjective benefit, and quality of life changes associated with traditional and direct-mail hearing aid use. *Hearing Review, 21*(1), 16–26.

Kochkin, S., Beck, D. L., Christensen, L. A., Compton-Conley, C., Fligor, B. J., Kricos, P. B., . . . Turner, R. G. (2010). MarkeTrak VIII: The impact of the hearing healthcare professional on hearing aid user success. *Hearing Review, 17*(4), 12–34.

Kochkin, S., & Tyler, R. (2008). Tinnitus treatment and the effectiveness of hearing aids: Hearing care professional perceptions. *Hearing Review, 15*(13), 14–18.

Kokx-Ryan, M., Cohen, J., Cord, M. T., Walden, T. C., Makashay, M. J., Sheffield, B. M., & Brungart, D. S. (2015). Benefits of nonlinear frequency compression in adult hearing aid users. *Journal of the American Academy of Audiology, 26*(10), 838–855.

Korhonen, P., Kuk, F., Lau, C., Keenan, D., Schumacher, J., & Nielsen, J. (2013). Effects of a transient noise reduction algorithm on speech understanding, subjective preference, and preferred gain. *Journal of the American Academy of Audiology, 24*(9), 845–858.

Korhonen, P., Kuk, F., Seper, E., Mørkebjerg, M., & Roikjer, M. (2017). Evaluation of a wind noise attenuation algorithm on subjective annoyance and speech-in-wind performance. *Journal of the American Academy of Audiology, 28*(1), 46–57.

Kramer, S. E., Allessie, G. H. M., Dondorp, A. W., Zekveld, A. A., & Kapteyn, T. S. (2005). A home education program for older adults with hearing impairment and their significant others: A randomized trial evaluating short- and long-term effects. *International Journal of Audiology, 44*(5), 255–264.

Kramer, S. E., Kapteyn, T. S., & Houtgast, T. (2006). Occupational performance: Comparing normally-hearing and hearing-impaired employees using the Amsterdam Checklist for Hearing and Work. *International Journal of Audiology, 45*(9), 503–512.

Kraus, N. (2012). Biological impact of music and software-based auditory training. *Journal of Communication Disorders, 45*(6), 403–410.

Kricos, P. B., & Holmes, A. E. (1996). Efficacy of audiologic rehabilitation for older adults. *Journal of the American Academy of Audiology, 7*(4), 219–229.

Kringlebotn, M. (1999). A graphical method for calculating the speech intelligibility index and measuring hearing disability from audiograms. *Scandinavian Audiology, 28*(3), 151–160.

Kroll, K., Grant, I. L., & Javel, E. (2002). The Envoy totally implantable hearing system, St. Croix Medical. *Trends in Amplification, 6*(2), 73–80.

Kuhn, G. (1979). The pressure transformation from a diffuse soundfield to the external ear and to the body and head surface. *Journal of the Acoustical Society of America, 65*(4), 991–1000.

Kuhn, G. F., & Burnett, E. D. (1977). Acoustic pressure field alongside a manikin's head with a view towards *in situ* hearing-aid tests. *Journal of the Acoustical Society of America, 62*(2), 416–423.

Kuhn, G. F., & Guernsey, R. M. (1983). Sound pressure distribution about the human head and torso. *Journal of the Acoustical Society of America, 73*(1), 95–105.

Kuk, F. K. (1994). Maximum usable real-ear insertion gain with ten earmold designs. *Journal of the American Academy of Audiology, 5*(1), 44–51.

Kuk, F. (2003). reconsidering the concept of aided of the aided threshold for nonlinear hearing aids. *Trends in Amplification, 7*(3), 77–97.

Kuk, F., Keenan, D., Lau, C. C., Dinulescu, N., Cortez, R., & Keogh, P. (2005). Real-world performance of a reverse-horn vent. *Journal of the American Academy of Audiology, 16*(9), 653–661.

Kuk, F., Keenan, D., Korhonen, P., & Lau, C. (2009). Efficacy of linear frequency transposition on consonant identification in quiet and in noise. *Journal of the American Academy of Audiology, 20*(8), 465–479.

Kuk, F., Ludvegsen, C., & Kaulberg, T. (2002). Understanding feedback and digital feedback cancellation strategies. *Hearing Review, 9*(2), 36–43.

Kuk, F., Schmidt, E., Jessen, A. H., & Sonne, M. (2015). New technology for effortless hearing: A "Unique" perspective. *Hearing Review, 22*(11), 32–36.

Ladefoged, P., & Broadbent, D. E. (1957). Information conveyed by vowels. *Journal of the Acoustical Society of America, 29*(1), 98–104.

Laitakari, K., Löppönen, H., Salmivalli, A., & Sorri, M. (1995). Brief communication: Objective real ear measures of bone conduction hearing aid performance. *Scandinavian Audiology, 24*(1), 53–56.

Laplante-Lévesque, A., Hickson, L., & Worrall, L. (2010). Factors influencing rehabilitation decisions of adults with acquired hearing impairment. *International Journal of Audiology, 49*(7), 497–507.

Laplante-Lévesque, A., Hickson, L., & Worrall, L. (2012). What makes adults with hearing impairment take up hearing aids or communication programs and achieve successful outcomes? *Ear and Hearing, 33*(1), 79–93.

Laplante-Lévesque, A., Jensen, L. D., Dawes, P., & Nielsen, C. (2013). Optimal hearing aid use: Focus groups with hearing aid clients and audiologists. *Ear and Hearing, 34*(2), 193–202.

Laplante-Lévesque, A., Pichora-Fuller, K. M., & Gagné, J. P. (2006). Providing an internet-based audiological counselling programme to new hearing aid users: A qualitative study. *International Journal of Audiology, 45*(12), 697–706.

Larsby, B., Hallgren, M. & Lyxell, B. (2005). Cognitive performance and perceived effort in speech processing tests; Effects of different noise background in normal-hearing and hearing-impaired subjects. *International Journal of Audiology, 44*(3), 131–143.

Latzel, M., & Appleton, J. (2013). Evaluation of a binaural speech in wind feature, Part 1: Verification in the laboratory. *Hearing Review, 20*(8), 32–34.

Lau, C., & Kuk, F. (2011). Enough is enough: A primer on power analysis in study designs. *Hearing Journal, 64*(4), 30–39.

Lau, C. C., Kuk, F., Keenan, D., & Schumacher, J. (2014). Amplification for listeners with a moderately severe high-frequency hearing loss. *Journal of the American Academy of Audiology, 25*(6), 562–575.

Leavitt, R., & Flexer, C. (2012). Speech degradation as measured by the Rapid Speech Transmission Index (RASTI). *Ear and Hearing, 12*(2), 115–118.

Lehiste, I., & Peterson, G. E. (1959). Linguistic considerations in study of speech intelligibility. *Journal of the Acoustical Society of America, 31*(3), 280–286.

Levitt, H. (2014). *Efficacy of ReadMyQuips (NIH sponsored research)*. SenseSynergy.com. Retrieved from http://www.sensesynergy.com/articles/research/initial

Levitt, H., Oden, C., Simon, H., Noack, C., & Lotze, A. (2011). Entertainment overcomes barriers of auditory training. *Hearing Journal, 64*(8), 40–42.

Lewis, J. D., Goodman, S. S., & Bentler, R. A. (2010). Measurement of hearing aid internal noise. *Journal of the Acoustical Society of America, 127*(4), 2521–2528.

Lewis, M. S., Crandell, C. C., Valente, M., Horn, J. E. (2004). Speech perception in noise: Directional microphones versus frequency modulation (FM) systems. *Journal of the American Academy of Audiology, 15*(6), 426–439.

Libby, E. R. (1982a). A new acoustic horn for small ear canals. *Hearing Instruments, 33*(9), 48.

Libby, E. R. (1982b). In search of transparent insertion gain hearing aid responses. In G. A. Studebaker & F. H. Bess (Eds.), *The Vanderbilt hearing aid report* (pp. 112–123). Upper Darby, PA: Monographs in Contemporary Audiology.

Libby, R. (1986). The 1/3–2/3 insertion gain hearing aid selection guide. *Hearing Instruments, 37*(3), 27–28.

Lichtenstein, M., Bess, F., & Logan, S. (1988). Validation of screening tools for identifying hearing-impaired elderly in primary care. *Journal of the American Medical Association, 259*(19), 2875–2878.

Lindley, G. A., & Palmer, C. V. (1997). Fitting wide dynamic range compression hearing aids: DSL [i/o], the IHAFF protocol, and FIG6. *American Journal of Audiology, 6*(3), 19–28.

Lindley, G. A., Palmer, C. V., Durrant, J., & Pratt, S. (2000). Adaptation to loudness and environmental stimuli in three newly fitted hearing aid users. *Journal of the American Academy of Audiology, 11*(6), 316–322.

Littmann V., Wu Y.H., Froehlich M., & Powers T.A. (2017). Multi-center evidence of reduced listening effort using new hearing aid technology. *Hearing Review, 24*(2), 32–34.

Liu, H., Zhang, H., Bentler, R. A., Han, D., & Zhang, L. (2012). Evaluation of a transient noise reduction strategy for hearing aids. *Journal of the American Academy of Audiology, 23*(8), 606–615.

Longwell, T., & Johnson, J. (1980). Estimating hearing aid insertion gain from coupler gain. *Hearing Instruments, 31*, 20–22.

Lowery, K. J., & Plyler, P. N. (2013). The effects of noise reduction technologies on the acceptance of background noise. *Journal of the American Academy of Audiology, 24*(8), 649–659.

Luce, P. A. (1986). *Neighborhoods of words in the mental lexicon. Research on speech perception* (Technical Report No. 6). Bloomington IN: Department of Psychology, Indiana University.

Luce, P. A., & Pisoni, D. B. (1998). Recognizing spoken words: The neighborhood activation model. *Ear and Hearing, 19*(1), 1–36.

Luetje, C. M., Brackmann, D., Balkany, T. J., Maw, J., Baker, R. S., Kelsall, D., . . . Arts, A. (2002). Phase III clinical trial results with the Vibrant® Soundbridge implantable middle ear hearing device: A prospective controlled multicenter study. *Otolaryngology-Head and Neck Surgery, 126*(2), 97–107.

Lundeen, C. (1996). Letter to the editor. *American Journal of Audiology, 5*(3), 57–58.

Lunner, T., Hellgren, J., Arlinger, S., & Elberling, C. (1997). A digital filterbank hearing aid: Three digital signal processing algorithms—User preference and performance. *Ear and Hearing, 18*(5), 373–387.

Lustig, L. R., Arts, H. A., Brackmann, D. E., Francis, H. F., Molony, T, Megerian, C. A., . . . Niparko, J. K. (2001). Hearing rehabilitation using the BAHA bone-anchored hearing aid: Results in 40 patients. *Otology and Neurotology, 22*(3), 328–334.

Luterman, D. (2004). Counseling families of children with hearing loss. *Volta Review, 104*(4), 215.

Lybarger, S. F. (1944). U.S. Patent application SN 5320 278. July 3, 1944.

Lybarger, S. F. (1947, November). Development of a new hearing aid with magnetic microphone. *Electric Manufacturing, 40*, 104–108.

Lybarger, S. F. (1953). U.S. Patent No. 2,656,421. Washington, DC: U.S. Patent and Trademark Office.

Lybarger, S. F. (1963). *Simplified fitting system for hearing aids*. Canonsburg, PA: Radioear.

Lybarger, S. (1985). Earmolds. In J. Katz (Ed.), *Handbook of clinical audiology* (3rd ed., pp. 885–910). Baltimore, MD: Lippincott Williams & Wilkins.

Lyons, R. G. (2010). *Understanding digital signal processing* (3rd ed.). Englewood Cliffs, NJ: Prentice Hall.

Lyregaard, P. (1982). Frequency selectivity and speech intelligibility in noise. *Scandinavian Audiology, 15*(Suppl.), 113–122.

MacKenzie, D. J. (2006). Open-canal fittings and the hearing aid occlusion effect. *Hearing Journal, 59*(11), 50–56.

Mackersie, C. L., & Cones, H. (2011). Subjective and psychophysiological indices of listening effort in a competing-talker task. *Journal of the American Academy of Audiology, 22*(2), 113.

Mackersie, C. L., Crocker, T. L., & Davis, R. A. (2004). Limiting high-frequency hearing aid gain in listeners with and without suspected cochlear dead regions. *Journal of the American Academy of Audiology, 15*(7), 498–507.

Macrae, J. (1986). *Relationships between the hearing threshold levels and aided speech discrimination of severely and profoundly deaf children* (Rep. No. NAL Report No. 107). Canberra, Australia: Australian Government Publishing Service.

Madaffari, P. L. (1974, November). *Pressure response about the ear*. Paper presented at the 88th meeting of the Acoustical Society of America, St. Louis, MO.

Magnusson, L., Claesson, A., Persson, M., & Tengstrand, T. (2013). Speech recognition in noise using bilateral open-fit hearing aids: The limited benefit of directional microphones and noise reduction. *International Journal of Audiology, 52*(1), 29–36.

Marcrum, S., & Ricketts T. A. (2011, March). *Assessment of modern feedback reduction systems*. Invited poster at the American Auditory Society Annual Meeting, Scottsdale, AZ.

Margolis, R. H. (2004a). Boosting memory with informational counseling: Helping patients understand the nature of disorders and how to manage them. *ASHA Leader, 28*, 10–11.

Margolis, R. H. (2004b). What do your patients remember? *Hearing Journal, 57*(6), 10–12.

Martin, M. (2007). Software-based auditory training program found to reduce hearing aid return rate. *Hearing Journal, 60*(8), 32–34.

Matkin, N., & Thomas, J. (1972). The utilization of CROS hearing aids by children. *Maico Audiological Library Series*, 10.

Matthews, L. J., Lee, F., Mills, J. H., & Dubno, J. R. (1997). Extended high-frequency thresholds in older adults. *Journal of Speech, Language, and Hearing Research*, 40(1), 208–214.

McArdle, R. A., Killion, M. C., Mennite, M. A., & Chisolm, T. H. (2012). Are two ears not better than one? *Journal of the American Academy of Audiology*, 23(3), 171–181.

McArdle, R. A., & Wilson, R. H. (2006). Homogeneity of the 18 QuickSIN lists. *Journal of the American Academy of Audiology*, 17(3), 157–167.

McArdle, R. A., Wilson, R. H., & Burks, C. A. (2005). Speech recognition in multitalker babble using digits, words, and sentences. *Journal of the American Academy of Audiology*, 16(9), 726–739.

McCandless, G. A., & Lyregaard, P. E. (1983). Prescription of gain/output (POGO) for hearing aids. *Hearing Instruments*, 34(1), 16–21.

McCreery, R. (2016). 20Q: Frequency lowering ten years later—Evidence for benefit. *Audiology Online*. Retrieved from https://www.audiologyonline.com/articles/20q-frequency-lowering-evidence-for-18370.

McCreery, R. W., Alexander, J., Brennan, M. A., Hoover, B., Kopun, J., & Stelmachowicz, P. G. (2014). The influence of audibility on speech recognition with nonlinear frequency compression for children and adults with hearing loss. *Ear and Hearing*, 35(4), 440.

McCreery, R.W., Venediktov, R.A., Coleman, J.J., & Leech, H.M. (2012). An evidence-based systematic review of frequency lowering in hearing aids for school-age children with hearing loss. *American Journal of Audiology*, 21(2), 313–328.

McDermott, H. J., Lech, M., Kornblum, M. S., & Irvine, D. R. (1998). Loudness perception and frequency discrimination in subjects with steeply sloping hearing loss: Possible correlates of neural plasticity. *Journal of the Acoustical Society of America*, 104(4), 2314–2325.

McFadden, B., & Pittman, A. (2008). Effect of minimal hearing loss on children's ability to multitask in quiet and in noise. *Language, Speech, and Hearing Services in Schools*, 39(3), 342–351.

McGarrigle, R., Munro, K. J., Dawes, P., Stewart, A. J., Moore, D. R., Barry, J. G., & Amitay, S. (2014). Listening effort and fatigue: What exactly are we measuring? A British Society of Audiology Cognition in Hearing Special Interest Group "white paper." *International Journal of Audiology*, 53(7), 433–440.

McLeod, B., Upfold, L., & Broadbend, C. (2001). An investigation of the applicability of the inventory, Satisfaction of Amplification in Daily Life, at 2 weeks post hearing aid fitting. *Ear and Hearing*, 22(4), 342–347.

McShefferty, D., Whitmer, W. M., & Akeroyd, M. A. (2014, August). *On meaningful increase in signal-to-noise ratio*. Podium presentation at International Hearing Aid Research Conference, Tahoe City, CA.

McShefferty, D., Whitmer, W. M., & Akeroyd, M. A. (2015). The just-noticeable difference in speech-to-noise ratio. *Trends in Hearing*, 19, 2331216515572316.

Mejia, J., Carter, L., Dillon, H., & Littmann, V. (2017). Listening effort, speech intelligibility, and narrow directionality. *Hearing Review*. Retrieved from http://www.hearingreview.com/2017/01/listening-effort-speech-intelligibility-narrow-directionality/

Mejia, J., Dillon, H., Van Hoesel, R., Beach, E., Glyde, H., Yeend, I., . . . & Sharma, M. (2015, December). Loss of speech perception in noise—causes and compensation. In *Proceedings of the International Symposium on Auditory and Audiological Research* (Vol. 5, pp. 205–216).

Meyers, M., & Smith, B. D. (1986). Hemispheric asymmetry and emotion: Effects of nonverbal affective stimuli. *Biological Psychology*, 22(1), 11–22.

Mid-Atlantic Addiction Technology Transfer Center. *Motivational interviewing*. Retrieved from http://motivationalinterview.org/

Miles, R. N., & Hoy, R. R. (2006). The development of a biologically-inspired directional microphone for hearing aids. *Audiology and Neurotology*, 11(2), 86–94.

Miller, C. W., Bates, E., & Brennan, M. (2016). The effects of frequency lowering on speech perception in noise with adult hearing-aid users. *International Journal of Audiology*, 55(5), 305–312.

Miller, J. D., Watson, C. S., Kewley-Port, D., Sillings, R., Mills, W. F., & Burleson, D. F. (2008). SPATS: Speech Perception Training and Assessment System. In *Proceedings of Meetings on Acoustics* (Vol. 2, No. 05005, p. 17).

Miller, J. D., Watson, C. S., Kistler, D. J., Preminger, J. E., & Wark, D. J. (2008b). Training listeners to identify the sounds of speech: II. Using SPATS software. *Hearing Journal*, 61(10), 29–33.

Miller, W. R., & Rollnick, S. (2002). *Motivational interviewing: Preparing people for change* (2nd ed.). New York, NY: Guilford Press.

Moncur, J. P., & Dirks, D. (1967). Binaural and monaural speech intelligibility in reverberation. *Journal of Speech and Hearing Research*, 10(2), 186–195.

Montgomery, A. (1995). Treatment efficacy in adult audiological rehabilitation. *Journal of the Academy of Rehabilitative Audiology*, 27(16), 317–336.

Moodie, K. S., Seewald, R. C., & Sinclair, S. T. (1994). Procedure for predicting real-ear hearing aid performance in young children. *American Journal of Audiology*, 3(1), 23–31.

Moore, B. C. (1989). *An introduction to the psychology of hearing*. London, UK: Academic Press.

Moore, B. C. J. (2007). Binaural sharing of audio signals: Prospective benefits and limitations. *Hearing Journal, 60*(11), 46–48.

Moore, B. C. J. (2010). Testing for cochlear dead regions: Audiometer implementation of the TEN (HL) test. *Hearing Review, 17*(1), 10–16, 48.

Moore, B. C. (2012). Effects of bandwidth, compression speed, and gain at high frequencies on preferences for amplified music. *Trends in Amplification, 16*(3), 159–172.

Moore, B. C. J., Creeke, S., Glasberg, B. R., Stone, M. A., & Sek, A. (2012). A version of the TEN test for use with the ER-3A insert earphones. *Ear and Hearing, 33*(4), 554–557.

Moore, B. C. J., Glasberg, B. R., & Stone, M. A. (2004). New version of the TEN test with calibrations in dB HL. *Ear and Hearing, 25*(5), 478–487.

Moore, B. C., Glasberg, B. R., & Stone, M. A. (2010). Development of a new method for deriving initial fittings for hearing aids with multi-channel compression: CAMEQ2-HF. *International Journal of Audiology, 49*(3), 216–227.

Moore, B. C. J., Huss, M., Vickers, D. A., Glasberg, B. R., & Alcántara, J. I. (2000). A test for the diagnosis of dead regions in the cochlea. *British Journal of Audiology, 34*(4), 205–224.

Moore, B. C., Stone, M. A., & Alcántara, J. I. (2002). Comparison of the electroacoustic characteristics of five hearing aids. *International Journal of Audiology, 41*(6), 371–373.

Moore, B. C. J., & Tan, C. T. (2003). Perceived naturalness of spectrally distorted speech and music. *Journal of the Acoustical Society of America, 114*(1), 408–419.

Morgan, S., & Raspet, R. (1992). Investigation of the mechanisms of low-frequency wind noise generation outdoors. *Journal of the Acoustical Society of America, 92*(2), 1180–1183.

Mormer, E., & Palmer, C. V. (2001, April). *Reliability of hearing aid expectation responses.* Paper presented at the annual meeting of the American Academy of Audiology. San Diego, CA.

Moryl, C. L., Danhauer, J. L., & DiBartolomeo, J. R. (1992). Real-ear unaided responses in ears with tympanic membrane perforations. *Journal of the American Academy of Audiology, 3*(1), 60–65.

MRC Institute of Hearing Research. (1999). *GHABP-information package.* Retrieved from http://www.ihr.mrc.ac.uk/index.php/products/display/questionnaires

Mueller, H. G. (1985). Evaluation of central auditory function: Monosyllabic procedures. In J. Katz (Ed.), *Handbook of clinical audiology* (3rd ed., pp. 355–382). Baltimore, MD: Lippincott Williams & Wilkins.

Mueller, H. G. (1990). Probe tube microphone measures: Some opinions on terminology and procedures. *Hearing Journal, 41*(1), 1–5.

Mueller, H. G. (1992). Terminology and procedures. In H. Mueller, D. Hawkins, & J. Northern (Eds.), *Probe microphone measures* (pp. 41–66). San Diego, CA: Singular.

Mueller, H. G. (1994a). CIC hearing aids: What is their impact on the occlusion effect? *Hearing Journal, 47*(11), 29–35.

Mueller, H. G. (1994b). Getting ready for the IHAFF protocol. *Hearing Journal, 47*(6), 10, 46–48.

Mueller, H. G. (1994c). Small can be good too! *Hearing Journal, 47*(11), 11–12.

Mueller, H. G. (1995). Probe-microphone measurements: Unplugged. *Hearing Journal, 48*(1), 10–34.

Mueller, H. G. (1999). Experts debate key fitting issues. *Hearing Journal, 52*(10), 21–32.

Mueller, H. G. (2001). Probe-mic assessment of digital hearing aids? Yes, you can!! *Hearing Journal, 54*(1), 10–12.

Mueller, H. G. (2003a). Fitting test protocols. *Hearing Journal, 56*(10), 19–26.

Mueller, H. G. (2003b). There's less talking in barrels, but the occlusion effect is still with us. *Hearing Journal, 56*(1), 10–18.

Mueller, H. G. (2003c). In the words of Shakespeare: Fitting test protocols are "more honored in the breach than the observance." *Hearing Journal, 56*(10), 19–20.

Mueller, H. G. (2005a). Fitting hearing aids to adults using prescriptive methods: An evidence-based review of effectiveness. *Journal of the American Academy of Audiology, 16*(7), 448–460.

Mueller, H. G. (2005b). Probe-mic measures: Hearing aid fitting's most neglected element. *Hearing Journal, 58*(10), 21–22.

Mueller, H. G. (2006). Hearing aid verification: Old concepts and new considerations. In C. Palmer & R. Staefa Seewald (Eds.), *Hearing care for adults* (pp. 155–165). Stäfa, Switzerland: Phonak AG.

Mueller, H. G. (2007). Data logging: It's popular, but how can this feature be used to help patients? *Hearing Journal, 60*(10), 19–26.

Mueller, H. G. (2009). A candid round table discussion on open-canal fittings. *Hearing Journal, 62*(4), 19–26.

Mueller, H. G. (2010). Three pre-tests: What they do and why experts say you should use them more. *Hearing Journal, 63*(4), 17–23.

Mueller, H. G. (2014a). 20Q: Real-ear probe-microphone measures—30 years of progress? *Audiology Online,* Article #12410. Retrieved from http://www.audiologyonline.com

Mueller, H. G. (2014b). Trainable hearing aids—Friend or foe for the clinician? *Audiology Online*, Article #12774. Retrieved from http://www.audiologyonline.com

Mueller, H. G. (2015). 20Q: Today's use of validated prescriptive methods for fitting hearing aids—What would Denis say? *Audiology Online*. Retrieved from http://www.audiologyonline.com

Mueller, H. G. (2016) Speech-in-noise testing for selection and fitting of hearing aids: Worth the effort? *Audiology Online*, Article 18336. Retrieved from http://www.audiologyonline.com

Mueller, H. G., Alexander, J. M., & Scollie, S. (2013). 20Q: Frequency lowering—The whole shebang. *Audiology Online*, Article #11913. Retrieved from http://www.audiologyonline.com/articles/20q-frequency-lowering-whole-shebang-11913

Mueller, H. G., & Bentler, R. A. (1994). Measurements of TD: How loud is allowed? *Hearing Journal*, 47(1), 10, 42–46.

Mueller, H. G., & Bentler, R. A. (2002). How loud is allowed? *Hearing Journal*, 52(1), 10–17.

Mueller, H. G., & Bentler, R. A. (2005). Fitting hearing aids using clinical measures of loudness discomfort levels: An evidence-based review of effectiveness. *Journal of the American Academy of Audiology*, 16(7), 461–472.

Mueller, H. G., & Bentler, R. A. (2008). How loud is allowed? It's a three-peat! *Hearing Journal*, 61(4), 10–15.

Mueller, H. G., Bentler, R. A., & Wu, Y. H. (2008). Prescribing maximum hearing aid output: Differences among manufacturers found. *Hearing Journal*, 61(3), 30–36.

Mueller, H. G., & Bright, K. E. (1994). Selection and verification of maximum output. In M. Valente (Ed.), *Strategies for selecting and verifying hearing aid fittings*. New York, NY: Thieme Medical.

Mueller, H. G., Bright, K. E., & Northern, J. L. (1996). Studies of the hearing aid occlusion effect. *Seminars in Hearing*, 17(1), 21–32.

Mueller, H. G., & Ebinger, K. A. (1996). CIC hearing aids: Potential benefits and fitting strategies. *Seminars in Hearing*, 17(1), 29–35.

Mueller, H. G., & Ebinger, K. A. (1997). Verification of the performance of CIC hearing aids. In M. Chasin (Ed.), *CIC handbook* (pp. 101–126). San Diego, CA: Singular.

Mueller, H. G., & Hall, J. W. (1998). *Audiologists' desk reference* (Vol. 2). San Diego, CA: Singular.

Mueller, H. G., & Hawkins, D. B. (1992). Assessment of fitting arrangements, special circuitry, and features. In H. G. Mueller, D. B. Hawkins, & J. L. Northern (Eds.), *Probe microphone measurements* (pp. 201–226). San Diego, CA: Singular.

Mueller, H. G., & Hawkins, D. B. (2006). Trouble-shooting hearing aid fitting issues: The case of the missing ping. *Hearing Journal*, 59(1), 10–17.

Mueller, H. G., Hawkins, D. B., & Northern, J. L. (1992). *Probe microphone measurements: Hearing aid selection and assessment*. San Diego, CA: Singular.

Mueller, H. G., & Hornsby, B. (2002). Selection, verification and validation of maximum output. In M. Valente (Ed.), *Strategies for selecting and verifying hearing aid fittings* (pp. 23–66). New York, NY: Thieme Medical.

Mueller, H. G., & Hornsby, B. (2014). Trainable hearing aids: The influence of previous use-gain. *Audiology Online*. Retrieved from http://www.audiologyonline.com/articles/trainable-hearing-aidsthe-influence--12764

Mueller, H. G., Hornsby, B. W., & Weber, J. E. (2008). Using trainable hearing aids to examine real-world preferred gain. *Journal of the American Academy of Audiology*, 19(10), 758–773.

Mueller, H. G., & Johnson, E. E. (2013). Hearing aids. In S. Kramer (Ed.), *Audiology: Science to practice* (2nd ed., pp. 287–320). San Diego, CA: Plural.

Mueller, H. G., Johnson, E. E., & Weber, J. (2010). Fitting hearing aids: A comparison of three pre-fitting speech tests (Article 2332). Retrieved from http://www.audiologyonline.com

Mueller, H. G., & Johnson, R. M. (1979). The effects of various front-to-back ratios on the performance of directional microphone hearing aids. *Ear and Hearing*, 5(1), 30–34.

Mueller, H. G., & Killion, M. C. (1990). An easy method for calculation the articulation index. *Hearing Journal*, 43(9), 14–17.

Mueller, H. G., & Palmer, C. V. (1998). The profile of aided loudness: A new "PAL" for '98. *Hearing Journal*, 51(1), 10–19.

Mueller, H. G., & Picou, E. M. (2010). Survey examines popularity of real-ear probe-microphone measures. *Hearing Journal*, 63(5), 27–28.

Mueller, H. G., & Powers, T. A. (2001). Consideration of auditory acclimatization in the prescriptive fitting of hearing aids. *Seminars in Hearing*, 22(2), 103–124.

Mueller, H. G., & Ricketts, T. A. (2005). Digital noise reduction: Much ado about something? *Hearing Journal*, 58(1), 10–18.

Mueller, H. G., & Ricketts, T. A. (2006). Open-canal fittings: Ten take-home tips. *Hearing Journal*, 59(11), 24–39.

Mueller, H. G., Ricketts, T. A., & Bentler, R. A. (2014). *Modern hearing aids: Pre-fitting testing and selection considerations*. San Diego, CA: Plural.

Mueller, H. G., Ricketts, T. A., & Bentler, R. A. (2017). *Speech mapping and probe microphone measurements*. San Diego, CA: Plural.

Mueller, H. G., & Strouse, A. L. (1995). Survey shows that user judgment remains dispensers' favorite fitting procedure. *Hearing Journal*, 48(10) 25–31.

Mueller, H. G., & Sweetow, R. W. (1987). A clinical comparison of probe microphone systems. *Hearing Instruments, 38*, 19–21, 57.

Mueller, H. G., Weber, J., Bellanova, M. (2011). Clinical evaluation of a new hearing aid anti-cardioid directivity pattern. *International Journal of Audiology, 50*(4), 249–254.

Mueller, H. G., Weber, J., & Hornsby, B. W. (2006). The effects of digital noise reduction on the acceptance of background noise. *Trends in Amplification, 10*(2), 83–93.

Munro, K. J., & Davis, J. (2003). Deriving the real-ear SPL of audiometric data using the "coupler to dial difference" and the "real ear to coupler difference." *Ear and Hearing, 24*(2), 100–110.

Munro, K. J, & Millward, K. E. (2006). The influence of the RECD transducer when deriving the real-ear sound pressure level. *Ear and Hearing, 27*(4), 409–423.

Munro, K. J., & Patel, R. (1998). Are clinical measurements of uncomfortable loudness levels a valid indicator of real-world auditory discomfort? *British Journal of Audiology, 32*(5), 287–293.

Munro, K. J., & Toal, S. (2005). Measuring the real-ear to coupler difference transfer function with an insert earphone and a hearing instrument: Are they the same? *Ear and Hearing, 26*(1), 27–34.

Munro, K. J., & Trotter, J. H. (2006). Preliminary evidence of asymmetry in uncomfortable loudness levels after unilateral hearing aid experience: Evidence of functional plasticity in the adult auditory system. *International Journal of Audiology, 45*(12), 684–688.

Munro, M. J., & Derwing, T. M. (2011). The foundations of accent and intelligibility in pronunciation research. *Language Teaching, 44*(3), 316–327.

Murray, M., Popelka, G. R., & Miller, R. (2011). Efficacy and safety of an in-the-mouth bone conduction device for single-sided deafness. *Otology and Neurology, 32*(3), 437–443.

Musiek, F. E. (1983). Assessment of central auditory dysfunction: The dichotic digit test revisited. *Ear and Hearing, 4*(2), 79–83.

Mynders, J. M. (2003). Essentials of hearing aid selection, Part 2: It's in the numbers. *Hearing Review, 10*(11).

Mynders, J. M. (2004). Essentials of hearing aid selection, Part 3: Perception is reality. *Hearing Review, 11*(2).

Nabelek, A. K., Freyaldenhoven, M. C., Tampas, J. W., Burchfield, S. B., & Muenchen, R. A. (2006). Acceptable noise level as a predictor of hearing aid use. *Journal of the American Academy of Audiology, 17*(9), 626–639.

Nabelek, A. K., Tampas, J. W., & Burchfield, S. B. (2004). Comparison of speech perception in background noise with acceptance of background in aided and unaided conditions. *Journal of Speech, Language, and Hearing Research, 47*(5), 1001–1011.

Nabelek, A. K., Tucker, F. M., & Letowski, T. R. (1991). Toleration of background noises: Relationship with patterns of hearing aid use by elderly persons. *Journal of Speech and Hearing Research, 34*(3), 679–685.

Nachtegaal, J., Kuik, D. J., Anema, J. R., Goverts, S. T., Festen, J. M., & Kramer, S. E. (2009). Hearing status, need for recovery after work, and psychosocial work characteristics: Results from an internet-based national survey on hearing. *International Journal of Audiology, 48*(10), 684–691.

Nair, E. L., & Cienkowski, K. M. (2010). The impact of health literacy on patient understanding of counseling and education materials. *International Journal of Audiology, 49*(2), 71–75.

Neel, A. T. (2008). Vowel space characteristics and vowel identification accuracy. *Journal of Speech, Language, and Hearing Research, 51*(3), 574–585.

Newman, C. W., Jacobson, G. P., Hug, G. A., & Sandridge, S. A. (1997). Perceived hearing handicap of patients with unilateral or mild hearing loss. *Annals of Otology, Rhinology, and Laryngology, 106*(3), 210–214.

Newman, C. W., Jacobson, G. P., & Spitzer, J. B. (1996). Development of the tinnitus handicap inventory. *Archives of Otolaryngology–Head and Neck Surgery, 122*(2), 143–148.

Newman, C. W., & Weinstein, B. E. (1986). Judgments of perceived hearing handicap by hearing-impaired elderly men and their spouses. *Journal of the Academy of Rehabilitative Audiology, 19*(2), 109–115.

Newman, C. W., Weinstein, B. E., Jacobson, G. P., & Hug, G. A. (1990). The Hearing Handicap Inventory for Adults: Psychometric adequacy and audiometric correlates. *Ear and Hearing, 11*(6), 430–433.

Newman, C. W., Weinstein, B. E., Jacobson, G. P., & Hug, G. A. (1991). Test-retest reliability of the Hearing Handicap Inventory for Adults. *Ear and Hearing, 12*(5), 355–357.

Ng, E. H. N., Rudner, M., Lunner, T., Pedersen, M. S., & Rönnberg, J. (2013). Effects of noise and working memory capacity on memory processing of speech for hearing-aid users. *International Journal of Audiology, 52*(7), 433–441.

Ng, E. H. N., Rudner, M., Lunner, T., & Rönnberg. J. (2015). Noise reduction improves memory for target language speech in competing native but not foreign language speech. *Ear and Hearing, 36*(1), 82–91.

NIDCD (2016). Quick statistics about hearing. *National Institute on Deafness and Other Communication Disorders*. Retrieved from https://www.nidcd.nih.gov/health/statistics/quick-statistics-hearing

Nielsen, H. B., & Rasmussen, S. B. (1984). New aspects in hearing aid fittings. *Hearing Instruments, 35*(1), 18–20.

Nilsson, M. J., & Soli, S. D. (1994). Norms for a headphone simulation of the hearing in noise test: Comparison of physical and simulated spatial separation of sound sources. *Journal of the Acoustical Society of America, 95*(5), 2994.

Nilsson, M., Soli, S. D., & Sullivan, J. A. (1994). Development of the hearing in noise test for the measurement of speech reception thresholds in quiet and noise. *Journal of the Acoustical Society of America, 95*(2), 1085–1099.

Niparko, J. K., Cox, K. M., Lustig, L. R. (2003). Comparison of the bone anchored hearing aid implantable hearing device with contralateral routing of signal of offside signal amplification in the rehabilitation of unilateral deafness. *Otology and Neurotology, 24*(1), 73–78.

Noble, W. (2002). Extending the IOI to significant others and nonhearing-aid-based intervention. *International Journal of Audiology, 41*(1), 27–29.

Noble, W., Byrne, D., & LePage, B. (1994). Effects on sound localization of configuration and type of hearing impairment. *Journal of the Acoustical Society of America, 95*(2), 992–1005.

Noble, W., & Gatehouse, S. (2006). Effects of bilateral versus unilateral hearing aid fitting on abilities measured by the speech, spatial and qualities of hearing scale (SSQ). *International Journal of Audiology, 45*(3), 172–181.

Noble, W., Jensen, N. S., Naylor, G., Bhullar, N., & Akeroyd, M. A. (2013). A short form of the speech, spatial and qualities of hearing scale suitable for clinical use: The SSQ12. *International Journal of Audiology, 52*(6), 409–412.

Norrix, L. W., Camarota, K., Harris, F. P., & Dean, J. (2016). The effects of FM and hearing aid microphone settings, FM gain, and ambient noise levels on SNR at the tympanic membrane. *Journal of the American Academy of Audiology, 27*(2), 117–25.

Nunley, J., Staab, W., Steadman, J., Wechsler, P., & Spenser, B. (1983). A wearable digital hearing aid. *Hearing Journal, 36*(10), 29–35.

O'Brien, A., Keidser, G., Yeend, I., Hartley, L., & Dillon, H. (2010). Validity and reliability of in-situ air conduction thresholds measures through hearing aids coupled to closed and open instant-fit tips. *International Journal of Audiology, 49*(12), 868–876.

Oliveira, R. J. (1997). The active earcanal. *Journal of the American Academy of Audiology, 8*(6), 401–410.

Olsen, S. Ø., & Brännström, K. J. (2014). Does the acceptable noise level (ANL) predict hearing-aid use? *International Journal of Audiology, 53*(1), 2–20.

Olson, A. D., Preminger, J. E., & Shinn, J. B. (2013). The effect of LACE DVD training in new and experienced hearing aid users. *Journal of the American Academy of Audiology, 24*(3), 214–230.

Owen, J. H. (1981). Influence of acoustical and linguistic factors on the SPIN test difference score. *Journal of the Acoustical Society of America, 70*(3), 678–682.

Padgett, D. K. (1998). *Qualitative methods in social work*. Thousand Oaks, CA: Sage.

Painton, S. W. (1993). Objective measure of low-frequency amplification reduction in canal hearing aids with adaptive circuitry. *Journal of the American Academy of Audiology, 4*(3), 152–156.

Palmer, C. V. (2009). Best practice: It's a matter of ethics. *Audiology Today, 21*(5), 31–35.

Palmer, C. V. (2012). Siemens Expert Series: Implementing a gain learning feature. *Audiology Online*, Article #11244. Retrieved from http://www.audiologyonline.com

Palmer, C., Bentler, R., & Mueller, H. G. (2006a). Evaluation of a second-order directional microphone hearing aid: II. Self-report outcomes. *Journal of the American Academy of Audiology, 17*(3), 190–201.

Palmer, C. V., Bentler, R., & Mueller, H. G. (2006b). Amplification with digital noise reduction and the perception of annoying and aversive sounds. *Trends in Amplification, 10*(2), 95–104.

Palmer, C. V., Killion, M. C., Wilber, L. A., & Ballad, W. J. (1995). Comparison of two hearing aid receiver-amplifier combinations using sound quality judgments. *Ear and Hearing, 16*(6), 587–598.

Palmer, C. V., & Lindley, G. (1998). Reliability of the contour test in a population of adults with hearing loss. *Journal of the American Academy of Audiology, 9*(3), 209–215.

Palmer, C. V., Mormer, E., Ortmann, A., Byrne, D., Ye, Y., & Keogh, L. (2008). Is it REAL? Research evaluation of audiology literature. *Hearing Journal, 61*(10), 17–28.

Palmer, C. V., & Mueller, H. G. (2000). Hearing aid selection and assessment. In J. G. Alpiner & P. A. McCarthy (Eds.), *Rehabilitative audiology, children and adults* (pp. 332–376). Baltimore, MD: Lippincott Williams & Wilkins.

Palmer, C. V., Mueller, H. G., & Moriarty, M. (1999). Profile of aided loudness: A validation procedure. *Hearing Journal, 52*(6), 34–42.

Palmer, C. V., Solodar, H. S., Hurley, W. R., Byrne, D. C., & Williams, K. O. (2009). Self-perception of hearing ability as a strong predictor of hearing aid purchase. *Journal of the American Academy of Audiology, 20*(6), 341–347.

Parbery-Clark, A., Strait, D. L., Anderson, S., Hittner, E., & Kraus, N. (2011). Musical experience and the aging auditory system: Implications for cognitive abilities and hearing speech in noise. *PLoS One, 6*(5), e18082.

Parsa, V. (2006). Acoustic feedback and its reduction through digital signal processing. *Hearing Journal*, 59(11), 16–23.

Parsa, V., Scollie, S., Glista, D., & Seelisch, A. (2013). Non-linear frequency compression: effects on sound quality ratings of speech and music. *Trends in Amplification*, 17(1), 54–68.

Partala, T., & Surakka, B. (2003). Pupil size variation as an indication of affective processing. *International Journal of Human-Computer Studies*, 59(1), 185–198.

Pascoe, D. (1975). Frequency responses of hearing aids and their effects on the speech perception of hearing-impaired subjects. *Annals of Otology, Rhinology, and Laryngology*, 84(Pt. 5, Suppl. 23), 1–40.

Pascoe, D. P. (1978). An approach to hearing aid selection. *Hearing Instruments*, 29(6), 12–16, 36.

Pascoe, D. P. (1980). Clinical implications of nonverbal methods of hearing aid selection and fitting. *Seminars in Hearing*, 1(3), 217–228.

Pascoe, D. P. (1988). Clinical measurements of the auditory range and their relation to formulas for hearing aid gain. In J. Jensen (Ed.), *Hearing aid fittings: Theoretical and practical views*. 13th Danavox Symposium. (pp. 129–152), Copenhagen, Denmark: Stongaard Jensen.

Pavlovic, C. V. (1984). Use of the articulation index for assessing residual auditory function in listeners with sensorineural hearing impairment. *Journal of the Acoustical Society of America*, 75(4), 1253–1258.

Pavlovic, C. V. (1987). Derivation of primary parameters and procedures for use in speech intelligibility predictions. *Journal of the Acoustical Society of America*, 83(2), 413–422.

Pavlovic, C. V. (1988). Articulation index predictions of speech intelligibility in hearing aid selection. *ASHA*, 30(6/7), 63–65.

Pavlovic, C. V. (1989). Speech spectrum considerations and speech intelligibility predictions in hearing aid evaluations. *Journal of Speech and Hearing Disorders*, 54(1), 3–8.

Pavlovic, C. V. (1991). Speech recognition and five articulation indexes. *Hearing Instruments*, 42(9), 20–24.

Pavlovic, C. V. (1993). Problems in the prediction of speech recognition performance of normal-hearing and hearing impaired individuals. In G. A. Studebaker & I. Hochberg (Eds.), *Acoustical factors affecting hearing aid performance* (2nd ed., pp. 221–234). Boston, MA: Allyn & Bacon.

Pavlovic, C. V., & Studebaker, G. A. (1984). An evaluation of some assumptions underlying the articulation index. *Journal of the Acoustical Society of America*, 75(5), 1606–1612.

Pavlovic, C. V., Studebaker, G. A., & Sherbecoe, R. (1986). An articulation index-based procedure for predicting the speech recognition performance of hearing-impaired individuals. *Journal of the Acoustical Society of America*, 80(1), 50–57.

Pearsons, K. S., Bennett, R. L., & Fidell, S. (1977). *Speech levels in various noise environments* (Report No. EPA-600/1-77-025). Washington, DC: U.S. Environmental Protection Agency.

Peterson, G. E., & Lehiste, I. (1962). Revised CNC lists for auditory tests. *Journal of Speech and Hearing Disorders*, 27(1), 62–70.

Peutz, V. (1971). Articulation loss of consonants as a criterion for speech transmission in a room. *Journal of the Audio Engineering Society*, 19(11), 915–919.

Pichora-Fuller, M. K. (2003). Processing speed and timing in aging adults: Psychoacoustics, speech perception, and comprehension. *International Journal of Audiology*, 42, S59–S67.

Pichora-Fuller, M. K., & Benguerel, A. P. (1991). The design of CAST (computer-aided speechreading training). *Journal of Speech, Language, and Hearing Research*, 34(1), 202–212.

Pichora-Fuller, M. K., Kramer, S. E., Eckert, M. A., Edwards, B., Hornsby, B. W., Humes, L. E., . . . Naylor, G. (2016). Hearing impairment and cognitive energy: The framework for understanding effortful listening (FUEL). *Ear and Hearing*, 37, 5S–27S.

Pichora-Fuller, M. K., Schneider, B. A., & Daneman, M. (1995). How young and old adults listen to and remember speech in noise. *Journal of the Acoustical Society of America*, 97(1), 593–608.

Picou, E. M., Aspell, E., & Ricketts, T. A. (2014). Potential benefits and limitations of three types of directional processing in hearing aids. *Ear and Hearing*, 35(3), 339–352.

Picou, E. M., Gordon, J., & Ricketts, T. A. (2016). The effects of noise and reverberation on listening effort for adults with normal hearing. *Ear and Hearing*, 37(1), 1–13.

Picou, E. M., Marcrum, S., & Ricketts, T. A. (2015). Evaluation of the effects of non-linear frequency compression on speech recognition and sound quality for adults with mild to moderate hearing loss. *International Journal of Audiology*, 54(3), 162–169.

Picou, E. M., Moore, T. M., & Ricketts, T. A. (2017). The effects of directional processing on objective and subjective listening effort. *Journal of Speech, Language, and Hearing Research*, 60(1), 199–211.

Picou, E. M., & Ricketts, T. A. (2011). Comparison of wireless and acoustic hearing aid-based telephone listening strategies. *Ear and Hearing*, 32(2), 209–220.

Picou, E. M., & Ricketts, T. A. (2013). Efficacy of hearing-aid based telephone strategies for listeners with moderate-to-severe hearing loss. *Journal of the American Academy of Audiology, 24*(1), 59–70.

Picou, E. M., & Ricketts, T. A. (2014). The effect of changing the secondary task in dual-task paradigms for measuring listening effort. *Ear and Hearing, 35*(6), 611–622.

Picou, E. M. & Ricketts, T. A. (2014). Increasing motivation changes subjective reports of listening effort and choice of coping strategy. *International Journal of Audiology, 53*(6), 418–426.

Picou, E. M., & Ricketts, T. A. (2017). How directional microphones affect speech recognition, listening effort and localisation for listeners with moderate-to-severe hearing loss. *International Journal of Audiology*. Advance online publication. Retrieved from http://www.tandfonline.com/doi/full/10.1080/14992027.2017.1355074

Pirzanski, C. (1998). The anatomy of a perfect ear impression. *Hearing Review, 5*(12), 2–24.

Pirzanski, C. Z. (2003). Issues in earmold fitting and troubleshooting. *Seminars in Hearing, 24*(4), 355–363.

Pittman, A. (2011). Age-related benefits of digital noise reduction for short-term word learning in children with hearing loss. *Journal of Speech, Language, and Hearing Research, 54*(5), 1448–1463.

Plomp, R. (1976). Binaural and monaural speech intelligibility of connected discourse in reverberation as a function of azimuth of a single competing sound source (speech or noise). *Acustica, 34*(3), 200–211.

Plomp, R. (1978). Auditory handicap of hearing impairment and the limited benefit of hearing aids. *Journal of the Acoustical Society of America, 63*(2), 533–549.

Plomp, R. (1984). Perception of speech as a modulated signal. In A. Cohen & M. P. R. van de Broecke (Eds.), *Proceedings of the Tenth International Congress of Phonetic Sciences* (pp. 29–40). Dordrecht, The Netherlands: Foris.

Plomp, R. (1986). A signal-to-noise ratio model for the speech-reception threshold of the hearing impaired. *Journal of Speech and Hearing Research, 29*(2), 146–154.

Plomp, R., & Mimpen, A. M. (1979). Speech-reception threshold for sentences as a function of age and noise level. *Journal of the Acoustical Society of America, 66*(5), 1333–1342.

Plyler, P. N. (2009). Acceptance of background noise: Recent developments. *Hearing Journal, 62*(4), 10–17.

Plyler, P. (2015). 20Q: Acceptable Noise Level Test—Supporting research and clinical insights. *Audiology Online.* Retrieved from http://www.audiologyonline.com/articles/20q-acceptable-noise-test-research-14692

Plyler, P. N., Reber, M. B., Kovach, A., Galloway, E., & Humphrey, E. (2013). Comparison of multichannel wide dynamic range compression and ChannelFree processing in open canal hearing instruments. *Journal of the American Academy of Audiology, 24*(2), 126–137.

Pols, L. C., van der Kamp, L. J., & Plomp, R. (1969). Perceptual and physical space of vowel sounds. *Journal of the Acoustical Society of America, 46*(2), 458–467.

Powers, T. A., & Burton, P. (2005). Wireless technology designed to provide true binaural amplification. *Hearing Journal, 58*(1), 25–34.

Powers, T., & Littmann, V. (2016). Benefits of binaural beamforming for individuals with severe hearing loss. *Hearing Review, 23*(5), 28.

Preminger, J. E. (2003). Should significant others be encouraged to join adult group audiologic rehabilitation classes? *Journal of the Acoustical Society of America, 116*(1), 49–50.

Preminger, J. E., (2009). Audiologic rehabilitation with adults & significant others: Is it really worth it? *Audiology Online.* Retrieved from http://www.audiologyonline.com/articles/audiologic-rehabilitation-with-adults-significant-882

Preminger, J. E., Carpenter, R., & Ziegler, C. H. (2005). A clinical perspective on cochlear dead regions: Intelligibility of speech and subjective hearing aid benefit. *Journal of the American Academy of Audiology, 16*(8), 600–613.

Preminger, J. E., & Yoo, J. K. (2010). Do group audiologic rehabilitation activities influence psychosocial outcomes? *American Journal of Audiology, 19*(2), 109–125.

Preminger, J. E., & Ziegler, C. H. (2008). Can auditory and visual speech perception be trained within a group setting? *American Journal of Audiology, 17*(1), 80–97.

President's Council of Advisors on Science and Technology. (2015, October 26). *PCAST recommends changes to promote innovation in hearing technologies.* Retrieved from https://obamawhitehouse.archives.gov/blog/2015/10/26/%E2%80%8Bpcast-recommends-changes-promote-innovation-hearing-technologies

Preves, D. A., & Curran, J. R. (2000). Hearing aid instrumentation and procedures for electroacoustic testing. In M. Valente, H. Hosford-Dunn, & R. J. Roeser (Eds.), *Audiology treatment* (pp. 1–58). New York, NY: Thieme Medical.

Preves, D. A., Sammeth, C. A., & Wynne, M. K. (1999). Field trial evaluations of a switched directional/omnidirectional in-the-ear hearing instrument. *Journal of the American Academy of Audiology, 10*(5), 273–284.

Pumford, J. (2005). Benefits of probe-mic measures with CROS/BiCROS fittings. *Hearing Journal, 58*(10), 34–40.

Pumford, J. M., Seewald, R. C., Scollie, S. D., & Jenstad, L. M. (2000). Speech recognition with in-the-ear and behind-the-ear dual-microphone hearing instruments.

Journal of the American Academy of Audiology, 11(1), 23–35.

Rabiner, L. R., & Gold, B. (1975). *Theory and Application of Digital Signal Processing.* Englewood Cliffs, NJ: Prentice-Hall.

Rankovic, C. M. (1991). An application of the articulation index to hearing aid fitting. *Journal of Speech and Hearing Research, 34*(2), 391–402.

Reed, N. S., Betz J., Kendig, N., Korczak, M., & Lin, F. R. (2017). Personal sound amplification products vs a conventional hearing aid for speech understanding in noise. *JAMA, 318*(1), 89–90.

Rehmann, J., Siddhartha, J., & Baumann, S. A. (2016). SoundRecover2—The adaptive frequency compression algorithm: More audibility of high frequency sounds. *Phonak Insight* (Phonak AG, Stäfa, Switzerland).

Resnick, D. M., & Becker, M. (1963). Hearing aid evaluation: A new approach. *ASHA, 5,* 695–699.

Revit, L. J. (1997). The circle of decibels: Relating the hearing test, to the hearing aid, to the real-ear response. *Hearing Review, 4*(11), 35–38.

Revit, L. J. (2000). Real-ear measures. In M. Valente, H. Hosford-Dunn, R. J. Roeser (Eds.), *Audiology treatment* (pp. 105–148). New York, NY: Thieme Medical.

Richards, V. M., Moore, B. C. J., & Lauer, S. (2006). Potential benefits of across-aid communication for bilaterally aided people: Listening in a car. *International Journal of Audiology, 45*(3), 182–189.

Ricketts, T. A. (1996). Fitting hearing aids to individual loudness-perception measures. *Ear and Hearing, 17*(2), 124–132.

Ricketts, T. A. (2000a). Directivity quantification in hearing aids: Fitting and measurement effects. *Ear and Hearing, 21*(1), 45–58.

Ricketts T. A. (2000b). The impact of head angle on monaural and binaural performance with directional and omnidirectional hearing aids. *Ear and Hearing, 21*(4), 318–329.

Ricketts, T. A. (2012, May). *What's new in directional hearing aid technology: Clinical applications and pitfalls.* Invited presentation for the New Zealand Audiological Society, Hamilton, NZ.

Ricketts, T. A., & Bentler, R. A. (1992). Comparison of two digitally programmable hearing aids. *Journal of the American Academy of Audiology, 3*(2), 101–112.

Ricketts, T. A., & Bentler, R. A. (1996). The effect of test signal type and bandwidth on the categorical scaling of loudness. *Journal of the Acoustical Society of America, 99*(4), 2281–2287.

Ricketts, T. A., & Dittberner, A. B. (2002). Directional amplification for improved signal-to-noise ratio: Strategies, measurement, and limitations. In M. Valente (Ed.), *Hearing aids: Standards, options, and limitations* (2nd ed., pp. 274–346). New York, NY: Thieme Medical.

Ricketts, T. A., Dittberner, A. B., & Johnson, E. E. (2008). High-frequency amplification and sound quality in listeners with normal through moderate hearing loss. *Journal of Speech, Language, and Hearing Research, 51*(1), 160–72.

Ricketts, T. A., & Galster, J. (2008). Head angle and elevation in classroom environments: Implications for amplification. *Journal of Speech, Language, and Hearing Research, 51*(2), 516–525.

Ricketts, T. A., Galster, J. A., & Tharpe, A. M. (2007). Directional benefit in simulated classroom environments. *American Journal of Audiology, 16*(2), 130–144.

Ricketts, T. A., & Henry, P. (2002). Low frequency gain compensation in directional hearing aids. *American Journal of Audiology, 11*(1), 29–41.

Ricketts, T. A., Henry, P., & Gnewikow, D. (2003). Full time directional versus user selectable microphone modes in hearing aids. *Ear and Hearing, 24*(5), 424–439.

Ricketts, T. A., Henry, P., & Hornsby, B. W. Y. (2005). Application of frequency importance functions to directivity for prediction of benefit in uniform fields. *Ear and Hearing, 26*(5), 473–486.

Ricketts, T. A., & Hornsby, B. W. Y. (2003). Distance and reverberation effects on directional benefit. *Ear and Hearing, 24*(6), 472–84.

Ricketts, T. A., & Hornsby, B. W. (2005). Sound quality measures for speech in noise through a commercial hearing aid employing digital noise reduction. *Journal of the American Academy of Audiology, 16*(5), 270–277.

Ricketts, T. A., & Hornsby, B. W. Y. (2006). Directional hearing aid benefit in listeners with severe to profound hearing loss. *International Journal of Audiology, 45*(3), 190–197.

Ricketts, T. A., Johnson, E. E., & Federman, J. (2008). Individual differences within and across feedback suppression hearing aids. *Journal of the American Academy of Audiology, 19*(10), 748–757.

Ricketts, T. A., Lindley, G., & Henry, P. (2001). Impact of compression and hearing aid style on directional hearing aid benefit and performance. *Ear and Hearing, 22*(4), 348–361.

Ricketts, T. A., McCardle, R., Smith, S., Chisolm, T., & Bratt, G. (2011, March). *Open canal hearing aids: Tips and tricks for the clinic.* Invited presentation to the Military Audiology Association JDVAC Annual Convention, San Diego, CA.

Ricketts, T. A., & Mueller, H. G. (2014). When is the best time to activate the "training" feature in hearing aids?

Audiology Online, Ask the Expert 12350. Retrieved from http://www.audiologyonline.com

Ricketts, T. A., & Picou, E. (2013). Speech recognition for bilaterally asymmetric and symmetric hearing aid microphone modes in simulated classroom environments. *Ear and Hearing, 34*(5), 601–609.

Ricketts, T. A., Picou, E. M., & Galster, J. (2017). Directional microphone hearing aids in school environments: working toward optimization. *Journal of Speech, Language, and Hearing Research, 60*(1), 263–275.

Robey, R. (2004). Levels of evidence. *The ASHA Leader, 9*(5), 12–18.

Rochlin, G. D. (1993). Status of sound field audiometry among audiologists in the United States. *Journal of the American Academy of Audiology, 4*(2), 59–68.

Rodemerk, K. S., & Galster, J. A. (2015). The benefit of remote microphones using four wireless protocols. *Journal of the American Academy of Audiology, 26*(8), 724–731.

Romanow, F. (1942). Methods for measuring the performance of hearing aids. *Journal of the Acoustical Society of America, 13*(3), 294–304.

Rönnberg, J. (2003). Cognition in the hearing impaired and deaf as a bridge between signal and dialogue: A framework and a model. *International Journal of Audiology, 42*, S68–S76.

Rönnberg, J., Lunner, T., Zekveld, A., Sörqvist, P., Danielsson, H., Lyxell, B., . . . Rudner, M. (2013). The Ease of Language Understanding (ELU) model: Theoretical, empirical, and clinical advances. *Frontiers in Systems Neuroscience, 7*. Advance online publication. doi:10.3389/fnsys.2013.00031

Rönnberg, J., Rudner, M., Foo, C., & Lunner, T. (2008). Cognition counts: A working memory system for ease of language understanding (ELU). *International Journal of Audiology, 47*(S2), S99–S105.

Ross, M. (2002b). Telecoils: The powerful assistive listening device. *Hearing Review, 9*(9), 22–26, 57.

Ross, M. (2011, Jan/Feb). Is auditory training effective in improving listening skills? *Hearing Loss Magazine*, 25–27.

Rubinstein, A., & Boothroyd, A. (1987). Effect of two approaches to auditory training on speech recognition by hearing-impaired adults. *Journal of Speech, Language, and Hearing Research, 30*(2), 153–160.

Rudmose, W. (1982). The case of the missing 6 dB. *Journal of the Acoustical Society of America, 71*(3), 650–659.

Ruscetta, M. N., Palmer, C. V., Durant, J. D., Grayhack, J., & Ryan, C. (2005). Validity, internal consistency, and test-retest reliability of a localization disabilities and handicaps questionnaire. *Journal of the American Academy of Audiology, 16*(8), 585–595.

Sachs, R. M., & Burkhard, M. D. (1972). *Earphone pressure response in ears and couplers*. Report No. 20021-2. Elk Grove Village, IL: Industrial Research Products.

Sackett, D. L., Rosenberg, W. M. C., Gray, J. A. M., Haynes, R. B., & Richardson, W. S. (1996). Evidence-based medicine: What it is and what it isn't. *British Medical Journal, 312*(7023), 71–72.

Sanders, D. A. (1971). *Aural rehabilitation*. Englewood Cliffs, NJ: Prentice Hall.

Sanders, J., Stoody, T. M., Weber, J. E., & Mueller, H. G. (2015). Manufacturer's NAL-NL2 fittings fail real-ear verification. *Hearing Review, 21*(3), 24.

Sandridge, S. A., & Newman, C. W. (2006). Improving the efficiency and accountability of the hearing aid selection process—Use of the COAT. *Audiology Online*. Retrieved from http://www.audiologyonline.com/articles/article_detail.asp?article_id=1541

Sarampalis, A., Kalluri, S., Edwards, B., & Hafter, E. (2009). Objective measures of listening effort: Effects of background noise and noise reduction. *Journal of Speech, Language, and Hearing Research, 52*(5), 1230–1240.

Saunders, G. H. (2009). Understanding in noise: Perception vs. performance. *Hearing Journal, 62*(5), 10–16.

Saunders, G. H., Chisolm, T. H., & Wallhagen, M. I. (2012). Older adults and hearing help-seeking behaviors. *American Journal of Audiology, 21*(2), 331–337.

Saunders, G. H., & Forsline, A. (2006). The performance perceptual test (PPT) and its relationship to aided reported handicap and hearing aid satisfaction. *Ear and Hearing, 27*(3), 229–242.

Saunders, G. H., Forsline, A., & Fausti, S. (2004). The performance-perceptual test (PPT) and its relationship to unaided reported handicap. *Ear and Hearing, 25*(2), 117–126.

Saunders, G. H., & Morgan, D. E. (2003). Impact on hearing aid targets of measuring thresholds in dB HL versus dB SPL. *International Journal of Audiology, 42*(6), 319–326.

Scarinci, N., Worrall, L., & Hickson, L. (2008). The effect of hearing impairment in older people on the spouse. *International Journal of Audiology, 47*(3), 141–151.

Schafer, E. C., Pogue, J., & Milrany, T. (2012). List equivalency of the AzBio sentence test in noise for listeners with normal-hearing sensitivity or cochlear implants. *Journal of the American Academy of Audiology, 23*(7), 501–509.

Schmitt, N. (2004). *National Acoustic Laboratories Research & Development annual report 2003/2004: A new speech test (BEST test). Practical training report*. Sydney, Australia: National Acoustics Laboratory.

Schow, R. L., & Nerbonne, M. A. (1976). *Research reports, 1*. Pocatello, ID: Idaho State University Press.

Schow, R. L., & Nerbonne, M. A. (1977). Assessment of hearing handicap by nursing home residents and staff. *Journal of the Academy of Rehabilitative Audiology, 10*(2), 2–12.

Schow, R. L., & Nerbonne, M. A. (2012). *Introduction to audiologic rehabilitation* (6th ed.). London, UK: Allyn & Bacon.

Schum, D. (1996). Speech understanding in background noise. In M. Valente (Ed.), *Hearing aids: Standards, options, and limitations* (pp. 368–406). New York, NY: Thieme Medical.

Schum, D. J. (1999). Perceived hearing aid benefit in relation to perceived needs. *Journal of the American Academy of Audiology, 10*(1), 40–45.

Schum, D. J. (2001). Adaptation management for amplification. *Seminars in Hearing, 22*(2), 173–182.

Schwartz, D., Lyregaard, P., & Lundh, P. (1988). Hearing aid selection for severe-to-profound hearing loss. *Hearing Journal, 41*(2), 13–17.

Schwartz, K., & Cox, R. (2011, March). *Relationship between acceptable noise levels and hearing aid success*. Presented at the American Auditory Society Convention, Scottsdale, AZ.

Schwartz, K., & Cox, R. (2012, March). *Does acceptable noise level predict hearing aid success?* Presented at the American Auditory Society Convention, Scottsdale, AZ.

Schweitzer, H. C., Sullivan, R. F., Beck, L. B., & Cole, W. A. (1990). Developing a consensus for "real ear" hearing aid terms. *Hearing Instruments, 41*(2), 28, 46.

Scollie, S. (2007). DSL version v5.0: Description and early results in children. *Audiology Online.* Retrieved from http://www.audiologyonline.com/articles/dsl-version-v5-0-description-959

Scollie, S. (2013). 20Q: The ins and outs of frequency lowering amplification. *Audiology Online,* Article #11863. Retrieved from http://www.audiologyonline.com

Scollie, S. (2016). New RECDs and a new ANSI standard: Revisiting RECD basics and applications. *Audiology Online.* Retrieved from http://www.audiologyonline.com/articles/new-recds-and-ansi-standard-16380

Scollie, S., Bagatto, M., Moodie, S., & Crukley, J. (2011). Accuracy and reliability of a real-ear-to-coupler difference measurement procedure implemented within a behind-the-ear hearing aid. *Journal of the American Academy of Audiology, 22*(9), 612–622.

Scollie, S., Ching, T. Y., Seewald, R., Dillon, H., Britton, L., Steinberg, J., & Corcoran, J. (2010). Evaluation of the NAL-NL1 and DSL v4. 1 prescriptions for children: Preference in real world use. *International Journal of Audiology, 49*(S1), S49–S63.

Scollie, S., Glista, D., Seto, J., Dunn, A., Schuett, B., Hawkins, M., . . . Parsa, V. (2016). Fitting frequency-lowering signal processing applying the American Academy of Audiology pediatric amplification guideline: Updates and protocols. *Journal of the American Academy of Audiology, 27*(3), 219–236.

Scollie, S., Levy, C., Pourmand, N., Abbasalipour, P., Bagatto, M., Richert, . . . Parsa, V. (2016). Fitting noise management signal processing applying the American Academy of Audiology Pediatric Amplification Guideline: Verification protocols. *Journal of the American Academy of Audiology, 27*(3), 237–251.

Scollie, S., Seewald, R., Cornelisse, L., Moodie, S., Bagatto, M., Laurnagaray, D., . . . Pumford, J. (2005). The desired sensation level multistage input/output algorithm. *Trends in Amplification, 9*(4), 159–197.

Scollie, S. D., & Seewald, R. C. (2002). Evaluation of electroacoustic test signals I: Comparison with amplified speech. *Ear and Hearing, 23*(5), 477–487.

Scollie, S. D., Seewald, R. C., Moodie, K. S., & Dekok, K. (2000). Preferred listening levels of children who use hearing aids: Comparison to prescriptive targets. *Journal of the American Academy of Audiology, 11*(4) 230–238.

Searchfield, G. D., Kaur, M., & Martin, W. H. (2010). Hearing aids as an adjunct to counseling: Tinnitus patients who choose amplification do better than those that don't. *International Journal of Audiology, 49*(8), 574–579.

Seewald, R. C., Cornelisse, L. E., Black, S. L., & Block, M. G. (1996). Verifying the real-ear gain in CIC instruments. *Hearing Journal, 49*(6), 25–26.

Seewald, R. C., Cornelisse, L. E., Richert, F. M., & Block, M. G. (1997). Acoustic transforms for fitting CIC instruments. In M. Chasin (Ed.), *CIC handbook* (pp. 83–100). San Diego, CA: Singular.

Seewald, R. C., Moodie, S., Scollie, S., & Bagatto, M. (2005). The DSL method for pediatric hearing instrument fitting: Historical perspective and current issues. *Trends in Amplification, 9*(4), 145–157.

Seewald, R. C., Moodie, K. S., Sinclair, S. T., & Cornelisse, L. E. (1996). Traditional and theoretical approaches to selecting amplification for infants and children. In F. H. Bess, J. A. Gravel, & A. M. Tharpe (Eds.), *Amplification for children with auditory deficits* (pp. 161–191). Nashville, TN: Vanderbilt University Press.

Seewald, R. C., Moodie, K. S., Sinclair, S. T., & Scollie, S. D. (1999). Predictive validity of a procedure for pediatric hearing instrument fitting. *American Journal of Audiology, 8*(2), 143–152.

Seewald, R. C., Ramji, K. V., Sinclair, S. T., Moodie, K. S., & Jamieson, D. G. (1993). *A computer-assisted implementation of the desired sensation level method for electroacoustic selection and fitting in children: User's manual.* London, ON: Hearing Health Care Research Unit.

Seewald, R. C., Ross, M., & Spiro, M. K. (1985). Selecting amplification characteristics for young hearing-impaired children. *Ear and Hearing, 6*(1), 48–53.

Seewald, R. C., Zelisko, D. L., Ramji, K., & Jamieson, D. (1991). *DSL 3.0: A computer-assisted implementation of the desired sensation level method for electroacoustic selection and fitting in children*. London, ON: University of Western Ontario.

Sessler, G. M. & West, J. E. (1962). Self-biased condenser microphone with high capacitance. *Journal of the Acoustical Society of America, 34*(11), 1787–1788.

Shapiro, I. (1976). Hearing aid fitting by prescription. *International Journal of Audiology, 15*(2), 163–173.

Shaw, E. A. G. (1966). Ear canal pressure generated by a free sound field. *Journal of the Acoustical Society of America, 39*(3), 465–470.

Shaw, E. A. G. (1974). The external ear. In *The auditory system* (pp. 455–490). Heidelberg, Germany: Springer.

Shaw, E. A. G. (1975). The external ear: New knowledge. Earmolds and associated problems—Proceedings of the seventh Danavox Symposium. *Scandinavian Audiology, 78*, 1120–1123.

Shaw, E. A. G. (1980). The acoustics of the external ear. In G. A. Studebaker & I. Hochberg (Eds.), *Acoustical factors affecting hearing aid performance* (pp. 109–126). Baltimore, MD: University Park Press.

Shaw, E. A. G., & Vaillancourt, M. M. (1985). Transformation of sound-pressure level from the free field to the eardrum presented in numerical form. *Journal of the Acoustical Society of America, 78*(3), 1120–1123.

Sherbecoe, R. L., & Studebaker, G. A. (2002). Audibility-index functions for the connected speech test. *Ear and Hearing, 23*(5), 385–398.

Shi, L. F., Doherty, K. A., Kordas, T. M., & Pellegrino, J. T. (2007). Short-term and long-term hearing aid benefit and user satisfaction. *Journal of the American Academy of Audiology, 18*(6), 482–495.

Shield, B. (2006, October). *Evolution of the social and economic costs of hearing impairment* [Report for Hear-It]. Retrieved from http://www.Hear-It.org

Shore, I., Bilger, R. C., & Hirsh, I. J. (1960). Hearing aid evaluation: Reliability of repeated measurements. *Journal of Speech and Hearing Disorders, 25*(2), 152–170.

Silman, S., Gelfand, S. A., & Silverman, C. A. (1984). Late-onset auditory deprivation: Effects of monaural versus binaural hearing aids. *Journal of the Acoustical Society of America, 76*(5), 1357–1362.

Simon, H. J. (2005). Bilateral amplification and sound localization: Then and now. *Journal of Rehabilitations Research and Development, 42*(4), 117–132.

Simon, H. J., Yund, E. W., & Levitt, H. (2008). Auditory localization with linear and compression hearing aids. *Journal of the Acoustical Society of America, 123*(5), 3168.

Simpson, A. (2009). Frequency-lowering devices for managing high-frequency hearing loss: A review. *Trends in Amplification, 13*(2), 87–106.

Sinclair, S., Cole, W., & Pumford, J. (2001). The Audioscan® RM500 real-ear hearing aid analyzer: Measuring for a successful fit. *Trends in amplification, 5*(2), 81–90.

Sindhusake, D., Mitchell, P., Smith, W., Golding, M., Newall, P., Hartley, D., & Rubin, G. (2001). Validation of self-reported hearing loss. The Blue Mountains Hearing Study. *International Journal of Epidemiology, 30*(6), 1371–1378.

Singh, G., & Pichora-Fuller, K. (2010). Older adults' performance on the speech, spatial, and qualities of hearing scale (SSQ): Test-retest reliability and a comparison of interview and self-administration methods. *International Journal of Audiology, 49*(10), 733–740.

Sivian, L. J., & White, S. D. (1933). On minimum audible soundfields. *Journal of the Acoustical Society of America, 4*(4), 288–321.

Sjoblad, S., & Warren, B. W. (2011). Myth busters: Can you unbundle and stay in business? *Audiology Today, 23*(5), 37–45.

Skinner, M. W., Holden, L. K., Holden, T. A., Demorest, M. E., & Fourakis, M. S. (1997). Speech recognition at simulated soft, conversational, and raised-to-loud vocal efforts by adults with cochlear implants. *Journal of the Acoustical Society of America, 101*(6), 3766–3782.

Skinner, M. W., Karstaedt, M. M., & Miller, J. D. (1982). Amplification bandwidth and speech intelligibility for two listeners with sensorineural hearing loss. *Audiology, 21*(3), 251–268.

Smeds, K., Wolters, F., & Rung, M. (2015). Estimation of signal-to-noise ratios in realistic sound scenarios. *Journal of the American Academy of Audiology, 26*(2), 183–196.

Smith, S. L. (2013). Self-efficacy theory in audiologic rehabilitation. In J. J. Montano & J. B. Spitzer (Eds.), *Adult audiologic rehabilitation* (2nd ed., pp. 219–232). San Diego, CA: Plural.

Smith, P., Davis, A., Day, J., Unwin, S., Day, G., & Chalupper, J. (2008). Real-world preferences for linked bilateral processing. *Hearing Journal, 61*(7), 33–38.

Smith-Olinde, L., Nicholson, N., Chivers, C., Highley, P., & Williams, D. K. (2006). Test-retest reliability of in situ unaided thresholds in adults. *American Journal of Audiology, 15*(1), 75–80.

Southall, K., Gagn., J. P., & Jennings, M. B. (2010). Stigma: A negative and a positive influence on help-seeking for adults with acquired hearing loss. *International Journal of Audiology, 49*(11), 804–814.

Souza, P. (2012). 20Q: Cognition measures—They might change the way you fit hearing aids! *Audiology Online*.

Retrieved from http://www.audiologyonline.com/articles/august-20q-by-pamela-souza-6925

Souza, P. E., Arehart, K. H., Kates, J. M., Croghan, N. B., & Gehani, N. (2013). Exploring the limits of frequency lowering. *Journal of Speech, Language, and Hearing Research*, *56*(5), 1349–1363.

Souza, P. E, & Sirow, L. (2014). Relating working memory to compression parameters in clinically fit hearing aids. *American Journal of Audiology*, *23*(4), 394–401.

Spahr, A. J., & Dorman, M. F. (2004). Performance of subjects fit with the advanced bionics CII and nucleus 3G cochlear implant devices. *Archives of Otolaryngology-Head and Neck Surgery*, *130*(5), 624–628.

Spahr, A. J., Dorman, M. F., Litvak, L. M., Van Wie, S., Gifford, R. H., Loizou, P. C., . . . Cook, S. (2012). Development and validation of the AzBio sentence lists. *Ear and Hearing*, *33*(1), 112–117.

Sperry, J. L., Wiley, T. L., & Chial, M. R. (1997). Word recognition performance in various background competitors. *Journal of the American Academy of Audiology*, *8*(2), 71–80.

Stach, B. D. (1998). *Clinical audiology: An introduction* (p. 72). San Diego, CA: Singular.

Steeneken, H. J. M., & Houtgast, T. (1980). A physical method for measuring speech-transmission quality. *Journal of the Acoustical Society of America*, *67*(1), 318–326.

Stelmachowicz, P. (1991). Clinical issues related to hearing aid maximum output. *Vanderbilt Hearing Aid Report II*, 141–145.

Stelmachowicz, P., Lewis, D., Hoover, B., Nishi, K., McCreery, R., & Woods, W. (2010). Effects of digital noise reduction on speech perception for children with hearing loss. *Ear and Hearing*, *31*(3), 345–355.

Stelmachowicz, P. G., Mace, A. L., Kopun, J. G., & Carney, E. (1993). Long-term and short-term characteristics of speech: Implications for hearing aid selection for young children. *Journal of Speech Language Hearing Research*, *36*(3), 609–620.

Stelmachowicz, P. G., Pittman, A. L., Hoover, B. M., & Lewis, D. E. (2001). Effect of stimulus bandwidth on the perception of/s/in normal-and hearing-impaired children and adults. *Journal of the Acoustical Society of America*, *110*(4), 2183–2190.

Stender, T., & Appleby, R. (2009). Occlusion effect measures: Are they all created equal? *Hearing Journal*, *62*(7), 21–24.

Stewart, M. A., Brown, J. B., & Weston, W. W. (1989). Patient-centered interviewing Part III: Five provocative questions. *Canadian Family Physician*, *35*(1), 159–161.

Stone, M. A., & Moore, B. C. (1992). Syllabic compression: effective compression ratios for signals modulated at different rates. *British Journal of Audiology*, *26*(6), 351–361

Stone, M. A., & Moore, B. C. (1999). Tolerable hearing aid delays. I. Estimation of limits imposed by the auditory path alone using simulated hearing losses. *Ear and Hearing*, *20*(3), 182–192.

Stone, M. A., & Moore, B. C. (2005). Tolerable hearing-aid delays: IV. effects on subjective disturbance during speech production by hearing-impaired subjects. *Ear and Hearing*, *26*(2), 225–235.

Stone, M. A., Moore, B. C., Meisenbacher, K., & Derleth, R. P. (2008). Tolerable hearing aid delays. v. estimation of limits for open canal fittings. *Ear and Hearing*, *29*(4), 601–617.

Storey, L., & Dillon, H. (2001). Estimating the location of probe microphones relative to the tympanic membrane. *Journal of the American Academy of Audiology*, *12*(3), 150–154.

Strom, K. (2013). Hearing aid sales up 2.9% in '12. *Hearing Journal*, *20*(2), 6.

Strouse, A., & Wilson, R. H. (1999). Recognition of one-, two-, and three-pair dichotic digits under free and directed recall. *Journal of the American Academy of Audiology*, *10*(10), 557–571.

Studebaker, G. (1974). The acoustical effect of various factors on the frequency response of a hearing aid receiver. *Journal of the Audio Engineering Society*, *22*(5), 329–334.

Studebaker, G. (1985). A "rationalized" arcsine transform. *Journal of Speech, Language, and Hearing Research*, *28*(3), 455–462.

Sullivan, R. F. (1988). Probe tube microphone placement near the tympanic membrane. *Hearing Instruments*, *39*(7), 43–44.

Summers, V., Molis, M. R., Müsch, H., Walden, B. E., Surr, R. K., & Cord, M. T. (2003). Identifying dead regions in the cochlea: Psychophysical tuning curves and tone detection in threshold-equalizing noise. *Ear and Hearing*, *24*(2), 133–142.

Surr, R. K., Cord, M., & Walden, B. (2001) Response of hearing aid wearers to the absence of a user-operated volume control. *Hearing Journal*, *54*(4), 32–36.

Surr, R. K., Walden, B. E., Cord, M. T., & Olson, L. (2002). Influence of environmental factors on hearing aid microphone preference. *Journal of the American Academy of Audiology*, *13*(6), 308–322.

Sussman, H. M., McCaffrey, H. A., & Matthews, S. A. (1991). An investigation of locus equations as a source of relational invariance for stop place categorization. *Journal of the Acoustical Society of America*, *90*(3), 1309–1325.

Sutter, A. H. (1985). Speech recognition in noise by individuals with mild hearing impairments. *Journal of the Acoustical Society*, *78*(3), 887–900.

Swan, I. R. C., Guy, F. H., & Akeroyd, M. A. (2012). Health-related quality of life before and after management in adults referred to otolaryngology: a prospective national study. *Clinical Otolaryngology, 37*(1), 35–43.

Swanepoel, D. W., Clark, J. L., Koekemoer, D., Hall III, J. W., Krumm, M., Ferrari, D. V., . . . Barajas, J. J. (2010). Telehealth in audiology: The need and potential to reach underserved communities. *International Journal of Audiology, 49*(3), 195–202.

Sweetow, R. (2009, April). *Integrating LACE into a busy clinical practice.* Presentation at the American Academy of Audiology AudiologyNOW! meeting, Dallas, TX.

Sweetow, R. W., & Sabes, J. H. (2006). The need for and development of an adaptive listening and communication enhancement (LACE) program. *Journal of the American Academy of Audiology, 17*(8), 538–558.

Sweetow, R. W., & Sabes, J. H. (2007). Listening and communication enhancement (LACE). *Seminars in Hearing, 28*(2), 133.

Taubman, L. B., Palmer, C. V., Durrant, J. D., & Pratt, S. (1999). Accuracy of hearing aid use time as reported by experienced hearing aid wearers. *Ear and Hearing, 20*(4), 229–305.

Taylor, B. (2007). Predicting real world hearing aid benefit with speech audiometry: An evidence-based review. *Audiology Online*. Retrieved from http://www.audiologyonline.com/articles/predicting-real-world-hearing-aid-946

Taylor, B. (2008). The acceptable noise level test as a predictor of real-world hearing aid benefit. *Hearing Journal, 61*(9), 39–42.

Taylor, B., & Hayes, D. (2015). Does current hearing aid technology meet the needs of healthy aging? *Hearing Review, 22*(2), 22–26.

Taylor, B., & Mueller, H. G. (2016). *Fitting and dispensing hearing aids* (2nd ed.). San Diego, CA: Plural.

Taylor, R. S., Paisley, S., & Davis, A. (2001). Systematic review of the clinical and cost effectiveness of digital hearing aids. *British Journal of Audiology, 35*(5) 271–288.

Tecca, J. (1991). Real-ear vent effects in ITE hearing instrument fittings. *Hearing Instruments, 42*(12), 10–12.

Thibodeau, L. (2007). Speech audiometry. In R. Roeser, M. Valente, & H. Hosford-Dunn (Eds.), *Audiology: Diagnosis* (pp. 281–309). New York, NY: Thieme.

Thibodeau, L. (2014). Comparison of speech recognition with adaptive digital and FM remote microphone hearing assistance technology by listeners who use hearing aids. *American Journal of Audiology, 23*(2), 201–210.

Thompson, S. C., & Dillon, H. (2002, April). *Wind noise in hearing aids: Causes and effects.* Presented at the 14th Annual Convention of the American Academy of Audiology, Philadelphia, PA.

Thompson, S. C., LoPresti, J. L., Ring, E. M., Nepomuceno, H. G., Beard, J. J., Ballad, W. J., & Carlson, E. V. (2002). Noise in miniature microphones. *Journal of the Acoustical Society of America, 111*(2), 861–866.

Thorén, E. S., Öberg, M., Wänström, G., Andersson, G., & Lunner, T. (2014). A randomized controlled trial evaluating the effects of online rehabilitative intervention for adult hearing-aid users. *International Journal of Audiology, 53*(7), 452–461.

Thorne, P. R. (2003). Evidence-based audiology and clinical practice. *Australian and New Zealand Journal of Audiology, 25*(1), 10–15.

Thornton, A. R., & Raffin, M. J. M. (1978). Speech discrimination scores modeled as a binomial variable. *Journal of Speech and Hearing Research, 21*(3), 507–518.

Thornton, A. R., & Raffin, M. J. M. (1982). Comment on "a quantitative examination of the sources of speech discrimination test score variability. *Ear and Hearing, 3*(6), 340.

Tillman, T. W., Carhart, R., & Wilber, L. (1963). *A test for speech discrimination composed of CNC monosyllabic words.* (Northwestern University, Auditory Test No. 4). SAM-TDR-62.

Tillman, T. W., & Olsen, W. O. (1973). Speech audiometry. In J. Jerger (Ed.), *Modern developments in audiology* (2nd ed., pp. 37–74). New York, NY: Academic Press.

Tremblay, K., Kraus, N., Carrell, T. D., & McGee, T. (1997). Central auditory system plasticity: Generalization to novel stimuli following listening training. *Journal of the Acoustical Society of America, 102*(6), 3762–3773.

Tremblay, K., Kraus, N., McGee, T., Ponton, C., & Otis, B. (2001). Central auditory plasticity: Changes in the N1-P2 complex after speech-sound training. *Ear and Hearing, 22*(2), 79–90.

Tremblay, K. L., & Kraus, N. (2002). Auditory training induces asymmetrical changes in cortical neural activity. *Journal of Speech, Language, and Hearing Research, 45*(3), 564–572.

Tuckett, D., Boulton, M., Olson, C., & Williams, A. (1985). *Meetings between experts: An approach to sharing ideas in medical consultations.* London, UK: Tavistock.

Turner, C. W., & Bentler, R. A. (1998). Does hearing aid benefit increase over time? *Journal of the Acoustical Society of America, 104*(6), 3673–3674.

Turner, C. W., & Cummings, K. J. (1999). Speech audibility for listeners with high-frequency hearing loss. *American Journal of Audiology, 8*(1), 47–56.

Tye-Murray, N. (2014). *Foundations of aural rehabilitation: Children, adults, and their family members.* Clifton Park, NY: Cengage Learning.

Tye-Murray, N., Sommers, M. S., Mauz., E., Schroy, C., Barcroft, J., & Spehar, B. (2012). Using patient perceptions of relative benefit and enjoyment to assess auditory training. *Journal of the American Academy of Audiology, 23*(8), 623.

Tyler, R. S., & Kuk, F. K. (1989). The effects of "noise suppression" hearing aids on consonant recognition in speech-babble and low-frequency noise. *Ear and Hearing, 10*(4), 243–249.

United States Department of Health and Human Services, Administration for Children and Families. (2003). Program announcement. *Federal Register, 68*(131).

Unitron. (2014). *Troubleshooting tips*. Retrieved from http://unitron.com/unitron/us/en/consumer/help/troubleshooting-tips.html

Upfold, L. J. (1980). The evaluation of CROS aids with the unilateral listener. *Scandinavian Audiology, 9*(2), 85–88.

Uziel, A., Mondain, M., Hagen, P., Dejean, F., & Doucet, G. (2003). Rehabilitation for high-frequency sensorineural hearing impairment in adults with the Symphonix Vibrant Soundbridge: A comparative study. *Otology and Neurotology, 24*(5), 775–783.

Vaisberg, J. M., Macpherson, E. A., & Scollie, S. D. (2016). Extended bandwidth real-ear measurement accuracy and repeatability to 10 kHz. *International Journal of Audiology, 55*(10), 580–586.

Valente, M. (2006). Guideline for audiologic management of the adult patient. *Audiology Online*. Retrieved from http://www.audiologyonline.com/articles/pf_article_detail.asp?article_id=1716

Valente, M., Fabry, D., Potts, L. G., & Sandlin, R. E. (1998). Comparing the performance of the Widex SENSO digital hearing aid with analog hearing aids. *Journal of the American Academy of Audiology, 9*(5), 342–360.

Valente, M., & Mispagel, K. M. (2008). Unaided and aided performance with a directional open-fit hearing aid. *International Journal of Audiology, 47*(6), 329–336.

Valente, M., Oeding, K., Brockmeyer, A., Smith, S., & Kallogjeri, D. (2017). Differences in Word and Phoneme Recognition in Quiet, Sentence Recognition in Noise, and Subjective Outcomes between Manufacturer First-Fit and Hearing Aids Programmed to NAL-NL2 Using Real-Ear Measures. *Journal of the American Academy of Audiology*. DOI: 10.3766/jaaa.17005

Valente, M., Potts, L. G., Valente, M., & Goebel, J. (1995). Wireless CROS versus transcranial CROS for unilateral hearing loss. *American Journal of Audiology, 4*(1), 52–59.

Valente, M., Potts, L. G., Valente, M., Vass, W., & Goebel, J. (1994). Intersubject variability of real-ear sound pressure level: Conventional and insert earphones. *Journal of the American Academy of Audiology, 5*(6), 390–398.

Valente, M., & Van Vliet, D. (1997). The independent hearing aid fitting forum (IHAFF) protocol. *Trends in Amplification, 2*(1), 6–35.

Van den Bogaert, T., Doclo, S., Wouters, J., Moonen, M. (2008). The effect of multimicrophone noise reduction systems on sound source localization by users of binaural hearing aids. *Journal of the Acoustical Society of America, 124*(1), 484–497.

Van den Bogaert, T., Klasen, T. J., Moonen, M., Van Deun, L., & Wouters, J. (2006). Horizontal localization with bilateral hearing aids: Without is better than with. *Journal of the Acoustical Society of America, 119*(1), 515–526.

Ventry, I. M., & Weinstein, B. E. (1982). The Hearing Handicap Inventory for the Elderly: A new tool. *Ear and Hearing, 3*(3), 128–134.

Ventry, I. M., & Weinstein, B. E. (1983). Identification of elderly people with hearing problems. *Journal of the American Speech Language Hearing Association, 25*(7), 37–42.

Vermiglio, A. J. (2008). The American English hearing in noise test. *International Journal of Audiology, 47*(6), 386–387.

Vestergaard, M. D. (2006). Self-report outcome in new hearing-aid users: Longitudinal trends and relationships between subjective measures of benefit and satisfaction. *International Journal of Audiology, 45*, 382–392.

Viemeister N. (1979). Temporal modulation transfer function based on modulation thresholds *Journal of the Acoustical Society of America, 66*(5), 1364–1380.

Vinay, & Moore, B. C. J. (2007). Prevalence of dead regions in subjects with sensorineural hearing loss. *Ear and Hearing, 28*(2), 231–241.

Vinay, Moore, B. C. J., & Baer, T. (2008). Speech recognition in noise as a function of high-pass filter cutoff frequency for people with and without low-frequency cochlear dead regions. *Journal of the Acoustical Society of America, 123*(2), 456–464.

Vorobyov, S. A. (2014). Adaptive and robust beamforming. In R. Chellappa & S. Theodoridis (Eds.), *Academic Press library in signal processing. Vol. 3, Array and statistical signal processing* (pp. 503–552). Chennai, India: Academic Press.

Vuorialho, A., Karinen, P., & Sorri, M. (2006). Counselling of hearing aid users is highly cost-effective. *European Archives of Oto-Rhino-Laryngology, 263*(11), 988–995.

Wade, P. S. (2002). Medical aspects of bone anchored hearing aids and middle ear implants. *Trends in Amplification, 6*(2), 39–44.

Walden, B. E. (1997). Toward a model clinical-trials protocol for substantiating hearing aid user-benefit claims. *American Journal of Audiology, 6*(2), 13–24.

Walden, B. E., Surr, R. K., Cord, M. T., & Dyrlund, O. (2004). Predicting hearing aid microphone preference in everyday listening. *Journal of the American Academy of Audiology, 15*(5), 365–396.

Walden, B. E., Surr, R. K., Cord, M. T., Edward, B., & Olson, L. (2000). Comparison of benefits provided by different hearing aid technology. *Journal of the American Academy of Audiology, 11*(10), 540–560.

Walden, B. E., & Walden, T. C. (2005). Unilateral versus bilateral amplification for adults with impaired hearing [Report]. *Journal of the American Academy of Audiology, 16*(8), 574–584.

Walden, E. E., Prosek, R. A., & Holum-Hardegan, L. L. (1984). Some principles of aural rehabilitation. *Hearing Instruments, 35,* 40–48.

Walden, T. C., & Walden, B. E. (2004). Predicting success with hearing aids in everyday living. *Journal of the American Academy of Audiology, 15*(5), 342–352.

Walker, E. A., Spratford, M., Moeller, M. P., Oleson, J., Ou, H., Roush, P., & Jacobs, S. (2013). Predictors of hearing aid use time in children with mild-to-severe hearing loss. *Language, Speech, and Hearing Services in Schools, 44*(1), 73–88.

Walker, G. (1979). Earphone termination and the response of behind-the-ear hearing aids. *British Journal of Audiology, 13*(2), 41–46.

Wallenfels, H. G. (1967). *Hearing aids on prescription.* Springfield, IL: Charles C. Thomas.

Wang, D. & Brown, G. J. (Eds) (2006). *Computational auditory scene analysis: Principles, algorithms, and applications.* Hoboken, NJ: Wiley-IEEE Press.

Ware, J. E., Jr., & Sherbourne, C. D. (1992). The MOS 36-item short-form health survey (SF-36): I. Conceptual framework and item selection. *Medical Care,* 473–483.

Warnaar, B., & Dreschler, W. (2012). Agreement between psychophysical tuning curves and the threshold equalizing noise test in dead region identification. *International Journal of Audiology, 51*(6), 456–464.

Warner, R. L., & Bentler, R. A. (2002). Thresholds of discomfort for complex stimuli: Acoustic and sound quality predictors. *Journal of Speech, Language, and Hearing Research, 45*(2), 1016–1026.

Watson, C. S., Miller, J. D., Kewley-Port, D., Humes, L. E., & Wightman, F. L. (2008). Training listeners to identify the sounds of speech: I. A review of past studies. *Hearing Journal, 61*(9), 26.

Watson, L., & Tolan, T. (1949). *Hearing tests and hearing instruments.* Baltimore, MD: Williams and Wilkins.

Watson, N. A., & Knudsen, V. O. (1940). Selective amplification in hearing aids. *Journal of the Acoustical Society of America, 11*(4), 406–419.

Wayner, D. S., & Abrahamson, J. E. (1996). *Learning to hear again: An audiolgical rehabilitation curriculum guide.* Austin, TX: Hear Again.

Wazen, J. J., Caruso, M., & Tjellstrom, A. (1998). Long-term results with the titanium bone-anchored hearing aid: The US experience. *American Journal of Otology, 19*(6), 737.

Wazen, J. J., Spitzer, J. B., Ghossaini, S. N., Fayad, J. N., Niparko, J. K., Cox, K., ... Soli, S. D. (2003). Transcranial contralateral cochlear stimulation in unilateral deafness. *Otolaryngology-Head and Neck Surgery, 129*(3), 248–254.

Wedenberg, E. (1951). Auditory training of deaf and hard-of-hearing children. *Acta Otolaryngologica, 94*(Suppl.), 114.

Weinstein, B. E. (1986). Validity of a screening protocol for identifying elderly people with hearing problems. *ASHA, 28*(5), 41–45.

Westerkull, P. (2002). BAHA®: The direct bone conductor. *Trends in Amplification, 6*(2), 45–52.

White, S. C. (2009). Third-party payment for auditory rehabilitation. *SIG 7 Perspectives on Aural Rehabilitation and Its Instrumentation, 16*(1), 4–7.

Wiener, F. M., & Ross, D. A. (1946). The pressure distribution in the auditory canal in a progressive sound field. *Journal of the Acoustical Society of America, 18*(2), 401–408.

Wiley, T. L., Cruickshanks, K. J., Nondahl, D. M., & Tweed, T. S. (2000). Self-reported hearing handicap and audiometric measures in older adults. *Journal of the American Academy of Audiology, 11*(2), 67–75.

Wilson, F. (2009). *Graduate medical education: Issues and options.* New York, NY: Radcliffe Medical Press.

Wilson, R. H. (2003). Development of a speech in multi-talker babble paradigm to assess word-recognition performance. *Journal of the American Academy of Audiology, 14*(9), 453–470.

Wilson, R. H. (2011). Clinical experience with the words-in-noise test on 3,430 veterans: Comparisons with pure-tone thresholds and word recognition in quiet. *Journal of the American Academy of Audiology, 27*(7), 405–423.

Wilson, R. H., Abrams, H. B., & Pillion, A. L. (2003). A word-recognition task in multitalker babble using a descending presentation mode from 24 dB to 0 dB signal to babble. *Journal of Rehabilitation Research and Development, 40*(4), 321–328.

Wilson, R. H., & Burks, C. (2005). Use of 35 words for evaluation of hearing loss in signal-to-babble ratio: A clinic protocol. *Journal of Rehabilitation Research and Development, 42*(6), 839–852.

Wilson, R. H., Carnell, C. S., & Cleghorn, A. L. (2007). The words-in-noise (WIN) test with multitalker babble and speech-spectrum noise maskers. *Journal of the American Academy of Audiology, 18*(6), 522–530.

Wilson, R. H, & Cates, W. B. (2008). A comparison of two word-recognition tasks in multi-talker babble: Speech recognition in noise test (SPRINT) and words-in-noise test (WIN). *Journal of the American Academy of Audiology, 19*(7), 548–556.

Wilson, R. H., Coley, K. E., Haenel, J. L., & Browning, K. M. (1976). Northwestern University Auditory Test

No. 6: Normative and comparative intelligibility functions. *Journal of the American Audiological Society, 1*(5), 221–228.

Wilson, R. H., Farmer, N. M., Gandhi, A., Shelburne, E., & Weaver, J. (2010). Normative data for the words-in-noise test for 6- to 12-year-old children. *Journal of Speech, Language, and Hearing Research, 53*(5), 1111–1121.

Wilson, R. H., & McArdle, R. (2008). A change is in the air. *The Hearing Review, 61*(10), 10–15.

Wilson, R. H., & McArdle, R. (2012). Speech-in-noise measures: Variable versus fixed speech and noise levels. *International Journal of Audiology, 51*(9), 708–712.

Wilson, R. H., McArdle, R. A., & Smith, S. L. (2007). An evaluation of the BKB-SIN, HINT, QuickSIN, and WIN materials on listeners with normal hearing and listeners with hearing loss. *Journal of Speech, Language, and Hearing Research, 50*(4), 844–856.

Wilson, R. H., McArdle, R., Watts, K. L., & Smith, S. L. (2012). The revised speech perception in noise test (R-SPIN) in a multiple signal-to-noise ratio paradigm. *Journal of the American Academy of Audiology, 23*(8), 590–605.

Wilson, R. H., & Watts, K. L. (2012). The words-in-noise test (WIN), list 3: A practice list. *Journal of the American Academy of Audiology, 23*(2), 92–96.

Wolfe, J., John, A., Schafer, E., Nyffeler, M., Boretzki, M., Caraway, T., & Hudson, M. (2011). Long-term effects of non-linear frequency compression for children with moderate hearing loss. *International Journal of Audiology, 50*(6), 396–404.

Wolfe, J., Mills, E., Schafer, E., John, A., & Hudson, M. (2014). Binaural hearing on the telephone for preschool children with hearing loss. *Hearing Review, 21*(6), 14–16. Retrieved from from http://www.hearingreview.com/2014/06/binaural-hearing-telephone-preschool-children-hearing-loss/.

Wolfe, J., Schafer, E., Martella, N., Morais, M., & Mann, M. (2015). Evaluation of extended-wear hearing technology for children with hearing loss. *Journal of the American Academy of Audiology, 26*(7), 615–631.

Wong, L. L., & Hickson, L. (2012). *Evidence-based practice in audiology: Evaluating interventions for children and adults with hearing impairment.* San Diego, CA: Plural.

Wright, B. A. (2007). Hearing lessons: Perceptual learning on basic auditory skills. *Hearing Journal, 60*(2), 10–14.

Wu, Y. H., & Bentler, R. A. (2010a). Impact of visual cues on directional benefit and preference: Part I Laboratory tests. *Ear and Hearing, 31*(1), 22–34.

Wu, Y. H., & Bentler, R. A. (2010b). Impact of visual cues on directional benefit and preference: Part II Field tests. *Ear and Hearing, 31*(1), 35–46.

Wu, Y. H., & Bentler, R. A. (2012). Do older adults have social lifestyles that place fewer demands on hearing? *Journal of the American Academy of Audiology, 23*(9), 697–711.

Wu, Y. H., & Bentler, R. A. (2012). The influence of audiovisual ceiling performance on the relationship between reverberation and directional benefit: Perception and prediction. *Ear and Hearing, 33*(5), 604–614.

Wu, Y. H., Stangl, E., Bentler, R. A., & Stanziola, R. W. (2013). The effect of hearing aid technologies on listening in an automobile. *Journal of the American Academy of Audiology, 24*(6), 474–485.

Wu, Y. H., Stangl, E., Chipara, O., Hasan, S. S., Welhaven, A., & Oleson, J. (2017). Characteristics of real-world signal to noise ratios and speech listening situations of older adults with mild to moderate hearing loss. *Ear and Hearing.* Advance online publication. Retrieved from http://homepage.divms.uiowa.edu/~ochipara/papers/EANDH.pdf

Wu, Y. H., Stangl, E. A., Pang, C., & Zhang, X. (2014). The effect of audiovisual and binaural listening on the acceptable noise level (ANL): Establishing an ANL conceptual model. *Journal of the American Academy of Audiology, 25*(2), 141–153.

Wu, Y. H., Stangl, E. A., & Perkins, J. (2014, March). *New insight regarding psychometric functions of dual-task paradigms.* Poster session presented at the annual meeting of the American Auditory Society, Scottsdale, AZ.

Wu, Y. H., Stangl, E., Zhang, X., & Bentler, R. A. (2015). Construct validity of the ecological momentary assessment in audiology research. *Journal of the American Academy of Audiology, 26*(10), 872–884.

Yanz, J. L., & Preves, D. (2003). Telecoils: Principles, pitfalls, fixes, and the future. *Seminars in Hearing, 24*(1), 029–042.

Yost, W. A. (2007). *Fundamentals of hearing: An introduction* (3rd ed.). New York, NY: Academic Press.

Yost, W. A., & Killion, M. C. (1997). Hearing thresholds. *Encyclopedia of Acoustics, 3*, 1545–1554.

Yueh, B., Souza, P. E., McDowell, J. A., Collins, M. P., Loovis, C. F., Hedrick, S. C., . . . Deyo, R. A. (2001). Randomized trial of amplification strategies. *Archives of Otolaryngology-Head and Neck Surgery, 127*(10), 1197–1204.

Yund, E. W., Buckles, K. M. (1995). Multichannel compression hearing aids: Effect of number of channels on speech discrimination in noise. *Journal of the Acoustical Society of America, 97*(2), 1206–1223.

Zakis, J. A., & Hawkins, D. J. (2015). Wind noise within and across behind-the-ear and miniature behind-the-ear hearing aids. *Journal of the Acoustical Society of America, 138*(4), 2291–2300.

Zekveld, A. A., Kramer, S. E., & Festen, J. M. (2010). Pupil response as an indication of effortful listening: The influence of sentence intelligibility. *Ear and Hearing, 31*(4), 480–490.

Index

Note: Page numbers in **bold** reference non-text material.

2-cc coupler, converting to, 114

A

AAA (American Academy of Audiology), 605
  audiologists in, 30
  board certification, 36
  code of ethics, 45–47, 607–608
  fitting guidelines, 39–40
  Guidelines for the Audiologic Management of Adult Hearing Impairment, 37
  scope of practice, 35–36
AAO (American Academy of Otolaryngology), 145
AARP (American Association of Retired (Persons), 34
Abbreviated Profile of Hearing Aid Benefit (APHAB), 2, 108, 198, 201, 206–212
  AV subscale of, **723**
  clinical application of, 210–212, 745–749
  hearing aid fitting, 614
  scoring, 738
  self reporting-outcomes, 745–749
Abel, Debbie, 44
Academy of Dispensing Audiology (ADA), 30
  complaints to FDA, 480
Acceptable Noise Level (ANL), 182–186, 397
Accessible and Affordable Hearing Health Care for Adults with Mild to Moderate Hearing Loss, 477
Acclimatization
  auditory, **731**
  defined, 730
Acoustic
  feedback, 718–722
    described, 233
    hearing aid selection and, 233–237
    internal, 236
    listening environment, described, 431
  mass, calculating, **302**
  positioning, 640–641
  shadow
    See Head shadow effect
  telephones, 726–728
Acoustical Society of America, 484, 648–649
  standards, 491
Acoustically assisted positioning, 641
Acoustics
  band-level, **81**
  dB
    adding, 789–790
    weighting, 790–791
  of earmolds, 288–291
  pressure vs. power, 789
  speech, 75–100, 457–459
    articulation/audibility index, 83–87
    audibility/speech recognition, 82–87
    long-term, 75–81
    short-term, 88–95
Acquired hearing loss, cochlea, 128
Acrylic earmolds, 282
Actual values, vs. theoretical, **307**
A/D (Analog to digital), conversion, 330–333
Ad Hoc Committee on Hearing Aid Selection and Fitting, 37
ADA (Academy of Dispensing Audiology), 30
  complaints to FDA, 480
Adaptation, defined, 730
Adaptive
  compression, described, 370
  SNR, vs. fixed, 138–139
  speech tests, 161–163
Additional gain before feedback (AGBF), 443
Addition-cure
  silicone impression materials, 277
  vinylpolysiloxane impression materials, 277

Adjustment
    defined, 730
    period, 729–730
        clinical relevance, 730–733
Administration and scoring
    ANL, 184–185
    APHAB, 208–210, 745
    BKB-SIN, 172–173
    COSI, 217–219, 767, **768**
    CST, 155–157
    DDT, 194–195
    DOSO, 760–761
    DSI, 191–192
    ECHO, 214–215
    GHABP, 750
    HASP, 220
    HHIE, 205–206
    HINT, 163–165
    IOI-HA, 764–766
    LDL, 110
    Maryland CNCs, 151
    NU#6, 142–148
    PAL, 770–771
    PPT, 187
    QuickSIN test, 169–170
    SADL, 754–755
    SPIN/R-SPIN, 153–155
    SPRINT, 159–161
    SSQ, 776
    TEN (HL), 130–131
    WIN, 177–180
ADRO, CI and, 371
Advertising, testimonials and, **479**
AGBF (Additional gain before feedback), 443
AGC (Automatic gain control), 365
AGCi (Automatic Gain Control Input), **107**, 369–370
AGCo (Automatic Gain Control-output), **107**
    multiple channels, 372
AGI (Automatic gain increase)
    advantages of, 430
    algorithms, 429–430
    training and, 438–439
AHAA, 31
AI (Articulation Index), 83, 95, **99**
    calculation of, 86
    frequency bands for, 86–87
    SII and, **84**
Aided
    audibility testing, 567, 569
    gain, **567**
    loudness judgments, 590–595
    loudness testing, 591–592

prefitting LDL, 119
soundfield threshold, 526
    verification, 567–569
speech recognition benefit, 569–583
verification threshold, **563**
Air-bone gap, LDL and, 118
Air conduction, hearing aids and, 258–260
Aid-to-aid connectivity, 446–448
Algorithms
    AGI, 429–430
    Camfit, **549**
    DFS, benefits/limitations of, 442–443
    feedback reduction, 719
    FL, 459–468
    gain increase, 733
    NAL, 611
    prescriptive, 781
    Visual Input/Output Locater Algorithm (VIOLA), 535–537
Alpha, defined, **5**
Ambient noise levels, 781–782
American Academy of Audiology (AAA), 604, 605
    audiologists in, 30
    board certification, 36
    code of ethics, 45–47 607–608
    complaints to FDA, 480
    fitting guidelines, 39–40
    Guidelines for the Audiologic Management of Adult Hearing Impairment, 37
    scope of practice, 35–36
American Academy of Otolaryngology (AAO), 145
American Association of Retired Persons (AARP), 34
American Engineering Standards Committee (ANSC), 483
American Medical Association, Council on Physical Therapy of, 473–475
American National Standards Institute (ANSI)*See* ANSI
American Speech-Language-Hearing Association (ASHA), 3, 34, 605
    Ad Hoc Committee on Hearing Aid Selection and Fitting, 37
    code of ethics, 30, 45–47, 608
    complaints to FDA, 480
    fitting guidelines, 39–40
    preferred practice patterns, **38**
AMI, **364**
Ampclusion, **239**
Amplification
    satisfaction with, 61–63
    selective, 518
        Watson and Knudsen, 522–523
    unilateral vs. bilateral, 226–233

Amplified stethoscopes, **499**, **500**
Amplifiers, 318–322
   Class A, 320
   Class B, 320
   Class D, 320, 322
   Class H, 320
   described, **310**
Amplifon, 31
Amplitude compression, 446
Analog
   clipping, **319**
   filters, **337**
Analog to digital (A/D), conversion, 330–333
Analyzers, hearing aid, 493–495
ANL (Acceptable Noise Level), 182–186, 397
ANSI (American Engineering Standards Committee), 483
ANSI (American National Standards Institute), 78, 491–493, 672
ANSI/ASA S1.1,
ANSI/ASA S3.7, **672**
ANSI/ASA 3.22, **672**
ANSI 1.1-1994, **91**, 793
ANSI C63.19, 481
ANSI S2.35-2010, 492
ANSI S3.1-2010, 781
ANSI 3.5-1997, 78, 83, 86, 104
ANSI S3.22, **107**, 368, 483–384, 495, 499, 501, 503, 507, 515, 566–567, 735
ANSI S3.22-2009, 494, **496**
ANSI S3.22-2014, 491–492
ANSI S3.25, 489
ANSI S3.25-1979, 488
ANSI S3.25-2009, 492
ANSI S3.35-2004, 349
ANSI S3.36-2012, 492
ANSI S3.42, 800
ANSI S3.42-1992, 492–493, 797
ANSI S3.42-2012 Part 2, 493
ANSI S3.461997, 648
ANSI S3.46-2013, 123, 631
ANSI S3.46-2014, 493
ANSI S3.5-1997, 797
ANSI S3.6-1989, 493, 787
ANSI S3.6-1996, 678
ANSI S3.6-2004, 114
ANSI 3.6-2010, 114, 782
ANSI S3.7-1995, 488, 493, 495
ANSI S3.8-1967
ANSI S3.46-1997, 648
ANSI S3.46-2013, 632, 649, **672**, **673**
Antikickback statue, 42

APHAB (Abbreviated Profile of Hearing Aid Benefit), 2, 108, 198, 201, 206–212, 745–749
   AV subscale of, **723**
   hearing aid fitting, 614
   obtaining, 211–212
   post fitting self-assessment, 744
   report card for, **741**
   scoring, 738
   self-reporting-outcomes, 745–749
Argosy Manhattan circuit, **389**
Arizona Biomedical Institute, 195
Arizona State University
   Arizona Biomedical Institute, 195
   Department of Speech and Hearing Science, 195
Armature, 360
Army Rehabilitation Centers, 518–519
Arrays, **404**
   microphone, traditional/high order, 407–409
   situation-specific microphones and, 423–426
Articulation Index (AI), 83–87, 95, **99**
   calculation of, 86
   clinical use of, 95–97
      procedures, 97–99
   frequency bands for, 84–85
   SII and, **84**
ASHA (American Speech-Language-Hearing Association), 3, 29, 34, 605
   Ad Hoc Committee on Hearing Aid Selection and Fitting, 37
   board certification, 36
   code of ethics, 30, 45–47, 608
   complaints to FDA, 480
   preferred practice patterns, **38**
Assessment tools, selecting, **744**
Asymmetric switching technique, **411**
Attack time, 368
   G-DNR, 391–392
Attenuation, defined, 226
Attribution, assessing patients, 70
Audibility, 82–87
   effective, 625
   excessive, **629**
   extender, 460, **461**
   feedback, 233
   hearing aids and, 571–577
   index, 83–87, **99**
   testing aided, 569
Audigy, 31
Audio deprivation, avoidance of, 230–231
Audiogram
   construct added, REIG and, **684**
   counseling using, 102–106

Audiogram *(continued)*
    flat aided, 523
    interpreting, for children, **123**
    techniques, mirroring, 523
Audiologic, counseling strategy, **59**
Audiologists
    defined, 41
    as middle man, 29
    in the workplace, 30
Audiology
    board certification, 36
    first use of term, 27
    licensure, 36
    scope of practice, 35–36
Audiology Today, **28**, 607
Audioscan Verifit®, 625
Auditec of St. Louis, 137, **149**, 591, 593
    dichotic digits tests, 193
    obtaining
        BKB-SIN, 175
        DDT, 195
        DSI, 193
        QuickSIN test, 172
        SPRINT test, 161
Auditory acclimatization, **731**
Auditory and Vestibular Research Laboratory, 181
Auditory localization, **242**
    improved, 228
Auditory pathways, crossed, 189
Auditory scene analysis, 385
AuDNET, 31
Australian National Laboratories (NAL)
    algorithm, 611
    Family of Prescriptive Methods, 530–531
        revised, 532–533
Automatic gain control (AGC), 365
Automatic gain increase (AGI)
    advantages of, 430
    algorithms, 429–430
    training and, 438–439
Automatic gain control input (AGCi), **107**, 370
Automatic gain control output (AGCo), **107**, 369
    multiple channels, 372
Automatic volume control (AVC), described, 370
Average values, 590
AzBio sentences, 195–196

B

Babble, 137
    AzBio and, 195
    competing signals and, 168

CST, 156
fixed condition, **162**
multitalker, 137–138, 159, 176–177
    ANL measurement and, 184
    BNL and, 182
    QuickSIN test and, **181**
noise in, 792
SPIN and, 153
two-talker, 397
Back volume, 360
Background noise, 172, 388
    acoustic telephones and, 726–728
Background Noise Level (BNL), 182
BAHA® Attract, 264
BAHA™, 262–263
BAI (Bone anchored implant), 262–265
Balance problems, 69
Balanced armature transducer, 360
Baltimore Longitudinal Study on Aging, dementia and, **61**
Bamford-Knowal-Bench Sentences in Noise (BKB-SIN), 137
    Hearing In Noise Test (HINT), 172–182
    speech noise test, 138
Band Importance Functions (BIFs), 84–86, **800**, 802
Band-level acoustics, **81**
Bandwidth, frequency, remote microphones, **406**
Base decrease for lower levels (BDHL), **389**
Bass increase for lower levels (BILL), **389**
Batteries, 357–359, **710**
    current drain, 505–506
    life of, **456**, 457
BDHL (Base decrease for lower levels), **389**
Beamformers, **404**
    bilateral, 414–415
    MDVR, 396
    remote microphones and, 412
Becker Library, **10**
Behavioral aided loudness measures, need for, 590–591
Behavioral
    measures, **561**
    outcomes, role of, 560–562
Behind the ear (BTE) hearing aids, 240, 241–247, 362
    couplers and, 485
    eyeglass, 244–247
    microphone locations and, 807–808
    omnidirectional, **409**
Beltone, hearing aids, 31
Beneficiaries, gifts or inducements to, 43–44
Berger, Ken, 27
Berger method, 524–526
Bergman, Albert, 385
Bergman, Joe, **28**

Best practice, 37–38
    compliance with guidelines, 605–607
    levels of, **38**
    vs. real practice, **109**
BiCROS hearing aids, 258
    air conduction and, 258–260
    applications of, 260
BIFs (Band Importance Functions), 84–86, 800, 802
Bilateral amplification
    perceived benefit of, 232–233
    potential contraindications of, 231–233
    speech understanding and, 228–229
    vs unilateral, 226–233
        advantages of, 226–227
        beamformers, 414–415
        data sharing, 445–448
            feature control and, 446
        fittings, **113**, 226–227
            clinical speech measures for, **229**
        hearing, vs binaural, **226**
        LDLs, **113**
        lobe-steering technologies, 425
        loudness testing, **592**
        processing, **226**
BILL (Bass increase for lower levels), **389**
Billing, 44
Binaural
    hearing, 226–227
        vs bilateral, **226**
    interference, 232
        screening for, **233**
    processing, **226**
        speech understanding and, 228–229
    redundancy, 228
    squelch, 228
    model, **147**
        NU#6, 146
Biocommunications Research Laboratory, 150
Bipolar transistors, **318**
BKB-SIN (Bamford-Knowal-Bench Sentences in Noise), 137, 172
    Hearing In Noise Test (HINT), 172–182
    speech noise test, 138
Block processing, 335
Bluetooth, Harald, **316**
Bluetooth, BLE, 326, 552
    remote microphones and, **406**
    RF and, 448
    streaming and, 453
    wireless streaming, 448
Bluetooth™, 323, **325**
    low energy, 326

protocols, 326
relay signals and, 452
technology, **316**
television streaming and, 450
Blu-Ray DVDs, 328
BNL (Background Noise Level), 182
Board certification, audiology, 36
Body hearing aids, 241–242
Body transformations, 804–805
Bone anchored implant (BAI), 262–265
Bone conduction
    hearing aids, 262–263
    hearing through, **264**
    implantable, 262–265
Boots, connecting, 553–554
Bordon General Hospital, 28
Boyle, Robert, 120
Boyle's Law, 120
Brain, hearing loss and, **61**
Broadband noise, signal classification system and, 90
Brown noise, 620, 627, 792, 794
BTE (Behind the ear) hearing aids, 240, 241–247, 362
    couplers and, 485
    eyeglass, 244–247
    microphone locations and, 807–808
    omnidirectional, **409**
Bump-and-pull, 641
Bundled approach, **32**
Bundling, 44–45
Button switches, 267, **710**
Buying groups, hearing aids, 31
Byrne, Denis, 530, 610
Byrne and Tonisson method, 531

C

Cafeteria noise, 137
Calibration, sound field, Speech-in-Noise Testing, 140–141
Camfit algorithms, **549**
Canal locks, 284, 286
Candidates
    amplification, satisfaction with, 61–63
    four habits model and, 67–73
    hearing aids, 53–74
        benefits of, 59–60
        effects of stigma, 58–59
        willingness to use, 56–57
    identifying, 64–66
    interviewing, 66–67
    understanding, 63–67
    See also Patients

Canfield, Norton, 27
Capacitance, **312**
   microphones and, 311–313
Capacitor, schematic of, **311**
Carhart, June, 421–422
Carhart, Raymond, 27, 28, 421–422, 518–519, 570
Carina®, 266
Carrot passage, 625
Case reports/series, evidence and, 6
Case-controlled studies, 6
Categorical scale, 585–589
Category scaling, **585**
   normative data applied to, **589**
Causey, Don, 150
Cavitt, Kim, 44
CBI (Counterbalanced intervention studies), 7–8
CCC-A, 36
CDs (Compact discs), 328
Central Institute for the Deaf (CID), 523
   prescriptive approach, 526
Central processing unit (CPU), **318**
Cerumen
   ear impressions and, 278
   limiting drainage of, 364
   receivers and, 363
CEUs (Continuing education evidence), 26
CFA (Continuous flow adaptor), 298
Change factors, **385**
Channel summation, 591
ChannelFree™, 371
Channels
   frequency, **337**
   frequency bands and, 336
Characteristic frequency, described, 128
Characteristics of Amplification Tool (COAT), 201
Checklist, use of, 714, **715**
Children, interpreting audiogram for, **123**
CI (Cochlear implant), 582
   ADRO and, 371
   AzBio sentences and, 195–196
   bilateral amplification and, 232
   BKB-SIN and, 173
   HAT and, 269
   high-frequency consonants, 458
   HINT and, 168
   low-frequency techniques and, 460
   Noah modules and, 552
   QuickSIN and, 174–175
   speech enhancement and, 457
CIC (Completely-in-the canal)
   coupler, 487
      microphone locations and, 809

CID (Central Institute for the Deaf), 523
   prescriptive approach, 526
CINAHL (Cumulative Index to Nursing and Allied Health Literature), **10**
Circle of Decibels, 114
CK (Compression kneepoint), 365
   AGCi and, 370
CL (Compression limiting), 39
   described, 370
Class A amplifiers, 320, 322
Class B amplifiers, 320, 322
Class D amplifiers, 322
Clayton Act of 1914, 475
Client Oriented Scale of Improvement (COSI), 201, 215–219
   excessive sound and, 724
   post fitting self-assessment, 744
   self-reporting-outcomes, 766–769
Clinical application, 124–125
   ANLs, 185–186
   APHAB, 745–749
   APHAD, 210–211
   BKB-SIN, 174–175
   COAT, 222–223
   COSI, 769
   CST, 157
   DDT, 195
   DOSO, 761–762
   DSI, 192–193
   ECHO, 214–215
   GHABP, 751–752
   HASP, 220–221
   HHIE/A, 206
   HINT, 166–167
   IOI-HA, 766
   LDL, 113–120
   listening effort/fatigue and, 596–600
   Maryland CNCs, 151
   PAL, 771–774
   PPDIS, 187–188
   QUICKSIN test, 170–172
   REAR, 666, 672
   RECD, 676
   RECDs, 124–125
   REDD, 678
   REIG, 670
   REUG, 654–655
   ROEG, 660
   R-SPIN, 151–152
   SADL, 755–758
   SNR-50, 180–181
   speech recognition in quiet, 148–151

SPRINT, 161
SSQ, 778–779
STI, 99
TEN, 131–133
Clinical Certificate of Competence in Audiology, board certification, 36
Clinical experience, 3
Clinical speech measures, for bilateral fittings, **229**
Clinical subjective ratings, **585**
Closed loop response, 233
CMOS (Complementary metal oxide semiconductor), **318**
COAT (Characteristics of Amplification Tool), 201, 222–223
Cochlea
   hearing loss and, acquired, 128
   TEN test, 128
   tuning capabilities of, 129
Cochlear Corporation, 263
Cochlear implant (CI), 582
   ADRO and, 371
   bilateral amplification and, 232
   BKB-SIN and, 173
   HAT and, 269
   high-frequency consonants, 458
   HINT and, 168
   low-frequency techniques and, 460
   Noah modules and, 552
   speech enhancement and, 457
Cochlear™ Carina®, 266
Cocktail party noise, 137
Code of ethics, 30, 45–47, 607–608
Coding, **43**
Cohort studies, 7
Cole, Bill, 604
ComDisDome, **10**
Committee on Accessible and Affordable Hearing Health Care for Adults, 33
Committee on Hearing Aid Selection and Fitting, Ad hoc, 37
Compact discs (CDs), 328
Compensation and Pension Evaluation Guidelines, 150
Complementary metal oxide semiconductor (CMOS), **318**
Completely-in-the canal (CIC)
   coupler, 487
   hearing aids, 241
      microphone locations and, 809
Composite noise, 620
Compression, 367
   applications, 370–372
   attack, 367

benefits/limitations of, 376–378
controlling, **367**
described, 365
dynamic, properties/audibility of, 375–376
effects of on speech, 372–373
   dynamic properties of, 373–375
input vs. output, 369–370
ratio, 366–367
training, 431
Compression kneepoint (CK), 365, 369
   AGCi and, 370
Compression limiting (CL), 39, 371–372
   described, 370
Compression threshold (CT), 39, 365
Computational auditory scene analysis, 385
Concerns, eliciting, 68–69
Condensation-cure silicone impression materials, 276–277
Condition for sale, 41
Conductive hearing loss, LDL and, 118
Conductor, described, 310
Confidence interval (CI), effect size (ES) and, 18–19
CONFIG (Coupler response for flat insertion gain), 811–813
   open-canal fittings and, **813**
Connected Speech Test (CST), 138, 155–158, 414, 536, 572
   band importance functions for, **804**
Connectivity, aid-to-aid, 446–448
Consonants, high-frequency, cochlear implant and, 458
Consultant on Audiometers and Hearing Aids, 473–475
Consumer Technology Association, 34
   directional, quality review, 15–16
Continuing education evidence (CEUs), 26
Continuous Flow Adaptor (CFA), 298
Contour Test, VIOLA and, 537
Contraction ratio, viscosity materials, **275**
Contralateral routing of signal (CROS) hearing aids, 258
   air conduction and, 258–260
   transcranial, 260–261
Conversational vocal effort, **77**
Cookie bite, **293**
CORFIG (Coupler response for flat insertion gain), 522
Corner audiogram, **293**
COSI (Client oriented scale of improvement), 201, 215–219
   excessive sound and, 724
   self-reporting-outcomes, 766–769
Costco, 31
Council on Physical Therapy of the American Medical Association, 473–475

Counseling, 729–730
  audiogram and, 102–106
  informational, 71–72
  strategy, **59**
Counterbalanced intervention (CBI) studies, 7–8
Coupler gain, **566**
Coupler response for flat insertion gain (CONFIG), 522, 811–813
Couplers
  CIC, 487
  clinical use of measures, **494**
  hearing aids, 485–488
  measurement, 484–485
  OFC, 487
  Zwislocki, 488–491
Coupling, streaming and, 450
Cox, Robyn, **8**, 111, 211, 528
Cox Contour Anchors, **723**
Cox Contour Test, 111, **113**, 543, 769
CPU (Central processing unit), **318**
Critical gain, measures, 234–235
CROS (Contralateral routing of signal) hearing aids, 258
  air conduction and, 258–260
    fittings, 703–705
    transcranial, 260–261
Crossed auditory pathways, 189
CST (Connected Speech Test), 138, 155–158, 536, 572
CT (Compression threshold), 39, 365
Cumulative Index to Nursing and Allied Health Literature (CINAHL), **10**
Current, described, 309–310
Current drain, batteries, 505–506
Custom hearing aids, 247–251
Cut-off frequencies, **337**

D

D/A (Digital to analog), conversion, 330–333
DAI (Direct audio input), 356
Dampers, described, 292–294
Damping
  effects, earhooks and, 291–294
  screens, 363
Danilewicz, Leonard, **325**
Data logging, 428–429
Davis, Hallowell, 27
DDD (Direct digital drive), **320–321**
DDT (Dichotic Digit Test), 193–195
Dead zones/regions, 128
Decibels
  adding, 789–790
  hearing loss and, **57**
  ratios of, **791**
  weighting, 790–791
Decision
  making, involving patients in, 72–73
  rules, 386
Deep canal hearing aids, 251–252
Delta convertors, 332
Dementia, hearing loss and, **61**
Department of Speech and Hearing Science, Arizona State University, 195
Deshon Army Hospital, 518–519
Deshon General Hospital, 28
Desired sensation level (DSL), 533–535, 540–543
  fitting software and, 119, **623**
  input/output (DSL [i/o]), 539, 539–540
  MPO (Maximum power output) and, 110
  RECD and, **675**
Device oriented subjective outcome (DOSO), 759–762
  post fitting self-assessment, 744
Devices, medical, FDA classification of, 476
DFS (Digital feedback suppression), 440–445, 509
  algorithms, benefits/limitations of, 442–443
  individualization of, 445
DFT (Discrete Fourier transform), **340**
DI (Directivity index), **409**, 508
  increasing, 414
Diabetes, opium and, 3
Diagnostic information, delivering, 71
Diaphragm, 360
Dichotic Digit Test (DDT), 193–195
Dichotic sentence identification test (DSI), 190
Dichotic speech tests, 189–195
  defined, **189**
Dielectric, described, **312**
DigiSpeech, 621
Digital amplifier, **320–321**
Digital delay, 334–335
Digital feedback suppression (DFS), 440–445, 509
  algorithms, benefits/limitations of, 442–443
  individualization of, 445
Digital filter banks, 336–339
Digital filters, 337
  coefficients, **338**
  quantifying, **338**
Digital noise reduction (DNR), 389–403, 695–697
  bilateral data sharing and, 446
  gain-reduction, 390–393
  limitations/clinical adjustment, 398
  nonspeech signals, 627
  quality control measures assessing, 512
  spatially-based, 396
Digital RF modulation, **325**

Digital signal processing (DSP), 333–340
    memory, 340–341
    sound, 326–330
Digital speech in noise, 621
Digital switches, **308**
Digital to analog (D/A), conversion, 330–333
Digital wireless telephones, FCC and, 481
Dillon, Harvey, 118, 530
Diotic, defined, **189**
Direct audio input (DAI), 356
Direct digital drive (DDD), **320–321**
Direct sequence spread spectrum (DSSS), **325**
Directional microphone, **397**, **404**, 508
    activating, 408
    effectiveness factors, 416–420
    gain equalization, 419
    insignificant factors, 420–421
    listening effort, 415
    localization/monitoring, 419–420
    orientation
        physical, 416
        port orientation, 416–418
    quality review, 15–16
    subjective benefit, 415–416
    technology, 691–695
    venting, 418–419
Directional processing, 446
Directionality, adjustment of, **409**
Directivity index (DI), **409**, 508
    increasing, 413–414
Direct-recall, described, 190
Dirks, Don, 639
Discrete Fourier transform (DFT), **340**
Dispensers
    defined, 41
    FDA regs and, 477
Display
    accuracy of software, 617
    output, 632
Distortion, described, **310**
DNR (Digital noise reduction), 389–403, 695–697
    attack time, 391–392
    limitations/clinical adjustment, 398
    nonspeech signals, 627
    quality control measures assessing, 512
    spatially-based, 396
Doerfler, Leo, 30
DOSO (Device oriented subjective outcome), 759–762
    post fitting self-assessment, 744
DRAM (Dynamic random access memory), **342**
Drive rod, 360
DSI (Dichotic sentence identification test), 190

DSL (Desired sensation level) method, 533–535
    Multistage Input/Output v5.0, 80, 540–543
        fitting software and, **623**
        MPO (Maximum power output) and, 110, 119
    RECD and, **675**
DSL i/o (Desired sensation level) input/output, 539–540
DSP (Digital signal processing), 326–341
    memory, 340–341
    sound, 326–330
DSPfactory, **364**
DSSS (Direct sequence spread spectrum), **325**
Dual compression, described, 370–371
Dual streaming, 448
Dubno data, 148
DVDs, Blu-Ray, 328
Dynamic compression, properties/audibility of, 375–376
Dynamic random access memory (DRAM), **342**
Dynamic range, 80–81
Dynamic Roving Tone, 621

E

Ear canal resonance, 650
Ear effect, unaided, avoidance of, 230–231
Ear impressions, 273–282
    contraindications of, 278
    good, 277–280
    material terms, **275**
    materials, 276–277
    for microphone port openings, **280**
    scanning, 280–282
    syringe/gun, 274–275
Eardrum
    perforated, ear impressions and, 278
    transformation, 805, 807
Earhooks, damping effects and, 291–294
Earlens Corporation, **469**
Earlens™, 468–469
The Earmold as Part of the Receiver Acoustic System, 288
Earmold plumbing, frequency response range and, **294**
Earmold tubing, NAEL sizes, **294**
Earmolds
    care of, **711**
    materials, 282–288
    modular fittings, 287–288
    plumbing, 286–291
        acoustics of, 288–291
    styles, 284–286
Earphones
    monosyllabic words, recognition scores, 148
    RETSPLs and, 785–789
    speech-in-noise testing and, 140

EarQ, 31
Eartips, **286**
   care of, **711**
   OC fittings and, **255**
Earwax
   ear impressions and, 278
   limiting drainage of, 364
   receivers and, 363
ECHO (Expected consequences of hearing aid ownership), 201, 211–215
   excessive sound and, 724
ECR (Effective compression ratio), 375
Educational Audiology, complaints to FDA, 480
EEG (Electroencephalpgram), 385
EEPROM (Electrically erasable programmable read-only memory), **342**
Effect size (ES), 16–18
   confidence interval (CI) and, 18–19
   defined, **5**
Effective audibility, 626
Effective compression ratio (ECR), 375
Effective eardrum volume, 490
Effectiveness
   hearing aids, 40
   of treatment, 40
Efficacy, hearing aids, 40
Efficiency
   hearing aids, 40
   of treatment, 40
Effort
   listening, 595–596
      objective measures of, 598–600
EHIMA (European Hearing Instrument Manufacturers Association), 56, 624
EIN (Equivalent input noise), 503–505
Elderly, age and, 119
Electrical transformers, T-coils and, 355
Electrically erasable programmable read-only memory (EEPROM), **342**
Electroacoustic measures, 495–507
   guide, 495–499
Electroencephalpgram (EEG), 385
Electromagnetic induction, 313
Electronic principles, hearing aids, 309–326
Empathy, demonstrating, 70–71
Empirical evidence, 3
Energetic masking, **137**
Enhanced audibility extender, **461**
Entific Medical Systems, 263
Environment, noise in, **575**
Envoy Esteem®, 266
EPROM (Erasable programmable read-only memory), **342**
Equivalent input noise (EIN), 503–505

Erasable programmable read-only memory (EPROM), **342**
Ericsson Telecommunications, **316**
ES (Effect size), 16–18
   confidence interval (CI) and, 18–19
   defined, **5**
"Essential" telephones, **481**
Ethics, 45–51
   behavior, unethical, 46–47
   code of, 30, 45–47, 607–608
   licensure and, 48–49
   manufacturers, 48–50
   medical centers, 50–51
   VA and, 50
Etymotic Design Incorporated, 604
Etymotic gain, **566**
Etymotic research, **364**
   BKB-SIN and, 175
   obtaining
      BKB-SIN, 175
      QuickSIN test, 172
European Hearing Instrument Manufacturers Association (EHIMA), 56, 624
Event-based training, **431**
Evidence
   based practice, 39–40
   case reports/series, 6
   grading, 16
   levels of, 12, 40
      pyramid, 5
   pyramid levels of, **5**
   terms used, **5**
   for verification/validation, 20–24
Evidence-Based Practice (EBP)
   defined, 2–3
   importance of, 1
   schematic of, **9**
Excessive sound, 720–722
Expected Consequences of Hearing Aid Ownership (ECHO), 201, 211–215
   excessive sound and, 724
Expert opinion, 4, 6
Extended wear technologies, 469–470
External devices, **449**
   wireless routing from, 450

F

Faceplates, recessed, 249–251
False claims act, 43
Family of Prescriptive Methods, 530–531
   revised, 532–533
      for severe and profound losses (NAL-RP), 532–533

Farad, **312**
Faraday, Mihael, 313
Faraday's law, 313
Fast Fourier Transform (FFT), 335–336, 340, 632
Fatigue, listening, 595–596
FBR (Measurement of front-to-back ratio), 508–510
FCC (Federal Communications Commission), 480–482
   complaints to, 481–482
FDA (Food and Drug Administration), 476–478
   1993 uprising, 477–478
   510(k), **480**
   BAI and, 263, 265
   complaints to, 479–480
   medical clearance, 41
   red flags, 41
   regulations, 40–41, 476–477
FDA Modernization Act, 478–479
Federal Communications Commission (FCC), 480–482
   complaints to, 481–482
Federal Food, Drug, and Cosmetic Act, 34
Federal Trade Commission (FTC), 226
   Red Flag Rules, 41, 42
Feedback
   acoustic, 718–722
      described, 233
      hearing aid selection and, 233–237
      internal, 236
   identifying/modeling, 440
   management, quality control of, 512–513
   path cancellation, 441–442
   reduction algorithms, 719
   stigma and, **236**
   suppression, 563
      assessment of, 700–703
      of digital, 440–445
FFT (Fast Fourier Transform), 335–336, 340, 632
FHSS (Frequency-hopping spread-spectrum), 323–324, **325**
Field tested best practice, **38**
Fifer, Bob, 44
FIFs (Frequency Important Functions), 83–84
FIG6, 537–538
Filter
   described, **310**
   bands, **337**
   length, **338**
   phase response, 338
   roving notch, 440
   slope, **337**
Filtering
   defined, **337**
   notch, 440–441
Fine tuning, automatically, **556**

Finite impulse response (FIR), 338
FIR (Finite impulse response), 338
Fitting
   appointment, 711, 713–714
      follow-up, short-term, 714–715
   guidelines, hearing aids, 39–40
   software
      clinical protocol, 110
      using, 105–106
   tolerances, 606
Fittings
   bilateral, **113**
   CROS, 703–705
   dilemma of, **231**
   eras, 518–520
   modular, earmolds, 287–288
   open-canal, 272, 615, **657**
      CONFIGS and, **813**
      loudness measures and, **593**
      MPO and, 118–119
      RCED and, 118
      RESR and, 118
   pre-fitting LDLs, 119
   proprietary, 610–614
   RECD and, 120–121
Fixed SNR, vs. adaptive, 138–139
FL (Frequency-lowering), 697–700
   algorithms, 459–468
   benefits/limitations of, 464–467
   goals, 467–468
   techniques, **461**
   technology, 129
Flash
   drives, **342**
   memory, **342**
Flat
   aided audiogram, 523
   response, 523
Flex strips, connecting, 554
Fluid discharge, ear impressions and, 278
Fluorescent lights, T-coils and, 355
FM (Frequency modulation), 323–324
   FCC and, 480–481
   testing, **623**
FOG (Full-on-gain), 501
Follow-up procedures, short-term, 714–715
Food and Drug Administration (FDA), 265, 476–478
   1993 uprising, 477–478
   510(k), **480**
   BAI and, 263
   complaints to, 479–480
   Federal Food, Drug, and Cosmetic Act and, 34
   on hearing aids and PSAPs, 33

Food and Drug Administration (FDA) *(continued)*
  medical clearance, 41
  Modernization Act, 478–479
  regulations, 40–41
Foreign objects, ear impressions and, 278
Four habits model, candidates and, 67–73
Fourier transform
  defined, **340**
  discrete, **340**
Frame processing, 335
Free-field eardrum transfer function, 650
Freeman, Barry, **456**
Free-recall, described, 190
Frequencies
  horn cutoff, 296–298
  testing
    best, 116
    how many, 116
Frequency
  bands for AI, 86–87
  bandwidth, remote microphones, **406**
  channels, **337**
  compression, **460**, **461**, 462–464
  domain, 335–336
  factors, **385**
  phase shifting, 442
  reinforcement, music playback and, **465**
  response, 502
    range, earmold plumbing and, **294**
    shape, described, **310**
Frequency importance functions (FIFs), perpetually relevant, 83–84
Frequency modulation (FM), 323–324
  FCC and, 480–481
  testing, **623**
Frequency transposition (FT), **460**, 462
Frequency-hopping spread-spectrum (FHSS), 323–324, **325**
Frequency-lowering (FL), 697–700
  algorithms, 459–468
  benefits/limitations of, 464–467
  goals, 467–468
  techniques, **461**
  technology, 129
Frequency-specific
  analysis, 335–336
  data, 338
  delay, 334–335
  functional gain, 562
  measures, pre-fitting tests using, 101–134
Front volume, 360
Frye Electronics, 151, 621

FT (Frequency transposition), **460**, 462
FTC (Federal Trade Commission), 226, 475–476
  Rear-ear saturation response (RESR), 42
  Red Flag Rules, 41
Full-on-gain (FOG), 501
Functional gain, **567**
  frequency specific, 562
  verification, 562–565
Fun-Tak, 485

G

Gain, 364–366
  controlling, **367**
  defined, 226
  equalization, directional microphone, 419
  formula
    coupled, **527**
    desired insertion, **527**
  high-frequency, 171
    open/closed, **256**
  increase algorithms, 733
  reduction, DNR and, 390–393
  terminology, **566–567**
  verification, 562–565
Gain reduction digital noise reduction (G-DNR), 390–393
  clinical quantification of, **392**
  evidenced-based benefits, 396–398
Game ear, 33
Gatehouse, Stuart, **731**, 749
  compression and, 376
  COSI and, 216
  SSQ and, 774
G-DNR (Gain reduction DNR), 390–393
  clinical quantification of, **392**
  evidenced-based benefits, 396–398
Geometric positioning, 640
Geotagged memories, 454
GHABP (Glasgow Hearing Aid Benefit Profile), 749–752
  post fitting self-assessment, 744
  self-reporting-outcomes, 745–749
Glasgow Hearing Aid Benefit Profile (GHABP), 749–752
  post fitting self-assessment, 744
  self-reporting-outcomes, 749–752
Global Coils SAGL, **364**
GN (Great Nordic), 30
Gnewikow, David, 2
Good Manufacturing Practices for Hearing Aids, 34
Good Practice Guidance for Adult Hearing Aid Fittings and Services, 37
  on fitting tolerances, 606
Google Scholar, 9

Great Nordic (GN), 30
Grief, stages of, 64
Guidelines for Hearing Aid Fitting for Adults, 37
Guidelines for the Audiologic Management of Adult Hearing Impairment, 37

H

HA-1 coupler, 485
HA-2 coupler, 485–486
HA-3 coupler, 486
HA-4 coupler, 486–487
HAC (Hearing Aid Compatibility) for Wireline Telephones, 481
HACTES (Hearing Aid Clinical Test Environment Standardization), 621
HAIC (Hearing Aid Industries Council), 482
Hand-mixed silicones, 277
Hang three approach, 29
Hardware
    hearing aids, 342–356
        microphones, 342–354
        T-coils, 354–356
HARL website, 537
Harmonic distortion measures, 503
The Harvard Report, 518
HASP (Hearing aid selection profile), 201, 219–222
HAT (Hearing assisted technology), 96, 269–270
Hawkins, David, 111
HCL (Highest comfortable level), **107**, 371
    MSU method and, 528
Head-shadow effect, 232, 804–805
    amplitude compression and, 446
    CROS and, 259, **272**, 703–704
    elimination of, 227–228
    hearing aids and, **259**
    high frequencies and, **242**, 261
    implantable bone stimulating devices, 265
    loudspeaker presentation and, 630, **636**
    unilateral beamformer and, **350**
Head transformations, 804–805
Headphones
    Bluetooth™ and, 326
    CID procedure and, 526
    directionality and, **513**
    feedback and, 513
    HINT and, 167
    monitor, 632
    QuickSIN test and, 172–173
    word-in-noise testing and, 177
Health Insurance Portability and Accountability Act (HIPPA), 41–42

gifts/inducements to beneficiaries, 43–44
Hearing
    hearing aids vs., **227**
    threshold measurement, 782–785
        factors affecting, **788**
Hearing aid candidate, 53–74
    MarkeTrak, 54–56
    willingness to use hearing aids, 56–57
Hearing Aid Clinical Test Environment Standardization (HACTES), 621
Hearing Aid Compatibility Act of 1988, 480
Hearing Aid Compatibility (HAC) for Wireline Telephones, 481
Hearing aid control
    bilateral data sharing and, 445–448
        feature control and, 446
Hearing Aid Industries Council (HAIC), 482
Hearing aid occlusion effect, assessing, 706–708
Hearing Aid Research Laboratory, 572, 758
Hearing aid selection profile (HASP), 201
Hearing aids, 572
    adjustment to, 729–730
        TEN test and, 132–133
    analyzers, 493–495
    assessment, ANSI standards used in, 491–493
    audibility/speech recognition, 571–577
    automatic fine tuning, **556**
    batteries for, 357–359
    benefits of, 59–60
        limitations of, **271–272**
    best setting, **496**
    BiCROS, 258
    bone conduction, 262–263
    candidates, identifying, 64–66
    care/maintenance of, 713
    connecting devices to, potential limitations, 456–457
    couplers, 485–488
    CROS, 258
    digital, filter banks and, 337
    directional, evidenced-based benefits, 411–416
    distribution channels, 30–35
    effectiveness, 40
    efficacy, 40
    efficiency, 40
    electronic principles of, 309–326
    extended wear, 469–470
    fitting, 1
        code of ethics, 45–46
        guidelines, 39–40
        terminology, 730
    government regulation of, 475–482
    grades of recommendation, **39**

Hearing aids (continues)
  hardware, 342–356
    T-coils, 354–356
  head-shadow effect and, **259**
  hearing vs., **227**
  input analysis, 384–388
  input ceilings of, **328**
  LDL and, 118
  licensure laws, 48–49
  limitations, 440–457
  manufacturers
    ethical behavior for, 46–47
    ethics and, 48–50
  moisture and, 713
  non-government regulation of, 482–484
  normalization process, 58
  open-canal, 440
  open-conduction, measurement methods, 491
  orientation of, **710–711**
  over-the-counter, 33
  plumbing and, **296**
  potential problems/solutions, **712–713**
  prescriptive approaches, 522–549
    Australian National Laboratories Family of Prescriptive Methods, 530–533
    Berger method, 524–526
    CID procedure, 526
    comparing, 545–549
    Desired sensation level (DSL), 533–535
    FIG6 and, 537–538
    input/output [i/o], 539–543
    LGOB, 535
    Libby, 529–530
    Lybarger half-gain rule, 523
    MSU, 528–529
    NAL-NL2
    Pascoe, 523–524
    POGO, 526–527, **528**
    Rickets and Bentler (RAB), 537
    VIOLA, 535–537
    Watson and Knudsen, 522–523
  programming of, 549–556
    adjusting, 557–558
    connecting boots, 553–554
    connecting FlexConnect strips, 554
    features/options, 556–557
    special features activation, 557–558
    user memories, 557
    wireless, 554
  reasons for not using, **57**
  receivers, 359–364
  recessed faceplates, 249–251
  selection of, 170–171
    testing, 781–789
  signal classification system, 90
  signal's path through, **381**
  signals to, 356
  smartphone pairing, 455–456
  stages of, 225
  state sales laws, **33**
  stigma, 58–59
  stigmatization process, 58
  style selection, acoustic feedback, 233–237
  styles, 240–258
    body, 241–242
    BTE, 242–244
    deep canal CIC, 251–252
    mimi, 257–258
    open canal fittings, 252–257
    special designs, 258–266
    traditional custom, 247–251
  table of evidence, **39**
  targeted interventions, 468–470
  telephone used with, 713
  trainable, 430–439
    advantages of, 432–433
    disadvantages of, 433
    gain increase algorithms, 733
    research with, 433–438
  unilateral vs. bilateral, 171–172
  user controls, 266–269
  VCS and, **268**
  willingness to use, 56–57
Hearing Aids 101, 611
Hearing assisted technology (HAT), 96, 269–270
Hearing Handicap Inventory for Elderly (HHIE), 780
  PPDIS and, 187
Hearing Handicap Inventory for Elderly/Adults (HHIE/A), 70, 201–206
  post fitting self-assessment, 744
  report card for, **741**
  scoring, 738
Hearing In Noise Test (HINT), **17**, **351**
  adaptive versus fixed SNR and, 138
  microphone technologies and, 411
  pediatric, 580
  Performance-Perceptual Test (PPT), 186, 188
  QuickSIN test, 169
  reception thresholds, 139, 162–168
  speech noise and, 137
  trainable hearing aids and, 434–435
  Words in Noise (WIN) Test, 172–182
Hearing In Noise Test-C (HINT-C), 413
Hearing Industries Association, 34

Hearing Industries Association (HIA)
  NFO panel and, 54–56
  task force, 1993 uprising and, 478–479
Hearing Instrument Manufacturers' Software Association (HIMSA), 551
Hearing Instruments, 55
The Hearing Journal, 55, 249, 648
Hearing loss
  acquired, cochlea, 128
  conductive, LDL and, 118
  deciles, **57**
  degree of, 231–232
  dementia and, **61**
Hearing Loss Association of America (HLAA), 355
Hearing Planet, 32
Hearing Tests and Hearing Instrument, 27
HearUSA, 31
Helmholtz resonator, **290**
Henry, defined, 313
Henry, Joseph, 313
HFA-FOG (High-frequency average full-on gain), 501
HFA-OSPL90, 501
HFE (High Frequency Emphasis), 171
  QuickSIN test and, 169
HHIE/A (Hearing Handicap Inventory for the Elderly/Adult), 70, 201–206
  post fitting self-assessment, 744
  report card for, **741**
  scoring, 738
HIA (Hearing Industry Association)
  NFO panel and, 54–56
  task force, 1993 uprising and, 478–479
High frequencies, individualization of extended, 459
High Frequency Emphasis (HFE),
  QuickSIN test and, 169
  Low Pass (HFE-LP), 171
High viscosity materials, **275**
Highest comfortable level (HCL), **107**
  MSU method and, 528
High-frequency
  consonants, cochlear implant and, 458
  gain, 171
    reinforcement, **460**, 464
  QuickSIN test and, 169
High-level compression (HLC), **107**, 371
High-level speech, limits of, 543
HIMSA (Hearing Instrument Manufacturers' Software Association), 551
HINT (Hearing in Noise Test), **17, 351**
  Acceptable Noise Level (ANL), 182
  adaptive versus fixed SNR and, 138
  microphone technologies and, 411
  pediatric, 580
  Performance-Perceptual Test (PPT), 186, 188
  QuickSIN test, 169
  reception thresholds, 139, 162–168
  speech noise and, 137
  trainable hearing aids and, 434–435
  Words in Noise (WIN) Test, 172–182
HINT-C, 413, 580
HIPPA (Health Insurance Portability and Accountability Act), 41–42
  gifts/inducements to beneficiaries, 43–44
HI-PRO, 551
HLAA (Hearing Loss Association of America), 355
Horn effects, sound bore tubing and, 296–298
Humes, Larry, 34
Hunter's ear, 33
Hyperacusis
  defined, 120
  LDL and, 119–120

I

ICRA (International Collegium of Rehabilitative) signals, 621, 625
  obtaining, **622**
Identity, stigma induced threat to, 58–59
IEC (International Electrotechnical Commission), 78, 482, 483–484
IEC 711 couplers, 491
IEC 711 real-ear simulator, 488–489, 493
IEC 60118, 797
IEC 60118-15, 800
IEC 60268-16, 94
IEC 60318, 489
IEC 60711, 489
IFFT (Inverse Fast Fourier Transform), 335
I/G (Input/gain), functions, 365–366
IHAFF (The Independent Hearing Aid Fitting Forum), 37, 111, 605
IID (Interaural Intensity Difference), **242**
IIR (Infinite impulse response), 338
ILD (Interaural Level Difference), **242**
  cues, 419–420
Impacted earwax, ear impressions and, 278
Implantable, bone conduction stimulation, 262–265
Implicit Association Test, 51
Impulse response, **338**
In situ
  gain, **566–567**
  testing, 125–127
Independent Hearing Aid Fitting Forum (IHAFF), 37, 111, 605

Inductance, 313–318
Induction
    coil response, 506–507
    electromagnetic, 313
    generators, 355
Infinite impulse response (IIR), 338
Inflammation, ear impressions and, 278
Informational masking, **137**
Input ceilings, of hearing aids, **328**
Input compression, vs. output compression, 369–370
Input levels
    loud, 732–733
    soft, 730–732
Input signal, intensity of, 431
Input/gain (I/G), functions, 365–366
Input/output (I/O), functions, 365–366
Insertion gain, **566**
Intelligibility subjective ratings, 584–589
Interaction effect, described, 193
Interaural Intensity Difference (IID), **242**
Interaural Level Difference (ILD), **242**
Interference
    binaural, 232
        screening for, **233**
Internal acoustic feedback, 236
International Collegium of Rehabilitative (ICRA) signals, 621, 625
    obtaining, **622**
International Electrotechnical Commission (IEC), 78, 483–484
International Outcome Inventory for Hearing (IOI-HA)
    post fitting self-assessment, 744
    self-reporting-outcomes, 762–766
International Society of Audiology, Good Practice Guidance for Adult Hearing Aid Fittings and Services, 37
International Speech Test Signal (ISTS), 493, 623–626
Internet sales, hearing aids, 31–32
Intertragal Notch Rule, 640
Interval scale, 585–589
In-the-canal (ITC) hearing aids, 241
    couplers and, 485
    microphone locations and, 809
In-the-ear (ITE) hearing aids, 240–241
    couplers and, 485
    microphone locations and, 807–808
Introduction to Research, 4
Inverse Fast Fourier Transform (IFFT), 335
I/O (Input/output), functions, 365–366
IOI-HA (International Outcome Inventory for Hearing)
    post fitting self-assessment, 744
    self-reporting-outcomes, 762–766

Ipsilateral suppression, 189
ISTS (International Speech Test Signal), 493, 623–626
ITC (In-the-canal) hearing aids, 241
    couplers and, 485
    microphone locations and, 809
ITD (Interaural Time Difference), **242**
ITE (In-the-ear) hearing aids, 240–241
    couplers and, 485
    microphone locations and, 808
"It's a Matter of Ethics", 607

J

Jadad scale, 15–16
Jerger, James, 30, 138, 189
Journal of Speech Disorders, 27
Journal of the American Medical Association, 474

K

Kahneman, Daniel, 4
Katz Clinical Audiology Handbooks, 288
KEMAR (Knowles Electronics Manikin for Acoustic Research), 229
Kessler, David, 477, 478
Killion, Mead, 537
Kimura, Doreen, 189
Kincaid, Gerald, 639
Knowledge-Attitude-Practices (KAP), 3
Knowles Electronics, 55–56, **364**, 489–491
    Manikin for Acoustic Research (KEMAR), 229
Knowles microphone, 618
Kochkin, Sergei, 779
Kowal-Bench, 172
Kubler-Ross's five stages of grief, 64

L

Lamarr, Hedy, **325**
LDL (Loudness discomfort level), 11, **107**, **528**, 732–733
    administration/scoring of, 110–120
    age and, 119
    air-bone gap and, 118
    audiometer limits and, 117–118
    bilateral, **113**
    clinical application, 113–120
    conducting, 117
    conductive hearing loss and, 118
    FAQs about, 115–120
    hearing aid use and, 118
    hyperacusis and, 119–120
    instructions, 111, **112**

measures, 546–547
prefitting, 119
test procedures, 111–113
testing, 106, 108
testing reliability, 117
variability measures, 108–109
LE Bluetooth, 326
   remote microphones and, **406**
   RF and, 448
   streaming and, 453
   wireless streaming, 448
Least Mean Square (LMS) filters, 402
Left ear deficit, described, 193
Level coding, of research design, **12–13**
Levels of evidence, 12, 40
   pyramid of, 5
LFL (Low-frequency limit), 460
LGOB (Loudness growth in one-half octave Bands), 535
Libby, E. Robert "Cy", 529
Libby horn, 298
Libby prescriptive approach, 529–530, 647
Licensure
   audiology, 36
   ethics and, 48–49
Light actuated amplification, 468–469
Likert scale, 21, 25, **758**
   COSI (Client Oriented Scale of Improvement) and, 219
   listening effort/fatigue and, 597
   MarkeTrak and, 61
Limitations, hearing aids, 440–457
Lin, Frank, **61**
Lincoln law, 43
Linear
   phase, 339
   window, sliding, 371
Lipitor, 51
Liquid impression material, 276
Listen in the gaps, 137
Listening
   effort, 415, 595–596
      objective measures of, 598–600
   effort/fatigue, 596–600
   environment, **412**
   fatigue, 595–596
   in noise, 545–546
LMS (Least Mean Square) filters, 402
Long-Term Average Speech Spectrum (LTASS), 76–78, 95, 102–103
   differences across, 78
   measurement bandwidths, **798**
   microphone systems and, 621–626
   NAL, 531

overall level for, **800**
proprietary fittings, 610
speech noise and, 137
speech signal and, 796–797
VIOLA and, 537
vocal effect on, **620**
Long-term speech acoustics, 75–81
Loud input levels, 732–733
Loudness
   anchors, 110–111, **723**
   excessive, 720–722
   monaural balancing, 523
   summation, 228–229
Loudness discomfort level (LDL), 11, **107**, **528**, 732–733
   administration/scoring of, 110–120
   age and, 119
   air-bone gap and, 118
   bilateral, **113**
   clinical applications, 113–120
   conducting, 117
   conductive hearing loss and, 118
   FAQs about, 115–120
   hearing aid use and, 118
   hyperacusis and, 119–120
   instructions, 111, **112**
   measures, 546–547
   prefitting, 119
   test procedures, 111–113
   testing, 106, 108
      reliability, 117
   variability measures, 108–109
Loudness equalization, vs. loudness normalization, **536**
Loudness growth in one-half octave bands (LGOB), 535
Loudness judgments
   aided, 590–595
   conducting, 592–593
Loudness measures
   behavioral aided, need for, 590–591
   open fittings and, **593**
Loudness normalization, vs. loudness equalization, **536**
Loudness testing
   conducting aided, 591–592
   unilateral/bilateral, **592**
Loudspeakers, 314–315
   correct placement of, **637**
   presentation, probe microphone and, 630
Low energy (LE) Bluetooth™, 326
Low-frequency limit (LFL), 460
Low-level
   expansion, gain and, 562–563
   noise reduction, 379
Low Pass (HFE-LP), High Frequency Emphasis, 171

Low threshold compression (LTC), described, 370
Lower frequency cutoff, **792**
Lower viscosity materials, **275**
LTASS (Long-Term Average Speech Spectrum), 76–78, 95, 102–103, 531, 604
  differences across, 78
  measurement bandwidths, **798**
  microphone systems and, 621–626
  overall level for, **800**
  proprietary fittings, 610
  speech noise and, 137
  speech signal and, 796–797
  VIOLA and, 536
  vocal effect on, **620**
LTC (Low threshold compression), described, 370
Lucite earmolds, 282
Lybarger, Samuel, 518, 523
Lybarger half-gain rule, 518, 523

M

Magnetic
  feedback, 361
    loop, 361
  flux, 313–314
  shielding, 361
Magnitude estimation, **585**
Maico Corporation, 27
Maintenance instructions, **711**
Manhattan II, **389**
Manikin for Acoustic Research (KEMAR) Knowles Electronics Manikin for Acoustic Research, 489–491
Manufacturers, ethical behavior for, 46–47
MarkeTrak
  hearing aid candidate, 54–56
  Likert scale, 61
  vs. SADL (Satisfaction with Amplification in Daily Life), **754**
MarkeTrak VIII, 21–24, 108, 401, 617
MarkeTrak9, new baseline, 56
Maryland CNCs, 150–151
Masking
  energetic/informational, **137**
  Tinnitus, 468
Maximum output, setting corrections, 814–816
Maximum permissible ambient noise levels (MPANL), 781
Maximum power output (MPO), **107**
  Berger method, 524–526
  comparative study of, 110
  fitting software and, 110
  LDL and, 109
  NAL-NL2 fitting and, 110, 118–119
  open-canal fittings and, 118–119
  POGO method, 527
  software adjustments, 114–115
  test signals and, 627
  verification of, 593–595, 688–691
Maxwell-Faraday equation, 313
MCL (Most Comfort Level), 182
  equal loudness curve, 522–523
  Lybarger half-gain rule, 523
  Pascoe method, 523–524
  Watson and Knudsen, 522–523
MDVR beamformers, 396
Mean sound pressure levels, in one-third octaves, **799**
Measurement
  couplers, 484–485
  errors, 590
  methods
    open-conduction hearing aid, 491
    RECD, 123
  microphone, 631
Measurement of front-to-back ratio (FBR), 508–510
Measurement of Performance Characteristics of Hearing Aids, 492
Measurement of Real-Ear Performance Characteristics of Hearing Aids, 493
Med-EL Bonebridge, 263
Med-El Vibrant®, 266
Medicaid, antikickback statue, 41
Medical centers, ethics and, 50–51
Medical devices, FDA classification of, 476
Medicare, antikickback statue, 41
Medicare and Medicaid Patient Protection Act of 1987, 42
MedRx, 619
MedTronic Sophono Alpha2™, 263
MEI (Middle ear implants), 265–266
Mel-Frequency-Cepstral Coefficients (MFCCs), **384**
Memories
  DSP, 340–341
  flash, **342**
  user, hearing aids, 557
  sticks, **342**
  VC, **269**
Memphis State University (MSU), prescriptive approach, 528–529
MEMS (Microelectro-mechanical system) microphone, 312–313
Meta-analysis, 11
Method for Coupler Calibration of Earphones, 493

Methods for Calculation of Speech Intelligibility Index, 104
Methods for Characterizing Signal Processing in Hearing Aid with Speech-like Signal, 797
MFCCs (Mel-Frequency-Cepstral Coefficients), **384**
Microelectro-mechanical system (MEMS) microphone, 312–313
Microphone arrays, traditional/high order, 407–409
Microphone location effect (MLE), 812
Microphones
    adjusting, **423**
    adjustment of directionality, **409**
    based, noise reduction, 403, 405
    calibration of, **486**
    capacitance and, 311–313
    directional, **397**, **404**, 508
        activating, 408
        effectiveness factors, 416–420
        gain equalization, 419
        insignificant factors, 420–421
        listening, effort 415
        localization/monitoring, 419–420
        measures, 632–634
        orientation: physical, 416
        orientation: port, 416–418
        quality review, 15–16
        subjective benefit, 415–416
        technology, 691–695
        venting effects, 418–419
    hearing aid hardware and, 342–354
    individualization of, 421
    measurement, 631
    MEMS, 312
    noise reduction, 379
    port openings, ear impressions and, **280**
    probe
        See Probe microphone
    reference/regulating, 630–631
    remote, 405–407, **725**
        beamformers and, 412
    situation-specific, 423–426
    technology tradeoffs, **422**
    transformations and, 807–809
Middle-ear implants (MEI), 265–266
Military
    audiology and, 27–28
    health care system, 244
Military Medical Retention Board (MMRB), 159
Miracle Ear, 31, 478
Mirroring, audiogram techniques, 523
Mix ratio, **406**
MLE (Microphone location effect), 812

MMRB (Military Medical Retention Board), 159
Modern Developments in Audiology, 189
Modular
    fittings, earmolds, 287–288
    transmission function (MTF), 93–95
Modulated Speech Noise, 621
Modulation, digital RF, **325**
Moisture
    hearing aids and, 713
    receivers and, 363
Monaural
    hearing, **226**
    loudness balancing, 523
    summation, 590
Monitor
    headphones, 632
    probe microphone and, 630–631
Monosyllabic word testing, 142, **143**
    APHAB and, 208
    DDT and, 194
    Maryland CNCs, 141, 150
    NU#6, 141
    procedural rules of, **151**
    recognition scores, 148
    R-SPIN and, 155
    SPRINT and, 159
        scoring, 160
Monotic, defined, **189**
Most Comfort Level (MCL), 182
    equal loudness curve, 522–523
    Lybarger half-gain rule, 523
    Pascoe method, 523–524
    Watson and Knudsen, 522–523
Motion detection systems, 454
MPANL (Maximum Permissible Ambient Noise Levels), 781
MPO (Maximum power output), **107**
    Berger method, 524–526
    comparative study of, 110
    DSL v5.0 and, 110
    fitting software and, 110
    LDL and, 109
    NAL-NL2 fitting and, 110, 118–119
    open-canal fittings and, 118–119
    POGO method, 527
    RETSPLs and, 814
    software adjustments, 114–115
    test signals and, 627
    verification of, 593–595, 688–691
MSU (Memphis State University), prescriptive approach, 528–529

MTF (Modular transmission function), 93–95
Multiple channels, AGCo and, 372
Multitalker babble, 137–138, 159, **166**, 172, 176–177
   ANL measurement and, 184
   BNL and, 182
   QuickSIN test and, **181**
Multitalkers, 137
Munich, 521
Music
   data logging and, 428
   signal classification system and, 90, 386, 388
   train gain independently and, **268**
Musiek, Frank, 193
Musiek Auditec, 193

N

NAEL (National Association of Earmold Laboratories), 294
NAL (Australian National Laboratories), 647
   algorithm, 611
   Family of Prescriptive Methods, 530–531
   National Acoustic Laboratories method, 531–533
NAL-NL1 (National Acoustic Laboratories Nonlinear), 538–539
NAL-NL2 (National Acoustic Laboratories Nonlinear), 543–545
NAL-NL2 fitting, 80, 304, 433–435, 539–540, 543–550
   fitting software and, 110, 610–618, **623**
   MPO (Maximum power output) and, 110
   RECD and, **675**
   SII and, 34
NAL-R (National Acoustic Laboratories method), 532–533, 647
NAL-RP (National Acoustic Laboratories method), for severe and profound losses, 532–533
"Name-The-Circuit" contest, **389**
NASEM (National Academies of Sciences, Engineering and Medicine), 33
National Academies of Sciences, Engineering and Medicine (NASEM), 33
National Acoustic Laboratories method, Family of Prescriptive Methods, 530–531
National Acoustic Laboratories Nonlinear (NAL-NL1), 538–539
National Acoustic Laboratories Nonlinear (NAL-NL2), 543–545
National Association of Earmold Laboratories (NAEL), 294
National Family Opinion (NFO)
   HIA and, 54–56
   panel, 53

National Institute of Neurological Disorders and Stroke, 152
National Institute on Deafness and Other Communication Disorders (NIDCD), 477
National Institutes of Health, 477
National Provider Identifier (NPI), 42
National Society of Professional Engineers, 30
NBC Dateline, 477
Near-field electromagnetic induction (NFEI)
   Bluetooth™ receivers and, 452–453
   wireless streaming, 448
Neck loops, 355
Newport Audiology, 31
Newsweek, **389**
NFEI (Near-field electromagnetic induction)
   Bluetooth™ receivers and, 452–453
   wireless streaming, 448
NFO (National Family Opinion)
   HIA and, 54–56
   panel, 53
NIDCD (National Institute on Deafness and Other Communication Disorders), 477
Noah software system, 551–553
NOAHlink™, 551–552
Noahlink™, 551–552
Noble, Bill, SSQ and, 774
Noise
   age and, 119
   ambient levels of, 781–782
   classifications, **390**
   competing noises, 136–138
   in environments, 575
   improved speech understanding in, 228–229
   limitations of performance in, 580–582
   low level reduction of, 379
   microphone reduction of, 379
   reduction, **389**
      microphone-based, 403, 405
   signal, 792
   signal classification system and, 386
   speech recognition in, 135, 151–155, 411–415
Non-ear test, eliminating, 562
Nonlinear gain, 365
Nonrecursive filters, 338
Normative data, applied to categorical scaling, **589**
North Dakota, Hearing Aid Dealers license, 48–49
Northwestern University, 28
   NU#6, 141–150, 208
Notch
   filtering, 440–441
   filters, 294
NPI (National Provider Identifier), 42

NU#6, 141–150, 208
Nyquist, Harold, 329
Nyquist rate, 329, **331**, 332
Nyquist Theorem, 329–330
Nyquist-Shannon Theorem, 329–330

O

OAD (Obscure auditory dysfunction), 182
Obscure auditory dysfunction (OAD), 182
OC (Open canal) fittings, 252–257
    eartips and, **255**
    occlusion effect and, 239–240
Occluded Ear Simulator, 492
Occlusion effect, 237–240, 715–718, **719**
    identifying/treating, 239–240
    magnitude of, 238–239
Octaves, 792
    frequencies/band limits of, **795**
OFC (Open-fit coupler), 487
Ohio Hearing Aid Internet Work Group, 32
Ohm, defined, 310
Ohm, Georg Simon, 310
Oktoberfest, 521
Omnibus Budget Reconciliation Act of 1989, 42
Omnidirectional BTE, **409**
One question assessment, 200
One-third octaves, 792
    frequencies/band limits of, **795**
    mean sound pressure levels in, **799**
    prescriptive fittings comparisons, **796**
ONsemi, **364**
Open canal (OC) fittings, 252–257, 272, 615, **657**
    CONFIGS and, **813**
    eartips and, **255**
    MPO and, 118–119
    occlusion effect and, 239–240
    RCED and, 118
    RESR and, 118
Open-canal hearing aid, 440
Open-conduction, hearing aids, measurement methods, 491
Open-fit coupler (OFC), 487
Open fittings, loudness measures and, **593**
Open loop
    described, 235
    gain, measures, 234–235
    response, 233
Opium, diabetes and, 3
Ordinal scale, 585–589
Orthotelephonic gain, **566**
OSPL90, **107**

OTC (Over the counter)
    devices defined, 34
    hearing aids, 33
    wearable hearing devices, 33
OTE (Over-the-ear) hearing aids, 240
Oticon, 30, **449**
    frequency-lowering techniques and, **461**
    FT and, 462
Oticon Medical, 263
Otoscopy, hearing aid selection during, **252**
Ototronix Maxum, 266
Outcome measures, need for, 735–737
Outcomes
    behavioral, role of, 560–562
    domains of, **736**
Output
    compression, vs. input compression, 369–370
    display, 632
    maximum, setting corrections, 814–816
    sound pressure level (OSPL), with 90 dB input, 499–501
Over-the-counter (OTC)
    devices defined, 34
    hearing aids, 33
    wearable hearing devices, 33
Over-the-counter Hearing Aid Act of 2017, 34
Over-the-ear (OTE) hearing aids, 240

P

p value, defined, **5**
Paired comparisons, **585**
PAL (Profile of Aided Loudness), **723**, 759–762
    self-reporting-outcomes, 769–774
Palmer, Catherine, 45, 607–608
Parade Magazine, **389**
Pascoe, David, 523–524
Pathways, crossed auditory, 189
Patient characteristics, 3
Patients
    assessing attribution, 69
    counseling, 729–730
        graphing QuickSIN, 578–579
    expectations, 713–714
    identifying requests, 70
    loyalty, 24–26
    positioning of, 637
    return visits, 23–24
    speech-in-noise test and, 572
    stages of grief, 64
    training, clinical implementation of, 439
    understanding, 63–67
    See also Candidates

Pavlovic, Chas, 97
PB-testing, 135
PC (Peak clipping), 39, 115, 319
PCAST (President's Council of Advisors on Science and Technology), 33
Peak clipping (PC), 39, 115, 319
Peaky response, 236
Pediatric, Hearing In Noise Test (HINT), 580
Perceived Value Measurement (PVM), 617–618
Percentage Articulation Loss of Consonants, 94–95
Percentile analysis, 625–626
Perceptions, professionalism and, 617–618
Perceptual, acclimatization, **731**
Percy, Charles, 476
Perforated eardrum, ear impressions and, 278
Performance-Perceptual Test (PPT), 186–188
Permanent Committee on Investigations, 476
Personal sound amplifier product (PSAP), 32–35
Perspective, eliciting patient's, 69
Phase shifting, 442
Philadelphia Naval Hospital, 28
Phon, 791
Phonak, 30, **449**
  frequency-lowering techniques and, 460, **461**
Phonemic compression, described, 370
Phonetically balanced words, **803**
Piconet, 326
Pink noise, 512, 620, 627, **655**, 695, 792–794
  RECD measurement and, 676
Pinna, landmarks, **284**
Placebo effect, 585
  groups, **20**
  labeling bias effect, 2
Plumbing
  earmolds, 286–291
    acoustics of, 288–291
POGO (Prescription of gain and output), 526–528, 647
Points to Ponder: A Brief History of Digital Hearing Aids, **308**
Polar response pattern, 510–512
Polyvinyl chloride earmolds, 282–283
Positive Venting Valve (PVV), 302
Post-fitting visits
  self-assessment scales, 743–744
  treating feedback problems, 719–720
Powder impression material, 276
Power
  analysis of, **13**
  cells, 357–359
  decibels ratio of, **791**
  defined, **5**
  lines, T-coils and, 355
  supply, described, **310**

vs. pressure, 789, **790**
PPDIS, 186–187, **188**
PPT (Performance-Perceptual Test), 186–188
Practical significance, defined, **5**
Practice
  guidelines, **38**
  scope of, 35–36
  statement, scope of, **38**
Preferred
  dynamic range, 537
  practice patterns, American Speech-Language-Hearing Association (ASHA), **38**
Pre-fitting tests
  self-assessment scales, 197–223
    APHAB, 206–211
    COAT, 222–223
    COSI, 215–219
    ECHO, 211–215
    HASP, 219–222
    HHIE/A, 201–206
    one question assessment, 200
    preview of, 200–201
    reasons for using, 197–199
  in situ, 125–127
  speech-in-noise, 135–141
  using frequency-specific measures, 101–134
Prescription
  fitting, described, 603
  of gain and output (POGO), 526–527, 647
Prescriptive
  algorithm, 781
  fitting, 518
  formulas, 520
  methods, correction factors, 520–522
Prescriptive approaches, 522–549
  Australian National Laboratories Family of Prescriptive Methods, 530–531
  Berger method, 524–526
  CID procedure, 526
  comparing of
    approaches, 545–547
    outcomes, 547–549
  Desired sensation level (DSL), 533–535
    input/output (DSL [i/o]), 539–543
  FIG6 and, 537–538
  Libby, 529–530
  Loudness growth in one-half octave bands (LGOB), 535
  Lybarger half-gain rule, 523
  MSU, 528–529
  National Acoustic Laboratories method, 531–533
  Pascoe, 523–524
  POGO, 526–527, **528**

Rickets and Bentler (RAB), 537
VIOLA, 535–537
Watson and Knudsen, 522–523
Presentation
  loudspeakers, probe microphone and, 630
  mode
    NU#6, 146
    terminology, **189**
President's Council of Advisors on Science and Technology (PCAST), 33
Pressure
  decibels ratio of, **791**
  vs. power, 789, **790**
Preves, David, 618
Probe microphone
  best practice guidelines compliance, 605–608
    not to use, 608–618
  binaural analysis and, **633**
  calibration of tube, 634–636
  equipment, 618–632
  is speech mapping, 605
  monitor and, 630–631
  vs. rear ear, speech mapping, 604–605
  REOG measures with, 716
  test procedures/conditions, 632–645
  testing, **77**
  tube placement, 638–643
    questions asked about, 643–644
  using, 105–106
Probe-tube microphone
  See Probe microphone
Problems
  troubleshooting
    acoustic feedback, 718–720
    excessive noise, 720–722
    occlusion effect and, 715–718
    speech noise, 722–725
    telephones, 725–729
  troubleshooting, 715–729
Processing
  based noise reduction, 389–403
  techniques, 335–336
Professionalism, perceptions and, 617–618
Profile of Aided Loudness (PAL), **723**
  post fitting self-assessment, 744
  self-reporting-outcomes, 769–774
Programmable read-only memory (PROM), **342**
Programming
  hearing aids, 553–556
    adjusting, 557–558
    connecting books, 553–554
    connecting wireless, 554
    features/options, 556–557
    FlexConnect strips, 554
    special features activation, 557–558
    user memories, 557
PROM (Programmable read-only memory), **342**
Promising practice, 37, **38**
Pronto, 263
Proprietary fittings, 610–614
Protocol for the provision of Amplification, University of Western Ontario (UWO), 627–629
PSAP (Personal sound amplifier product), 32–35
PsychINFO, **10**
Public phones, T-coils and, 355
PubMed, **10**
PULHES, 159
Pulse-density modulation, **320**
Purdue University, 28
Pure tones
  NU#6, 148
  testing for, 117
Push-pull amplifier
  See Amplifiers, Class D
PVM (Perceived Value Measurement), 617–618
PVV (Positive Venting Valve), 302

Q

Quality
  control, 473
    of feedback management scheme, 512–513
    measures assessing digital noise reduction (DNR), 512
  markers, 15
  of life, 779–780
  subjective ratings, 584–589
Quasi-experimental studies, 12
QUEASY experiment, 12
QuickSIN, 137, 168–172, 172
  excessive sound and, 724
  graphing, patient counseling and, 578–579
  Hearing In Noise Test (HINT), 169, 176, 180
  proprietary fittings and, 611
  reliability of, **172**
  speech recognition and, 376–377
  speech-in-noise tests, 138
  WIN vs, **181**
Quiet, speech recognition in, 141–151

R

RAB (Rickets and Bentler), 537
Radio frequency (RF) transmissions, 323–326
  digital modulation, **325**
  streaming, 448–449

Radioear Company, 518, 523
Rainbow Passage, **79**
RAM (Random access memory), **342**
Random access memory (RAM), **342**
Randomized controlled trial (RCT), 8–9
Rapid Speech Transmission Index (RASTI), 95
Rapport, creating, 68
Rasmussen, Steen, 618
RASTI (Rapid Speech Transmission Index), 95
Rastronics, 619
    CCI-10, 618
Ratings
    speech-based subjective, 182–188
        ANL, 182–188
RCT (Randomized controlled trial), 8–9
Reading Span Test, 196
Read-only memory (ROM), **342**
REAG (Rear-ear aided gain), 647–648, 660–666
    predicted, 676
Reagan, Ronald, **389**
Real practice, vs best practice, **109**
Real-ear aided response
    (REAR), 633
    (REAR85), 633
    (REAR90), 633
Real-ear coupler difference (RECD), **107**, 634, 812
Real-ear dial difference (REDD), **107**, 522, 634
Real-ear insertion gain (REIG), 633
Real-ear occluded response (REOR), 632, 656–660
Real-ear saturation response (RESR), **107**, **114**, 120–125, 633, 670
    open-canal fittings and, 118
    predicted, 676
Real-ear unaided response (REUR), 632, 649–655
Real-speech signal
    REUG and, **655**
REAR (real-ear aided response), 633, 660–666, 669–670
    AGBF and, 443
    clinical application of, 672
    MSU method verification, 528
    verification test protocols, 663–665
    verifying with REIG, 650
    VIOLA and, 537
REAR85 (Real-ear aided response), 633, **662**, 688
Rear-ear aided gain (REAG), 647–648
Rear-ear aided response (REAR), 633, 660–666, 670–672
    AGBF and, 443
    clinical application of, 672
    MSU method and, 528
    verification test protocols, 663–665
    verifying with REIG, 650
    VIOLA and, 537

Rear-ear coupler difference (RECD), 521–522, 672–676, 809–810
    clinical application of, 676
    described, 121–122
    measurement methods, 123
    variability, 122
Rear-ear dial difference (REDD), **107**, 522, 634, 677–682
    clinical application of, 678
Rear-ear insertion gain (REIG), 647–648, **662**, 666–670
    VIOLA and, 537
Rear-ear measurements (REM), 604
Rear ear simulators, 488–489
Rear-ear occluded gain (REOG), 656–660
    measurement of, 659–660
        with probe microphone, 716
    occlusion effect and, 717
Rear-ear saturation response (RESR), adult applications of, 121–122
Rear-ear unaided gain (REUG), 647–648, 649–655
    clinical application of, 654–655
    TM perforation and, **654**
Recall patterns, 190
RECD (Real-ear coupler difference), **107**, **114**, 521–522, 634, 672–676, 809–810, 812
    adult applications of, 121–122
    clinical application of, 676
    fitting and, 120–121
    measurement methods, 123
    open-canal fittings and, 118
    variability, 122
Receiver-in-the-aid (RITA), 244
    hearing aids, 241, 719
    OFC and, 487
    vs. RIC, **246**
Receiver-in-the-canal (RIC), 244–245, 362
    hearing aids, 241
    OFC and, 487
    vs. RITA, **246**
Receiver-in-the-ear (RITE) hearing aids, hearing aids, 241
Receivers, 359–364
Reception threshold for speech (RTS), 138
Reception thresholds, speech-in-noise testing, 161–162
Recessed faceplates, 249–251
Rechargeable batteries, 358–359
Recursive filter, 338
Red Flag Rules, 41, 42
    FDA, 41
REDD (Real-ear dial difference), **107**, 522, 634, 677–682
    clinical application of, 678
    described, 121–122
    RETSPLs and, 677–678

Redundancy principle, 189
Reference equivalent threshold in SPL (RETSPLs), 6, **107**, 114, **114**, 121–122, 785–786
   earphones and, 785–789
   REAR85/90 and, 670
   RECD and, 634
   REDD and, 677–678
   RETSPLs and, 814
   in SPL, 521–522
Reference microphone, 630–631
Reference test gain (RTG), 501–502
Regulating microphone, 630–631
REIG (real-ear insertion gain), 633, 647–648, **662**, 666–670
   real speech and, 667–668
   REUR verification and, 650
   VIOLA and, 537
Reimbursement, 44
REIR
   See REIG (Real-Ear Insertion Gain)
Release time, 368
Reliability
   ANL measure, 185
   BKB-SIN, **175**
   measures of, 669
   PPT, 188
   of quickSIN test, **172**
Remote
   controls, 267
   microphones, 405–407
      beamformers and, 412
      frequency bandwidth, **406**
      type, **406**
   switches, **710**
REOG (Rear-Ear Occluded Gain), 656–660
   measurement of, 659–660
      with probe microphone, 716
      occlusion effect and, 717
REOR (Real-Ear Occluded Response), 632, 656–660
Requests, identifying patients, 70
Research
   design
      level-coding of, **12–13**
      subject selection, **14–15**
      described, 310
      evaluating, **8**
      validated best practice, **38**
Resonance, 650
   ear canal, 650
Resonator, Helmholtz, **290**
ReSound, 30, **449**, 535
   frequency-lowering techniques and, **461**

Response, flat, 523
RESR (Real-ear saturation response), **107**, **114**, 120–125, 633, 670
   open-canal fittings and, 118
   predicted, 676
Retail outlets, hearing aids, 31
Retrolental fibroplasia, 3
RETSPL (Reference equivalent thresholds in SPL), 6, **107**, 114, **114**, 121–122, 785–786
   earphones and, 785–789
   MPO and, 814
   REAR85/90 and, 670
   RECD and, 634
   REDD and, 677–678
   in SPL, 521–522
REUG (Rear-ear unaided gain), 647–648, 649–655
   clinical application of, 654–655
   real-speech signal and, **655**
   TM perforation and, **654**
REUR (Real-ear unaided response), 632, 649–655
   real-speech signal and, **655**
Reverberation, 95
   effects of, 90–93
   suppression, 399–400
Reverse
   cookie bite, **293**
   slope, **293**
"Revised Estimates of Minimum Audible Pressure: Where Is the Missing 6 dB?", **785**
Revised speech-In-noise (R-SPIN), 137, 151–152
   monosyllabic words and, 155
Revit, Larry, 114
RF (Radio frequency) transmissions, 323–326
   digital modulation, **325**
RIC (Receiver-in-canal), 244–245, 362
   hearing aids, 241
   OFC and, 487
   vs. RITA, **246**
Rickets and Bentler (RAB), 537
Right ear effect, 189
RITA (Receiver-in-the-aid), 244
   hearing aids, 241, 719
   OFC and, 487
   vs. RIC, **246**
RMS (Root mean square), 528
ROC curves, **204**
ROEG (Rear ear occluded gain), 656–660
ROM (Read-only memory), **342**
Room
   loops, 355
   masking, gain and, 562
Root mean square (RMS), 528

Routing, wireless, from external devices, 450
Roving notch filter, 440
R-SPIN (Revised speech-in-noise), 137, 151–152
   monosyllabic words and, 155
RTG (Reference test gain), 501–502
RTS (Reception threshold for speech), 138

S

SAAVC (Slow acting automatic volume control), described, 370
Sackett, David L., 39
SADL (Satisfaction with Amplification in Daily Life), 752–758
   vs. Marketrak, **754**
   normative data for, **755, 756–757**
   post fitting self-assessment, 744
The Saga of Barry Elpern, 30
SALD/A, downloading, 758
Sample size
   defined, **5**
   ES in *t*-test, **14**
Sam's Club, 31
Satisfaction with Amplification in Daily Life (SADL), 752–758
   vs. Marketrak, **754**
   normative data for, **755**
   post fitting self-assessment, 744
SAV (Select-a-Vent), 302
Scopus, **10**
Screens, damping, 363
SDRAM (Synchronous dynamic random-access memory), **342**
Search engines, systematic reviews, **10**
Select-a-Vent (SAV), 302
Selective amplification, 518
   Watson and Knudsen, 522–523
Self-assessment scales
   post-fitting, 743–744
   pre-fitting tests, 197–223
     APHAB, 206–211
     COAT, 222–223
     COSI, 215–219
     ECHO, 211–215
     HASP, 219–222
     HHIE/A, 201–206
     one question assessment, 200
     preview of, 200–201
     reasons for using, 197–199
Self-report measures, 738–742
Sensitivity calculations, **132**
Sequential processing, 335

Shannon, Claude, 329–330
Shielding, magnetic, 361
Shore value, viscosity materials, **275**
Shortest Balanced Passage, **79**
Short-term
   follow-up procedures, 714–715
   speech acoustics, 88–95
Shouted vocal effort, **77**
Siemens ASP, **389**
Sigma-Delta A/D conversion, 332
Signal analysis, 631–632
Signal
   classification, **388**
     system, hearing aids, 90
   processing, potential benefits of, 454
Signals, test
   See Test signals
Signal-to-babble ratio, 177, 179
Signal-to-noise ratio (SNR), 93–94, **575**
   adaptive vs. fixed, 138–139
   audibility and, **574**
   excessive sound and, 724
   improving, 577–580
   remote microphones and, **725**
Signia, 30, **449**
   frequency-lowering techniques and, **461**
SII (Speech Intelligibility Index), 83
   AI and, **84**
Silhouette induction generator, 355
Silicone
   addition-cure, 277
   based microphones, 312
   condensation-cure, impression materials, 276–277
   ear molds, 283
Simulated gain, **566**
Simulators, rear ear, 488–489
Single-sided deafness, 258
Sinusoidal test signals, 620
Situational Hearing Aid Response Profile (SHARP), 98–99
Sivantos, 31, **449**
Sivantos Audiologische Technik, 521
Ski-slope, **293**
Slider switches, 267
Sliding linear window, described, 371
Slit leak, 236
Slow acting automatic volume control (SAAVC), described, 370
Smartphone, **409, 428,** 439
   connecting devices to, potential limitations, 456–457
   connectivity, 454–457
   hearing aid control and, **409, 410**

hearing aid paring, 455–456
integration, 452–455
RF transmission and, 323
streaming, 449, 451
SNR (Signal-to-noise ratio), 93–94, 140–141, **575**
adaptive vs. fixed, 138–139
audibility and, **574**
excessive sound and, 724
improving, 577–580
remote microphones and, **725**
Social Security Act, gifts/inducements to beneficiaries, 43–44
Soft
input levels, 730–732
squelch, 379
vocal effort, **77**
Software
accuracy of display, 617
adjustments to MPO, 114–115
fitting, 105–106, 610–618
clinical protocol, 110
Noah software system, 551–553
Sones, 791
Sonova, 30, 31, **449**
Sonus, 31
Sophono Alpha™, 264
Sound
amplifier, personal, 32–35
bore tubing, 294–303
diameter of, 294–296
horn effects, 296–298
venting effects, 298–303
clarity, 1
classifying inputs to, **384**
design technologies, **364**
digital representation of, 326–330
excessive, 720–722
field,
calibration, speech-in-noise testing, 140–141
testing, 140
hearing aid stages and, 225
quality, improved, 229–230
relax, 398
smoothing, 398
Sound Shaper, **461**
Soundbridge™, 266
Soundfield
aided testing, **568**, 604
considerations for, 571–583
calibration, **568**
SoundRecover, 460, **461**
Sounds, too loud, 720–722

Souza, Pam, 196
SPAMfest, 521
Spatial
balance, improved, 229–230
factors, **385**
Spatially-based DNR, 396
Specification for a Manikin for Simulated In Situ Airborne Acoustic Measurements, 492
Specification of Hearing Aid Characteristics, 491
Specificity, calculations, **132**
Spectral
enhanced contrast, 457
flux, **384**
sharpening, 457
subtraction, 395–396
SpectralIQ, **461**
Speech
acoustics, 75–100, 457–459
articulation/audibility index, 83–87
audibility/speech recognition, 82–87
long-term, 75–81
short-term, 88–95
babble, speech in quiet and, 586
banana, 102–103
with dots, 103–105
based subjective ratings
ANL, 182–188
PPT, 186–188
change in understanding, 733
compression effects on, 372–373
dynamic properties of, 373–375
dynamic range of, 624–626
dynamics of, 80–81
enhancement, 457
in noise, 395
ANL and, 182
AzBio sentences and, 182
bilateral beamformers and, **422**
binaural squelch and, 228
clinical speech measures and, **229**
data logging and, 428–429
dichotic speech tests and, 182
digital, 621
directional microphone and, 408
FBR measures and, 509
FDA Modernization Act and, 478–479
hearing aid programs and, 557
HINT and, 162, 167
LAL-R and, 533
OAD and, 182
patient
satisfaction and, 22

Speech *(continued)*
  in noise *(continued)*
    testing and, 572
    problems understanding, 722–725
    revised, 207
    self-reporting outcomes measures, 740
    sentence test, 139
    signal classification system and, 90, 267, 386, 388
    SNR and, 110, 138
    SNR-50 and, 172–173
    soft, 34
    sound field and, 140
    speech recognition in, 151
    standardized tests and, 577
    testing, 135–141
      adaptive vs. fixed, 138–139
      competing noises, 136–138
      earphones or field effect, 140
      in clinic, 93
      presentation level, 139–140
      reception thresholds, 161–162
      sound field calibration, 140–141
      words/sentences, 136
    train gain independently and, **268**
    trainable hearing aids and, 432, 435
    venting effects and, 418–419
    WIN test and, 176, 177, 181
    words/sentences, 136
  in quiet, 261, 388, **411**, 428, 466
    APHAB and, 614
    audibility and, 572
    directional microphone and, 408
    fitting tips and, 695
    for high frequencies, 435
    independent training and, 431–432
    MCL and, 182
    NAL-R and, 533
    pre-fitting testing and, 135
    signal classification system and, 90
    speech babble and, 586
    speech recognition in, 151
    SSQ12 and, 778
    train gain independently and, **268**
    WIN and, 177
  limits of high-level, 543
  noise in, 388
  shaped noise, 136–137
  signal, 794800
  spectrum level, **797**
  tests
    adaptive, 161–163
    one-third octave and, **802–803**
  understanding in noise, 228–229
  in verification stage, 800–802
  weighted signals, 620–621
  levels, **77**
  mapping, 122
    described, 604
    microphone, probe vs. rear ear, 604–605
    probe microphone and, 605
  noise, 136–137
  recognition, 82–87
    50-word list, **149**
    Monosyllabic words and, 159
    aided, 569–583
    described, 192–193
    hearing aids and, 571–577
    in noise, 135, 138, 158–161, 411–415
    QuickSIN and, 376–377
Speech Intelligibility Index (SII), 83
  AI and, **84**
Speech intelligibility ratings, obtaining in CST, 156–157
Speech reception in noise test (SPIN), 151–155
Speech reception threshold (SRT), 138, 141–151
Speech recognition in noise test (SPRINT), 138,
Speech Rescue[θ], **461**
Speech, Spatial, and Qualities of Hearing Scale (SSQ), 447, 597
  post fitting self-assessment, 744
  self-reporting-outcomes, 774–779
Speech Transmission Index (STI), 94–95
Speechmap™, 604
Speech-to-babble ratio, 159
SPIN (Speech Perception in Noise Test), 151–155
SPL-O-gram, 105, **535**, **568**
  DSL and, 540
  REAR and, 660
  REDD and, 677
  REUG and, 655
Spondee
  threshold method, **170**
  words, 116
Spread-spectrum RF modulation, **325**
SPRINT (Speech Recognition in Noise Test), 138, 158–161
  50-word list, **149**
  monosyllabic words and, 159
    scoring, 160
SRAM (Static random access memory), **342**
SRT (Speech reception threshold), 138
SSI (Synthetic Sentence Identification Test), 138
SSQ (Speech, Spatial, and Qualities of Hearing Scale) of Hearing Scale, 447, 597

post fitting self-assessment, 744
self-reporting-outcomes, 774–779
SSSPL90, 499–501
Standard for Specification of Hearing Aid Characteristics, 507
Starkey, 30, **449**, 521
frequency-lowering techniques and, **461**
high-frequency reinforcement, 464
Static random access memory (SRAM), **342**
Statistical significance, defined, **5**
Stethoscopes, **499**, **500**
listening, 508
STI (Speech Transmission Index), 94–95
clinical procedures, 97–99, 99
Stigma
effects of, 58–59
feedback and, **236**
induced identity threat, 58–59
Stigmatization process, 58
Stored equalization calibration, 637
Streaming
devices, 705–706
dual, 448
radio frequency, 448–449
smartphone, 449, 451
smartphones, 452
television, Bluetooth™ and, 450
wireless, 448
"Streamlining Regulations for Good Manufacturing Practices for Hearing Aids, 34
Stress relaxation, viscosity materials, **275**
Subcommittee on Government Regulations of the Select Committee on Small Business, 476
Subject selection, **14–15**
Subjective
judgements, conducting, 584–589
ratings
clinical, **585**
speech-based, 182–188
Summation effects, 228
SumSearch, **10**
Support ring, 360
Suprathreshold levels, summation at, 228
Supreme Court, ruling against the National Society of Professional Engineers, 30
Swimmer's ear, ear impressions and, 278
Switches, slider, 267
Switching technique, asymmetric, **411**
Syllabic compression, described, 370
Synchronous dynamic random-access memory (SDRAM), **342**

Synthetic Sentence Identification Test (SSI), 138
Systematic reviews, 9–11
search engines, **10**

T

Table of evidence, hearing aids, **39**
Taiwan Semiconductor Manufacturing Corporation (TSCM), **364**
Talking in a barrel, 715
Target verification, test signals, 620–627
Task deficit, described, 193
T-coils, 354–356
TCR (Traditional custom instruments), with recessed faceplates, 249–251
TD (Threshold of discomfort), 39, **107**
T-DNR (Traditional DNR), 393–396
Telefunken, **325**
Telephone listening, 452
Telephones
acoustic, 726–728
balancing environmental monitoring and, 728–729
labeling requirements, **482**
placement of, 725–726
streaming, 705–706
understanding problems, 725–729
use of, 713
wireless, FCC and, 481–482
Television streaming, Bluetooth™ and, 450
TEN (Threshold-equalizing noise) test, 128–133
TEREO (Transform for estimating rear-ear output), 810–811
Terms, ending in G or R, 649
Test
booths, **583**
conducting, loudness judgments outside, 592–593
hearing aids
with a broad-band noise signal, 492–493
methods
protocols, 679–680
HINT and, 168
for REAR verification, 663–665
REDD, 680–682
REIG, 683
signals, 619–630
categories of, 620
for counseling purposes, 629–630
for demonstration, 629–630
noise, 792
prescriptive target verification, 620–627
specific features evaluation, 627–629

Testimonials, advertising and, **479**
Testing hearing aids
  with a broad-band noise signal, 492–493
  methods, 493
Test-retest reliability, **161**
Theoretical values, vs. actual, **307**
THI (Tinnitus Handicap Inventory), 201
Thibodeau, Linda, 148
Thinking Fast and Slow, 4
Third-party reimbursement, **37**
Threshold
  measurement
    factors affecting, **788**
    hearing, 782–785
  summation at, 228
  verification, aided soundfield, 567–569
Threshold of discomfort (TD), 39, **107**
Threshold of kneepoint (TK), 365
Threshold-equalizing noise (TEN) test, 128–133
Thumb drives, **342**
Tibbets Industries, **364**
Timbre factors, **385**
Time, **389**
Time
  based training, defined, **431**
  domain, 336–339
  waveforms, interpreting, **88**
Timing factors, **385**
Tinnitus, 69, **145**
  masking, 468
Tinnitus Handicap Inventory (THI), 201
TK (Threshold of kneepoint), 365
TNR (Transient noise reduction), 398–399
Toggle switches, 267, **710**
Tolan, Thomas, 27
Tolerance training, 118
Tolstoy, Leo, **609**
Traditional custom instruments (TCR), with recessed faceplates, 249–251
Traditional DNR (T-DNR), 393–396
Trainable hearing aids, 430–439
  advantages of, 432–433
  disadvantages of, 433
  research with, 433–438
Training
  event-based, **431**
  patient, clinical implementation of, 439
  poor, 609
  time-based, **431**
Transcranial CROS, 260
Transducers, 342–343
  balanced armature, 360
  described, **310**
  influence of, **810**
Transform for estimating rear-ear output (TEREO), 810–811
Transformers, T-coils and, 355
Transient noise reduction (TNR), 398–399
Transistors, 318–322
Transmission, radio frequency, 323–326
Treatment
  effectiveness, 40
  efficiency of, 40
Troubleshooting, 715–729
  acoustic feedback, 718–720
  excessive noise, 720–722
  occlusion effect and, 715–718
  speech noise, 722–725
  telephones, 725–729
TSCM (Taiwan Semiconductor Manufacturing Corporation), **364**
Tubing
  sound bore, 294–303
    diameter, 294–296
    horn effects, 296–298
    venting effects, 298–303
Tuning curves, 129
Turning Research Into Practice Database (TRIP), **10**
Two-talker babble, 397

U

UCL (Uncomfortable loudness), **107**
UDI (Unidirectional index), 508
UFL (Upper-frequency limit), 460
ULC (Upper level of comfort), **107**
ULCL (Upper limit of comfortable loudness), 528
Unaided ear effect, avoidance of, 230–231
Unaided soundfield measures, **113**
Unbundling, 44–45
Uncomfortable loudness (UCL), **107**
Unethical behavior, **47**
Unidirectional index (UDI), 508
Unilateral amplification, vs. bilateral, 226–233
Unilateral loudness testing, **592**
University of Cambridge, **549**
University of Iowa, 28
University of Maryland, 150
University of Memphis, 572, 758
  Contour Test and, 537
University of Miami, 51
University of Minnesota, Medical School, 27
University of Pennsylvania, 51
University of Tennessee, 185

University of Western Ontario, 70, 533
University of Western Ontario (UWO), Protocol for the provision of Amplification, 627–629
Upcoding, **43**
Upper frequency cutoff, **792**
Upper level of comfort (ULC), **107**
Upper limit of comfortable loudness (ULCL), 528
Upper-frequency limit (UFL), 460
UWO (University of Western Ontario), Protocol for the provision of Amplification, 627–629

V

VA (Veterans Affairs), 28
   Auditory and Vestibular Research Laboratory, 181
   CD
      DDT, 195
      DSI, 193
      Speech Recognition and Identification Materials, 177
   Compensation and Pension Evaluation Guidelines, 150
   Military health care system, 244
Valente, Mike, 609
Validation
   evidence for, 20–24
   measures, types of, 737–738
   outcomes, need for, 735–737
   vs. verification, 559–560
Vanderbilt Report II, 605
Vanderbilt University, 414, 421
Vanderbilt/VA Hearing Aid Conference, 37
VCs (Volume controls), 267
   AGCi and, 370
   using memories as, **269**
Venting, **406**
   charts, **300**
   directional microphone, 418–419
   effects, sound bore tubing and, 298–303
Verification
   aided soundfield threshold, 567–569
   evidence for, 20–24
   functional gain, 562–565
   MPO, 688–691
   stage, speech in, 800–802
   vs. validation, 559–560
Veterans Affairs (VA), 28, 244
   Compensation and Pension Evaluation Guidelines, 150
   ethics and, 50
Vibration, reducing, 361
Vinylpolysiloxane, addition-cure, impression materials, 277

VIOLA (Visual Input/Output Locater Algorithm), Visual Input/Output Locater Algorithm 535–537
Virtual earmold, 281
Viscosity materials, **275**
Visual Input/Output Locater Algorithm (VIOLA), 535–537
Visually assisted positioning method, 640
Vocal efforts, **77**
Volatile memory, **342**
Volta, Alessandro, 310
Volta Review, 27
Voltage, described, 309
Volume
   back, 360
   front, 360
   switches, **710**
Volume controls (VCs), 267, **268**, 370

W

Walter Reed Army Medical Center, 28
   SPRINT and, 159
Warble tone, 117
Washington Post, **389**
Watson, Leland A., 27
Waveforms, time, interpreting, **88**
Wax guards, **253**, 364
WDRC (Wide dynamic range compression), 40, 372, 457
   audio expansion and, 379–380
   FIG6 and, 537–538
Wearable hearing devices, over-the-counter, 33
White noise, 512, 627, 695
   described, 792–793
Wide dynamic range compression (WDRC), 40, 372, 457
   audio expansion and, 379–380
   FIG6 and, 537–538
Widex, **449**
   frequency-lowering techniques and, 460, **461**
   FT and, 462
   hearing aids, 30
Wiener, Norbert, 394–395
Wiener filtering, 394–395
William Demant (Oticon), 30
Willingness to pay (WTP), 617–618
Wilson, Frank C., 39
Wilson, Richard, 177, 193
WIN (Words in Noise) test, 176–182
   excessive sound and, 724
   vs QuickSIN, **181**
Wind noise reduction (WNR), 400–403
Window, sliding linear, 371
Windowing, 335

Wireless
   microphones, 405–407
   programming, connecting, 554
   receivers, 355
   routing, from external devices, 450
   streaming, 448, **449**
   telephones
      FCC and, 481
      HAC for, 481
WNR (Wind noise reduction), 400–403
Woof, attack/release and, **368**
Word recognition, scores, 1
Word-rec testing, 135
Words in Noise (WIN) Test, 176–182
   excessive sound and, 724

World War II, audiology and, 27–28
WPT (Willingness to pay), 617–618

Y

"You Want Me to Put My Loudspeaker WHERE?," 630

Z

Zarlink Semiconductor, **364**
Zeta Noise Blocker™, 390
Zinc-air batteries, 357–359
Zocor, 51
Zwislocki coupler, 488–491

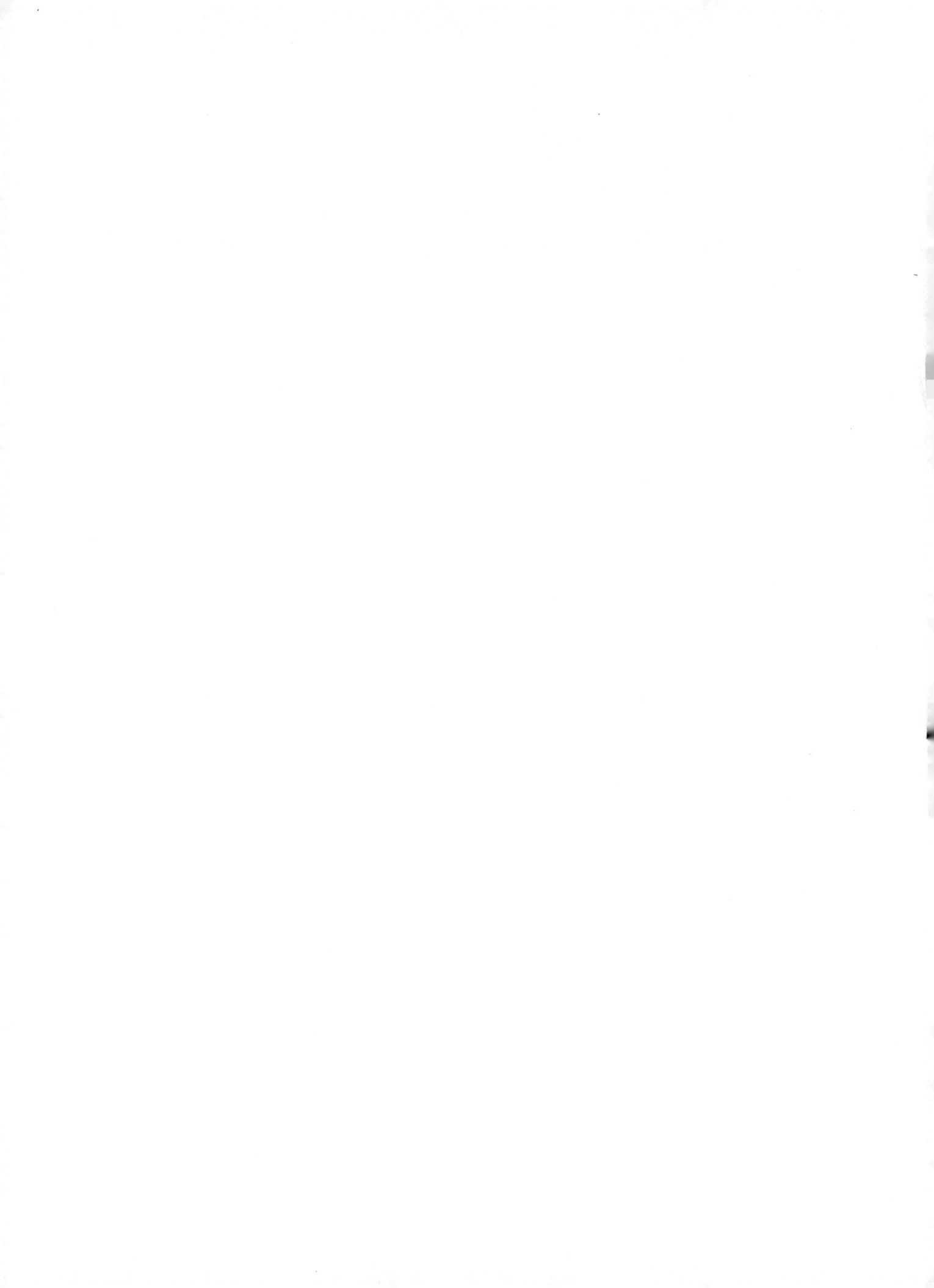